HUMAN SEXUALITY

ROGER R. HOCK

Mendocino College

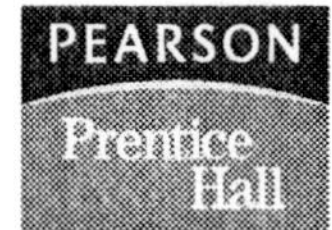

Upper Saddle River, New Jersey 07458

Library of Congress Cataloging-in-Publication Data

Hock, Roger R.
Human sexuality / Roger R. Hock.
p. cm.
Includes bibliographical references and index.
ISBN 0-13-198699-6
1. Sex. 2. Sex (Psychology) 3. Sex (Biology) 4. Sexual disorders. I. Title.
HQ21.H54 2007
613.9071--dc22 2006021599

Editorial Director: Leah Jewell
Executive Editor: Jessica Mosher
Editorial Assistant: William Grieco
Editor-in-Chief, Development: Rochelle Diogenes
Development Editor: Joanne M. Tinsley
Supplements Editor: Richard Virginia
Media Editor: Brian Hyland
Director of Marketing: Brandy Dawson
Senior Marketing Manager: Jeanette Moyer
Assistant Managing Editor (Production): Maureen Richardson
Production Liaison: Maureen Richardson
Manufacturing Manager: Nick Sklitsis
Manufacturing Buyer: Sherry Lewis
Creative Design Director: Leslie Osher
Interior/Cover Design: Ximena Tamvakopolous
Design Liaison: Nancy Wells
Manager, Rights & Permissions: Zina Arabia
Interior Image Specialist: Beth Brenzel
Cover Image Specialist: Karen Sanatar
Image Permission Coordinator: Joanne Dippel
Photo Researcher: Elaine Soares
Art Coordinator: Gail Cocker-Bogusz
Line Art: Precision Graphics
Composition/Full-Service Project Management: Rosaria Cassinese, Prepare, Inc.
Printer/Binder: RR Donnelley & Sons

Cover Images: *Front (L to R)*: Getty Images Inc.—Image Source; Stuart McClymont/Getty Images, Inc.; Fotosearch.Com, LLC; Index Stock Imagery, Inc.; Emely/zefa/Corbis; *Spine:* Eric Schmidt/Masterfile Stock Image Library; *Back (L to R)*: Dimitri Vervits/Photonica/Getty Images, Inc.; Stockbyte/Getty Images, Inc.; image: Kelvin Murray/Getty Images, Inc.; WireImageStock/Masterfile Stock Image Library; Norbert Schaefer Corbis-NY.

Credits and acknowledgments borrowed from other sources and reproduced, with permission, in this textbook appear on appropriate page within text (or on page 628).

Pearson Education, Ltd.
Pearson Education Australia PTY, Limited
Pearson Education Singapore, Pte., Ltd.
Pearson Education North Asia Ltd.
Pearson Education, Canada, Ltd.
Pearson Educación de Mexico, S.A. de C.V.
Pearson Education–Japan
Pearson Education Malaysia, Pte., Ltd.
Pearson Education, Upper Saddle River, NJ

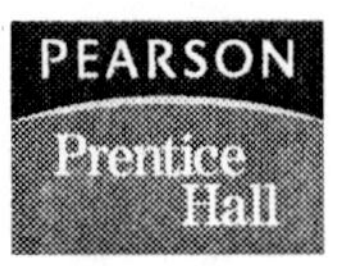

10 9 8 7 6 5 4 3 2 1
ISBN 0-13-198699-6

1

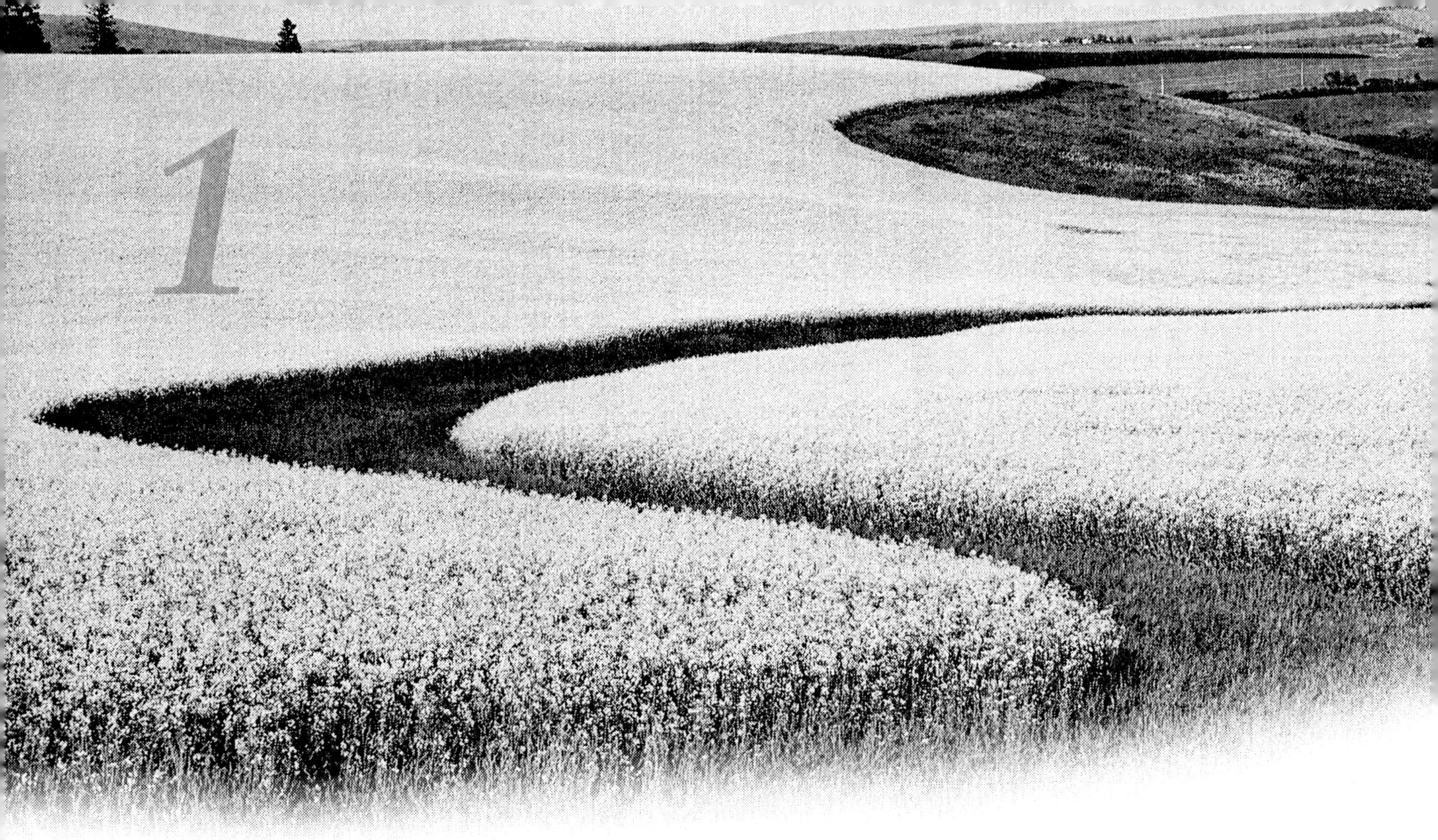

Studying Human Sexuality

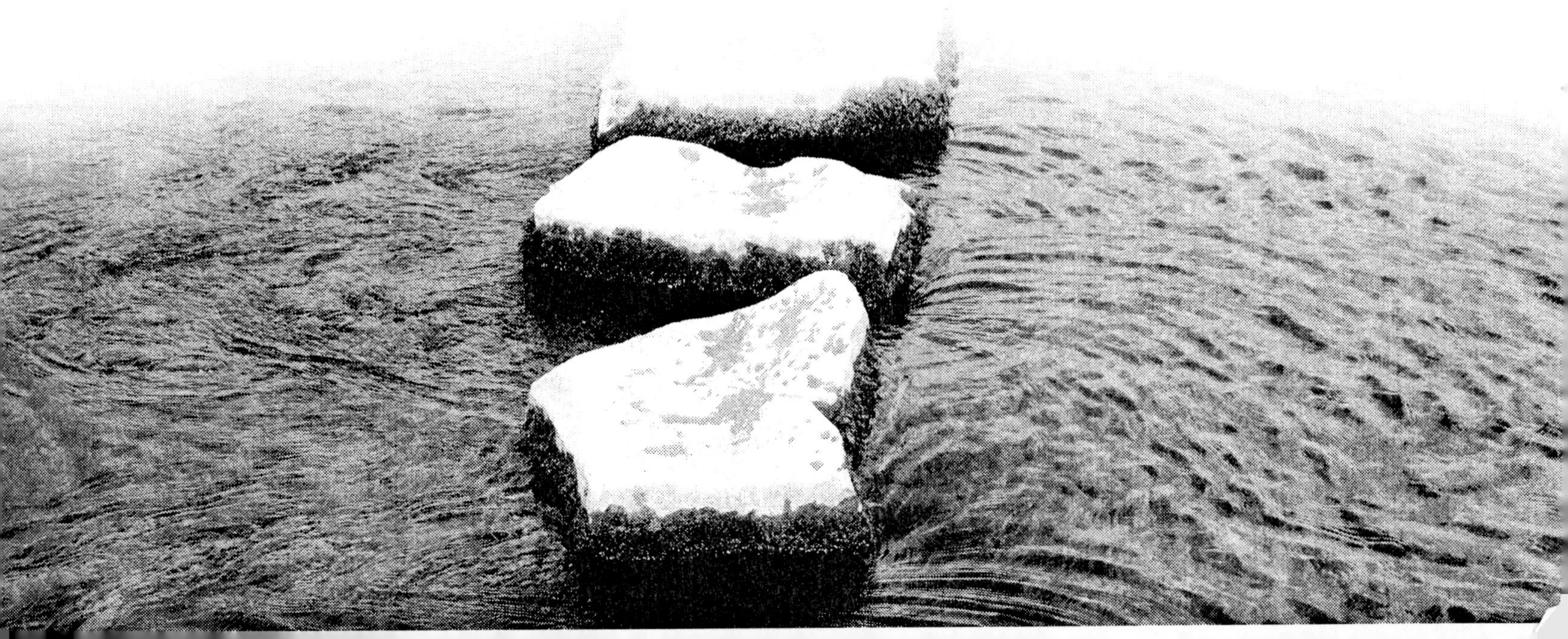

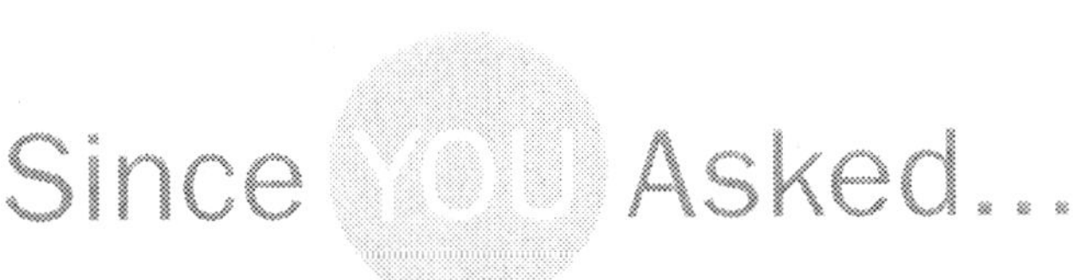

Since YOU Asked...

1. Do we really need a course about sex? Isn't sex just something that happens naturally? (see page 4)

2. My partner wants to perform oral sex on me, but I think it's gross. Should I let him do it just to please him? (see page 8)

3. Is it normal to have an orgasm by masturbating but not during sex with a partner? (see page 12)

4. I am 21 years old and had a "wet dream" two weeks ago. Is that normal at my age? (see page 12)

5. Is it normal for a guy to want to wait until marriage to have sex? I'm determined, but sometimes I have major doubts. (see page 12)

6. My parents have never had "the talk" with me. Are they just embarrassed, or did they think I would learn on my own? (see page 15)

7. How is it possible to study people's sexual behavior when it's such a private, personal experience? (see page 16)

8. Has anyone scientifically studied average penis size? If so, what is it? (see page 22)

9. I read in a checkout-stand magazine that a survey of readers found that most men and women (like 90 percent) do not like their own bodies. Could this be true? (see page 22)

10. Is it really ethical to study people's actual sexual behaviors? (see page 31)

Have you given much critical thought to your personal knowledge, desires, or identity as a sexual being? Most people haven't. Yet there are few areas in your life where this self-reflection is more important. Do you have a sense of what you want or don't want in terms of sexual intimacy with another person now or in the future? Under what conditions and with whom will you feel comfortable allowing that intimacy to grow? What is your vision of a healthy and fulfilling romantic relationship? Can you be sure that you will make choices and decisions that are right for you when sexual situations arise? How will you keep yourself safe from unwanted pregnancy, sexually transmitted infections, and sexual violence? How will you interact with others who are sexually different from you? How can you ensure for yourself a physically and emotionally gratifying sexual life?

The answer to all of these questions, and to many others, lies in your willingness to establish your own **personal sexual philosophy**—your unique foundation of knowledge, attitudes, and actions relating to what you want and who you are as a sexual person. This is not something that "just comes naturally"; it requires study and self-reflection. The worst time to try to make difficult decisions about sexual events is at the moment you are faced with them (especially if the moment is a steamy sexual one or if you are under the influence of some mind-altering substance). Better to take some time now to develop your knowledge of human sexuality and to think about who you are and what you want sexually; then, when difficult or confusing situations arise, you will be more confident and capable of making the choices that are right for you. In other words, *you* will be in charge of the sexual situations in your life rather than the situations taking charge of you.

Since YOU Asked...

1. Do we really need a course about sex? Isn't sex just something that happens naturally?

We will return to the theme of building your self-knowledge, attitudes, and actions at the close of this chapter—and every other chapter in this text—and offer you the opportunity to incorporate what you have learned in the chapter into your sexual philosophy. Remember, studying human sexuality is about far more than "getting the facts." It is about knowing who you are and what you want or don't want, and planning ahead.

Human sexuality is a complex area of study that focuses on all aspects of humans as sexual beings. This includes such topics as sexual anatomy and responses, sexual feelings and behaviors, intimate relationships, sexual identity and desires, sexual health and well-being, and how we perceive and express our individual sexual selves. Each chapter in this text is just one piece of the rich and challenging puzzle of human sexuality. In this chapter, we will examine the ways in which people learn about human sexuality. In the most basic sense, these learning experiences may be divided into two categories: (1) *experiencing* your sexuality for yourself and (2) deepening your *understanding* of human sexuality issues. On the experiential side, we will explore your emotional reactions relating to sexuality, getting to know yourself as a sexual person, developing your personal set of sexual morals and values, making responsible choices about sexual activities, discovering the full range of sexually intimate behaviors, and enhancing your lifelong sexual fulfillment and satisfaction.

In order to attain a deeper understanding of sexuality, we will focus on its surprising complexity, rejecting sexual myths and misconceptions you may hold about sexuality, developing tolerance and respect for sexual diversity, acquiring a sense of what is sexually "normal" and "abnormal," staying sexually healthy, preparing to talk to your own children about sex if and when the time comes, and becoming a critical, educated consumer of the mass of research and reporting about human sexuality.

personal sexual philosophy A person's unique foundation of knowledge, attitudes, and actions relating to what the person wants and who he or she is as a sexual being.

human sexuality An area of research and study focusing on all aspects of humans as sexual beings.

Table 1.1 GUIDING PRINCIPLES FOR THIS TEXT

It's no secret that most students never read the prefaces in textbooks. You know who you are! In this book's Preface, I have described seven principles for presenting human sexuality information correctly, effectively, and understandably. Because these principles have influenced me every step of the way in my teaching and writing about human sexuality and because many of you may have missed them, I summarize them here. R.H.

PRINCIPLE (FROM THE PREFACE)	HOW IT APPLIES TO THIS TEXT
Real-life relevancy	Every effort has been made to ensure that this text is relevant and meaningful to you.
Authoritative information	The content of this text is based on the most recent, up-to-date, scientific, and accurate research available.
Personal choice and responsibility	The assumption throughout this text is that you are in charge of your personal sexual choices throughout your adult life, with the goal of making decisions that are right for you, that you can feel good about, and that do not harm anyone else.
Awareness, tolerance, and respect for sexual diversity	The information in this text will assist you in understanding the world around you and how and where you fit into it; this mosaic of diversity plays a major role in making human sexuality such a rich and fascinating study.
Physical and emotional health and wellness	This text is designed to focus on specific as well as general sexual health issues and to decrease your discomfort in seeking care and treatment for sexual problems, if necessary.
Comfort with and acceptance of your own sexuality	This text highlights the importance of developing your personal sexual philosophy, so that you are in charge of the sexual situations in your life instead of the other way around.
Critical analysis of research and information about sexuality	This text will give you the ability to evaluate intelligently and critically the vast amount of sexual information you are receiving—both from the media and from your social interactions with others.

Later in this chapter, we will review the scientific methods researchers use to study human sexual behaviors, attitudes, and emotions. We will then consider the importance of ethics as it relates to sexuality research. As you read this chapter and throughout this text, keep in mind the guiding principles for this book, discussed in the Preface and summarized again for you in Table 1.1.

Historical Perspectives

A Human Sexuality Time Line

Many of the topics covered in this book are rooted in ancient history, some dating back millennia and others even to the very beginning of humankind (or humankind might no longer exist!). We touch on many of these events in greater detail in the Historical Perspective section early in each chapter. For this first chapter, the section offers you a glimpse of the major events over the recent past, the 150 years or so that have shaped our sexual history in the United States and much of the Western world. Each event on the time line on the front endsheets of this book notes the number of the chapter in which you will find a more detailed discussion of that topic in its current context. Enjoy the trip through sexual time!

Experiencing Human Sexuality

We experience sexuality in many personal and subjective ways. Our individual experiences regarding sexuality vary greatly from negative to positive, painful to joyful, traumatic to sublime. The factors that determine how we experience our sexuality may include any of the issues discussed next.

Sex Is Emotional

Students' personal experiences in a human sexuality course can often trigger emotional reactions, sometimes very strong ones. These feelings may include general discomfort, confusion, anxiety, embarrassment, anger, arousal, surprise, nervousness, and even fear. Because these emotions make some people uncomfortable about the study of human sexuality, we will spend a moment near the beginning of each chapter, in a feature called Focus on Your Feelings (see p. 7), to comment on and prepare you for possible emotional reactions you may experience as you read and learn.

Enriching Self-Knowledge

First and foremost, we are born to be sexual beings. This does not imply that we all engage in any particular sexual activity or that we all have the same or even similar sexual feelings and desires. But sexuality will always be a part of what makes each of us a unique individual. From infancy through old age, we have the capacity to experience both physical and emotional sexual feelings.

It follows, then, that your perception of your own sexuality is a major part of your self-identity. To demonstrate this, imagine that you wake up tomorrow morning and have no idea whether you are a man or a woman. How would this make you feel? Confused? Probably. Disoriented? At least! You would very likely be thinking, "I no longer know who I am!" Your **gender identity**—your concept of yourself as a man or woman—is one of the most important components of your sexual identity. And you probably do not need to study human sexuality to know what yours is. Most likely, you are already very clear about that, and it is not likely to change as you read this book.

However, other components of your sexual self may not be so clear to you. For example, some people are confused, at least at some point in their lives, about their **sexual orientation**, whether they are more attracted to members of the same sex or the opposite sex romantically, emotionally, and sexually. Others may be unsure about what qualities they desire in an intimate relationship or confused about their comfort level with specific sexual activities. This book and this course will help you find answers and better understand yourself.

Developing Morals and Values

Part of discovering yourself sexually usually involves developing your personal set of morals and values as they relate to sexual issues. You probably already have a sense of the morals and values that were instilled in you by your parents, your religious teachings, your peers, or other factors that have influenced you throughout your early life (Eyre, Davis, & Peacock, 2001). As you have grown into adulthood, however, you may have begun to question those beliefs and wonder if they still apply to you as an

gender identity A person's view of himself or herself as a man or a woman.

sexual orientation A person's primary sexual, social, romantic, and emotional attraction with respect to gender.

independent, mature individual. Some of you may feel the need to make modifications in your system of values and morals that are more in line with how you choose to live your life. Whether this is true for you or not, morality and personal values play a central role in how you experience most, if not all, of the issues discussed in this book.

It is not the job or intention of this book to infuse into you anyone else's sexual morals or values (including the author's). As you study human sexuality, you will acquire or enhance the knowledge and awareness you need to develop your own sexual standards and belief systems that make sense and feel right to *you* in *your* life (R. Hawkins, 1993). Consider the value in taking the time to weigh these issues and make some conscious decisions about how you want to live your sexual life (Feigenbaum, Weinstein, & Rosen, 1995). In this way, your values and moral beliefs can help guide you through the complexities of life as a sexual being, clearly an important part of your "sexual philosophy." At any time, you may find yourself faced with difficult decisions to make about your sexual behavior and your interactions, without time for thought or reflection. Without your personal moral compass, you may make choices that you later regret. In other words, the situation may take charge of you rather than the other way around.

Focus on Your Feelings

Sex is emotional. The study of human sexuality often activates in students unexpected emotional reactions to the subjects being discussed. At times during your reading or class discussions, you may find yourself feeling uncomfortable, embarrassed, aroused, shocked, offended, angry, confused, fearful, amused, or various combinations of these and other emotions. Your individual reactions will depend on your attitudes about sexual issues, your family and religious background, and your past and present sexual and relationship experiences. For example, here are two journal entries from students in the author's human sexuality classes:

> I was raised in a very strict religious household. Sex was never discussed, and even mentioning sexual topics was not allowed. I'm learning a lot in this course, but I find it very difficult to read the material and participate in the class discussions. I'm embarrassed and feel that I am doing something wrong (guilt!). This is why I have missed so many classes.
>
> *Tricia, first-year student*

> I've never told anyone this before, but from the time I was 8 until I was 12, I was sexually molested by my father. When we were in class discussing sexual abuse, it brought all this back to me. I don't know if I should get some counseling. I never thought it really bothered me, but now I'm not so sure.
>
> *Rick, sophomore*

Although you may or may not have had experiences such as these, you should expect to experience emotions that you would not usually feel in other courses. *These emotions are completely normal.* However, if you find that they are bothering you too much, or if they interfere with your ability to enjoy and do well in this course, it would be a good idea to discuss them in private with your instructor or perhaps with a professional counselor (usually available through your college's counseling services). Remember, you should never feel *forced* to read material or attend classes that would be emotionally painful for you. Your sexuality professor should be willing and open to discussing with you ways of reducing your discomfort.

Making Responsible Choices

Having a clear sense of your sexual morals and values is one factor in making responsible sexual choices throughout your life. Freely choosing to be sexually active in today's world requires you to make an almost overwhelming number of crucial decisions. For example, how will you protect yourself and your partner from HIV and other sexually transmitted infections? How can you be sure to avoid an unwanted pregnancy? How can you keep yourself safe from sexual violence and coercion? What are your expectations of dating and relationships? How can you and your partner communicate your needs and desires openly and honestly to each other? How will you handle a sexual problem with your partner?

At some point in life, almost everyone must answer at least some of these or other important questions about sexual issues that arise in their lives. If you make the wrong decisions due to lack of knowledge, misinformation, or poor judgment, the consequences can be extremely serious. But you already know that. How do you find the answers that are right for you? First, you are off to an excellent start because you are taking this course and reading this book. Research has shown that people who take a human sexuality course tend to make better, more informed, and more thoughtful choices. For example, high school seniors who received education about HIV and AIDS were found to engage in fewer high-risk sexual activities (Klitsch, 1994).

In another study, college students enrolled in a freshman seminar focusing on sexual health were more likely to use condoms and other forms of contraception (Turner et al., 1994). Also, students who complete a human sexuality course have been shown to be significantly less tolerant of rape in general, and date rape specifically, and less likely to believe common rape myths such as "most rapes are committed by strangers" and "some women ask to be raped by the way they dress" (Dallager & Rosen, 1993; Fischer, 1986; Flores & Hartlaub, 1998; Patton & Mannison, 1994).

As adults, the more accurate information you have, the more able you are to make responsible choices about your behavior. As mentioned earlier, choice and responsibility are recurring themes throughout this book.

Sex Is *More* than Intercourse

Yes, you read it right: sex is *more* than intercourse. This theme runs throughout this book and plays a role in many of the topics in various chapters. Why? Because equating sex to intercourse neglects the full range of sexual experience and pleasure that is available to us as human beings. Western cultures often tend to take *sex* as a synonym for *intercourse* (Goodson, et al., 2003). Consequently, any other pleasurable, arousing, and satisfying sexual behaviors, such as kissing, touching, massage, masturbation (solo and mutual), and oral sex, become lumped together into a single category called "foreplay" or "that which leads up to intercourse." But in reality, many behaviors can be sexually fulfilling in themselves, and for some individuals or couples, they may be more satisfying than intercourse.

Most of today's sexual problems, such as unwanted pregnancy, transmission of sexually transmitted infections, and sexual dysfunctions, stem from *insertive sexual practices*, especially vaginal and anal intercourse. Many of these problems could be reduced if people were more comfortable with the idea of sexual intimacy *without* intercourse. This does not imply abstinence, as most people interpret it—forgoing all sexual intimacy and activities—but may involve a decision to engage in only "safe" or "preferred" sexual behaviors. In addition, many situations may arise in one's life that make vaginal or anal intercourse uncomfortable, difficult, or medically inadvisable, but this does not mean that sexual intimacy must stop (Hatcher et al., 1994; Kowal, 1998a). Other intimate, sexually fulfilling activities can still be enjoyed fully.

Sex is more than intercourse

Although many people have discovered the pleasures of sex without intercourse, to others this is a new and strange idea. Culturally, especially for heterosexual couples, it is not a widely accepted concept. On the contrary, many if not most people will argue that you haven't really had sex if you haven't had intercourse (Bogart et al., 2000). Look for the "Sex is more than intercourse" icon throughout the text for discussions highlighting that sexual behaviors include far more than intercourse.

Enhancing Sexual Fulfillment

It is no secret that nearly all of you will, at some point in your life, choose to be sexually active and to share sexual intimacy with a partner. Once that decision is made, you will desire and deserve a healthy, satisfying, and fulfilling sex life.

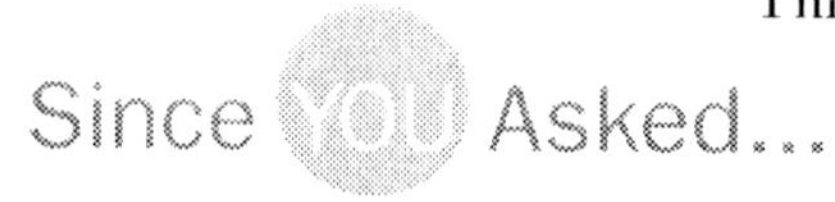

2. My partner wants to perform oral sex on me, but I think it's gross. Should I let him do it just to please him?

This text in no way intends to recommend, encourage, or promote any particular sexual behavior, feeling, or attitude. You should never feel pressured to do anything sexually that makes you feel uncomfortable. As discussed in the next section, sexuality is complex, and consequently, a fulfilling sex life is not always easy to achieve. One route to this goal, however, involves acquiring accurate and authoritative information, such as is provided in this text, about as many aspects of sexuality as possible. This foundation of knowledge will provide you with the tools to experience and maintain an enhanced, enriched, and exciting sexual life for yourself and your partner.

That said, it is important to add that you should be very clear that your body belongs to you and that your sexual behavior is, or should be, completely in your control. This principle, of course, refers to consensual, honest, and responsible sexual behavior between adults. Behaviors such as rape, telling someone you are using birth control when you are not, or not warning a partner about having a sexually transmitted infection are contrary to this premise, because these activities are nonconsensual, dishonest, and irresponsible.

Understanding Human Sexuality

Your education in human sexuality is only partly about your *experience* of being a sexual person. Other specific topics are essential for your *understanding* of human sexuality, which we will consider here.

It's More Complex than You Think

One of the most important (and obvious) reasons to study sexuality is to increase your knowledge of the subject. This will not be difficult, because human sexuality is a huge field! For example, in the next two chapters, you will be introduced to sexual anatomy and physiology. Right away, you'll begin to see that even our sexual bodies are wonderfully complex in form and function. But in many ways, the biology of sex is far simpler than the psychological and social intricacies of sexual feelings, desires, choices, interactions, and behaviors.

To acquire a general idea of how much you already know about the range of topics this book will cover, take a few minutes to complete and score "Self-Discovery: Sexual Knowledge Self-Test". When you finish this textbook, many weeks from now, you may wish to take the test again. You will have a significantly higher score—guaranteed.

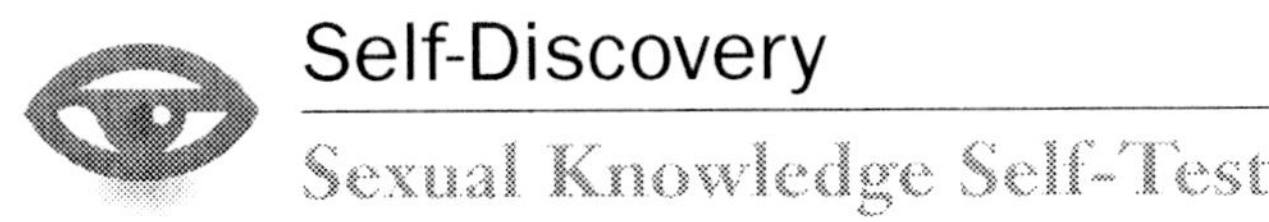

Self-Discovery

Sexual Knowledge Self-Test

Mark each of the statements *True* or *False*. If you know someone you would like to pass the self-test along to, you may want to answer on a separate sheet of paper. Scoring instructions and interpretations are at the end of the test.

TRUE OR FALSE?

Chapter 1: Studying Human Sexuality

____ **1.** Because of ethical and personal privacy considerations, it is not possible to conduct first-hand scientific research on human sexuality.

____ **2.** The average length of a man's penis when erect is about 7.5 inches.

____ **3.** Devices used to electronically measure signs of penile and vagina arousal are sometimes used by sexuality researchers.

Chapter 2: Sexual Anatomy

____ **4.** Erection of the penis is caused by contracting muscles and the build-up of semen.

____ **5.** Semen is produced by the testicles.

____ **6.** When a girl is born, her ovaries contain over 400,000 immature eggs.

Continued. . .

Chapter 3: The Physiology of Human Sexual Responding

____ 7. The clitoris and penis both become erect during sexual stimulation.

____ 8. Women generally say that intercourse is the most reliable and satisfying method for achieving orgasm.

____ 9. A man who carries a sexually transmitted infection may transmit the infection even without ejaculating.

Chapter 4: Love, Intimacy, and Sexual Communication

____ 10. Physical attractiveness is a relatively unimportant factor in the formation of romantic relationships.

____ 11. In abusive or violent relationships, the victim often remains in the relationship in spite of the abuse.

____ 12. Physical violence is virtually always present in abusive relationships.

Chapter 5: Contraception: Planning and Preventing Pregnancy

____ 13. All hormonal forms of contraception currently on the market are for women.

____ 14. The female condom has been shown to be as effective in preventing pregnancy as the male condom.

15. A woman cannot get pregnant if the man successfully withdraws his penis before he ejaculates.

Chapter 6: Sexual Behaviors: Experiencing Sexual Pleasure

____ 16. Most sexual behaviors fall into one of three categories: (a) heterosexual, (b) gay, or (c) lesbian.

____ 17. Research shows that about the same percentage of males and females masturbate.

____ 18. Most women do not experience orgasm routinely during heterosexual intercourse.

Chapter 7: Sexual Problems and Solutions

____ 19. Problems with erection for men and orgasm for women are rare.

____ 20. Nearly all sexual problems are easily treated and solved.

____ 21. Lack of sexual desire is one of the most common sexual problems couples face.

Chapter 8: Sexually Transmitted Infections

____ 22. Bacterial sexually transmitted infections are generally curable; viral STIs are generally not.

____ 23. Many sexually transmitted infections may be spread through oral sexual activities.

____ 24. The human papilloma virus (HPV) that causes genital warts has been shown also to be the primary cause of cervical cancer.

Chapter 9: Conception, Pregnancy, and Birth

____ 25. A woman can get pregnant during her period.

____ 26. During each menstrual cycle, there are about 7 to 10 days during which unprotected intercourse can cause a woman to become pregnant.

____ 27. A miscarriage is another term for a spontaneous abortion.

Chapter 10: Gender: Expectations, Roles, and Stereotypes

____ 28. A person's femininity or masculinity is directly related to their sexual orientation.

____ 29. A small percentage of infants are born with genitals that are ambiguous—neither fully male nor female.

____ 30. Androgyny refers to males who are highly masculine and females who are highly feminine.

Chapter 11: Sexual Orientation

____ 31. The love between gay and lesbian couples is similar in quality to the love between heterosexual couples.

____ 32. In reality, "bisexuality" refers to people who are actually gay, but have not yet fully acknowledged their true sexual orientation.

____ 33. Research has shown that parenting styles do not appear to influence the sexual orientation of the children.

Chapter 12: Sexual Development throughout Life

____ 34. If a young child masturbates, it is usually a sign that he or she is being sexually abused.

____ 35. The male sexual peak is at about 18, while the female peaks at around 35, causing serious difficulties in many intimate relationships.

____ 36. Most women begin to care less about sex when they become menopausal (around their mid 40s to mid 50s).

Chapter 13: Sexual Aggression and Violence: Rape, Child Sexual Abuse, and Harassment

____ 37. Most rapes are committed by someone the victim knows.

____ 38. Women can resist being raped if they really want to.

____ 39. Men who sexually abuse boys are usually gay.

Chapter 14: Paraphilias: The Extremes of Sexual Behavior

____ 40. Sadomasochism (giving and receiving pain for sexual arousal) is clinically defined as sexual perversion.

____ 41. If a man frequently uses women's shoes for sexual stimulation during masturbation and orgasm, this would likely be called a fetish.

____ 42. Exhibitionism and voyeurism are non-coercive paraphilias in that neither involves a victim.

Chapter 15: The Sexual Marketplace: Prostitution and Pornography

____ 43. With few exceptions, most male prostitutes are gay.

____ 44. "Sex trade worker" is a phrase often used in place of "prostitute."

____ 45. Explicit sexual materials are no longer censored in the U.S.

Continued. . .

Now, score your self-test using the answer key below. You might wish to compare your score with the scores from students on the first day of several past human sexuality classes which are divided into five categories described below.

Correct Answers:

1. F, 2. F, 3. T, 4. F, 5. F, 6. T, 7. T, 8. F, 9. T, 10. F, 11. T, 12. F, 13. T, 14. F, 15. F, 16. F, 17. F, 18. T, 19. F, 20. T, 21. T, 22. T, 23. T, 24. T, 25. T, 26. T, 27. T, 28. F, 29. T, 30. F, 31. T, 32. F, 33. T, 34. F, 35. F, 36. F, 37. F, 38. F, 39. T, 40. F, 41. T, 42. F, 43. F, 44. T, 45. F

INTERPRETING YOUR SCORE

41–45: ***Sexual Wizard!*** However, you still have a great opportunity to learn the finer points and can probably contribute a great deal to class discussions. You should find much of the text and course material somewhat more familiar than many others in the class.

36–45: ***Very sexually knowledgeable.*** You should be fairly comfortable participating in class discussions and may be able to add interesting insights. However you will be quite surprised at how many new discoveries you will make in this book and course.

30–35: ***Average level of knowledge for those taking this class.*** Most students score around this range at the beginning of the course. You will pick up many new concepts as you go through this book. You probably came into the class with some misconceptions about human sexuality, but those will be corrected soon!

25–29: ***Still a lot to learn about human sexuality.*** Like many people, you probably believe in some myths and misconceptions about sexuality that you learned from friends or parents. Perhaps you grew up in a sexually restricted household where talking and learning about sex was frowned upon or forbidden. For you, this will be an extra valuable course.

Under 25: ***You need this course!*** This is not a criticism. You are the person who will benefit the most from this book and this course. For whatever reason, you simply have not yet had much opportunity to acquire accurate knowledge about human sexuality. This course will give you the information you need to help you live a healthy and fulfilling sexual life.

People Know a lot about Sex—And Much of It Is Wrong

Each of you is unique in your level of sexual knowledge and experience. As you may have discovered if you answered the questions on "Self-Discovery: Sexual Knowledge Self-Test", all of you come into this course with a base of knowledge, a starting point for your study of human sexuality. You may also have discovered that there are some significant gaps in your knowledge that this book can fill.

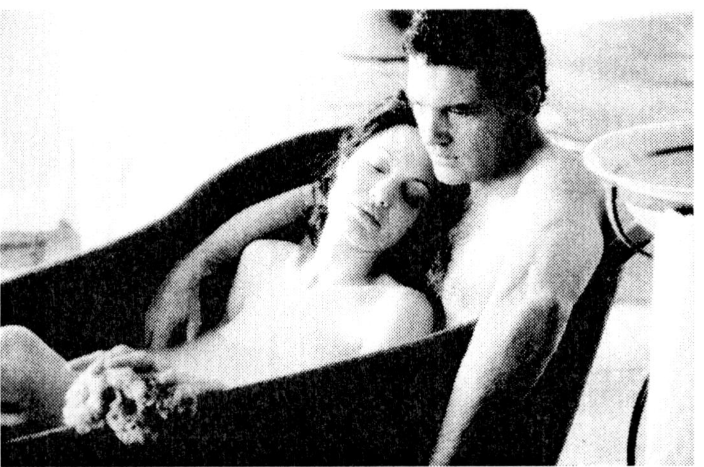

Images from movies and TV often provide an exaggerated or mythical view of sexuality.

That said, can you think of any other course that you began with as much "advance information" as this one? But consider for a moment the *sources* of your information. A great deal of your sexual knowledge probably came from parents, friends and acquaintances, books, magazines, movies, TV shows, and the Internet—what might be called your "informal sex education network." Although some of you may have had some more formal sex education in high school, most of the sexual knowledge you possess probably came from your personal collection of casual, nonscientific sources. Unfortunately, all of these sources are subject to error, misinformation, and the perpetration of myths and falsehoods (yes, even parents can be wrong about sex at times).

Personal experience can be a poor teacher as well. Among teens and young adults, early sexual experimentation tends to be awkward, embarrassing, not necessarily pleasurable, and even frightening or painful. These experiences may lead to expectations and conclusions about sexual behavior that are fundamentally incorrect.

In this book, you have a source of information about human sexuality that is as accurate, up-to-date, and scientifically based as possible. Your challenge in reading and learning the material in these pages is not only to gain new information and develop a comprehensive base of accurate knowledge about human sexuality but also to *unlearn* any faulty ideas and preconceptions you may currently have about sex. Don't expect this to be easy. Unlearning is often more difficult than learning, because many misconceptions are reinforced through your informal sex education network. It's not easy to accept that something you thought was true about sex—even something you may have used to make decisions about your behavior—may stem from faulty information from all those well-meaning but misinformed sources (Farrington, 2002).

The main point here is that as you read this book, be open to knowledge and ideas that may be new or different from what you thought was true.

Tolerance and Respect for Sexual Diversity

The fabric of human sexuality is one of the most diverse of all human attributes. People's sexual "personalities" can include cultural, ethnic, and religious differences; differences in family background; differences in sexual orientation; differences in sexual attitudes, morals, and values; differences in sexual behavior preferences, experiences, and sexual role expectations; and differences in personal comfort about sexual issues (see "Sexuality and Culture: Sex Education in China").

Humans have a tendency to fear and reject people perceived as different, especially when the differences appear strange and even extreme. Your study of human sexuality will increase your knowledge and awareness of humans' sexual richness and diversity and develop further your understanding and tolerance of those who may be sexually different from you. Research has demonstrated that students who take human sexuality courses increase their comfort level with various diverse groups, such as those with gay, lesbian, and bisexual orientations (Patton & Mannison, 1994; Waterman, Reid, Garfield, & Hoy, 2001; Weiss, Rabinowitz, & Ruckstuhl, 1992). Furthermore, in the author's own courses, when guest speakers who represent sexual diversity—for example, people from the gay, lesbian, and bisexual community; guests from sexual abuse and rape crisis centers; people living with HIV or AIDS; transgender individuals—come to speak to classes about their experiences, students frequently report profound changes in their awareness, empathy, and tolerance for these diverse groups and often refer to these visits as among their most enlightening learning experiences of the semester.

What Is "Normal" Sexuality?

As indicated by several questions from the Since You Asked feature at the beginning of this chapter, one of the most common concerns people have about their sexuality, especially in young adulthood, is whether or not they are "normal." But the concept of "normal" is a slippery one. It is difficult to define exactly what we mean when we say something or someone is normal or abnormal, especially when it comes to sexuality. Furthermore, when people worry that their sexual feelings, desires, behaviors, or body are not normal, they are usually too embarrassed or fearful to discuss it with anyone else. Consequently, they may believe that they are the only one who has their particular concern. The truth is that just about anything people feel might be abnormal about themselves is probably a common concern held by many others—which in a sense makes it normal! One of the most important and most reassuring benefits of studying human sexuality is that nearly everyone who feels that he or she is abnormal in some way discovers that that is not the case. For more on this issue, see "Self-Discovery: Am I Sexually Normal?" on page 14. By the way, the answers to Since You Asked questions 3, 4, and 5 are *yes*, *yes*, and *yes*. These issues are all discussed in greater detail elsewhere in this text.

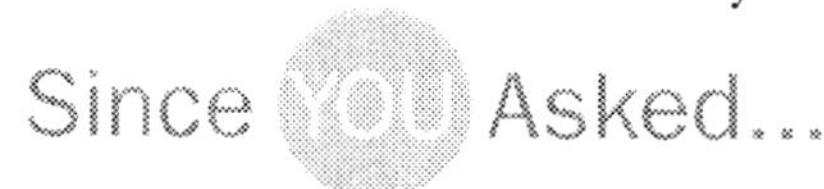

3. Is it normal to have an orgasm by masturbating but not during sex with a partner?

4. I am 21 years old and had a "wet dream" two weeks ago. Is that normal at my age?

5. Is it normal for a guy to want to wait until marriage to have sex? I'm determined, but sometimes I have major doubts.

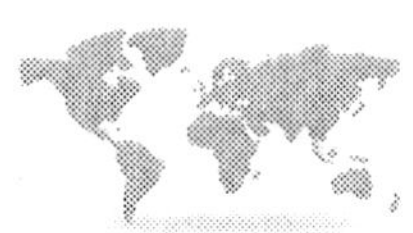

Sexuality and Culture

Sex Education in China

China is one of many countries that has traditionally placed taboos on sex education in virtually any form. Nearly half of all college students in China have received no education in school about sexual behavior and health (Li et al., 2004), and sex is not generally discussed in the home. Recently, however, China began efforts to educate the country's young people about sex and especially sexual health. In 2003, with financial and social backing from the United Nations, the Chinese government created a first-of-its-kind Web site for that country, called "You and Me," with the intention of engaging and informing youth on a variety of sexual topics. Although the Web site covers a wide range of issues, sexual and otherwise, it places an extra emphasis on such subjects as HIV/AIDS, unwanted pregnancies, and unsafe abortion practices. Through this Web site, people are not only able to read about sexuality but are also able to communicate with each other about matters of interest.

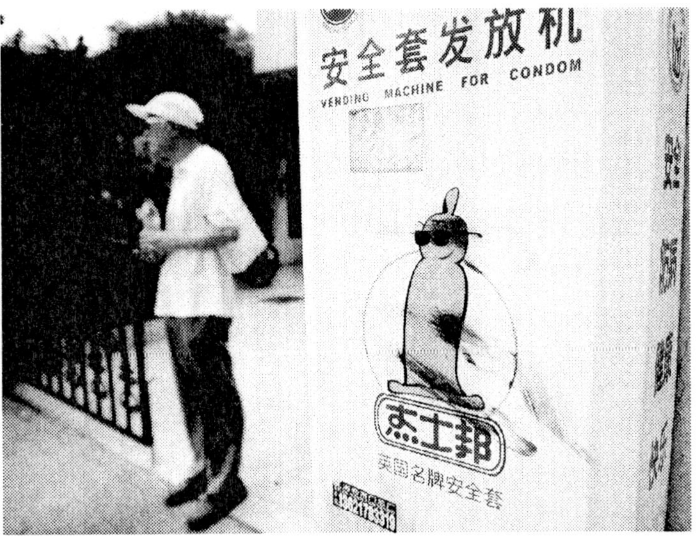

A condom vending machine in Beijing.

In addition to the Web site, three major cities in China—Shanghai, Beijing, and Chongqing—are experimenting with a sexual education program aimed at middle school girls. The program was established by China's State Education Commission in conjunction with the Chinese branch of Procter & Gamble. If all goes well, the program will be instituted in more than 300 additional cities around the country (Harvard Medical School, 2004).

Several factors have prompted China's newfound interest in sexual education. One of these is the increasingly younger ages at which girls reach puberty. China's growing economy has led to healthier diets, and girls in China are now reaching puberty, on average, at age 11, two years earlier than previously. Chinese officials have recognized that although young girls may be physically ready to have sex at earlier ages, they may not be emotionally ready or have all of the information they need to make safe, responsible choices about their sexual behavior.

China is also becoming increasingly concerned about the growing public health issues of sexually transmitted infections (STIs), particularly HIV, within its borders. At least a million people in China are estimated to be HIV positive, and the UN predicts the number of cases could grow to over 10 million by 2010. Other STIs are also becoming a problem in China; adults are becoming infected with chlamydia as often as those in industrialized countries in the West, though few Chinese seem to know what chlamydia is or how it is transmitted (BBC, 2003).

In China, as in most Western countries, young people are at greater risk of STIs as they become more sexually active than in past generations. They are having more sex before marriage, due in part to the earlier onset of puberty among girls, which creates a longer span of time between the onset of puberty and marriage (BBC, 2003).

Despite signs of sexual liberation in China, openly discussing sex is still considered socially unacceptable. For instance, although condoms are freely sold, a recent ad that depicted a condom was deemed indecent and banned there. Moreover, China's ministry of communication routinely blocks Web sites from other countries that discuss STIs and other sexual health topics. Despite these attitudes, China is beginning to recognize the health dangers inherent in sexual activity. In Beijing beginning in 2004, condom vending machines were being installed in restrooms throughout the city.

Younger generations in China are eager to learn about sex. In 2003, a new textbook on sexual education was put on sale and was already in its third printing within a week. Though still in its earliest stages of educating its population of over a billion in matters of sex, China has begun to take some small steps in this direction.

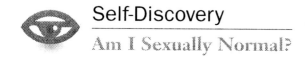

Self-Discovery

Am I Sexually Normal?

Professional sex therapist Marty Klein has noted that Americans are concerned—virtually obsessed—with the normality of their sexual fantasies, preferences, responses, secrets, turnoffs, and problems; the normality of their bodies; and the frequency with which they have sex. The fear of being sexually abnormal interferes with—and can even prevent—pleasure and intimacy (1993, p. 49). As we grow and develop in our culture the subtle (or not-so-subtle) messages most people receive during childhood and adolescence imply that sexuality is something we shouldn't talk about. This denial of our natural sexuality interferes with learning about what is considered sexually normal. In turn, this causes the development of "normality anxiety," which can negatively affect our intimate sexual relations with our partners.

Klein lists some of the most commonly asked questions about what is "normal":

1. Are my sexual fantasies normal?
2. Are my genitals the normal shape, size, color?
3. Unlike my friends, I like/don't like watching X-rated videos. Am I normal?
4. I want sex a lot more often than my partner. Am I normal?
5. I enjoy lovemaking, but my biggest orgasms are from masturbation. Am I normal?

Klein says (and most sexuality researchers and educators would agree), "I tell them time and time again, not one of these facts or feelings is *abnormal* (in fact in a more sexually enlightened world, the question of their *normality* would not even arise)" (pp. 50–51).

Source: Klein, M. (1993) Am I sexually normal? *New Woman, May, 1993,* 49–52.

Sexual Health

Sexual health is a significant part of your overall health, yet it is the part that is hidden and neglected the most (Baber & Murray, 2001). Sexual health refers to a wide range of physical, psychological, and emotional issues relating to your sexuality and discussed in various chapters in this book, including the following:

- Sexually transmitted infections (i.e., HIV, genital warts, herpes, hepatitis B, gonorrhea, chlamydia, and pubic lice)
- Problems with sexual functioning (i.e., premature ejaculation, erectile difficulties, problems with arousal or orgasm, loss of sexual desire)
- The health of your sexual anatomy (i.e., cancer of the breast, cervix, ovaries, testicles, or prostate; painful sex; urinary and reproductive tract infections)
- Emotional and psychological sexual health issues (i.e., abusive or controlling relationships, past sexual traumas, sexual violence, fear or guilt about sex)

One of the recurring features in all the other chapters of this text, "In Touch with Your Sexual Health," is designed to highlight and draw your attention to important issues of sexual health as they arise throughout the text. An awareness and understanding of these health concerns is crucial to maintaining healthy sexual functioning for yourself and your partner.

Parenting

Most of you who are reading this have or will have children of your own. One of your important responsibilities in raising them will be to teach them about sex. Although *you* may or may not have learned about sex from your parents, most people agree that parents are the most appropriate source of this knowledge. This assumes, however, that parents are willing to talk to each other and their kids about sex and are able to impart complete and accurate information. Studying human sexuality will help prepare you for this aspect of parenthood, should you choose to become a parent, by providing you with

sexual health Overall physical and psychological health relating to sexuality.

Table 1.2 EFFECT OF A HUMAN SEXUALITY COURSE ON PARENTS' DISCUSSIONS OF SEXUALITY WITH THEIR CHILDREN

QUESTIONS PARENTS WERE ASKED	PERCENTAGE WHO TOOK SEXUALITY COURSE ANSWERING YES	PERCENTAGE WITHOUT SEXUALITY COURSE ANSWERING YES
Have you had discussions about sexuality with your children?	45	9
Do you use correct anatomical words for genitals?	24	6
Have you discussed where babies come from? (children age 5–11)	24	5
Have you discussed inappropriate touching by others? (age 5–11)	29	22
Have you discussed menstruation? (age 12+)	30	16
Have you discussed masturbation? (age 12+)	14	2
Have you discussed intercourse and reproduction? (age 12+)	30	4
Have you discussed birth control? (age 12+)	30	6
Have you discussed homosexuality? (age 12+)	25	5
Have you discussed sexual abuse? (age 12+)	26	11
Have you discussed sexually transmitted diseases? (age 12+)	30	6

Note: All differences are statistically significant

Source: Adapted from King, Parisi, and O'Dwyer (1993).

the knowledge, resources, and degree of comfort you need to teach your children about sex. Research clearly supports the advantages of this knowledge to parents and their children. In a study by King, Parisi, and O'Dwyer (1993), parents who had taken a human sexuality class in college were compared to those who had not. The results indicated a striking difference between the groups. Parents who had taken the human sexuality course were found to be much more likely to discuss various aspects of sexuality with their children and to use correct terminology when doing so. Table 1.2 summarizes some of their findings.

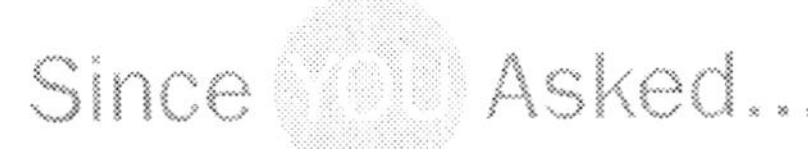

6. My parents have never had "the talk" with me. Are they just embarrassed, or did they think I would learn on my own?

Evaluating Sexual Research

You are constantly deluged by sexual messages and information in the form of advice columns, rumors, gossip, stories, pictures, TV shows, movies, Internet sites, advertisements, catalogs, and all the other audio or visual media you can imagine. How do you know what to do with such an excess of information? Your ability to sort, analyze, and interpret sexual material is becoming increasingly important as more and more information becomes available in this electronic age (Cooper, McLoughlin, & Campbell, 2000). In the next section, we will focus on how human sexuality research is conducted so that you will be able to understand better how to analyze and interpret what gets reported in the media. Moreover, this book will give you information about sexuality based on the best solid, systematic research available. As you study what is contained in these pages, you will begin to think critically about the issues and apply what you learn to assess the world around you. In short, you will become a more educated and knowledgeable consumer in the marketplace of sexual information.

Whether taken individually or together, all of these experiential and understanding factors should make it clear that studying human sexuality may be one of the most valuable endeavors you will undertake (see Table 1.3). Many of the benefits are immediate and will affect your life now. But you will likely discover that you will be putting the information in this book to work for you, your relationships, and your family years and even generations into the future.

Table 1.3 EXPERIENCING AND UNDERSTANDING HUMAN SEXUALITY

EXPERIENCING SEXUALITY

People who take a course in human sexuality . . .

- Are more comfortable with the many and sometimes conflicting emotions that surround sexual issues
- Have greater knowledge and awareness of who they are as sexual individuals
- Are more confident and clear about their personal sexual morals and values
- Make more informed, responsible, and healthy choices about their sexual behavior and relationships
- Know that sex is more than intercourse and appreciate a wider range of intimate sexual behaviors
- Enjoy more overall satisfying sex lives

UNDERSTANDING SEXUALITY

People who take a course in human sexuality . . .

- Understand that human sexuality is complex
- Are more likely to reject common sexual myths, falsehoods, and misconceptions
- Are more tolerant of others' sexual preferences, orientations, morals, values, customs, and differences
- Are less likely to worry about being sexually "strange" or "abnormal"
- Maintain better physical, emotional, and sexual health
- Have a greater level of skill and comfort in discussing sexual issues with their partners and their own children
- Are better able to analyze and evaluate critically sexual research and information

Methods for Studying Human Sexuality

Imagine for a moment that you are a researcher in a field that studies human sexuality, say a psychologist, sociologist, biologist, physician, or nurse. You want to study some aspect of sexuality to answer a question that might further our understanding of this complex field. What sort of question might you ask? Here are some possibilities:

- On average, at what age do people first have sexual intercourse?
- How often do married couples make love?
- What percentage of college students are sexually active?
- What are the differences in sexual arousal for men and women?
- What type of therapy works best for sexual problems?
- Does an herbal aphrodisiac (sex stimulant) advertised in the tabloids really work?
- Does HIV awareness education in high schools reduce high-risk sexual behaviors?
- What is the most effective form of birth control?

You can probably think of many other questions (and many students have, as you will see in the Since You Asked section at the beginning of each chapter in this book).

Our focus here is on how you would go about answering these questions in ways that are accurate and meaningful. The study of human sexuality is a science, and it follows the methods of research used by all scientists. These methods include scientific surveys, careful behavioral observation, correlational research, and experiments. Which of these methods might researchers use to address the questions posed in the preceding paragraph? Could they (1) ask people to tell about their personal sex lives, (2) observe people engaging in sexual behavior, (3) analyze the relationships among various aspects

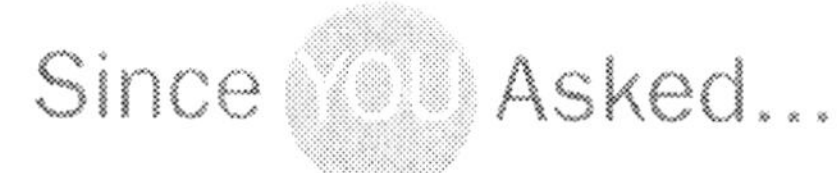

7. How is it possible to study people's sexual behavior when it's such a private, personal experience?

of people's sexuality, or (4) perform actual experiments involving sexuality? The answer to all four is *yes!* However, we're dealing with a very intimate topic here, so you can imagine the difficulties that might be encountered when trying to carry out such studies in accurate, unbiased, and ethical ways.

In this section, we will examine scientific research methods as they apply to the study of human sexuality and consider the advantages, disadvantages, potential for error and bias, and ethical considerations associated with each.

No matter what research method a researcher chooses, information and data gathering must be planned carefully and carried out systematically. Participants to be studied should be chosen to represent, as closely as possible, the larger population of interest. All research volunteers should be treated in similar ways. Researchers must be trained to interact with participants consistently and to avoid introducing their own biased attitudes into the study. Information should be gathered so that it can be analyzed using statistical methods. Participants must be made to feel comfortable, safe, and assured of complete confidentiality when participating in a study involving their personal sexual attitudes and behaviors. Any reliable and valid scientific study should be able to be *replicated*—repeated using the same methodology on the same or a different sample of participants—with virtually identical results. Finally, strict ethical guidelines must be followed when engaging in any research involving humans, especially when engaging in studies related to sexuality.

Surveys

The most common form of sexual research is the **survey**. A survey is the process of collecting information from volunteer **respondents** for the purpose of explaining, describing, or comparing people's knowledge, attitudes, beliefs, and behaviors. Large-scale surveys of sexual behavior and attitudes were pioneered by Dr. Alfred Kinsey in the 1940s. His approach and methodologies provided the foundation for most of the survey research about sexuality that has followed for over half a century. Today, the Kinsey Institute at Indiana University is one of the leading centers promoting and carrying out scientific research on human sexuality.

Conducting a survey seems simple enough, right? Just put together a list of questions, send it out to a lot of people, and ask them to fill it out and send it back! That may sound easy on the surface, but survey research is actually extremely difficult to carry out and end up with results that we can trust to be consistent and accurate. All surveys (and measuring devices of all kinds) must possess two basic requirements: reliability and validity.

Reliability refers to a survey's ability to measure a characteristic consistently over time. This simply means that if I give you a survey designed to measure, say, your attitudes about sex education in high schools, I should be able to give you that same survey next week or next month and obtain similar results (unless, of course your attitude has changed drastically, which is unlikely). If, on the other hand, your results were to vary significantly each time you take it, I would not be able to count on the accuracy of the survey. To understand this concept more clearly, imagine you have a tape measure you are using to find the dimensions of a doorway. Every time you measure the same doorway, the tape shows a different dimension: first, the door is 5 feet 6 inches tall; you measure it again, and the tape reads 6 feet 3 inches; so you measure it again, and the tape shows 4 feet 9 inches. You would probably throw the tape measure in the trash because you are unable to count on it for accuracy—it is unreliable. The same principle applies to surveys.

survey The scientific collection of data from a group of individuals about their beliefs, attitudes, or behaviors.

respondents Individuals selected to respond to a researcher's request for information.

reliability The ability of any measuring instrument, such as a questionnaire or personality scale, to provide consistent responses over repeated administrations.

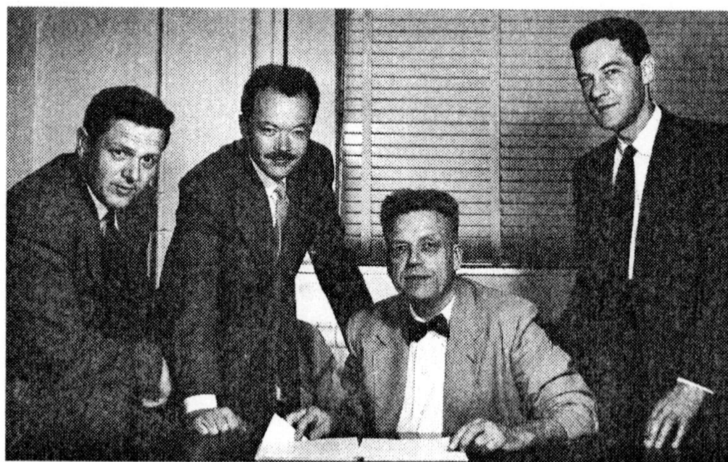

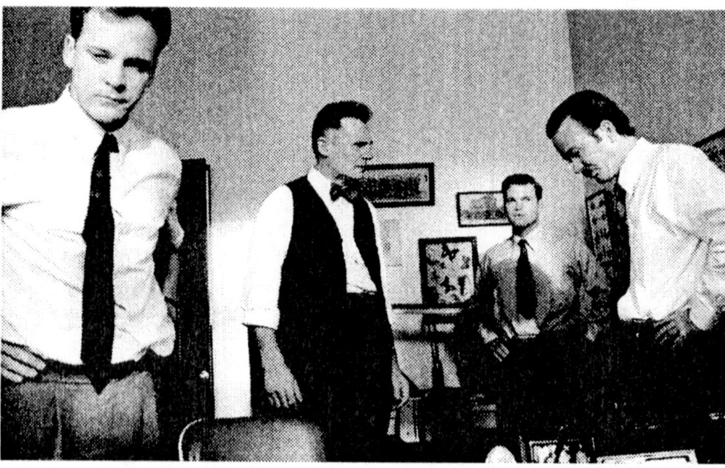

The 2004 film Kinsey *(photo right) reintroduced the world to the life and work of pioneering sex survey researcher, Alfred Kinsey seated in the real-life photo (left). Although we must always be cautious about interpreting Hollywood's version of historical events,* Kinsey *provides a fascinating glimpse into one of the most influential figures in the history of sexuality research. In the late 1940s and early 1950s when Kinsey was gathering his data about the sexual behavior of men and women in the United States, attitudes about sex were generally quite restrictive. A scene in the film shows government agents seizing a package of Kinsey's research materials, claiming they were "obscene." Not only did Kinsey pioneer the survey method of sexuality research, but he did so with conviction—some might say courage—in the highly nonsupportive social and political environment of the time.*

Validity is the extent to which your survey measures what it is intended to measure. In other words, to be valid, the results of a survey (or any measuring device) must be a "truthful" representation of the underlying characteristic being measured. For many reasons, that is often not as easy as it sounds. First, the questions must truly tap into the characteristic. Second, the wording of survey items must not allow for more than one interpretation or hint at a desired response. Third, the sample of participants who respond to the survey must accurately represent the larger group that you are trying to study. And fourth, researchers must be reasonably sure that participants have not been biased in their responses to the survey items.

Because surveys have been so common in research on human sexuality, it is important to discuss reliability and validity in greater detail. First we will look at various types of surveys and then examine potential problems that must be avoided if a survey is to provide accurate, scientific information.

Types of Surveys

Four basic types of surveys are most often used by researchers: the self-administered written questionnaire, face-to-face interviews, interviews conducted over the telephone, and Internet surveys. Each method has inherent advantages and disadvantages (Binik, Mah, & Kiesler, 1999; Epstein, Klinkenberg, Wiley, & McKinley, 2001; Nachmias & Nachmias, 1987).

When dealing with sensitive issues relating to a person's sexual attitudes and behaviors, which survey method do you think would yield the most honest answers from participants? The written questionnaire offers the greatest anonymity and privacy for the respondent and may therefore produce more honest responses. However, the face-to-face interview allows the interviewer to establish a friendly, trusting rapport with the participants and to have more flexibility in asking planned and follow-up questions, which may lead to greater honesty in the answers (Nachmias & Nachmias, 1987). The telephone survey may fall somewhere in between these methods, allowing for both anonymity and flexibility in questioning. However, the possibility exists that some people may not take telephone interviews seriously or may be annoyed at the intrusion into their lives, thereby reducing the completeness or accuracy of their answers. Surveys conducted over the Internet offer the possibility of a large number of responses from a wide geographical area over a relatively short time span. However, Internet surveys also pose new and troubling concerns over research ethics and validity. Some of these concerns relate to the following questions: Is it possible to inform people about the survey so that they are aware of the nature of the items before they

validity The extent to which a measuring instrument is a true assessment of the characteristic it is intended to measure.

agree to participate? Are the data truly confidential? Are all the participants of legal age (Binik et al., 1999)? Are they all whom they claim to be relative to age, gender, attitudes, and experiences? To what extent does the Internet provide a nonrepresentative, self-selected sample of participants (Bradley, 1999; Epstein et al., 2001)? Will Internet respondents take the survey seriously? Will they respond honestly? The answers to these questions are not yet clear, but most researchers agree that the Internet offers far-reaching and powerful opportunities for all psychological research, including studies of human sexuality. For an overview of some of the most important survey studies since the 1940s in the field of human sexuality, see Table 1.4 on pages 20–21.

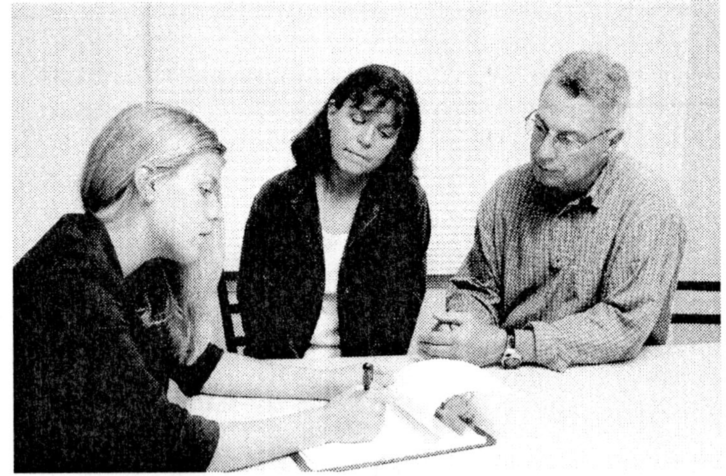

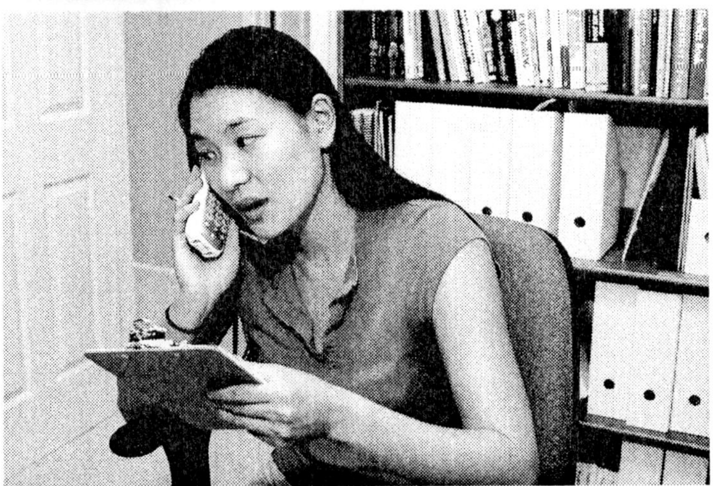

Surveys may be conducted in various formats, including in-person and telephone surveys.

Wording of Survey Questions

The reliability and validity of a survey require that the questions be unbiased and clearly worded so that each person responding to the survey will interpret the items in the same way and will not be led into any particular response. For example, consider the following seemingly simple, straightforward question: *How often do you and your partner make love?* Someone answering this question might wonder, During what period of time? Last week? Last month? On average through our entire relationship? And what is meant by "make love"? Some people would probably interpret this to mean sexual intercourse, but what if a couple sometimes likes to just kiss and touch—is that making love? Does oral sex count as making love? You can see that questions must be carefully designed to avoid this sort of confusion, or we can never be sure what the respondents' answers really mean. To achieve such clarity, the question might be changed to *On average, how many times per week have you and your partner had sexual intercourse during the past six months?* Many other potential problems may arise on the road to clear, effective wording of questionnaire items, and a great deal of education and training is required before someone is qualified to develop valid and reliable survey instruments (for a more detailed discussion of survey item construction, Anastasi & Urbina, 1997, or Nachmias & Nachmias, 1987).

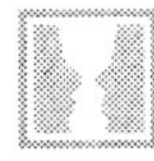

Sex is more than intercourse

Participant Sample

The entire group of people being studied in a survey is called the **target population**. Typically, this is a very large group, such as "college students," "teenagers," "adult males," "adult females," or "students in human sexuality classes." However, it is usually not possible to survey an entire target population, so researchers select a smaller group, called a **sample**, from the population. To maximize the validity of a survey, the sample of people selected to participate should represent as closely as possible the larger population that is being studied. For example, if you were interested in studying the sex lives of college students, you would not ask people at the local mall to fill out your surveys, because they would probably not be representative of your target population (students are not at the mall; they're in the library studying, right?).

The best way to ensure a representative sample would be to select respondents randomly from the entire population of interest. This process is called **random sampling**. To illustrate the importance of this idea, suppose you are doing a study on the sexual experiences of first-year American college students. You send a survey

target population The entire group of people to which a researcher is attempting to apply a study sample's findings.

sample A subset of the target population selected by researchers to represent the entire population under study.

random sampling A method of selecting a sample of participants in such a way that each member of the population has an equal chance of being selected.

Table 1.4 LARGE-SCALE SCIENTIFIC SURVEYS OF HUMAN SEXUALITY SINCE 1948

SURVEY	REPORTING AUTHORS	YEAR OF PUBLICATION	SUBJECTS	TYPE	NOTES
Sexual Behavior in the Human Male ("The Kinsey Report")	Kinsey, Pomeroy, & Martin	1948	5,300 white males	Face-to-face interview	Scientific question construction; well-trained interviewers; large number of questions (300+); nonrepresentative sample; did not include nonwhite ethnic groups and underrepresented rural residents and the elderly.
Sexual Behavior in the Human Female	Kinsey et al.	1953	5,940 white females	Face-to-face interview	Same criticisms as first Kinsey study.
Sexual Behavior in the 1970s ("The Hunt Report")	Hunt	1974	982 males and 1,044 females, age 18+	Panel discussion and written questionnaire	Random selection from telephone books created reasonably representative mix of subgroups; serious volunteer bias: 20 percent agreed to participate, 80 percent refused.
Hite Report on Female Sexuality	Hite	1976	3,019 women	Written essay questionnaire	Demonstrated diversity of sexual experience; nonrepresentative samples obtained through feminist and college women's groups; serious volunteer bias: 3 percent return rate; poorly constructed questions.
Hite Report on Male Sexuality	Hite	1981	7,239 men	Written essay questionnaire	Same comments as first Hite study; 6 percent return rate of questionnaires
Women and Love: A Cultural Revolution	Hite	1987	4,500 women	Written questionnaire	Same prior Hite study; 4.5 percent return rate.
American Couples	Blumstein & Schwartz	1983	6,071 heterosexual, gay, and lesbian couples	Questionnaire and Interviews	First study to focus on couples; included gay and lesbian couples; included nonsexual aspects of relationships; sample not representative: underrepresents elderly, minorities, and lower socioeconomic groups.
National Survey of Men	Billy, Tanfer, Grady, Klepinger; Tanfer; Tanfer, Grady, Klepinger, & Billy	1993	3,321 men, age 20–39	Face-to-face interviews	Males only; good representation of minorities; excellent volunteer rate of 70 percent; possible social desirability response bias on some items.
Janus Report on Sexual Behavior	Janus & Janus	1993	1,347 men; 1,418 women	2,765 questionnaires and 125 face-to-face interviews	Scientific random sampling used; attempt to obtain sample reflecting population distributions in 1990 census data.
National AIDS Behavioral Survey	Dolcini	1993	Over 10,000 heterosexual adults	Face-to-face interviews	Very large sample with variation in ethnic groups, income level, marital status, age and sex; good return rate of 70 percent; interview offered in Spanish as well as English.

Table 1.4 (*Continued*)

SURVEY	REPORTING AUTHORS	YEAR OF PUBLICATION	SUBJECTS	TYPE	NOTES
National Health and Social Life Survey	Michael, Gagnon, Laumann, & Kolata; Laumann; Gagnon, Michael, & Michaels	1994	3,432 adults, age 18–59	Face-to-face interviews	Excellent response rate of 79 percent; reasonably representative sample; 90-minute time limit on interviews; probable response bias due to presence of spouse or children during 21 percent of interviews; interviewers minimally trained.
Advocate Sex Poll	*The Advocate* (national gay and lesbian news magazine)	2002	1,438 gay men, 391 lesbians; and 18 transsexuals	Online survey	Nonrandom, self-selected sample; primarily limited to readers of the *Advocate*; conducted on the publication's Web site; rare survey focusing on nonheterosexual respondents.
International Sexuality Description Project	Schmidt et al.	2003	Over 16,000 men and women worldwide	Anonymous written self-report survey	Only large-scale multinational survey to date; relied on anonymous written questionnaires.
Durex Global Sex Survey	Durex Corp.	2005	Over 50,000 men and women worldwide	Online survey	Nonrandom, self-selected, "youth-oriented sample" (primarily Caucasian Americans) conducted on the company's Web site.

to 1,000 students at, say, the University of Nebraska and Texas A&M University. Do you suppose their responses represent first-year American college students in general? How different do you think their experiences might be from first-year students at, say, NYU or UC Berkeley? This is not to assume that students at any of these particular universities are strange or abnormal (probably not, anyway), but it points out that for your sample to be random, you would need to include participants from colleges and universities of various sizes, types, and locations throughout the country or else narrow the target population you are studying (Gliner, Morgan, & Harmon, 2000; Kantowitz, Roediger, & Elmes, 1994).

Another important point about sampling and validity is that the larger your sample, the more representative of your population it is likely to be. If your population is 10,000 people, a sample of 1,000 respondents will almost certainly represent your overall population significantly more accurately than if you have only 100 participants.

Finally, the point needs to be made that in actual research studies, these requirements for selecting a sample of participants are often not met. You can imagine how difficult, time-consuming, and expensive it would be to survey a very large random sample of a target population containing hundreds of thousands or millions of people. Therefore, many studies are published using potentially nonrepresentative samples of subjects (such as, say, first-year psychology students at a single university). Although these studies can be informative and helpful in our understanding of human nature, they must be viewed with a critical eye, recognizing possible weaknesses in the sample of subjects selected.

Self-Selection of Participants

A common problem with sexuality research is that some individuals will agree to participate (volunteers) and others will refuse (nonvolunteers). Do you think these two groups might be fundamentally different in some important ways? It may be that those who refuse to participate in a survey about sexuality might feel uncomfortable or embarrassed about revealing personal sexual issues, believe that such information is nobody else's business, believe that such research is morally wrong, or feel more guilt about sex than the volunteers. On the other hand, if a study focused on an aspect of sexuality most people considered positive, such as sexual attractiveness or skill as a lover, you would expect people who felt proud of possessing that quality to be more likely to volunteer for the study. If either of these situations occurs, your sample may be nonrandom and biased.

Since YOU Asked...

8. Has anyone scientifically studied average penis size? If so, what is it?

For example, in 2001, a condom company wanted to do a study to determine average penis length. The company set up a "penis-measuring tent" outside a popular nightclub in Cancun, Mexico, during spring break. Researchers invited men to come in, look at some sexy literature, become erect, and be measured. The researchers found that the average erect penis length of the 300 volunteers was 5.877 inches. This was slightly longer than had been found in previous studies (more about this in Chapter 2, "Sexual Anatomy"). Why the difference? *Self-selection.* If you think about it, wouldn't you logically assume, considering the value placed on penis size in our culture (however misguided this emphasis may be), that men with larger penises would be more likely to volunteer to be measured? This demonstrates how self-selection may lead to unreliable findings.

Research has uncovered a number of differences between volunteer sex research participants and those who are randomly selected. These differences between volunteers and nonvolunteers, summarized in Table 1.5, may create what is referred to as a **self-selection bias** in the conclusions drawn from the data gathered in sexual research. This implies that the very nature of the people who agreed to be studied places them in a group that may not accurately represent the population as a whole.

Since YOU Asked...

9. I read in a checkout-stand magazine that a survey of readers found that most men and women (like 90 percent) do not like their own bodies. Could this be true?

"Evaluating Sexual Research: 'What Men and Women Really Want in Bed: Take Our Reader's Survey'" on page 24 focuses on how this self-selection bias renders most surveys in popular magazines seriously flawed and invalid. Of course, we cannot *force* people to participate in research about sex (or on any topic, for that matter) if they choose not to, so no easy solution exists to the self-selection bias. However, such built-in biases must be kept in mind whenever you are studying the findings of human sexuality research.

Self-Report Data

A potential problem with most surveys is that the information gathered is based on participants' reporting of their own behavior or attitudes. This means that the data are subjective without any way of verifying if the answers given by participants are accurate or if their answers truly reflect their actual behavior. For one thing, humans are notoriously poor at accurately remembering specific events and behaviors (Loftus, 1980; Schachter, Norman, & Koutstall, 1998). But beyond faulty memory, people may be motivated to give incorrect information, especially on sexuality surveys, due to embarrassment, fear of appearing immoral or abnormal, or general discomfort with discussing their sexual lives.

One common source of misinformation in survey research is called the **social desirability bias**. Most of us, whether we are talking to friends, making comments in a class, or responding to a survey, want to express ourselves in ways that are socially acceptable

self-selection bias The effect of allowing members of a target population under study to volunteer to participate in the study; it may compromise the randomness and validity of the research.

social desirability bias The tendency of individuals to answer survey questions in socially desirable and culturally approved ways.

Self-Selection of Participants

A common problem with sexuality research is that some individuals will agree to participate (volunteers) and others will refuse (nonvolunteers). Do you think these two groups might be fundamentally different in some important ways? It may be that those who refuse to participate in a survey about sexuality might feel uncomfortable or embarrassed about revealing personal sexual issues, believe that such information is nobody else's business, believe that such research is morally wrong, or feel more guilt about sex than the volunteers. On the other hand, if a study focused on an aspect of sexuality most people considered positive, such as sexual attractiveness or skill as a lover, you would expect people who felt proud of possessing that quality to be more likely to volunteer for the study. If either of these situations occurs, your sample may be nonrandom and biased.

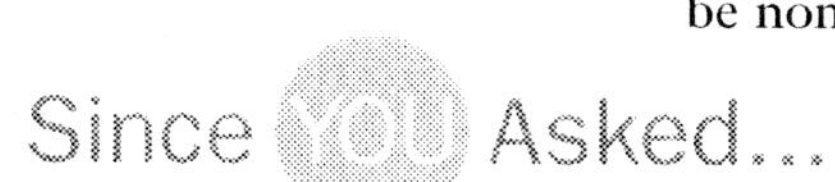

8. Has anyone scientifically studied average penis size? If so, what is it?

For example, in 2001, a condom company wanted to do a study to determine average penis length. The company set up a "penis-measuring tent" outside a popular nightclub in Cancun, Mexico, during spring break. Researchers invited men to come in, look at some sexy literature, become erect, and be measured. The researchers found that the average erect penis length of the 300 volunteers was 5.877 inches. This was slightly longer than had been found in previous studies (more about this in Chapter 2, "Sexual Anatomy"). Why the difference? *Self-selection.* If you think about it, wouldn't you logically assume, considering the value placed on penis size in our culture (however misguided this emphasis may be), that men with larger penises would be more likely to volunteer to be measured? This demonstrates how self-selection may lead to unreliable findings.

Research has uncovered a number of differences between volunteer sex research participants and those who are randomly selected. These differences between volunteers and nonvolunteers, summarized in Table 1.5, may create what is referred to as a **self-selection bias** in the conclusions drawn from the data gathered in sexual research. This implies that the very nature of the people who agreed to be studied places them in a group that may not accurately represent the population as a whole. "Evaluating Sexual Research: 'What Men and Women Really Want in Bed: Take Our Reader's Survey'" on page 24 focuses on how this self-selection bias renders most surveys in popular magazines seriously flawed and invalid. Of course, we cannot *force* people to participate in research about sex (or on any topic, for that matter) if they choose not to, so no easy solution exists to the self-selection bias. However, such built-in biases must be kept in mind whenever you are studying the findings of human sexuality research.

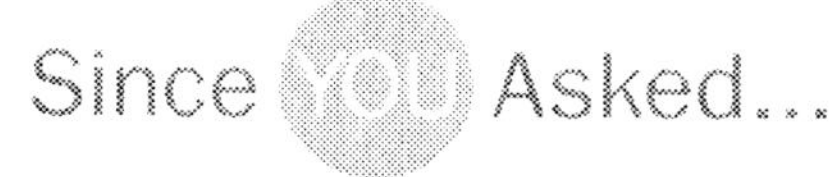

9. I read in a checkout-stand magazine that a survey of readers found that most men and women (like 90 percent) do not like their own bodies. Could this be true?

Self-Report Data

A potential problem with most surveys is that the information gathered is based on participants' reporting of their own behavior or attitudes. This means that the data are subjective without any way of verifying if the answers given by participants are accurate or if their answers truly reflect their actual behavior. For one thing, humans are notoriously poor at accurately remembering specific events and behaviors (Loftus, 1980; Schachter, Norman, & Koutstall, 1998). But beyond faulty memory, people may be motivated to give incorrect information, especially on sexuality surveys, due to embarrassment, fear of appearing immoral or abnormal, or general discomfort with discussing their sexual lives.

One common source of misinformation in survey research is called the **social desirability bias**. Most of us, whether we are talking to friends, making comments in a class, or responding to a survey, want to express ourselves in ways that are socially acceptable

self-selection bias The effect of allowing members of a target population under study to volunteer to participate in the study; it may compromise the randomness and validity of the research.

social desirability bias The tendency of individuals to answer survey questions in socially desirable and culturally approved ways.

Table 1.4 (*Continued*)

SURVEY	REPORTING AUTHORS	YEAR OF PUBLICATION	SUBJECTS	TYPE	NOTES
National Health and Social Life Survey	Michael, Gagnon, Laumann, & Kolata; Laumann; Gagnon, Michael, & Michaels	1994	3,432 adults, age 18–59	Face-to-face interviews	Excellent response rate of 79 percent; reasonably representative sample; 90-minute time limit on interviews; probable response bias due to presence of spouse or children during 21 percent of interviews; interviewers minimally trained.
Advocate Sex Poll	*The Advocate* (national gay and lesbian news magazine)	2002	1,438 gay men, 391 lesbians; and 18 transsexuals	Online survey	Nonrandom, self-selected sample; primarily limited to readers of the *Advocate*; conducted on the publication's Web site; rare survey focusing on nonheterosexual respondents.
International Sexuality Description Project	Schmidt et al.	2003	Over 16,000 men and women worldwide	Anonymous written self-report survey	Only large-scale multinational survey to date; relied on anonymous written questionnaires.
Durex Global Sex Survey	Durex Corp.	2005	Over 50,000 men and women worldwide	Online survey	Nonrandom, self-selected, "youth-oriented sample" (primarily Caucasian Americans) conducted on the company's Web site.

to 1,000 students at, say, the University of Nebraska and Texas A&M University. Do you suppose their responses represent first-year American college students in general? How different do you think their experiences might be from first-year students at, say, NYU or UC Berkeley? This is not to assume that students at any of these particular universities are strange or abnormal (probably not, anyway), but it points out that for your sample to be random, you would need to include participants from colleges and universities of various sizes, types, and locations throughout the country or else narrow the target population you are studying (Gliner, Morgan, & Harmon, 2000; Kantowitz, Roediger, & Elmes, 1994).

Another important point about sampling and validity is that the larger your sample, the more representative of your population it is likely to be. If your population is 10,000 people, a sample of 1,000 respondents will almost certainly represent your overall population significantly more accurately than if you have only 100 participants.

Finally, the point needs to be made that in actual research studies, these requirements for selecting a sample of participants are often not met. You can imagine how difficult, time-consuming, and expensive it would be to survey a very large random sample of a target population containing hundreds of thousands or millions of people. Therefore, many studies are published using potentially nonrepresentative samples of subjects (such as, say, first-year psychology students at a single university). Although these studies can be informative and helpful in our understanding of human nature, they must be viewed with a critical eye, recognizing possible weaknesses in the sample of subjects selected.

Table 1.5 COMPARISON OF VOLUNTEERS AND NONVOLUNTEERS FOR SEXUALITY RESEARCH

PARTICIPANT CHARACTERISTIC	VOLUNTEERS	NONVOLUNTEERS
Age	Younger	Older
Education	Slightly more years	Slightly fewer years
Income level	Higher	Lower
Experienced past sexual trauma	More likely	Less likely
Masturbation	More often	Less often
Exposure to sexual erotica	More	Less
Sexual experience	More	Less
Attitudes about sex	More positive	Less positive
Attitudes about sexual research	More positive	Less positive
Sexual fear	Less	More
Sexual guilt	Less	More
Sexually permissive	More	Less
Political views	More liberal	More conservative

Sources: Adapted from Clement (1990); Morokoff (1986); Strassberg & Lowe (1995); Wiederman (1993); and Wolchik, Spencer, & Lisi (1983).

and allow us to be seen in a positive light by others. Questions about very personal issues, such as number of sexual partners or the frequency of certain sexual behaviors (i.e., masturbation, oral sex, same-sex encounters), may lead to inaccurate answers because participants feel that a truthful response would be judged socially unacceptable (Anastasi & Urbina, 1997; Bolton & Nardi, 1993; Ingall, 1995). Social desirability bias may also lead to inaccuracies in participants' responses due to exaggeration or denial. For example, researchers have found that in U.S. culture, men tend to "enhance" their level of sexual experience, while women tend to minimize theirs (Havemann & Lehtinen, 1990).

It is interesting to note that this tendency to respond to survey items in socially desirable ways is not necessarily a deliberate attempt to deceive the researchers. The desire to avoid criticism or embarrassment and gain social approval in our interactions with others may be a tendency of which we are largely unaware (Anastasi & Urbina, 1997). However, this bias is another important factor to consider when interpreting sexual research findings.

Case Studies

The **case study** has been a popular method of research by professionals in such fields as medicine, psychology, and sexuality. In a case study, a single individual (or occasionally a small group) with a particular illness, problem, or unusual set of life circumstances is followed closely over time. Data may be gathered from direct observation and interaction with the subject or through analysis of medical records, journals, diaries, or other historical records of the individual being studied.

In the past, sexuality researchers often relied on individual case studies to gather information about specific sexual topics. Sigmund Freud in the late 1800s and early 1900s relied heavily on individual case histories of his patients in psychoanalysis to develop, demonstrate, and defend his theories of personality and the psychosexual stages of development (for example, Freud, 1965). During the same

case study An in-depth study and analysis of one person or group who demonstrates specific characteristics of interest to a researcher.

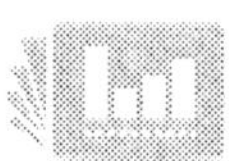

Evaluating Sexual Research

"What Men and Women Really Want in Bed! Take Our Reader's Survey"

How much of your sexual knowledge have you obtained from newsstand magazines? One of the favorite features often found in magazines such as *Redbook*, *Cosmopolitan*, *New Woman*, *Playboy*, *McCall's*, and *Esquire* are surveys that ask readers to respond by mail or online and then report the findings from the survey in a subsequent issue a month or two later. Can you see a flaw in this survey methodology? Even if the items on the survey are constructed properly (and usually they are not), the responses are bound to be seriously biased. First off, all respondents are readers of that particular magazine and would not, therefore, represent the general population. In fact, all magazines are intentionally targeted at a very specific audience, such as single working women, professional men between the ages of 20 and 45, or parents. Second, only a small percentage of readers will take the time and energy to respond to the questionnaire (see Table 1.5 on page 23 comparing volunteers to nonvolunteers in sexual research). These eager participants certainly were not typical of the overall population. Their responses may not even be representative of the readers of that magazine, much less you or me or most other people.

The bottom line is that surveys such as these can be fun and titillating and may, on occasion, offer some interesting information for conversation or gossip, but they should not be considered scientific and cannot be relied on for meaningful sexual knowledge.

The surveys summarized in Table 1.4 on page 20–21 are some of the larger scientific and relatively valid sexuality surveys conducted over the past 60 years or so. Most of them made a major effort to avoid the problems discussed in this box. You will see references to these surveys, along with other smaller survey studies that have been published in professional, scientific journals, throughout this book.

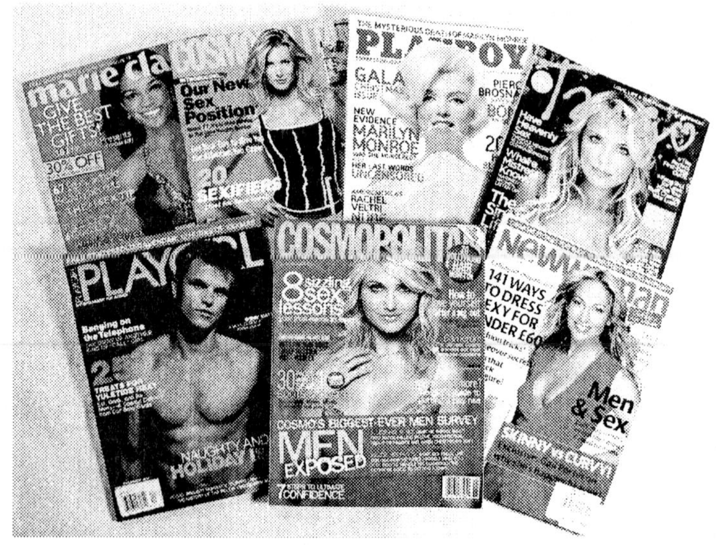

Most surveys in popular magazines rely on biased samples and lack validity.

period in history, Havelock Ellis wrote extensively about sexuality, using hundreds of autobiographical case histories written by his friends, colleagues, and other volunteers (Ellis, 1936).

More recently, Skeen (1991) reported on ten case studies to examine in detail various aspects of sexual experience such as lesbianism, celibacy in the Catholic priesthood, sexual promiscuity, prostitution, incest, and HIV infection and AIDS. And Chopin-Marce (2001) used a case study to examine the effectiveness of psychotherapy for a man who engaged in compulsive exhibitionism. However, relying on a single case to draw conclusions about people in general is risky at best.

Obviously, a single case, especially if it involves unusual or atypical behavior of some kind, is unlikely to represent the majority, or even a small percentage, of people in general. In addition, some researchers may become overly focused on a single subject during an extended study period and lose objectivity. Finally, since this method of research typically involves only one subject and one researcher, the data-gathering process may be biased. This can happen when researchers unintentionally focus on the evidence that supports their theories and ideas and fail to see other evidence that may refute them. This bias, which can occur in any type of research, is referred to as **researcher expectancy effects** (Anastasi & Urbina, 1997; J. D. Evans, 1985).

researcher expectancy effects The influence of the researchers' personal biases on participants' responses and consequently on the study's findings.

Because of these problems, the results of case studies are often referred to as **anecdotal evidence**, meaning individual stories rather than scientifically gathered data. An example of the various pitfalls of the case study method can be seen in "Evaluating Sexual Research: A Case Study of a Case Study" on page 26.

Observational Studies

A great deal can be learned about the behavior of humans simply by observing them directly or by correlating information already known about them. You probably engage in "direct observational research" often and can name several of your favorite "people-watching places." When you people-watch, however, you are doing it in a casual way, for fun. When social scientists engage in **observational research**, they use methods that are systematic and organized in order to obtain the most accurate and precise data possible from their observations. Many human behaviors related to sexuality can be studied using observational techniques. For example, in the 1980s, a group of researchers wanted to study flirting behavior among adults in the United States (Perper, 1985; Perper & Fox, 1981; Perper & Weiss, 1987). They went to public places such as singles bars, college pubs, and nightclubs where single people were likely to meet and flirt. Through careful observation, they identified a sequence of five steps that most people progress through when they flirt. The researchers labeled the steps, "The Approach," "Talk," "Swivel or Turn," "Touch," and "Synchronization." We will examine this research in greater detail in Chapter 4, "Love, Intimacy, and Sexual Communication," but I mention it here to highlight how observational research can offer revealing insights into human sexuality.

Masters and Johnson's Observational Research

Arguably, among the most famous and most important research contributions to the field of human sexuality have been the observational studies conducted by William Masters and Virginia Johnson in the 1960s and described in their groundbreaking book *Human Sexual Response* (1966). In their research center at Washington University's School of Medicine in Saint Louis, Missouri, Masters and Johnson's research team was able to observe hundreds of volunteer participants engage in thousands of actual sexual behaviors. The researchers' goal was to determine how the human body responds during sexual stimulation and arousal and to apply their findings to help people achieve satisfying and fulfilling sexual lives (Hock, 2005). Masters and Johnson have been at the forefront of sexuality research for decades and have published books on a wide range of topics dealing with sex and relationships (1970, 1976, 1979, 1994). You will see their work cited throughout this book.

Masters and Johnson believed that to understand human sexuality, we must go beyond surveys that simply ask people what they do sexually (which was the focus of nearly all prior sexuality research) and study actual physical responses to sexual stimulation. Their research objective was a therapeutic one: to help people overcome sexual problems. They expressed this goal in the following way:

> [The] fundamentals of human sexual behavior cannot be established until two questions are answered: What physical reactions develop as the human male and female respond to effective sexual stimulation? Why do men and women behave as they do when responding to sexual stimulation? If human sexual inadequacy ever is to be treated successfully, the medical and behavioral professions must provide answers to these basic questions. (1966, p. 4)

Masters and Johnson proposed that the only method by which such answers could be obtained was direct systematic observation and physiological measurements of men and women in all stages of sexual responding.

anecdotal evidence Research information gathered through informal stories of people's experiences, which cannot be relied on to draw scientific conclusions.

observational research Gathering behavioral data through direct or indirect observation using scientific techniques.

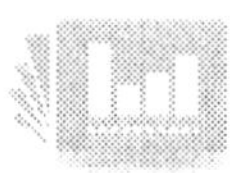

Evaluating Sexual Research

A Case Study of a Case Study

Imagine that you are waiting to check out at the supermarket, and you notice on the cover of a popular magazine a headline for an article about a sex therapist from Chicago, Dr. Sylvia Jenkins, who has developed a new therapeutic technique for assisting couples who are seeking help for what is called "hypoactive [low] sexual desire" (HSD), a chronic loss of enthusiasm and appetite for sex within a relationship (read more about this sexual problem in Chapter 7, "Sexual Problems and Solutions"). You eagerly snatch up the magazine and turn to the article. Through her own experiences and conversations with friends, the article explains, Dr. Jenkins believes that if a couple who has diminished sexual desire begins to engage in a nightly pattern of mutual foot massage, focusing on a spot in the center of the arch of each foot, their sexual passion will be reawakened.

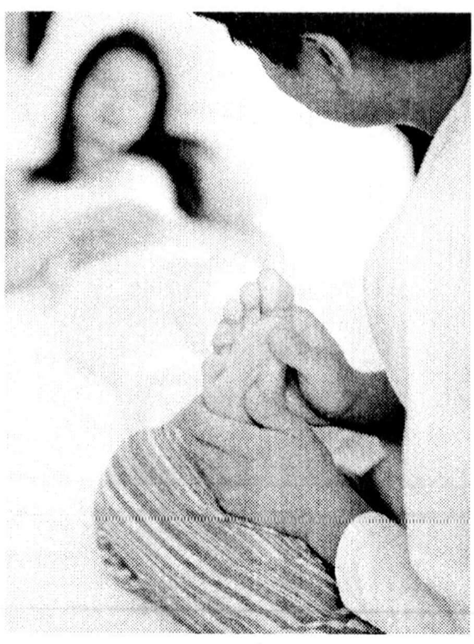

Can sensual massage restore sexual passion?

To test her new technique, she suggests to a couple who have recently begun counseling with her that they try the "foot-rub path to passion." After trying the nightly foot rub for six weeks, Dr. Jenkins finds that although their sexual activity has not changed very much, the couple has noticed a steady increase in sexual desire and in satisfaction with their relationship in general. This outcome leads Dr. Jenkins to publish the article you are reading, titled "Lost Your Sexual Zest? It's in Your Feet!" proclaiming the success of her new therapeutic technique.

Do you see any problems with Dr. Jenkins's conclusions based on her case study? Here are several:

1. Dr. Jenkins's recording of the couple's reports may have been biased to support her theory. After all, the main objective was to increase sexual *activity*, which did not happen. Why did sexual activity not increase even though desire apparently did? Was Dr. Jenkins only recording the data she wanted and expected?
2. How does she really know sexual desire increased if she was only taking the clients' word for it? She did not report any other, more objective measures of sexual desire.
3. How could she be sure the increase in sexual desire (if it really occurred) was due to the foot massages? Maybe any type of touching would have had the same results. Or perhaps this couple would have become sexier over the six weeks with no treatment at all.
4. Maybe a foot massage worked for this couple, but this does not predict whether it will work for you or me or anyone else.

What this case study really does is offer some interesting facts about a *single* case, some anecdotal evidence that foot massage *may* be helpful in treating HSD in *some* people. It does not offer proof of effectiveness and is not scientific enough to be published in a professional journal (which supermarket magazines clearly are not). The study may have some value in that it might stimulate interest in further research that might demonstrate in more reliable and valid ways that foot massage really does turn people on (see "Experimental Research" later in this chapter).

To study in detail these physiological responses during sexual activity and stimulation, various methods of measurement and observation were used. These included standard measures of physiological responses such as pulse, blood pressure, and respiration rate. In addition, specific sexual responses were to be observed and recorded. Sometimes participants were observed and measured while having intercourse in various positions, and other times they were observed and measured during masturbation either manually or with mechanical devices specially designed to allow for internal observation.

You can imagine that all the expectations, observations, and devices might create emotional difficulties for many of the participants. Masters and Johnson were acutely aware of these potential difficulties. To help place participants at ease with the research procedures, they ensured that

> Sexual activity was first encouraged in privacy in the research quarters and then continued with the investigative team present until the study subjects were quite at ease in their artificial surroundings. No attempt was made to record reactions . . . until the study subjects felt secure in their surroundings and confident of their ability to perform. . . . This period of training established a sense of security in the integrity of the research interest and in the absolute anonymity embodied in the program. (1966, pp. 22–23)

The results of Masters and Johnson's early work established a basic foundation and language for understanding and discussing human sexual response. This, in turn, allowed for great strides to be made in the treatment of sexual problems. Even now, four decades later, their findings relating to the sexual response cycle, sexual anatomy, and differences in sexual response between men and women form the basis for most discussions (and many controversies) about basic human sexuality.

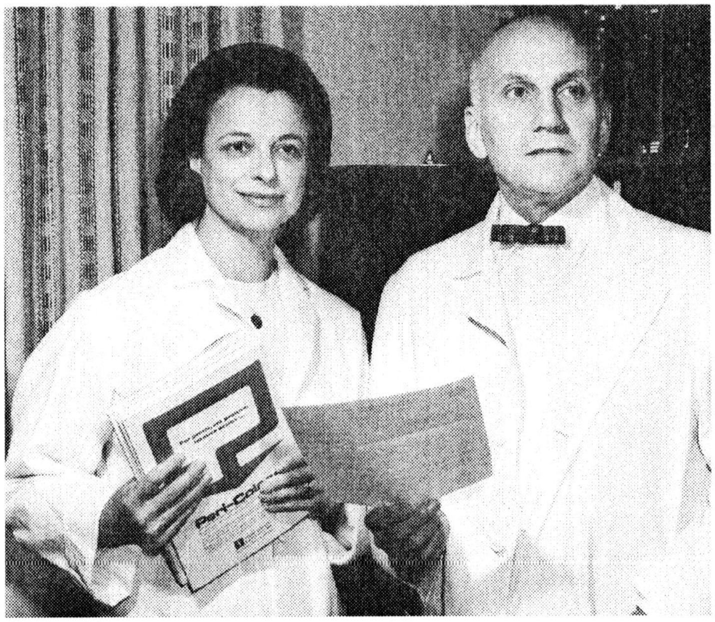

William Masters and Virginia Johnson are among the most influential researchers in the history of the study of human sexuality.

Related and Competing Theories

You will see as you read this text that the processes and theories proposed by Masters and Johnson are not the only views of human sexual response. Several related and competing theories have developed since Masters and Johnson published their early findings. These include a theory set forth by Helen Singer Kaplan, who in the 1970s proposed three stages of sexual response—desire, excitement, and orgasm—and focused far more than Masters and Johnson on the desire component of sexual arousal and satisfaction (Kaplan, 1974). More recently, researcher and psychiatrist David Reed has suggested an Erotic Stimulus Pathway Model of sexual response, which makes use of evocative terms such as *seduction*, *sensations*, and *surrender* (Greenberg, Bruess, & Haffner, 2002).

A significant departure from Masters and Johnson's theory has become known as the "new view" model of sexual response; it strives to delineate the sexual responses and feelings of women as distinct from those of men (Tiefer, 2001). This new view model clearly states that women's sexual responses generally do not fit well into the Masters and Johnson mold and, to be understood, must take into account additional issues such as the relationship in which the sexual behavior occurs, cultural and economic factors, psychological issues, and medical factors. The Masters and Johnson model and these competing theories will be discussed in greater detail in Chapter 3, "The Physiology of Sexual Responding."

Correlational Research

Another type of research methodology often used when scientists study human sexuality, as well as many other issues, is **correlational research**. Correlational research is similar to observational research in that we are observing how two variables relate to each other (how they "co-relate"). If you know two facts about each member in a group of people, you can probably determine if those two facts are correlated, that is, if they are interrelated in a predictable and consistent way. To use a nonsexual example, height is correlated with shoe size: As one is larger, the other is larger as well. In other words, tall people tend to have larger feet than short people, and vice versa. You

correlational research A scientific research methodology that determines the extent to which two variables are systematically related to each other (how they "co-relate").

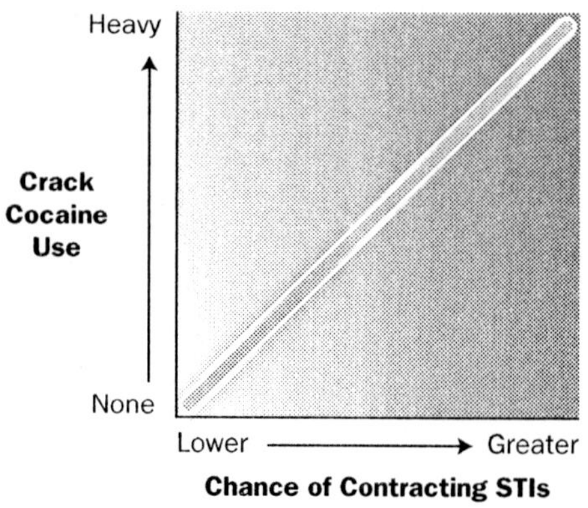

FIGURE 1.1 Positive Correlation between Crack Cocaine Use and Sexually Transmitted Infections

may find a few exceptions to this rule, but in general, this correlation holds true (except perhaps for clowns in the circus).

Three types of correlation exist among variables. A *positive correlation* indicates that we can predict that the two variables will change together in the same direction (such as shoe size and height; as one increases, the other does as well). A *negative correlation* tells us that the variables move predictably in the opposite direction. An example of a negative correlation might be amount of alcohol consumed and driving ability; as one increases, the other decreases. The third type of correlation is, simply, *no correlation* at all. That is, no consistent, predictable relationship exists between the two variables, such as the relationship between shoe size and driving ability (except perhaps among clowns in the circus).

The reason correlational research is so common in studies of sexuality is that researchers typically cannot control people's sexual behavior as would be necessary for an experiment (discussed in the next section). Instead, what people *report* about their sexual behavior or other relevant variables that we can ethically discover about them can be studied by examining how the variables relate to each other in a predictive way; this is correlational research.

Many, if not most, of the studies conducted in the field of human sexuality use correlational research. That is because researchers must usually take data that are already associated with their research participants and look for predictive links between them. Such relationships, when revealed, are important because scientists and clinicians are then able to predict one variable from another. An example from actual scientific studies is the correlation found between drug abuse and the spread of sexually transmitted infections (STIs). As you will read later in this text, one of the risk factors for contracting and transmitting STIs is the abuse of certain drugs, especially crack cocaine (Ross & Williams, 2001; Word & Bowser, 1997). This connection is graphically illustrated in Figure 1.1. You can see that the relationship is a positive correlation, and as one increases, the other climbs as well. Of course, exceptions to any correlational finding will exist (some people use crack and never contract an STI; some people contract STIs and never abuse drugs), but the graph represents the general trend of the correlational finding.

Can you conclude from this connection that researchers have demonstrated a *causal* link between the use of crack and STIs? The answer is no. All they know—and this is abundantly clear—is that the use of crack and STIs are *linked*. They are correlated. The exact factors creating this connection are not fully understood and are not revealed by the correlational finding itself. Perhaps crack cocaine reduces the brain's normal inhibitions, causing people to engage in more risky sexual behaviors when under its influence. Or maybe crack interferes in some way with the immune system, making people more susceptible to all infections, including STIs. Another explanation of the correlation, and this is probably most likely, is that some people who are addicted to crack engage in risky sexual behaviors to obtain money to feed their habit. The point is, you cannot be sure about cause and effect from a correlational finding. In other words, *correlation does not equal causation*.

Again, keep in mind that this is not to imply that correlational research is unscientific or invalid. What it does mean is that you must interpret correlational findings critically and not jump to an unwarranted conclusion that one variable is causing the other. In science, only one research method allows researchers to assume a cause-and-effect relationship with some degree of certainty: the experiment. And as we discuss experiments in the next section, you will see that they may only be conducted when it is possible, both ethically and practically, for the researcher to control or manipulate various aspects of the participants' behavior. Although ethically no one would ever be able to manipulate people's crack use or sexual practices for the sake of research, many other sexually related experiments can be, and have been, done.

Experimental Research

Surveys, case studies, observational research methods, and correlations can tell us a great deal about *what* people do and how various characteristics are interrelated. However, none of these methods offer very much, if any, information about *why* people do what they do. In other words, as noted earlier, they do not reveal *cause-and-effect* relationships. If we really want to understand cause and effect—what behaviors are actually triggered by certain experiences—it is necessary to do an *experiment*.

Unlike the methods discussed thus far, experiments do not rely on information about people's lives and behavior as they already exist in the world. Instead, when researchers undertake an experiment, they stage events, set up situations, and carefully measure responses in order to determine how behavior is affected by specific conditions under the researchers' control.

In experiments, researchers employ the **experimental method**. In its most basic form, this method involves bringing together a group of participants and dividing them into two groups (subjects may be divided into more than two groups, but for simplicity's sake, we will use just two in our discussion here). One group is given some kind of **treatment**, and the other receives a different treatment or no treatment at all. Finally, the average difference (if any) between the groups on some behavior of interest is analyzed statistically. If the experiment is done carefully and correctly, the researchers can conclude that differences found in the groups' behavior were *caused* by the treatment. The group receiving the treatment is referred to as the **experimental group**, and the group receiving no treatment or a different treatment is the **control group** or *comparison group*. The treatment administered is the **independent variable**, and the resulting behavior is the **dependent variable**.

As an example of the experimental method, let's return to our hypothetical example of Dr. Sylvia Jenkins and her theory of foot massage as a treatment for hypoactive sexual desire. Imagine that she has hired you as her research assistant to discover if her treatment truly causes an increase in sexual appetite. She asks you to conduct an experiment, and you agree. Your experimental design would resemble the illustration in Figure 1.2. Here are the steps you would take. First, you recruit a group of 60 or so couples who have volunteered to participate in an experiment on massage and sexual arousal. You divide them randomly (say, with a flip of a coin) into two groups of 30 couples each. You meet with each couple individually and provide training in massage techniques. To one group you teach Dr. Jenkins's foot massage technique, and to the other group you teach a simple shoulder rub. All the couples are instructed that the massages should take exactly 20 minutes, 10 minutes for each partner. Each couple then enters a private room where the massage takes place. They then view an erotic movie (the same movie for all couples) while their level of sexual arousal is recorded using special devices designed to measure blood flow to the genitals (see Figure 1.3).

When you analyze all the data using established statistical techniques, you find that the group employing Dr. Jenkins's foot massage technique experienced a higher level of arousal than the shoulder rub group. This difference was *statistically significant* (this means that a large enough difference was found that we can be almost certain that it did not occur simply by chance). Since all the couples in both groups had the same treatment except for the type of massage, you may conclude that Dr. Jenkins's "foot rub path to passion" probably does cause an increase in sexual arousal.

experimental method A type of scientific research in which variables of interest are changed while all other unrelated variables are held constant to determine cause-and-effect relationships among variables.

treatment The action performed on or by a group in an experiment.

experimental group The participants in an experiment who are subjected to a variable of research interest.

control group The participants in an experiment who receive no treatment and are allowed to behave as usual, for the purposes of comparison to an experimental group; also known as the *comparison group*.

independent variable The variable of interest in an experiment that is allowed to change between or among groups while all other variables are held constant.

dependent variable The result of an experiment, evaluated to determine if the independent variable actually caused a change in the experimental group of participants.

FIGURE 1.2 Experimental Design for Dr. Jenkins's "Foot Rub Path to Passion"

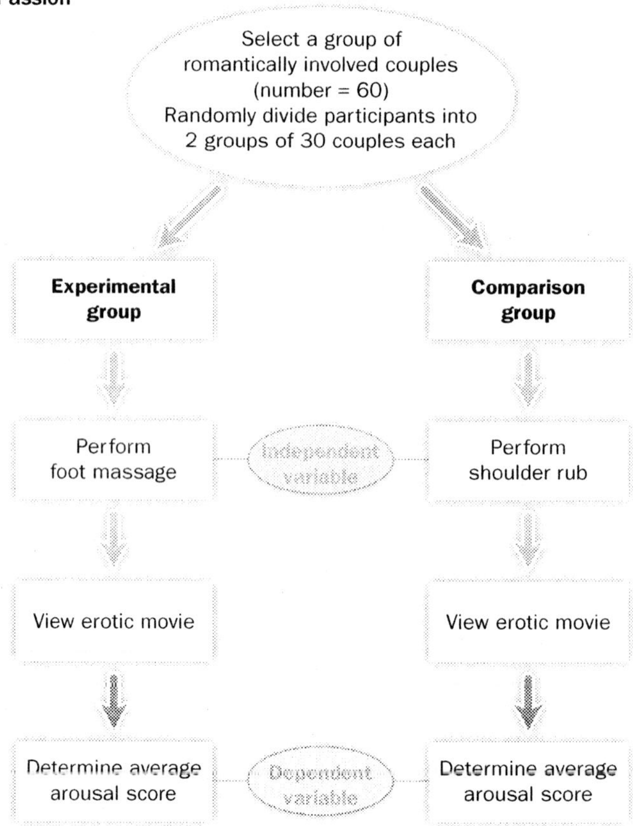
Select a group of romantically involved couples (number = 60) Randomly divide participants into 2 groups of 30 couples each
Experimental group
Comparison group
Perform foot massage
Independent variable
Perform shoulder rub
View erotic movie
View erotic movie
Determine average arousal score
Dependent variable
Determine average arousal score
Analyze the average scores to determine if the difference between the groups is statistically significant

Are you convinced that Dr. Jenkins's method works? Are there any problems in the experimental methods you used? The answer is that there might be some problems. Although it is true that the experiment is the only way we can determine cause and effect with a reasonable degree of confidence, several potential drawbacks to all experiments must be taken into account when interpreting the results:

1. *Gaining control sacrifices realism*. People are very likely to behave and respond differently in an artificial setting than they would in the real world. You can not be sure that couples using the foot massage technique in an experimental setting would actually increase their desire and arousal in the privacy of their own home under more natural conditions.
2. *The act of observing changes the behavior*. Simply knowing that they are part of a study and that you are analyzing their responses could alter the couples' usual behavior.
3. *The subject sample is not representative*. As discussed earlier in regard to surveys, the participants chosen for your experiment may not represent the general population you wish to study. To the extent that your sample of couples does not represent *all* couples, your ability to apply your findings to couples in general may be limited.

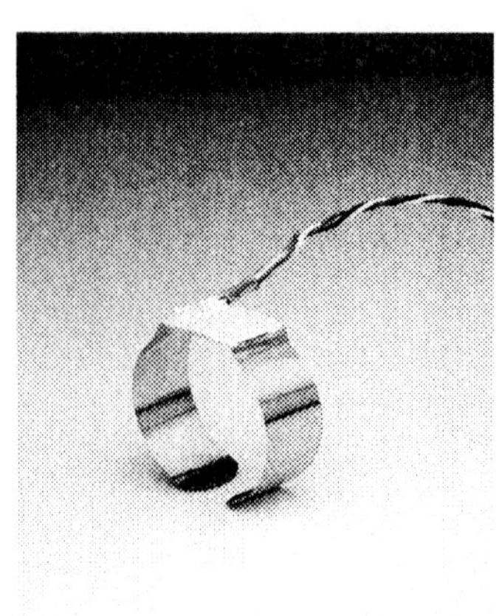

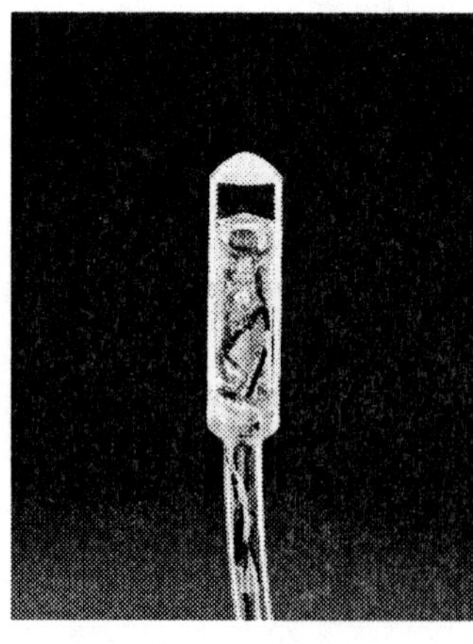

FIGURE 1.3 Measuring Sexual Arousal: The Penile Strain Gauge (Plethysmograph) and the Vaginal Photoplethysmograph

The devices shown here detect and measure slight changes in blood flow indicative of sexual arousal. Both devices are placed in position in private by the participants themselves following precise instructions.

Ethics And Sexuality Research

Since YOU Asked...

10. Is it really ethical to study people's actual sexual behaviors?

All research in any field involving human participants must be carried out with careful attention to ethical standards and principles. It's not difficult to see that when doing research in human sexuality, ethical guidelines relating to the safety, dignity, and anonymity of participants must be followed with extra care. Various professional groups—including the American Psychological Association (APA), the American Medical Association (AMA), and the Society for the Scientific Study of Sexuality (SSSS)—have developed guidelines for the ethical treatment of human participants, which are summarized in Table 1.6. These directives apply to all research with humans and are especially important in sexuality research.

Protection from Harm

This is the first rule for all studies employing human participants and is especially important in studies in sexuality. Researchers have the duty to protect their subjects from all physical and psychological harm. Even sexual studies that appear totally harmless on the surface may involve the potential for hidden or delayed emotional difficulty for the participants. For example, an anonymous written survey seems harmless enough, right? But what if the participant's boyfriend, girlfriend, spouse, or parent happens to see and read the answers before it is returned? Suddenly it might not seem so harmless.

Sometimes it is possible for unexpected future harm to occur from research that appears harmless in the present. To illustrate this, imagine you have volunteered as a subject in a study involving observation of sexual activity. The study is conducted in a completely professional and ethical manner. You feel you are helping to increase our knowledge of sexuality and are completely comfortable with your decision to participate. However, suppose a few years later, you become romantically involved with someone, but upon learning of your past sexual research involvement, your partner becomes uncomfortable and distant. Or perhaps worse, imagine later in your life, you are in the middle of divorce proceedings and during the child custody hearings, as a

Table 1.6 ETHICAL SAFEGUARDS IN SEXUALITY RESEARCH

All researchers conducting studies in human sexuality (and virtually any other field) are required to adhere to the principles for the ethical treatment of their human participants summarized in the table.

PRINCIPLE	SUMMARY
Protection from harm	Participants must be protected from all types of harm: physical and psychological, present and future.
Informed consent	Participants must receive an explanation of research procedures so that they may make informed choices about agreeing to participate.
Freedom to withdraw	Participants must never be coerced into participating and must be aware that they are free to withdraw from the study at any time without penalty.
Debriefing	Participants must be informed following their participation of the true purposes and goals of the study and told of any deception that may have been employed for the purposes of research validity.
Confidentiality	Participants must be guaranteed that the results of their participation will be either anonymous or kept in strict confidence.

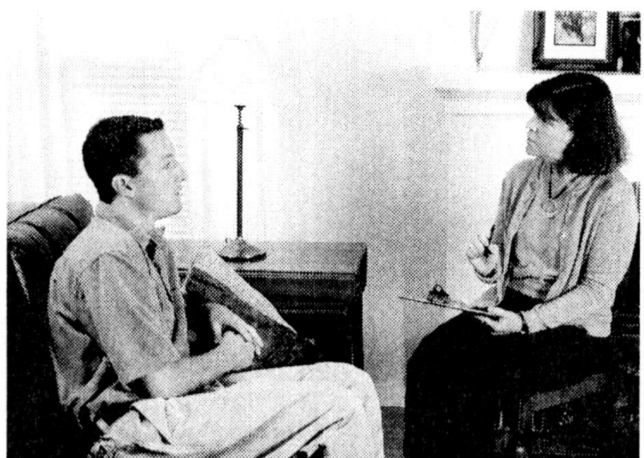

Researchers must inform potential participants of a study's procedures so that consent may be obtained.

legal ploy to malign your character, your spouse reveals that you participated in sex research (Masters, Johnson, & Kolodny, 1977a). This is not to say that protecting research participants from harm is impossible, but it illustrates how careful researchers must be to consider all the possibilities. One common way researchers try to reduce the chance of emotional distress that might arise during or following a study is to provide participants with telephone and e-mail access to the research team so that subjects may contact them at any time with questions or concerns.

Informed Consent

Researchers must explain to potential participants what the study is about, what procedures will be used, what possible risks are involved, and what benefits the study might have to the participants or to society. They must assure participants that the records are to be kept confidential or, if that is not possible, to explain exactly who will have access to the records and why. For sexuality research, it is also important to advise participants in advance if sensitive or potentially embarrassing topics will be part of the study (Ringheim, 1995). All this information provided to potential participants ensures that the individual is able to make an *informed* decision about whether to participate. If the person then agrees to participate, this is called **informed consent**. If a study involves a written questionnaire and then a follow-up interview, a potential participant must be told of this before the questionnaire is administered. This is because a participant might be willing to fill out a questionnaire but unwilling to be interviewed. It would not be ethical to ask individuals to complete the written survey and then spring the interview on them. One of the criticisms of the survey conducted by Hunt in 1975 (see Table 1.4) was that volunteers had been recruited to participate in a panel discussion about sexual topics, but after the discussion, they were asked to fill out a questionnaire. Even though everyone agreed to complete the questionnaire and no one was harmed by this, the ethics of not informing the participants of the written follow-up prior to their consenting to participate in the study is questionable.

If minors are to be part of a study, informed consent must be obtained from their parents or legal guardian. If the minor is old enough to give consent, respect for the minor as a person requires that his or her consent be obtained as well (Ringheim, 1995).

Freedom to Withdraw

All human participants in research projects must understand that they have the freedom to remove themselves from the study *at any time*. This may seem like an unnecessary rule, since it probably appears rather obvious to you that anyone in the study who becomes too uncomfortable with the procedures can simply leave. However, this is not always so straightforward. Many people feel that since they agreed to participate, it would be wrong to withdraw and risk ruining the study, so they continue even when they do not feel comfortable. Another problem with freedom to withdraw arises when participants are paid for their participation, which is a common practice. If participants are made to feel that their completion of the study is required for payment, this may produce an unethical inducement to avoid withdrawing even if they wish to do so. A common, though not universally used, solution to this problem is to pay participants at the beginning of each research session "just for showing up."

Debriefing

Another important safeguard against potential harm to research participants is the ethical obligation called **debriefing**, which occurs after participants have completed their role in the study. During debriefing, the researchers explain the goals and pro-

informed consent Agreeing to participate in an experiment only after having been provided with complete and accurate information about what to expect in the study.

debriefing Explanations of the purpose and potential contributions of the findings given to participants at the end of a study.

cedures of the study to the participants and allow them the opportunity to ask questions or make comments about their experiences. If deception was employed in any way during the study, participants must be fully counseled about the form of the deception and why it was necessary and be assured that they were not foolish in any way to have been deceived. The debriefing is also an opportunity for researchers to determine if any lingering negative aftereffects from the study should be addressed with the participants. This is the time when the researchers may reassure participants of the confidentiality of the data and give them phone numbers or e-mail addresses for further contact, if needed at any time in the future.

Confidentiality

All results from research participants, especially those who agree to take part in sexuality research, must be kept in complete confidence unless permission has been given by participants to share their data with certain other specific individuals (such as another research team). This does not mean that *results* cannot be reported and published, but reporting of findings must be done in such a way that individual data cannot be identified. Often no individual identifying information at all is obtained from participants, and the resulting anonymous data are combined to arrive at overall statistical findings. Today, the widespread use of computer databases and electronic storage and transfer of information have created new challenges for maintaining the confidentiality of research data. It is crucial that researchers develop methods of guarding against any possible breach of confidentiality *before* they begin to gather data. If records of individual participant data are kept for follow-up or additional analysis, confidentiality must be guaranteed.

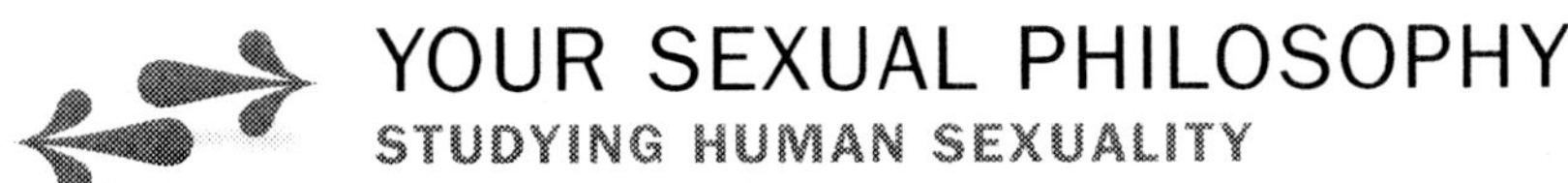

YOUR SEXUAL PHILOSOPHY
STUDYING HUMAN SEXUALITY

As mentioned at the beginning of the chapter, you will have the opportunity to integrate the material throughout this text into *your own personal sexual philosophy*. You will see this feature at the close of every chapter, along with a brief explanation of how the chapter's information fits into the sexual philosophy you are developing and will continue to develop for yourself throughout your life.

The basic idea behind this feature is to encourage you to do some thinking about and preparation for your life as a sexual being, now and in the future. As noted early in this chapter, your sexual philosophy is about knowing who you are, what you want and don't want, and planning ahead. If you take the time now to consider and explore your sexual feelings, attitudes, desires, and preferences and to form your sexual "rules for life," you will be far better equipped to be in control of your sexual life and to make healthy, informed choices about your sexual behaviors. Although no one can plan for every future event in life, having your sexual philosophy in place helps you take charge of sexual situations when they arise, rather than the situations taking charge of you.

Chapter 1 contributes to your sexual philosophy in two ways. First, it is crucial for you to gather as much accurate information as possible, now and in the future, about experiencing and understanding human sexuality, so that the choices and decisions you make about sex and relationships are based on a solid foundation of knowledge. Second, learning to analyze sexuality research *critically* will enable you to evaluate what you hear, see, and read about sex. Then you will be equipped to incorporate into your personal life the best information that will enhance your sexual enjoyment, satisfaction, health, and fulfillment. Many students have remarked that their human sexuality course was one of the most fascinating and personally useful courses of their college career.

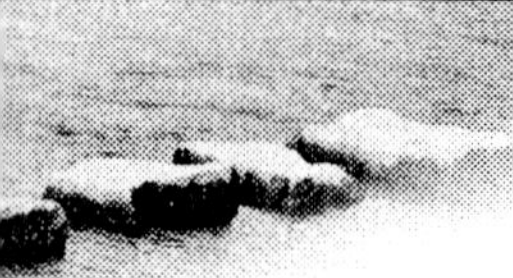

Summary

HISTORICAL PERSPECTIVES A Human Sexuality Time Line

- The world of human sexuality has been marked by many influential historical events. To illustrate, on the inside covers of this book, we journey back over 150 years of significant events that have changed our views of human sexuality.

Experiencing Human Sexuality

- Sexuality is a crucial part of what makes us each unique. Learning to deal effectively with the wide range of topics that comprise the study of human sexuality is a basic foundation for living a healthy sexual life. Although we are all born to be sexual beings, knowledge of our sexuality is vital for overall understanding of ourselves and of others.
- The development of clear sexual morals and values is critical for making responsible choices. Along with self-understanding should come an exploration of your sexual morals and values—your personal "sexual philosophy." This knowledge allows for planning ahead and helps you make responsible decisions about your sexual behaviors and attitudes.
- Sex is far more than intercourse, and many people's sexual lives are enriched through an awareness of the range of activities that comprise sex. Learning about sexuality and sexual behaviors enhances sexual satisfaction throughout our lives.

Understanding Human Sexuality

- Human sexuality is far more complex than most people think. Students often enter a human sexuality class with inaccurate knowledge and various erroneous beliefs about sex. By studying and absorbing accurate information about sexuality, these misconceptions can usually be cleared up.
- Understanding of human sexuality also increases tolerance and respect for sexual diversity and allows for a clearer appreciation of what is "normal" sexually. Perhaps even more important, learning about sexuality is vital in staying sexually healthy, which includes knowing how to prevent contracting or spreading sexually transmitted infections.
- Accurate understanding of human sexuality provides the tools necessary for assessing sexual research. When it comes to sexuality, as in most areas of life, the ability to separate fact from fiction is one of our most important skills as critical thinkers. And the best way to do that is to learn as much as we can about humans as sexual beings.

Methods for Studying Human Sexuality

- Sex researchers use many methods to study human sexual behavior scientifically. Developing and administering scientific, unbiased, valid surveys requires extensive training and expertise. Scientific surveys must be reliable, providing consistent measurement over repeated administrations, and they must be valid, measuring truthfully the characteristic being studied. The respondents should represent the population being studied as closely as possible.
- Research relying on case studies of only one individual may provide valuable information but often fails to represent the larger, overall population.
- Observational research may provide useful information about sexual behavior but does not indicate the cause of the behaviors. The work of Masters and Johnson in the 1960s was a landmark example of observational research in human sexuality. However, several diverse and competing theories of human sexual functioning have developed since then.
- Correlational research allows researchers to show relationships between variables. However, two variables may be strongly related but not necessarily causally related.
- Experimental research can demonstrate cause-and-effect connections among variables by holding constant all possible influences except those under study. Although experimental methods provide additional control of the variables under study, this control is usually at the expense of the realism of other research methods.

Ethics and Sexuality Research

- Formal ethical guidelines have been established that govern research involving human participants. Researchers must adhere to these ethical precepts, which include protecting participants from harm, obtaining participants' informed consent prior to beginning the research, ensuring participants' freedom to withdraw from the study at any time, the promise of confidentiality of all findings, and offering a full debriefing for all participants following the study.

YOUR SEXUAL PHILOSOPHY: Studying Human Sexuality

- Developing your personal sexual philosophy is the key to living a fulfilling sexual life. Building this philosophy requires thinking about and preparing for your life as a sexual person, now and in the future. Ultimately your sexual philosophy is about knowing who you are, what you want and don't want, and planning ahead. Your sexual philosophy allows you to take charge of sexual situations rather than allowing those situations to take charge of you.

Have You Considered?

1. Imagine that you have been selected to give a talk about sexuality to high school juniors and seniors who probably think they already know it all. One of your goals is to convince them that they do *not* know it all and that it is important for them to learn as much as they can. What arguments would you use to convince them of the importance of being educated about human sexuality?
2. In the question-and-answer portion of your talk to the high school students, several students ask you about unusual sexual situations and practices they have learned about on TV talk shows. What would you want to tell them about drawing conclusions about sex based on this kind of information?
3. A friend confides in you that she has been having some sexual fantasies recently that she thinks are unconventional and strange. She is feeling a lot of anxiety about these fantasies and is beginning to feel depressed about having them. She believes that these fantasies indicate that she is sexually abnormal. What would you say to try to help her?
4. Do you feel that the moral values and principles taught to you by your parents and others as you were growing up still apply to your life now as an independent adult? If so, are you comfortable living by them? If not, how have you and your values changed?
5. Do you think you will be comfortable talking about sex with your children in the future? Why or why not?
6. How do you feel about sexually explicit materials? Do you feel that a textbook on human sexuality containing sexually explicit language and pictures would be difficult for you to read or study? Why or why not?
7. Suppose you want to study the progression of sexual intimacy in dating couples. You are interested in knowing how long, on average, the two people have known each other or have been dating when they first engage in various intimate behaviors (kissing, erotic touching, nudity, genital touching, oral sex, intercourse). What kind of study would you propose? How would you obtain subjects? Exactly how would you go about gathering your data? What methodological problems do you think you might encounter?
8. In your study of dating and sexual behaviors in question 7, how would you ensure that your study does not violate ethical considerations?

Companion Website Resources

For further chapter resources go to **www.prenhall.com/hock**. This robust text website includes polling questions for you to vote on, regular news updates, quizzes, sample tests, suggested reading lists, and more.

SCENARIOS USA Also on the website are links to videos. *Scenarios USA*'s films portray real-life narratives that explore the non-biological aspects of relationships and sexual health. The films will help you consider how the themes of the text affect your own life and the lives of those around you.

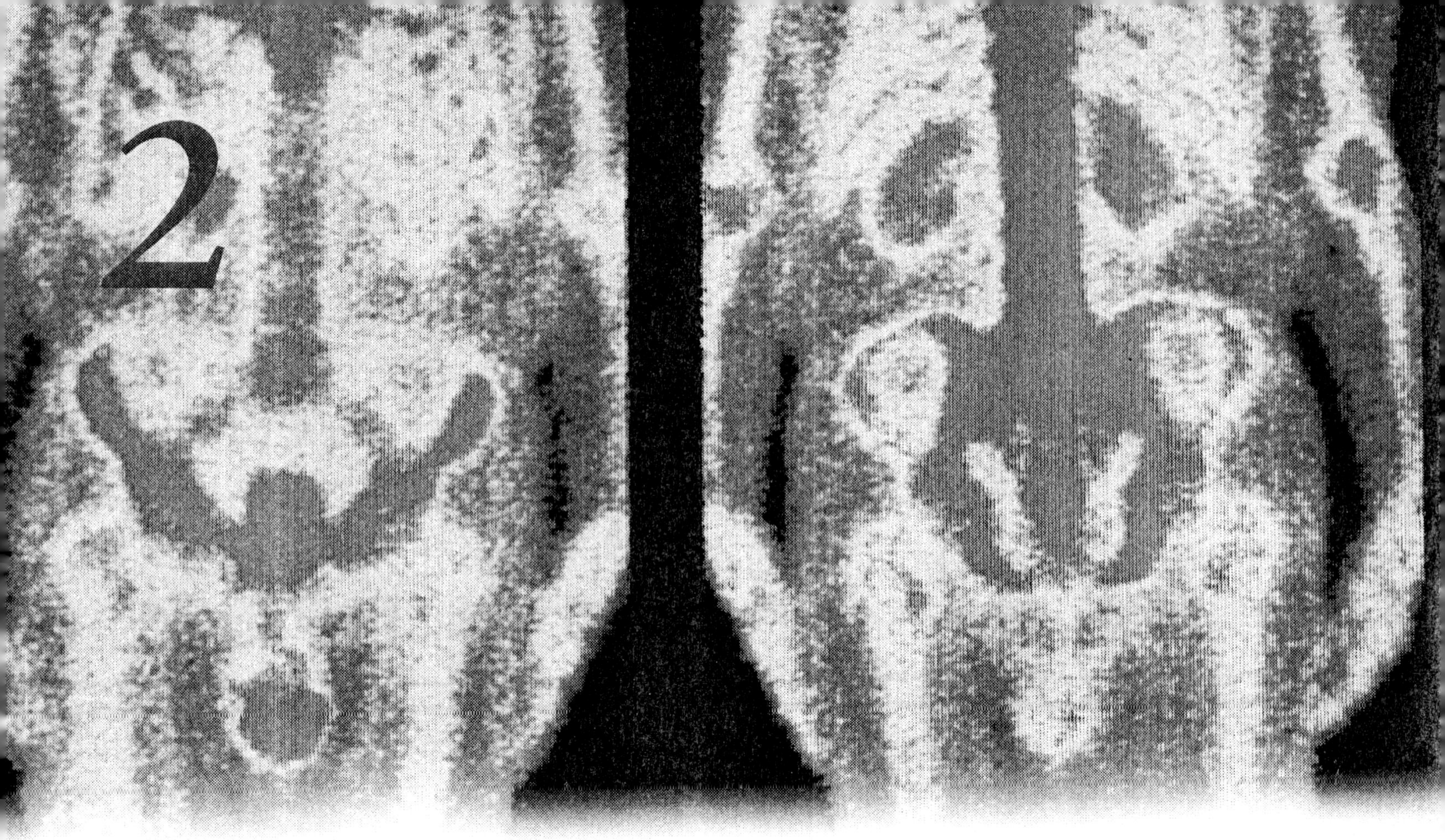

2

Sexual Anatomy

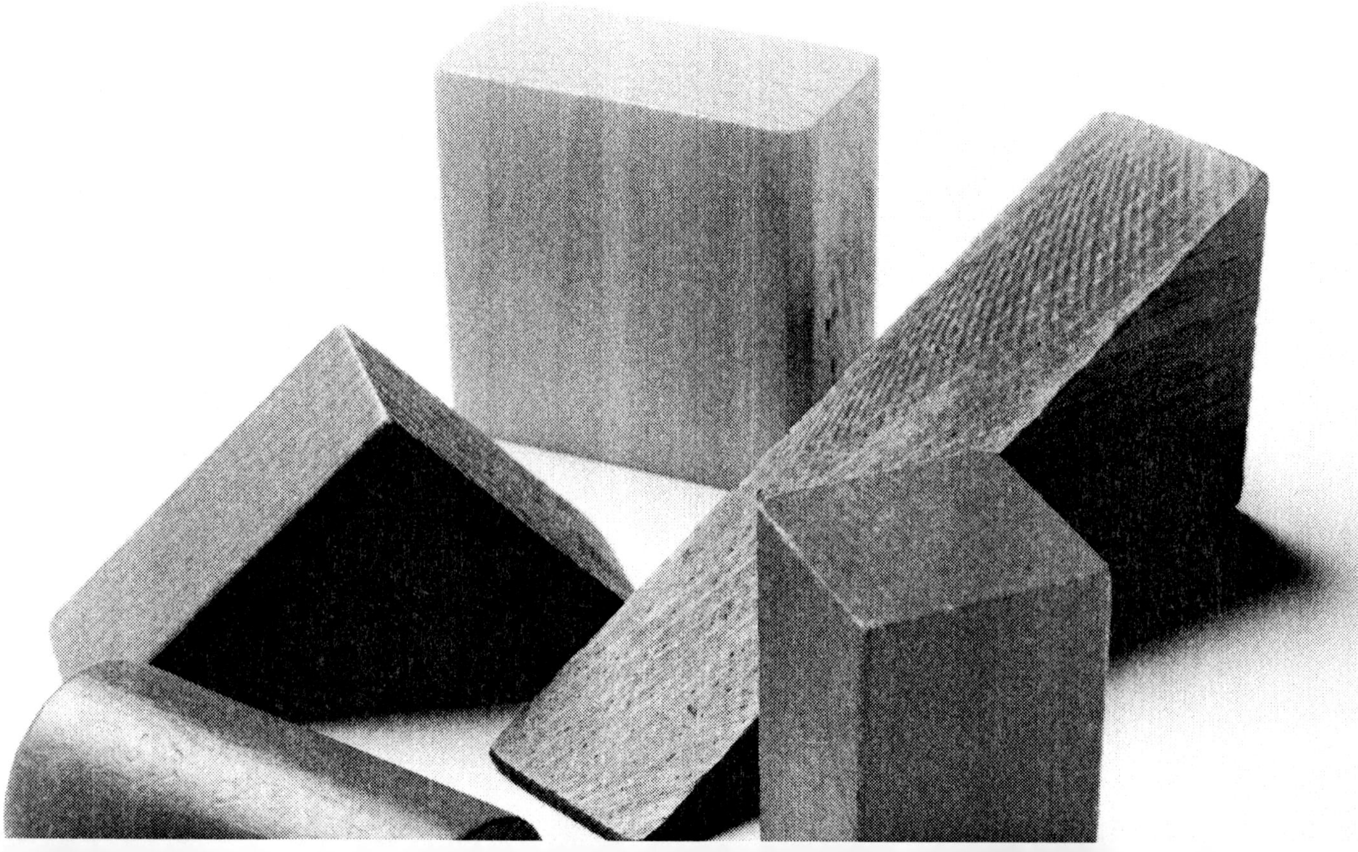

Since YOU Asked...

1. How common is male circumcision in the United States? (see page 41)
2. A lot of magazines advertise for penis-increasing creams or exercises. Do any of these really work? (see page 43)
3. What is the average penis size? Can a man be too small or too large? (see page 44)
4. How do the sperm get from the testicles to the penis? (see page 48)
5. I feel that my genitals don't look right. The lips are sort of large and not pink like I see in pictures. They're more grayish. Is this normal? (see page 51)
6. I've heard that the clitoris is the same as the penis, but they seem totally different to me. Why do people say they are the same? (see page 53)
7. Lately I've been getting bladder infections a lot, like once or twice a month. They are awful. Why am I getting so many, and how can I prevent them? (see page 56)
8. Is there any sure way to tell if a woman is a virgin before (or after) you have intercourse with her? Is there actually something you "break" inside the vagina? (see page 56)
9. Are larger breasts more sensitive than smaller ones? (see page 59)
10. Once a condom came off during sex and we couldn't find it. Is it possible for a condom to get "lost" up inside a woman? (see page 62)
11. If a Pap test is negative, can you be sure you are completely free of disease? (see page 62)
12. My sister told me she has endometriosis, which is why she has such bad cramps during her period. What exactly is endometriosis? (see page 63)

This chapter is going to be far more interesting than you may think. Why? For several reasons. First, the more you know about your sexual anatomy, the more enjoyment you will be able to derive from the many sexual activities discussed throughout this book. Of course, many sexual feelings and sensations are preprogrammed from birth, but the more you learn about your body (and your sexual responses, covered in the next chapter), the more comfortable you will feel exploring your own personal sexuality. This, in turn, will enhance your sexual enjoyment and satisfaction, both solo and with a partner, throughout your life. Sexuality may seem to be a wondrous and mysterious gift from nature, and you may feel it should remain a mystery and not be spoiled by examining it too closely. But the truth is, with knowledge and education, sex is better in nearly every way imaginable.

Second, at the risk of sounding like a bad advertisement in the back of an equally bad magazine, "You too can be a better lover!" But without a solid foundation in sexual anatomy and physiology, satisfying a partner or helping a partner satisfy you is difficult at best and frustrating and disappointing at worst. Even if you have a pretty good idea about what feels good and what turns you on, you need to be able to communicate that effectively and correctly to someone with whom you are sexually intimate. The more you know about sexual anatomy, the better prepared you will be to satisfy your partner and respond to his or her sexual desires. One of the most frequently cited reasons for sexual problems in relationships is poor knowledge and communication about sexual anatomy and physiology. This chapter and those that follow offer you the information you need now or in the future to be a loving and caring sexual partner.

Third, as you explore the topics throughout this book, you will discover that many of them involve issues of health and disease. You'll be reading about various sexually transmitted infections, other bacterial infections relating to sexual anatomy and function, self-examinations of sexual parts of the body to help prevent diseases or detect them early for more effective treatment, and many other topics relating to the health of your sexual body. And because your sexual self is the most personal and private part of you, your awareness of the signs and symptoms of any potential health problems in yourself or in an intimate partner is crucial to staying well. The information in this chapter is fundamental to recognizing a possible problem, detecting abnormal changes in various sexual structures that may indicate illness or disease, and knowing when to visit a health care professional either for routine preventive care or treatment of a condition you may discover.

Fourth, as is obvious by now, this chapter's topics, along with those in Chapter 1, will serve as an indispensable foundation for what is to follow in this text. What you are about to explore here will provide you with the knowledge, insights, vocabulary, and understanding necessary to benefit from the material in *every* chapter throughout this book. But don't worry: This is a human sexuality text, so this chapter is *not* your typical anatomy lesson. This is, first and foremost, about you and your partner (present or future) as sexual beings.

In this chapter, after a brief look back at the history of sexual anatomy, we will explore in some detail the most important structures that comprise the male and female sexual bodies. For both sexes, we will take an "outside-in" route; that is, first we will examine the external anatomy and then

Focus on Your Feelings

Probably the most common emotion experienced by students when reading and discussing the topics in this chapter is embarrassment. We live in a paradoxical culture that is immensely preoccupied with sex but at the same time is uncomfortable with frank, straightforward sexual discussion and education. For many, perhaps most, people, discussing and looking at drawings and photographs of sexual anatomy makes them more than a little uneasy.

Feeling embarrassed about these issues is normal and understandable. However, we hope, as you have the chance to read and discuss them, you'll feel somewhat less uncomfortable. Why? Because the embarrassment people feel about sex contributes to many sexual problems. For example, embarrassment over sexual anatomy causes couples to avoid talking about sexual difficulties they may be experiencing, which only makes them worse; it causes people to avoid examining their own sexual bodies, which is crucial for early detection of health problems; it causes people to avoid seeing the doctor about potential sexual medical problems that, left untreated, can become much more serious; it causes parents to fail to provide their kids with correct and much needed information about sex, which may lead to unsafe sexual behaviors and unwanted pregnancy; it causes many people to suffer from insecurities about their bodies that are based in falsehoods rather than facts; the list goes on and on.

Sexual anatomy is simply a normal, natural part of your body and your life—one of the most important parts. The more you can move past your embarrassment or uneasiness and help others do so as well, the more we can look forward to a world in which people are sexually happy and healthy.

proceed logically inward to the various internal structures. This is not intended to be an exercise in memorization of "sexual parts" but rather a conceptual clarification of the purpose and function of sexual structures and their roles in reproduction and sexual responding (to be discussed in Chapter 3).

With that, you should be aware that humans have not always been as enlightened as we are now about sexual anatomy. In fact, in earlier times, people held some pretty strange ideas about the sexual body, as you will see in the next section.

Historical Perspectives

Anatomy in the Dark Ages

Throughout history, and even today, to some extent, human sexual anatomy was seen as a shameful subject for study or discussion. Why? Because such topics might excite people to engage in "impure acts." Consequently, the study of sexual anatomy prior to the nineteenth century was typically wildly misguided (Stolberg, 2003). Here is a partial list of early beliefs about human sexual anatomy—all of them erroneous and some widely held as late as the seventeenth century (we will be discussing our *current* knowledge of all these structures next):

- Men and women have the same sexual body (the *one-sex model*), but in men the genitals have been pushed out of the body, while in the woman they have been retained inside.
- The male body was the "norm;" the female body is merely a "variation."
- The uterus is an internal scrotum.
- The cervix is an internal penis.
- The vagina is an inwardly inverted penile foreskin.
- The ovaries are retained testicles.
- A sudden violent physical movement such as jumping over a stream can turn a girl into a boy by forcing her genitals to the outside of her body.
- The "testicles" in men and women both generate sperm.
- The uterus was seen as unclean and poisonous, able to wander through the woman's body causing illness and even suffocation, a condition referred to as *hysteria* (from the Greek word for *uterus*).
- The clitoris was not "discovered" until the mid-1500s.
- The uterus is divided into two halves (like the scrotum) and consists of seven *cells*—three on the left, three on the right, and one in the middle (see Figure 2.1); males are born from the right side, females from the left.
- A woman has two uteri (wombs), corresponding to her two breasts.
- The penis is situated in front of the pubic bone so that it will not collapse inward during intercourse. (Leonardo da Vinci wrote, "If this bone did not exist, the penis in meeting resistance would turn backwards and would often enter more into the body of the operator than into that of the operated.")
- Sperm comes directly from the male brain.
- The fallopian tubes, discovered by Gabriel Fallopius, have no known function.
- Menstrual fluid flows directly from the uterus to the breasts, generating breast milk.
- Reproduction is similar to the manufacture of cheese: The woman's "sperm" is the milk, and the male sperm is the "clotting agent."

Even without the benefit of the wisdom you are about to obtain from this chapter, you can tell that our knowledge of human sexual anatomy has come a long way in the last few hundred years. We will now examine in detail our current and far more accurate understanding of male and female sexual anatomy.

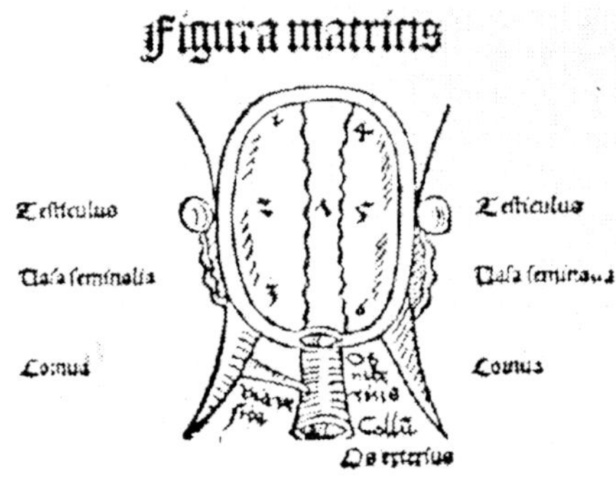

FIGURE 2.1 Historical View of the Uterus

An early drawing of the uterus showed seven "cells." It was thought that the location of the male sperm would determine the sex of the child: right side, male; left side, female; and middle, "hermaphrodite."

The Male Sexual Body

Our discussion of the male sexual body begins with an examination of the external sexual anatomy—structures on the outside of the body—primarily the penis, scrotum, testicles, and anus, along with some interesting related issues. Then we move inward to the internal male structures—located inside the body cavity—including the prostate gland, seminal vesicles, urethral bulb, bladder, Cowper's glands, ejaculatory duct, and urethra. We will discuss these structures as they relate to the production of semen and its journey through a man's sexual anatomy.

Male External Structures

If you are looking at a naked male standing facing you, his genitals are right out there with nowhere to hide. However, if you assume the same view of a naked woman, you see virtually nothing of her genitals; they are hidden between her legs and partly, mostly, or completely concealed by the structures called the labia majora—but more on that later in this chapter. The external male sexual anatomical organs include the penis, the scrotum, the testicles, and the epididymis (the testicles and epididymis, although located inside the scrotum, are external relative to the man's body).

The Penis

The **penis**, the primary male sexual organ, has two jobs: to ejaculate semen and to transport urine from the inside of the body to the outside. There are wide variations in penis appearance, as is true of all human body parts.

Part (b) of Figure 2.2 shows the basic external components of the penis. As you can see (and probably already knew), it's not particularly complex, consisting of the penile shaft, the foreskin (in uncircumcised men), the penile glans, the corona, the frenulum, and the urethral opening. A very sexually sensitive area of the penis, and of the male body, is the tip, or **penile glans** or glans. Stimulation to this glans is primarily responsible for male orgasm and ejaculation. This is not to say that the glans is the only sexually sensitive area on a man's body; men are sexually aroused through stimulation of many body parts, but typically, the penile glans must be stimulated directly or indirectly for most men to reach orgasm. The **corona** is the raised ridge at the base of the penile glans where the tip of the penis joins the shaft. Most men report that the corona is somewhat more sexually sensitive than the rest of the tip of the penis. The **frenulum**, an area of tissue at the base of the underside of the penile glans, is typically reported to be even more sexually sensitive than the glans.

The skin on the **penile shaft** is loose to allow for expansion during **erection**. All males are born with skin covering the penile glans, called the **foreskin**. As infants, this is a small amount of skin, but in an adult male it averages approximately 3 by 5 inches, or 15 square inches. Beneath the foreskin, small glands secrete *smegma*, a substance

penis The primary male anatomical sexual structure.

penile glans The end or tip of the penis, its most sexually sensitive part.

corona The raised edge at the base of the penile glans.

frenulum The band of tissue connecting the underside of the penile glans with the shaft of the penis.

penile shaft The area of the penis between the glans and the abdomen.

erection Rigidity of the penis or clitoris resulting from an inflow of blood during sexual arousal.

foreskin A layer of skin covering the glans of the penis.

FIGURE 2.2 The Penis

The penis varies in shape, color, and appearance, just like any part of the male body. Shown here are an uncircumcised penis (right) and a circumcised penis (left).

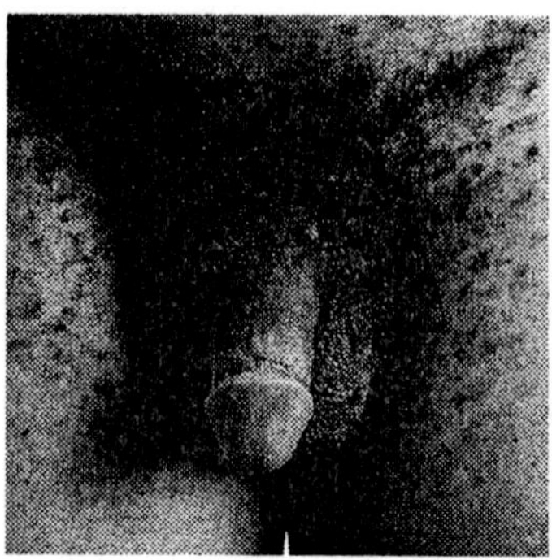

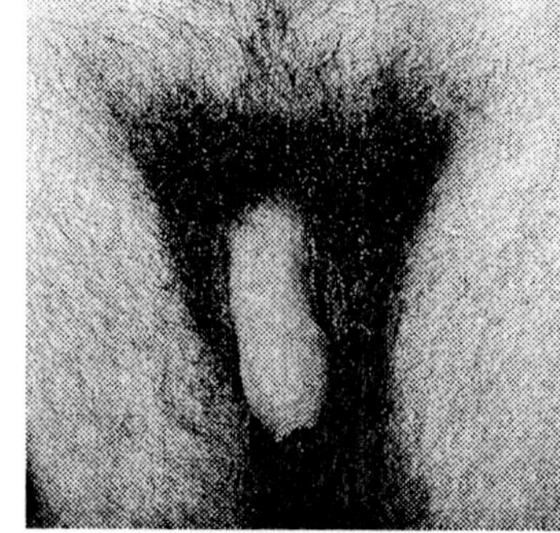

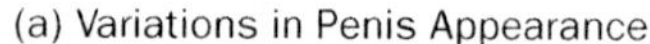

(a) Variations in Penis Appearance

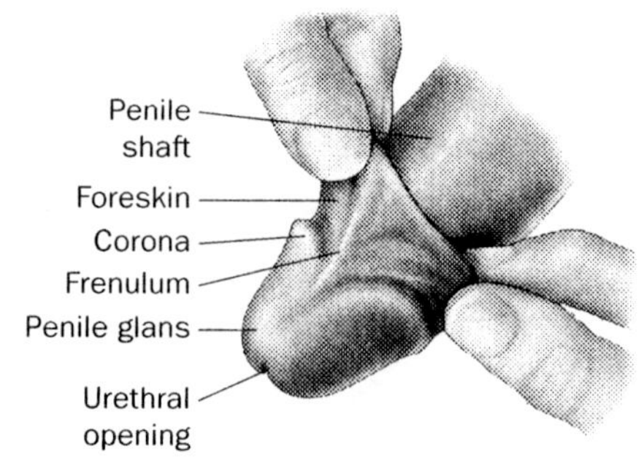

(b) External Structures of the Penis

The Male Sexual Body

Our discussion of the male sexual body begins with an examination of the external sexual anatomy—structures on the outside of the body—primarily the penis, scrotum, testicles, and anus, along with some interesting related issues. Then we move inward to the internal male structures—located inside the body cavity—including the prostate gland, seminal vesicles, urethral bulb, bladder, Cowper's glands, ejaculatory duct, and urethra. We will discuss these structures as they relate to the production of semen and its journey through a man's sexual anatomy.

Male External Structures

If you are looking at a naked male standing facing you, his genitals are right out there with nowhere to hide. However, if you assume the same view of a naked woman, you see virtually nothing of her genitals; they are hidden between her legs and partly, mostly, or completely concealed by the structures called the labia majora—but more on that later in this chapter. The external male sexual anatomical organs include the penis, the scrotum, the testicles, and the epididymis (the testicles and epididymis, although located inside the scrotum, are external relative to the man's body).

The Penis

The **penis**, the primary male sexual organ, has two jobs: to ejaculate semen and to transport urine from the inside of the body to the outside. There are wide variations in penis appearance, as is true of all human body parts.

penis The primary male anatomical sexual structure.

penile glans The end or tip of the penis, its most sexually sensitive part.

corona The raised edge at the base of the penile glans.

frenulum The band of tissue connecting the underside of the penile glans with the shaft of the penis.

penile shaft The area of the penis between the glans and the abdomen.

erection Rigidity of the penis or clitoris resulting from an inflow of blood during sexual arousal.

foreskin A layer of skin covering the glans of the penis.

Part (b) of Figure 2.2 shows the basic external components of the penis. As you can see (and probably already knew), it's not particularly complex, consisting of the penile shaft, the foreskin (in uncircumcised men), the penile glans, the corona, the frenulum, and the urethral opening. A very sexually sensitive area of the penis, and of the male body, is the tip, or **penile glans** or glans. Stimulation to this glans is primarily responsible for male orgasm and ejaculation. This is not to say that the glans is the only sexually sensitive area on a man's body; men are sexually aroused through stimulation of many body parts, but typically, the penile glans must be stimulated directly or indirectly for most men to reach orgasm. The **corona** is the raised ridge at the base of the penile glans where the tip of the penis joins the shaft. Most men report that the corona is somewhat more sexually sensitive than the rest of the tip of the penis. The **frenulum**, an area of tissue at the base of the underside of the penile glans, is typically reported to be even more sexually sensitive than the glans.

The skin on the **penile shaft** is loose to allow for expansion during **erection**. All males are born with skin covering the penile glans, called the **foreskin**. As infants, this is a small amount of skin, but in an adult male it averages approximately 3 by 5 inches, or 15 square inches. Beneath the foreskin, small glands secrete *smegma*, a substance

FIGURE 2.2 The Penis

The penis varies in shape, color, and appearance, just like any part of the male body. Shown here are an uncircumcised penis (right) and a circumcised penis (left).

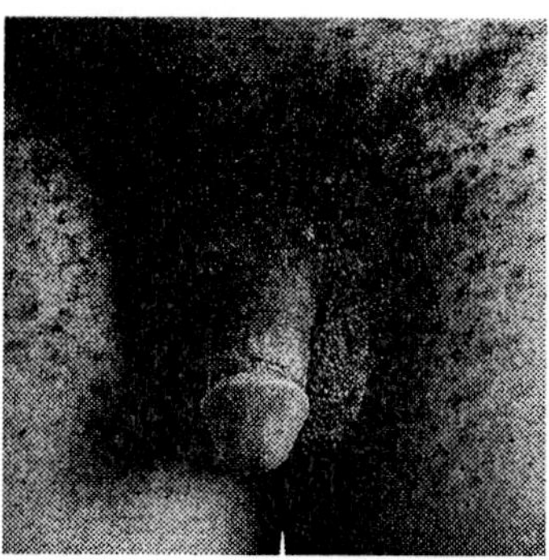

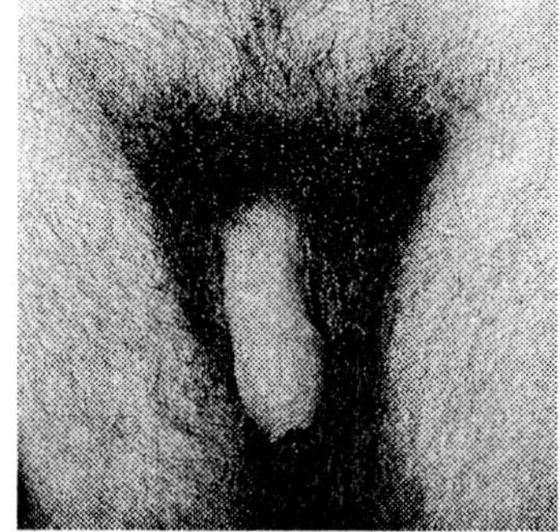

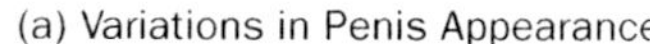

(a) Variations in Penis Appearance

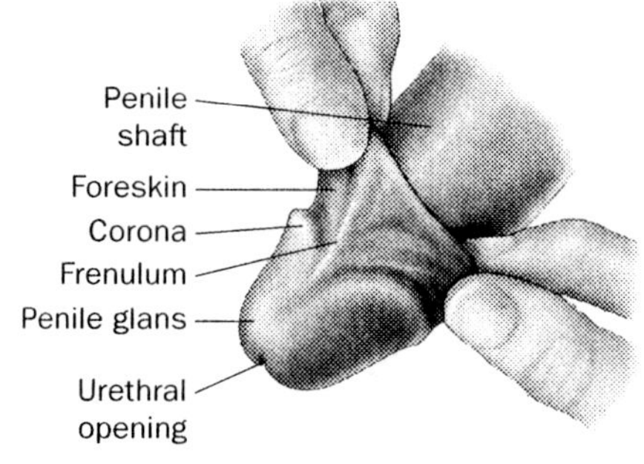

(b) External Structures of the Penis

proceed logically inward to the various internal structures. This is not intended to be an exercise in memorization of "sexual parts" but rather a conceptual clarification of the purpose and function of sexual structures and their roles in reproduction and sexual responding (to be discussed in Chapter 3).

With that, you should be aware that humans have not always been as enlightened as we are now about sexual anatomy. In fact, in earlier times, people held some pretty strange ideas about the sexual body, as you will see in the next section.

Historical Perspectives

Anatomy in the Dark Ages

Throughout history, and even today, to some extent, human sexual anatomy was seen as a shameful subject for study or discussion. Why? Because such topics might excite people to engage in "impure acts." Consequently, the study of sexual anatomy prior to the nineteenth century was typically wildly misguided (Stolberg, 2003). Here is a partial list of early beliefs about human sexual anatomy—all of them erroneous and some widely held as late as the seventeenth century (we will be discussing our *current* knowledge of all these structures next):

- Men and women have the same sexual body (the *one-sex model*), but in men the genitals have been pushed out of the body, while in the woman they have been retained inside.
- The male body was the "norm;" the female body is merely a "variation."
- The uterus is an internal scrotum.
- The cervix is an internal penis.
- The vagina is an inwardly inverted penile foreskin.
- The ovaries are retained testicles.
- A sudden violent physical movement such as jumping over a stream can turn a girl into a boy by forcing her genitals to the outside of her body.
- The "testicles" in men and women both generate sperm.
- The uterus was seen as unclean and poisonous, able to wander through the woman's body causing illness and even suffocation, a condition referred to as *hysteria* (from the Greek word for *uterus*).
- The clitoris was not "discovered" until the mid-1500s.
- The uterus is divided into two halves (like the scrotum) and consists of seven *cells*—three on the left, three on the right, and one in the middle (see Figure 2.1); males are born from the right side, females from the left.
- A woman has two uteri (wombs), corresponding to her two breasts.
- The penis is situated in front of the pubic bone so that it will not collapse inward during intercourse. (Leonardo da Vinci wrote, "If this bone did not exist, the penis in meeting resistance would turn backwards and would often enter more into the body of the operator than into that of the operated.")
- Sperm comes directly from the male brain.
- The fallopian tubes, discovered by Gabriel Fallopius, have no known function.
- Menstrual fluid flows directly from the uterus to the breasts, generating breast milk.
- Reproduction is similar to the manufacture of cheese: The woman's "sperm" is the milk, and the male sperm is the "clotting agent."

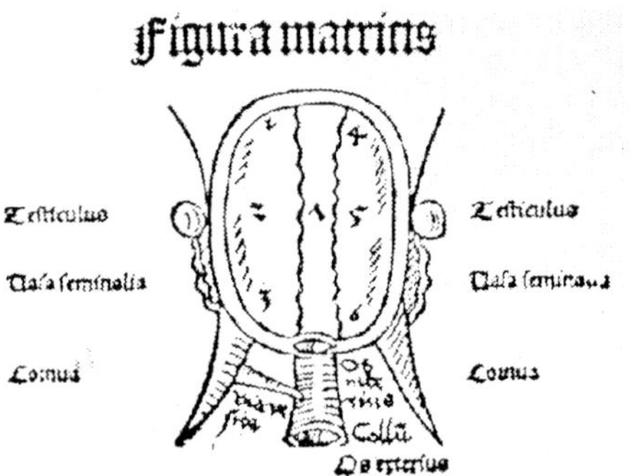

FIGURE 2.1 Historical View of the Uterus

An early drawing of the uterus showed seven "cells." It was thought that the location of the male sperm would determine the sex of the child: right side, male; left side, female; and middle, "hermaphrodite."

Even without the benefit of the wisdom you are about to obtain from this chapter, you can tell that our knowledge of human sexual anatomy has come a long way in the last few hundred years. We will now examine in detail our current and far more accurate understanding of male and female sexual anatomy.

that provides lubrication between the foreskin and the glans and assists in the separation of the foreskin from the glans in infants.

Male **circumcision** involves the removal of the foreskin covering the glans of the penis. Looking back at Figure 2.2, you can see both a circumcised and uncircumcised penis. Until late in the twentieth century, most male infants born in the United States were circumcised as a matter of course. Over the past 20 years or so, however, the practice of circumcision has declined dramatically and is no longer routine by any means. "Sexuality and Culture: Male Circumcision in the United States" summarizes the current controversy about male circumcision.

As the practice of circumcision in the United States has declined, education about caring for an intact penis has been slow to keep pace. Many parents, boys, and even some doctors are unclear about what to expect as the uncircumcised penis develops. Proper care of the intact penis can be summarized in one sentence: *Leave it alone*. The biggest mistake parents make is assuming that the foreskin should be able to be retracted before it has separated from the penile glans. Attempting to retract the foreskin too early in the boy's development can cause tears, which then heal incorrectly and adhere to the penile glans. These adhesions can lead to serious problems later on in life that may require surgery, usually circumcision, to resolve (Camille, Kuo, & Wiener, 2002; NOCIRC, 1997). The age at which full retraction of the foreskin from the penile glans occurs varies greatly from a few years of age to 18 years old. Until that happens and the boy is able to retract his foreskin himself, the only hygiene necessary is gentle washing of the outside of the foreskin with soap and water (in infants, water alone is usually sufficient).

The penis consists of three spongy, cavernous tubes running along its length as shown in Figure 2.3. The two tubes located on the top side of the penis are the **corpora cavernosa**, meaning "cavernous bodies." The third tube that runs along the underside of the penis is the **corpus spongiosum**, meaning "spongy body," and it surrounds the urethra. During sexual arousal, these spongy, cavernous tubes become engorged with blood, which results in erection of the penis. When sexual excitement diminishes, blood flows back out of these structures and the erection subsides. The **urethra** is the tube that runs the length of the penis and on into the body to carry semen or urine from the inside to the outside of the body.

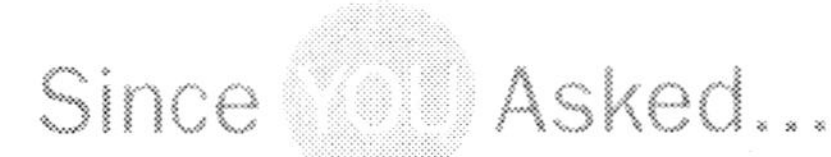

1. How common is male circumcision in the United States?

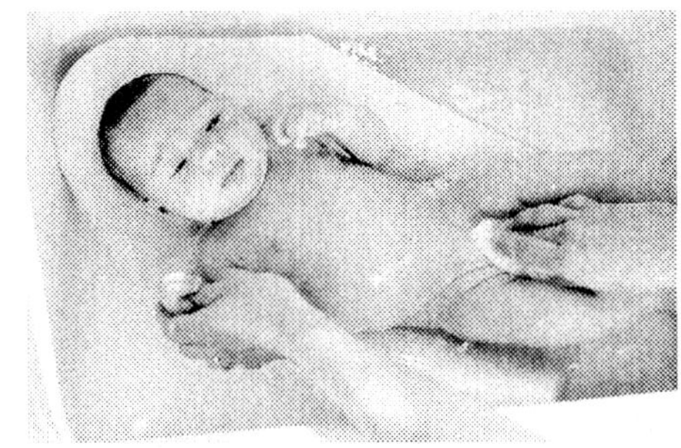

A baby's intact penis requires very little care other than gentle washing of the outside of the foreskin. No attempt should be made to retract the foreskin until it separates naturally from the penile glans years later.

circumcision Removal of the foreskin of the penis.

corpora cavernosa Two parallel chambers that run the length of the penis and become engorged with blood during erection.

corpus spongiosum A middle chamber running the length of the penis into the glans that engorges with blood during erection.

urethra The tube extending from the bladder to the urethral opening, which carries out of the body urine in women and men and semen as well in men.

FIGURE 2.3 The Penis: Internal view

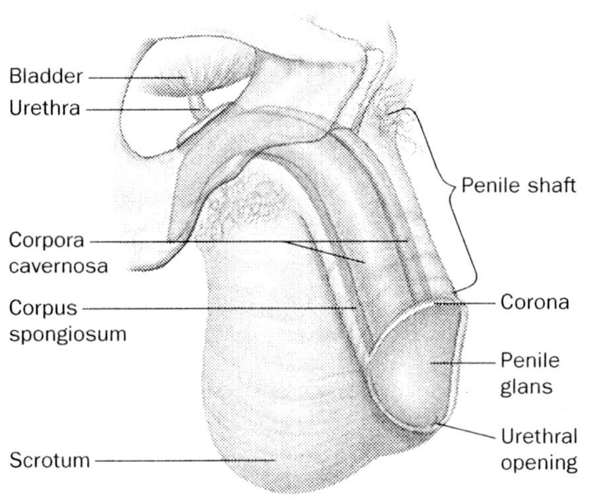

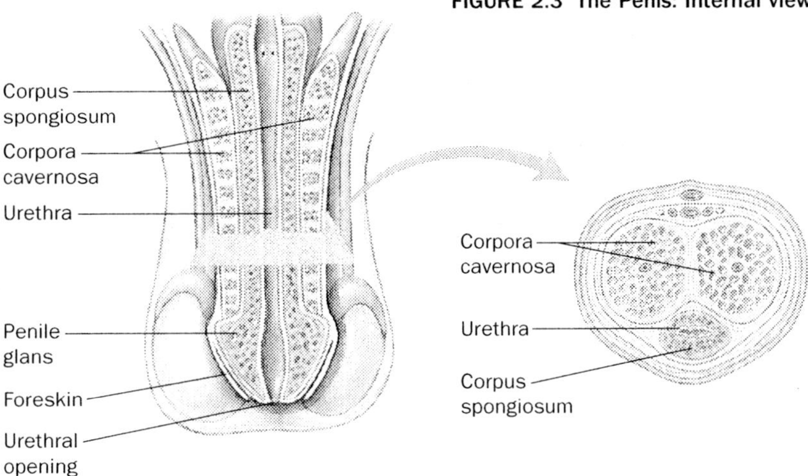

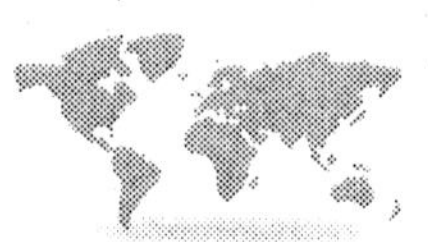

Sexuality and Culture

Male Circumcision in the United States

The Practice of Male Circumcision

Male circumcision is the surgical removal of the foreskin covering of the glans of the penis. In an infant this is a rather small area of skin, but if left intact, it will grow to become 15 square inches of skin covering the glans of an adult male. Circumcisions have usually been performed on infant boys before two weeks of age and often without anesthesia. The reasoning for the lack of pain medication has been based on the erroneous belief that very young infants do not feel much pain and that anesthesia can be dangerous to infants. It should be noted that the United States is one of a very few countries worldwide that has routinely performed male circumcisions, and over the past 20 years or so, the practice has become quite controversial.

Although some variations exist among racial, ethnic, and religious groups, nearly all male babies born in the United States before 1980 were routinely circumcised. Since that time the practice has been on the decline, with the most recent estimates placing the circumcision rate at about 60 percent nationwide (Camille, Kuo, & Wiener, 2002). Most of these procedures are carried out for health, rather than religious, reasons. The controversy centers around whether a valid medical reason exists for male circumcision. Prior to 1980, the prevailing belief was that uncircumcised, or intact, males were more prone to various diseases, including urinary tract infections, penile irritations, penile cancer, and various sexually transmitted diseases. However, no solid scientific literature exists to support these claims.

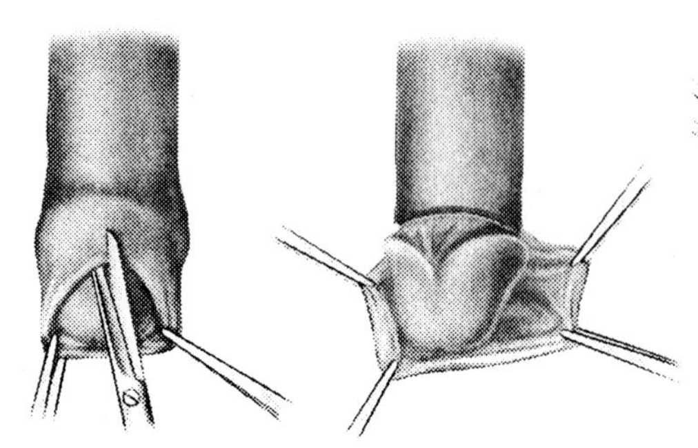

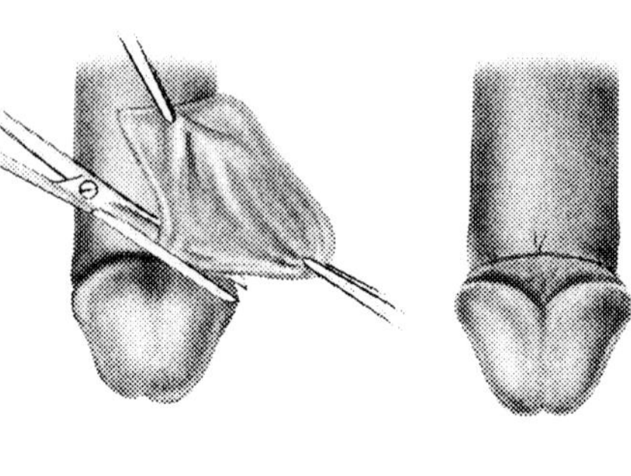

In 1999, the American Academy of Pediatrics, the primary governing board for medical decisions involving children in the United States, reviewed all the available literature on male circumcision and incidence of disease and concluded that there is *no medical justification for routine circumcision of newborn males*. It also added that if parents choose to have their baby circumcised, anaesthesia should be used. (For more information on male circumcision, see the *Circumcision Information Resource Page* at http://www.cirp.org/.)

The Procedure

Several procedures exist for circumcision surgery. The goal is to remove the foreskin that covers the tip, or glans, of the penis (see diagram). Methods for circumcision vary from freehand techniques, in which the foreskin is stretched away from the glans and cut away with a scalpel, to the use of various clamp devices that reduce bleeding and ensure a more even surgical result. The figure illustrates one method of circumcision.

The Results

The penile glans, protected by the foreskin of a natural, intact penis, is a moist mucous membrane, one skin layer thick, much like the inside of your mouth, and just as sensitive. When a penis is circumcised, the glans grows additional layers of skin as it heals from the loss of the foreskin. The glans of a circumcised penis eventually develops 10 to 15 layers of skin, more like the back of your hand. Therefore, the glans of a circumcised penis is less sensitive to sexual stimulation than the glans of an intact penis.

It should be noted that among some religious groups, especially in Conservative and Orthodox Judaism, circumcision is considered a necessary religious ritual for all male infants. The surgery is typically performed a week following the child's birth by a *mohel* (pronounced "moyl"), a Jewish official (a mohel is usually a man, but there are a small number of female mohels, called *mohelets*). Although this religious custom is typically not part of the larger cultural debate over male circumcision, a parallel debate is occurring within some Jewish groups as well.

Penis Size

You may be surprised to learn that penises are more similar in size than they are different. Many people *think* penises vary in size more than they actually do. In fact, the large number of myths about the penis is quite remarkable, and most of them relate to penis size (see Table 2.1).

2. A lot of magazines advertise for penis-increasing creams or exercises. Do any of these really work?

Throughout modern and ancient history, a great deal of attention has been paid to penis size. This attention has been based on erroneous beliefs that a bigger penis represents a more masculine man and that men with bigger penises are better able to satisfy their sexual partners. Historically, and still today, many men worry about the size of their penis—usually that it is too small—and men are significantly more concerned about this issue than women are. These myths are not based on any scientific evidence, and yet they persist. Part of the reason for these beliefs is that while growing up, most boys and young men rarely, if ever, have the opportunity to see other penises erect. The exception to this is when they are able to view sexually explicit materials such as so-called pornographic videos. But if you think about it, you'll immediately see the flaw in this "education" about penis size. The men in those videos are clearly not hired because they are normal or average. They are "porn stars" precisely because they have penises that perpetuate the myths: abnormally large ones. In addition, prosthetic

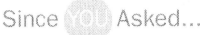

Table 2.1 PHALLIC FALLACIES: COMMON MYTHS ABOUT PENIS SIZE

FALLACY	FACT
Penis size increases with frequent sexual activity and decreases with lack of sex.	Penis size changes only temporarily with sexual activity, during erection.
Penis size can be increased with exercises, pumps, or surgery.	So far, no proven method exists for increasing penis size. Exercise of the penis (whatever that might be) does nothing for size; penis pumps simply draw blood into the penis, which makes it appear bigger temporarily as with an erection. No surgical technique has shown consistent enough results to be approved by any professional medical association (no matter what you see online), and some can cause serious deformities.
Erect human penises have been documented from 1 inch to 18 inches in length.	A rare congenital (inborn) disorder called *micropenis,* usually requiring surgical intervention, may cause a penis to be an inch or less in length. However, nothing close to a penis 18 inches long has ever been documented. Overall, erect penises are between 5 and 7 inches long, and average about $5\frac{1}{2}$ inches.
A small flaccid (unerect) penis predicts a small erect penis.	Actually, the opposite is usually true. Research has shown that smaller flaccid penises tend to grow more than larger flaccid penises upon erection. There is a significantly greater range of lengths in flaccid penises than in erect penises, which is why some analysts have called erection "the great equalizer."
The size of a man's penis can be predicted from other physical characteristics.	This has no basis in scientific fact. Contrary to popular belief, penis size is not meaningfully related to overall build, height, nose size, foot size, middle finger size, race, or ethnicity. The only possible predictor of a man's penis size might be the size of his father's penis.
Large penises provide greater sexual satisfaction for a partner during intercourse.	In heterosexual intercourse, nearly all of the pleasure nerve endings in the vagina are located along the outer one-third of its length (the portion closest to the opening). Moreover, the vagina is a very elastic structure that can accommodate a penis of any size. Penises of any length are able to reach this part of the vagina. Also, for both gay and straight couples, depth of penetration depends more on sexual position than on penile length.
Most partners prefer larger penises.	Actually, most partners of men don't think or care very much about penis size. Men are much more concerned about their own penis size than their partners are. In fact, some people worry more about a partner with a very large penis than a smaller one in terms of comfort during penetration.

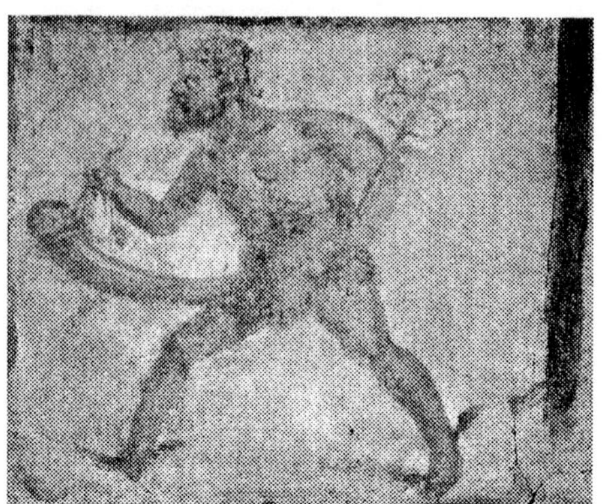

Throughout history, exaggerated penis size has been a preoccupation in many cultures.

or even computer-generated oversized penises are sometimes used in these videos. If computer-generated images can make dinosaurs look real or the *Titanic* appear to sink into the sea, a computer-generated, larger-than-life penis should be a snap. Nevertheless, when men see these exaggerated penises on the screen and do a quick self-comparison, it is difficult for many of them not to feel inadequate.

In reality, some relatively accurate, scientific statistics exist about penis size, starting with Masters and Johnson's research in the 1950s and 1960s. They found that the normal range for flaccid (meaning not erect) penile length for their research subjects was between 2.8 inches and 4.3 inches, with an average length of about 3 inches. The average length of erect penises ranged from about 4.9 inches to 6.9 inches, with an average of 5.1 inches. These measurements are significantly smaller than the commonly held beliefs about what constitutes a large versus a small penis. Furthermore, when Masters and Johnson (1966) measured the size of erect penises, they found that a larger flaccid penis does not predict a larger erect penis. They discovered that smaller flaccid penises tend to enlarge proportionately more upon sexual excitement than do larger flaccid penises. Looking at averages, a flaccid penis of 3 inches increased to a length of 6 inches, while a 4 inch flaccid penis only added about 2.5 inches to reach a length of 6.5 inches.

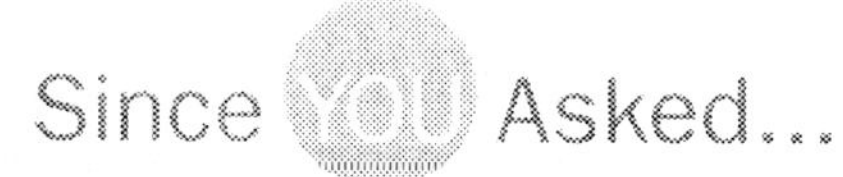

3. What is the average penis size? Can a man be too small or too large?

Masters and Johnson's findings about penis size have been confirmed in other studies with only slight variations. Another study of 80 ethnically diverse men found an average flaccid penile length of 3.7 inches, with a range from 1.97 to 6.1 inches, and an average erect length of 5.07 inches, with a range from 2.95 inches to 7.48 inches (Wessells & McAninch, 1996). As mentioned in Chapter 1, a 2001 study by a condom manufacturer, Lifestyles, asked college men on spring break in Cancun, Mexico, to volunteer to have their penises measured by health professionals in exchange for a T-shirt and free condoms (Edell, 2001). In a private setting, with erotic material available for the men to use to achieve erections, each volunteer was measured by two health care professionals supervised by a physician. A total of 300 men participated. In this study, the average erect penis length was 5.877 inches and the average girth, or circumference, was 4.972 inches (less than the circumference of a "D" battery). Moreover, the variation in size among all 300 men was inconsequential. Length varied less than an inch (0.83 inch) and girth varied only 0.5 inch from the smallest to the largest penis among the 300 men. You should be aware that the data from the Lifestyles study showing slightly greater penile length may be biased due to subject self-selection, and this probably accounted for the slightly longer average finding (in other words, men with smaller penises might have been less likely to volunteer to be measured). The bottom line of all these findings is that penises are much more similar than different (see "Evaluating Sexual Research: Self-Reports of Penis Size" for an interesting look at other, less scientific studies on penis size).

What is more important than all these measurements of penises is the notion that a partner's sexual enjoyment and satisfaction depends on penis size. For heterosexual intercourse, Masters and Johnson's research found that idea to be without merit. In their careful observations, they determined that the vagina is an extremely elastic organ capable of accommodating penises of any size and that during intercourse with a man, a woman's sexual satisfaction is typically *not* related to the size of her partner's penis (Masters & Johnson, 1966). Furthermore, as you will see later in this chapter, most of the nerve endings in the vagina are concentrated in the outer third of its length, the third closest to the opening. Therefore, depth of penetration during intercourse is not a major factor in the sensations most women feel during intercourse.

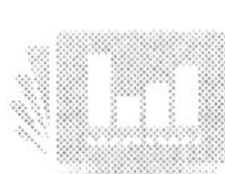

Evaluating Sexual Research

Self-Reports of Penis Size

In addition to the studies cited here, several other projects have been carried out to determine penis size. Some of these, rather than using trained researchers to do the measuring, asked men to measure their own penises and submit their findings (Durex, 2002b; Kinsey, Pomeroy, & Martin, 1948). Well, guess what: All those studies found larger averages. Kinsey's study found an average erect penis size of 6.3 inches, and the average self-report length in a study by the condom company came in at 6.5 inches in length with a girth of 5.0 inches. Not very surprising, is it? Because of the value placed (or misplaced) on penis size, men in the self-report studies either fudged their answers, unconsciously measured in ways to maximize their findings, or perhaps just made something up. We should note that these studies provided directions for proper penis measurement; had they not done so, the results might have been much more distorted.

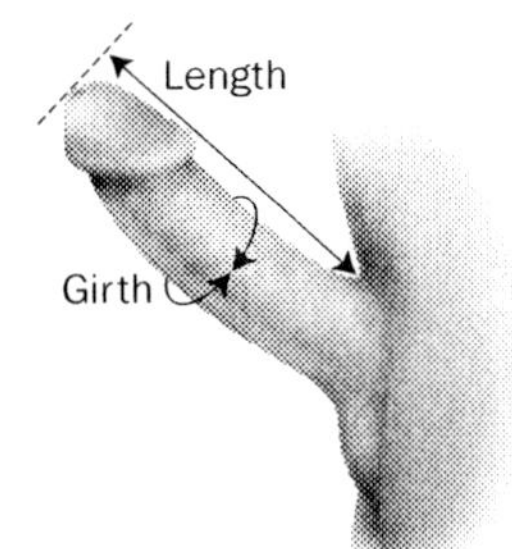

If you are so inclined (even though it really doesn't matter), here is the correct method for measuring a penis. When erect, place a ruler where the top of the penis meets the pubic bone and measure to the tip of the penis, as shown in the diagram. If uncircumcised, the foreskin should be retracted. This is the correct length of the penis as reported in the studies discussed in this chapter. If you want to measure girth (circumference), wrap a tape measure snugly, but not tightly, around the shaft of the penis about midway down.

If you decide to measure your (or your partner's) penis, what should you do with that information? Well, sex educators would probably tell you to *forget about it*; it makes no difference. However, if you are concerned about your penis being abnormally small or large, it is perfectly reasonable to talk to your doctor about your concerns.

This is not to say that some people prefer, psychologically, a partner with a smaller or larger penis, just as everyone tends to be turned on by different physical characteristics in a sexual partner. However, in terms of the *anatomy* and *physiology* of sexual satisfaction, penis size appears to play no role (more about this issue in Chapter 3, "The Physiology of Human Sexual Responding").

scrotum The sac of thin skin and muscle containing the testicles in the male.

spermatic cords Supporting each testicle and encasing the vas deferens, nerves, and muscles.

The Scrotum and Testicles

The **scrotum** is a pouch of two layers of skin that hangs below and behind the penis. Its function is to house and protect the *testicles* (also called *testes* or *male gonads*) and help provide them with the best possible conditions to produce sperm cells. The scrotum is divided into two sacs, one for each testicle. Men are acutely aware that the scrotal skin is not passive tissue that just hangs there in the same form all the time. On the contrary, the scrotum has an active role in male sexuality and reproduction. Two small muscles, one located in the walls of the scrotum and one in each of the **spermatic cords**, move the scrotum and the testicles up and down, depending on specific situations, especially external temperature. The testicles require a temperature that is slightly lower than normal body temperature to maximize production of sperm cells (about 94 degrees rather than average body temperature of around 98.6). This is why when a man's scrotum is hot, say, after a shower or a soak in the hot tub, the scrotal skin is very loose and the testicles are hanging down away from the body. The scrotum is cooling the testicles by moving them as far away from body heat as possible. Conversely, after a swim in cold water, the scrotum skin is very tight and is holding the testicles up closely under the penis in an attempt to maintain the ideal temperature for sperm production (see Figure 2.4).

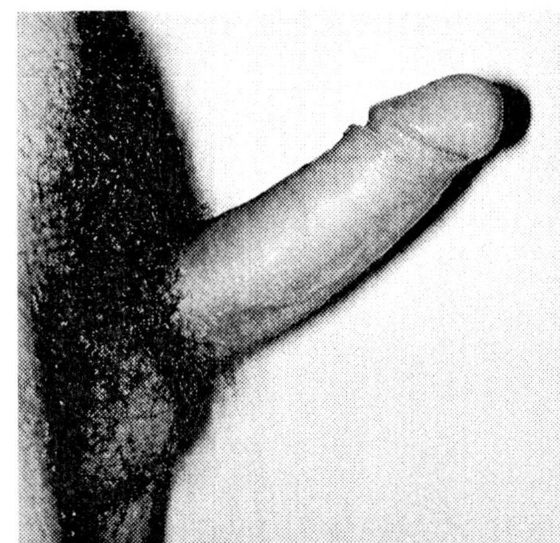

FIGURE 2.4 Changes in Tightness of Scrotal Skin

The scrotum tightens or relaxes in an effort to maintain a constant temperature for sperm production by the testicles. It also tightens to lift the testicles close to the body during sexual arousal, as shown here.

FIGURE 2.5 Internal View of Testicles

Each testicle is suspended by the spermatic cord, which also encases the vas deferens, the tube that carries sperm into the penis for ejaculation.

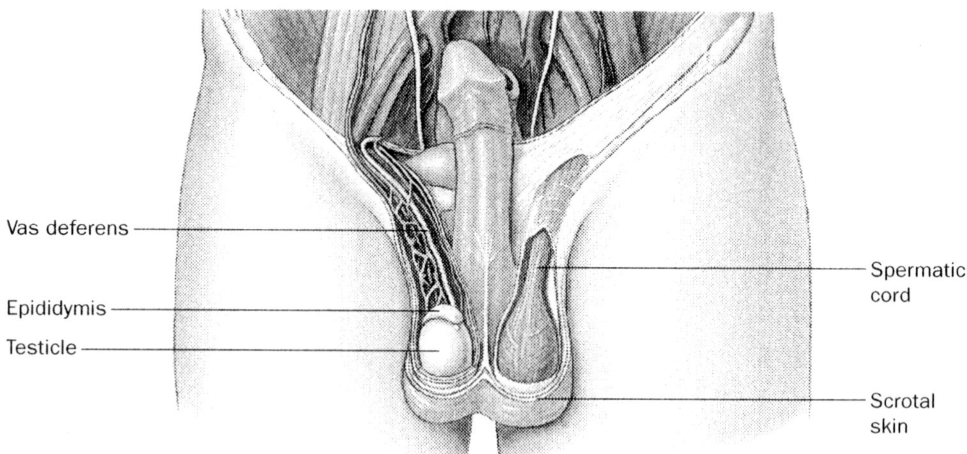

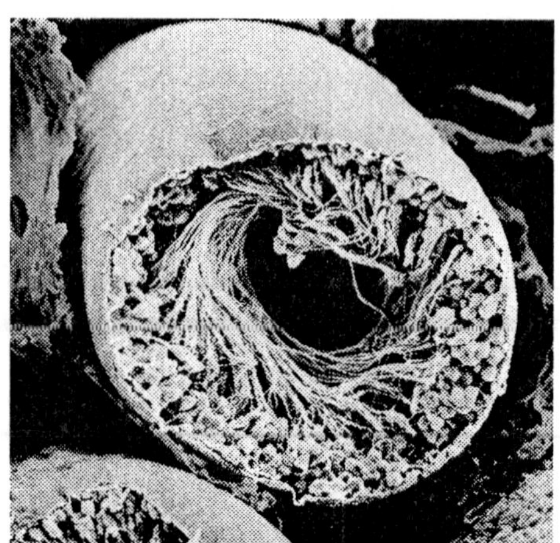

FIGURE 2.6 Development of Sperm Cells

Sperm cells are produced continuously in the hundreds of feet of seminiferous tubules that comprise the testicles.

testicles Oval structures approximately 1.0 to 1.5 inches in length made up of microscopic tubes in which sperm cells and testosterone are produced in the male.

gonads Organs that produce cells (ova or sperm) for reproduction.

testosterone The male sex hormone responsible for male sexual characteristics and the production of sperm cells.

seminiferous tubules Tightly wound microscopic tubes that comprise the testicles in the male, where sperm cells are generated.

epididymis A crescent-shaped structure on each testicle where sperm cells are stored as they mature.

ejaculation Expulsion of semen through the penis.

vas deferens A tube extending from the testicle (epididymis) into the male's body for the transport of mature sperm cells during ejaculation.

The scrotum also tightens and pulls the testicles up toward the underside of the penis during sexual arousal. As we will discuss more in the next chapter, when the testicles are drawn as far up as possible, it is a signal that orgasm is quickly approaching.

The **testicles** float freely, one in each sac, within the scrotum as shown in Figure 2.5. They are glands referred to as **gonads**, which produce cells for reproduction (in common usage, the word *gonads* usually refers to the testicles, but females have gonads too—the *ovaries*, to be discussed later). The testicles' primary function is to manufacture sperm cells and secrete the male sex hormone, **testosterone**.

Each testicle is composed of tightly packed microscopic **seminiferous tubules**, or "sperm-forming" tubes. To get an idea of the small size of these tubules, if they could be removed and stretched out end to end, they would be nearly 1,000 feet long. It is in these tubules that sperm cells are continuously formed throughout a man's life. Figure 2.6 shows (under powerful magnification) actual sperm cells forming in the seminiferous tubules.

When sperm cells are formed, they migrate in an immature state to the **epididymis**, which is the long, narrow structure attached to the back of each testicle. In the epididymis, the sperm cells mature and wait to be ejaculated. Sperm cells require approximately 70 days to mature before they are ready for **ejaculation**. Cells that are not ejaculated are simply reabsorbed by the man's body. Attached to each epididymis is a tube, called the **vas deferens**, through which mature sperm cells travel to the man's internal reproductive system, where they are mixed with semen and ejaculated through the penis and out the urethral opening.

The testicles are among the sites in the human sexual anatomy that are subject to cancer. Testicular cancer, although not a common cancer overall, is the most frequently diagnosed cancer in men between the ages of 15 and 35, with approximately 9,000 new cases identified in the United States in 2004 (American Cancer Society, 2004a). In addition, the incidence of testicular cancer worldwide has increased more than 50 percent since the mid-1900s (Pinkowish, 2000), and the average age at which it is diagnosed has been steadily decreasing from 30 to under 25 years of age. The exact causes of this increase are not fully understood. However, the greater incidence of testicular cancer among men who work in certain professions—including agricultural workers, miners, firefighters, and utility workers—has led some researchers to suspect that exposure to environmental toxins may play an important role (American Cancer Society, 2004b; Guillette, 2002).

As the incidence of testicular cancer has grown, so has medicine's ability to treat it. Today the average cure rate for testicular cancer is 85 percent, with much greater success when the disease is diagnosed early (Pinkowish, 2000). Therefore, all men should

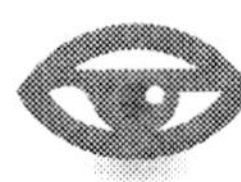

Self-Discovery
Testicular Self-Examination

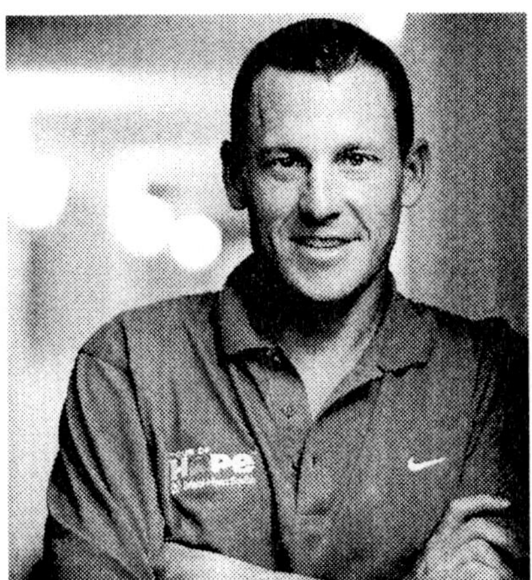

Lance Armstrong, who had testicular cancer has worked to increase awareness and early detection of the disease.

Many people are surprised to learn that the most common form of cancer in males between the ages of 15 and 35 is testicular cancer. In 2004, approximately 9,000 new cases of testicular cancer were diagnosed in the United States (American Cancer Society, 2004a). The three most important issues relating to this form of cancer are (1) most young men are unaware of their risk; (2) they do not know that they should be examining their own testicles once each month for lumps, irregularities, swelling, and other changes that may be an early sign of cancer; and (3) they have no idea how to perform a testicular self-exam (TSE). The cure rate for testicular cancer approaches 100 percent with early detection. Some well-known celebrities who have been diagnosed, treated, and cured of testicular cancer—cyclist Lance Armstrong and comedian Tom Green, for example—have gone public with their experiences in recent years to increase awareness of this disease and of the importance of TSE. Males should begin a monthly habit of examining their own testicles starting at about age 15 (Hock, 2003). It is a very simple procedure.

A testicular self-exam is best performed after a warm bath or shower. Heat relaxes the scrotum, making it easier to feel anything abnormal. The National Cancer Institute recommends following these steps every month:

1. Stand in front of a mirror. Check for any swelling on the scrotum skin.
2. Examine each testicle with both hands. Place the index and middle fingers under the testicle with the thumbs placed on top. Roll the testicle gently between the thumbs and fingers. Don't be alarmed if one testicle seems slightly larger than the other. That's normal.
3. Find the epididymis, the soft structure behind the testicle where sperm cells mature. If you become familiar with this structure, you won't mistake it for a suspicious lump. Cancerous lumps are usually found on the sides of the testicle but can also show up on the front or at the bottom.
4. If you find a lump, see a doctor right away. It may not be cancer, but if it is, you'll want to have it treated as soon as possible to prevent it from spreading. Only a physician can make a positive diagnosis.

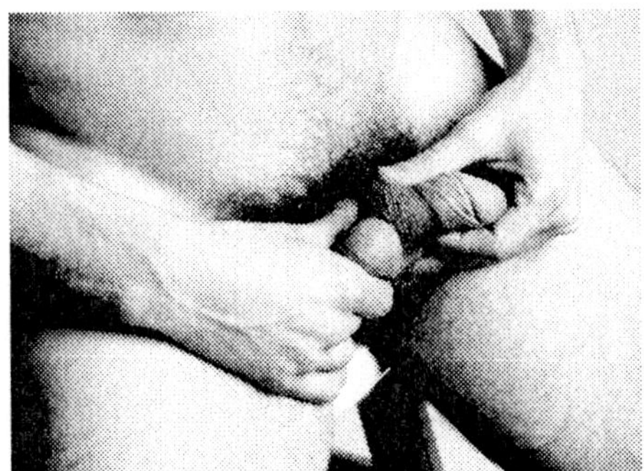

Men should perform a testicular self-exam once a month starting at age 15.

learn to examine their testicles to help detect testicular cancer early and maximize the chances of a full cure and recovery. How to do a testicular self-exam is explained in "Self-Discovery: Testicular Self-Examination."

The Anus

The **anus** and the area around it contain nerve endings that are sensitive to stimulation and are considered by some men (and women) to be part of their sexual anatomy, providing pleasurable feelings when stimulated or penetrated. Some men, regardless of sexual orientation, enjoy having their anal area caressed manually, stimulated orally, or penetrated during sexual activities (see Chapter 6, "Sexual Behaviors," for more information about anal sexual activities). Some men find caressing or massaging of the surface of the prostate gland (to be discussed shortly) through the wall of the rectum to be sexually stimulating. These positive views of the anus are far from universal, and

anus The end of the digestive tract and outlet for bodily excretions. It is also a sexually stimulating area for some people.

many people are repulsed by the idea that this area would even be considered part of sexual anatomy or behaviors.

It should be noted that the anal area and the walls of the rectum consist of delicate tissues and the risk is that membranes can be easily damaged during sexual activity, creating an easy route of transmission for bloodborne sexually transmitted infections. In addition, bacteria that exist normally and harmlessly in the anal area and rectum may cause infections if they are transferred to other parts of the anatomy, such as the urethra or digestive tract.

Male Internal Structures

Mature sperm cells enter the inside of the male sexual body. Although male internal reproductive anatomy is fairly complex, we will simplify the discussion by focusing on the structures most important for laying the groundwork for the many other topics throughout this book. These structures are diagrammed in Figure 2.7.

The Vas Deferens

The vas deferens is the tube connecting each testicle and epididymis with the male internal reproductive structures. Upon sexual arousal and orgasm, the sperm cells cross from the external to the internal anatomical structures as they travel up each vas deferens, where they will eventually be expelled through the urethra during orgasm and ejaculation. When a man chooses to have a vasectomy so that he will no longer be fertile, each vas deferens is severed and sealed off. Obviously, if sperm cells cannot travel from the epididymis up either vas deferens, they will never be ejaculated and never be able to fertilize an ovum. The man will still ejaculate, however, because *semen* is produced by the seminal vesicles and prostate gland, to be discussed next. The process of sperm production and function are discussed in greater detail in Chapter 9, "Conception, Pregnancy, and Birth."

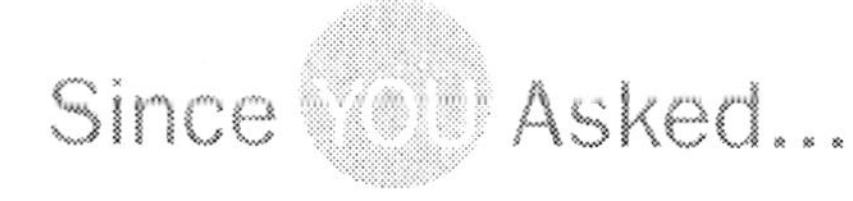

4. How do the sperm get from the testicles to the penis?

Semen

During sexual arousal and ejaculation, as the sperm cells are moving through the vas deferens from each epididymis, other anatomical organs are producing fluid, or *ejaculate*, that will mix with the sperm and carry them out of the man's body. This fluid is called **semen**. Semen is a whitish or yellowish, viscous fluid composed of water, salt,

semen The fluid produced primarily by the prostate gland and seminal vesicles that is ejaculated with the sperm cells by men during orgasm.

FIGURE 2.7 Male Internal Sexual Anatomy

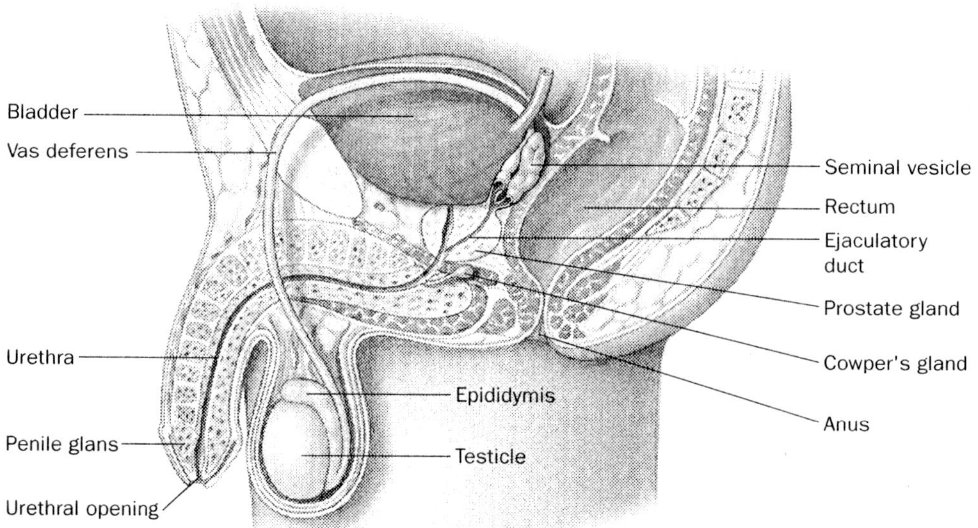

and fructose sugars designed by nature to nourish and sustain sperm cells for their journey from the vagina through the cervix, along the walls of the uterus, and into the fallopian tubes, where, if the timing is right, they may encounter and fertilize an ovum (the process of conception is covered in Chapter 9, "Conception, Pregnancy, and Birth"). Semen is primarily a mixture of secretions from the *seminal vesicles* and the *prostate gland*, which we will discuss next.

The Seminal Vesicles

The **seminal vesicles** are small glands that are located at the upper, (internal) end of each vas deferens just as they feed into the **ejaculatory duct**, which directs semen into the urethra. They are connected to each vas deferens by a series of small tubules that carry fluids from the seminal vesicles to mix with the sperm cells during ejaculation. The secretions from the seminal vesicles contain high concentrations of fructose, a type of sugar that provides energy and nourishment to the sperm cells so they will be prepared to survive the arduous journey to rendevous with the egg. Fluid from the seminal vesicles makes up about 70 percent of the volume of the semen.

The Prostate Gland

Next, the gathering ejaculate passes through the **prostate gland**, which adds most of the remaining liquid, called *prostatic fluid*. This fluid is quite thick, giving the semen its typical viscous texture. It is also very alkaline to help counteract the normally acidic environment of the vagina, making it more hospitable to sperm and enhancing the odds of conception. You can see from Figure 2.7 that the urethra extends from the bladder and also passes through the prostate gland. When a man is sexually aroused and approaching ejaculation, the prostate contracts, shutting off the possible flow of urine from the bladder so that both cannot normally occur at the same time. This is why, for a brief time following ejaculation, many men find it difficult or even slightly painful to urinate.

A common health problem for older men is noncancerous enlargement of the prostate (called *benign prostatic hyperplasia*, or BPH). Fifty percent of men in their 60s and nearly 90 percent of men in their 70s will experience this health problem (National Institute of Health [NIH], 2002). If the prostate enlarges too much, it can squeeze the urethra, making urination slow, difficult, painful, or even impossible. This condition is usually successfully treated with medication or surgery to open up the passageway through the prostate gland. Also, the prostate is a very common site for cancer in older men. It is the second most common form of cancer in men (skin cancer is number one) and is even more common than breast cancer in women. Most men who live to be 80 or older will develop prostate cancer, but it may be found in men in their 50s or 60s. Prostate cancer is diagnosed by a digital (finger) rectal exam and a blood test.

Usually, prostate cancer grows very slowly and usually does not metastasize, or spread, beyond the gland itself. If it does spread, however, it can be deadly, which is why all men over 40 should be routinely screened for signs of prostate cancer. Depending on a man's age at the time of diagnosis and the type of cancer, treatment options range from complete surgical removal of the prostate to chemotherapy and radiation and sometimes no treatment at all. This last choice, called "watchful waiting," relates to the slow-growing nature of prostate cancer; and for most men diagnosed in their 70s or older, it will not be fatal. In other words, they will almost certainly die of other causes before the prostate cancer becomes life-threatening (Zepf, 2003b).

The prostate is also prone to bacterial infections, called **prostatitis**, in men of any age. The symptoms of prostatitis include chills; fever; pain in the lower back and genital area; urinary frequency and urgency, often at night; burning or painful urination; body aches; and white blood cells and bacteria in the urine (Shoskes, Katske, & Kim, 2001).

seminal vesicle A structure that produces fluid that becomes part of the semen that is expelled during ejaculation.

ejaculatory duct A continuation of the tube that carries semen into the urethra for ejaculation.

prostate gland A gland in males surrounding the urethra that produces the largest proportion of seminal fluid (ejaculate).

prostatitis An uncomfortable or painful inflammation of the prostate gland, usually caused by bacteria.

orgasm The peak of sexual arousal.

urethral bulb The prostatic section of the urethra that expands with collected semen just prior to expulsion, creating the sensation of ejaculatory inevitability.

Cowper's glands Small glands near the penile urethra that produce a slippery mucus-like substance during male sexual arousal (also referred to as the *bulbourethral glands*).

pre-ejaculate The fluid produced by the Cowper's glands.

Prostatitis may be either acute, lasting a relatively short period of time, or chronic, coming and going over a period of months or years. The antibiotic *levofloxicin* appears to be quite successful in the treatment and cure of prostatitis ("Antibiotic," 2003).

The Urethral Bulb

At **orgasm**, the peak of sexual arousal, the semen that has been gathering from these various structures is forced into the **urethral bulb**, a portion of the urethra surronded by the prostate gland, causing the man to experience the feeling of impending ejaculation. Muscle contractions force the semen out through the urethra in the final stage of ejaculation. This two-stage process of ejaculation will be discussed in greater detail in Chapter 3, "The Physiology of Human Sexual Responding."

The Cowper's Glands

As the semen passes through the urethra, the **Cowper's glands**, one on each side of the urethra, also add a small amount of fluid to the semen (see Figure 2.7). Of greater importance, however, is that the Cowper's glands often secrete fluid into the urethra and out through the penis well *before* ejaculation. This fluid is called **pre-ejaculate**. During sexual arousal, a small amount of clear, thick, slippery fluid from the Cowper's glands may appear at the urethral opening at the tip of the penis. The exact function of these secretions is not fully understood, although they may, along with the other components in semen, help nourish and protect sperm cells and lubricate the urethra prior to ejaculation. However, the fluid may contain live sperm cells left over from a recent ejaculation, capable of causing pregnancy even in the absence of a new ejaculation. Moreover, if the man has a sexually transmitted infection such as HIV or gonorrhea, the infectious microbes can be transmitted by the Cowper's gland fluid (Garbo, 2002; Kowal, 1998b). These are important reasons why the withdrawal method ("pulling out") is *not* recommended as a means of contraception (see Chapter 5, "Contraception: Planning and Preventing Pregnancy," for more on this).

In "Historical Perspectives" at the beginning of this chapter, you learned how the male body was once, centuries ago, thought to be the norm for sexual anatomy throughout ancient history. The sexual anatomy of women was seen as merely a variation on that of men. Today, of course, we know that this is inaccurate. However, as you will see as we begin to discuss female sexual anatomy, certain similarities between women and men do exist, in addition to many fundamental differences.

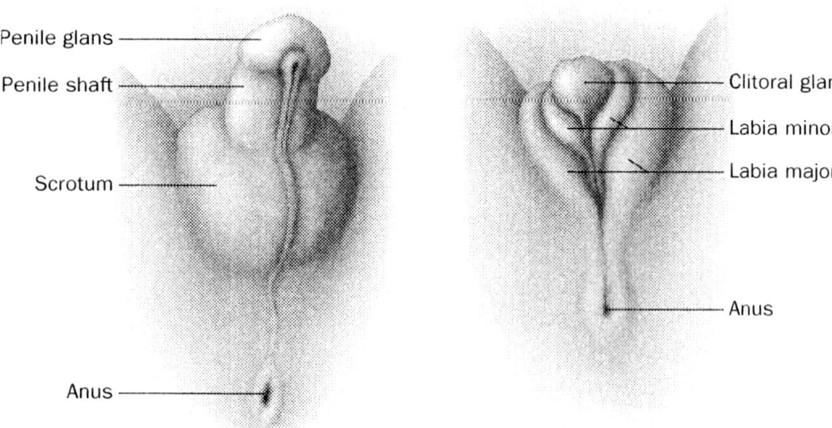

FIGURE 2.8 Origins of Male and Female Sexual Anatomy

If you could look carefully at a developing fetus, you would be unable to tell by looking at its genitals whether it is a boy or a girl until about the twelfth week of pregnancy. Prior to that stage of development, all fetal external genitalia resemble female structures. Normally, these genital areas only begin to develop into male external genitals when a male fetus's testicles begin to secrete androgens, or male hormones. In a female fetus, the absence of these hormones causes the genitals to continue to develop as female. This means that male and female genitalia are homologous, or *originate from* the very same fetal cells, but due to the presence or absence of hormones, they grow into either boy or girl sexual anatomical structures. The correspondence between the sexes is much more evident than most people realize. The list below shows which male and female genitals develop in the womb from the same underlying structures.

MALE	FEMALE
Testicles	Ovaries
Penile glans	Clitoral glans
Foreskin	Clitoral hood
Penile shaft	Clitoral shaft
Scrotum	Labia majora
Underside of penis	Labia minora

The Female Sexual Body

Male and female sexual anatomical organs are, of course, different but equally complex overall. However, as mentioned earlier, the *external* genitals of women are a bit more complicated to explain fully than those of men. In addition, fewer people are as familiar with female genitals simply because they are not as readily visible. For women to examine their own sexual anatomy typically requires some bodily contortions and the use of a mirror. Nevertheless, as for men, it is a good idea for women to become familiar with their genitals, just as they might for any other part of the body. Why? Because an intimate knowledge of your sexual body enhances sexual satisfaction, sexual intimacy, and sexual health. Interestingly, many of the sexual anatomical organs for men and women grow from the very same cells and tissue and begin to differentiate as the fetus develops in the uterus. Figure 2.8 illustrates how male and female anatomical structures are homologous prior to this process of differentiation in appearance and function.

vulva The female external genitals.

mons veneris A slightly raised layer of fatty tissue on the top of a woman's pubic bone, usually covered with hair in the adult.

labia majora Folds of skin and fatty tissue that extend from the mons down both sides of the vulva, past the vaginal opening to the perineum.

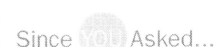

Female External Structures

Taken together, the female external genitals are referred to as the **vulva** (see Figure 2.9). Components of the vulva, identified in part (a) of the figure, are the *mons veneris*, the *labia majora*, the *labia minora*, the *urethral opening*, the *clitoral glans* (or tip) of the clitoris, the *vaginal opening*, the *hymen*, the *perineum*, and the *anus*, each of which we will discuss in turn.

Although both men and women have breasts and nipples that may be sensitive to sexual stimulation, we are discussing them here only because in most Western cultures the breasts are more frequently associated with female sexual anatomy.

The Mons Veneris

The **mons veneris** (meaning "mount of Venus" and sometimes called the *mons pubis*) is typically the only part of female sexual anatomy easily seen when looking at a woman's body, legs together, from the front. It is simply a slightly raised layer of fatty tissue on the top of the pubic bone and is usually covered with pubic hair. Part of its function is to cushion impact with the pubic bone during sexual intercourse.

The Labia Majora

Just below the mons veneris are the **labia majora**, meaning "major lips." These structures are folds of skin and fatty tissue and extend from the mons down both sides of the vulva, past the vaginal opening to the perineum. The labia majora close over and protect the more sensitive and delicate genital structures underneath them. As you can see in Figure 2.9, the labia majora vary in size, shape, amount of hair, and skin tone.

5. I feel that my genitals don't look right. The lips are sort of large and not pink like I see in pictures. They're more grayish. Is this normal?

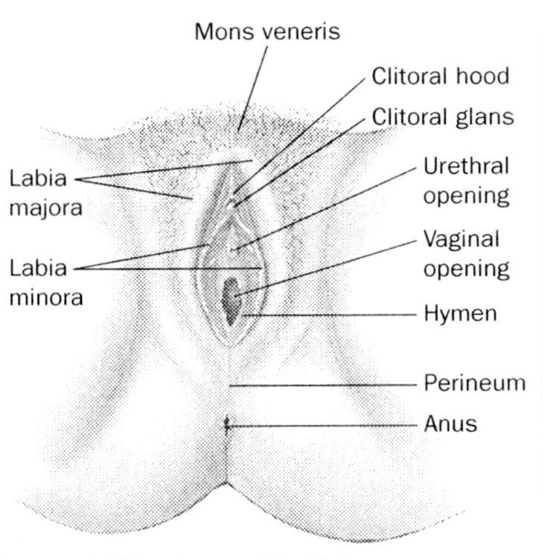

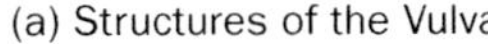
(a) Structures of the Vulva

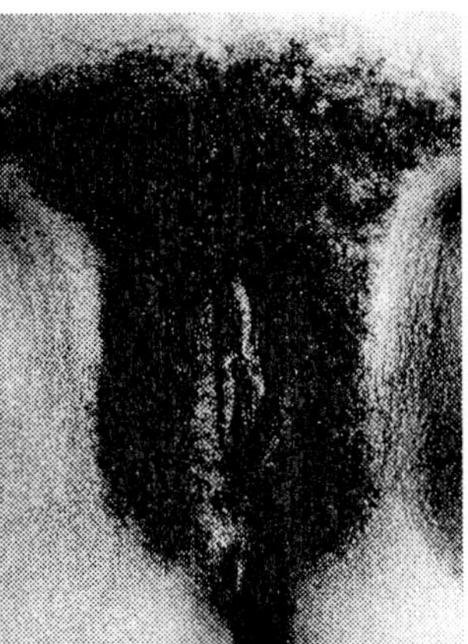

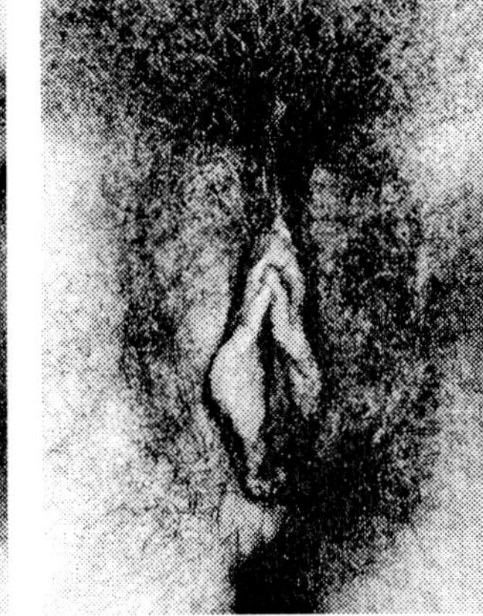

(b) Variations in the Appearance of the Vulva

FIGURE 2.9 The Female External Genitals, or Vulva

The female vulva varies normally in shape, color, and appearance, just like other parts of the female body.

labia minora The smooth, hairless, inner lips of the vulva.

clitoral glans The outer end or tip of the clitoris.

clitoris An erectile sexual structure consisting of the clitoral glans and two shafts (*crura*) that is primarily responsible for triggering orgasm in most women.

clitoral hood Tissue that partially or fully covers the clitoral glans.

The Labia Minora

As can be seen in part (a) of Figure 2.9, the labia majora must be parted to allow us to see and study the rest of the vulva. Immediately inside the labia majora are the **labia minora**, or "minor lips." These are smooth, hairless, and, again, vary in size and shape from woman to woman as you can see in Figure 2.9. Many women are insecure about this part of their anatomy because, like men concerned about penis size, they have very little opportunity for comparison. However, with rare exceptions, all labia minora fall within perfectly normal ranges. The labia minora are sexually sensitive; during sexual arousal, they become engorged with blood and darken in color.

The Clitoral Glans and Hood

At the top of the labia minora is the **clitoral glans**, which is the tip of the **clitoris** and the part that can usually be seen and is typically covered partly or completely by the **clitoral hood**. These are analogous, in terms of the fetal origin of the cells, to the penile glans, penis, and foreskin of the male, respectively. Stimulation of the clitoral glans, either directly or indirectly, is primarily responsible for triggering orgasm in most women. Some of you may be wondering why we are referring to this structure as the clitoral glans rather than simply as the clitoris. It is true that most people, and most anatomical references throughout history, refer to this small, visible structure as the clitoris, but that is incorrect. Such a characterization of the clitoris would be analogous to defining the male penile glans as if it were the entire penis and disregarding the rest of it. The difference is that the rest of the clitoris is inside the woman's body. As shown in Figure 2.10, we now know that the clitoris is a much larger and more complex organ than has been acknowledged in the past.

The Clitoris

Researchers have learned the true nature of the clitoris only recently, in the 1990s (O'Connell et al., 1998; Williamson & Nowak, 1998). It turns out that the clitoral shaft is about 0.5 inch in diameter and divides into two legs called *crura* as it extends 3 to 4 inches into the woman's body. These shafts of the clitoris pass on either side of the urethra. Between the crura are two clitoral bulbs, one on each side of the vagina. The clitoris, seen in its entirety, has a similar structure to the male penis, which also consists of three "sections" (the corpus spongiosum and corpora cavernosa), as shown in part (b) of Figure 2.3. Furthermore, we now know that the clitoris, just like the penis, engorges with blood along its entire length, straightens out, and becomes erect during sexual arousal. This typically causes the glans of the clitoris to pull up under the clitoral hood as a woman becomes increasingly sexually excited (this will be dis-

FIGURE 2.10 The Clitoral Truth

The clitoris is a significantly larger and more complex organ than previously thought. As seen in (b), during sexual arousal the clitoris, just like the penis, engorges with blood and becomes erect.

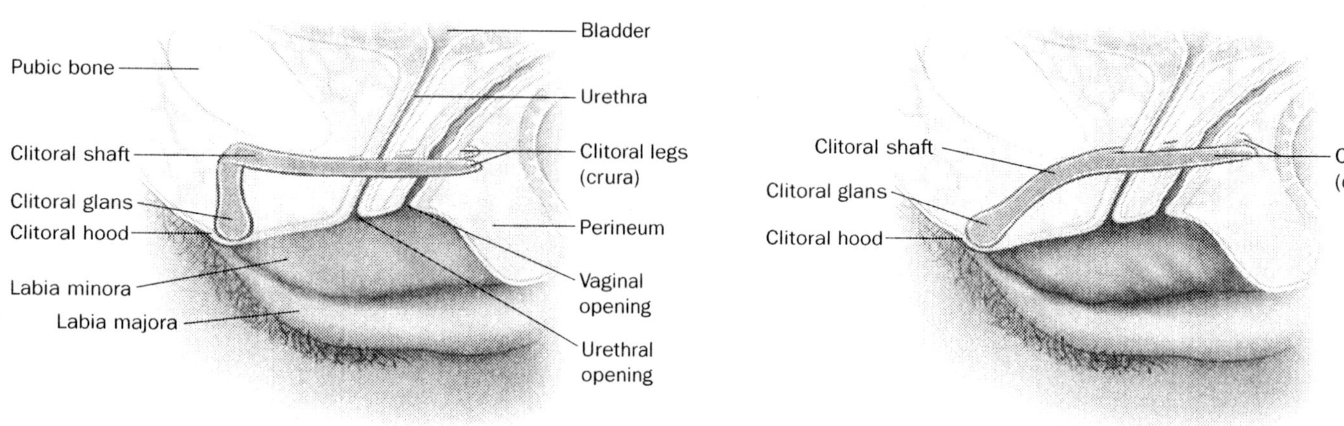

(a) The Clitoris: Unaroused

(b) The Clitoris: Aroused

cussed in more detail in Chapter 3). Figure 2.10 depicts the correct anatomy of the clitoris, unaroused (flaccid) and aroused (erect).

Why are we only finding this out now, you ask? Good question! The most common explanations relate to cultural hesitancy over careful exploration of female sexuality and anatomy. One article states, "The fact that this had only been discovered in the 1990s reveals much of anatomists' prudish reluctance to accurately study female genitalia" (Williamson & Nowak, 1998). In the past, the clitoris was often thought of as just a bit of extra tissue. Since the clitoris is not essential to reproduction, no one worried about it much. Instead, more emphasis was placed then on female anatomical organs in terms of their importance in child bearing (Australian Broadcasting Corporation, 1998).

The discovery of the true anatomical complexity and size of the clitoris is comparable to scientists suddenly finding that the penis is several times larger than first thought. That would be big news. However, these studies about the clitoris, which took place in the late 1990s, have been barely a blip on the news media's radar screens. Now, at least *you* have accurate information.

Earlier in this chapter, we noted the controversy surrounding male circumcision, the surgical removal of the penile foreskin. As you may know, a much more drastic practice of female genital cutting occurs in many countries throughout the world, sometimes called *female circumcision* but more frequently, and more appropriately, referred to as **female genital mutilation, or FGM**. Found mostly in parts of Africa and the Middle East, FGM bears little resemblance to male circumcision in the procedure itself or the reasons underlying it. Male circumcision is performed because many parents believe that it promotes a healthier sexual life for the child as he grows up and will enhance his sexual pleasure; in contrast, female genital mutilation is performed with the expressly *opposite* intention of *preventing* normal sexual functioning in women, and the practice is known to lead to various health complications, infections, and even death. Typically, FGM is performed when a girl is about to enter puberty. It entails the cutting off of the clitoral glans and part or all of the labia minora, lacerating (scraping) the labia majora, and then sewing together the labia majora, leaving only a small opening for the passage of urine and menstrual fluid. This ancient and continuing cultural practice is drawing increased awareness and outrage from the United States and many countries of the world and is now seen as a human rights issue. This controversy is discussed in greater detail in "Sexuality and Culture: Female Genital Mutilation" on pages 54–55.

The Urethral Opening

About halfway down the vulva, between the clitoris and the vagina, is the **urethral opening**, the outside end of the tube leading from the bladder. This is a sensitive structure and can provide pleasurable sexual sensations for some women when stimulated. The location of the urethral opening in women is important for specific health reasons. If you compare male and female anatomy, one of the marked differences is the length of the urethra, the tube from the bladder to the outside of the body; it is considerably shorter in women than in men. The short distance from the vulva to the bladder in women means that bacteria have an easier time reaching the bladder and causing infection. This is why women are significantly more prone than men to **urinary tract infections (UTIs)**. Moreover, many women suffer from recurring UTIs, sometimes as often as once every few months. Urinary tract infections may occur anywhere in the urinary system, but they are usually centered in the bladder. They are caused when common bacteria travel from the outside world up the urethra and into the

Since YOU Asked...

6. I've heard that the clitoris is the same as the penis, but they seem totally different to me. Why do people say they are the same?

female genital mutilation (FGM) Removing part or most of the vulva to prevent sexual stimulation or pleasure; a cultural practice in many countries, especially in Africa.

urethral opening An opening in the mid section of the vulva, between the clitoral glans and the vagina, that allows urine to pass from the body.

urinary tract infection (UTIs) An infection of the urethra, bladder, or other urinary structure, usually caused by bacteria.

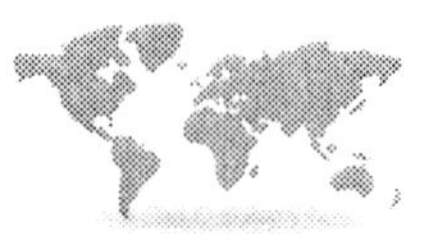

Sexuality and Culture

Female Genital Mutilation

In some countries and cultures in the Middle East, Asia, and Africa (see map), ritualistic cutting of female genitals is performed on infants, girls, and women of any age, but it is usually done as a girl approaches puberty. It is a centuries-old practice rooted in strong cultural beliefs that place a high value on female virginity prior to marriage and hold that it is immoral for women to enjoy sexual pleasure (Abusharaf, 1998). The procedure is referred to as "female circumcision" among those who engage in the practice, but this is recognized as a medically incorrect characterization in most of the rest of the world, where it is now referred to as *female genital mutilation*, or FGM (Morris, 1996). It is estimated that 2 million girls undergo some form of FGM each year throughout the world, and that percentage varies among the countries where the practice exists. However, in some countries such as Somalia and Egypt, the rates exceed 90 percent (Barber, 2003; Ford, 2001). The practice of FGM is illegal in the United States, Canada, and many other countries.

Traditional FGM procedures vary in the degree of mutilation inflicted and are generally divided into three types (Morris, 1996). All the procedures are typically performed without anesthesia, using nonsterile, primitive instruments such as pieces of broken glass, pocket knives, razor blades, or scissors. Type I involves removal of the clitoral hood and part or all of the external clitoris (called a *clitorectomy*). In Type II, the most common form of FGM, the clitoral hood and visible portion of the clitoris are removed and part or all of the labia minora are cut away. Type III is the most extreme form but is also quite common in some countries, mainly Somalia, Sudan, Mali, and Nigeria. Here the clitoris and labia minora are removed as in Type II, but in addition, the labia majora are also cut or scored. Then the labia majora are stitched together or, in some rituals, stuck together with paste or thorns, with only a small opening left near the bottom of the vaginal opening for the passage of menstrual blood and urine. This procedure is called *infibulation*. The cutting or scoring of the outer labia causes them to fuse together during the healing process. When the woman later marries, the vulva is reopened, sometimes by the new husband, so that intercourse becomes possible. The diagrams on page 55 detail these three types of FGM.

As you can imagine, women who have been subjected to such procedures suffer great pain. In addition, medical complications stemming from the unsanitary and primitive nature of the process are extremely common. These complications include infection, tetanus, hemorrhage, impaired urinary and menstrual function, incontinence, infertility, various problems in childbirth for both the mother and fetus, and sexual dysfunction (Ford, 2001).

Worldwide awareness of and opposition to FGM has been growing rapidly in recent decades. This is due in part to greater global intercultural awareness in general but also because FGM

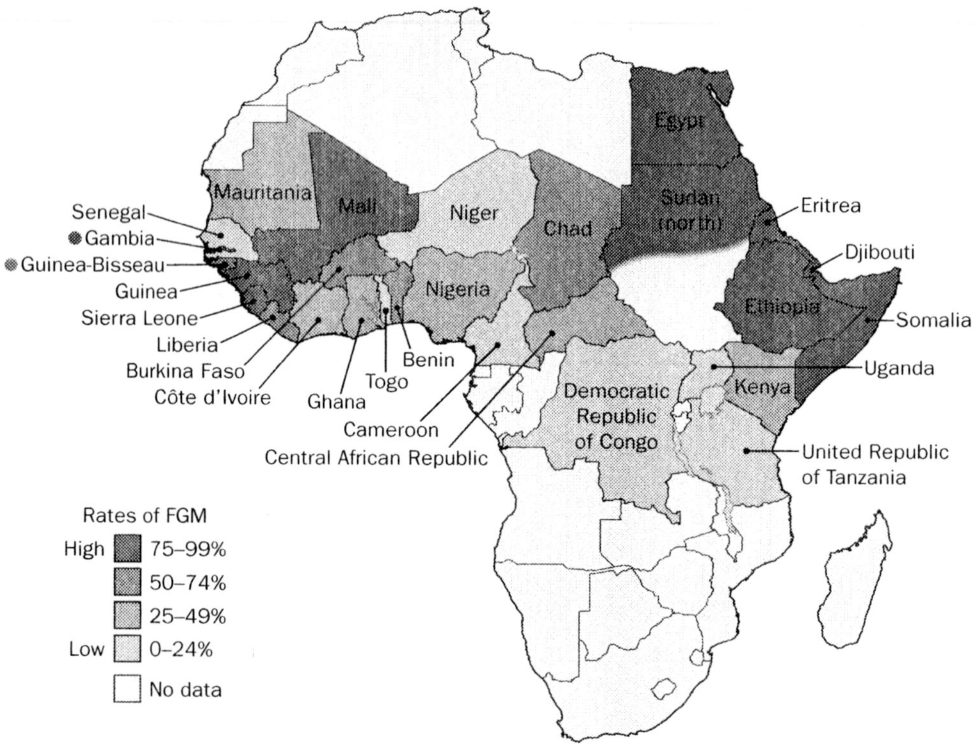

Countries Practicing Female Genital Mutilation

Female genital mutilation is a common practice in many countries in the world, most of which are located in Africa.

Source: Map, p. 43 from *Female Genital Mutilation*: Integrating the Prevention and the Management of the Health Complications into the Curricula of Nursing and Midwifery, A Teacher's Guide, World Health Organization. (http://www.who.int/gender/other_health/en/teachersguide.pdf). Reprinted by permission of WHO.

and its consequences are being encountered increasingly in the West as people from cultures where it is performed emigrate in larger numbers to Western nations.

Although the practice is deeply embedded and continues unabated in some countries, many groups are working to educate people in those countries to reduce or eliminate FGM. This includes professional medical organizations, women's groups, and human rights groups. Numerous countries, including the United States and Canada, now offer political asylum to girls and women who would face mutilation if they were to return to their homelands. Most see that the social changes necessary to eradicate the practice of FGM will not happen quickly, but as worldwide awareness, condemnation, and efforts to educate grow, we are likely to see the practice slowly diminish. In 1996, the World Health Organization issued the following position statement on FGM:

Female genital mutilation is a deeply rooted, traditional practice. However, it is a form of violence against girls and women that has serious physical and psychosocial consequences which adversely affect health. Furthermore, it is a reflection of discrimination against women and girls.

The World Health Organization is committed to the abolition of all forms of female genital mutilation. It affirms the need for the effective protection and promotion of the human rights of girls and women, including their rights to bodily integrity and to the highest attainable standard of physical, mental and social well-being.

WHO strongly condemns the medicalization of female genital mutilation, that is, the involvement of health professionals in any form of female genital mutilation in any setting, including hospitals or other health establishments.

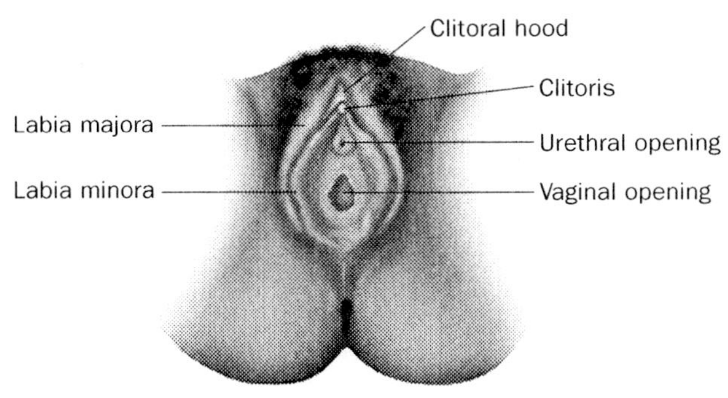

(a) Normal female genital anatomy

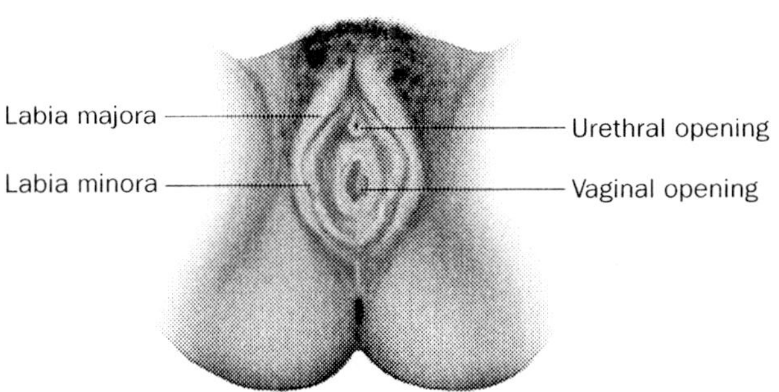

(b) Type I: Removal of clitoral hood and part or all of external clitoris

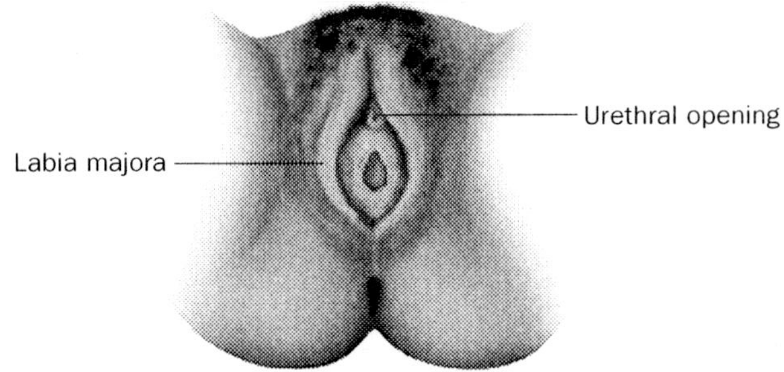

(c) Type II: Removal of external portion of clitoris and part or all of the labia minora

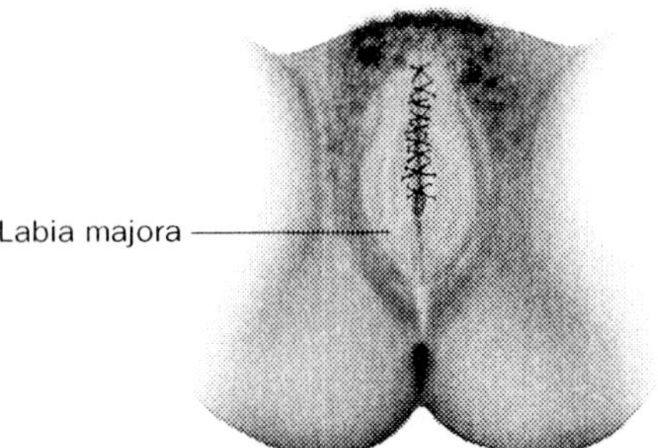

(d) Type III: Removal of external genitalia (clitoris, clitoral hood, labia minora, and inside of labia majora) followed by stitching of the remaining skin surrounding the vulva (a process called infibulation), leaving only a small opening for urine and menstrual blood to pass

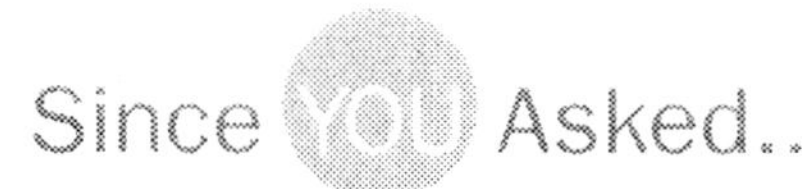

7. Lately I've been getting bladder infections a lot, like once or twice a month. They are awful. Why am I getting so many, and how can I prevent them?

bladder, where they find ideal (moist, dark, warm) conditions in which to grow and proliferate. However, the good news is that UTIs are usually fairly easy to treat, and various measures exist to help prevent them or reduce their frequency. "In Touch with Your Sexual Health: Urinary Tract Infections" provides more detailed information about the causes, treatment, and prevention of UTIs.

The Hymen and the Vaginal Opening

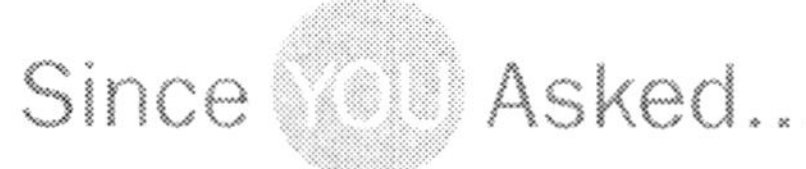

8. Is there any sure way to tell if a woman is a virgin before (or after) you have intercourse with her? Is there actually something you "break" inside the vagina?

Near the lower end of the vulva is the *vaginal opening*. And at the entrance to the vagina is a structure known as the **hymen**. The hymen is a thin layer of tissue that partly covers or surrounds the vaginal opening. Although its true anatomical purpose is unclear, the hymen, in its own way, has drawn nearly as much attention as the penis in terms of sexual mythology because it is so closely tied to the notion of female virginity. Many of the most common delusions worldwide about female sexuality concern the hymen. Here is a partial list of some of the most common myths about the hymen—all of them false.

1. *Myth: The condition of a woman's hymen is indicative of whether or not she is a virgin* (meaning that she has never engaged in penile-vaginal intercourse). This belief is false because the appearance of the hymen relates to many factors; for example, some girls are born without a hymen; nearly all hymens are at least partially separated naturally to allow for passage of normal vaginal discharge and menstrual fluid; the hymen may be separated due to strenuous athletic movements such as bicycle or horseback riding, gymnastics, or even dancing (Azam, 2000); the hymen may be perforated due to tampon insertion; it may be separated during behaviors during masturbation; or some women's hymens are separated or perforated for no apparent reason other than normal variations among humans. Figure 2.11 shows some common, normal configurations of the hymen.
2. *Myth: Upon first sexual intercourse, the hymen will "break" and bleed.* For some women, having intercourse for the first time may indeed cause some tearing of the hymen, and this may include some minor bleeding, which typically stops quite quickly (DiscoveryHealth.com, 2002). However, for many women, first intercourse causes little or no damage to the hymen and no bleeding. In rare cases, the hymen completely covers the vaginal opening and must be opened slightly by a doctor when a girl begins to menstruate.
3. *Myth: Intercourse is very painful the first time due to the rupturing of the hymen.* As was just mentioned, the hymen often does not tear at all with intercourse, and even if it does, the trauma to the structure is minor and usually not particularly painful. In reality, the most common reason for painful intercourse, whether the first time or

hymen A ring of tissue surrounding, partially covering, or fully screening the vaginal opening.

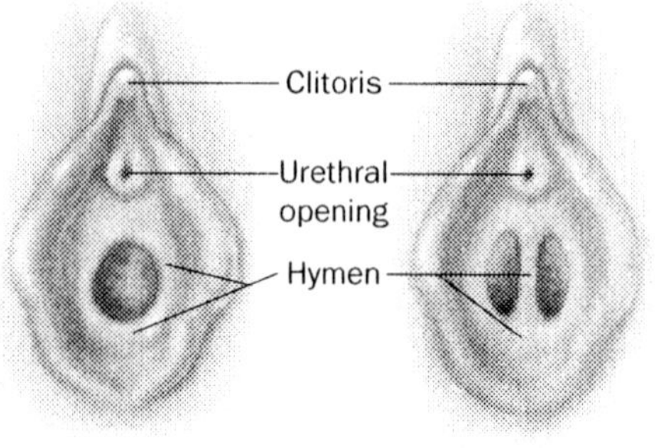

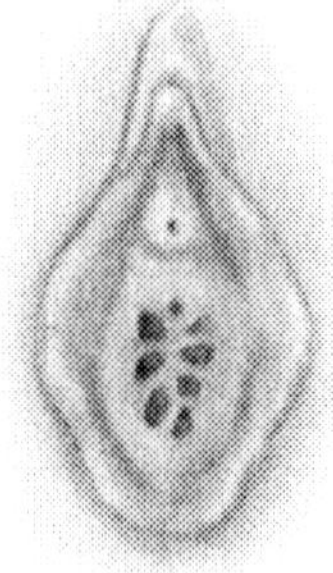

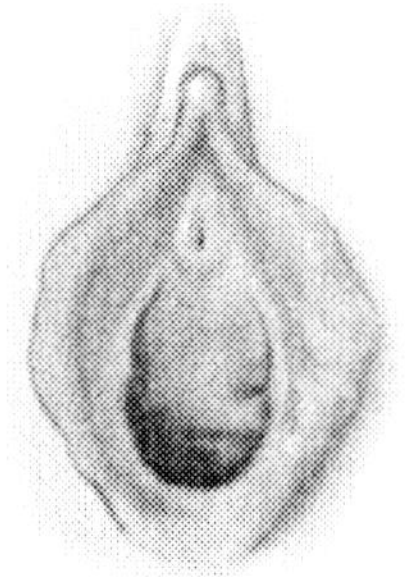

FIGURE 2.11 Normal Variations in Appearance of the Hymen

The hymen varies in appearance and degree of intactness, often regardless of a female's sexual experience.

In Touch with Your Sexual Health

Urinary Tract Infections: Causes, Treatment, and Prevention

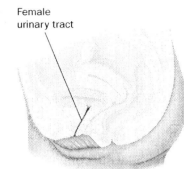

Anyone who has ever had a urinary tract infection (UTI) knows how unpleasant such infections can be. Typical symptoms include pain and stinging, often intense, during urination; the persistent feeling of a strong need to urinate even though the bladder has just been emptied; frequent urination; darker and bad-smelling urine; the sensation of pressure and pain in the lower back or abdomen; and sometimes slight fever, chills, nausea, or blood in the urine (Walling, 1999).

Women are more than 40 times more likely than men to be diagnosed with a UTI. Approximately 20 to 40 percent of women, compared to 0.5 percent of men, will contract a UTI at least once in their lifetime, and some women have frequent, recurring cases numerous times a year (Walling, 1999). UTIs account for nearly 10 million doctor visits each year in the United States (Medical Network, 2000). The huge difference in incidence is due to the fact that bacteria have a much easier time reaching the bladder in women. As you can see in the diagram, the urethra in women is relatively short (about 1.5 inches) from the opening at the vulva to the bladder. In men, however, the urinary tract extends the full length of the penis and into the body before reaching the bladder (about 7 to 8 inches). In addition, this physiological difference also places the opening to the urethra in women in close proximity to the anus and rectum, which contain certain bacteria that are harmless in the rectum, especially *Escherichia coli*, which is the cause of nearly all (85 to 90 percent) cases of UTIs. These bacteria are relatively easy to transfer accidentally from the anal area to the vulva during sexual activity or when wiping the anal area following bowel movements. This by no means implies that women are less hygienic (they're not) or harbor more bacteria than men do (they don't); it's just a natural anatomic difference. By the way, one widespread myth is that sitting in hot tubs causes UTIs, but this is rarely, if ever, the case (Medical Network, 2000).

Fortunately, UTIs are typically easy to cure with antibiotics that target the pathogenic bacteria. In addition to antibiotics, UTI treatments often include the recommendation to drink large amounts of water or other nonirritating fluids when symptoms appear (avoiding alcohol, tea, coffee, or citrus juices) to flush bacteria out of the urinary system. Also, many people believe that cranberry juice has certain chemical properties that help change the acidity of the urine to fight and prevent UTIs, and some scientific evidence supports this notion (Johannsen, 2001).

Of course, it is always better to prevent illness than to treat it, especially if you are prone to recurring UTIs. So with this in

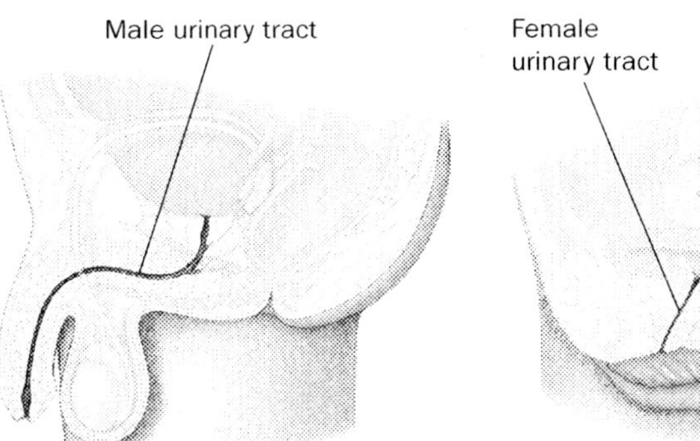

mind, what can women do to prevent or reduce the number of UTIs? Here is a list of common suggestions: (NIH, 2003).

- Always wipe from the front toward the back after a bowel movement so that bacteria will not be accidentally spread to the vulva area.
- Urinate soon after intercourse or other sexual activity that might introduce bacteria to the urethra area of the vulva.
- Try to urinate soon after you realize you need to. Avoid "holding it" for long periods, as this may allow bacteria to establish themselves.
- When you urinate, empty your bladder completely so that any bacteria that might be present are washed out as fully as possible.
- Avoid scented feminine hygiene products and douches, as these appear to encourage bacterial growth.
- In general, take showers instead of baths because bacteria may migrate via bath water (usually not a problem in chlorinated hot tubs).
- Drink lots of water every day to keep your urinary system flowing so that bacteria are less able to get a foothold.
- Drink cranberry juice frequently.
- Avoid coffee, alcohol, and spicy foods, as these may increase urinary irritation.
- Avoid tight-fitting, synthetic clothing and underwear, as they trap heat and moisture, allowing bacteria near the urethral opening to grow more easily.

Finally, on a hopeful note, a new vaccine that may prevent most UTIs altogether is working its way through the approval process (Stephenson, 2002). It's not a shot but a body-heat-activated vaginal suppository. Early studies have shown the vaccine to be extremely effective in preventing new UTIs over a six-month period in women who had between 3 and 20 infections in the previous year, and no significant negative side effects were found. If you suffer from frequent UTIs, be sure to try all the precautions listed, but if nothing works, this vaccine may be exactly "what the doctor ordered" for you.

not, is insufficient lubrication of the vagina due to rushing the experience or lack of arousal on the part of the woman for various reasons (see Chapter 7, "Sexual Problems and Solutions," for more information about painful intercourse).

4. *Myth: If a woman has an intact hymen, she cannot become pregnant.* Even if no penetration occurs due to what is perceived as an intact hymen or for any other reason, pregnancy can still occur. If semen is ejaculated near the vaginal opening, some sperm cells may make their way past the hymen into the vagina.

While all of these beliefs are false, the importance attached to the hymen and its role in presuming virginity persists in many cultures throughout the world. In fact, in a few cultures some women are obtaining a procedure called **hymenorraphy**, or *hymenoplasty*, which surgically restores the hymen to an intact-appearing state so that the women will not be deemed "unmarriagable" or in some countries even subject to torture and death (Azam, 2000; DiscoveryHealth.com, 2002; Paterson-Brown, 1998).

The Perineum

The **perineum** is the area of skin, rich in nerve endings, between the vaginal opening and the anus. Men have a perineum as well, located between the underside of the scrotum and the anus. Some women and men find that manual stimulation of the perineum during sexual activity enhances feelings of sexual arousal. The reason the structure is discussed under the heading of female external genitals is because it has been historically involved in childbirth. The perineum is the area that may be cut during delivery in a procedure called an **episiotomy**. This procedure was a relatively routine part of the hospital childbirths because doctors believed it allowed more room for the baby's head to move through the birth canal and reduced the chances for an unplanned tearing of the perineum. Today, this procedure has become far less routine, and many health professionals now believe it is unnecessary during a routine birth. You can read more about the newest thinking about the episiotomy in Chapter 9, "Conception, Pregnancy, and Birth."

The Anus

As is true for men, discussed earlier, the anus is considered by some women to be a sexually responsive part of their anatomy. Some women find manual or oral stimulation of the anal area to be sexually arousing, and some enjoy anal penetration with a finger or penis. Statistics show that approximately a fifth of women have engaged in anal intercourse at some point in their lives (Baldwin & Baldwin, 2000; Laumann et al., 1994). It is important to stress once again that anal intercourse is one of the riskiest sexual activities for the spread of sexually transmitted infections, especially HIV and hepatitis. Also, we should reiterate here that some bacteria normally found in the anal area and rectum may cause infections if they are transferred to other parts of the female sexual anatomy such as the vagina or urethra.

The Breasts

Breasts are part of the sexual anatomy of both males and females. However, the sexual focus placed on the female breast is significantly greater in most cultures, so we include the discussion here, as part of female external sexual anatomy. Breasts have three major functions: They may supply nourishment for newborn infants, they may provide sexual pleasure for both the woman and her partner, and in most Western cultures, they play a role in a woman's perceived attractiveness and self-image. Breasts vary greatly in size, shape, coloring, and symmetry. The nipples are typically somewhat darker in pigmentation than the surrounding skin of the breast. The normal size and shape of the nipples vary greatly from woman to woman. They may protrude, lie flat, or even turn inward, referred to as *inverted nipples*. The darker skin encircling each nipple is called the **areola** and is actually part of the skin of the nipple. The size and color of the are-

hymenorraphy A medical procedure, common in some cultures, to reconstruct or repair the hymen to allow a woman to appear "virginal"; also known as *hymenoplasty*.

perineum The area of skin in the female between the vulva and the anus and in the male between the scrotum and the anus.

episiotomy Surgical cutting of the perineum during childbirth, a procedure that was believed to allow for easier passage of the infant and less tearing of the vaginal opening. Found to be ineffective, it is rarely performed today.

areola The darker skin encircling each nipple; actually part of the skin of the nipple.

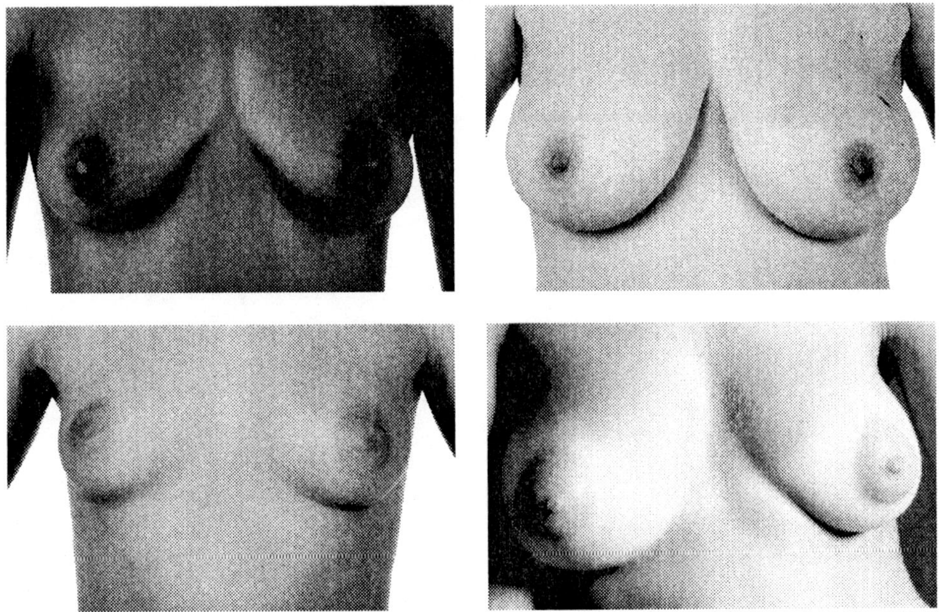

(a) Variations in Breast Shape, Size and Appearance

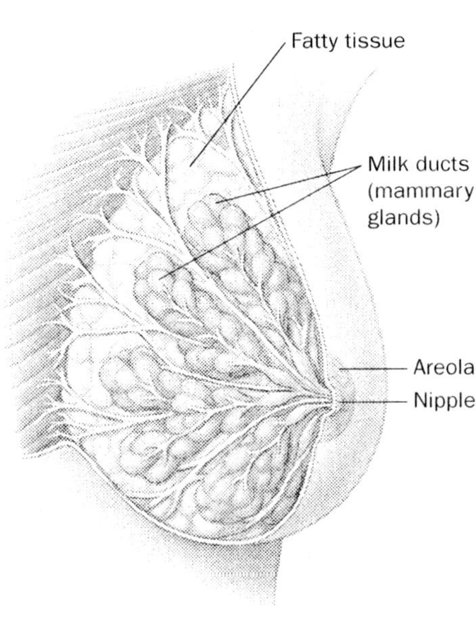

(b) Anatomy of the Female Breast

FIGURE 2.12 The Female Breast

Female breast shape, size, and appearance vary greatly, just like other parts of the female body.

olas also vary from woman to woman. Virtually all of these differences in the appearance of the breasts are normal human variations—see part (a) of Figure 2.12.

Internally, the female breast is a relatively simple anatomical structure consisting primarily of milk glands, milk ducts, connective tissue, and fat, as shown in part (b) of Figure 2.12. During *lactation*, the milk glands produce milk, which flows through the milk ducts to the nipple when the women is breast-feeding.

The breasts are usually a sexually responsive part of the human anatomy. Sexual stimulation of the breasts and the nipples cause most women and some men to become sexually aroused. Both the nipples and areolas contain erectile tissues that engorge with blood, causing them to become erect during sexual arousal and stimulation.

The size and shape of a woman's breasts, nipples, and areolas are unrelated to how sexually sensitive her breasts are or to her level of sexual desire and responsiveness. Women vary greatly in the amount of pleasure they experience from breast and nipple stimulation regardless of their breast size or shape. Some women do not find breast and nipple stimulation particularly arousing at all, while other women are able to experience orgasm from nipple stimulation alone. Most women fall somewhere between these extremes.

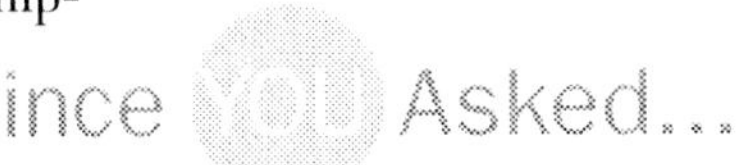

9. Are larger breasts more sensitive than smaller ones?

Just as men's sexuality is culturally (and mistakenly) linked to penis size, women's sexuality is often judged based on the size of their breasts. This preoccupation with breasts in most Western cultures causes many women to worry that their breasts, nipples, or areolas are too small, too large, or "incorrectly" shaped. Women's perception of their own breasts is a major determining factor in their overall body image and self-esteem (Koff & Benavage, 1998; Tantleff-Dunn, 2001). For proof of this, you need only consider the booming worldwide industry in breast augmentation and breast reduction surgery. In the United States in 2001, women underwent 220,000 breast augmentations and nearly 100,000 breast reductions. These procedures were exceeded in frequency only by liposuction (fat extraction) and rhinoplasty (nose reshaping) as the most common cosmetic surgeries (American Society of Plastic Surgeons, 2002).

The breasts are one of many parts of our sexual anatomy that are prone to cancer. A diagnosis of breast cancer is a very frightening and sometimes devastating event in a

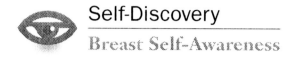

Self-Discovery

Breast Self-Awareness

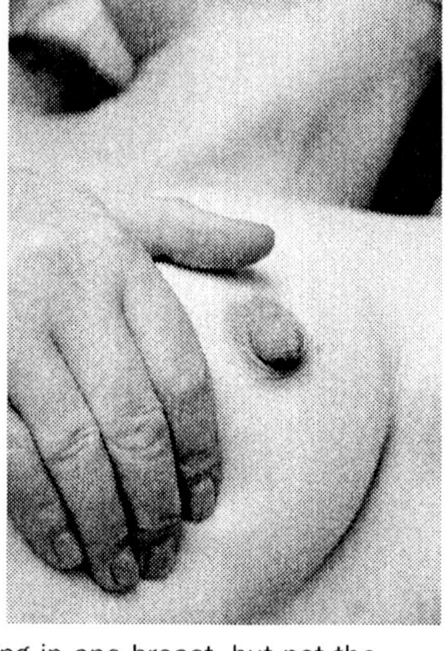

The American Cancer Society and other health groups have recommended that all women over the age of 20 perform monthly breast self-examinations as part of a program designed to detect breast cancer as early as possible. Early detection is key to surviving breast cancer as well as helping ensure the least invasive treatment. However, the percentage of women who actually perform monthly exams has always been quite small, because women tend to be unsure about when to do them, worried about doing them correctly, or afraid of finding a suspicious lump (Brett & Austoker, 2002). Nevertheless, breast self-examination, done correctly, is an effective means of detecting cancer in its earliest stages ("Early Detection," 2002; Hackshaw & Paul, 2003). For more information on breast self-exams and illustrated instructions on how to do them, go to www.breastcancer.org.

Recently, the focus has shifted away from routine, monthly self-exams to a more overall *breast awareness* approach. The idea behind breast awareness is that every woman should become familiar with her own breasts to learn what is normal for her, which will in turn allow her to be more skilled at recognizing any small changes that may occur. Here are the five guiding principles of breast awareness (Brett & Austoker, 2002).

1. *Know what is normal for you.* No two women are identical, and no two breasts are identical. So it is crucial for women to become intimately familiar with their bodies in general and their breasts specifically. This will increase the chances that if something changes relating to the health of the breast, it will be detected early by the woman herself.
2. *Look and feel.* Many women are hesitant to touch or look carefully at their own bodies, especially sexual areas, due to cultural expectations or taboos. Such teachings and beliefs work against maintaining a healthy body. Women should take the opportunity when showering, bathing, or dressing to feel and look at their breasts closely and in detail. This way they can learn how breast tissue changes normally during their menstrual cycle and be better able to spot abnormal changes if they occur.
3. *Become aware of breast changes that may signal a problem.* These include the following:
   - A new, clearly defined lump that has not been there all along
   - Unusual (not merely cyclic) changes in the outline, shape, or size of a breast
   - Lumps, bumps, or swelling in one breast, but not the other, that appear early in the menstrual cycle and do not go away
   - Unusual, atypical pain or discomfort that is focused in one part of a breast
   - Nipple discharge, especially if it is thin and watery or bloody
   - Persistent discharge, especially if it is from only one breast
   - A nipple that has begun to pucker or retract inward
4. *Report any such changes immediately to your health care professional.* Odds are very much in your favor that whatever change you detect is not cancer, but if it is, you'll be in the best possible position to treat it early and recover completely.

In addition to a woman's personal level of breast self-awareness, women between the ages of 20 and 40 should have checkups by a health care professional every three years; for women over 40, these professional exams should be annual. Finally, women over 40 should have yearly **mammograms,** low-dose breast X-rays that can detect tumors too small to be felt or noticed through self-awareness or a professional breast exam.

woman's life. The good news is that treatments for breast cancer have become increasingly effective, and five-year survival rates have reached 98 percent when the cancer is detected and treated before it has spread beyond the breast ("Early Detection," 2002). Diagnosing cancer early, through breast self-awareness, regular doctor visits, and mammograms, is the key to our ability to cure it. "Self-Discovery: Breast Self-Awareness" explains the latest overall approach to breast health and breast cancer prevention.

Female Internal Structures

mammogram Low dose X-ray of the breast to detect tumors.

The internal sexual anatomy of women is rather complex, but as we did for male sexual anatomy, we will limit our discussion here to structures that are essential to understanding the various topics explored throughout this book. Figure 2.13 shows the internal reproductive anatomy of the human female. We will begin our discussion with the vaginal opening and proceed inward, structure by structure, to the ovaries.

The Vagina

The **vagina** is a flexible, muscular canal or tube, normally about 3 to 4 inches in length when a woman is not sexually aroused. The vagina extends into the woman's body at an angle toward the small of the back, from the vulva to the cervix, as shown in part (a) of Figure 2.13. This is where the penis is inserted during penile-vaginal intercourse. When not sexually aroused, the walls of the vagina lie very close together and collapse upon one another along most of its length (the vagina is not an open "tunnel" as many people visualize it and as it is often shown, erroneously, in diagrams). During sexual arousal, the tissues lining the vagina become engorged with blood and secrete a clear, slick fluid along its entire length. This lubrication is part of nature's design to facilitate insertion of the penis for intercourse and reproduction, but it occurs during sexual excitement regardless of the particular sexual behavior a woman is engaged in, including fantasy, masturbation, or same-sex interactions. The vagina is

vagina A flexible, muscular canal or tube, normally about 3 to 4 inches in length, that extends into the woman's body at an angle toward the small of the back, from the vulva to the cervix.

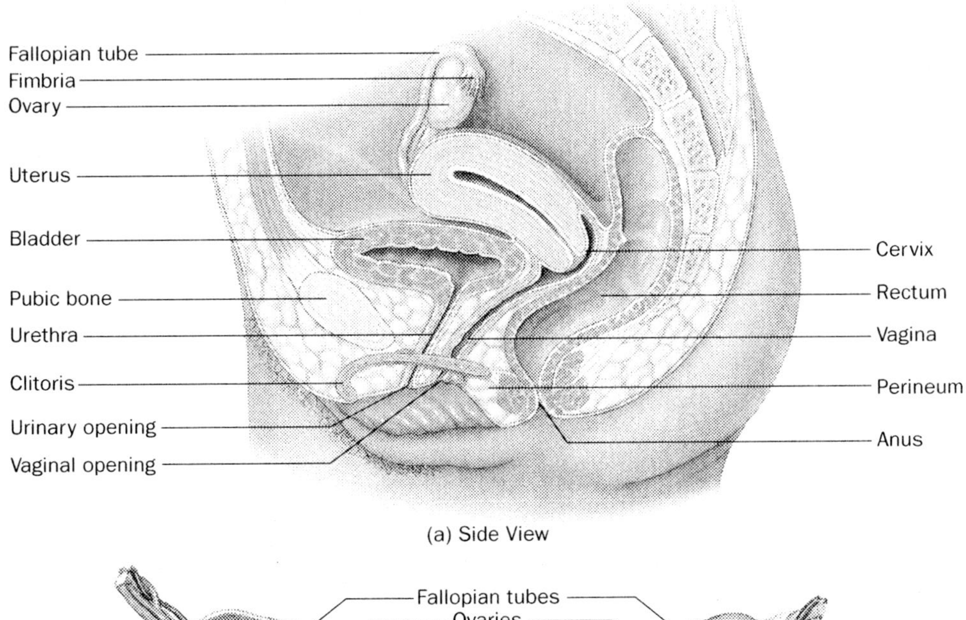

(a) Side View

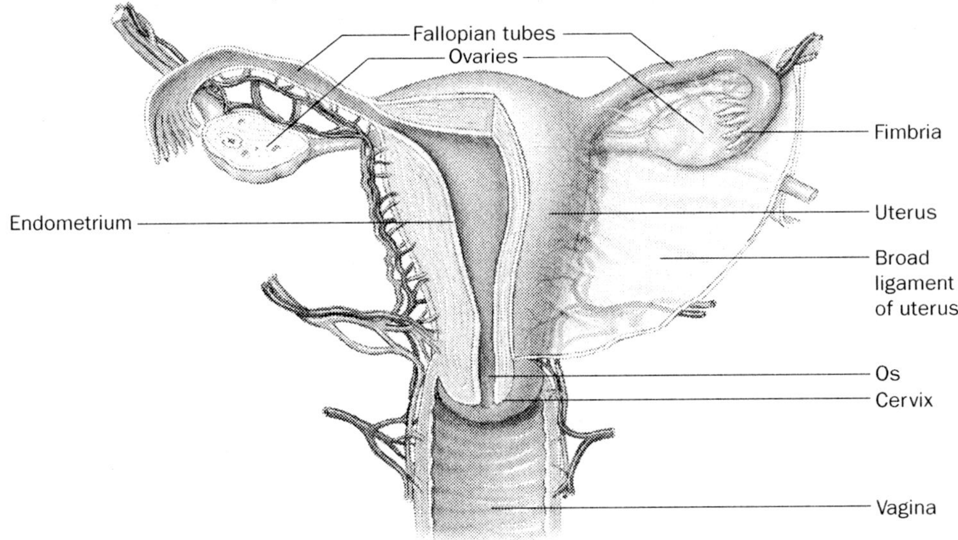

(b) Front View

FIGURE 2.13 Female Internal Sexual Anatomy

G-spot An especially sensitive area inside the vagina that some but not all women have identified and credit with enhancing sexual arousal.

cervix The lower end of the uterus that connects it to the vagina.

os The very narrow passageway through the cervix from the vagina to the uterus.

Pap test A routine test in which cells from the cervix are examined microscopically to examine them for potentially cancerous abnormalities.

human papilloma virus (HPV) A sexually transmitted infection, some strains of which are believed to cause cervical cancer.

an extremely elastic organ capable of molding itself around an object as small as a finger or allowing the passage of something as large as a baby's head. During childbirth, the vagina in often referred to as the *birth canal.* Most of the vagina's nerve endings that respond to sexual stimulation are located in the lower one-third, the portion closest to the vaginal opening.

Some women and researchers claim that located within the vagina is a structure that has become known as the Grafenberg spot or **G-spot** (so named after the researcher who first discovered the structure in the 1950s). The function and even the existence of the G-spot is controversial. Evidence suggests that it is an area of tissue located about a third of the way in from the opening of the vagina in the anterior vaginal wall (the "upper" wall if the woman is lying on her back). Some women find that this area is sexually responsive and enhances arousal and orgasm when stimulated during sexual activities. The reasons for the controversy surrounding the G-spot relate to the fact that not all women report being able to locate a G-spot, and researchers are still unclear as to how it functions physiologically, if it does indeed exist as a structure separate from the female sexual anatomy in general. The purported location and sexual role of the G-spot, as currently understood in the research on female sexual response, is discussed in greater detail in Chapter 3, "The Physiology of Human Sexual Responding."

The Cervix

Since YOU Asked...

10. Once a condom came off during sex and we couldn't find it. Is it possible for a condom to get "lost" up inside a woman?

11. If a Pap test is negative, can you be sure you are completely free of disease?

At the inner or upper end of the vagina is the **cervix.** A woman may feel (and even see) her own cervix by inserting a finger into the vagina while her hips are fully flexed. The cervix connects the vagina with the uterus. The passageway through the cervix, called the **os,** is very small, about as wide as the thickness of the lead inside a pencil, on average, but it becomes slightly larger or smaller on different days during the menstrual cycle. Contrary to sexual myths, an object in the vagina, such as a tampon, a "lost" condom, or a diaphragm, cannot accidentally migrate higher up into the reproductive tract and cause a medical emergency because they are all far too large to pass through the cervical os. That said, the cervix is capable of expanding greatly, a process called *dilation,* to allow for childbirth (more on this process is found in Chapter 9, "Conception, Pregnancy, and Birth").

The cervix is a relatively common site in the female body for the formation of abnormal cells that may, if not treated, lead to cervical cancer. The medical test that is used to check the cervix for any signs of abnormal cells is called a **Pap test** or *Pap smear* In this simple procedure, the vagina is held open with a device called a *speculum* and a few cells are gently subbed or brushed from the cervix. The cells are then sent to a lab to be examined microscopically for any abnormalities (see Figure 2.14). The

FIGURE 2.14 The Pap Test

The Pap test detects abnormal cells in the cervix so that cervical cancer may be prevented or treated.

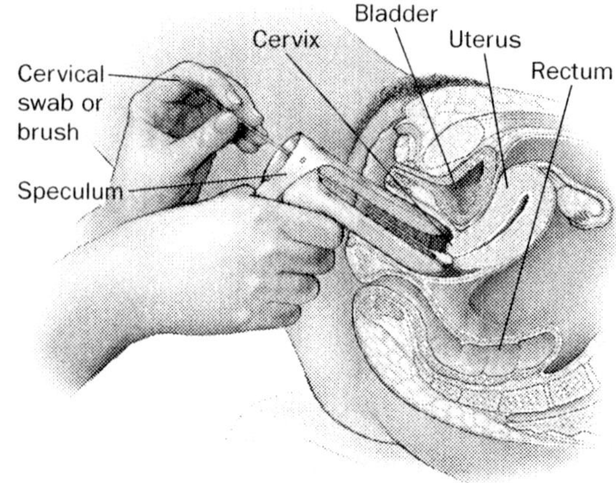

(a) Internal View of the Pap Test Procedure

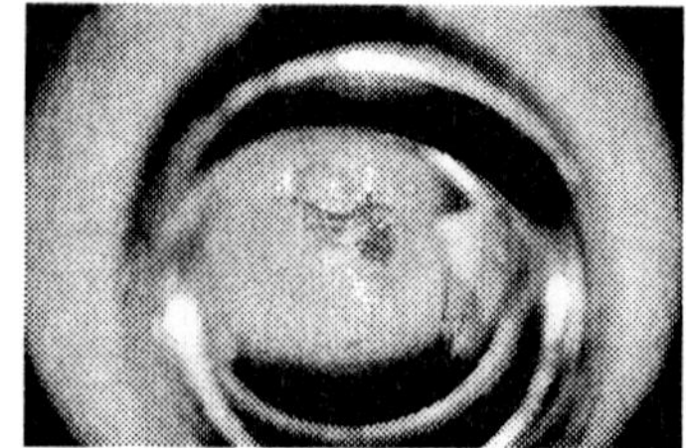

(b) Abnormal Cervix

American Cancer Society recommends that all girls and women have a Pap test every one to two years starting three years after they become sexually active, or at age 21 regardless of sexual activity (Erieden, 2003). The Pap test is fairly accurate, but it is possible for it to miss abnormal cells or produce a false positive result. This is why it is important that the test be done on a regular basis. In general, cervical cancer, when it is found, is a very slow-growing cancer and rarely spreads beyond the cervix in the interval between tests.

The primary cause of cervical cancer is a sexually transmitted infection, the **human papilloma virus (HPV)**, which causes certain strains of genital warts (for more information on HPV, see Chapter 8, "Sexually Transmitted Infections"). HPV is a very common virus that is found in a high percentage of women regardless of whether they have ever had noticeable symptoms of genital warts. No cure yet exists for the virus. Because of the connection between HPV and cervical cancer, combined with the fact that some infected people may never experience an outbreak of warts, many health professionals are calling for routine HPV screening to accompany the standard Pap test (Erieden, 2003; Oliver, 2002). HPV does not always lead to cancer, and Pap tests showing abnormal cells usually do not indicate cancer. However, if a woman tests positive for HPV, she will then have the information she needs to be extra vigilant about her cervical health and to have regular Pap tests at more frequent intervals.

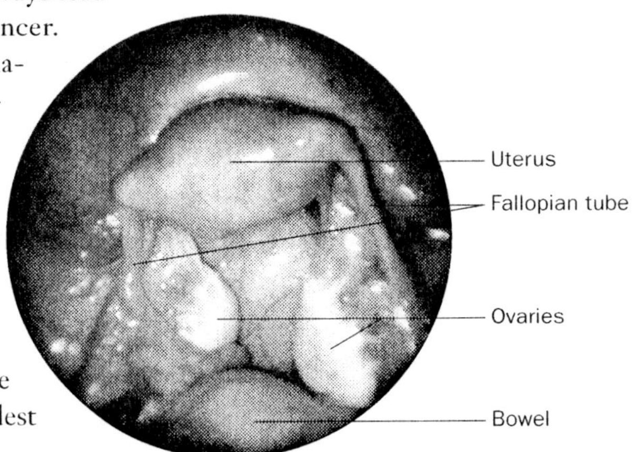

FIGURE 2.15 The Uterus

The Uterus

The **uterus**, or womb, is the organ in which a fertilized egg implants itself and an embryo and fetus grow from a few days after fertilization until birth (see Figure 2.15). The uterus is a very flexible organ with strong muscle fibers that allow it to expand greatly during pregnancy and push the infant out during labor and delivery. In its nonpregnant state, the uterus is about the size and shape of a small pear, about 3 inches long and 1.5 inches at its widest point.

During pregnancy, the capacity of the uterus increases as much as 1,000 times its nonpregnant size (Rodriguez, 2004). The uterus also undergoes major changes every month during a woman's menstrual cycle. Under the influence of monthly hormonal changes in a woman's body, the lining of the uterus, the **endometrium**, builds up an extra layer of blood and tissue, preparing to receive and nourish a fertilized egg. If fertilization and pregnancy do not occur, the uterus sheds this extra lining, which flows through the cervix and down the vagina as menstrual fluid (menstruation is discussed in more detail later in this chapter).

In some women, cells and tissue from the endometrium migrate to outside the uterus and begin to grow in the abdominal cavity or other areas in the body. This condition, called **endometriosis**, often referred to simply as "endo," has been on the increase over recent decades. The exact cause of endometriosis is not fully understood, but women with the condition are also more likely than average to experience illnesses relating to the immune system such as allergies, asthma, and autoimmune disorders including lupus, rheumatoid arthritis, and chronic fatigue syndrome. This link has lead many researchers to suspect that increases in toxins in the environment may be at least partly responsible for the development of endometriosis (Boschert, 2002).

Endometriosis is typically a painful and potentially serious health condition for women. The misplaced uterine cells, triggered by a woman's monthly hormone cycle, build up and bleed each month just like normal endometrial tissue in the uterus. The symptoms of endometriosis include severe pain before and during periods, pain during sexual intercourse, difficulty conceiving or complete infertility,

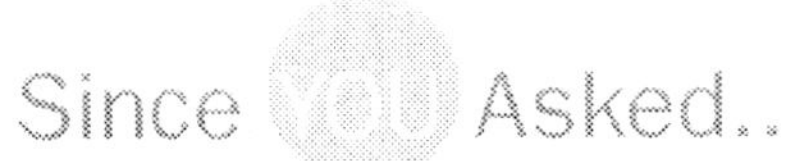

12. My sister told me she has endometriosis, which is why she has such bad cramps during her period. What exactly is endometriosis?

uterus A very flexible organ with strong muscle fibers where a fertilized egg implants and an embryo and fetus grow from a few days after fertilization until birth.

endometrium The tissue lining the uterus that thickens in anticipation of pregnancy and is sloughed off and expelled during menstruation.

endometriosis A potentially painful and dangerous medical condition caused by endometrial cells migrating outside the uterus into the abdominal cavity.

general fatigue, painful urination during periods, painful bowel movements during periods, and other gastrointestinal problems such as diarrhea, constipation, or nausea (National Endometriosis Society, 2002). Typically, endometriosis becomes worse over time if not treated. Treatment usually involves medications or surgery to remove the patches of endometrial tissue within the abdominal cavity. If you or someone you know is experiencing symptoms of endometriosis, it is important to seek medical care and treatment sooner rather than later (go to http://www.endometriosisassn.org/index.html for more detailed information on this condition).

The Fallopian Tubes

At the top of the uterus, two **fallopian tubes** extend from the uterus up to the ovaries, as shown in part (b) of Figure 2.13. Each fallopian tube is about 4 inches long and quite narrow, about 2 millimeters across, or the diameter of cooked spaghetti, for most of its length. At the uterus, the passageway inside each tube is even smaller, no more than the width of a sewing needle. As the fallopian tubes approach the ovaries, they become somewhat wider and branch into many finger-like tendrils called *fimbriae* (singular *fimbria*) that float next to and drape against the ovary. The fallopian tubes are not connected to the ovary, but the fimbria move and create currents that draw in the **ovum**, or egg, released by the ovary, and direct it down into the fallopian tube.

Fertilization of the ovum by a sperm cell occurs in the one-third of the fallopian tube nearest each ovary. The newly released ovum is available in that section of the fallopian tube for only about a day; if no sperm cells are present, or if none is successful in penetrating the ovum, pregnancy will not occur during that cycle.

In one out of every 50 potential pregnancies, the fertilized egg becomes lodged in the fallopian tube, implants there, and begins to grow (Tay, Moore, & Walker, 2000). This is called a *tubal pregnancy* and is the most common type of **ectopic pregnancy**, meaning the growth of a fertilized egg outside of the uterus. Tubal pregnancies result in the loss of the embryo and may pose a serious health risk to the mother. If the embryo grows to the point of rupturing the fallopian tube, internal bleeding and, in about 0.5 percent of cases, death of the woman may result (see Chapter 9, "Conception, Pregnancy and Birth").

If the fallopian tubes are blocked or damaged, the egg and sperm will be less able to rendezvous at an appropriate location, and fertility will be impaired. Fallopian tube problems are the most common reason for infertility in women. The most common causes of fallopian tube obstruction is *pelvic inflammatory disease* (PID), usually the result of an untreated sexually transmitted infection (see Chapter 8, "Sexually Transmitted Infections") and endometriosis, discussed earlier.

fallopian tubes The tubes that carry the female ovum from the ovaries to the uterus and in which fertilization occurs.

ovum The female reproductive cell stored in the ovaries; usually, one ovum is released approximately every 28 days between menarche and menopause. The plural is *ova*.

ectopic pregnancy A pregnancy complication in which a fertilized ovum attaches and begins to grow outside the uterus, most commonly in the fallopian tube, called a *tubal pregnancy*.

ovaries The female organs that produce sex hormones such as estrogen and progesterone and where follicle cells are stored and mature into ova.

The Ovaries

The **ovaries** are *gonads*, like the testicles. In popular usage, the word *gonads* is used as a euphemism for the testicles, but the word *gonad* just means a sex organ that produces cells for reproduction. The testicles produce sperm, and the ovaries produce eggs, or *ova* (*ovum* is the singular, meaning one egg). However, a major difference between male and female gonads is that the testicles manufacture sperm cells continuously throughout a man's adult life at the average rate of nearly 1,000 per minute, while the ovaries contain their full supply of immature ova at birth, about 400,000 of them. When a girl enters puberty, hormonal changes in her body trigger the maturation of, on average, one ovum each month, a process that will continue for the next 40 years or so. If you do the math, you will see that the average woman needs only about 500 eggs during her fertile lifetime, but nature has given her a huge backup supply.

The ovaries are also responsible for production of the female hormones **estrogen** and **progesterone**. These hormones are responsible for girls developing physically into mature women, inducing changes in the breasts, vagina, and uterus during puberty. They also play crucial roles in the woman's fertility cycle by signaling the woman's body to produce mature eggs, release eggs, and prepare the uterus for a possible pregnancy by building up the lining of the endometrium. The role of and functions of female hormones will be discussed more in the next section and in Chapter 9, "Conception, Pregnancy, and Birth."

Menstruation

As you already know, when a girl enters puberty, hormonal secretions cause her body to undergo many changes. One of these changes is called **menarche**, the onset of her **menstrual cycle**. This signals that her body is preparing to begin **ovulation**, the releasing of a mature ovum about once each month. The first sign of menarche is a girl's first period, the passing of menstrual fluid from her uterus, through the cervix, and out the vagina. This typically occurs between the ages of 11 and 16. In the beginning, menstruation is likely to be quite irregular and may occur only once every two or three months. During this initial phase, ovulation may or may not occur. Then, over the next year or two, ovulation and menstruation will become more regular, and the young woman will settle into her normal menstrual cycle.

The purpose of the menstrual cycle is to create conditions in a woman's body that allow for conception and pregnancy. The menstrual cycle corresponds to a woman's *fertility cycle*, the times during each menstrual cycle when she is more likely or less likely to be able to conceive. The fertility cycle and menstruation are discussed in greater detail in Chapter 9, "Conception, Pregnancy, and Birth," and Chapter 12, "Sexual Development throughout Life," respectively. However, as these processes are so closely linked to our discussion about anatomy and physiology, we will summarize some of the basics of menstruation here.

The Menstrual Cycle

The menstrual cycle starts on the first day of a woman's period. The average menstrual cycle is 28 days long; however, women's cycles can vary a great deal, from as few as 23 days to 35 days or longer. As noted earlier, regularly fluctuating levels of hormones are responsible for the changes associated with the menstrual cycle. The female hormones involved in the regulation of the menstrual cycle include estrogen, progesterone, **follicle-stimulating hormone (FSH)**, and **luteinizing hormone (LH)**.

In the first half of the menstrual cycle, called the *follicular* or *proliferative phase*, levels of estrogen rise, causing the lining of the uterus to thicken. In response to follicle-stimulating hormone, an ovum in one of the ovaries starts to mature. At about day 14 of a typical 28-day cycle, in response to a surge of luteinizing hormone, ovulation occurs; the egg leaves the ovary and enters the fallopian tube.

In the second half of the menstrual cycle, referred to as the *luteal* or *secretory phase*, the ovum travels through the fallopian tube to the uterus. Progesterone levels rise and help prepare the uterine lining for pregnancy (see Figure 2.16). Conception occurs if the egg in the upper region of the fallopian tube is fertilized by a sperm cell. If the fertilized ovum subsequently attaches itself to the uterine wall, pregnancy has begun. If pregnancy does not occur, the ovum moves down the fallopian tube, estrogen and progesterone levels drop, and the thickened lining of

estrogen The female hormone responsible for regulating ovulation, endometrial development, and the development of female sexual characteristics.

progesterone The female hormone responsible for the release of ova and implantation of the fertilized egg in the uterine wall.

menarche In girls, the onset of the menstrual cycle in puberty.

menstrual cycle The hormone-controlled reproductive cycle in the human female.

ovulation The release of an egg, or ovum, from the ovary into the fallopian tube.

follicle-stimulating hormone (FSH) A hormone that stimulates the development of a mature ovum.

luteinizing hormone (LH) A hormone that acts in concert with follicle-stimulating hormone to stimulate ovulation and the release of estrogen and progesterone.

FIGURE 2.16 The Uterus during the Menstrual Cycle

During the first half of the menstrual cycle (a), estrogen causes the lining of the uterus (the endometrium) to grow and thicken. In the second half of the cycle (b), if no pregnancy occurs, the lining of the uterus is shed and excreted in the form of menstrual fluid.

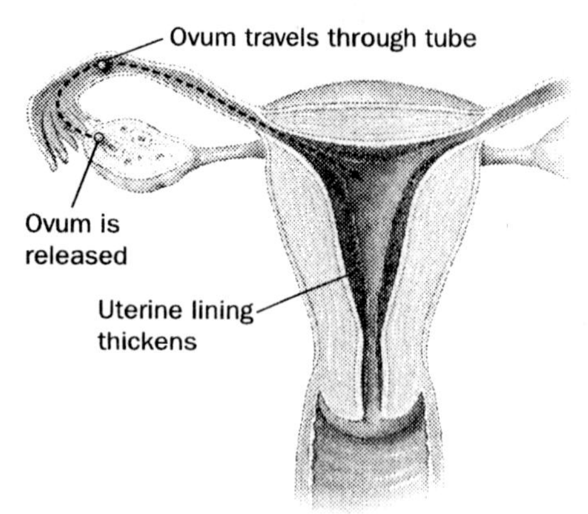
Ovum travels through tube
Ovum is released
Uterine lining thickens

(a) Follicular Phase
(First Half of Menstrual Cycle)

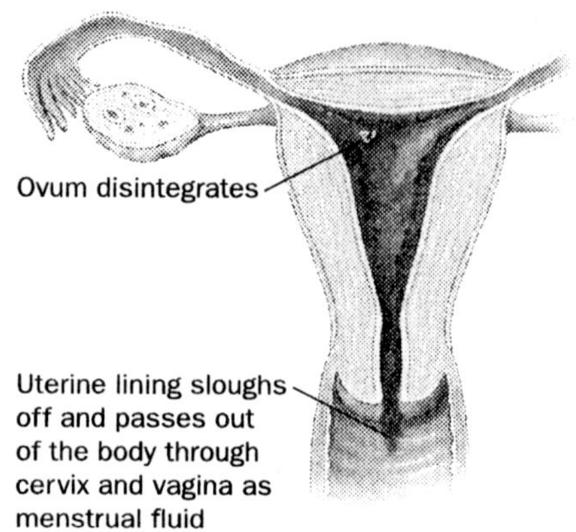
Ovum disintegrates
Uterine lining sloughs off and passes out of the body through cervix and vagina as menstrual fluid

(b) Luteal Phase
(Second Half of Menstrual Cycle)

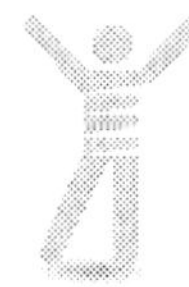

In Touch with Your Sexual Health

PMS or PMDD?

Almost everyone knows about premenstrual syndrome, or PMS. The old joke goes something like this: "Why does it take five women with PMS to change a lightbulb? Because it just *does*! Now leave me alone!" The point of the joke is that a woman with PMS may be tense and irritable. But that's far from the whole story. For some women, physical and emotional changes accompanying menstruation can be quite serious and debilitating.

In 2000, the American Psychiatric Association, in its *Diagnostic and Statistical Manual*, proposed a psychological diagnosis termed *premenstrual dysphoric disorder*, or *PMDD*. Although attempts have been made to distinguish the more commonly known PMS from the proposed clinical diagnosis of PMDD, they are in reality quite similar, the major distinction being the number and severity of symptoms. Also, it is estimated that as many as 70 percent of women suffer some symptoms of PMS during their fertile years, while PMDD, by definition, affects only about 5 percent of women, and the diagnosis applies to those with the most serious and most debilitating symptoms (Dell, Moskowitz, & Sondheimer, 2001).

- **What are the symptoms of PMDD?** A diagnosis of PMDD requires that *five or more* of the following symptoms (including at least one of the first four) be present during the week before the start of menstruation and must have occurred for nearly every menstrual period over the past year. In addition, the diagnosis suggests that the combination of symptoms must seriously impair the woman's relationships with others and her ability to function effectively in activities of daily life (Nguyen, 2001).
  - Serious depression (especially feelings of low self-worth and hopelessness)
  - Serious anxiety, tension, a sense of being "on edge" much of the time
  - Radical mood swings, such as sudden sadness or crying or increased sensitivity in social situations
  - Persistent, extreme anger, irritability, or increased interpersonal conflicts
  - Loss of interest in usual or favorite activities
  - Poor concentration
  - Fatigue, general lack of energy
  - Changes in appetite such as overeating or cravings for specific foods
  - Difficulty sleeping or sleeping too much
  - Feeling overwhelmed or out of control
  - Physical symptoms such as bloating, breast tenderness, headaches, and muscle pains

Remember that a diagnosis of PMDD must include at least five of these signs (including at least one of the first four), and symptoms must clearly interfere with social relationships (e.g., avoiding social activities) or with performing daily activities (e.g., a marked decrease in productivity and efficiency at work or school). It is also important to point out that the symptoms must be linked to the menstrual cycle; if the uterus is shed, along with the ovum, during the menstrual period (see Chapter 9, "Conception, Pregnancy, and Birth").

Menstrual Problems

During each menstrual cycle, the cells from the thickened uterine lining and extra blood are shed through the cervix and vagina. This flow is referred to as the women's *period*. A woman's period may be quite regular from month to month or may vary considerably. The amount of menstrual fluid expelled may be light, moderate, or heavy. On average, menstrual periods last from three to five days, but anywhere from two to seven days is considered normal.

As is true of all human anatomical functions, menstruation is not free of health and medical difficulties. Usually these problems are mild and little cause for concern, but some women encounter various difficulties with their periods, including skipped periods (*amenorrhea*), pain (*dysmenorrhea*), and heavy or abnormal bleeding. In addition, a rare, but potentially serious complication, called *toxic shock syndrome*,

they are not, they may signal a different disorder, such as serious depression.

- **How is PMDD diagnosed?** PMDD is formally diagnosed by a medical professional in partnership with the patient using a method called a daily symptom checklist. This is a special chart itemizing symptoms such as those listed that is completed by the patient over two consecutive months. A woman who suspects PMDD carefully charts her symptoms and their severity each day, beginning with the first day of her period and continuing for at least two full menstrual cycles. The pattern of the timing and severity of symptoms that emerges from this charting process allows PMDD to be diagnosed with a reasonable degree of certainty.
- **How is PMDD treated?** Numerous effective treatments exist for PMDD (many of which are effective for milder forms of PMS as well). The treatment chosen by a woman and her doctor will depend on many issues relating to her specific symptoms, the seriousness of the overall symptomology, the individual patient's profile, and the treatment preferences of the doctor (Thys-Jacobs, et al., 1998; Yonkers, 2004; Young, 2001). Treatments that have been shown to be at least somewhat beneficial include increased exercise, dietary changes (especially avoiding sugar, caffeine, and alcohol; decreasing dietary fat; and increasing daily calcium intake), and various relaxation and stress-reduction strategies. However, for severe cases of PMDD, and often for milder PMS, the treatment of choice is one of the selective serotonin reuptake inhibitors (SSRIs). These drugs, with trade names such as Prozac, Zoloft, and Paxil, were originally developed to treat depression, but some of them appear to be effective in relieving the symptoms of PMDD as well (in fact, in 2000, the makers of Prozac began marketing the very same drug, fluoxetine, under the name of Sarafem for the treatment of PMDD). Apparently, as the ovaries produce varying levels of hormones during a woman's normal reproductive cycle, they trigger changes in the brain's balance of neurotransmitter chemicals, primarily serotonin. Numerous studies have confirmed that most of the SSRIs can significantly reduce both the psychological and the physical symptoms commonly associated with PMDD (Dimmock et al., 2000; Yonkers, 2004; Young, 2001).

These drugs are now considered by many in the medical community to be first-line drug therapy for PMDD for the simple reason that they work to relieve the symptoms with few negative side effects for most users (Skolnik & Cohen, 2004). However, as is the case with most prescription drugs, they are not completely free of side effects, and any woman considering drug therapy for premenstrual symptoms should consult with her health care provider and become educated about the medication before taking it.

The primary message today about PMS and PMDD is that it can be treated effectively so that women need not suffer the potentially severe effects of these conditions. If you find yourself cycling through the symptoms discussed in this section, talk to your health care professional; help is available.

has been associated with improper use of tampons. Problems that can occur during the menstrual cycle include (National Women's Health Information Center, 2002):

- **Amenorrhea** This term is used to describe the absence of a period in women who haven't started menstruating by age 16 or the absence of a period in women who used to have a regular period. Causes of amenorrhea include pregnancy, breast-feeding, and extreme weight loss caused by serious illness, eating disorders, excessive exercising, or stress. Hormonal problems (involving the pituitary, thyroid, ovary, or adrenal glands) or problems with the reproductive organs may be involved.
- **Dysmenorrhea** *Dysmenorrhea* is the term applied to painful periods, including severe menstrual cramps. In younger women, there is often no known disease or condition associated with the pain. A hormone called *prostaglandin* is responsible for the symptoms. Some pain medicines available over the counter, such as ibuprofen, can help with these symptoms. Sometimes a disease or condition, such as uterine fibroids or endometriosis, causes the pain. Treatment depends on what is causing the problem and how severe it is.
- **Abnormal Uterine Bleeding** Vaginal bleeding that is different from normal menstrual periods would include very heavy bleeding or unusually long periods (also called *menorrhagia*), periods too close together, and bleeding between periods. In adolescents and women approaching menopause, hormone imbalance problems often cause menorrhagia and irregular cycles. Sometimes this is called *dysfunctional uterine bleeding* (DUB). Other causes of abnormal bleeding include uterine fibroids and polyps. Treatment for abnormal bleeding depends on the cause and may include medication or surgery.
- **Toxic Shock Syndrome** Women who use tampons to absorb the menstrual flow are advised to follow specific guidelines to avoid toxic shock syndrome, or TSS. TSS is a rare but potentially deadly bacterial infection that has been associated with tampon use. Symptoms include high fever, muscle aches, diarrhea, dizziness or fainting, sunburnlike rash, sore throat, and bloodshot eyes. Using any kind of tampon—cotton or rayon of any absorbency—puts a woman at greater risk for TSS than using menstrual pads. The Food and Drug Administration (FDA) recommends the following tips to help avoid tampon problems:
    - Follow package directions for insertion.
    - Choose the lowest effective absorbency.
    - Change tampons at least every four to eight hours.
    - Consider alternating pads with tampons.
    - Know the warning signs of toxic shock syndrome.
    - Avoid using tampons between periods.
- **When to call a Doctor** Consult with your health care provider if you experience any of the following menstrual problems:
    - If you have not started menstruating by the age of 16
    - If your period has suddenly stopped
    - If you bleed for more days than usual
    - If you bleed excessively
    - If you suddenly feel sick after using tampons
    - If you bleed between periods (more than just a few drops)
    - If you have severe pain during your period

The cycling of hormones in a woman's body, in addition to forming the basic physiological foundation for fertility, conception, and pregnancy, may also affect some women emotionally and psychologically. The best known of these effects is a set of symptoms that may occur during the days leading up to the start of a woman's period, including cramping and feelings of bloating, which often lead to irritability and depressed mood. These symptoms are commonly known as **premenstrual syndrome**, or **PMS**. A relatively rare but significantly more intense form of PMS has been identified by health professionals and is now a proposed clinical diagnosis, called **premenstrual dysphoric disorder**, or **PMDD**. Both of these are discussed in detail in "In Touch with Your Sexual Health: PMS or PMDD?"

Women usually continue having regular periods until menopause, when ovulation and menstruation cease. On average, **menopause** occurs around the age of 51, but menopause-related physiological changes, referred to as **perimenopausal changes**, occur gradually over a time frame of ten years or more. These changes may begin in a woman's early to mid-40s and extend into her mid-50s (see Chapter 12, "Sexual Development throughout Life"). Also, some women may experience menopausal changes earlier in life due to surgery, illness, or medications.

premenstrual syndrome (PMS) A set of symptoms that may occur during the days just before and during the start of a woman's period including irritability, depressed mood, and feelings of physical bloating or cramping.

premenstrual dysphoric disorder (PMDD) A significantly more intense and debilitating form of PMS.

menopause The time in a woman's life when menstruation and the reproductive cycle cease to occur.

perimenopausal changes The physical and psychological changes many women experience during the decade leading up to menopause.

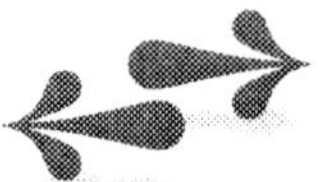

YOUR SEXUAL PHILOSOPHY

SEXUAL ANATOMY

As discussed in Chapter 1, your personal sexual philosophy is about making choices that are right for you and planning ahead so that you are in control of your sexual life. The development of a healthy sexual philosophy depends on your willingness to become educated and comfortable about all areas of human sexuality. This comfort level begins with an accurate and reasonably complete working knowledge of the sexual anatomy of both sexes. As you will see, sexual anatomy relates to virtually every topic throughout this book, so it follows that it also relates to nearly all facets of your life as a sexual person. Many people are uneasy, embarrassed, or even ashamed to study and learn about the sexual aspects of the human body. Overcoming discomfort and being open to developing and maintaining an accurate working knowledge of sexual anatomy will assist you in living a healthy and satisfying life as a sexual person.

Most people want and expect to have a satisfying and fulfilling sexual life with their chosen partner or partners. Often one barrier to that fulfillment is a lack of knowledge about sexual anatomy. When both partners are educated about their bodies, their ability to please each other is enhanced. Knowledge of our sexual bodies allows for effective, sensitive, and meaningful sexual communication. Furthermore, this knowledge may be even more important when sexual problems arise relating to sexual responding or sexual health. Identifying, discussing, and resolving sexual difficulties or illnesses is greatly facilitated by an understanding of the physical structures that may be involved.

These are just a few of the many reasons to make an understanding of sexual anatomy a central feature in who you are as a sexual person—your sexual philosophy. That so many people resist and avoid studying sexual anatomy is rather ironic. After all, your sexual body, as a primary force in reproduction, sexual pleasure, and human intimacy, is arguably your most important anatomical system of all.

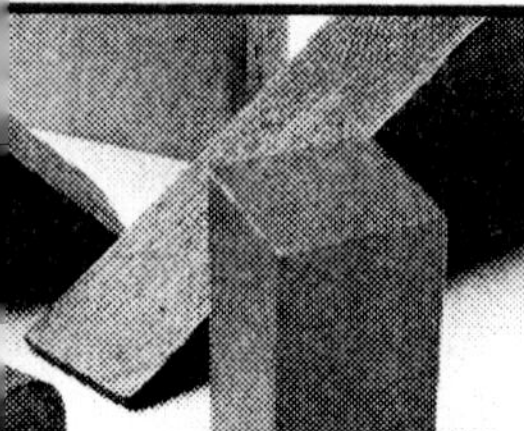

Summary

HISTORICAL PERSPECTIVES Sexual Anatomy in the Dark Ages

- Early conceptualizations of sexual anatomy were highly inaccurate. False beliefs included the notion that the male and female bodies were the same, but the male's genitals had simply been "pushed out"; the uterus was an internal scrotum: a girl could be "turned into" a boy by a sudden jarring motion, forcing the genitals to pop out; the uterus consisted of two halves—boys were born from the right half, girls from the left; and the source of sperm was the male brain.

The Male Sexual Body

- Penis size has been the central focus of male anatomy for centuries. Despite, or perhaps because of, this preoccupation among many men throughout history, most people are surprised to find that the length of the average erect penis is about 5.5 inches and varies little among the majority of men. Self-reports of penis size are larger but are probably not accurate due to inflated self-reporting or faulty measurement.
- Sperm starts its journey in the testicles, which produce sperm cells and testosterone. Sperm cells mature and are stored adjacent to the testicles in the epididymis before traveling through both vas deferens into the man's body, where they mix with semen for ejaculation. Semen is produced primarily by the seminal vesicles and the prostate gland.

The Female Sexual Body

- The female external sexual anatomy, the vulva, is more complex than the male's. The female genitals vary normally in size, shape, and color. The clitoris is a significantly larger and more complex organ than once thought; it extends several inches inside the woman's body. Women are more prone than men to urinary tract infections (UTIs) due to the shorter urethral length and its proximity to anal bacteria. Women who experience frequent UTIs should become knowledgeable about prevention techniques. A vaccine to immunize women against UTIs is under development.
- Breast augmentation is the third most common cosmetic surgery procedure in the United States. Breast augmentation chosen for purely cosmetic purposes, as opposed to reconstruction of the breast follow surgery or injury, reflects the value Western cultures place on that particular aspect of female sexual anatomy.
- Female internal sexual anatomy is designed primarily to serve the purpose of pregnancy. The passageway between the vagina and the uterus is the cervix. Certain strains of the human papilloma virus (HPV) that cause genital warts have been found to be the primary cause of cervical cancer. Many doctors and health organizations are recommending that HPV screening be done in conjunction with the yearly Pap test.
- The ovaries produce estrogen and progesterone and typically release one mature ovum during each fertility cycle of 28 days, on average.

Menstruation

- A young woman's menstrual cycle typically begins between the ages of 11 and 16 and ceases during menopause in her late 40s or early 50s.
- For conception to occur, the egg, or ovum, must be fertilized in the upper third of the fallopian tube. If the fertilized egg implants successfully in the uterine wall, pregnancy begins. If neither of these events occurs, the ovum is expelled along with the uterine lining during menstruation.

YOUR SEXUAL PHILOSOPHY: Sexual Anatomy

- Accurate knowledge plays an important role in sexual health and satisfaction. A clear understanding of both male and female sexual anatomy enhances a couple's ability to communicate about sexual issues, which in turn helps promote a satisfying and fulfilling sexual life. In addition, feeling comfortable with your own sexual anatomy contributes to maintaining sexual health and wellness and seeking medical attention when it is needed.

Have You Considered?

1. Imagine that you have a close friend who confides in you that he is worried and embarrassed because he thinks his penis is too small. Discuss at least three responses you could give him that might help him feel better about himself.
2. Discuss why you think men worry more than women do about penis size.
3. If you were the parent of a new baby boy, would you have him circumcised? Give three reasons for your answer.
4. Explain why the Cowper's glands are an important part of male sexual anatomy.
5. What, in your opinion, are some reasons that the true structure of the clitoris was not known until recently?
6. The practice of female genital mutilation (FGM), called female circumcision by some, is deeply ingrained in many cultures throughout the world. Do you feel that members of cultures such as the United States that disapprove of the practice have a right to interfere in those cultures and attempt to put a stop to it? Explain your answer.
7. Many groups around the world are working to stop FGM. If they asked for your help, what three strategies might you suggest to reduce the incidence FGM?
8. Breast augmentation is a thriving industry in the United States. Discuss your opinion of the procedure and how you feel about women who choose to undergo breast enlargement for cosmetic reasons.

Companion Website Resources

For further chapter resources go to **www.prenhall.com/hock**. This robust text website includes polling questions for you to vote on, regular news updates, quizzes, sample tests, suggested reading lists, and more.

SCENARIOS USA Also on the website are links to videos. *Scenarios USA's* films portray real-life narratives that explore the non-biological aspects of relationships and sexual health. The films will help you consider how the themes of the text affect your own life and the lives of those around you.

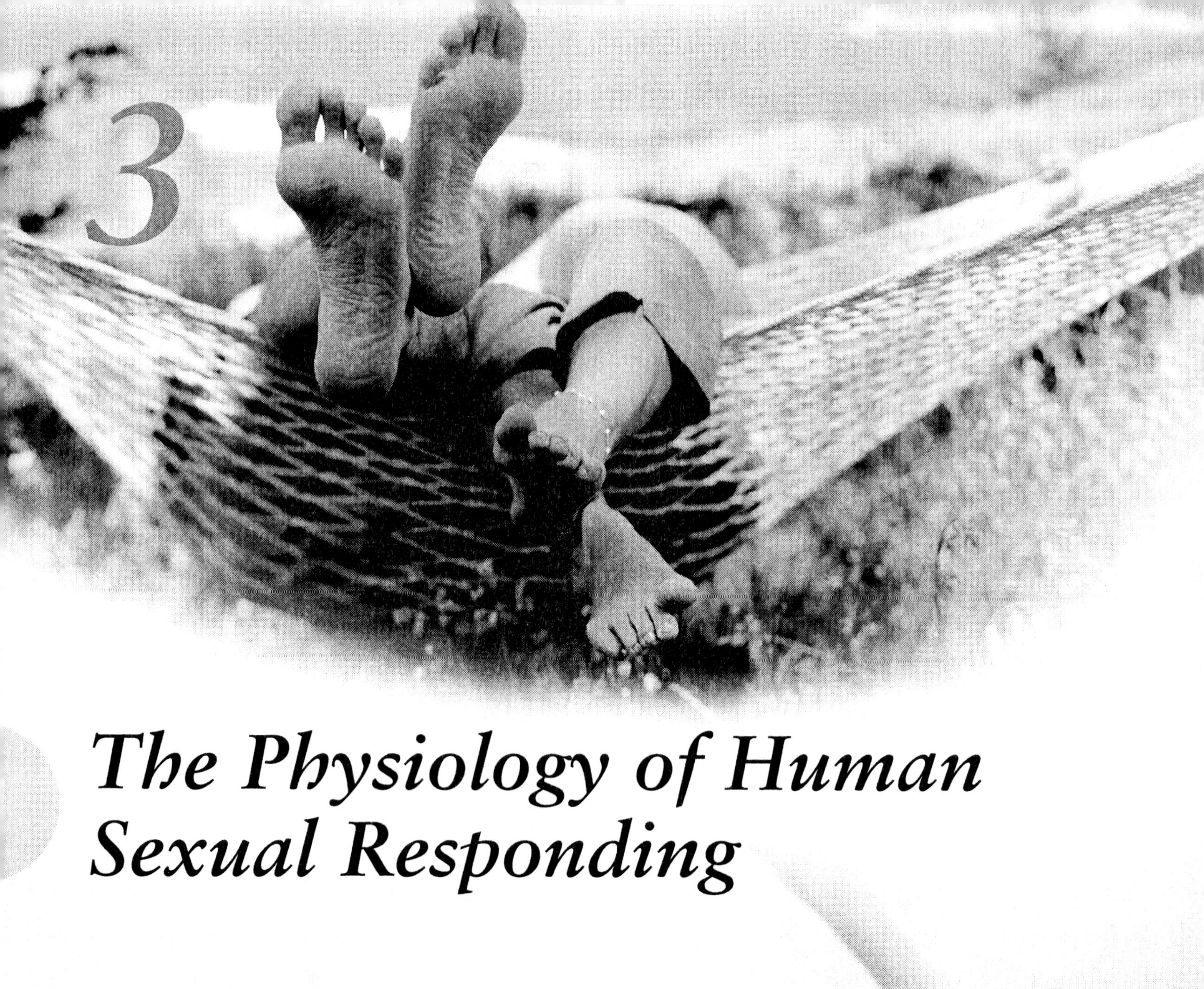

3

The Physiology of Human Sexual Responding

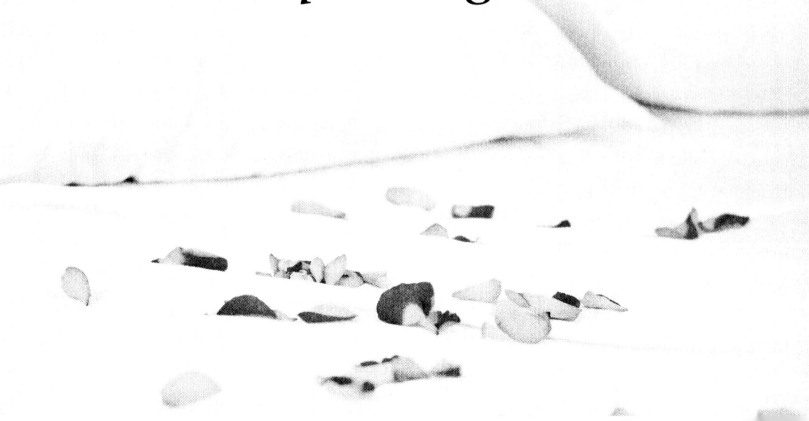

Since YOU Asked...

1. How can we know for sure what happens during sex? You can't exactly study people while they're doing it, right? (see page 75)

2. What really goes on inside the body during sex? (see page 77)

3. I'm a woman. During intercourse, why does it take so long for me to have an orgasm? Is it unusual for women not to have orgasms at all during sex? (see page 80)

4. What is "pre-cum," and why does it appear? (see page 80)

5. Do orgasms feel the same to men and women? Are men's stronger or more intense? (see page 83)

6. Are too many orgasms dangerous to your health? How many are too many? (see page 83)

7. I'm a man. After I have an orgasm, I can get another erection pretty fast, but I can't seem to orgasm again. Is this normal or a problem of some kind? (see page 85)

8. I've heard that some women ejaculate like men. Is this true? How is it possible? (see page 86)

9. Exactly what and where is the "G-spot"? My boyfriend and I can't seem to find it! (see page 87)

10. I've heard that there is a new pill for women that works like Viagra for men. Is this true? What does it do? (see page 90)

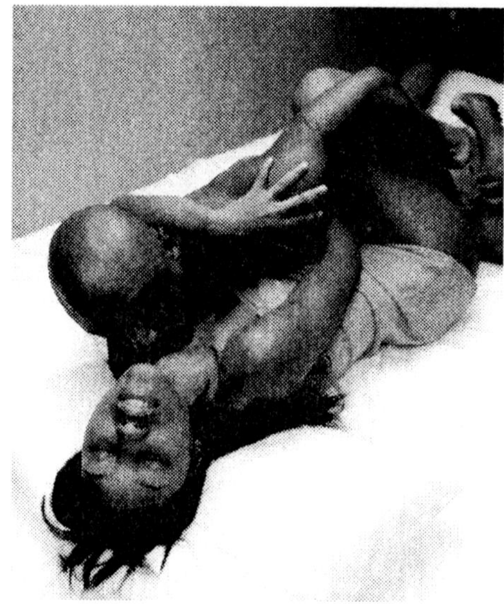

Our sexual anatomy plays an important role in sexual pleasure and intimacy.

Your sexual anatomy is inextricably linked to sexual activities, sexual feelings, sexual interactions, sexual pleasure, and sexual intimacy. For a full understanding of the male and female sexual bodies, we must turn our attention away somewhat from the parts themselves (which we explore in Chapter 2) and refocus on the *physiology* of sex—on how our sexual structures function and relate to our ability to respond physically and emotionally to sexual stimulation. In other words, *anatomy* and *physiology* are not the same, although many people use the words interchangeably. If we use another physical system as an example, this difference will become clearer. The *anatomy* of, say, your digestive system includes the mouth, esophagus, stomach, intestines, and anus. Knowing that, however, tells us nothing about how digestion actually works and what role each of those structures plays in the digestive process. To understand that, we would have to study the *physiology* of digestion. And so it is with our sexual anatomy.

In this chapter, we move to a new and higher level of appreciation of the unique complexities of human sexuality through an examination of the physiology of the body's sexual responses. We will examine what happens to the body before, during, and after sexual activities (with or without a partner). We will examine various researchers' theories and conceptualizations of human sexual responding. Through these theories, we will explore the many physical changes that accompany sexual desire, excitement, orgasm, and resolution (the body's process of returning to its unaroused state), and we will clarify the similarities and differences in the responses of men and women.

To start us off, let's go back more than 40 years, to a time when one of the most important studies in the history of sex was being conducted in a research center in Saint Louis, Missouri. Much of what we know today about sexual anatomy and response, we owe to the pioneering studies of William Masters and Virginia Johnson.

Focus on Your Feelings

Topics relating to how the human body responds during sex can trigger an immense range of emotional responses, both positive and negative. These emotions are probably largely why most people tend to avoid sexual response as a popular topic of casual conversation. "Hi Lucy! Orgasms OK lately?" "Super, Pete, how about you? No more erectile difficulties?" Not a likely conversation starter, right? It's probably safe to say that people are generally more uncomfortable studying and discussing the functioning of their sexual anatomy than learning about the parts themselves. In some ways, this discomfort makes complete sense; after all, your sexual activities are intensely personal and are really nobody's business but your own.

Studying and thinking about your own or your partner's sexual responses may evoke pleasurable, happy, intimate, loving, or arousing feelings. There's certainly nothing wrong with this; sexual fantasy is the most common human sexual activity! On the other hand, issues relating to sexual functioning may also prompt negative emotions such as guilt, anxiety, or embarrassment. The particular emotions you experience while reading this chapter will depend on many personal factors, including your sexual experiences; your family's attitudes about sex as you were growing up; past sexual abuse or trauma; and your overall comfort level with yourself as a sexual being. No matter what emotions may arise from the material in this chapter, rest assured that they are almost certainly normal and that you are not the only one feeling them. The information you gain in these pages will help enhance the positive feelings about your sexual life and help you to find ways of overcoming the negative ones.

Historical Perspectives
Sexual Pioneers

Prior to the 1960s, the definitive published work on the sexual behavior of humans consisted primarily of large-scale surveys, most notably, those by Alfred Kinsey in the late 1940s and early 1950s. The renowned Kinsey Reports offered a rare glimpse into the sexual activities of humans. Kinsey and his associates (Kinsey, Pomeroy & Martin, 1948; Kinsey et al., 1953) surveyed thousands of men and women about their sexual behavior and attitudes and reported on topics ranging from frequency of intercourse and masturbation habits to homosexual experiences. Data from the Kinsey Reports are still cited today as a source of statistical information about sexual behavior. Although Kinsey's research provided information about what people *say* they do sexually, a conspicuous information gap remained about how the human body functions anatomically when we engage in sexual behavior.

In the 1960s, William H. Masters (1915–2001) and Virginia E. Johnson (b. 1925) changed all that. Their research into human sexual physiology and response (beginning with Masters's earlier research in the mid-1950s) is largely credited with revealing to the world how our sexual bodies function during sexual activity (Hock, 2003). As the 1960s began, the United States launched into what has become known as the *sexual revolution*, a time of sweeping social changes marked by the introduction of the birth control pill, a greater openness about sexuality, and the "free love" movement. This provided an ideal historical opportunity for candid and definitive scientific exploration of our sexuality that would not have been possible previously. Until the 1960s, lingering Victorian messages that sexual behavior is something secretive, hidden, and certainly not a topic of discussion, much less study, would have precluded virtually all support, social and financial, from Masters and Johnson's research. But as men and women began to acknowledge more openly that we are sexual beings, with strong sexual feelings and desires, the social climate became ready not only to accept the explicit research of Masters and Johnson but to demand it. Statistics were no longer enough. People were ready to learn about their sexual bodies and their physical responses to sexual stimulation.

It was within this social context that Masters and Johnson set about studying human sexual anatomy and physiology. Their early work culminated in the publication of their first book, *Human Sexual Response* (1966). Although, as you will read shortly, their work created its share of controversy, and more recent research has drawn some of their findings into question, Masters and Johnson's discoveries continue to form the foundation of our current knowledge of the physiology of sexual response.

To study in detail the physiological responses during sexual activity and stimulation, Masters and Johnson's team of researchers developed elaborate methods of measurement and observation. These included standard measures of physiological response, such as pulse, blood pressure, and rate of respiration. In addition, the researchers observed and recorded specific sexual responses. For this the "sexual activity of study subjects included, at various times, manual and mechanical manipulation, natural coition [intercourse] with the female partner in supine, superior, or knee-chest position, and, for many female study subjects, artificial coition in the supine or knee-chest positions" (Masters & Johnson, 1966, p. 21). In other words, sometimes subjects were observed and measured having intercourse in various positions or during masturbation, either manually or with mechanical devices specially designed to allow for clear recording of changes in external and internal sexual anatomy, such as erection, vaginal lubrication, and orgasmic contractions. In their initial studies, Masters and Johnson's team of researchers observed an estimated 10,000 complete sexual response cycles.

Since YOU Asked...

1. How can we know for sure what happens during sex? You can't exactly study people while they're doing it, right?

It is impossible to overestimate the contributions of Masters and Johnson in our understanding and study of human sexuality. For nearly 30 years following the publication of *Human Sexual Response*, Masters and Johnson continued to study human sexual responding and apply their findings to helping people achieve sexual fulfillment. Four years after the publication of their first book, they released *Human Sexual Inadequacy* (1970), which took their earlier research and applied it directly to solutions for sexual problems (as we discuss in Chapter 7, "Sexual Problems and Solutions"). Their decades of research and writing on various topical issues in the field of sexuality may be seen in the titles of some of their subsequent books: *The Pleasure Bond* (1974), *Homosexuality in Perspective* (1979), *Masters and Johnson on Sex and Human Loving* (1986), and *Crisis: Heterosexual Behavior in the Age of AIDS* (1988).

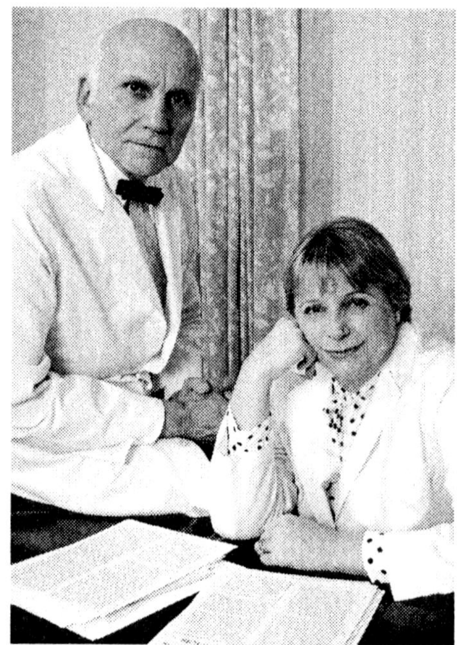

William Masters and Virginia Johnson were pioneers in the study of human sexual anatomy and response.

An interesting side note in this story is that during their early years of research collaboration, William Masters and Virginia Johnson were married to other people, but they eventually married each other and remained together for more than 20 years before their divorce in 1993. Johnson left the research clinic prior to their divorce, and Masters retired in 1995, six years before his death in 2001. Their last published work together was *Heterosexuality* (Masters, Johnson, & Kolodny, 1994).

Throughout our discussion of the physiology of human sexual response, you will be able to see how the early work of Masters and Johnson allows us to talk about human sexual responding in systematic, organized, and understandable ways.

Biology, Psychology, and Human Sexual Responding

For most nonhuman mammals, sexual behavior is governed primarily, or in some cases exclusively, by the biological forces of reproduction. When the female of many nonhuman species is fertile, she sends out strong signals to the males of the species, announcing her readiness to mate. The males get the message clearly and respond to it with mating behavior. You know this if you have ever seen the behavior of male dogs around a female during *estrus*, when she is "in heat." At other times, however, their interest in sexual behavior is minimal or nonexistent.

Although humans are animals, too, and many aspects of our sexual responses rest on shared biological foundations, numerous differences exist between humans and other animals. Our willingness to engage in mating behavior is not clearly linked to the female's fertility cycle to ensure reproduction. Our reasons for engaging in sexual behavior are far more varied and complicated, because *psychological* processes play a role at least as great as, or arguably greater than, biology.

Why do humans become sexually aroused? In addition to the impulse toward reproduction, the reasons may include feeling pleasure, giving pleasure, expressing feelings of closeness and love, relieving stress, feeling valued by another person, expressing how much another person is valued, feeling more or less dominant or submissive, and many other reasons that you can probably think of. These are not purely biological reasons for sexual desire; they are, essentially, psychological and as such are fundamentally human. As we discuss what we know about the physical side of human sexual responding, we must always keep in mind how intricately connected it is to our psychological triggers and motivations (Bancroft, 2002; Bozeman & Beck, 1991).

Masters and Johnson: The Excitement-Plateau-Orgasm-Resolution Model

As we begin this discussion, you should be aware that not all of Masters and Johnson's observations and conclusions are universally accepted, nor have they endured without some valid criticism. Some specifics of their findings have been drawn into question or even shown to be less than completely accurate. Masters and Johnson made some errors, jumped to some conclusions that have been shown to be flawed, and have been criticized on several fronts. We will discuss three alternative views of the human sexual response cycle later in this chapter. However, Masters and Johnson's basic observations and conceptualizations of how humans respond physically to sexual stimulation are still applied almost universally to this day when these functions are studied.

In their extensive observations of people engaged in various sexual activities, Masters and Johnson's team of researchers found certain predictable consistencies in human sexual responding. Although we are all sexually unique in terms of the choices we make about sexual behaviors and what kinds of stimulation each of us finds most exciting, our physical patterns of sexual responses are much more similar than they are different. To facilitate explanations of how our bodies change during sexual stimulation, Masters and Johnson (1966) divided the process into four phases of sexual response—*excitement, plateau, orgasm*, and *resolution*—often called simply the **EPOR model**. Masters and Johnson never intended for these four phases to be conceptualized as four separate and distinct events. They were careful to explain that their model was an "arbitrary four-part division of the sexual response cycle [that] provides an effective *framework* for detailed description" (1966, p. 4). As they readily noted, it is fundamentally impossible to identify exactly when excitement stops and plateau begins or the precise instant orgasm starts or ends. Sexual responding is a much more seamless process. However, the four-phase model was simple to understand; it made sense for many people when they thought about their own sexual reactions and converted the complex experience of sexual responding into a more clearly defined phenomenon (Hock, 2005).

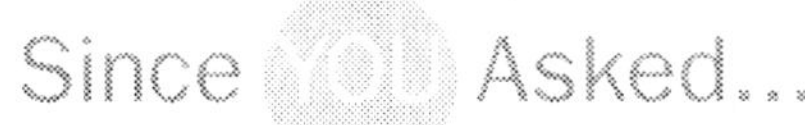

2. What really goes on inside the body during sex?

To this day, most people study sexual responding against the backdrop of Masters and Johnson's four-phase model, which is summarized in Figure 3.1. Keep in mind that sexual responses are designed by nature to be pleasurable, to "feel good," and thus enhance the odds of reproduction. But these responses typically occur in men and women in reaction to many forms of sexual stimulation, whether the setting involves a man and woman having intercourse; a same-sex couple making love; a couple sharing manual, oral, or anal sex; an individual masturbating; or an erotic dream.

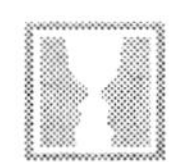

Sex is more than intercourse

EPOR model Masters and Johnson's approach to explaining the process of human sexual response, encompassing four arbitrarily divided phases: excitement, plateau, orgasm, and resolution.

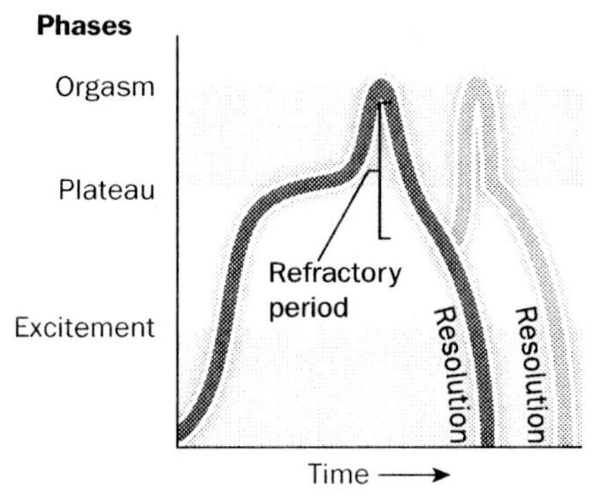

(a) The Male Sexual Response Cycle

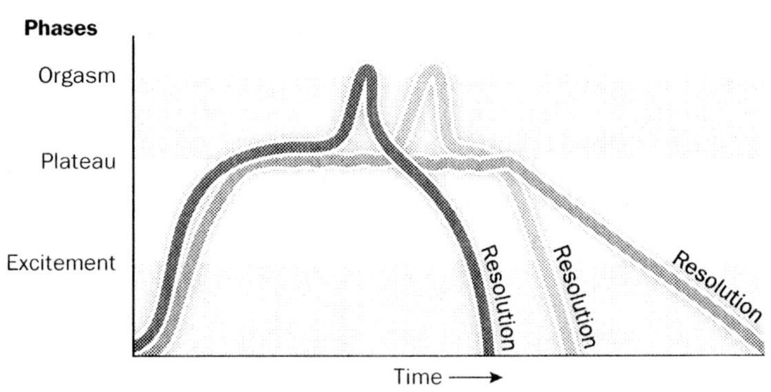

(b) The Female Sexual Response Cycle

FIGURE 3.1 Masters and Johnson's Four-Phase Model of the Sexual Response Cycle

Masters and Johnson proposed that human sexual responding was more understandable when conceptualized in four phases: excitement, plateau, orgasm, and resolution. This diagram, adapted from their theory, shows how the female response cycle tends to be more varied than that of the male. Men generally progress fairly predictably through the four stages red line) and require some time between orgasms, called a refractory period, before another orgasm (green line) is possible. In contrast, women may follow a similar pattern (red line) or may experience multiple orgasms without a refractory period (green line) or, as is quite common during heterosexual intercourse, may progress from excitement to plateau to resolution without experiencing an orgasm (blue line).

Source: Adapted from Masters and Johnson (1966).

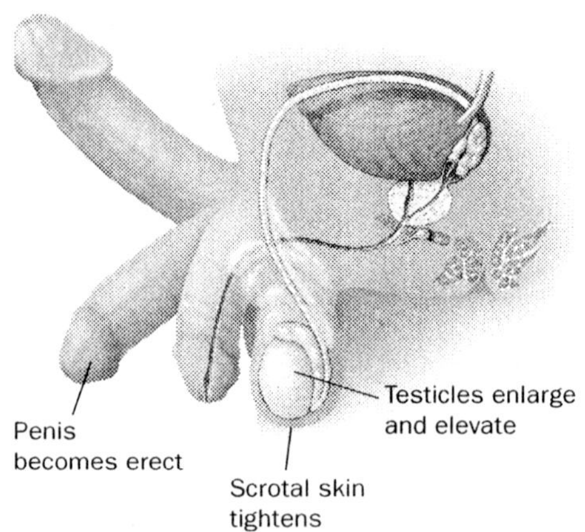

FIGURE 3.2 Physical Changes in the Male during the Excitement Phase

Excitement

Masters and Johnson referred to the beginning stage of the sexual response cycle as the **excitement phase**. Early physical responses can occur to any type of pleasurable sexual stimulation, for example, kissing, touching, sexual fantasy, sexually arousing visual materials, or masturbation. Exactly what triggers sexual arousal depends on many factors, including each person's sexual history and cultural beliefs about sexuality. "Sexuality and Culture: Tantric Sexual Techniques" illustrates some of these differences.

For both sexes, blood begins to circulate into all the erectile structures throughout the body, causing them to expand and stiffen, a process called **vasocongestion**. A **sex flush** or reddening of the skin of the chest and abdomen may occur in some people, the nipples become erect, breathing becomes heavier, heart rate increases, and voluntary muscles tense in a process called *myotonia.*

For men, the first and most obvious sign that sexual excitement has started is erection of the penis. The scrotal skin tightens, the testicles begin to rise up toward the underside of the penis, and the testicles themselves enlarge somewhat (see Figure 3.2). At this early stage, the man may not achieve a full erection, and his erection is easily lost if stimulation ceases or some sort of distraction occurs. Losing an erection during the excitement stage is completely normal, and it is usually easily regained. However, many men become concerned if they lose their erection at *any* time during sexual

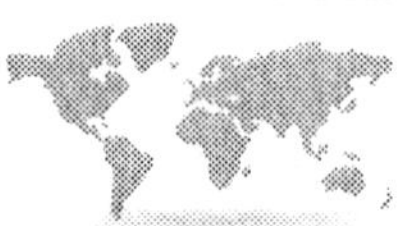

Sexuality and Culture

Tantric Sexual Techniques

Tantra is a spiritual practice that originated in India thousands of years ago. Those who practice Tantrism work to achieve enlightenment, the totality of the development of their potential as humans (Shaw, 1998). Tantra involves learning to release the mind and body from their usual limited space on earth and allowing them to soar, boundlessly reaching cosmic heights of existence. More recently, Western cultures have latched on to one particular Tantric practice, commonly referred to as *Tantric sex*, which refers to a set of sexual exercises and activities that are said to transform pleasurable sex acts into ecstatic, rapturous, spiritual experiences.

Tantra relates to another Eastern religious teaching that energy flows through the body, just as blood runs though our vascular systems. In Tantric beliefs, this spiritual or psychic energy joins together seven main energy centers, called *chakras*, throughout the body, from the base of the spine to the scalp. Although no physiological studies have ever confirmed the existence of *chakras*, followers of Tantra and other Eastern religions believe not only that they exist but that they are also in large part responsible for human energy, healing, and sexual pleasure (Driedger, 1996).

During the practice of Tantric sex, the goal is to open up the *chakras* and move the sexual energy, or *kundalini*, from the *chakras* nearest the genitals up to the heart, which is the "feeling *chakra*." From there the sexual energy unites with the partner's energy channel before flowing to the crown *chakra* at the top of the head, creating a sensation of oneness and ecstasy.

Both partners must be committed to learning and practicing the techniques of Tantric sex. A great deal of the emphasis is on breathing exercises, meditation, yoga, massage, and even dance as part of the process leading up to making love. Other exercises are more sexual, including the woman learning to receive pleasure from stimulation of the so-called sacred spot, which appears to be what is commonly referred to in the west as the G-spot, and the man learning to have orgasms without necessarily ejaculating.

In the Tantric tradition, the joining of two people is considered a spiritual rite and leads to a unity between them that is a stronger force than the sum of their individual spiritual energy. Prolonging lovemaking serves to further increase this energy and maximize sexual pleasure for both partners. Moreover, as mentioned in "In Touch with Your Sexual Health: The Health Benefits of Orgasm" later in this chapter, Tantric philosophy suggests that lovers who have practiced these ancient techniques can learn to move sexual energy to the body's *chakras*, which is thought to create sensations of ecstasy throughout the body and enhance overall health.

FIGURE 3.3 Physical Changes in the Female during Excitement Phase

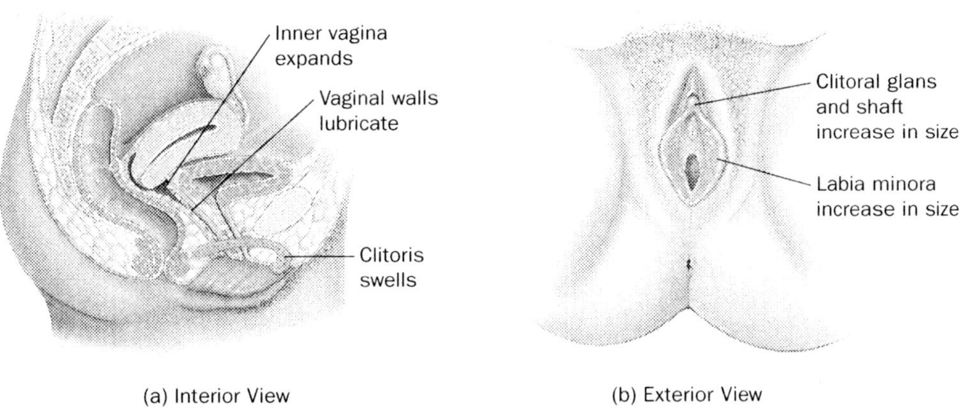

activity. This worry over a normal fluctuation in penile erection can become a self-fulfilling prophecy in that the anxiety itself can prevent the return of the erection.

For women, the first and most marked sign that sexual excitement has begun is vaginal lubrication. However, the woman's clitoris is also beginning to become erect along its full length (see Figure 3.3). During this phase, the shaft of the clitoris increases in size and the labia minora swell and may separate slightly from around the opening to the vagina. Various internal changes are occurring as well. The uterus engorges with blood, enlarges, and moves slightly upward in the abdominal cavity, and it may exhibit fibrillations. The vagina begins to change shape, becoming longer and widening out along the inner two-thirds of its length. Also the breasts, nipples, and areolas enlarge slightly (in men as well as women).

Plateau

In their early studies, Masters and Johnson noticed that for many individuals and couples, a leveling off of arousal seemed to occur at some point in the excitement phase, during which both men and women continued to be very aroused but did not appear to be experiencing much additional elevation in their level of arousal. They called this the **plateau phase**.

For both sexes during this phase, all erectile tissues throughout the sexual anatomy are now fully engorged with blood. Respiration, heart rate, blood pressure, and muscle tension are all at high levels as orgasm approaches. The sexual flush in some people spreads and darkens.

For women, nipples maintain their erect state, but the areolas continue to become larger, which may cause the nipple to appear less erect in comparison (see Figure 3.4). The walls of the outer one-third of the vagina become engorged with blood and thicken, reducing the size of the vaginal opening (see Figure 3.5). This may be nature's way of increasing stimulation to the penis during intercourse to ensure male orgasm and

excitement phase The first phase in the EPOR model, in which the first physical changes of sexual arousal occur.

vasocongestion The swelling of erectile tissues due to increased blood flow during sexual arousal.

sex flush A darkening or reddening of the skin of the chest area that occurs in some people during sexual arousal.

plateau phase The second phase in the EPOR model, during which sexual arousal levels off (reaches a plateau) and remains at an elevated level of excitement.

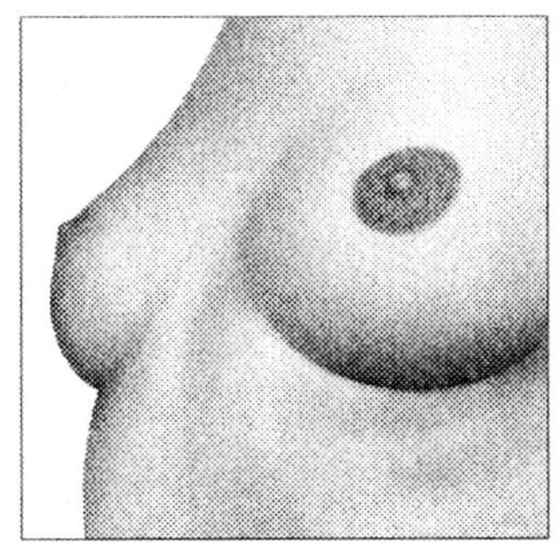

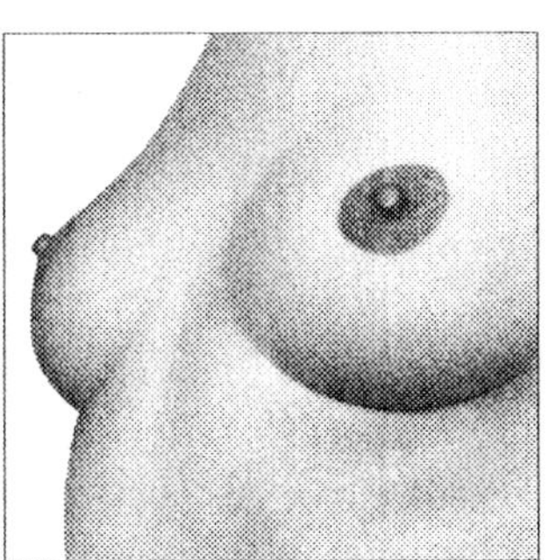

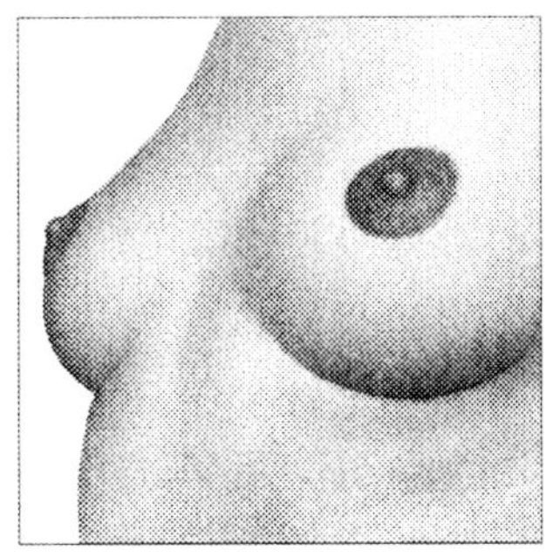

FIGURE 3.4 Sexual Arousal in the Female Breast

During the plateau stage, the breasts, nipples, and areolas typically enlarge due to engorgement of erectile tissues.

FIGURE 3.5 Physical Changes in the Female during the Plateau Phase

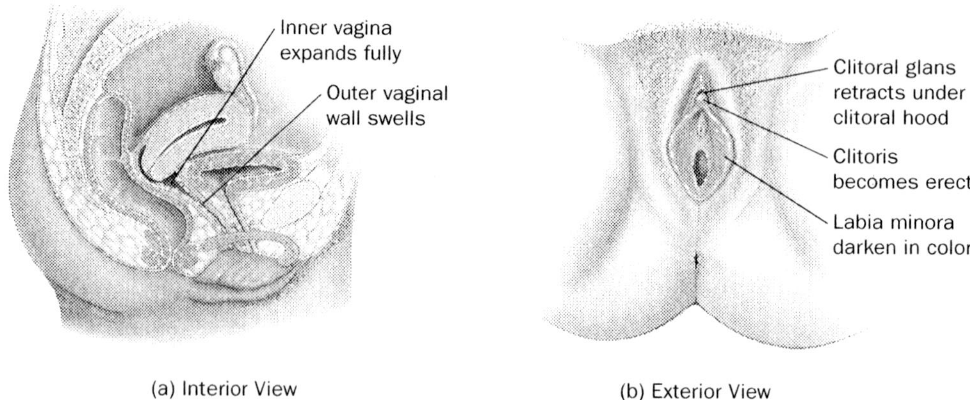

ejaculation, but it happens whether or not intercourse is taking place. The inner two-thirds of the vagina continues to expand in a process called **tenting**. Most researchers agree that tenting creates a place for semen to pool directly under the cervix and stimulate it with hormones in the seminal fluid to suck sperm into the uterus on their journey to the fallopian tubes.

Since YOU Asked...

3. I'm a woman. During intercourse, why does it take so long for me to have an orgasm? Is it unusual for women not to have orgasms at all during sex?

As the clitoris continues to engorge with blood, it straightens out along its length. This causes the glans of the clitoris in most women to retract closer to the body and under the clitoral hood. This is an important point in that if you picture the changes in the clitoris at this point, you can see that the clitoral glans actually becomes *less* available for stimulation. Therefore, as explained and illustrated in "Self-Discovery: Clitoral Erection and the Myth of Female Orgasms during Heterosexual Intercourse," most women do not reach orgasm from intercourse by itself and may want additional stimulation of the clitoral area either before, during, or after intercourse if they desire an orgasm. This is also why many women report that they find activities *other* than intercourse more sexually satisfying.

As the plateau stage continues, the labia minora deepen in color as they become increasingly engorged with blood, indicating that orgasm is approaching.

Since YOU Asked...

4. What is "pre-cum," and why does it appear?

For men, the penis now becomes fully erect, and the erection is unlikely to be lost due to anything short of a major distracting event (see Figure 3.6). The corona enlarges further, and the Cowper's glands by now have usually secreted enough pre-ejaculate fluid ("pre-cum") that it can be seen and felt at the opening to the urethra. This fluid is believed to add additional lubrication for intercourse and may serve to flush out or cleanse the urethra prior to the ejaculation of semen. It is important to stress that pre-ejaculate fluid may contain live sperm cells or infection-causing microbes, if the man has a sexually transmitted infection.

The scrotal skin is tight, and the testicles are now pulled up very closely against the body at the underside of the penis, an indication that orgasm is approaching.

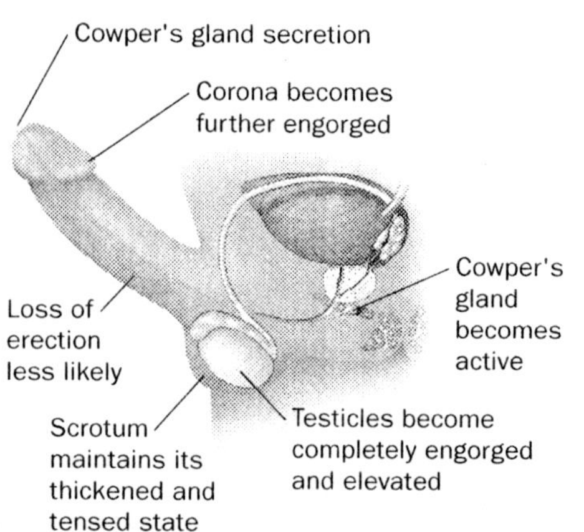

FIGURE 3.6 Physical Changes in the Male during the Plateau Phase

Orgasm

The climax of sexual arousal is the **orgasmic phase**. Although this is the shortest of the four phases, usually lasting less than 15 seconds, most people would agree that orgasm is the most intensely pleasurable experience of sexual responding. Orgasms vary in character and intensity from person to person, from one sexual experience to the next, and among various sexual acts that may lead to orgasm, including intercourse, oral sex, manual or vibrator stimulation, anal sex, and masturbation (these sexual activities are discussed in greater detail in Chapter 6, "Sexual Behaviors: Experiencing Sexual Pleasure").

As noted, women tend to require a somewhat longer period of stimulation than men do to achieve orgasm with a partner, and the majority of women do not routinely experience orgasm through intercourse exclusively. Although penile penetration may feel pleasurable for most women, it does not generally produce orgasm, nor is orgasm necessarily a woman's goal for intercourse (Nicolson & Burr, 2003). Most women require additional manual or oral stimulation of the clitoral area either before, during, or after intercourse. For many women, orgasm is the result of direct or indirect stimulation of the clitoris by a partner, manually or orally, or through masturbation. For some women, direct stimulation of the highly sensitive clitoral glans may be too intense and can actually inhibit orgasm.

Among the factors influencing the intensity and duration of orgasm are the length of arousal prior to orgasm, the length of time since the previous orgasm, alcohol or

tenting A widening of the inner two-thirds of the vagina during sexual arousal.

orgasmic phase The third stage in the EPOR model, during which sexual excitement and pleasure reach a climax.

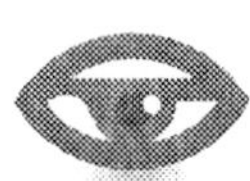

Self-Discovery

Clitoral Erection and the Myth of Female Orgasms during Heterosexual Intercourse

When Masters and Johnson wrote about the human sexual response cycle in the 1960s, they placed their discussion within a framework of male-female sexual intercourse. Of course, all the phases of sexual response occur during any form of sexual stimulation, whether it's between a man and a woman, two men, two women, or just yourself alone. However, one of the most common sexual myths that grew out of Masters and Johnson's assumption of penile-vaginal sex was the *expectation* that when a man and a woman are engaging in sexual intercourse, they both can and *should* experience an orgasm. Still today, 40 years or so later, many, if not most, heterosexual couples continue to believe that an orgasm for both is the "normal and natural" culmination of intercourse. The problem is that most of the time, this simply does not happen. Don't misunderstand: It nearly always happens for the man, but for the majority of women, sexual intercourse, by itself, does not result in an orgasm, no matter how long that man is able to "last." In fact, only about 30 percent of women experience orgasms routinely through sexual intercourse (Laumann et al., 1994; "His and Hers," 2001). Of the 70 percent who do not have orgasms during intercourse, most are orgasmic through manual stimulation, oral sex, or masturbation (or some combination of these). So, what is going on?

Sex therapists and researchers have found many factors that may interfere with a person's sexual arousal, sexual pleasure, and orgasm. But one of the most common reasons why women do not experience orgasm during intercourse relates simply to differences in sexual anatomy. As you will recall, orgasm is usually achieved through stimulation of the penile glans in men and the clitoral glans in women. The figure shows the position of the male and female sexual anatomy during sexual intercourse. If you imagine the activity of intercourse, which primarily involves the penis moving back and forth within the vagina, you can easily see that the glans of the penis receives a great deal of stimulation. Indeed, as the woman becomes increasingly aroused, the walls of her vagina swell, reducing the size of the vaginal opening and providing even greater friction to the penis.

Now notice the position of the clitoral glans. You can see that it is far less likely to receive adequate stimulation from intercourse alone. Usually the clitoris is stimulated when the pubic bone of the man hits it when the penis is deep in the vagina or when the motion of the penis in the vagina moves the minor labia, which in turn move the clitoral hood over the clitoris. However, as discussed in Chapter 2 (p. 52), the clitoris has been moving up under the hood and closer to the woman's body, so it's even less available for such stimulation. Even if the man is able to delay his orgasm for long periods of thrusting, most women find this form of stimulation insufficient for orgasm.

This is not to imply that orgasm is or should be the goal of lovemaking. Many women are satisfied without an orgasm during intercourse or enjoy orgasms through other forms of stimulation, as mentioned earlier. However, if a couple feels somehow incomplete if orgasm isn't shared during intercourse, the easiest solution is to incorporate some additional clitoral stimulation during intercourse. Various sexual positions discussed in Chapter 7, "Sexual Problems and Solutions," allow for easier access to the clitoral area so that the man or the woman herself can provide the extra stimulation that she may want.

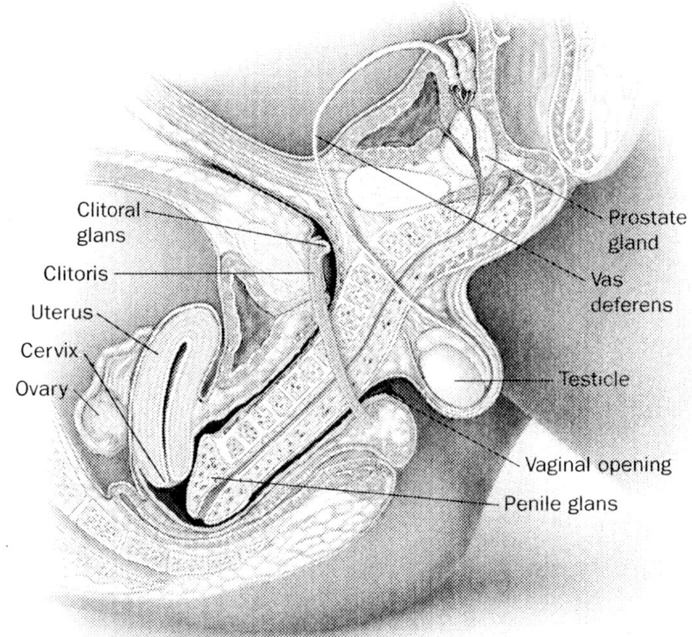

Positions of Male and Female Anatomy during Heterosexual Intercourse

FIGURE 3.7 Physical Changes in the Female during Orgasm

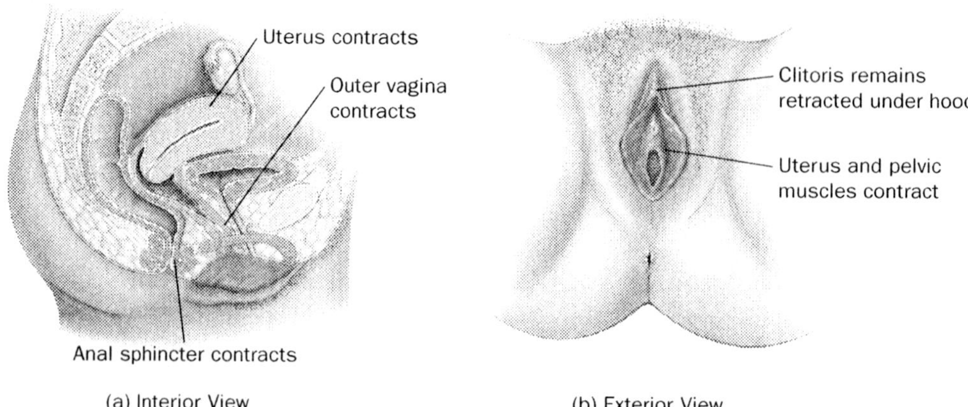

other drug use, and feelings of comfort and intimacy with a partner. Virtually everyone is capable of having an orgasm, although a small percentage of adults have not experienced orgasm for various reasons. Those who have never experienced an orgasm are referred to as preorgasmic, and although this is relatively uncommon overall, it is more common among women than men (see Chapter 7, "Sexual Problems and Solutions," for more about this).

For both sexes, as orgasm approaches, respiration increases dramatically, and pulse rate and blood pressure continue to rise. Any existing sexual flush spreads over more of the body. Usually, a loss of control over voluntary muscles results in muscle contractions and spasms, especially in the hands and feet. Muscles in the pelvic area begin to contract rhythmically at the rate of once every 0.8 second (however, you would find it quite a challenge to try to time these as they are happening).

For women, the anus, uterus, muscles of the pelvic floor, and walls of the outer third of the vagina all contract at intervals of 0.8 second during orgasm (see Figure 3.7). The number of these contractions varies from 3 to about 15.

For men, orgasm involves similar contractions of the anus but also involves ejaculation (we will discuss female ejaculation a little later). Ejaculation occurs in two stages (see Figure 3.8). The first stage, **emission**, is when semen builds up in the urethral bulb, creating the subjective sensation that ejaculation has begun and nothing can stop it. This sensation of having reached the "point of no return" is called the moment of **ejaculatory inevitability** because once the semen has collected in the urethral bulb, the rest of the ejaculatory process is reflexive and cannot be controlled voluntarily. Immediately after emission, the prostate gland, urethra, and muscles at the base of the penis contract at intervals of 0.8 second, pushing the semen through the urethra and out of the penis in the second stage of ejaculation, called **expulsion**.

Explaining the physiological events that occur during male and female orgasm is not terribly difficult, but asking people to describe how orgasm *feels* is more difficult. Most people agree that the experience of orgasm is too intense and all-encompassing to describe adequately in words. Also, people's conscious awareness of the experience of orgasm tends to be clouded by the event itself, so detailed descriptions are rare. Although people's characterizations of orgasm vary a great deal, they usually include accounts of intense pleasurable sensations centered in the genitals and emanating out through the pelvic area and sometimes throughout the entire body. During orgasm, the person is usually very self-focused and, at the climactic peak, typically experiences a loss of awareness of his or her surroundings. Orgasm typically brings about an immense release of psychological and physical tension, leading to satisfied, warm sensations of emotional well-being, sometimes called **afterglow**, which may be facilitated by an increase in the hormone oxytocin, released during orgasm.

Contractions force semen out through urethra
Semen builds up in urethral bulb
Contractions of penile urethra
Contractions of muscles around base of penis

FIGURE 3.8 Physical Changes in the Male during Orgasm and Ejaculation

emission In males, the buildup of sperm and semen in the urethral bulb just prior to being expelled through the urethra.

ejaculatory inevitability In males, the sensation produced during the emission phase of ejaculation that expulsion of semen is imminent, reflexive, and cannot be stopped; often referred to as the "point of no return."

expulsion In males, the contraction of pelvic muscles that force semen through the urethra and out of the body through the penis.

afterglow The emotional and physical feeling of satisfaction, relaxation, and intimacy that follows the act of making love.

FIGURE 3.7 Physical Changes in the Female during Orgasm

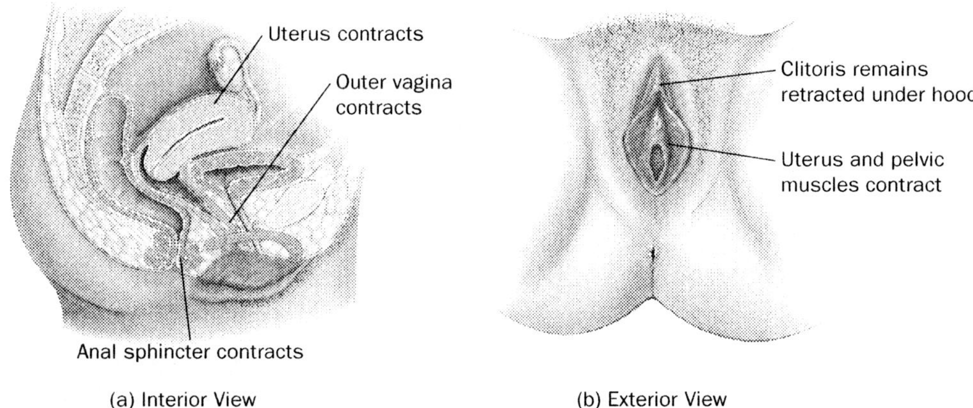

other drug use, and feelings of comfort and intimacy with a partner. Virtually everyone is capable of having an orgasm, although a small percentage of adults have not experienced orgasm for various reasons. Those who have never experienced an orgasm are referred to as preorgasmic, and although this is relatively uncommon overall, it is more common among women than men (see Chapter 7, "Sexual Problems and Solutions," for more about this).

For both sexes, as orgasm approaches, respiration increases dramatically, and pulse rate and blood pressure continue to rise. Any existing sexual flush spreads over more of the body. Usually, a loss of control over voluntary muscles results in muscle contractions and spasms, especially in the hands and feet. Muscles in the pelvic area begin to contract rhythmically at the rate of once every 0.8 second (however, you would find it quite a challenge to try to time these as they are happening).

For women, the anus, uterus, muscles of the pelvic floor, and walls of the outer third of the vagina all contract at intervals of 0.8 second during orgasm (see Figure 3.7). The number of these contractions varies from 3 to about 15.

For men, orgasm involves similar contractions of the anus but also involves ejaculation (we will discuss female ejaculation a little later). Ejaculation occurs in two stages (see Figure 3.8). The first stage, **emission**, is when semen builds up in the urethral bulb, creating the subjective sensation that ejaculation has begun and nothing can stop it. This sensation of having reached the "point of no return" is called the moment of **ejaculatory inevitability** because once the semen has collected in the urethral bulb, the rest of the ejaculatory process is reflexive and cannot be controlled voluntarily. Immediately after emission, the prostate gland, urethra, and muscles at the base of the penis contract at intervals of 0.8 second, pushing the semen through the urethra and out of the penis in the second stage of ejaculation, called **expulsion**.

Explaining the physiological events that occur during male and female orgasm is not terribly difficult, but asking people to describe how orgasm *feels* is more difficult. Most people agree that the experience of orgasm is too intense and all-encompassing to describe adequately in words. Also, people's conscious awareness of the experience of orgasm tends to be clouded by the event itself, so detailed descriptions are rare. Although people's characterizations of orgasm vary a great deal, they usually include accounts of intense pleasurable sensations centered in the genitals and emanating out through the pelvic area and sometimes throughout the entire body. During orgasm, the person is usually very self-focused and, at the climactic peak, typically experiences a loss of awareness of his or her surroundings. Orgasm typically brings about an immense release of psychological and physical tension, leading to satisfied, warm sensations of emotional well-being, sometimes called **afterglow**, which may be facilitated by an increase in the hormone oxytocin, released during orgasm.

Contractions force semen out through urethra
Semen builds up in urethral bulb
Contractions of penile urethra
Contractions of muscles around base of penis

FIGURE 3.8 Physical Changes in the Male during Orgasm and Ejaculation

emission In males, the buildup of sperm and semen in the urethral bulb just prior to being expelled through the urethra.

ejaculatory inevitability In males, the sensation produced during the emission phase of ejaculation that expulsion of semen is imminent, reflexive, and cannot be stopped; often referred to as the "point of no return."

expulsion In males, the contraction of pelvic muscles that force semen through the urethra and out of the body through the penis.

afterglow The emotional and physical feeling of satisfaction, relaxation, and intimacy that follows the act of making love.

ence orgasm through intercourse exclusively. Although penile penetration may feel pleasurable for most women, it does not generally produce orgasm, nor is orgasm necessarily a woman's goal for intercourse (Nicolson & Burr, 2003). Most women require additional manual or oral stimulation of the clitoral area either before, during, or after intercourse. For many women, orgasm is the result of direct or indirect stimulation of the clitoris by a partner, manually or orally, or through masturbation. For some women, direct stimulation of the highly sensitive clitoral glans may be too intense and can actually inhibit orgasm.

Among the factors influencing the intensity and duration of orgasm are the length of arousal prior to orgasm, the length of time since the previous orgasm, alcohol or

tenting A widening of the inner two-thirds of the vagina during sexual arousal.

orgasmic phase The third stage in the EPOR model, during which sexual excitement and pleasure reach a climax.

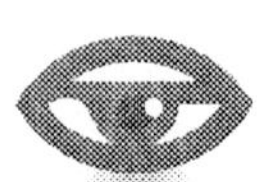

Self-Discovery

Clitoral Erection and the Myth of Female Orgasms during Heterosexual Intercourse

When Masters and Johnson wrote about the human sexual response cycle in the 1960s, they placed their discussion within a framework of male-female sexual intercourse. Of course, all the phases of sexual response occur during any form of sexual stimulation, whether it's between a man and a woman, two men, two women, or just yourself alone. However, one of the most common sexual myths that grew out of Masters and Johnson's assumption of penile-vaginal sex was the *expectation* that when a man and a woman are engaging in sexual intercourse, they both can and *should* experience an orgasm. Still today, 40 years or so later, many, if not most, heterosexual couples continue to believe that an orgasm for both is the "normal and natural" culmination of intercourse. The problem is that most of the time, this simply does not happen. Don't misunderstand: It nearly always happens for the man, but for the majority of women, sexual intercourse, by itself, does not result in an orgasm, no matter how long that man is able to "last." In fact, only about 30 percent of women experience orgasms routinely through sexual intercourse (Laumann et al., 1994; "His and Hers," 2001). Of the 70 percent who do not have orgasms during intercourse, most are orgasmic through manual stimulation, oral sex, or masturbation (or some combination of these). So, what is going on?

Sex therapists and researchers have found many factors that may interfere with a person's sexual arousal, sexual pleasure, and orgasm. But one of the most common reasons why women do not experience orgasm during intercourse relates simply to differences in sexual anatomy. As you will recall, orgasm is usually achieved through stimulation of the penile glans in men and the clitoral glans in women. The figure shows the position of the male and female sexual anatomy during sexual intercourse. If you imagine the activity of intercourse, which primarily involves the penis moving back and forth within the vagina, you can easily see that the glans of the penis receives a great deal of stimulation. Indeed, as the woman becomes increasingly aroused, the walls of her vagina swell, reducing the size of the vaginal opening and providing even greater friction to the penis.

Now notice the position of the clitoral glans. You can see that it is far less likely to receive adequate stimulation from intercourse alone. Usually the clitoris is stimulated when the pubic bone of the man hits it when the penis is deep in the vagina or when the motion of the penis in the vagina moves the minor labia, which in turn move the clitoral hood over the clitoris. However, as discussed in Chapter 2 (p. 52), the clitoris has been moving up under the hood and closer to the woman's body, so it's even less available for such stimulation. Even if the man is able to delay his orgasm for long periods of thrusting, most women find this form of stimulation insufficient for orgasm.

This is not to imply that orgasm is or should be the goal of lovemaking. Many women are satisfied without an orgasm during intercourse or enjoy orgasms through other forms of stimulation, as mentioned earlier. However, if a couple feels somehow incomplete if orgasm isn't shared during intercourse, the easiest solution is to incorporate some additional clitoral stimulation during intercourse. Various sexual positions discussed in Chapter 7, "Sexual Problems and Solutions," allow for easier access to the clitoral area so that the man or the woman herself can provide the extra stimulation that she may want.

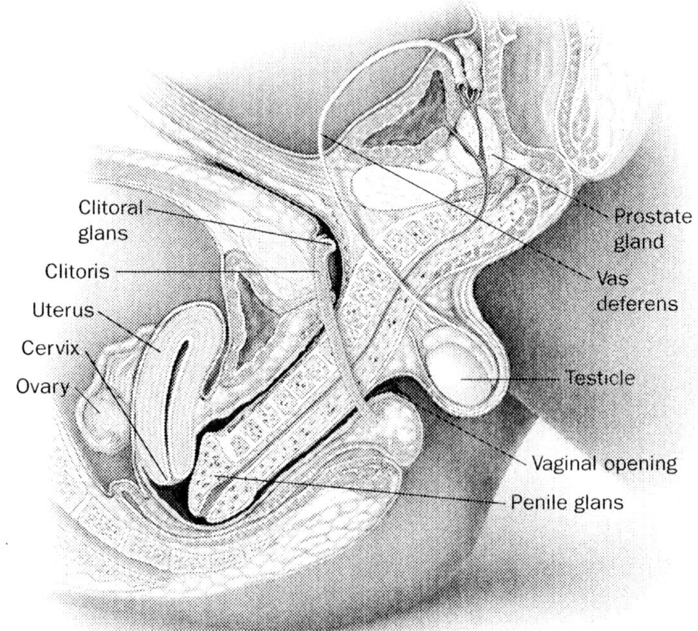

Positions of Male and Female Anatomy during Heterosexual Intercourse

You may be surprised to learn that men's and women's descriptions of their orgasms are quite similar. In one often-cited study, 48 written descriptions of orgasm, 24 from men and 24 from women, with all the sex-specific terms removed, were submitted to health care and psychological professionals, who were asked to judge whether each description was written by a man or a woman. The 70 male and female judges were unable to distinguish between men's and women's descriptions of orgasm (Vance & Wagner, 1976). In a more recent study, researchers asked men and women to rate various factors of the experience of orgasm, including satisfaction (with partner and alone), emotional intimacy, relaxation, ecstasy, and various bodily sensations (Mah & Binik, 2002). Figure 3.9 summarizes the study's results. As you can see, most rating scores, on average, were similar for the male and female participants, with women rating several of the bodily sensations only slightly higher than men. The exception was "shooting sensations," which was rated far higher by men than by women, probably due to the nature of male ejaculation.

Since YOU Asked...

5. Do orgasms feel the same to men and women? Are men's stronger or more intense?

That said, it appears that orgasms not only provide great physical and emotional pleasure but may actually be biologically healthy as well. "In Touch with Your Sexual Health: The Health Benefits of Orgasm" lists a number benefits that have been linked to orgasms for men and women. However, most sex educators and sex therapists stress that although orgasm is a natural part of human sexual response, it should not be the goal of sexual interactions. In fact, focusing on orgasm as the main objective of lovemaking may detract, rather than enhance, the intimate experience.

Since YOU Asked...

6. Are too many orgasms dangerous to your health? How many are too many?

When couples value and embrace the entire lovemaking process, they often discover new and deeper levels of closeness and intimacy. An orgasm-as-the-goal approach to sexual intimacy often leads to repetitive, mechanical sexual interactions that are targeted at that goal but may fail to produce the expressions of love and intimacy couples seek. Moreover, if one partner does not experience orgasm, the sexual encounter may be

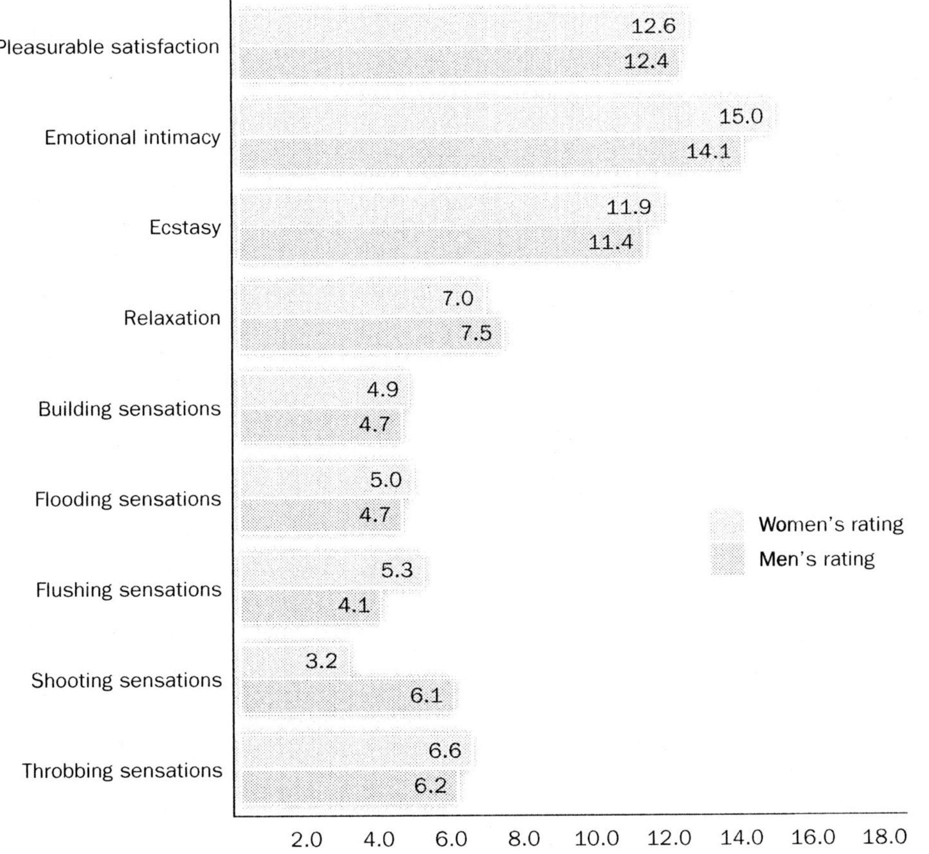

FIGURE 3.9 Average Ratings by Men and Women of Various Components of Orgasm

This graph illustrates that most of the perceived sensations accompanying orgasm are rated similarly by women and men. Ratings indicate how well each component described participants' most recent orgasm experience with a partner; higher ratings indicate greater descriptive accuracy and were based on mean component scale scores adjusted for co-variates for each gender.

Source: Based on data in Mah & Binik, 2002, p. 110.

Sex is more than intercourse 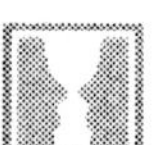

interpreted as a failure. Instead, sexuality educators and therapists try to assist couples in learning to experience all sexual activities as pleasurable in and of themselves. As one well-known sex researcher suggests:

> If the sexual experience does not lead to the achievement of the goal [orgasm], then the couple or the person who is goal-oriented does not feel good about all that has been experienced. The alternative view is *pleasure-directed*, which can be conceptualized as a circle, with each expression on the perimeter of the circle considered an end in itself. Whether the experience is kissing, oral sex, holding, etc., each is satisfying to the couple. There is no need to have this form of expression lead to anything else. If one person in a couple is goal-directed . . . and the other person is pleasure-directed . . . problems may occur if they fail to realize their goals or to communicate their goals to their partner. (Whipple, 1999)

Resolution

The **resolution phase**, also referred to as *detumescence* ("reduction in swelling"), is the completion of the cycle when the body returns to its nonaroused state. Typically, this process happens fairly rapidly following orgasm but takes somewhat longer if orgasm has not occurred.

For both sexes, heart rate, blood pressure, and muscle tension drop quickly. The body may be covered with perspiration. If a sexual flush was present, it now fades. Both men and women usually feel relaxed, warm, content, and sleepy. Masters and Johnson (1966) found that if a woman receives additional stimulation following orgasm, she may be capable of returning to the plateau phase and have one or more

resolution phase The fourth and last stage in the EPOR model, during which sexual structures return to their unaroused state; also referred to as *detumescence*.

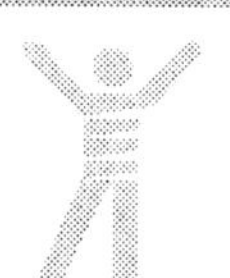

In Touch with Your Sexual Health

The Health Benefits of Orgasm

Recent research has revealed a number of health benefits associated with orgasm. Note that the findings cited here are based primarily on correlational research that has shown a *connection* between orgasm and these health benefits. The extent to which orgasm *causes* the benefit will require additional research.

HEALTH BENEFIT	RESEARCH FINDINGS
General health	An orgasm at least once or twice per week appears to strengthen the immune system's ability to resist flu and other viruses
Pain relief	Some women find that an orgasm's release of hormones and muscle contractions help relieve the pain of menstrual cramps and raise pain tolerance in general
Lower cancer rate	Men who have more than five ejaculations per week during their 20s have a significantly lower rate of prostate cancer later in life
Mood enhancement	Orgasms increase estrogen and endorphins, which tend to improve mood and ward off depression in women
Longer life	Men who have two or more orgasms per week live significantly longer than men who have fewer
Greater feelings of intimacy	The hormone oxytocin, which may play a role in feelings of love and intimacy, increases fivefold at orgasm
Less heart disease	Studies have shown that men who have at least three orgasms per week are 50 percent less likely to die of heart disease
Better sleep	The neurotransmitter dopamine, released during orgasm, triggers a stress-reducing, sleep-inducing response that may last up to two hours
Younger appearance	People who have the most frequent orgasms in conjunction with lovemaking are judged to look younger than their less sexually active counterparts

Sources: Giles et al. (2003); "His and Hers" (2001); Komisaruk and Whipple (1995); Resnick (2002); G. Smith, Frankel, and Yarnell (1997); Weeks & James (1999); Whipple (2000).

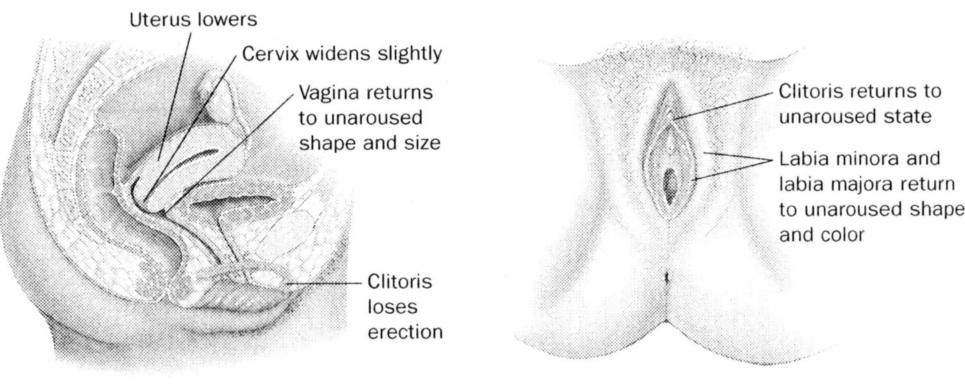

FIGURE 3.10 Physical Changes in the Female during the Resolution Phase

additional orgasms (**multiple orgasms**) without ever entering the resolution phase. We will explore this a bit more in the next section.

For women, blood flows back out of erectile tissues throughout the genitals and breasts. The breasts and areolas diminish in size, and the nipples return to their unerect state. The clitoris resumes its prearousal position and shrinks slightly (see Figure 3.10). The labia minora return to their normal size and position over the vaginal opening. The walls of the vagina relax and fold in on one another. Also, the cervix widens slightly to facilitate the passage of semen into the uterus (assuming heterosexual intercourse) and narrows again about a half hour after orgasm. The uterus drops back down to just above the cervix, where the semen is pooled if ejaculation has occurred in the vagina (Engender Health, 2004).

For men, nipples lose their erection; the penile glans lightens in color, and the penis becomes softer and smaller, returning to its unaroused state. The scrotum relaxes, and the testicles drop down, away from the body (see Figure 3.11). Masters and Johnson found that unlike women, when men enter the resolution phase, they must take a break prior to becoming aroused again and reaching another orgasm. They called this break the **refractory period**. In other words, they contended that men are not capable of multiple orgasms. Depending on a number of factors (including age), the refractory period in men may last anywhere from a few minutes to 24 hours or more (Engender Health, 2004). Masters and Johnson's claim of a refractory period in all men, along with some of their other findings, have been questioned, as we will discuss shortly.

Masters and Johnson's EPOR model is fairly complex. For an overview of the physical changes that accompany the four phases of their model, see Table 3.1.

Erection loss begins
Unstimulated state (erection loss completed)
Testicles descend and return to unstimulated size
Scrotum thins and resumes wrinkled appearance

FIGURE 3.11 Physical Changes in the Male during the Resolution Phase

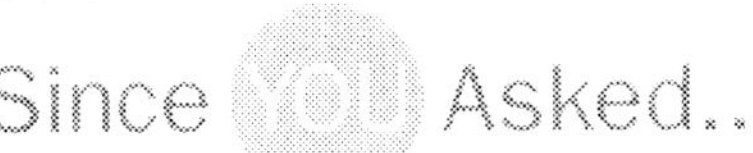

7. I'm a man. After I have an orgasm, I can get another erection pretty fast, but I can't seem to orgasm again. Is this normal or a problem of some kind?

Variations in Orgasm

Masters and Johnson were quite clear in their claim that women are capable of multiple orgasms but men must pass through a refractory period in between orgasms. However, this particular conclusion of theirs has been found to be oversimplified. Several studies have found that some men are capable of experiencing multiple orgasms without loss of erection or a distinct break in between them (Dunn & Trost, 1989; Whipple, Myers, & Komisaruk, 1998). Furthermore, ejaculation does not necessarily occur with each orgasm: Some men may ejaculate with each sequential orgasm, others may have several orgasms and then ejaculate; and some men may ejaculate during the first orgasm and then go on to have more orgasms without ejaculation. It is important to note, however, that the number of documented cases of multiple orgasms in men is quite small, and overall, this phenomenon appears to occur primarily in women (Dunn & Trost, 1989; Whipple

multiple orgasms More than one orgasm at relatively short intervals as sexual stimulation continues without a resolution phase or refractory period in between orgasms.

refractory period A period of time following orgasm when a person is physically unable to become aroused to additional orgasms.

Table 3.1 SUMMARY OF PHYSICAL CHANGES ACCOMPANYING MASTERS AND JOHNSON'S FOUR PHASES OF SEXUAL RESPONSE

STAGE	FEMALE RESPONSE	MALE RESPONSE
Excitement	First sign: vaginal lubrication. Clitoral glans becomes erect. Nipples become erect; breasts enlarge. Vagina increases in length and inner two-thirds of vagina expands.	First sign: erection of penis. Time to erection varies (with person, age, alcohol or drug use, fatigue, stress, etc.). Skin of scrotum pulls up toward body, and testicles rise. Erection may be lost if distracted but is usually regained readily.
Plateau	Outer third of vagina swells, reducing opening by up to 50 percent. Inner two-thirds of vagina continues to balloon or "tent." Clitoris retracts toward body and under hood. Lubrication decreases. Minor lips engorge with blood and darken in color, indicating orgasm is near. Muscle tension and blood pressure increase.	Full erection is attained and is not lost easily if distracted. Corona enlarges further. Cowper's gland secretes pre-ejaculate fluid. Testicles elevate farther and enlarge, indicating orgasm is near. Muscle tension and blood pressure increase.
Orgasm	Begins with rhythmic contractions in pelvic area at intervals of 0.8 second, especially in muscles behind the lower vaginal walls. Uterus contracts rhythmically as well. Muscle tension increases throughout body.	Begins with pelvic contractions 0.8 second apart. Ejaculation, the expelling of semen, occurs in two phases. (1) Emission: Semen builds up in the urethral bulb, producing a sensation of ejaculatory inevitability. (2) Expulsion: Genital muscles contract, forcing semen out through the urethra.
Resolution	Clitoris, uterus, vagina, nipples, etc., return to unaroused state in less than one minute. Clitoris often remains very sensitive to touch for five to ten minutes. This process may take several hours if woman has not experienced an orgasm.	Approximately a 50 percent loss of erection within one minute; more gradual return to fully unaroused state. Testicles reduce in size and descend. Scrotum relaxes.

Source: Adapted from Hock (2005b).

& Komisaruk, 1998). Nevertheless, several books on the market claim to teach men how to have multiple orgasms, but none has been scientifically validated (Chia & Arava, 1997).

On the other hand, although some women may be capable of multiple orgasms during heterosexual intercourse, this ability does not appear to be universal—or universally desired. As mentioned earlier, the majority of women do not routinely have orgasms at all through intercourse exclusively. That said, women who do have multiple orgasms during penile-vaginal intercourse tend to report similar overall levels of sexual satisfaction as those who have single orgasms. In the same vein, most women who have multiple orgasms on some intercourse occasions and single orgasms on others tend to find both experiences equally satisfying. Also, some women may experience multiple orgasms through one type of stimulation, say, masturbation, oral stimulation, or vibrator use, and single orgasms (or no orgasm at all) during heterosexual intercourse (Darling, Davidson, & Jennings, 1991).

The "G-Spot" and Female Ejaculation

Since YOU Asked...

8. I've heard that some women ejaculate like men. Is this true? How is it possible?

Another purported flaw in Masters and Johnson's conclusions involves something that most people take for granted: men ejaculate and women do not. However, beginning in the 1970s, reports began appearing of women who claimed to ejaculate fluid from the urethra upon orgasm. In the early 1980s, new research on women's sexual anatomy claimed to have found (or "rediscovered") a structure linked to the intensity of female orgasm, called the *Grafenberg spot* or **G-spot**, named for Ernst Grafenberg, a physician who first described this structure in the 1950s (Belzer, Whipple, & Moger, 1984). Since 1981, when the findings were first published, the G-spot and female ejaculation have often been linked because many women who report ejaculating also say that stimulation of the G-spot during sexual activity enhances the like-

G-spot An area of tissue on the anterior (upper) wall of the vagina that, when stimulated, causes many women to experience enhanced sexual arousal and more intense orgasms.

lihood of ejaculation during orgasm (Whipple, 2001). The G-spot, as identified in most of the relevant literature, is an area located on the anterior wall of the vagina (the upper wall as the woman lies on her back) about 1 to 2 inches in from the vaginal opening. It is often described as a slightly raised area about the size of a dime that increases in size during sexual stimulation. This spot is often difficult to find, and some women do not perceive that they have one. The easiest way to explore the G-spot is to place one or two fingers inside the vagina and press firmly but gently against the upper wall in a massaging motion (see Figure 3.12). Many women report that when their G-spot is first stroked, they feel a sensation similar to that of having to urinate, but that feeling passes quickly and with continued stimulation is replaced with sexually pleasurable responses.

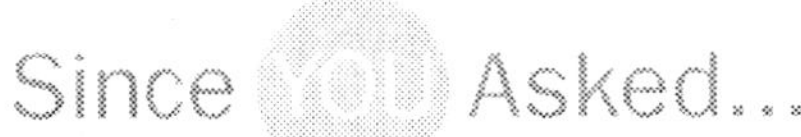

9. Exactly what and where is the "G-spot"? My boyfriend and I can't seem to find it!

The phenomenon of female ejaculation has been the subject of much debate but not much study. The research so far has tried to answer two questions: Do some women truly ejaculate upon orgasm, and if so, what does the female ejaculate consist of?

Many women report that stimulation of the G-spot (usually in conjunction with clitoral stimulation) produces deeper, more intense orgasms, in some cases leading to ejaculation of fluid from the urethra. If semen is produced by the seminal vesicles and prostate gland in men, as we discussed in Chapter 2, then what is it that women ejaculate? This is not yet fully understood, but the debate over the years has been between those who claim that the fluid expelled by women during orgasm is identical to urine (Hines, 2001) and those who argue that it is not urine but something more akin to semen. If it is urine, this leads to the conclusion that the intense muscular activity during orgasm can, in some women, lead to some slight incontinence, in the same way that some people will urinate slightly when laughing too hard. However, several other studies have found that female ejaculate actually resembles male prostatic fluid in chemical composition and is not similar at all to urine (Belzer et al., 1984; Cabello Santamaría, 1997; Whipple & Zaviacic, 1993).

The majority of current thinking on this by most researchers is that female ejaculate is made up mostly of a fluid secreted by two *paraurethral glands* (*para*-means "alongside") that lie on either side of the female urethra, known as **Skene's glands** (see Figure 3.12) (Cabello Santamaría, 1997; Chalker, 2002; Zaviacic, 2002b). In the

Skene's glands In the female, a pair of glands on either side of the urethra that in some women may produce a fluid that is expelled during orgasm; also known as the *paraurethral glands*.

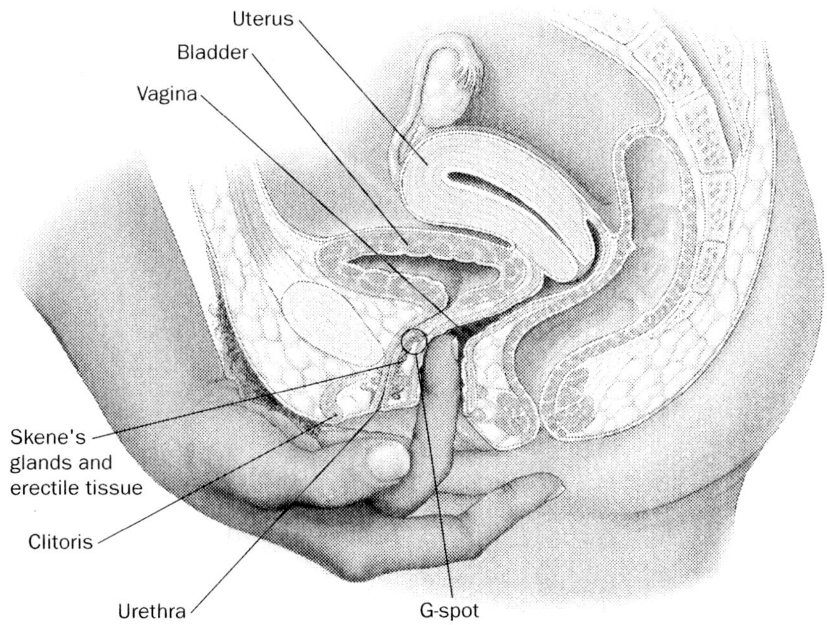

FIGURE 3.12 The G-Spot

Some women report that stimulation of the G-spot enhances sexual arousal. For some women, especially those who have identified a G-spot, ejaculation accompanies orgasm. The fluid is theorized to come from Skene's glands, located along the urethra.

past, these glands were thought to be very small and nonfunctional in humans. However, more recent findings indicate that they are larger, running along the length of the urethra, and are quite active in some women (Zaviacic, 2002b). Because these glands may secrete fluid into the urethra at the moment of orgasm, some researchers are making the case that they may be thought of as a female equivalent, in terms of function, of the prostate gland in males (Whipple, 2002; Zaviacic, 2002a). The purpose of the fluid these glands secrete is unclear. It is expelled through the urethral opening, not the vagina, and does not appear to add significantly to sexual lubrication or enhance the odds of conception. Women who report ejaculating describe the sensation as extremely pleasurable, and researchers are suggesting that sexual pleasure may be the only reason for female ejaculation (Well-Woman, 2001).

It is important to note that not all women ejaculate, nor do most women who do not ejaculate particularly care about it. Studies have indicated that about 40 percent of women report being aware of ejaculation during orgasm (Darling, Davidson, & Conway-Welch, 1990; Zaviacic et al., 1988). Furthermore, women who ejaculate are no more satisfied overall with their sexual lives than those who do not (Darling et al., 1990). Lack of ejaculation is not a sign *in any way* that a woman is somehow deficient in her sexual responses, and female ejaculation should not be seen by women or their partners as a goal in sexual interactions. It is just one more example of how men and women, who seem so sexually differentiated on many levels, may be more similar physiologically than we ever realized.

Alternatives to Masters and Johnson

Although Masters and Johnson's EPOR model of sexual response has formed the foundation for discussions and explanations of human sexual responding, it has not been without its critics and several competing conceptualizations. Criticisms have included the contention that Masters and Johnson neglected emotional components of sexuality, especially desire; that any valid conceptualization of human sexual response must emerge from psychological interpretations of sexuality, rather then purely physical reactions; and that the EPOR model was far too *androcentric*—that is, it relies too heavily on a one-size-fits-all male sexual response and fails to acknowledge many fundamental differences in female sexuality. In this section, we will explore each of these criticisms and some of the alternative theories that have been proposed. One popular alternative was developed in the 1970s, about ten years after Masters and Johnson's EPOR model was published; another began to make its way into the literature in the 1990s; and a third, focusing on women's sexual problems, is currently emerging and encouraging new discussion and debate.

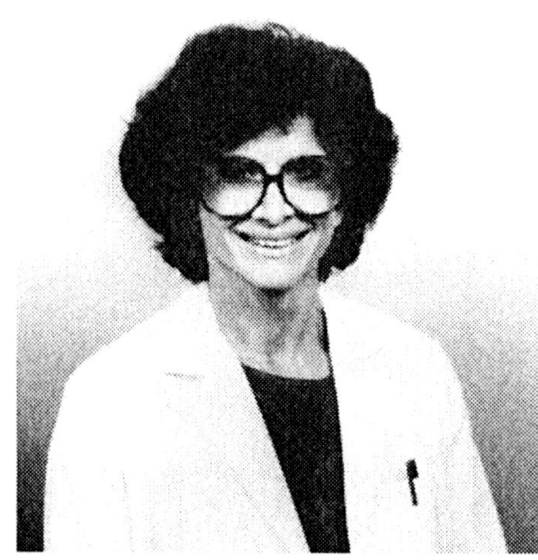

Helen Singer Kaplan (1929–1995) added the stage of desire *to human sexual response cycle.*

Kaplan's Three-Stage Model An alternative to Masters and Johnson's EPOR model of human sexual response developed by Helen Singer Kaplan that features the three stages of desire, excitement, and orgasm.

Kaplan's Three-Stage Model of Sexual Response

Helen Singer Kaplan (1929–1995) followed in the footsteps of Masters and Johnson in developing many effective forms of sexual therapy and became one of the best-known sex therapists in the world. She published numerous books designed to help people enjoy sexually satisfying lives, including *The New Sex Therapy: Active Treatment of Sexual Dysfunctions* (1974) and *The Sexual Desire Disorders: Dysfunctional Regulation of Sexual Motivation* (1995). Her approach to sexual response mirrored that of Masters and Johnson, but she felt they had left out one crucial factor and had divided the response process into too many rigid, sequential stages. Kaplan proposed a more fluid model consisting of *desire*, *excitement*, and *orgasm* that is known as **Kaplan's Three-Stage Model** (see Figure 3.13).

Kaplan argued that sexual responding is unlikely unless someone wants to be sexual; therefore, she conceived that the first stage of sexual response is *desire*. Because of her focus on sex therapy, she also jettisoned Masters and Johnson's notions of plateau and resolution from her theory. Kaplan interpreted the plateau phase as simply a part of excitement; and resolution, while it obviously occurs, rarely poses any sexual problems and is therefore of minimal clinical interest. By contrast, difficulties with *sexual desire*, called *inhibited* or **hypoactive sexual desire** are extremely common (this disorder and Kaplan's contributions are discussed in greater detail in Chapter 7, "Sexual Problems and Solutions"). According to Kaplan, among the many factors that may interfere with sexual desire are stress, fatigue, depression, pain, fear, prescribed medication, recreational drugs, negative past sexual experiences, power and control issues in a relationship, loss of interest in a partner, low self-image, and hormonal influences. By adding desire at the beginning of the stages and streamlining the sexual response cycle, Kaplan's Three-Stage Model became a popular alternative approach to Masters and Johnson's EPOR model for understanding, evaluating, and treating problems with sexual responding.

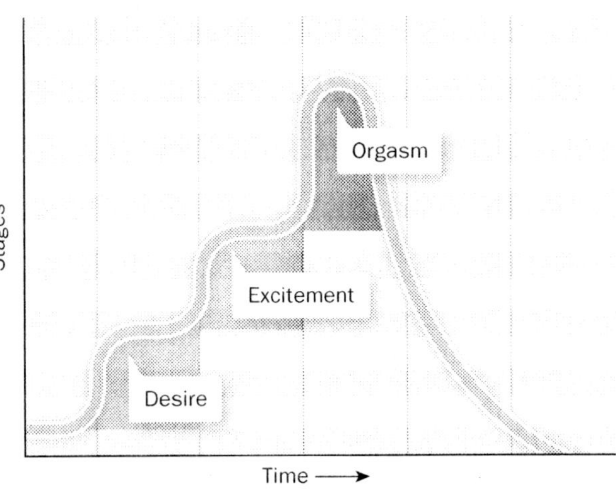

FIGURE 3.13 Kaplan's Three Stage Model of Sexual Response

Over time, some of Kaplan's notions about human sexual response have been criticized for being overly simplified and for making the assumption that desire must always be present for sexual responding to occur. Some individuals and couples find that even if they are lacking in sexual desire initially, as they begin to engage in sexual activity, desire may awaken and flow out of the sexual behavior rather than necessarily preceding it.

Reed's Erotic Stimulus Pathway Theory

Psychiatrist David Reed has taken the popular theories of Masters and Johnson and Kaplan and reinterpreted them from a more psychological and interpersonal perspective that he calls the **Erotic Stimulus Pathway Theory** (Greenberg, Bruess, & Haffner, 2002). He has labeled his four stages using the more psychological terms *seduction*, *sensations*, *surrender*, and *reflection* (see Figure 3.14). His first stage, *seduction*, corresponds to Kaplan's desire stage, but in Reed's model, desire is created by the behaviors people engage in that they believe will attract another person and make themselves sexually attractive to others. These rituals may include wearing cologne and perfumes, using makeup, dressing in alluring ways, flirting, making eye contact, touching, sending love notes, buying flowers, arranging dates, engaging in self-disclosure, and signaling a desire for sex.

The seduction behaviors then move into the *sensation* phase, when sexual behavior and sexual arousal begin (akin to excitement and plateau in the EPOR model). Reed suggests that during this phase, our heightened senses, fantasy, and imagination combine to feed the arousal and motivate us to make it continue. Reed conceptualizes the peak of sexual arousal, orgasm, as a giving over of oneself, a *surrender*, as he calls it, to the culmination of sexual intimacy.

hypoactive sexual desire A loss or lack of sexual desire; also known as *inhibited sexual desire*.

Erotic Stimulus Pathway Theory A model of human sexual response based on the psychological and cognitive stages of seduction, sensations, surrender, and reflection.

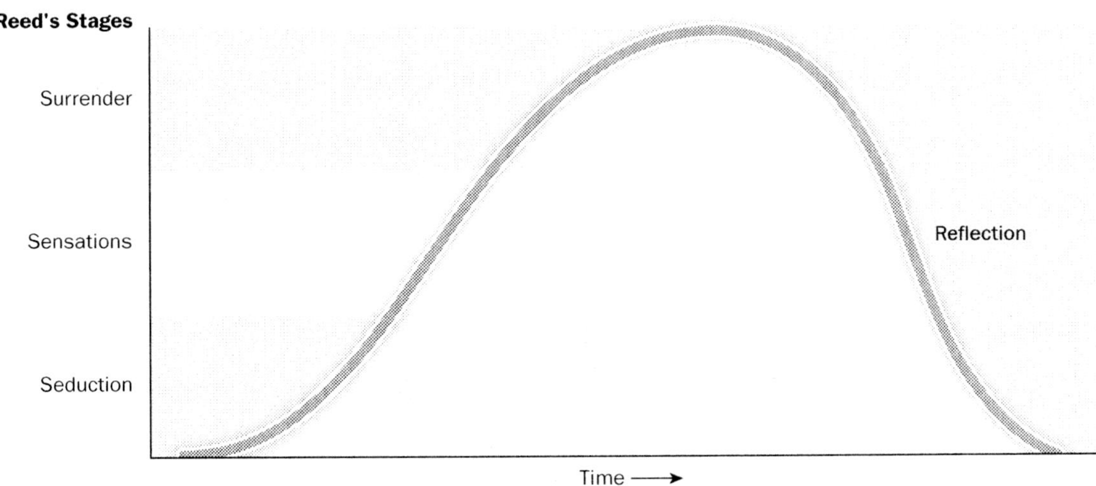

FIGURE 3.14 Reed's Erotic Stimulus Pathway Model

Finally, Reed proposes that the after-orgasm phase is a time when both partners reflect on the experience and bring meaning to it. The importance of the *reflection* phase is that it provides an opportunity for partners to interpret the sexual encounter in positive or negative terms, and this helps us make choices about whether or not to engage in the activity again, under the same circumstances or with the same partner.

Although Reed's Erotic Stimulus Pathway model reflects Masters and Johnson's and Kaplan's stages, the focus in each phase is placed on the cognitive and psychological, rather than on or in addition to the physical. A great deal of current thinking about human sexual response is slowly yielding to a more holistic approach to understanding the complexities of human sexual responding. In this vein, some researchers are suggesting that male and female sexual responses are significantly less similar than the traditional EPOR model implies. In general, this view contends that the Masters and Johnson model applies reasonably well to male sexual response, but to understand *female* sexual response, we must consider a range of different factors.

A "New View" of Women's Sexual Response

Since YOU Asked...

10. I've heard that there is a new pill for women that works like Viagra for men. Is this true? What does it do?

In 2000, a new approach to understanding female sexual problems was developed by a working group of 12 women scientists, researchers, and clinicians. Out of this collaboration has come a new conceptualization of female sexual responding in general, explained in a joint statement proclaiming a "**new view of women's sexual problems**" (FSD Alert, 2000; Tiefer, 2001). This *manifesto*, as it is referred to by the authors, emerged as a response to the increasing trend to "medicalize" sexual problems, to view them as illnesses and treat them with drugs. The best-known examples of this trend are reflected in the widespread use of Viagra, Cialis, and Levitra, all drugs for the treatment of male impotence.

Because sexual problems tend to be viewed by the medical and pharmaceutical communities through the lens of Masters and Johnson's EPOR model, attention is now focused on a new pill, sometimes referred to as "pink Viagra," to enhance women's sexual response. Because of this trend, the "new view" working group and other researchers who had previously argued against the validity of the EPOR model for women felt an urgency to differentiate between male and female sexual responding. They contend that the EPOR model reduces sexual responding to mere physiological processes similar to breathing or digestion when in reality women's sexuality is far too complex to be "fixed" with a pill. The manifesto contends that "women's accounts do not fit neatly into the Masters and Johnson model; for example, women generally do not separate 'desire' from 'arousal,' [and] women care less about physical than [about] subjective arousal" (Tiefer, 2001, p. 93). The document goes on to what the authors considered to be the most serious flaws in applying the traditional Masters and Johnson model to women (FSD Alert, 2000):

1. *The incorrect assumption that male and female sexuality are fundamentally the same.* As you may remember from earlier in this chapter, the four-stage model assumes many similarities between men's and women's responses, so sex therapists and researchers have tended to assume that their sexual problems must be similar as well.
2. *An exaggerated focus on physiology of sexual response to the exclusion of the relationship context in which it occurs.* This focus has led to assumptions that sexual response can be understood and enhanced without regard for the larger issues of the interpersonal sexual relationship.
3. *The minimization of individual differences in sexual responding among women.* The working group proposed that women vary more than men do in their sexual responses and therefore do not fit neatly into the desire-arousal-plateau-orgasm pattern.

New view of women's sexual problems A model of female sexual response incorporating a larger variety of factors than previous models, including physical, cognitive, social, and relationships issues.

Finally, Reed proposes that the after-orgasm phase is a time when both partners reflect on the experience and bring meaning to it. The importance of the *reflection* phase is that it provides an opportunity for partners to interpret the sexual encounter in positive or negative terms, and this helps us make choices about whether or not to engage in the activity again, under the same circumstances or with the same partner.

Although Reed's Erotic Stimulus Pathway model reflects Masters and Johnson's and Kaplan's stages, the focus in each phase is placed on the cognitive and psychological, rather than on or in addition to the physical. A great deal of current thinking about human sexual response is slowly yielding to a more holistic approach to understanding the complexities of human sexual responding. In this vein, some researchers are suggesting that male and female sexual responses are significantly less similar than the traditional EPOR model implies. In general, this view contends that the Masters and Johnson model applies reasonably well to male sexual response, but to understand *female* sexual response, we must consider a range of different factors.

A "New View" of Women's Sexual Response

Since YOU Asked...

10. I've heard that there is a new pill for women that works like Viagra for men. Is this true? What does it do?

In 2000, a new approach to understanding female sexual problems was developed by a working group of 12 women scientists, researchers, and clinicians. Out of this collaboration has come a new conceptualization of female sexual responding in general, explained in a joint statement proclaiming a "**new view of women's sexual problems**" (FSD Alert, 2000; Tiefer, 2001). This *manifesto*, as it is referred to by the authors, emerged as a response to the increasing trend to "medicalize" sexual problems, to view them as illnesses and treat them with drugs. The best-known examples of this trend are reflected in the widespread use of Viagra, Cialis, and Levitra, all drugs for the treatment of male impotence.

Because sexual problems tend to be viewed by the medical and pharmaceutical communities through the lens of Masters and Johnson's EPOR model, attention is now focused on a new pill, sometimes referred to as "pink Viagra," to enhance women's sexual response. Because of this trend, the "new view" working group and other researchers who had previously argued against the validity of the EPOR model for women felt an urgency to differentiate between male and female sexual responding. They contend that the EPOR model reduces sexual responding to mere physiological processes similar to breathing or digestion when in reality women's sexuality is far too complex to be "fixed" with a pill. The manifesto contends that "women's accounts do not fit neatly into the Masters and Johnson model; for example, women generally do not separate 'desire' from 'arousal,' [and] women care less about physical than [about] subjective arousal" (Tiefer, 2001, p. 93). The document goes on to what the authors considered to be the most serious flaws in applying the traditional Masters and Johnson model to women (FSD Alert, 2000):

1. *The incorrect assumption that male and female sexuality are fundamentally the same.* As you may remember from earlier in this chapter, the four-stage model assumes many similarities between men's and women's responses, so sex therapists and researchers have tended to assume that their sexual problems must be similar as well.
2. *An exaggerated focus on physiology of sexual response to the exclusion of the relationship context in which it occurs.* This focus has led to assumptions that sexual response can be understood and enhanced without regard for the larger issues of the interpersonal sexual relationship.
3. *The minimization of individual differences in sexual responding among women.* The working group proposed that women vary more than men do in their sexual responses and therefore do not fit neatly into the desire-arousal-plateau-orgasm pattern.

New view of women's sexual problems A model of female sexual response incorporating a larger variety of factors than previous models, including physical, cognitive, social, and relationships issues.

resolution, while it obviously occurs, rarely poses any sexual problems and is therefore of minimal clinical interest. By contrast, difficulties with *sexual desire*, called *inhibited* or **hypoactive sexual desire** are extremely common (this disorder and Kaplan's contributions are discussed in greater detail in Chapter 7, "Sexual Problems and Solutions"). According to Kaplan, among the many factors that may interfere with sexual desire are stress, fatigue, depression, pain, fear, prescribed medication, recreational drugs, negative past sexual experiences, power and control issues in a relationship, loss of interest in a partner, low self-image, and hormonal influences. By adding desire at the beginning of the stages and streamlining the sexual response cycle, Kaplan's Three-Stage Model became a popular alternative approach to Masters and Johnson's EPOR model for understanding, evaluating, and treating problems with sexual responding.

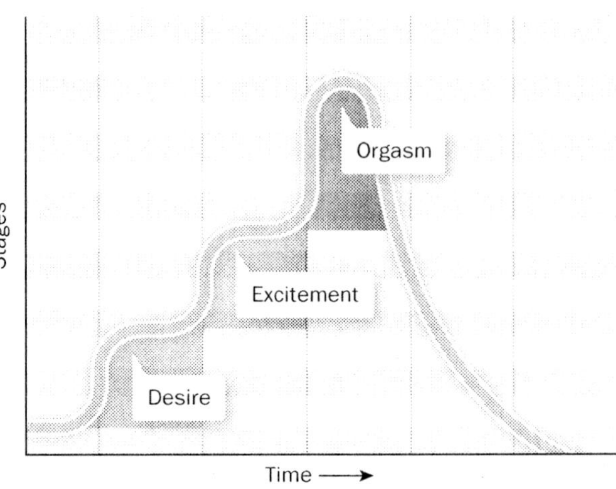

FIGURE 3.13 Kaplan's Three Stage Model of Sexual Response

Over time, some of Kaplan's notions about human sexual response have been criticized for being overly simplified and for making the assumption that desire must always be present for sexual responding to occur. Some individuals and couples find that even if they are lacking in sexual desire initially, as they begin to engage in sexual activity, desire may awaken and flow out of the sexual behavior rather than necessarily preceding it.

Reed's Erotic Stimulus Pathway Theory

Psychiatrist David Reed has taken the popular theories of Masters and Johnson and Kaplan and reinterpreted them from a more psychological and interpersonal perspective that he calls the **Erotic Stimulus Pathway Theory** (Greenberg, Bruess, & Haffner, 2002). He has labeled his four stages using the more psychological terms *seduction*, *sensations*, *surrender*, and *reflection* (see Figure 3.14). His first stage, *seduction*, corresponds to Kaplan's desire stage, but in Reed's model, desire is created by the behaviors people engage in that they believe will attract another person and make themselves sexually attractive to others. These rituals may include wearing cologne and perfumes, using makeup, dressing in alluring ways, flirting, making eye contact, touching, sending love notes, buying flowers, arranging dates, engaging in self-disclosure, and signaling a desire for sex.

The seduction behaviors then move into the *sensation* phase, when sexual behavior and sexual arousal begin (akin to excitement and plateau in the EPOR model). Reed suggests that during this phase, our heightened senses, fantasy, and imagination combine to feed the arousal and motivate us to make it continue. Reed conceptualizes the peak of sexual arousal, orgasm, as a giving over of oneself, a *surrender*, as he calls it, to the culmination of sexual intimacy.

hypoactive sexual desire A loss or lack of sexual desire; also known as *inhibited sexual desire*.

Erotic Stimulus Pathway Theory A model of human sexual response based on the psychological and cognitive stages of seduction, sensations, surrender, and reflection.

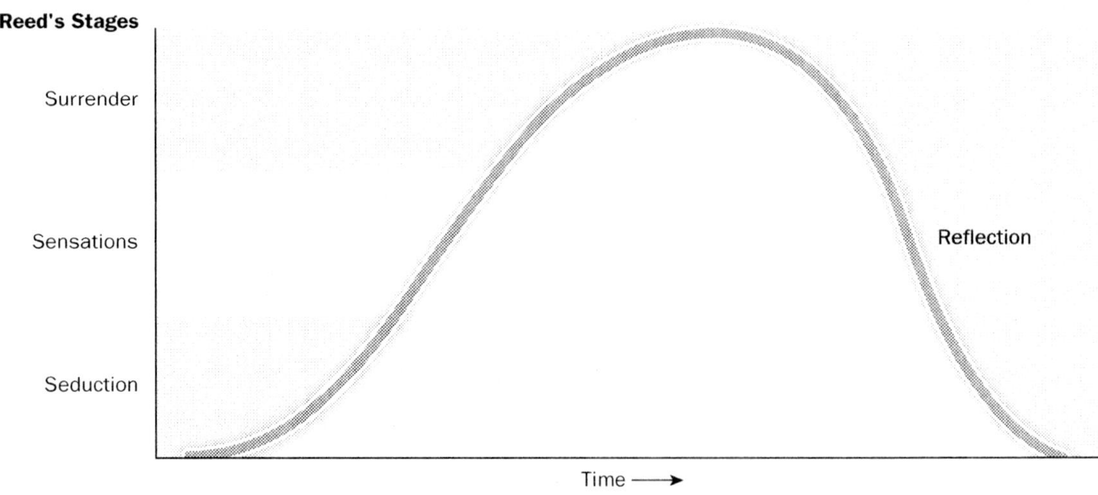

FIGURE 3.14 Reed's Erotic Stimulus Pathway Model

How do the members of the working group propose to overcome the difficulties they see in past and current thinking about female sexuality? Here is their proposal from the manifesto:

> We propose a new and more useful classification of women's sexual problems, one that gives appropriate priority to individual distress and inhibition arising within a broader framework of cultural and relational factors. . . . We call for research and services driven not by commercial interests but by women's own needs and sexual realities. (FSD Alert, 2000; Teifer, 2001, p. 94)

More specifically, they suggest that women's sexuality, sexual response, and sexual difficulties require a radical revision of classification that takes into account cultural, political, and economic factors (i.e., lack of sexuality education or access to contraception); a woman's partner and the relationship between them (i.e., fear of abuse, imbalance of power, overall discord); psychological factors (i.e., past sexual trauma, depression, anxiety); and medical factors (i.e., hormonal imbalances, sexually transmitted infections, medication side effects) (C. Graham, 2003). This approach to women's sexuality will be discussed further in Chapter 7, "Sexual Problems and Solutions".

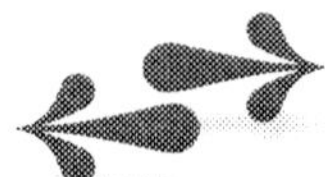

YOUR SEXUAL PHILOSOPHY
THE PHYSIOLOGY OF HUMAN SEXUAL RESPONDING

You can see how theories, approaches, and practices relating to the physiology of human sexual response continue to evolve and change over time. These changes stimulate discussion, debate, and research. Although studying the various theories, both old and new, can be confusing at times, this variety is beneficial to the overall study of human sexuality. It requires researchers and clinicians to stay alert and active in their fields and, in the final analysis, enriches our understanding of the complexities of humans as sexual beings.

As noted at the beginning of this chapter, your knowledge of sexual anatomy from Chapter 2 is of little use without also understanding how that anatomy functions. Consequently, Chapters 2 and 3 go hand in hand to provide you with the foundation for understanding the human sexual body. You will probably find that you will be looking back at these discussions as you read the remaining chapters in this book. In fact, before moving on to our discussion of love, intimacy, and sexual communication in Chapter 4, take a look at Table 3.2, which offers some hints about how the material you've learned in Chapters 2 and 3 applies to the topics in the remaining chapters.

With this in mind, you can see how developing a clear understanding of human sexual responding is a central feature in your sexual philosophy. Moreover, this understanding helps extend your knowledge of sexual anatomy to enhance sexual satisfaction and enjoyment. Your philosophical commitment to developing an awareness of how the human body typically reacts to sexual stimulation will allow you to become more aware of your own body's responses and acquire a greater sensitivity to your partner's responses. This knowledge, in turn, will allow you to communicate more clearly about sexual issues with a partner or health care professional and will enhance sexual intimacy, enjoyment, and satisfaction throughout your life.

At the beginning of this chapter, we noted that a basic understanding of sexual anatomy is connected to how your body functions during sexual stimulation. Sexual functioning, or *response*, is in turn intertwined with your sexual activities, sexual pleasure, and sexual intimacy. An appreciation of and familiarity with human sexual response is fundamental to living a satisfied and healthy sexual life. That is what your sexual philosophy is all about—knowing who you are as a sexual person, what you want and don't want sexually, and planning ahead for a fulfilling sexual life.

Table 3.2 APPLICATION OF MATERIAL IN CHAPTERS 2 AND 3 TO OTHER TEXT CHAPTERS

CHAPTER	APPLICATION OF KNOWLEDGE OF SEXUAL ANATOMY AND RESPONSE
Chapter 4, "Love, Intimacy, and Sexual Communication"	Effective communication about love and sex often requires an awareness and understanding of your own and your partner's anatomy and how you and your partner respond to each other sexually.
Chapter 5, "Contraception: Planning and Preventing Pregnancy"	Choosing an effective method of birth control for yourself and, more important, using it correctly require a working knowledge of anatomy, hormones, and how the body responds during sexual arousal.
Chapter 6, "Sexual Behaviors: Experiencing Sexual Pleasure"	Developing an awareness of the sexual body will allow you to become more aware of your own body's responses and acquire a greater sensitivity to your partner's responses as well.
Chapter 7, "Sexual Problems and Solutions"	Many sexual difficulties are caused or exacerbated by a basic lack of understanding of sexual anatomy and sexual response.
Chapter 8, "Sexually Transmitted Infections"	Knowing how STIs are transmitted and how to identify the symptoms relies on your familiarity with sexual anatomical structures.
Chapter 9, "Conception, Pregnancy, and Birth"	Virtually every topic of discussion on sexual anatomy and response relates to how conception occurs, the process of pregnancy, and the birth of a baby.
Chapter 10, "Gender: Expectations, Roles, and Behaviors"	Expectations about certain anatomical structures and about male and female sexual response play a significant role in gender roles and expectations.
Chapter 11, "Sexual Orientation"	When studying sexual orientation, it is very important to understand that a satisfying, healthy sexual life is the goal of nearly everyone, regardless of sexual orientation. A knowledge of anatomy and response helps all of us achieve this.
Chapter 12, "Sexual Development throughout Life"	Understanding and appreciating the physical side of sexual development from childhood through old age requires a clear understanding of the anatomical and sexual response changes that occur normally throughout our lives.
Chapter 13, "Sexual Aggression and Violence: Rape, Child Sexual Abuse, and Harassment"	Understanding what constitutes sexual violence and aggression and its aftereffects often requires a clear conception of sexual anatomy and physiology.
Chapter 14, "The Paraphilias: The Extremes of Sexual Behavior"	When studying these unusual sexual behaviors, it often helps to know how they affect the sexual responding and functioning of the people engaging in them.
Chapter 15, "The Sexual Marketplace: Prostitution and Pornography"	How erotica and pornography are defined involves issues of sexual anatomy and response, as does an understanding of the activities and dangers of prostitution.
Epilogue, "Exploring Your Sexual Philosophy"	A knowledge of sexual anatomy and sexual responding forms the foundation for virtually everything in your sexual philosophy of life.

Summary

HISTORICAL PERSPECTIVES Sexual Pioneers

- Although surveys had previously shed light on people's self-reported sexual activities, it was the pioneering studies of Masters and Johnson in the 1960s that revealed much of the physiological functioning of the human body during and after sexual activity.

Biology, Psychology, and Human Sexual Responding

- It is the psychological aspects of human sexuality that primarily differentiate humans from nonhuman animals in sexual functioning and behavior. Although biological factors play important roles in the sexual functioning of all animals, human sexual desire and activity are at least as strongly influenced by psychological forces such as feeling pleasure, giving pleasure, expressing feeling of closeness and love, relieving stress, feeling valued by another person, and expressing how much another person is valued.
- Many people mistakenly equate "sex" with sexual intercourse. However, human sexual responding, from a physical perspective, follows similar patterns for all kinds of sexual behavior including a man and a woman having intercourse, a man and a woman sharing manual or oral sex, a same-sex couple making love, an individual masturbating, or even an erotic dream.

Masters and Johnson: The Excitement-Plateau-Orgasm-Resolution Model

- Masters and Johnson's conceptualization of four phases—excitement, plateau, orgasm, and resolution (EPOR)—continues to dominate research and discussions about sexual physiology. It suggests that men and women typically proceed through these four predictable stages of response. Over the decades since Masters and Johnson first proposed their theory, various exceptions to their findings have been suggested, but the EPOR model continues to provide a valuable framework for discussions on human sexual responding.
- The excitement and plateau phases involve a building of sexual arousal. During these stages, the penis and clitoris become erect, the clitoral glans withdraws under the clitoral hood, the Cowper's glands in men secrete pre-ejaculate fluid (which may contain live sperm cells or sexually transmitted infectious microbes).
- A common myth of sexual responding in humans is that both partners should achieve orgasm during heterosexual intercourse. However, research has demonstrated that most women do not routinely reach orgasm through intercourse exclusively, no matter how long it lasts, and require additional genital stimulation for orgasm.
- Masters and Johnson claimed that women, but not men, are capable of multiple orgasms and that men, but not women, are capable of ejaculation. However, newer research has found that some men are able to experience multiple orgasms and some women ejaculate upon orgasm.
- Although the existence, structure, and function of the G-spot remains embroiled in controversy, many women find that stimulation of the G-spot during sexual activity enhances and deepens the sensation of orgasm and, for some, leads to ejaculation.
- Variations in the physiology of orgasm may exist between men and women, but their subjective descriptions and perceptions of their orgasms appear to be quite similar.
- Numerous health benefits of orgasm are theorized. Various studies have suggested that orgasm, either with a partner or through masturbation, may provide many health benefits, from reduced cancer risk to pain reduction and even to an increased life span.

Alternatives to Masters and Johnson

- Several variations and alternatives have been proposed to Masters and Johnson's EPOR model of sexual response.
- Helen Singer Kaplan's Three-Stage Model is designed to apply more closely to treating sexual problems than the EPOR model. It adds the pre-excitement stage of desire and drops the stages of plateau and resolution.
- David Reed's Erotic Stimulus Pathway model of sexual response takes a more emotional and psychological approach, focusing on the emotional experiences of *seduction*, *sensations*, *surrender*, and *reflection* during sexual responding.
- A recent theory known as the new view of women's sexual problems seeks to redefine the sexual responses of women as fundamentally distinct from those of men and argues that a one-size-fits-all approach to human sexual responding is an invalid approach.

YOUR SEXUAL PHILOSOPHY: The Physiology of Human Sexual Responding

- Familiarity with human sexual anatomy and response is crucial for understanding the complexities of human sexuality. The information contained in this chapter, along with the material in Chapter 2, "Sexual Anatomy" lays the foundation for appreciating and understanding the topics throughout this book and for applying them in meaningful ways to your life and your sexual fulfillment. Your sexual philosophy is about knowing who you are, what you want and don't want, and planning ahead for a fulfilling sexual life.

Have You Considered?

1. Would you ever volunteer to be a participant in a study such as Masters and Johnson's research in the 1960s? Why or why not? Discuss your opinion about the ethics of such research.
2. Explain why many women do not routinely experience orgasm during heterosexual intercourse.
3. What are the three similarities and three differences between male and female sexual response that you believe are the most important? Explain your answers.
4. Discuss your opinions of and reactions to the topic of female ejaculation.
5. Which of the various models of human sexual response discussed in the chapter do you feel is most accurate? Which seems most questionable to you? Explain your answers.
6. In your opinion, what is the most important reason for people to study and understand the process of human sexual responding? Why?
7. Which of the various models of human sexual response do you feel best describes what really happens? By combining any of the components of the various models and adding any features of your own that you feel are missing, design a new model of human sexual response. Explain why you think your design is better.
8. For many couples, the goal of lovemaking is orgasm. Why do some sex researchers and therapists claim that this detracts from a satisfying sexual experience?

Companion Website Resources

For further chapter resources go to **www.prenhall.com/hock.** This robust text website includes polling questions for you to vote on, regular news updates, quizzes, sample tests, suggested reading lists, and more.

SCENARIOS USA Also on the website are links to videos. *Scenarios USA*'s films portray real-life narratives that explore the non-biological aspects of relationships and sexual health. The films will help you consider how the themes of the text affect your own life and the lives of those around you.

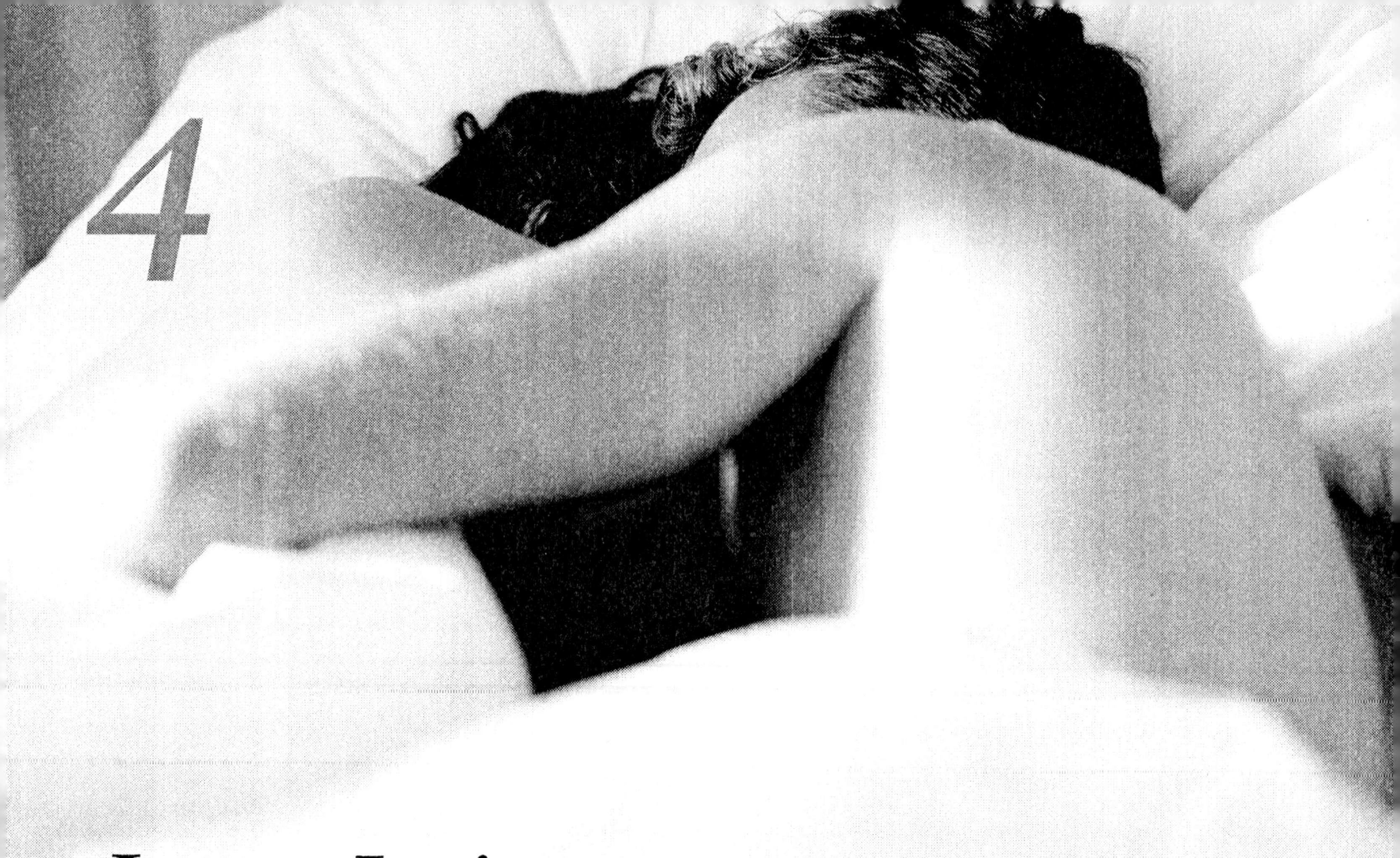

4

Love, Intimacy, and Sexual Communication

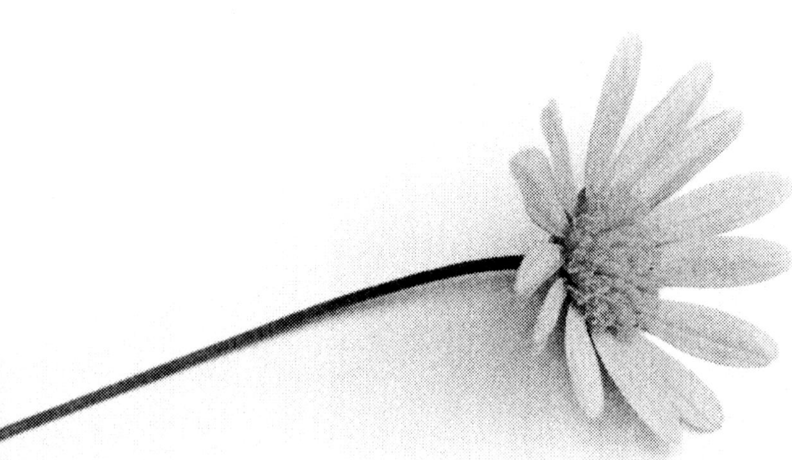

Since YOU Asked...

1. My boyfriend and I broke up almost a year ago, but I haven't been able to get involved with anyone since. In fact, I don't even like most of the guys I've met. What's going on? (see page 98)
2. My girlfriend (of two months) and I are very different. We disagree and argue about politics, religion, and nearly everything else. Is this going to be a problem, or is it true that opposites attract? (see page 102)
3. I feel I love my partner far more than he loves me. Is there some way to get him to love me more? (see page 106)
4. Why do people cheat? Is it because they just need a new conquest? (see page 108)
5. When a couple is having sex on a regular basis, does the emotional side fade or grow over time? Does it mean the relationship is not going well if it is just for the physical release? (see page 112)
6. How do you know when things are going wrong or if things are right between you and your partner? (see page 115)
7. My partner and I fight a lot. We yell at each other, and sometimes one of us will storm out of the house for several hours. But we love each other very much and are totally committed to each other. Is this normal? (see page 119)
8. Why is it so difficult to explain what does and does not feel good sexually? (see page 125)
9. How can I get my girlfriend to trust me? She's jealous all the time, and accuses me of cheating when I'm not doing anything. She's convinced I don't love her, but I do—I think. (see page 129)
10. Can someone who has been in an abusive relationship ever have a normal relationship again? Is it really possible to forgive and forget? (see page 137)

For most people, sexual behavior, love, and intimacy are closely linked. Research has shown that the most physically and emotionally satisfying sexual interactions occur in the context of a long-term, committed romantic relationship (Hill, 2002; Sprecher, 2002). We all know or have heard about people who are comfortable engaging in casual sex, without the need for any deep emotional investment, but these individuals appear to be the exception rather than the rule. One national survey conducted in the 1990s found that over 65 percent of respondents said they would not have sex with someone unless they were in love with that person (Michael et al., 1994). When people choose to engage in casual sex, such as "hooking up" at a party or participating in sexually permissive social settings during spring break, most will readily admit that someday they want a more meaningful emotional context for their sexual lives.

Sex, love, and intimate communication usually go hand in hand, and we would have difficulty separating them even if we wanted to, which we do not. In this chapter, we will focus on the emotional and relationship issues that typically surround sexual behaviors rather than on the behaviors themselves. This is not to say that we ignore the emotional side of sexuality in the other chapters in this book; the connection between sexual behavior and emotional reactions is apparent throughout this text. Even in Chapter 2, "Sexual Anatomy," the most biologically based chapter in the book, many of the topics are infused with references to emotions and attitudes. In this chapter, however, the emotional and interpersonal components of human sexuality, the good and the bad, will be our primary themes.

We will discuss the factors involved in early intimacy and love relationships. We will then turn to the meaning of love, exploring how intimacy and commitment between partners grows over time, how sex and intimacy intertwine, and how love relationships change as time goes on. We will consider what many people would say is the most important component of love relationships: communication. We will also explore factors involved in the decline and ending of romantic relationships and take a clear-eyed look at the tragedy and terror of abuse and violence in intimate relationships. As odd as it may sound to many of you to discuss relationship abuse and violence in a chapter on love and intimacy, it is important that we do so. Sometimes what begins as a seemingly loving, wonderful relationship turns controlling, abusive, and violent in ways that make escaping from the abusive partner extremely difficult. One effective way to prevent this from happening to you or to others you know is to learn as much as possible about these abusive relationships, which virtually never end happily. Finally, we will look at how all these issues fit into your sexual philosophy.

As we begin our journey though the complexities of love, intimacy, and sexual communication, ask yourself these questions: Are love and romance timeless processes that

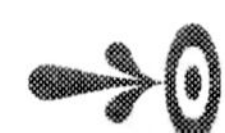

Focus on Your Feelings

In a way, this chapter is *all* about feelings. Many of you, as you read through its varied and complex topics relating to love, intimacy, and passion, may experience a wide range of emotional responses. Why? Because, most of you either are or have been in an intimate relationship, and some of you may have experienced more than one. Therefore, at least some of the issues discussed in this chapter are likely to be familiar to you—in some cases, perhaps too familiar.

If nothing else, this chapter is likely to make you think about past, present, and future love relationships. It is difficult to read this chapter without holding your own up for comparison to see how they fare. You may find yourself transported back to past relationships that were, in retrospect, mismatched, unhealthy, or even abusive. The frustration and pain of those relationships may be reactivated as you read this chapter. If this happens, you should know that it is a normal reaction to the memory of an unhealthy relationship and perhaps provides an opportunity for you to work through some of those lingering negative emotions. On the other hand, some of you may feel compelled to face suspicions you have about your current relationship. However, many of you, if not most of you, will find validation and confirmation that your current love relationship, if you are in one, is strong and healthy.

Regardless of where this chapter leads you emotionally, it should help you sort out and better understand your feelings about your romantic relationships. Keep in mind that love relationships are not easy; in fact, they are probably the most complex and mysterious of all human connections. However, through your basic awareness, sensitivity, and insight, combined with the knowledge and understanding of the issues discussed in this chapter, they can also be the most wondrous and rewarding.

flow naturally from human nature? Or are they products of the influence of time and culture? Let's take a glimpse back to love and romance in early colonial America by asking the question, how did George and Martha "hook up"?

Historical Perspectives

George and Martha in Love and Marriage

How different are love and relationships today compared to, say, in the years approaching U.S. independence? If you said very different, you would be correct. For one thing, marriage agreements "in the old days" were often arranged between the potential bride's and groom's fathers, not the couple themselves. A "good match" was considered one that increased the wealth of both families, through the professional "prospects" of the young man to earn a good living and the young woman's dowry, usually money, land, or other property given to the groom's parents in exchange for "allowing" the woman to marry their son. With all that out of the way, the "courtship" could begin.

And once begun, courting tended to move quickly to marriage. This was due in part to the fact that life expectancy was significantly shorter in the 1700s (only about 35 or 40 years on average), so if a couple did not marry relatively young and begin a family, they could end up courting for their entire lives (Dugan, 2001). Unmarried women acquired the dubious status of unmarriageable "old maid" between the ages of 22 and 27; and in many of the colonies, unmarried men were forced to pay a "bachelorhood tax."

One method for hurrying the courtship process along was a practice called *bundling*, in which the "engaged" couple was allowed, and even encouraged, by both sets of parents to sleep in the same bed on a regular basis in one of their homes. Before you think how awesome and open-minded of your ancestors, there were restrictions: The couple must be fully clothed and were sometimes actually sewn into their respective bedding, with a board placed vertically between them. The idea here was to allow long stretches of time, sometimes all night, for couples to talk and become emotionally intimate relatively quickly. Nothing of a sexual nature was allowed. Bundling as an integral part of courtship was practiced in New England for nearly a century until it was noticed (especially by the clergy) that many babies were being born much sooner than nine months after the couple married. As a result, bundling fell out of favor.

No evidence exists that George Washington and Martha Custis bundled before they married. However, they did have what today would be considered a whirlwind romance (Dugan, 2001). They became engaged after meeting only twice, for a total of about 20 hours. George had had two previous unrequited amorous attractions to women. Martha was a 26-year-old widow, something quite common in those years, when men could die early due to battle injuries or infections. However, it is said that she was one of the most sought-after women in Virginia, owing largely to her much desired dowry of 17,000 acres of prime tobacco farmland.

George and Martha Washington's wedding at Mount Vernon, Virginia, though a major social event, was primarily a marriage of convenience.

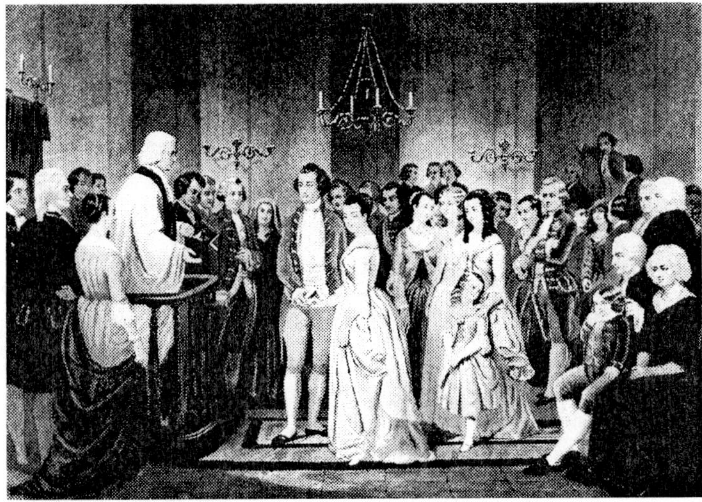

George and Martha's wedding was a major social event in Virginia in 1758. As was often true in those years, this was a marriage of convenience—George acquired land and a more lofty social standing, while Martha gained a husband to run the plantation and handle business dealings. Still, the couple appeared to have a harmonious relationship and to be caring toward each other. Although they never had children of their own, George and Martha raised the two surviving children from her first marriage. Early in the marriage, Washington wrote to a friend, saying, "I am now believed fixed at this seat [Mount Vernon] with an agreeable consort for life" (Dugan, 2001, p.1).

Today in many Western cultures, marriages (with some exceptions) are motivated by love and intimacy between two people and their desire to make a lasting commitment to each other, not usually by business advantages and dowries. Moreover, in these cultures, the decision to be together nearly always ultimately rests with the couple themselves.

Establishing Early Intimacy

Most of you can probably think back to the exact moment a romantic relationship began. The first contact with a potential partner or the initial realization that someone might become more than "just a friend" are usually fixed in our memories, regardless of how the relationship eventually turns out. The specific circumstances of that first flash of attraction or potential romance vary greatly, and people have their own unique stories of "how it all began." That said, some factors involved in the establishment of early intimacy appear to be more common than others and have been the subject of numerous studies. As you read on, think about your own relationships or those of friends or relatives—you are bound to recognize the role some of these factors played at, during, or even before the beginning of a romantic connection.

Field of Eligibles

Since YOU Asked...

1. My boyfriend and I broke up almost a year ago, but I haven't been able to get involved with anyone since. In fact, I don't even like most of the guys I've met. What's going on?

Each of us has a set of criteria that determines whether a person is a possible candidate for an intimate relationship. Those who meet our criteria—that is, those we perceive as having *potential* as a romantic partner—are referred to as our **field of eligibles** (Kerckhoff, 1962). To demonstrate this concept, think for a moment about how many people you meet in your life and yet how few of them you would even consider for a love relationship.

field of eligibles All the individuals who meet a person's criteria as a potential romantic partner.

We may not be consciously aware of our own "romantic attraction criteria," but we all have them, and they are functioning all the time as we interact with others in our lives. Most of us typically "filter out" those outside our field of eligibles before we even meet them. For example, you might be willing to consider someone older than you as a potential romantic partner. But how much older? One year? Five years? Ten years? Twenty? At some age difference, nearly everyone draws the line and eliminates people from consideration as potential romantic partners, regardless of who they are. In other words, people of a certain age or older would likely be outside your field of eligibles. That's just one example of a prerequisite that might be part of your field of eligibles, but many others exist. Here's another easy one—sex: Most of us filter out of our field of eligibles about half of all humans, either males or females. You may find it interesting to examine more closely the requirements you have in your own field of eligibles. "Self-Discovery: Your Field of Eligibles" lists some of the most common criteria, which you can rate in terms of their importance to you. You can also add criteria that you may see in yourself but may be of a more personal and less universal nature.

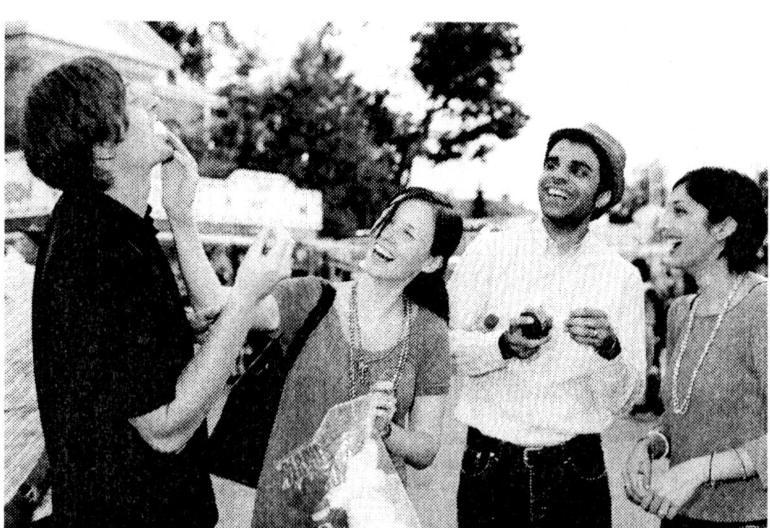

Your field of eligibles determines whom you rule out or rule in as a potential romantic partner.

The fact that you have a unique field of eligibles does not necessarily imply that you are shallow, narrow-minded,

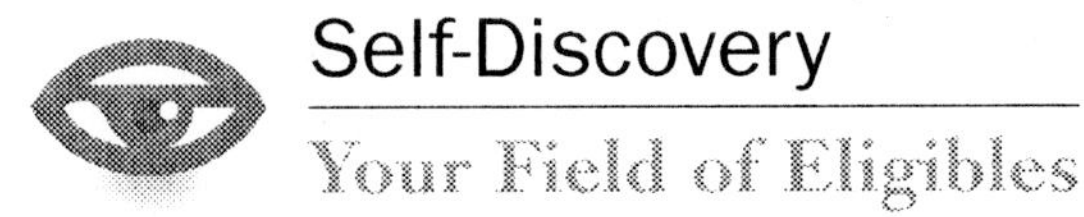

Self-Discovery

Your Field of Eligibles

Here is a list of criteria that are often included in people's field of eligibles. These criteria may determine whether you include or exclude certain individuals in your field of potential romantic partners *even before you get to know them or even meet them*. Feel free to add and rate other factors that are important to you. *Rate each item on its importance to you as a criterion in your own field of eligibles using the following scale*:

1 = Not at all important; I would not take this characteristic into account when considering someone for a potential romantic relationship.
2 = Of minor importance—it might make a small difference; I would prefer that the person fall within my requirements, but I'm flexible.
3 = Somewhat important; I'd definitely take this into account, but it would not make or break my decision.
4 = Quite important; I doubt that I would consider someone who did not meet my requirements.
5 = Extremely important; I would never consider someone who does not meet my requirements on this factor.

Factor	**Rating (1–5)**
Sex: Must be either male or female?	______
Race/ethnicity: Same racial or ethnic background as yours? Certain races or ethnicities included or excluded?	______
Age: Limit on number of years older or younger than you?	______
Height: Limit on how much taller or shorter than you?	______
Religion: Must be same religion as you? Certain religions included or excluded?	______
Socioeconomic background: Must be from a family of similar income or social status?	______
Education: Must have equal or similar educational level?	
Job or career: Must have a minimum level or specific type of job or career? Must *not* have certain jobs or careers?	______
Weight: Must be within certain limits in terms of weight (overweight or underweight)?	______
Body type: Must have (or not have) a certain body type?	______
Personality: Must have (or not have) specific personality characteristics?	______
Other: ______	______
Other: ______	______
Other: ______	______
Other: ______	______

or prejudiced. Instead, your field of eligibles enables you to direct your energy into those relationships that are most likely to succeed in satisfying your needs. Keep in mind that you have an active, functioning field of eligibles even if you are not currently looking for a romantic partner. If you are in an intimate relationship, your current partner may fit your criteria so well that you feel no need whatsoever for anyone else romantically, but psychologically, your field-of-eligibles criteria remain intact.

Finally, a person's field of eligibles is not cast in stone. It can change, and for many people it does change throughout their lives. Often it is difficult to imagine a major change in our basic requirements for a potential romantic partner, but meeting people and getting to know them often leads to a relationship with someone who is, shall we say, unexpected. You have probably heard someone say about a partner something like "I never expected this; when we first met he (or she) was not my type at all!" What the person is really saying is that the partner with whom a relationship developed did not originally fall within the criteria in her (or his) field of eligibles. It is not difficult to see how such an experience would change your criteria, probably forever. Moreover, experiences with a current partner can change your criteria in terms of a future partner.

Physical Attractiveness

For most of us, one prerequisite in our field of eligibles is physical appearance—our perception of the attractiveness of a potential partner. Many of us may want to deny that we base romantic attraction on others' physical appearance, but research has consistently shown that attractiveness plays a key role in the early formation of a potential intimate relationship. The truth is, you probably already have your personal criteria for the level of physical attractiveness you consider necessary in a possible romantic partner for you; this is already part of your field of eligibles.

The "Beautiful Is Better" Bias

The influence of physical attractiveness goes well beyond how drawn you may be to someone. Consider the following summary of just some of the research findings about the effects of physical attractiveness (K. Fox, 1997):

- Attractive children are more popular with both classmates and teachers. Teachers give higher evaluations to the work of attractive children and have higher expectations of them (which has been shown to improve future performance).
- Attractive applicants have a better chance of getting jobs and of receiving higher salaries. (One U.S. study found that taller men earned around $600 more a year per inch of height than shorter executives.)
- In court, attractive people are found guilty less often. When found guilty, they receive more lenient sentences.
- The bias for beauty operates in almost all social situations—experiments consistently show we react more favorably to physically attractive people.
- We also believe in the "what is beautiful is good" stereotype, an irrational but deep-seated belief that physically attractive people possess other desirable characteristics such as intelligence, competence, social skills, confidence, and even moral virtue. (The good fairy or princess is always beautiful; the wicked stepmother is always ugly.)

You can see from this list of research findings that physical attractiveness is deeply embedded in our cultural values and attitudes. With such a strong bias bombarding us throughout life, it is no wonder that physical attractiveness plays such a prominent role in the formation of romantic relationships.

The ideal of physical beauty conveyed by the mass media has changed noticeably over time.

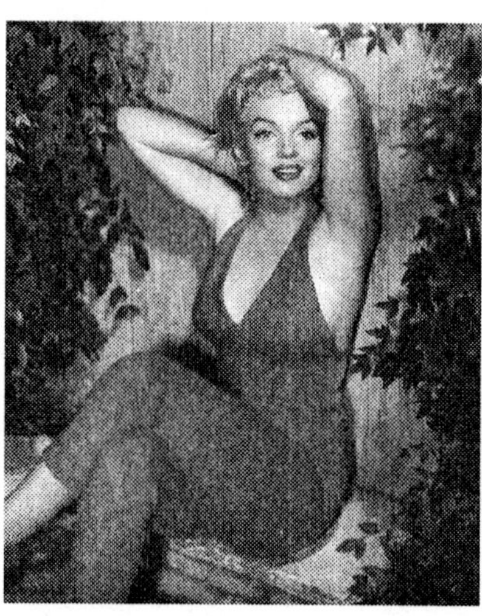

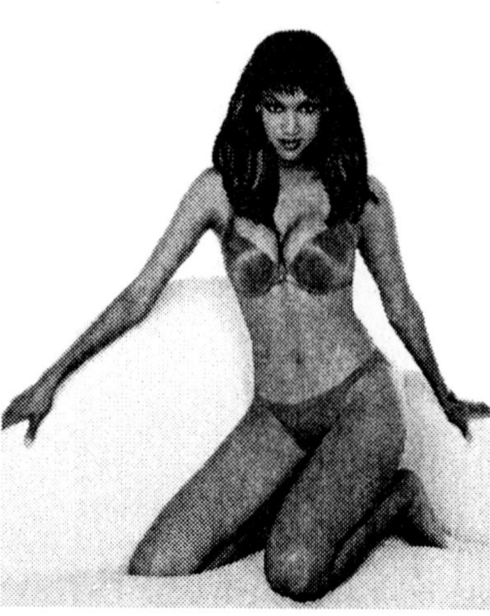

The Effect of Media

Media influences on attitudes and behavior are stronger now than in the past. TV, movies, magazines, and the Internet are constantly conveying today's standards of beauty and attractiveness in a particular culture. This repeated exposure causes the standards to become more rigid and widespread, so that even slight variations in physical appearance may fall outside of a particular culture's standard of attractiveness. The more we see these images, the more normal and attainable they seem to us. But for most of us, they are not attainable. To illustrate this, the current U.S. media ideal for how a woman's body "should" look is attainable by only about 5 percent of all women (Owen & Laurel-Seller, 2000). This media body ideal has changed drastically over time. In the early 1900s, the ideal female body was 5 feet 4 inches tall and weighed 140 pounds. In the 1970s, top fashion models weighed about 8 percent less than the average American woman; today the difference is 23 percent!

Men appear to be much less self-critical of their physical appearance. As many as eight out of ten women express dissatisfaction with their bodies. However, in general, men are mostly pleased with their bodies and may actually overestimate their attractiveness and fail to see physical flaws (Fox, 1997; Garcia, Khersonsky, & Stacey, 1997). In fact, one study found no change in men's self-rated physical attractiveness following a six-week physical and strength training program (Anderson et al., 2004). Nevertheless, recent research is showing an increase in the number of men seeking cosmetic surgery; however, it appears that men seek facial cosmetic procedures (such as Botox injections and microdermabrasion) for career reasons—to increase their professional potential and marketability in youth-focused professions (Palmquist, 2004).

matching hypothesis The theory that people tend to seek romantic and sexual partners who possess a level of physical attractiveness similar to their own.

proximity effect The theory that the closer we are to another person in geographical distance, the greater the probability that we will grow to like or even love the person.

The Matching Hypothesis

Although on a cultural level we appear to favor a certain standard of physical attractiveness when it comes to intimate partners, beauty is clearly in the eye of the beholder. According to the **matching hypothesis**, people tend to seek romantic and sexual partners who possess a similar level of physical attractiveness to their own (Feingold, 1988). When dating or married couples are analyzed, they tend to be fairly well matched on most measures of physical attractiveness (Kalick, 1988). This may be due to the expectation that someone of similar attractiveness is an emotionally "safer" choice and is a boost to each partner's self-esteem. On the other hand, a partner of much greater physical attractiveness may be seen as more likely to reject someone who is not as attractive. How well couples are matched on physical attractiveness is also related to the success of the relationship. Matched couples tend to become closer and their relationships tend to last longer than couples who differ significantly in physical attractiveness (Tucker & O'Grady, 1991).

Proximity

Proximity, in this context, refers to how close in physical distance we are to another person. Various studies have shown that as we spend more time in close proximity to other people, whether by living close by, working in the same office, taking many of the same classes, sitting near each other in class, and so on, we are more likely to develop positive feelings toward them. The closer we are in geographical distance, the greater the probability that we will grow to like or even love someone (assuming that the person does not violate too many criteria of our field of eligibles). Of course, there are exceptions to this basic theory; sometimes the more we see someone the less we like them. However, all things being equal, we tend to grow fonder of someone around whom we spend more time. Three reasons have been suggested for this **proximity effect**; consider how they might relate to your own situation.

First, it stands to reason that if you are sharing the same physical space with another person, you will

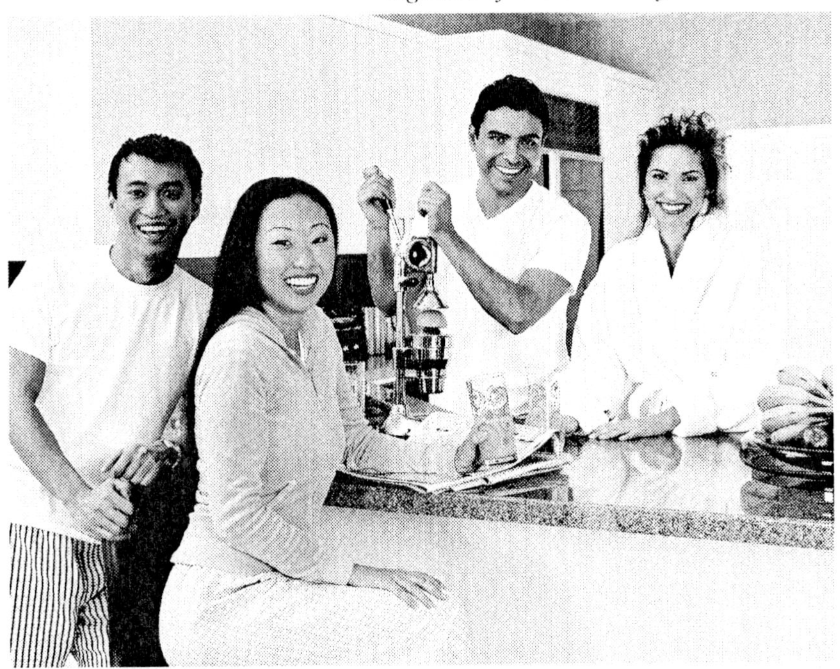

The matching hypothesis says that we tend to select romantic and sexual partners who are similar in physical attractiveness to ourselves, regardless of race or ethnicity.

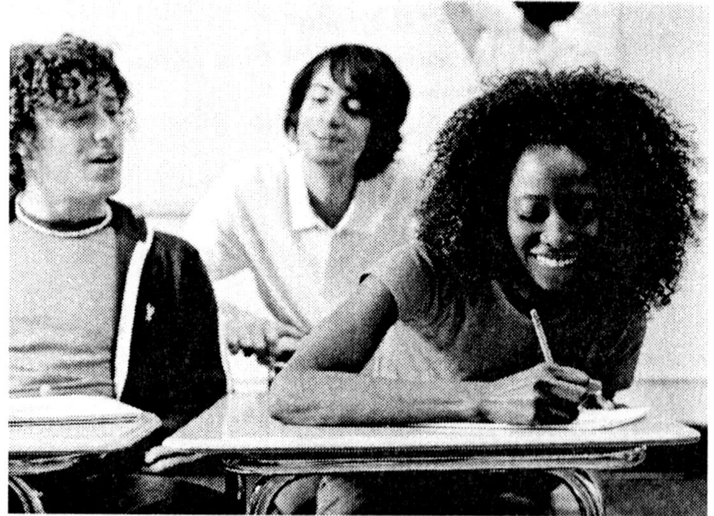

The proximity effect suggests that romantic relationships are more likely to occur when two people spend more time together in the same physical space.

have more opportunity to meet and get to know each other. By its very nature, this fact increases the chances of forming a romantic relationship.

Second, the more you find yourself in the same situation with another person, the more likely it is that the two of you have interests in common. Common interests pave the way for mutually interesting topics of conversation and shared activities, all of which enhance the probability that a romantic relationship may develop. To support this idea, the National Health and Social Life Survey of sexuality and relationships in the 1990s found that the two common locations where people meet and form romantic relationships are school and work. The survey's authors contend that these two settings are particularly conducive to the formation of relationships for two reasons, both relating to the proximity effect. First, both situations provide numerous opportunities for frequent contact with the same groups of people, which increases the odds that romantic relationships may develop. Second, both settings naturally involve people with similar backgrounds, goals, and interests, which further increases the potential for the formation of intimate partnerships (Laumann et al., 1994). In other words, your college or work environment typically contains an exceptionally large number of people who qualify for your field of eligibles.

A third explanation proposed for the influence of proximity on relationships is a psychological principle called the **mere exposure effect**. Research has shown that humans appear to have a natural and usually unconscious tendency to grow fonder of a "novel stimulus" as they see it more often (Bornstein, 1989; Zajonc, 1968, 2001). This is true of nearly anything we come across—a new model of car, an architecturally unusual building, a product in a TV commercial—and it's true for people as well. If we use the mere exposure effect to explain the impact of proximity on relationships, simply encountering a person more often, without even talking or acknowledging each other, will lead to greater liking, which in turn increases the probability of forming an intimate connection. One important exception to this theory is that if upon first encountering a new person, your initial reaction is profoundly negative, the mere exposure effect may not occur, and instead your dislike may increase with repeated encounters.

Similarity

Since YOU Asked...

2. My girlfriend (of two months) and I are very different. We disagree and argue about politics, religion, and nearly everything else. Is this going to be a problem, or is it true that opposites attract?

Are you more attracted to people who are similar to you or to those who are more complementary, that is, those who possess the characteristics you lack? Do "birds of a feather flock together," or do "opposites attract?" If you rely on your personal experience and common sense to answer these questions, you might be led down the wrong path. Many people believe in the saying that "opposites attract" and can point to instances in their own or others' lives when it appeared to be true. But in reality, the opposite is true: People are more likely to become romantically involved with and marry others who possess attitudes, interests, and personality characteristics similar to their own (Caspi, Herbener, & Ozer, 1992; Klohnen & Mendelsohn, 1998).

Upon reflection, this makes sense. Interpersonal similarity allows two people to enjoy the same activities, to agree on most of life's major issues and decisions, to feel a mutual understanding, to reinforce and support each other's attitudes and opinions, and to feel that they form a united front in dealing with the world around them. All of these shared characteristics and behaviors combine to produce a stronger bond between two people than would be possible if the similarities did not exist.

mere exposure effect The psychological principle that humans appear to have a natural and usually unconscious tendency to grow fonder of a "novel stimulus" the more often they are exposed to it.

Have you ever been in a relationship with someone who has many basic characteristics that complement or are the opposite of yours? If not, have you ever known such a couple? If you have, there is a good chance that the relationship was a stormy one and may not have lasted very long. Many people believe that opposites do attract and that they are looking for someone with qualities that are missing in themselves. When they meet such a person, they are fascinated by the other's differences and may be drawn into a relationship. In time, however, the very same differences that were so attractive early on typically begin to clash and cause friction and turmoil, often leading to the demise of the relationship.

This does not imply that people are looking for a relationship with their twin or clone. Although perceived similarity appears to be important in satisfying relationships, people still seek potential partners who offer at least a few contrasts and differences to themselves (W. Wilson, 1989). For example, someone who is a submissive person might feel more comfortable with a more dominant partner and vice versa, even when the partners consider themselves to be quite similar in other respects (Dryer & Horowitz, 1997).

Similarity appears to be a far more important and more powerful force than complementarity in successful, happy relationships. It is so important, in fact, that we will even make the assumption that our partners are more similar to ourselves than they actually may be. A study of dating and married couples found that "people in satisfying and stable relationships assimilated their partners to themselves, perceiving similarities that were not evident in reality" (Murray et al., 2002, p. 563).

Flirting

Most of you reading this have flirted with someone, have been flirted with, or both. You may have even engaged in flirtatious activities without being fully aware that it was happening. **Flirting** may be defined as subtle behaviors designed to signal sexual or romantic interest in another person. But flirting is not reserved for humans. Most nonhuman animals engage in complex behaviors to pique the interest of and attract a potential mate. Seeing that humans across all cultures share this tendency, flirting may be seen, to some extent, as a biologically based, genetically programmed behavior that increases the ability of the human species to survive. Flirting communicates mutual sexual interest but virtually no commitment. It allows us to "check someone out" as a potential sexual partner or mate at the earliest possible stage in a potential relationship, when rejection carries very little risk or pain (Rodgers & Veronsky, 1999).

What is most interesting about flirting is that the behaviors are quite similar in all humans and tend to follow fairly predictable patterns. For heterosexual individuals, these behaviors send signals not just about sex but also about the larger question of who will be the best person for mating and reproduction. Most probably, you have not always been aware of your own or others' behaviors while flirting. After reading this, however, you will be an informed observer of the flirting world around you. Although we will discuss flirting in heterosexual settings (where most of the research to date has been carried out), most of the behaviors and patterns are similar for gay and lesbian couples, although the individual who takes the initiative in the various flirting behaviors are typically more flexible (Lott & Veronsky, 1999).

The main messages male humans want to send is strength, trustworthiness, and good genes. The behaviors observed when men flirt are designed to get these ideas across in mostly nonverbal ways (Lott & Veronsky, 1999; Perper, 1986; Rodgers &

flirting Subtle behaviors designed to signal sexual or romantic interest in another person.

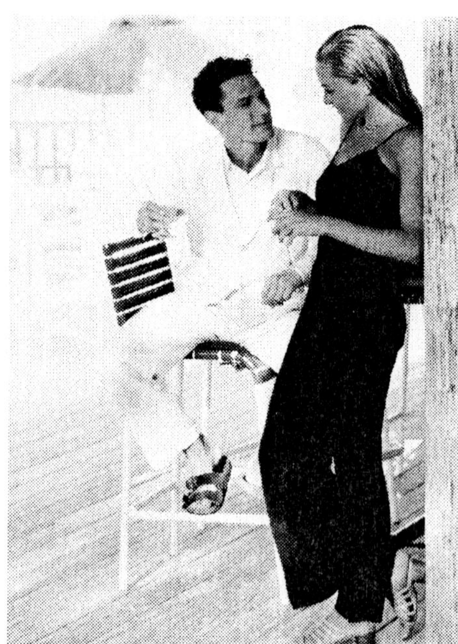

Considerable research has explored the variety of flirting behaviors humans use to signal romantic or sexual interest in another person.

Veronsky, 1999). Typically, the man can be observed arching his back (to puff out the chest), leaning back in his chair and tucking his hands behind his head (same effect), pointing his chin in the air, smiling a lot, strutting when he walks, laughing in loud bursts, and using large, grandiose gestures for lighting a cigarette or signaling a server. However, at times, he may also signal a more gentle or passive side by bowing his head lower than the woman's.

For her part, the woman wants to communicate that she is interested in a particular man and that she offers a clear advantage over other women for sex, intimacy, and potential reproduction. The nonverbal behaviors the woman may employ to attract a man include repeated short glances at the man in whom she is interested, prolonged gazing toward him, swaying her hips, smiling, licking her lips, twirling her hair, tossing her head, perhaps covering her mouth and giggling, and stretching and exposing her neck (Lott & Veronsky, 1999; Perper, 1986; Rodgers & Veronsky, 1999).

To study exactly how and when these behaviors occur in actual flirting situations, researchers have spent many hours in bars, lounges, restaurants, clubs, and other locales where people are likely to be flirting (M. Moore, 2002; Perper, 1986; Perper & Fox, 1980). Through these observations, not only have the behaviors of flirting been identified, but a predictable pattern of flirtation has also been revealed. The five steps in a typical flirting episode have been labeled *the approach*, *talk*, *swivel and turn*, *touch*, and *synchronization* (Perper & Fox, 1980). At each step, one member of the couple makes a subtle gesture designed to take the developing intimacy to the next level. It is then up to the other person to respond appropriately if the flirtation is to continue. If this back-and-forth "dance" is interrupted by either partner, the developing relationship will likely fail to materialize.

Imagine that you are observing people at a bar, lounge, or large party where people go to check out, meet, and potentially hook up with others. Here are the typical steps of flirting you are likely to see in a heterosexual setting within the space of about one hour (Martin, 2001; Perper, 1986; Perper & Fox, 1980).

1. **The Approach.** The initial contact between potential partners begins with a look by the woman. The cliché "their eyes met across a crowded room" appears to contain a grain of truth. A woman will scan a room of potentially desirable men and settle on one who piques her interest the most. When he returns the eye contact, she will either glance down and back up or maintain her gaze toward him. At this point, the man is expected to move toward her. He will follow a somewhat meandering pattern to "test the waters" and not appear too eager or aggressive, all the while maintaining the visual connection. Within a few minutes he should be positioned next to her. As he approaches, she may encourage him with a smile or a flick of her hair or by moving slightly to a location that is easier to reach. You can imagine that if either party deviates much from this scenario—if she looks away for an extended time or he becomes sidetracked on the way—the process may end before it has even begun.

2. **Talk.** Obviously, the next step is for someone to say something. Both flirting participants would be very uncomfortable if he were to go to the effort to reach her and then they just stood next to each other without speaking. But who talks first? Usually, he does. He engages in small talk (too much self-disclosure at this point is a turnoff), and he typically asks a question of some sort, requiring an

answer. Here is where the proverbial pickup line enters the flirting scene. However, most people do not respond well to "canned" or silly introduction lines ("Bond. James Bond" or "I didn't know angels could fly this low!"). Most women say they prefer a smile and authentic, simple introductory questions, such as "Hi, how are you? Are you having a good time? My name is Rex." Again, the woman must say something in return, or as you can imagine, the interaction may wind down rather quickly.

3. **Swivel and Turn.** Body language plays a role in most human communication, but at this stage in the flirting process, it becomes more pronounced than usual. Typically, the flirting pair will be standing or sitting side by side rather than face to face. This is because a face-to-face position feels far more intimate than a side-by-side stance. As the couple continue to talk and become acquainted, they will begin to shift their stances, little by little, toward each other. One person will swivel and turn slightly, and within a short time the other will reciprocate. Then they will take turns swiveling a bit more each time until, *voilà!* they are face to face. This is a very special and sensitive communication process. If one fails to swivel and turn in response to the other, or if one swivels and turns too quickly, the rhythm of the flirtation may be lost.

4. **Touch.** If all has been going well up to now, this next step is a clear escalation in the flirtation game: touching. Who do you think initiates the first touch? It's the woman. The first touch will be a subtle, seemingly "accidental" brief touch of his hand when she laughs at something witty he has said, picking a piece of lint from his shoulder, or touching his arm as she whispers in his ear. This also must be reciprocated either by a subtle touch in return, a thank-you, or a smile. If her touch is not returned, or if he appears startled by the touch and recoils involuntarily, this may be seen as rejection (or at least pretty darn uncool) and will not bode well for the continuation of the relationship.

5. **Synchronization.** Once again, body language becomes the focus of the final stage of flirtation. Synchronization means that the couple, who are now face to face, have established an easy, flowing unison of movement. They begin in concert to turn their heads at the same time, pick up and put down their drinks together, shift their weight if standing, or lean forward with their chins in their hands if sitting, and they even begin to breathe in the same rhythm in a virtual dance of flirtation. Research has shown that this synchronicity appears to happen naturally and cannot be faked. When acting students are asked to mimic this stage of flirting, they have great difficulty appearing realistic and natural.

After a couple completes these five steps of flirting, has a new intimate relationship been born? At this point we cannot know. A couple who has reached this point in flirting still know very little about each other and may or may not take the relationship to the next, more intimate and private level. In heterosexual settings, the male usually makes such a suggestion. If he does not do so at this point, the relationship will usually end here.

Exceptions to this flirtation pattern may occur (especially if the flirting individuals are under the influence of alcohol or other drugs). But if you think back over situations in which you or others have been flirting, and if you keep these steps in mind when you next find yourself in a flirtatious environment, you will likely see how accurate they are.

Reciprocity of Attraction

Have you ever been in love with someone who did not share your feelings no matter what you did? Feels terrible, doesn't it? Such relationships (if they can even be called that) are unsatisfying for both people and typically do not last very long. A long-established principle of successful interpersonal relationships is that they are based on *balance* (Bagarozzi, 1990; Zimmerman et al., 2003): balance of power, balance of control, balance in money matters, balance in decision making, and so on. This type of balance does not mean that the couple must be equal in all relationship matters but that the relationship should not be overly controlled by either partner. One type of balance, in particular, is very important at the earliest stages of a potential relationship. This balance is called **reciprocity of attraction**, which simply means that if you like or love someone, you need to feel that the other person likes or loves you back approximately the same amount—that he or she reciprocates your feelings. Knowing that someone we like likes us back is one of the key factors in the formation and continuation of new romantic relationships (Giles, 1994).

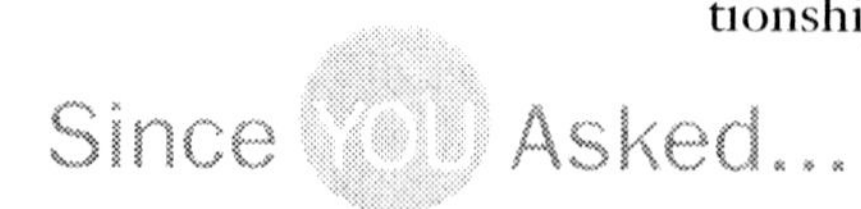

3. I feel I love my partner far more than he loves me. Is there some way to get him to love me more?

Psychologically, this makes perfect sense. When you like or love others, you usually want to support and share their beliefs, feelings, and favorite activities, and you are more willing to disclose your personal self to them. When you receive the same support and openness back from a potential partner, it is much more likely that a budding relationship will deepen and grow into a romance. However, when this reciprocity is lacking, both people may experience negative feelings such as anger, resentment, frustration, anxiety, sadness, and guilt, depending on which side of the unrequited love you are on.

Interestingly, reciprocity of attraction may help explain why individuals with poor self-esteem and high self-doubt have trouble forming lasting romantic relationships. The reason appears to be in part because people who doubt themselves also doubt that a partner they love could ever love them back equally. They feel unworthy and dubious of their partner's love, even when the partner really does reciprocate the love (Murray et al., 2001).

Love

Ask 100 people to define romantic love, and you'll probably get 100 different answers. If love is such a personal and individual phenomenon, it must be impossible to study it scientifically, right? Well, not really. Researchers have attempted to develop theories of love that can encompass everyone's individual definitions into an organized set of interrelated categories or types. Two of these theories have received considerable attention and research support: John Allen Lee's "styles of love" and Robert J. Sternberg's "triangular theory of love."

Styles of Love

One early theory about love has attempted to measure what kind of lover you are. No, this is not referring to your skills and talents in the bedroom but rather your approach to and style of relating to a partner when you are in a romantic relationship. Developed by the Canadian sociologist John Allen Lee in the 1970s, this theory of love suggests that people follow various psychological motifs in relating to a love partner. Lee divided these love patterns into six major categories he called **styles of love** (1973, 1977, 1988). Over the years, Lee's conceptualization of these styles of love has served as the basis for a great deal of research on intimate relationships (Kunkel &

reciprocity of attraction The idea that someone you like or love likes or loves you back—reciprocates your feelings—with approximately the same degree of intensity.

styles of love Lee's theory that people follow individual psychological motifs or styles in relating to a love partner.

Burleson, 2002; Worobey, 2001). Lee used concepts from Greek mythology and language to name his six styles. We will briefly describe each of them here. If you would like to discover which style reflects yourself and your partner, pause now and fill out the assessment scale in "Self-Discovery: Styles of Love," and then read the description of each style, including yours.

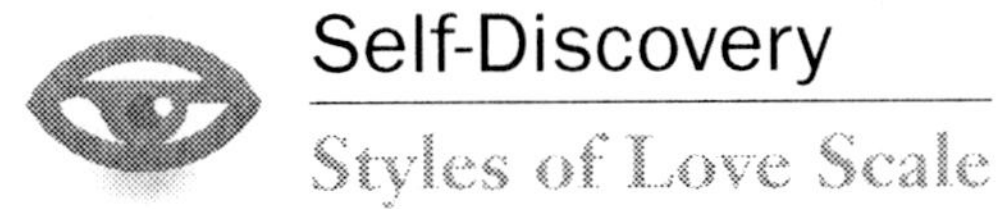

Self-Discovery

Styles of Love Scale

For each of the following statements, write T for *true* or F for *false* to reflect how the statement applies to you in your love relationships. If you are not in a love relationship, answer based on how you were in your last significant one. If you have never been in a love relationship, first, don't worry, the right person is out there somewhere, and second, respond to the items based on how you imagine you will be when you do fall in love. Try not to overthink your answers. If you are not sure how to answer, respond according to how you feel *most* of the time. Respond to all the items. Instructions for scoring follow the scale.

True or False?

____ **1.** My partner and I were attracted to each other immediately when we first met.

____ **2.** My partner and I have great physical chemistry between us.

____ **3.** I feel that my partner and I were meant to be together.

____ **4.** I have sometimes had to prevent two of my partners from finding out about each other.

____ **5.** Sometimes I enjoy playing "love games" with several partners at once.

____ **6.** I believe it's a good idea to keep my partner a little uncertain about my commitment to him or her.

____ **7.** I find it difficult to pinpoint exactly when my partner and I fell in love.

____ **8.** The most fulfilling love relationship grows out of a close friendship.

____ **9.** It is necessary to care deeply for someone for a while before you can truly fall in love.

____ **10.** When I am in love, I am sometimes so excited about it that I can't sleep.

____ **11.** I am constantly worried that my partner may be with someone else.

____ **12.** When my partner is busy or seems distant, I feel anxious and sick all over.

____ **13.** It is best to find a partner who has similar interests to your own.

____ **14.** I try to make sure my life is in order before I choose a partner.

____ **15.** A person's goals, plans, and status in life are very important to me in choosing a partner.

____ **16.** I would rather suffer myself than allow my partner to suffer.

____ **17.** I cannot be happy unless my partner's happiness needs are met first.

____ **18.** I am usually willing to sacrifice my own needs and desires to allow my partner to achieve his or hers.

Scoring: The six styles of love discussed in the chapter are measured by each successive group of three statements. If you divide the scale into sets of three items, the six styles are as follows (refer to the chapter's discussion for a detailed explanation of the various styles):

Statements 1, 2, and 3 reflect *Eros* love.
Statements 4, 5, and 6 reflect *Ludus* love.
Statements 7, 8, and 9 reflect *Storge* love.
Statements 10, 11, and 12 reflect *Mania* love.
Statements 13, 14, and 15 reflect *Pragma* love.
Statements 16, 17, and 18 reflect *Agape* love.

Continued. . .

To determine your style, see if you have answered "True" for all three statements in any of these sets. If so, that is the style that best reflects your approach to love relationships. If you do not have any sets of three items to which you answered "True," look for sets where you have answered "True" to two items. Though not quite as strongly as three "Trues" would indicate, these sets reflect your preferred style of love. Finally, see if you have any style for which you answered "False" to all three questions. This indicates the love style you most strongly reject.

What if you have indicated that you agree with more than one style? This is possible, and it implies one of several possibilities. First, you may have shifted your style over time and behaved according to one style in a past relationship but are now behaving differently. You might want to try the scale again, focusing closely on your one most important or longest relationship. Second, some relationships can change and grow over time, and you may have changed and grown with it. Your love style earlier in a relationship may have been different than it is now, but you responded to the scale with both in mind. Third, you may simply not know your own love style yet, either because you have never been in love or because you have just not thought about it very much. And fourth, some people may simply possess more than one love style that they may call on as needed in a particular relationship. Agreeing with a number of love styles on this scale might be a sign that more self-knowledge about yourself and your relationships is yet to come.

Source: Adapted from Hendrick and Hendrick (1986).

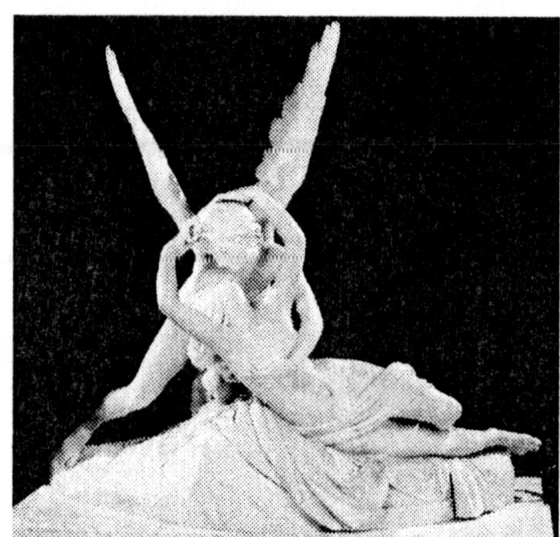

The eros style of love emphasizes passion, eroticism, and sexual energy.

Eros Love

You have no doubt heard of Cupid, the god of love in Roman mythology. Cupid's counterpart in Greek mythology is Eros. In his theory of love styles, Lee conceptualized **eros love** as erotic, passionate love. Eros lovers tend to place great emphasis on romance and physical beauty. They tend to feel an urgent sexual desire and strong physical attraction to their potential partners. They probably believe in love at first sight and have experienced it often. Eros lovers desire sexual intimacy earlier in a new relationship than those embracing other styles, and they value tactile (touch) sensations above the other senses. This style of love is very romantic and highly sexually charged, but typically that level of passion cannot be maintained for long, and relationships based on eros love tend to burn out quickly.

Ludus Love

Ludus is Greek for "play," and **ludus love** is characterized by game playing. Ludus lovers enjoy the excitement of forming a relationship more than the relationship itself—they like the "chase." They love to flirt and seduce their partners. They "play the field," typically moving rapidly from one relationship to another or juggling several partners at once. They enjoy the "conquest" of sex but grow bored quickly once a relationship becomes sexual. As you might imagine, ludus lovers are very unlikely to form a lasting commitment and tend to avoid serious relationships altogether. Often they will end a relationship just when it appears to be at its closest and most satisfying stage; they do so because that is the point at which the relationship seems secure and committed, and they simply do not want security and commitment. At times, they will even begin a new relationship before ending the current one so that they are never without the rush and excitement of the pursuit.

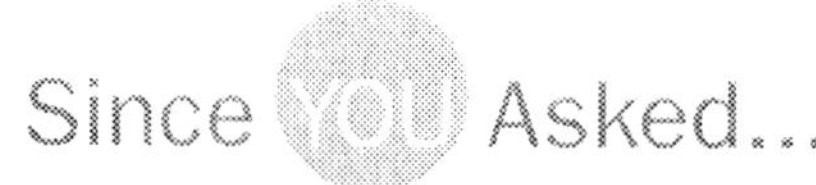

4. Why do people cheat? Is it because they just need a new conquest?

Storge Love

In Greek, *storge* ("STOR-gay") means "natural affection." **Storge love** is characterized by the central theme of friendship. Those who adhere to this style of romantic relationship usually begin with a close friendship and take a long time to develop feelings of love. In contrast to ludus and eros lovers, the sexual side of storge relationships arrives late and tends to take a back seat to the emphasis on friendship. Although passion is not a central feature, storge relationships offer peace, security, and stability, all of which are greatly valued. For storge lovers, more than for any other style, if love ends, the friendship usually returns and continues over time.

eros love An erotic, passionate style of love often characterized by short-lived relationships.

ludus love A style of love that focuses on the excitement of forming a relationship more than the relationship itself and typically moves rapidly from one relationship to another.

storge love A love style characterized by caring and friendship.

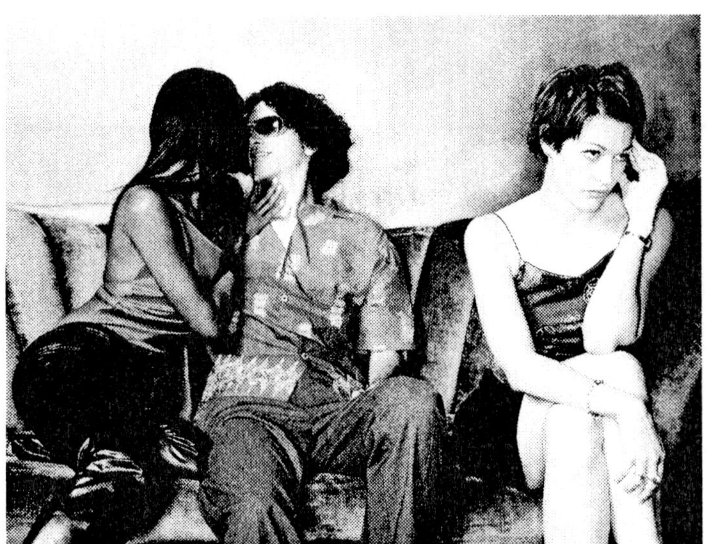

Ludus lovers enjoy playing the field and seek many sexual conquests.

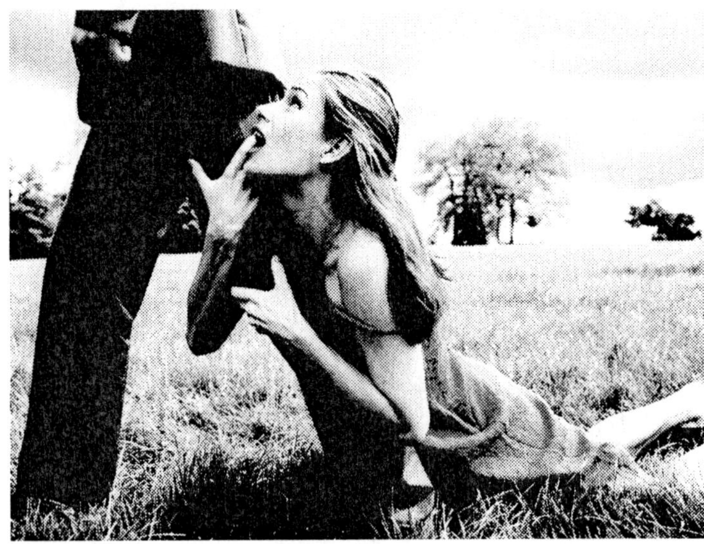

Mania lovers are insecure in love and obsessively cling to their partners.

Mania Love

Mania is Greek for "madness." You can probably conjure up an image in your mind of a "manic" lover (good examples are Glenn Close's character in *Fatal Attraction* or the teen female stalker in *Swimfan*). **Mania love** is possessive, dependent, and often controlling. Mania lovers are constantly fearful that their partner will leave and must be constantly reassured that the relationship is intact. These relationships are characterized by turmoil, extreme, unrealistic jealousy, and sometimes true obsession. Partners of mania lovers may feel excited at first that they are so intensely loved and needed, but they soon find that they are being emotionally smothered by a clinging, insecure partner. When mania lovers feel that a partner is drifting away, they may resort to such drastic measures as stalking, threats of suicide, actual suicide attempts, or physical violence to prevent the partner from leaving.

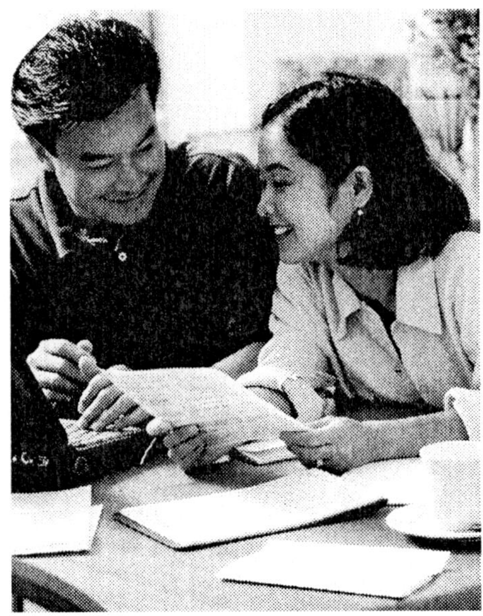

Individuals favoring the pragma style of love select romantic partners based on rational, practical criteria.

Pragma Love

Pragma means "business" in Greek, and **pragma love** is appropriately characterized as a practical love. Pragma lovers go about selecting their partners in a businesslike way based on rational, practical criteria. You can't really say that pragma lovers fall in love; rather, they decide to love the partner who best fits their requirements. These requirements include some of the factors included in most people's field of eligibles discussed earlier in the chapter, but the pragma lover focuses on the most down-to-earth, *pragmatic* aspects for compatibility, such as education level, profession, social status, income, common interests, potential as a parent, and material possessions. Although on its face this may sound like an effective way to build a strong relationship, it turns out that these partnerships tend to be less mutually satisfying and often unsuccessful. You can probably see why: Pragma lovers have a tendency to place too little importance on the emotional aspects of love that are so basic to bonding and forming strong attachments between people.

mania love A possessive, dependent, and often controlling style of love.

pragma love A love style in which partners are selected in a businesslike way on the basis of rational, practical criteria.

agape love A style of love focused on giving the partner whatever he or she may want or need without the expectation of receiving anything in return.

Agape Love

Agape ("uh-GAH-pay") is the Greek word for "brotherly love" or "divine love." **Agape love** is a selfless love, and agape lovers offer their partners a self-sacrificing, altruistic love. This means that they strive to give to their partner whatever he or she may want or need without any expectation of receiving anything in return. The word

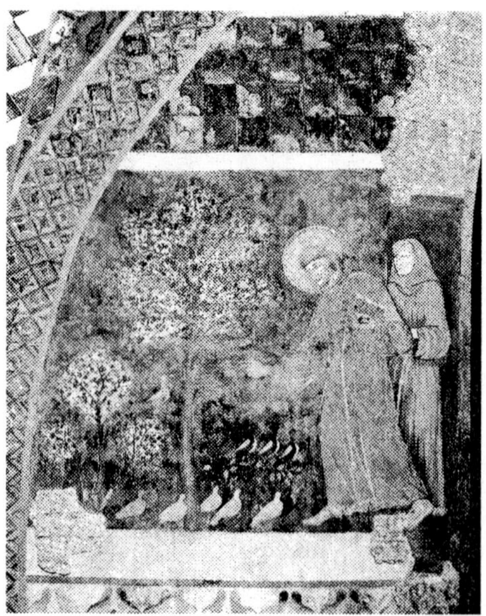

The agape love style is a selfless, all-giving, divine love.

agape has often been used to describe the love of God, of saints, and of martyrs. This style of love is patient and nondemanding. As described in 1 Corinthians 13 of the New Testament, agape love "suffers long; is kind; does not envy; does not parade itself; is not puffed up; does not behave rudely, does not seek its own; is not provoked; thinks no evil; does not rejoice in iniquity, but rejoices in truth; bears all things; believes all things; hopes all things; endures all things." Sounds wonderful, right? In many ways it is, but the problem is that although agape love may be wonderful as a way to love "all humankind" or as a way to describe the love between, say, a parent and a child, it turns out to be a rather weak form of romantic love between two adults. Why? Because agape love is all about giving, while romantic love involves a balance of giving and receiving.

Combining Love Styles

What combinations of love styles do you think would work best together in a relationship? In general, research has indicated that people prefer to partner with others who have the same love style as their own (Hahn & Blass, 1997). But what if two people with different love styles become romantically involved? Looking back over the descriptions of the six styles, you can see that some might fit together better than others, some combinations just would not work well at all, and some might be downright dangerous. For example, a storge lover and a pragma lover might get along just fine: one focused on establishing a close friendship and the other finding the perfect qualifications in the partnership. On the other hand, just imagine someone who embodies a strong mania style getting together with a pure ludus: One is manically in love, insecure, and clinging; the other is playing love games. What outcome might you expect from that? ("Homicide" might not be too far from the truth!) Table 4.1 illustrates how successful various matches among the six love styles are likely to be. Research has shown that love relationships are extremely complex, and a couple's individual love styles tell only part of the overall story of intimacy and overall satisfaction (Hendrick, 2004; Lacy et al., 2004). Therefore, exceptions always exist, and some couples with incompatible love styles may create a successful relationship through skillful communication, clear agreements, and mutual respect.

Table 4.1 COMPATIBILITY OF LOVE STYLES IN RELATIONSHIPS

This table graphically illustrates which combinations of the love styles are more likely to result in compatible relationships, which may be successful if the relationship is strong overall, which might work despite some difficulties, and which are potentially dangerous due to the level of dissatisfaction and discord such diverse styles are likely to produce.

	EROS	LUDUS	STORGE	MANIA	PRAGMA	AGAPE
Eros						
Ludus						
Storge						
Mania						
Pragma						
Agape						

GREEN = Good match BLUE = Possible match ORANGE = Difficult match RED = Dangerous match

The Triangular Theory of Love

No, this does not refer to the familiar "love triangle" in which three people are intimately and sexually entwined. Rather, Robert Sternberg calls his model the **triangular theory of love** because he conceptualizes the three fundamental components of love—intimacy, passion, and commitment—positioned at the three corners of a triangle, forming various combinations that define the qualities of a relationship (Sternberg, 1986, 1988, 1997, 1998; Leumieux & Hale, 2002). A relationship may consist of any one of these components, any combination of two, or all three.

Sternberg's *intimacy* component does not refer to sexual intimacy but rather to the emotional closeness two people feel. This includes such factors as wanting what is best for the partner, feeling the partner's happiness, holding the partner in very high regard, feeling able to count on the partner in times of need, sharing a sense of mutual understanding, giving and receiving emotional support, and being able to share private and personal thoughts and feelings with the partner.

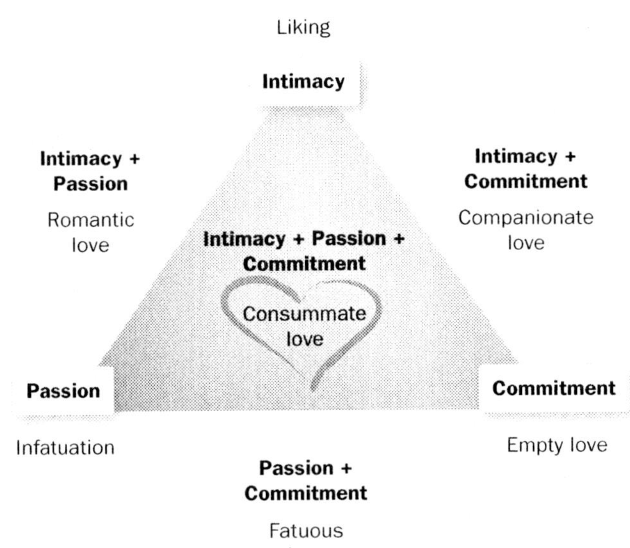

FIGURE 4.1 The Triangular Theory of Love

Sternberg's theory of love includes three fundamental components—intimacy, passion and committent—which, in various combinations, define seven types of love relationships.

Source: Figure from *The Triangle of Love* by Robert J. Sternberg. Copyright © 1998. Published by Basic Books. Reprinted by permission of Dr. Robert J. Sternberg.

Passion, Sternberg explains, is the physical arousal side of relationships. Passion is manifested in the increased heart rate when you are with your partner, the desire to be near your partner as much as possible, the sexual and romantic attraction you feel for your partner, the frequency of thinking about your partner, and the need to express your desire for your partner through touching, kissing, and making love.

The *commitment* component of Sternberg's model is a more rational aspect of a love relationship. It is determined by the strength of your decision to be with and to stay with your partner. It is your chosen desire to be loyal and faithful and to commit to working on creating and maintaining a loving, mutually satisfying, and lasting relationship.

According to Sternberg, these three components may exist in any combination, from none of them, which is *nonlove*, to all of them, which is *consummate love*. Overall, seven possible combinations can help couples see their relationship more clearly and explore what is working well or what might be causing the difficulties they have been experiencing. The combinations of the components of love are summarized in Figure 4.1; we will discuss each of these briefly. (Nonlove, as noted, reflects a lack of all three components.)

Intimacy Only = Liking

If you imagine a relationship in which two people feel intimacy but do not experience passion or a strong sense of commitment, what sort of relationship do you see? Most people see two people who like each other quite a lot and are probably good friends. Sternberg agrees and characterizes a relationship containing intimacy only as *liking*.

Passion Only = Infatuation

Now think of two people who are just bursting with passion and sexual heat for each other but who do not feel particularly intimate and are not committed to any sort of short- or long-term relationship. What would you call this type of love? Spring break, right? In a way, yes. When you experience **infatuation** with someone, you are usually very attracted and focused on that person, usually in a sexual way, and you may desire to spend all your time with him or her. But the relationship does not go much beyond that. It's very sexually charged, but at the same time, it's shallow. You may know (or care) little about the other person, so you don't experience much intimacy

triangular theory of love Sternberg's theory that three fundamental components of love—intimacy, passion, and commitment—in various combinations, define the qualities of a relationship.

infatuation Love based on passion but lacking intimacy and commitment; usually very sexually charged but shallow and devoid of much meaning.

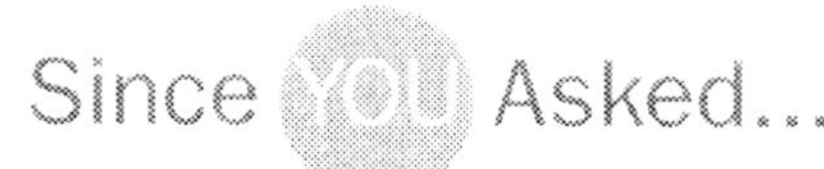

5. When a couple is having sex on a regular basis, does the emotional side fade or grow over time? Does it mean the relationship is not going well if it is just for the physical release?

and you aren't even thinking in terms of a commitment. It's simply a passionate connection that might be fun and sexy, but it exists only in the moment.

Commitment Only = Empty Love

This corner of the triangle is a little more difficult to imagine. Can you imagine being committed to someone without feeling any intimacy or passion? This may happen when attraction is not reciprocated. Imagine that you love someone with whom you have not established any intimacy and no real passion exists between you. How would that love feel to you? That's right, it would feel empty. Such **empty love** relationships are unlikely to have much of a future, unless a person becomes too focused on the other and develops an unhealthy "fatal attraction" or "stalker" sort of obsession. However, not many would define that as love at all. Some couples with children who are experiencing empty love might stay together "for the sake of the kids," but this is typically an unsatisfactory solution for everyone involved.

Intimacy + Passion = Romantic Love

This side of the triangle connects intimacy and passion. If you get to know someone well, establish a deep level of intimacy, and then add passion to that, the result is probably going to feel very romantic. And it will probably feel romantic regardless of whether or not you have established a commitment with that person. A good example of this is the so-called "shipboard romance," that short-term, intensely romantic relationship that sometimes develops between two people who meet on a cruise or at a resort or have a brief affair outside of their primary relationships. It is more than mere passion because they connect on an emotional and personal level in addition to the physical attraction. But due to the circumstances of the situation or other involvements in their lives, they do not choose to commit to one another. This is **romantic love**.

Passion + Commitment = Fatuous Love

Now imagine, if you can, two people who are very physically attracted to each other and share a strong sexual bond between them. In addition to having the hots for each other, they also feel a strong commitment to making the relationship last over the long term. However, they lack intimacy. That is, they don't really like each other all that much, they don't hold each other in especially high regard (except perhaps in terms of sexual skills), and they have never achieved close, private, intimate communication with each other. Sternberg labeled this side of the triangle **fatuous love**. *Fatuous* is a fairly uncommon word that means "absurd," "foolish," or "pointless."

Commitment + Intimacy = Companionate Love

Companionate love is a relationship characterized by two people who are truly in love and are committed to each other and who enjoy all or most of the characteristics relating to intimate love or liking. What's missing is the heat, the sexual arousal, the physical longing when apart, the *passion*. How might we describe such a couple? Without passion, it is difficult to see them as lovers, but rather they are companions, hence the term *companionate love*.

Intimacy + Passion + Commitment = Consummate Love

Finally, what if a couple is fortunate enough to possess all three of Sternberg's basic components of love? They will have what he termed **consummate love**, meaning the most complete, most fulfilling, most ideally perfect love two people can achieve. Sternberg believes—and research has borne him out—that consummate love is not only rare but also difficult to attain and perhaps even harder to maintain over time.

empty love Love based on commitment but lacking intimacy or real passion.

romantic love Love based on intimacy and passion but lacking commitment.

fatuous love Love based on passion and commitment but lacking intimacy; a foolish, or pointless love.

companionate love Love based on true intimacy and commitment but lacking passion; the couple are companions more than lovers.

consummate love Love that encompasses intimacy, passion, and commitment simultaneously.

Applying the Triangular Theory

Sternberg's theory can be helpful in relationships in which one or both partners feel dissatisfied or sense that something is missing. Sometimes couples find it difficult to put their finger on exactly what is causing their feelings of discontent or discord with their partner. If they examine their relationship from the perspective of the triangular theory, they may make two important discoveries. First, they may feel encouraged and relieved to find that they are quite strong on one or two of the components. This often helps validate their positive feelings for each other and motivates them to work on other areas in the relationship. Second, they will be able to identify more specifically the aspects of their relationship that may be weak, missing, or in need of work. This, then, will enable them to establish a mutual focus for enhancing and improving the bond between them.

Most people in love relationships tend to feel unhappy at times if any one of the three components—intimacy, passion, or commitment—is weak or missing. You can be in a committed relationship and feel lonely and disconnected if you do not feel that special intimacy with your partner. You can feel angry, frustrated, and betrayed if your relationship lacks commitment. And many couples find themselves dissatisfied and longing for the passion that has faded over time from their relationship, although they continue to experience a strong sense of commitment and intimacy (this loss of sexual desire is discussed in greater detail in Chapter 7, "Sexual Problems and Solutions").

Are you curious about *your* love triangle? "Self-Discovery: The Triangle of Your Love" offers you the opportunity to assess where your relationship (current or past) might fall withing Sternberg's theory. Take the scale yourself or with your partner (gently, as a basis for meaningful discussion, not as an argument starter!), or you and your partner might complete the assessment separately and then discuss your results.

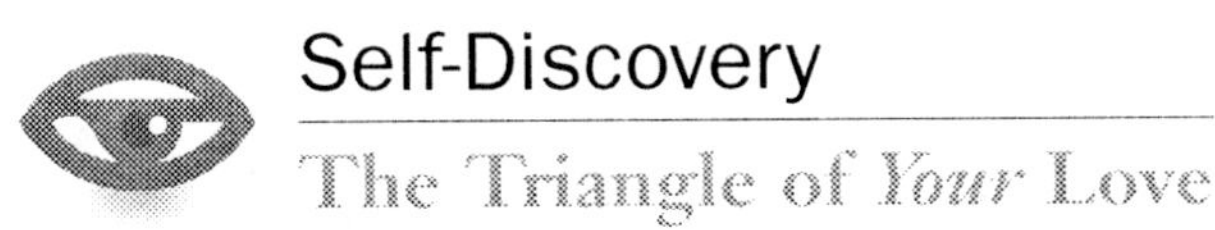

Self-Discovery
The Triangle of *Your* Love

Each component in Sternberg's triangular theory of love is measured by your responses on 15 items, for a total of 45 items. For each statement, *fill in the long blank with your current (or past or potential) partner's name*, and respond in the short blank using the following key:

1——2——3——4——5——6——7——8——9
"Not at all" "Moderately" "Extremely"

The scoring key is at the end of the scale. You can take the scale on your own, with your partner, or separately before discussing your results. (Be aware that some responses may be unexpected or displeasing, so exercise caution when sharing this assessment with your partner.)

Intimacy Component

____ **1.** I am actively supportive of my partner's well-being.

____ **2.** I have a warm relationship with my partner.

____ **3.** I am able to count on my partner in times of need.

____ **4.** My partner is able to count on me in times of need.

____ **5.** I am willing to share myself and my possessions with my partner.

____ **6.** I receive considerable emotional support from my partner.

____ **7.** I give considerable emotional support to my partner.

____ **8.** I communicate well with my partner.

____ **9.** I value my partner greatly in my life.

____ **10.** I feel close to my partner.

____ **11.** I have a comfortable relationship with my partner.

____ **12.** I feel that I really understand my partner.

Continued. . .

____ **13.** I feel that my partner really understands me.

____ **14.** I feel that I can really trust my partner.

____ **15.** I share deeply personal information about myself with my partner.

Passion Component

____ **16.** Just seeing my partner excites me.

____ **17.** I find myself thinking about my partner frequently during the day.

____ **18.** My relationship with my partner is very romantic.

____ **19.** I find my partner to be very personally attractive.

____ **20.** I idealize my partner.

____ **21.** I cannot imagine another person making me as happy as my partner does.

____ **22.** I would rather be with my partner than with anyone else.

____ **23.** There is nothing more important to me than my relationship with my partner.

____ **24.** I especially like physical contact with my partner.

____ **25.** There is something almost magical about my relationship with my partner.

____ **26.** I adore my partner.

____ **27.** I cannot imagine life without my partner.

____ **28.** My relationship with my partner is passionate.

____ **29.** When I see romantic movies and read romantic books, I think of my partner.

____ **30.** I fantasize about my partner.

Commitment Component

____ **31.** I know that I care about my partner.

____ **32.** I am committed to maintaining my relationship with my partner.

____ **33.** Because of my commitment to my partner, I would not let other people come between us.

____ **34.** I have confidence in the stability of my relationship with my partner.

____ **35.** I could not let anything get in the way of my commitment to my partner.

____ **36.** I expect my love for my partner to last for the rest of my life.

____ **37.** I will always feel a strong responsibility for my partner.

____ **38.** I view my commitment to my partner as a solid one.

____ **39.** I cannot imagine ending my relationship with my partner.

____ **40.** I am certain of my love for my partner.

____ **41.** I view my relationship with my partner as permanent.

____ **42.** I view my relationship with my partner as a good decision.

____ **43.** I feel a sense of responsibility toward my partner.

____ **44.** I plan to continue my relationship with my partner.

____ **45.** Even when my partner is hard to deal with, I remain committed to our relationship.

Scoring Key

Add your ratings for each of the three sections—intimacy, passion, and commitment—and write the totals in the blanks. Divide each score by 15 to get an average scale score or *rating*.

Intimacy score ____ ÷ 15 = ____ Intimacy *rating*.

Passion score ____ ÷ 15 = ____ Passion *rating*.

Commitment score ____ ÷ 15 = ____ Commitment *rating*.

A score of 5 on a particular scale indicates a moderate level of the component represented by the scale; for example, an average rating of 5 on the intimacy scale indicates a moderate amount of intimacy in the relationship you chose to measure. Following this example further, a higher average rating would indicate a higher level of intimacy, and a lower average rating would indicate a lesser amount of intimacy. Examining your ratings for each of the three scales will give you an idea of how *you perceive* the amount of intimacy, passion, and commitment in your love relationship.

Source: Scale, "The Triangle of Your Love" from *The Triangle of Love* by Robert J. Sternberg.

One final note about the triangular theory: When college students in my human sexuality classes were asked if they thought Sternberg's theory had omitted any fundamental components of love relationships, many felt that effective *communication* was at least as important as intimacy, passion, and commitment. Upon further examination and discussion, the students concluded that communication was not really a separate component but an inherent part of the other three. Without mutually satisfying communication, they believed that intimacy would never be attained, passion would be less than satisfying, and neither partner would ever be sure of the other's commitment to the relationship. The students contended, therefore, that communication affects all seven types of love described by Sternberg (and even perhaps nonlove). Figure 4.2 shows how they decided to redraw Sternberg's model. The importance and the challenges of effective communication in love relationships will be our next topic of discussion.

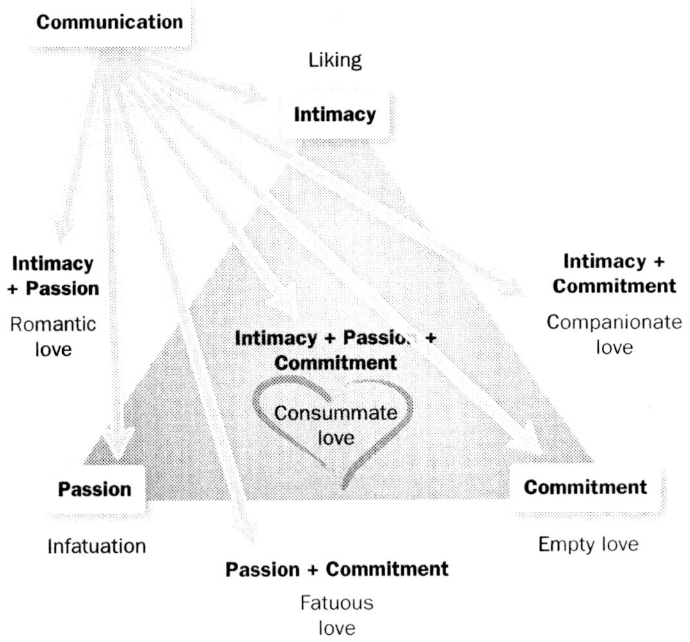

FIGURE 4.2 A Modified Triangular Theory of Love, Incorporating Communication

This is a depiction of a modified triangular theory of love that includes a fourth component, *communication*, as an inherent part of the other three components—passion, commitment, and intimacy—and, therefore, of all seven types of love described by Sternberg.

Communication in Love Relationships

How often have you heard someone say after a relationship has ended, "We just couldn't communicate?" The ability of both partners to communicate in clear, understandable, and meaningful ways is key to the happiness and long-term success of romantic relationships. Good communication skills allow couples to express the positive aspects of their relationship to each other, which tends to lead to more good feelings and a stronger connection. Equally important is the role communication plays in dealing with relationship problems and negative emotions when they arise.

Look again at Figure 4.2. You can see how the students who formulated this model envisioned communication as fundamental to love relationships. This conclusion is supported by research: The effectiveness of the pattern of communication in a relationship is one of the most accurate predictors of its future success or failure (Clements, Stanley, & Markman, 2004; Gottman & Carrere, 2000). The body of research on communication in relationships is too vast to discuss in detail here. However, examining several areas of study can provide some interesting and useful insights into effective or ineffective communication among couples and how they can learn to communicate better.

Since YOU Asked...

6. How do you know when things are going wrong or if things are right between you and your partner?

Self-Disclosure: How Much Should You Reveal about Yourself?

Most of you have probably had the experience of someone revealing personal information to you that seemed too private and made you uncomfortable—the "more than I wanted to know" phenomenon. You felt uncomfortable because you didn't think you were close or intimate enough with that person for such personal information to be disclosed to you. On the other hand, many people in love relationships become frustrated with what they perceive to be the opposite problem: Their partner seems unwilling to disclose his or her innermost thoughts and feelings, even though their relationship is intimate and such information sharing is expected and necessary for the relationship to grow and flourish. Opening up personally to each other is a major factor in building intimacy in love relationships, and some

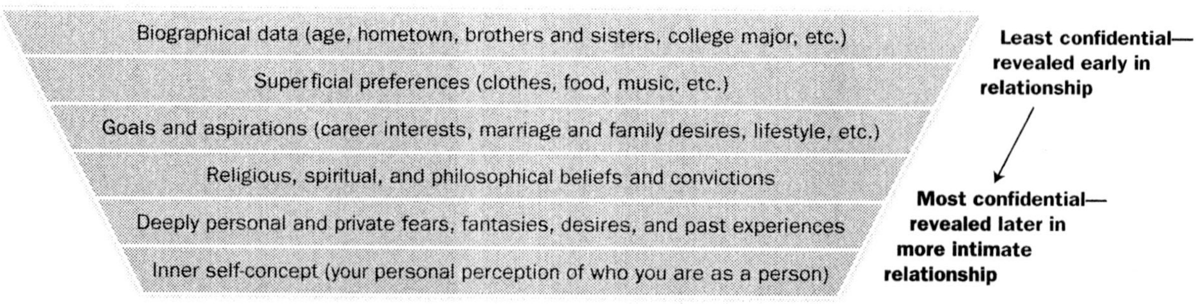

FIGURE 4.3 Levels of Self-Disclosure in Intimate Relationships

Deeper levels of self-disclosure typically occur as a love relationship matures.

Source: Based on *Social Penetration: The Development of Interpersonal Relationships* by I. Altman and D. Taylor, 1973, Holt.

researchers have suggested that it is the most important factor (Altman & Taylor, 1973; Collins & Miller, 1994).

Self-disclosure is the process of revealing personal, private, and intimate thoughts, feelings, and information to another person. How much a person reveals to a partner is usually a function of the perceived closeness of a relationship (Derlega et al., 1993; Fehr, 2004). Obviously, when you first meet a prospective romantic partner, you are unlikely to open up completely about your most personal self. In fact, if you did, the other person might be put off by your candor and back away. As a relationship continues over time and emotional intimacy deepens, self-disclosure typically increases (Byers & Demmons, 1999; Rubin et al., 1980). Conversely, gradually increasing self-disclosure tends to deepen intimacy and increase relationship satisfaction (Byers & Demmons, 1999; Derlega et al., 1993). This effect of self-disclosure in romantic relationships is due to various factors (Collins & Miller, 1994; Fehr, 2004; Parker & Parrott, 1995). One is that we tend to like people more who are willing to reveal some personal information about themselves. Another is that we are more willing to disclose our inner selves to someone to whom we feel romantically attracted. Third, when we disclose personal information to someone, we tend to become attracted even more to that person. Figure 4.3 details the widening and deepening topics of self-disclosure that typically occur as a relationship becomes increasingly intimate.

Many of you can remember a time early in a relationship when mutual self-disclosure moved the intimacy you felt to a significantly higher level. Perhaps it was just the two of you talking into the early morning hours by candlelight, an afternoon in a park with a picnic, a leisurely dinner at a secluded table in a restaurant, or any private setting. You talked and your conversation traveled to topics that revealed personal and private inner thoughts, feelings, and even secrets about your lives that neither of you had shared with anyone else or told very few others. When this mutual self-disclosure begins, many people report a significant and gratifying leap forward in the closeness of the relationship. It is at this point, when you might hear yourself say, "I think I'm falling in love."

Finally, it is important to note that although self-disclosure is concerned primarily with the verbal aspects of communication in relationships, our behaviors send strong messages between intimate partners as well. How a couple interprets each other's relationship-related behaviors can play a major role in the quality and satisfaction of the relationship. This behavioral-interpretation component of intimate communication is discussed next.

self-disclosure Revealing personal, private, and intimate thoughts, feelings, and information to another person.

Behavioral Attributions: Why Did You Do That?

In all aspects of life, one of the ways in which we judge the behavior of others and decide how we should respond to their behavior is by trying to determine why the behavior happened. For example, if someone says to you, "Leave me alone now; I just need to rest," you will interpret and react to those words far differently if you believe the person may be ill or tired as opposed to, say, angry with you. How partners in romantic relationships place blame or give credit—that is, to what they *attribute* each other's negative and positive actions—accurately reflects whether their relationship is happy or unhappy overall (Bradbury, et al., 1996; Bradbury & Fincham, 1992; Fincham & Bradbury, 1992; Karney et al., 1994). Happy couples engage in a pattern of *relationship-enhancing* attributions, whereas unhappy couples use more *distress-maintaining* attributions. Here's how attribution theory works in this context.

Imagine a couple who are generally enjoying a healthy, content relationship. On one particular occasion, one partner does something that makes the other feel upset, angry, sad, or inconvenienced. How is the aggrieved partner likely to interpret this behavior? According to attribution theory, a couple using relationship-enhancing attributions will probably (1) assume that the negative behavior is due to something external, such as being under a lot of stress lately; (2) perceive the negative behavior as an unusual and uncharacteristic event; or (3) focus on all the other positive aspects of the relationship and not dwell on the negative event. Now, what if one partner says or does something positive, something that pleases and makes the other feel good? In this case, happy couples will tend to (1) attribute the behavior to something internal about the partner, such as his or her being a wonderful person; (2) see the positive behavior as part of a stable pattern that happens often; and (3) perceive this behavior as consistent with other positive behaviors that have occurred between them in the past. You can see that whether the behavior is positive or negative, the attributions about the behavior lead to conclusions that *enhance* the relationship.

Couples in unhealthy relationships reverse this pattern and make distress-maintainig attributions. They tend to assume that negative behaviors are (1) due to something internal about the basic nature of the partner, such as the partner being an inconsiderate oaf; (2) typical of his or her usual pattern of negative behaviors, and (3) consistent with other negative behaviors that have occurred in the past. Conversely, positive behaviors are perceived as (1) caused by something external such as attempting to make-up some transgression, (2) atypical and probably temporary, and (3) inconsistent with past behaviors and performed for a self-serving reason, such as wanting something from the partner. These attributions lead the couple into patterns that maintain relationship *distress*. Figure 4.4 illustrates this theory.

If you think carefully about this apparent link between a couple's attributions for each other's positive and negative behaviors and the health of their relationship, you might wonder which is causing which. That is, do healthy relationships lead to relationship-enhancing attributions and unhealthy ones to distress-maintaining attributions, or does the attributional style of each partner produce healthy or unhealthy couples? Although the answer to this complex question is not completely clear, research suggests that it is the attributions that influence relationship health and happiness and not the other way around (Fincham & Beach, 1999). If this is true, learning more positive attribution strategies might offer a potential therapeutic route that unhappy couples might pursue to improve their unhealthy relationships.

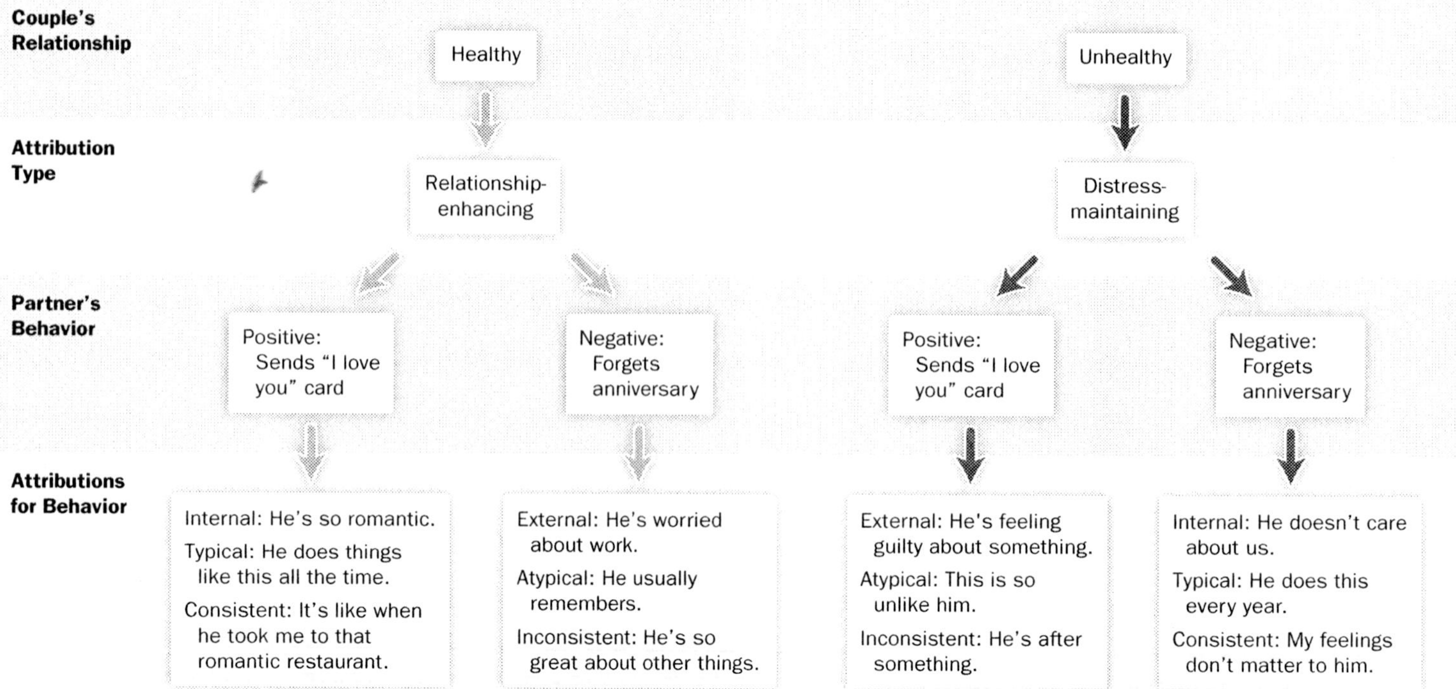

FIGURE 4.4 Relationship-Enhancing Versus Distress-Maintaining Attributions of Partner's Behavior in Healthy and Unhealthy Relationships

Partners in healthy and unhealthy relationships tend to attribute each other's positive and negative behaviors to very different motives.

Source: Adapted from Brehm, Kassin, and Fein (1999), Fig. 9.10.

Patterns of Effective Communication

Consider the words of John Gottman, one of the leading researchers on why relationships fail and how couples can repair a deteriorating relationship:

> In pursuit of the truth about what tears a [relationship] apart or binds it together, I have found that much of the conventional wisdom . . . is either misguided or dead wrong. For example, some marital patterns that even professionals often take as a sign of a problem—such as having intense fights or avoiding conflict altogether—I have found can signify highly successful adjustments that will keep a couple together. Fighting, when it airs grievances and complaints, can be one of the healthiest things a couple can do for their relationship. . . . Many couples tend to equate a low level of conflict with happiness and believe the claim "we never fight" is a sign of marital health. But I believe we grow in our relationships by reconciling our differences. That's how we become more loving people and experience the fruits of marriage. . . . Here's the surprise: There are couples whose fights are as deafening as thunder, yet who have long-lasting, happy relationships. (1994, pp. 38–39)

Gottman's research has demonstrated that it is not how much a couple fight and argue but rather their *style* of fighting that determines the happiness and success of their relationship. In fact, Gottman claims that by examining a couple's communication and conflict styles, he can predict a relationship's outcome with around 90 percent accuracy (Gottman & Carrere, 2000; Gottman & Levinson, 2002). This prediction is based on the presence of healthy communication patterns versus specific warning signs that the couple have slipped into destructive modes of interaction. Interestingly, some of the effective communication patterns Gottman has identified may not sound very healthy on the surface, but they allow relationships to maintain a fundamental balance and closeness. Gottman (in Gottman & Silver, 2000) has defined three patterns of effective communication most often seen in healthy relationships: *validating*, *volatile*, and *conflict-avoiding*.

Validating Communication

In *validating communication*, conflicts are resolved through calm discussion and compromise. Both partners listen and seek to understand each other's problems, feelings, and points of view. Even when these couples are "fighting," they each make a point of acknowledging and respecting the validity of the other's position and emotions. Because of this mutual respect, couples with this communication style typically have fewer fights than others. Here is a brief description from Gottman of such a couple:

> Bert and Betty, both 30, both came from families that weren't communicative, and they were determined to make communication a priority in their relationship. Although they squabbled occasionally, they usually addressed their differences before their anger boiled over. Rather than engaging in shouting matches, they dealt with their disagreements by having "conferences" in which each aired his or her perspective. Usually, they were able to arrive at a compromise. (1994, p. 39)

This may sound like the ideal relationship style and one that most or all successful relationships would endorse. However, research indicates that communication and conflict resolution patterns that are less validating may be just as effective in keeping a relationship together.

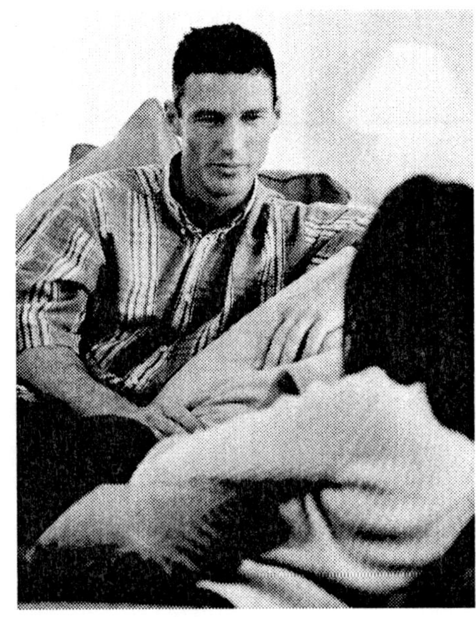

A couple with a validating communication style resolve differences through quiet discussion and mutually respectful agreements.

Volatile Communication

You have probably known couples (or been part of one) for whom conflict arises frequently; they seem to fight, bicker, and squabble and even explode into shouting matches significantly more often than average. Although some of these couples split up, others stay together over the long term and seem quite happy in the relationship. Gottman calls those who stay together *volatile couples. Volatile* means "explosive," "flammable," and "unpredictable," and that is exactly what these relationships are. The couples don't hold back and readily express their feelings in strong terms. They see themselves as equals in the relationship and feel that they possess approximately equal abilities to defend their points of view. They solve their conflicts by fighting them out (although they avoid fighting tactics that devalue or belittle the partner) until they reach some conclusion both can accept (Gottman, 1998). On the flip side of the intense conflicts, however, is an equally passionate and exciting love life. Here is an example from Gottman's research of such a couple who have a solid marriage:

Since YOU Asked...

7. My partner and I fight a lot. We yell at each other, and sometimes one of us will storm out of the house for several hours. But we love each other very much and are totally committed to each other. Is this normal?

> Max, 40, and Anita, 25, admitted that they quarreled far more than the average couple. They also tended to interrupt each other and defend their own point of view rather than listen to what their partner was expressing. Eventually, however, they would reach some sort of accord. Despite their frequent tension, they seemed to take much delight in each other. (1994, p. 39)

You can see from this example that peace and quiet is not a prerequisite for relationship success. For some couples, even a seemingly stormy relationship may be strong and loving.

Volatile couples stay together by openly and vigorously airing their feelings and fighting out their differences until they reach a mutually agreeable conclusion. They also tend to have a passionate and exciting love life.

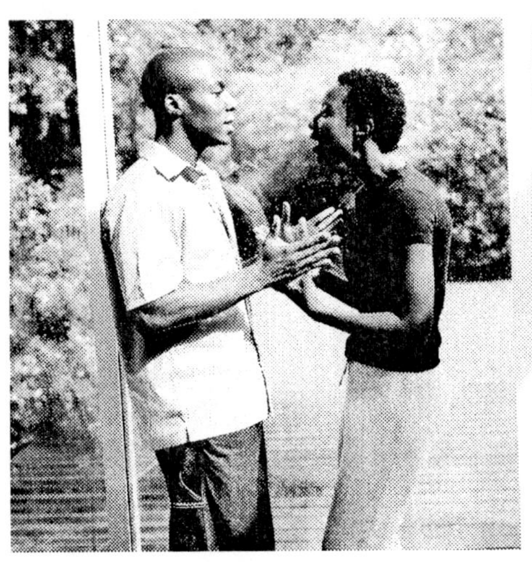

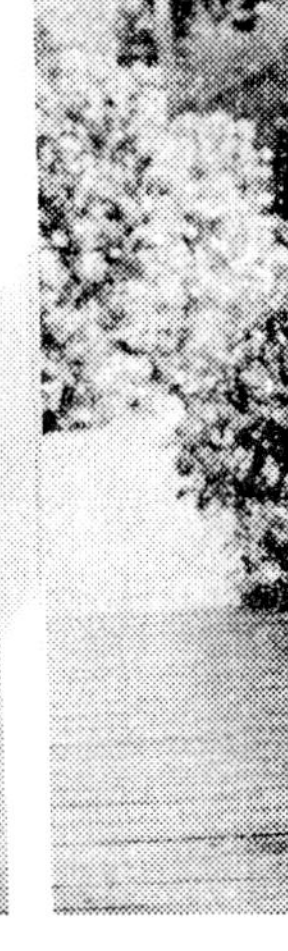

Conflict-Avoiding Communication

What about couples that are the opposite of volatile, the ones whose main goal is to avoid conflict altogether? Sound like a bad idea? Not necessarily. Couples referred to by Gottman as *conflict avoiders* may also find happiness and long-term success through the shared perception of a strong similarity between them and the apparent lack of importance they place on any differences or disagreements when they do occur. This might be called the "no big deal" approach in that they downplay conflicts they encounter and

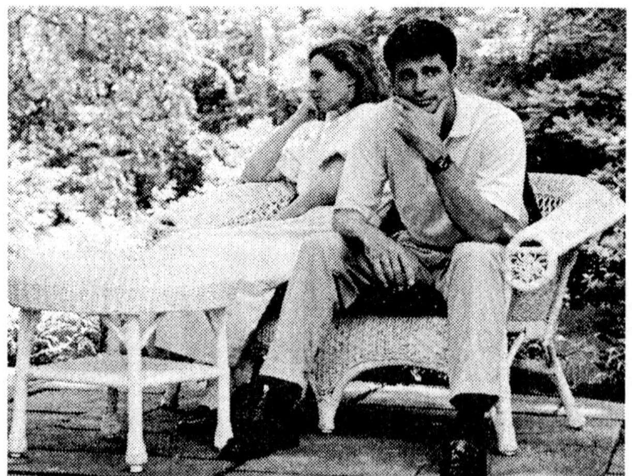

Conflict-avoiding couples would rather downplay conflicts and avoid fights and discussions altogether.

are not particularly concerned with reaching a mutual resolution. Although many people think this would only cause unresolved problems to fester and grow until they threaten the relationship itself, conflict-avoiding couples appear comfortable with this lack of resolution and truly seem able simply to "let it go," as Gottman exemplified as follows:

> Joe, 29, and Sheila, 27, said they thought alike about almost everything and felt "an instant comfort" from the start. Although they spent a good deal of time apart, they still enjoyed each other's company and fought very rarely. When tension did arise, both considered solo jogging more helpful in soothing the waters than talking things out or arguing. (1994, p. 39)

Remember, all three of these communication styles allow couples to adjust to conflicts and problems in their relationships and, according to Gottman's findings, increase the likelihood for happiness and long-term success. Some research has indicated that Gottman may have overestimated the predictiveness of the various communication patterns he has examined. One study found that relationships with validating styles of communication were, overall, more successful than those with volatile styles (Holman & Jarvis, 2003). Such conflicting findings serve as an indicator of the complexities of communication in intimate relationships and remind us that much research remains to be done. That said, ineffective communication and conflict resolution are not the only reason relationships fail; other important reasons will be discussed later in this chapter.

Communication Warning Signs

Along with the three effective communication patterns just discussed, Gottman and his research teams have also identified four communication warning signs that are common to most couples who find themselves drifting apart: criticism, contempt, defensiveness, and stonewalling. The goal in identifying these was not simply descriptive; rather it was *prescriptive:* By understanding how relationships deteriorate, couples will be better able to intervene in the process and rekindle happiness and romance. Here is a brief description of Gottman's four warning signs, which he called the "four horsemen of the relationship apocalypse" (Gottman & Silver, 2000).

Criticism

Gottman's research draws a clear distinction between complaining and criticizing. **Complaining** is an expression of an unmet need, something a person desires but is not receiving. **Criticism**, however, involves an attack on the partner's actions. The unmet need begins to be blamed on the partner. Complaining, Gottman maintains, is healthy because it expresses each partner's needs, which allows for the need to be met. But if the needs expressed by the complaints are never met, they pile up, frustration builds, and it is then only a small step from complaints to criticisms. For example, a complaint might be "I wish we could spend more time alone, just the two of us." If the complaint is not acknowledged and dealt within some way, over time it may become a criticism: "You don't want to be alone with me." This concept relates to the common relationship advice you have probably heard about fighting fairly: Use "I" statements, not "you" statements. If you find that many of the complaints between you and your partner begin with "you," this is a sign that you may have slipped from complaining to criticizing.

complaining Expressing an unmet need, something a person desires but is not receiving from a partner.

criticism Verbal fault-finding, such as commenting on a character flaw in the partner.

contempt Disrespect, disgust, or hate expressed when the positive feelings partners once had for each other have dissipated.

Contempt

If criticism is increasing in the relationship and is not averted in some way, it will eventually lead to contempt. **Contempt** implies that the true feelings the partners once had for each other have moved from liking and love to disgust, disrespect, and even hate: "You're so lazy and irresponsible; you don't even know what love is! I don't know why anyone would *want* to be with you." The difference between criticism and contempt is that criticism targets what a person does, while contempt is aimed at the person's character; comments are intentionally designed to insult and cause pain in ways only an intimate partner could know. These tactics may include specifically painful insults, name-calling, hostile humor, mockery, sneering at the partner's actions, indicating disgust for the partner, or curling the upper lip in the classic expression of contempt. Continuing our example, contempt might sound something like "You're such a jerk—I'm glad you're not around much!" As contempt builds, the couple lose the love and attraction they once felt for each other. They no longer complement each other or interact as two people who are part of an intimate partnership; instead, their focus turns to abusiveness toward one another (Gottman, 1994; Gottman & Notarius, 2002).

Defensiveness

If someone treats you with contempt or criticism, you are likely to become defensive. As natural and normal as that may be, it is bad news in a love relationship, because *defensiveness* allows each partner to deny responsibility for whatever problems are causing friction. You can see that this sets up a nearly impossible obstacle for overcoming problems: If neither partner is at fault, then all that's left is blame. It is a good idea to get to know if your own or your partner's response to disagreements is becoming defensive, so that if this is happening in your relationship, you can be aware of it and try to reverse it. Imagine one partner says to the other, "You're late again. You don't care about my schedule at all, do you?" Here are some signs of defensive tactics, along with an example of a defensive response to each criticism.

- Denying responsibility and blame for any problem your partner brings up: "*It's not my fault I'm late—class got out late.*"
- Making excuses and claiming external forces out of your control made you behave in some way that upset your partner: "*What was I supposed to do? I had to eat lunch, didn't I?*"
- Disagreeing with your partner's attempt to attribute negative thoughts to you: "*What makes you think you know what I care about?*"
- Cross-complaining—when your partner makes a complaint or criticism, you respond with one of your own, relevant or not: "*Well, you always get upset when I want to go out with my friends.*"
- Repeating yourself and your position over and over rather than trying to reach a compromise: "*I've told you before, this is about as punctual as I can get.*"

Stonewalling

Finally, as the relationship sinks deeper and deeper into hopelessness, the partners begin to give up on trying to make it work. One or both may stop engaging altogether when problems arise. This is called **stonewalling**—turning oneself into a "stone wall" when disagreements and disputes begin. In a way, stonewalling is a passive form of power and aggression. If you have ever tried discussing a personal problem with someone who simply shuts down, will not interact, and won't even offer a "hmmm" or a nod of the head, you know how powerful that silence can be. Gottman contends that stonewalling is the culmination of the three previous danger signs of criticism, contempt, and defensiveness. By stonewalling, the person is saying, "I don't care enough about you or this relationship anymore even to *try* to work things out." Stonewalling is the final event in a deteriorating relationship that leads one or both partners to say, "So, I guess it's over."

stonewalling Relying on a passive form of power and aggression by being unresponsive (erecting a metaphorical "stone wall") when disagreements and disputes erupt.

However, even when a relationship reaches a seemingly unsalvageable state, Gottman believes that all hope is not lost. He says, "If you learn to recognize what is happening to your once happy [relationship], you can still develop the tools you need to regain control of it" (1994, p. 45). Helping couples learn how to communicate their true feelings, attitudes, and desires is one of the primary paths to renewing a collapsing love relationship. That said, we now turn our attention to strategies couples can use to improve communication patterns.

Improving Communication

One strategy that couples can use to maintain positive communication is to work on preventing any of the "four horsemen"—criticizing, contempt, defensiveness, and stonewalling—from occurring. That's easy to say, but without specific techniques to develop, preserve, and renew effective communication, it may be a daunting task for some troubled couples. What does research have to offer in the way of specific suggestions to help couples communicate in ways that enhance intimacy?

Couples need to acknowledge that words are powerful and play a crucial role in building intimacy as well as destroying it. Consequently, then, couples must understand the verbal communication process and make an effort to incorporate that understanding into their interactions so that their patterns of communication bring their relationship closer rather than tearing it apart.

Understanding Intimate Communication: Six "Simple Truths"

Effective communication should be an integral part of a successful, happy relationship, not simply something a couple make a stab at when a big problem arises. In more than two decades of research into relationship conflict and communication processes, researchers Clifford Notarius and Howard Markman have observed how partners in intimate relationships either lack or lose effective communication skills and what they can do to develop or rebuild them. Notarius and Markman have condensed their findings into six basic communication principles they refer to as "simple truths." Although exceptions to general findings such as theirs always exist, their truths have, at their core, the goal of effective communication in love relationships (Markman, Stanley, & Bloomberg, 2001; Notarius & Markman, 1994).

Truth 1: Each relationship contains a reservoir of hope. Notarius and Markman contend that most relationships, even many of those that are in deep trouble and in which communication is failing, have a hidden pool, a reservoir of good intentions and hope. This pool can be used to help the couple regain good communication and intimacy if they can find where the good intentions lie and tap into them.

Truth 2: One zinger will erase 20 acts of kindness. You know what a zinger is, don't you? It's a put-down, a criticism, an unfair verbal attack on a partner. According to Notarius and Markman's research, one zinger can counteract many hours of kindness and tenderness partners give to each other. Consequently, couples must learn how to control these kinds of angry outbursts and to approach conflicts constructively and at the right time and place.

Truth 3: Small changes in you can lead to huge changes in the relationship. Improving the quality of a relationship sometimes requires only small changes, and often in only one partner. When a relationship is deteriorating, many couples often think that fixing it is insurmountable, that the amount of work and change required is overwhelming. Often, however, seemingly small adjustments can make a very positive difference. For example, Notarius and Markman suggest adding simple acts of kindness on a regular basis, such as complimenting your partner's looks or briefly stroking your partner's shoulder or back as you walk by. Conversely, they advocate that couples work to subtract thoughtless negative acts, such as ignoring your partner when you are upset or angry or resorting to name-calling, even in fun.

Truth 4: It's not the differences between partners that cause problems but how the differences are handled when they arise. No two people are exactly alike, and differences between partners are bound to cause problems in any relationship. However, in successful relationships, those differences are handled through careful listening to each other, understanding the differences, and learning to accept them. Notarius and Markman liken these listening and communication skills to being each other's best friend, not a judge or a counselor.

Truth 5: Men and women fight using different weapons but suffer similar wounds. According to Notarius and Markman, men and women are usually striving for the same goals in intimate relationships: acceptance, support, and affection. However, they use different strategies to obtain them. They claim that men are less comfortable with conflict, while women have more difficulty with emotional distance. Men have a greater tendency to withdraw from or avoid uncomfortable discussions about problems in the relationship, while women are more likely to need to resolve relationship conflicts through discussion as soon as possible.

Truth 6: Partners need to practice relationship skills in order to become good at them. This may seem simplistic or obvious. But a common misconception is that when we fall in love with someone, we should somehow just magically know how to make it work out. Clearly, that's not the case, or we would see a much higher percentage of successful relationships. In truth, happy, successful relationships require many learned communication abilities.

> Unfortunately, partners enter into relationships with no agreed-upon rules or skills for handling the strong negative feelings that are an inevitable part of all relationships. Without rules, in the face of conflict, partners often resort to forms of guerrilla warfare with random sniping that can seriously wound their mates. Instead of taking control of their conflict, partners let the conflict take control of them. (Notarius & Markman, 1994, p. 25)

Enhancing Intimate Communication: Five "Rules"

What sorts of rules and skills will help couples develop and preserve loving, happy relationships or repair them when they run into serious trouble? With their six "simple truths" in mind, Notarius and Markman have suggested a strategy they call *couple meetings* that partners can incorporate into their relationships to help keep them open, on track, and communicating well. Couple meetings require an agreement between partners to meet on a regular schedule to discuss specific instances of conflict-producing behaviors.

You may think at first glance that a couple meeting is a silly notion because most intimate couples spend a lot of time together anyway, right? Maybe, but the point of a couple meeting is not so much about the time together but rather about how that time is spent. The idea here is for the couple to agree to set aside at least 30 minutes per week, and more if needed, for open and honest communication during which it is each partner's responsibility to speak and listen as clearly and attentively as possible. Notarius and Markman (1993) offer five rules for making these couple meetings effective.

Rule 1: Make a date. Set up a regular weekly time for half an hour that goes on each partner's calendar of very important appointments. This assures both of you that no matter how busy your week becomes, this special time has been reserved for the two of you and your relationship. If problems come up at other times during the week, either discuss them immediately or allow each partner the right to decline to talk right then but schedule time for the discussion within the next 24 hours.

Rule 2: Focus on the problem. The scheduled meeting must be at a time and location that allow both partners to give their full attention to the issue at hand. If this crucial time is interrupted or disturbed by TV, telephone calls, children, or other distractions, the purpose and goals of the meeting will not be met. The couple must try to stay on one topic at a time and not allow the conversation to drift to unrelated issues.

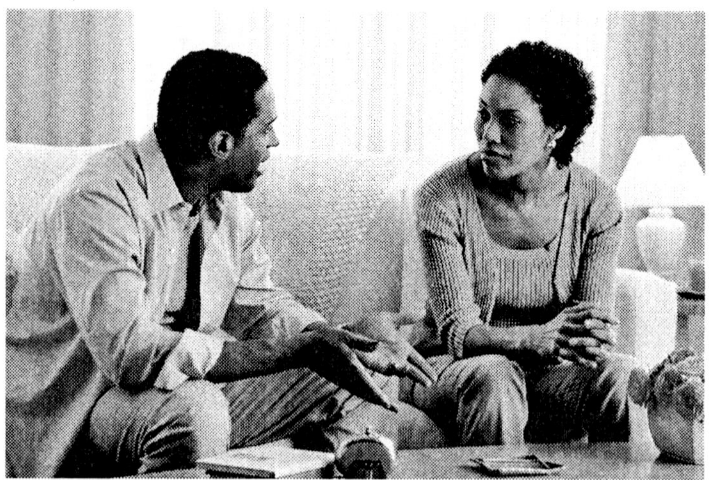

Establishing a regular, weekly meeting time when a couple can discuss their problems or concerns helps to create effective, intimate communication patterns.

Rule 3: Use the "speaker-listener tool." This is an ingenious idea in which the couple simply writes the word *floor* on an index card and passes it back and forth during the meeting. This serves as a reminder that only the partner who has the floor may speak, and the other must listen attentively. This also means that comments must be kept short and to the point and that long speeches should be avoided so that the "floor card" gets passed back and forth often.

Rule 4: Do not blame or attack. The point of the meeting is to discuss relationship problems. By definition, this means that both partners share the problem and share at least some of the responsibility for solving it. Each person must focus on his or her feelings and role in the problem, not the partner's. Blaming and attacking the other will do nothing except cause the meeting to fall apart.

Rule 5: Reserve the right to take a break. Nothing says that the meeting has to go straight through to a solution without a pause of any kind. Each partner needs to know that he or she can call for a break at any time. In fact, a break might be a good idea if anger, hostility, blaming, or attacking begins to arise. It is much better and more effective to stop the meeting and agree to pick up again later or the next day than to have the meeting deteriorate into negative feelings that cause both of you to avoid future meetings.

Couples who follow these five rules may find that such meetings can become an effective and rewarding way to communicate and iron out problems before they have a chance to escalate and threaten the relationship itself.

Finally, Notarius and Markman note that one of the most fundamental attributes of happy and successful relationships is *politeness*. Interestingly, politeness is often one of the first casualties of romantic relationships. Have you ever noticed how long-term "intimate" couples often treat each other far more disrespectfully than they would ever dream of treating a friend (or even an acquaintance). Why do you suppose this is? It probably has something to do with the assumption that in a committed relationship, you will be loved even if you ignore rules of common courtesy. Although that may be true in some relationships, the loss of politeness often causes or exacerbates existing problems, whereas behaving politely to each other is a sign of love and respect between the partners and may help prevent or diminish problems that arise.

Sexual Communication

Communicating effectively about sexual issues is one of the most difficult tasks in most relationships. People have a tendency to assume that the sexual side of an intimate relationship will take care of itself, naturally. Much of this assumption may be wishful thinking due to the fact that although most Western cultures may appear somewhat obsessed with sex, they are, paradoxically, uncomfortable with open and straightforward discussion of sexual feelings and behaviors in relationships. Partners often make the assumption that they are just supposed to know, through body language or ESP or some other sort of "lover's intuition," what the other likes and wants sexually. However, these forms of pseudocommunication rarely lead to a clear understanding of *any* important or complex issue, least of all sex. The result is that many couples experience sexual problems that increase in severity over time, in part because the partners are not willing or able to discuss them.

Research reveals that good sexual communication enhances both overall satisfaction and sexual satisfaction in intimate relationships (Byers & Demmons, 1999; MacNeil & Byers, 1997; Russell, 1990). In addition, effective sexual communication has been found to reduce unsafe sexual practices, increase sharing of information about sexually transmitted infections, and lead to more consistent use of contraception in teens and young adults (Poppen, 1994; Quina et al., 2000).

Two factors regarding sexual communication are central to this discussion: sexual self-disclosure and sexual communication. First, recall our earlier discussion of the role of self-disclosure in intimate relationships in general. One important subcategory of that relationship issue is **sexual self-disclosure**—the extent to which the partners in a love relationship are comfortable with and willing to reveal their sexual desires, backgrounds, fears, fantasies, and preferences. Second, the challenge of learning how to communicate about sexual issues with a partner is crucial. Let's briefly examine each of these issues.

Sexual Self-Disclosure

As we discussed earlier in this chapter, self-disclosure—confiding personal information and private feelings to a partner—is one of the factors that tends to increase intimacy and closeness in a growing love relationship. *Sexual self-disclosure* is an important component of intimacy with a partner and relates in significant ways to relationship success, happiness, sexual satisfaction, and sexual health (Byers & Demmons, 1999; Keller et al., 2000; MacNeil & Byers, 1997). Specifically, sexual self-disclosure is the process of revealing to your partner, in open and honest ways, any or all of the following:

- Sexual likes and dislikes, turn-ons and turnoffs
- Sexual needs and desires
- Sexual fears and concerns
- Questions about sexually transmitted infections
- Past positive sexual experiences
- Past negative sexual experiences or traumas
- Personal sexual values and morals
- Personal conditions for a sexual relationship

Some people believe that if you love your partner, sexual activities should automatically feel mutually wonderful and satisfying. However, the number and frequency of sexual problems reported by couples demonstrates all too conclusively that there is nothing automatic about it (see Chapter 7, "Sexual Problem and Solutions"). Communicating effectively about sex can pose a huge barrier, even for couples who communicate well about every other topic. It often feels emotionally risky to reveal yourself in that way. Consider some of the reasons people give for avoiding or feeling uncomfortable about confiding to their partner about personal sexual issues, and you will be better able to get a feel for why sexual self-disclosure is such a big stumbling block (in the next section, we will discuss ways of overcoming these barriers). Chances are good that you have, at some point in a relationship, felt some of these yourself.

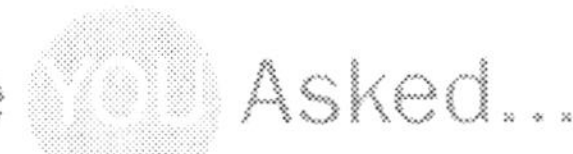

8. Why is it so difficult to explain what does and does not feel good sexually?

Lack of information. Of course, part of being able to discuss sexual topics is for both partners to possess a reasonable amount of knowledge and education about human sexuality. You will find that studying this book and taking a human sexuality course will help immensely with any future sexual discussions you may have. Virtually all sexual self-disclosure relates to one or more of the topics covered in this book and in your human sexuality course. Moreover, couples often possess varying degrees of sexual knowledge. When one member of a couple has a more extensive knowledge and education about sex, that person must take an understanding and gentle approach when discussing sexual issues to avoid making the partner feel ignorant and inferior.

sexual self-disclosure Revealing private sexual thoughts and feelings to another person.

Embarrassment. Most people feel at least some embarrassment when talking about explicit sexual topics, especially when the topic relates to themselves. For some, the embarrassment is so great that they would sooner end a relationship than try to disclose personal sexual information. However, as most love relationships grow and mature, and when people are mutually supportive and willing to work at communicating sexually, this embarrassment typically begins to decrease, and two-way sexual self-disclosure gradually becomes an integral part of the relationship.

Insecurity about using the right words. Related to these feelings of embarrassment, many people do not have a great deal of experience with sexual self-disclosures and worry about how, exactly, to say what they want to express. If the disclosure involves a sexual part of the body or a sexual act, many people are unsure what terms to use. Most of the time, a partner may know what the anatomical part or the behavior is called but feels confused or unsure about whether to use a formal, scientific term (*penis, vulva, intercourse, cunnilingus*) or more common slang terms (I'm sure you're familiar with these). To some, the formal terms may seem too clinical or stuffy, while to others, the slang may sound shocking or degrading. Again, as you will see, the solution to this problem is to take sexual communication slowly and develop mutually agreed modes of discussion.

Sexual taboos. Many people were brought up in families in which discussion of anything even hinting at sex was discouraged or forbidden. These individuals, as adults, often have a hard time talking about sexual issues with a romantic partner and an even greater difficulty initiating such conversations. This can be especially frustrating for a couple in which one partner comes from a sexually repressed background and the other grew up in a family more comfortable with discussions of sexual topics. As trust and closeness build, often the more sexually comfortable partner can help the other open up and become more at ease with sexual self-disclosure. However, couples in which both partners are from sexually inhibited backgrounds are sometimes unable to talk about their sexual relationship at all. This is a problem that, if not addressed, may lead to dissatisfaction and even failure of the relationship.

Fear of judgment. Even if partners are secure enough about their relationship not to fear rejection upon disclosing personal sexual information, one or both may still be concerned about negative judgments from the other. Often this fear stems from a reluctance to share sexual secrets until the relationship is well established. As discussed earlier, as relationships progress and deepen, other intimate self-disclosure has likely occurred, but sexual disclosures have been held back. The fear that a partner might be surprised, offended, shocked, or disbelieving upon learning something of a private sexual nature is understandable. However, as you will read in the next section, learning how to approach the discussion of sensitive sexual issues can relieve much of the anxiety about negative judgments.

Fear of rejection. Individuals who feel they can tell their partner just about anything often stop short of exposing the most personal sexual side of themselves. Many people feel guilty and uncomfortable about their own private sexual feelings, so you can imagine how afraid they would be to tell someone else about them. Why? Because no one is ever completely sure exactly how a partner might react. Although the real impact of sexual self-disclosure on a partner is frequently overestimated, the fear of rejection is real. However, love relationships that are unable to establish clear sexual communication are unlikely to succeed anyway, so the benefits of sexual self-disclosure are usually well worth the risks.

Strategies for Improving Sexual Communication

With so many potential barriers to sexual self-disclosure and sexual communication in general, how can a couple ensure that they will be able to enjoy the many benefits of an open and honest dialogue about sexuality? Many of the general guidelines for intimate communication discussed earlier in this chapter—such as avoiding criticism,

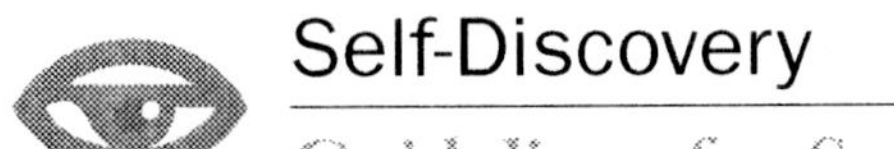

Self-Discovery

Guidelines for Sexual Communication

1. Know What You Want
   - Decide what you want and don't want in a relationship before becoming sexually involved.
   - Evaluate your personal sexual expectations and needs.
   - Behave in a manner that is consistent with your sexual philosophy and value system.
   - Be open with your partner by communicating your sexual philosophy to him or her.
   - Understand that two people can want different things and have differing sexual values and philosophies without one of them being "wrong."
2. Insist on Your Right to Postpone a Sexual Relationship
   - Set your own pace, one that is comfortable for you as the relationship progresses.
   - Wait until trust, comfort, and open communication exist in the relationship.
   - Be open and honest with your partner about your desires if you want to proceed slowly.
3. Be Responsible if You Decide to Engage in "Casual Sex"
   - Be honest with yourself and your partner if your commitment is limited to mutual enjoyment.
   - Consider whether or not this type of activity fits your personal sexual philosophy.
   - Be sure both partners want to be sexual.
   - Be sure neither partner feels coerced in any way by the other.
   - Respect your own and each other's feelings of self-worth.
   - Be sure that the responsibility to use precautions against sexually transmitted infections and unwanted pregnancy is mutually agreed on.

Source: Adapted from Michigan State University Counseling Center (2003).

contempt, stonewalling, and defensiveness; practicing the six "simple truths" of love relationships; and holding couple meetings—can be applied to sexual communication as well. However, because sexual communication has its own unique set of challenges, additional specific strategies may be valuable for those conversations. "Self-Discovery: Guidelines for Sexual Communication" offers suggestions for additional strategies when the discussion turns to sex.

Losing Love: Why Relationships End

Love relationships are among the most complex of all human connections and are rarely without conflict, stress, and periods of dissatisfaction. When a couple are unable to work through their difficulties or to find other ways of resolving friction and discord when they arise, the result, all too often, is the end of the relationship. If you were to look closely at failed relationships, you would probably be able to categorize the many explanations for their breakups into specific behaviors (or lack of them) and into certain common themes. For the purposes of our discussion here, we will consider some of the more common pitfalls couples experience that are important reasons that relationships fail.

Ten Reasons Why Relationships Fail

Lack of Self-Knowledge

If you don't know yourself, how can you expect someone else to know you? Self-knowledge about preferred lifestyle, interests, favorite activities, morals, values, sexual attitudes and preferences, field of eligibles (discussed earlier in this chapter), and expectations about love and relationships allows you to enter into a new relationship with a conscious awareness of what you want and what is best for you. Self-knowledge also allows you to communicate who you are and what you want to potential partners, so that both of you are in the best position to decide if the relationship is right.

Acceptance of Sexual Myths and Stereotypes

Men are dominant; women are passive. Men make more money than women. Women are in charge of the household. All women are multiorgasmic. All men want sex all the time. Men can have an erection whenever and for as long as they want. The man should always initiate sex. Men like sex more than women. Men are from Jupiter; women are from Saturn—or is that Mars and Venus? These are all examples of sexual myths and stereotypes in many Western cultures. As you read them, you may have been disagreeing with them and were perhaps even annoyed or angry because they sound so unfair and untrue. And you would have been correct. However, true or not, many people subscribe to these stereotypes about men, women, and sex. Relationships can easily be sabotaged by these beliefs, because they create false expectations. If a couple who has such beliefs becomes romantically involved, they are bound to end up disappointed and disillusioned.

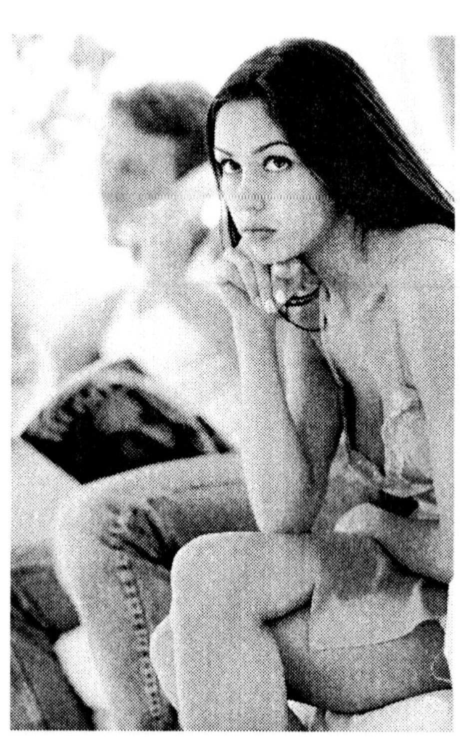

When romantic partners are unable to communicate their feelings and concerns to each other, they lose any opportunity to resolve conflicts that may eventually threaten the relationship.

Ineffective Communication

We have discussed the importance of communication in love relationships throughout this chapter. When partners fail to share with each other their feelings, concerns, frustrations, needs, and desires, they have no opportunity to address them and to repair any damage that may be occurring because of them. As problems grow without resolution through effective communication, they typically lead to behaviors that may destroy the relationship. For example, if a partner is dissatisfied about the sexual side of the relationship yet is unable to communicate this to his or her partner, what would you imagine might be the eventual outcome? One of the most common outcomes in this situation is infidelity, which eventually leads to the end of the relationship.

Imbalances of Decision-Making Power

Healthy, successful relationships are characterized by a balance between partners in money and finance matters, choices of friends, everyday activities, issues of family and children, and decision making in general. When a relationship is marked by an imbalance of power, it means that one partner has most or all of the power to make decisions that affect both partners (Blanc, 2001). You can see that such a lack of balance would render a relationship unstable. Eventually, lack of balance of power tends to lead to resentment in the lower-power partner and increasingly unhealthy levels of control by the more powerful partner.

A healthy power balance does not imply that every activity and decision must be exactly equally balanced. Partners always have different skills and preferences for dealing with various aspects of the relationship. For example, one may be good at financial details, while the other might enjoy planning social events. That partners divide up the "duties" in their relationship does not necessarily imply a lack of balance as long as such divisions are by mutual agreement and neither partner feels unwillingly excluded from the decision-making process.

Low Self-Esteem, Insecurity, and Lack of Self-Confidence

People with low self-esteem often feel that they are unworthy of being loved and may constantly look to their partner for validation and proof of love. This insecurity and lack of self-confidence typically leads to overdependence and possessiveness. Few relationships can bear the weight of one partner leaning so heavily on the other. The stronger partner is made to feel responsible for the weaker one's emotional well-being and begins to feel more like a parent or counselor than a lover. No matter how much the stronger partner may give to the weaker partner, it is never enough because the weaker partner's insecurity is typically not a product of external events but rather due to an internal disposition or basic personality characteristic. Moreover, the weaker partner is not in a position to give much to the relationship, so the stronger partner receives little support in return. Unless this lack of self-confidence and self-esteem are overcome, these relationships are usually doomed to eventual failure.

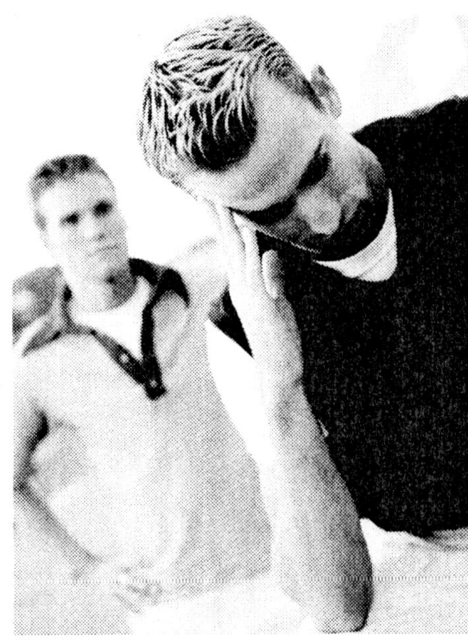

A partner's insecurity and low self-esteem can lead to over-dependency and possessiveness, creating a fundamental weakness in the relationship.

Isolation

Have you ever had a good friend with whom you got together frequently who then met someone, began a romantic relationship, and seemingly just disappeared? When a couple fall in love and then proceed to isolate themselves from the rest of the world, it is usually a red flag for potential relationship problems. Romantic love is a very strong force, and sometimes it can seem to block out everybody else in the couple's lives. However, no two people can meet all of each other's needs. We all need friends, family, colleagues, coworkers, and others who comprise a network of people who help us through life's complex challenges. Couples in healthy relationships understand that need in themselves and each other and encourage those outside connections. Usually, when a couple isolate themselves from others, it is not a sign of a deep, complete love (although that is what they may claim) but rather arises out of fear and insecurity. Eventually, this overdependence on each other may cause the relationship to be crushed under its own weight.

Failing to Keep Promises, Lying, or Cheating

This one seems obvious, doesn't it? Failing to keep promises, lying, or cheating, especially relating to infidelity, are blatant betrayals of the basic trust necessary for a relationship to survive and thrive. But even more subtle forms of deception can gradually unravel the fabric of an intimate relationship. Why? Because partners in healthy relationships tend to use rational problem-solving strategies to reconcile difficulties, disputes, disagreements, and other problems as they arise. All of these effective strategies rely on both partners *agreeing* to modify certain behaviors to resolve whatever problem they may be facing. Those agreements then become the basis for renewed happiness and satisfaction in the relationship. But these strategies are only as good as each partner's promise to carry through on them and his or her trust in the other to do the same. If one or both partners fail to keep their promise, they lose the most effective tool for solving their problems. The question then becomes "Why should I bother working out our differences when my partner won't do what he or she agrees to anyway?" Unless that basic trust can be recaptured, it is probably only a matter of time until one too many unresolved problems accumulate and the relationship dissolves.

Excessive Jealousy

Jealousy is a common reaction in romantic relationships that stems from losing all or certain aspects of a partner's exclusive love (or the fear of such a loss). Jealousy is cited as one of the most frequent causes of the breakup of romantic relationships (Knox et al., 1999). Jealousy appears to exist in similar forms in many cultures throughout the world (Buunk & Hupka, 1987). Perhaps most significant, jealousy is frequently the precipitating event in relationship abuse and violence, which will be discussed later in

Since YOU Asked...

9. How can I get my girlfriend to trust me? She's jealous all the time, and accuses me of cheating when I'm not doing anything. She's convinced I don't love her, but I do—I think.

this chapter (Moore, Eisler, & Franchina, 2000; Puente & Cohen, 2003). Jealousy may be divided into two main types—normal and delusional—and the distinction between them is important in understanding the effect jealousy can have on a love relationship (Pines & Bowes, 1992). **Normal jealousy** is based on a real threat to the relationship, as when one partner discovers that the other is attracted to, is in love with, or has been unfaithful sexually with someone else. **Delusional jealousy** is a reaction that emanates from within the jealous person when no threat or infidelity actually exists. Often called the "green-eyed monster," delusional jealousy is the form that is more likely, in itself, to destroy an intimate relationship. Normal jealousy is a reaction to factors that already indicate that a relationship is in trouble, although the intensity of the reaction may play a role in whether the couple is able to work through the episode and stay together.

Delusional jealousy typically stems from low self-esteem and overdependence in one or both partners. People with a low opinion of themselves and who look to a partner for validation, strength, and legitimacy are, understandably, terrified of losing that partner. In their eyes, without the partner, they see themselves as unworthy members of society. In these cases, it makes no difference how devoted and faithful a partner might be; delusionally jealous partners are incessantly suspicious. This is a no-win situation for their partners. They are forced to live in an atmosphere of suspicion and distrust when they have done nothing to cause or deserve it.

Ironically, delusional jealousy is often a self-fulfilling prophecy. The beleaguered, persecuted partner usually gives up trying to prove his or her fidelity and innocence because nothing ever seems to convince the jealous partner. Some individuals may eventually decide to stray from the relationship, saying to themselves, "My partner is convinced I'm guilty anyway, so why not?" Probably more commonly, the relationship cannot withstand the pressure of the constant suspicion, and the couple breaks up. The breakup then confirms the jealous partner's fears and strengthens the tendency for similar delusional jealousy patterns in subsequent relationships.

Jealousy, like most other relationship problems, can be overcome, but doing so requires a strong desire and commitment to work on the jealousy issue specifically. This may require individual and joint counseling to help the jealous partner gain the self-confidence and trust to overcome the fear and overdependence that underlies the jealous delusions.

Control Issues

A student in one of my human sexuality classes once remarked with a laugh, "My boyfriend got really mad at me last night because he said that there were 20 miles on the odometer of my car that I hadn't accounted for. Is that really weird?" No one else in the class laughed. Instead, most were shocked that anyone would keep such close tabs on someone they ostensibly love and uncomfortable that this student was laughing about it. This is an example of a controlling behavior in a potentially dangerous controlling relationship.

When one partner seeks to control the other, the relationship becomes weak at best and dangerous at worst. The need to control is actually inextricably linked to many of the other factors we have been discussing in this section, including belief in gender myths, lack of communication, unequal power, low self-esteem, isolation, overdependence, and jealousy. A relationship can remain healthy and happy only when both partners know that they have freely chosen to be in the relationship and are free to be who they are. In a controlling relationship, one partner attempts to

normal jealousy Jealousy based on a real threat to the relationship, as when one partner discovers that the other has been sexually unfaithful.

delusional jealousy Jealousy felt despite the fact that no threat to the relationship actually exists.

take that freedom away from the other and control the other's behavior. This controlling behavior may take many forms, including dictating where, when, and with whom the partner may go out; requiring the partner to report every detail of every minute whenever they are apart; demanding that the partner never deviate from an expected schedule and never arrive home late; threatening the partner with property damage or physical injury for any "disobedience"; frequently checking up on the partner at work, in the dorm, or in classes; taking charge of all the couple's money; using intimidation to prevent the partner from leaving; and name-calling, put-downs, or sudden explosions of anger.

Controlling partners are weak individuals with low self-worth who believe that the only chance they have of keeping their partners is to prevent them from having any opportunity to meet anyone else who might be a relationship possibility. They are convinced that if their partner does meet someone else, he or she will choose that person over the controlling partner.

As with delusional jealousy, relationships in which one partner is excessively controlling often fall victim to the self-fulfilling prophecy. No one wants to be controlled in these ways by another person. Eventually, the partners of controlling individuals will want out. The problem is that as a controlling partner becomes more controlling, the other partner becomes more unhappy, which makes the controlling partner more insecure and therefore more likely to exert stronger and more dangerous control until the relationship begins to resemble that of a prisoner and warden.

The most serious outcome of a controlling relationship is crossing the line from control to violence. In fact, as you will see, many behaviors that constitute relationship abuse fall under the heading of control. Not all controlling relationships become violent, but you can imagine that if a controlling partner feels that nonviolent control tactics are becoming less effective, it is a small step to violence.

Violence

Obviously, violence is a sure way to destroy a relationship. Unfortunately, violence does not usually destroy relationships fast enough, and victims are often trapped in abusive relationships for long periods of time; years, or even decades. The violence in intimate relationships is used for one purpose: to acquire total control over the victim. When that control is enforced with violence and the threat of violence, the victim's fear alone is often enough to prevent any attempt at escape. Sadly, many violent relationships end in the death of the victim. Both men and women may be victims of relationship violence, but violence by men against women is significantly more common. Statistics show that one-third of all women who are murdered are killed by their male partners (U.S. Bureau of Justice Statistics, 2002).

Many people believe that as soon as a relationship becomes violent, the victims should simply leave. However, leaving an abusive relationship is typically far from simple. Violence in intimate relationships is a very serious and complex matter to which we now turn.

Abusive and Violent Relationships

Domestic violence and relationship abuse are the dark side of love and intimacy, and unfortunately, they are an all-too-common part of intimate relationships. That is why these topics are being discussed here in greater detail than in Chapter 13, "Sexual Aggression and Violence." Everyone needs to be aware of these dangerous and destructive aspects of relationships to increase their chances of recognizing them as early as possible for themselves or for those they care about who may not perceive the risks.

For people who have never experienced an abusive or violent relationship, it is nearly impossible to imagine how a relationship that begins with love and happiness can transform into such horror and despair. As noted earlier, violence between partners not only destroys their relationship but may also devastate the victim's well-being.

If you or someone you know is caught in the trap of a violent relationship, help is available. Anyone in North America may call the National Domestic Violence Hotline (NDVH) at (800) 799-SAFE (799-7233). The hotline is staffed 24 hours a day by trained counselors who can provide crisis assistance and information about local shelters, legal assistance, health care resources, and counseling. This resource is also available on the Internet at http://www.ndvh.org, and internationally, the NDVH may be contacted via e-mail at ndvh@ndvh.org (with access to translators of 139 languages).

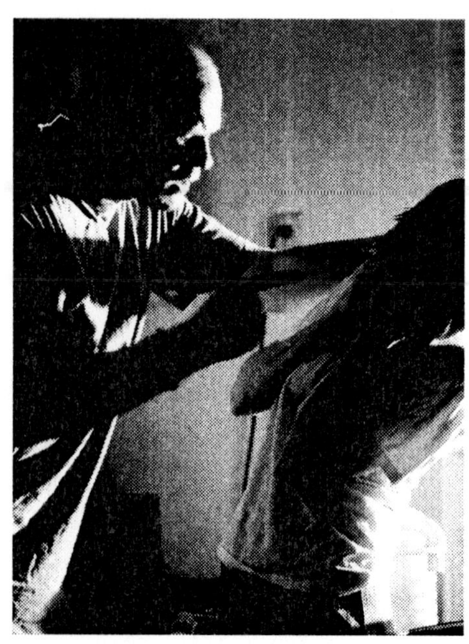

Relationship abuse may include physical violence, intimidation, or restraint, or it may involve verbal or emotional attacks such as threatening, ridiculing, or humiliating. An abuser's goal, however, is the same—to gain complete control over the partner and relationship.

Types of Relationship Abuse

No all-encompassing definition of relationship abuse exists. Each intimate relationship is unique, and so each abusive relationship is unique as well. However, if you suspect that you may be in an abusive relationship, you will notice certain signs that demonstrate clearly that your relationship is unhealthy and abusive. Two of these signs are common to nearly all cases of relationship abuse (Dugan & Hock, 2006).

First, abusive relationships are all about the use of power and control that is achieved through a wide range of tactics. The abuser's goal is to take complete control of the partner and of the relationship. The controlling tactics may be subtle and not easily recognized. It may seem to the victim that the gradual taking control over time, friends, and daily activities is a sign of love and caring. As time goes by, however, the abuser is able to render the partner totally powerless and acquire complete control of the relationship.

Second, relationship abuse usually involves a *pattern* of abusive events. A single abusive or violent act may or may not constitute abuse. However, abusive relationships are generally defined by a pattern of destructive behaviors that are cyclical and escalate over time.

Although nearly all abusive relationships share these two characteristics, the specific behaviors used by abusers to achieve these goals vary greatly and are not limited to physical violence. We will examine the three most common abuse strategies: physical, verbal, and emotional (Dugan & Hock, 2006). It is important to remember that at the beginning of most abusive relationships, the potential victim may not notice the negative behaviors. Some of the behaviors may even seem loving and caring. The jealousy may seem extreme, but it feels endearing and protective. The constant attention and togetherness may seem like a sign of the intensity of the love. However, paradoxically, these may also be signs of the violence to come.

Physical Abuse

It seems hard to believe, but some victims have experienced physical violence that they didn't label as abuse at the time. It is quite common when a woman describes a past relationship and is asked if it was abusive to reply, "Well, he never hit me." But not all physical abuse entails punching, broken bones, bleeding, or stitches. Most relationship violence causes damage that others cannot see, so they don't even know it has occurred if the victim does not choose to talk about it or does not label it as violence.

Violent partners may hit hard enough to leave bruises, but only on parts of the victim's body where others would not see them. Or the violence might entail grabbing and twisting an arm sufficiently to cause real pain without leaving a noticeable mark. If an abuser's partner is thrown against a wall, pushed to the floor, or strangled without leaving marks or bruises, no one else may ever know.

Any of these behaviors could be considered physical abuse: pushing, hitting, grabbing, choking, slapping, punching, biting, cutting, hitting with objects, pinching, physically restraining (holding partner down, pinning partner against a wall, etc.), rape or other sexual abuse, or physical intimidation (blocking partner's exit, waving a fist or a weapon, etc.). Although these behaviors may be easy for the victim to identify, some other forms of abuse, such as verbal or emotional, may not be so easy to recognize.

Verbal Abuse

Abusers may attack with words instead of—or more commonly, in addition to—physical violence. Attacks of verbal abuse may be directed at the victim or may take the form of belittling or humiliating comments or untrue accusations said to others about the victim.

Verbal abuse is extremely painful, and its effects are long-lasting. As with physical violence, verbal abuse can take many different forms, but its goal, once again, is to gain control over the victim, to crush the victim's self-image, and to cause fear and powerlessness. It often is designed to create feelings of worthlessness in the partner and transfer blame onto the victim for the abuser's attacks.

Behaviors that can be characterized as verbal abuse include yelling, threats, intimidation, ridiculing, name-calling, criticizing, accusing, insulting, humiliating, swearing, blaming, belittling, mocking, sarcasm, put-downs, and trivializing the victim's ideas, opinions, or wishes.

Emotional Abuse

Physical and verbal abuse take a terrible psychological toll. However, another category of abuse focuses on the victim's feelings themselves. This is referred to as *emotional abuse*. Emotional abuse is so insidious and psychologically devastating, it can take the longest time to identify and heal. Bruises, cuts, broken bones, or hurt feelings almost always mend faster than the wounds of emotional abuse. Abusers use many tactics to take control of and manipulate the partner's feelings and emotions. They attempt to make the victim feel unworthy of being loved, unattractive, sexually unskilled, and at fault for causing the abuse that is occurring. They intimidate and threaten their victims with bodily harm, damage to personal property, and injury to loved ones and pets.

Abusers also tend to minimize the extent of their abuse in numerous ways, trying to make the victim feel discounted, as though the seriousness of the abuse was not really so bad. Often this includes an implied or overt threat that the abuse could get much worse.

Actions that may constitute emotional abuse include entitlement ("I expect you to do what I say"); withholding information ("Why should I tell you what I'm thinking or feeling?"); withholding sex ("Why would I want to make love with someone like you?"); emotionally misrepresenting the victim's feelings ("You're not hurt—stop complaining"); risk taking (doing drugs, engaging in high-risk behaviors such as driving recklessly, not seeking medical care when needed); withholding help from the partner; excessive jealousy; threats of suicide; threatening to hurt or kill the partner, friends, relatives, or pets; and taking charge of all the decisions in the relationship.

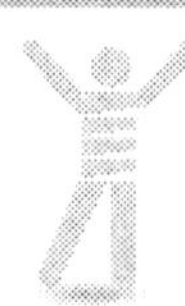

In Touch with Your Sexual Health

Signs of Relationship Abuse

Signs That You May Have an Abusive Partner

If you think you may be the victim of a violent relationship, ask yourself the following questions:

Are you . . .

- Frightened at times by your partner's behavior?
- Afraid to disagree with your partner?
- Often apologizing to others for your partner's behavior toward you?
- Verbally degraded by your partner?
- Unable to see your friends or family due to your partner's jealousy or control over you?
- Afraid to leave your partner because of threats to hurt you or commit suicide if you do?

Do you . . .

- Sometimes feel as if you have to make up excuses and justify your behavior to avoid your partner's anger?
- Avoid attending family or social function because you are afraid of how your partner will behave?

Have you been . . .

- Hit, shoved, thrown down, choked, grabbed, physically restrained, threatened, intimidated, humiliated, put down, ridiculed, or attacked by your partner with thrown objects?
- Forced by your partner to engage in sexual acts against your will?

If you answer yes to even *one* of these questions, you may be in an abusive relationship. Help is available: Call (800) 799-SAFE (799-7233) at a time and place unknown to your abuser.

Signs That You May Be an Abusive Partner

If you think you are being abusive to your partner, ask yourself the following questions:

Do you . . .

- Frequently check on your partner's whereabouts, friends, or activities?
- Criticize or insult your partner?
- Believe that you are permitted to hit, shove, or slap your partner for actions you do not like?
- Believe that your inappropriate or violent behaviors are caused by your partner's actions?

Have you . . .

- Threatened or broken things to frighten your partner?
- Threatened to leave or actually left your partner in a dangerous or unknown place?
- Driven too fast or recklessly to frighten your partner?
- Hit, shoved, thrown down, choked, grabbed, physically restrained, threatened, intimidated, humiliated, put down, ridiculed, or attacked your partner with thrown objects?
- Blamed your violent or abusive behavior toward your partner on alcohol or other drugs?
- Intimidated your partner to get your way?
- Threatened to harm yourself if your partner leaves or breaks up with you?
- Forced or coerced your partner into unwanted sexual acts?

If you answer yes to even *one* of these questions, you may very well be abusing your partner. Help is available: Call (800) 799-SAFE (799-7233) before the violence and abuse become more serious and more dangerous.

Source: Adapted from publications of Project Sanctuary, Ukiah and Fort Bragg, California.

How can you know if you are in an abusive relationship? The answer may not be as obvious as it seems. Many levels and types of violence exist, and some are not as immediately recognizable as others. "In Touch with Your Sexual Health: Signs of Relationship Abuse" will help you assess if you are in an abusive relationship or if you are engaging in behaviors commonly seen in abusers.

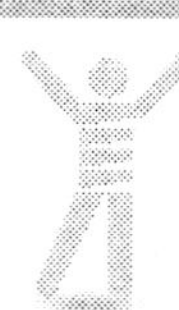

In Touch with Your Sexual Health

Signs of Relationship Abuse

Signs That You May Have an Abusive Partner

If you think you may be the victim of a violent relationship, ask yourself the following questions:

Are you . . .

- Frightened at times by your partner's behavior?
- Afraid to disagree with your partner?
- Often apologizing to others for your partner's behavior toward you?
- Verbally degraded by your partner?
- Unable to see your friends or family due to your partner's jealousy or control over you?
- Afraid to leave your partner because of threats to hurt you or commit suicide if you do?

Do you . . .

- Sometimes feel as if you have to make up excuses and justify your behavior to avoid your partner's anger?
- Avoid attending family or social function because you are afraid of how your partner will behave?

Have you been . . .

- Hit, shoved, thrown down, choked, grabbed, physically restrained, threatened, intimidated, humiliated, put down, ridiculed, or attacked by your partner with thrown objects?
- Forced by your partner to engage in sexual acts against your will?

If you answer yes to even *one* of these questions, you may be in an abusive relationship. Help is available: Call (800) 799-SAFE (799-7233) at a time and place unknown to your abuser.

Signs That You May Be an Abusive Partner

If you think you are being abusive to your partner, ask yourself the following questions:

Do you . . .

- Frequently check on your partner's whereabouts, friends, or activities?
- Criticize or insult your partner?
- Believe that you are permitted to hit, shove, or slap your partner for actions you do not like?
- Believe that your inappropriate or violent behaviors are caused by your partner's actions?

Have you . . .

- Threatened or broken things to frighten your partner?
- Threatened to leave or actually left your partner in a dangerous or unknown place?
- Driven too fast or recklessly to frighten your partner?
- Hit, shoved, thrown down, choked, grabbed, physically restrained, threatened, intimidated, humiliated, put down, ridiculed, or attacked your partner with thrown objects?
- Blamed your violent or abusive behavior toward your partner on alcohol or other drugs?
- Intimidated your partner to get your way?
- Threatened to harm yourself if your partner leaves or breaks up with you?
- Forced or coerced your partner into unwanted sexual acts?

If you answer yes to even *one* of these questions, you may very well be abusing your partner. Help is available: Call (800) 799-SAFE (799-7233) before the violence and abuse become more serious and more dangerous.

Source: Adapted from publications of Project Sanctuary, Ukiah and Fort Bragg, California.

How can you know if you are in an abusive relationship? The answer may not be as obvious as it seems. Many levels and types of violence exist, and some are not as immediately recognizable as others. "In Touch with Your Sexual Health: Signs of Relationship Abuse" will help you assess if you are in an abusive relationship or if you are engaging in behaviors commonly seen in abusers.

Violent partners may hit hard enough to leave bruises, but only on parts of the victim's body where others would not see them. Or the violence might entail grabbing and twisting an arm sufficiently to cause real pain without leaving a noticeable mark. If an abuser's partner is thrown against a wall, pushed to the floor, or strangled without leaving marks or bruises, no one else may ever know.

Any of these behaviors could be considered physical abuse: pushing, hitting, grabbing, choking, slapping, punching, biting, cutting, hitting with objects, pinching, physically restraining (holding partner down, pinning partner against a wall, etc.), rape or other sexual abuse, or physical intimidation (blocking partner's exit, waving a fist or a weapon, etc.). Although these behaviors may be easy for the victim to identify, some other forms of abuse, such as verbal or emotional, may not be so easy to recognize.

Verbal Abuse

Abusers may attack with words instead of—or more commonly, in addition to—physical violence. Attacks of verbal abuse may be directed at the victim or may take the form of belittling or humiliating comments or untrue accusations said to others about the victim.

Verbal abuse is extremely painful, and its effects are long-lasting. As with physical violence, verbal abuse can take many different forms, but its goal, once again, is to gain control over the victim, to crush the victim's self-image, and to cause fear and powerlessness. It often is designed to create feelings of worthlessness in the partner and transfer blame onto the victim for the abuser's attacks.

Behaviors that can be characterized as verbal abuse include yelling, threats, intimidation, ridiculing, name-calling, criticizing, accusing, insulting, humiliating, swearing, blaming, belittling, mocking, sarcasm, put-downs, and trivializing the victim's ideas, opinions, or wishes.

Emotional Abuse

Physical and verbal abuse take a terrible psychological toll. However, another category of abuse focuses on the victim's feelings themselves. This is referred to as *emotional abuse*. Emotional abuse is so insidious and psychologically devastating, it can take the longest time to identify and heal. Bruises, cuts, broken bones, or hurt feelings almost always mend faster than the wounds of emotional abuse. Abusers use many tactics to take control of and manipulate the partner's feelings and emotions. They attempt to make the victim feel unworthy of being loved, unattractive, sexually unskilled, and at fault for causing the abuse that is occurring. They intimidate and threaten their victims with bodily harm, damage to personal property, and injury to loved ones and pets.

Abusers also tend to minimize the extent of their abuse in numerous ways, trying to make the victim feel discounted, as though the seriousness of the abuse was not really so bad. Often this includes an implied or overt threat that the abuse could get much worse.

Actions that may constitute emotional abuse include entitlement ("I expect you to do what I say"); withholding information ("Why should I tell you what I'm thinking or feeling?"); withholding sex ("Why would I want to make love with someone like you?"); emotionally misrepresenting the victim's feelings ("You're not hurt—stop complaining"); risk taking (doing drugs, engaging in high-risk behaviors such as driving recklessly, not seeking medical care when needed); withholding help from the partner; excessive jealousy; threats of suicide; threatening to hurt or kill the partner, friends, relatives, or pets; and taking charge of all the decisions in the relationship.

The Cycle of Violence and Abuse

Relationship abuse and violence typically increase gradually over time, often causing the victim to be unsure of exactly when the abuse began. This is in part because no violent relationship is violent all the time. Even if a relationship is violent on a frequent and ongoing basis, the couple still experience many moments, hours, or even days or weeks when no overt violence occurs. This pattern can make it difficult for a victim to recognize the abusiveness of the relationship until the violence becomes extreme (Dugan & Hock, 2006). Nevertheless, the abuse usually follows a fairly predictable pattern, often called the *cycle of violence*.

cycle of violence The repetitive pattern of stages that define most abusive and violent relationships, cycling through the honeymoon stage, the tension-building phase, and the explosion of violence, followed by a return to the honeymoon stage, and the beginning of a new cycle.

The **cycle of violence** describes how a violent relationship typically develops unless something is done to intervene. For most relationships, even potentially violent ones, the early stages are happy, exciting, even idyllic. Everything seems wonderful. Partners are loyal, devoted, and caring and seem to have eyes only for each other. It feels like a dream come true. This is the *honeymoon phase* of an intimate relationship.

In all relationships (healthy and unhealthy), after a while, something happens that creates tension between the partners. It may be a simple difference of opinion, a disagreement over a purchase, an activity, or just an argument about a controversial subject. Whatever the issue is, even it is relatively trivial, it temporarily disrupts the harmony of the new relationship. This is completely normal. In healthy relationships, the problem is typically resolved by talking about it and working it out between the partners.

In contrast, in abusive relationships, this rational, problem-solving approach fails, and the tension persists and builds. Soon one partner realizes that the only way to regain the harmony is to give in to the other's position. Although giving in may cause this partner to feel resentful and discounted, he or she usually decides that if giving in relieves the tension, it is worth doing so that the loving, harmonious atmosphere of the honeymoon phase can return. However, at some point, another event occurs that once again creates tension between the couple. This is the *tension-building* phase of the cycle. This time, instead of one partner surrendering, an abusive or violent explosion occurs. Typically, the abusive partner yells, ridicules, threatens, insults, or engages in other acts of bullying and intimidation. Now the victim is afraid and does whatever is necessary to calm things down. Then, again, for days, weeks, or even months, relations return to a happy, loving, honeymoonlike period.

As time passes, this cycle continues, but typically the explosive events become more extreme and dangerous, and the buildup of tension nearly always ends in abuse. What began as insults and threats may now become physical violence. But still, after the violence, the honeymoon begins again. The abuser is sorry, promises it will never happen again, asks forgiveness, is repentant, perhaps buys gifts for the victim. The victim, in turn, tries to make things better and does everything humanly possible to make the relationship happy and tension-free. As the relationship reenters the honeymoon phase, emotions are soothed, but by now the victim lives in fear of another explosion and goes to great lengths (characterized as "walking on eggshells") to avoid any behavior that might trigger more violence. Compared to the other phases of the cycle, this time between outbursts truly feels like another honeymoon, and the victim hopes it will last. But it does not, and sooner or later the abuse and violence return. Figure 4.5 illustrates this cycle of violence and abuse.

FIGURE 4.5 The Cycle of Violence and Abuse in Intimate Relationships

Violent and abusive relationships tend to progress in a predictable cycle of repeating and increasing volatility.

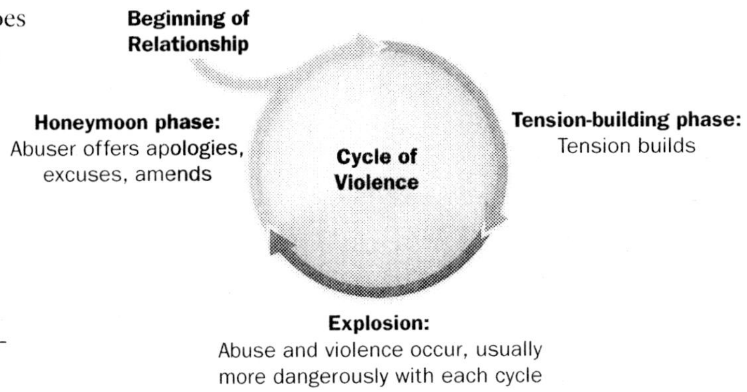

Beginning of Relationship

Honeymoon phase: Abuser offers apologies, excuses, amends

Cycle of Violence

Tension-building phase: Tension builds

Explosion: Abuse and violence occur, usually more dangerously with each cycle

Leaving a Violent Relationship

Relationship abuse is far more complex a problem than most people realize. Strange as it may seem to many people, those caught up in a violent or abusive relationship may not even realize what is happening until the abuse has escalated to the point of real physical danger. Even then, a victim may find escape from the violent setting nearly impossible because of overdependence on the abuser, fear of being left alone and without financial means, terrified of worse or even deadly violence, or concern for children who may be part of the relationship.

Unfortunately, relationship violence tends not to diminish or go away over time; on the contrary, it is more likely to become worse. Usually, the only way to stop relationship violence is for the victim to leave. Ironically, however, a victim of an abusive relationship is at the greatest risk of violence when trying to leave the abuser. The vast majority of serious assaults and murders in violent relationships occur while the victim is attempting to leave the relationship or has already left the abuser (Anderson, 2003). If you think about it, this makes a great deal of sense. Remember, the goal of the abuse is control over the other person, and typically this control stems from the fear that the victim will leave the abuser. When that fear becomes a reality, the only recourse an abuser knows is to become more violent in a desperate attempt to regain control over the departing partner.

What should a victim do to be reasonably safe after leaving an abusive relationship? There are no guarantees of safety, but several guidelines can help (Dugan & Hock, 2006):

1. Assess the abuser's danger level. Analyze past violent behavior, threats made about the consequences for attempting to leave, possession or past use of weapons, and so on.
2. Have an escape plan. Develop a route of escape if the abuser attempts access at home, at work, at relatives' homes, or anywhere else a violent approach might be attempted. Know how to get away and where to go. This helps a victim stay one step ahead of an abuser out for control and revenge.
3. Create a safety network of trusted people. Keep their phone numbers handy at all times. Work out how they can provide a place to hide or other forms of shelter from the abuser.
4. Obtain a court-ordered restraining order that legally requires the abuser to stay away from you. Even this is no guarantee of safety, but many abusers will not violate a restraining order because they can be arrested and jailed if they do.

These measures may sound drastic, but severe violence and even murder are very real possibilities in the aftermath of violent relationships.

The Temptation to Go Back

It is difficult for anyone who has not experienced an abusive relationship to understand how a survivor would ever consider, even for a moment, returning to the abusive partner. When survivors consider returning and try to discuss it with friends or family, they may encounter shock, astonishment, disbelief, anger, and recriminations. Some survivors become very upset with themselves at the thought of returning to their abuser. They may wonder if they are crazy to contemplate such a seemingly irrational act.

But returning can be very tempting. The vast majority of women victims of relationship violence return to their abusing partner at least once, and nearly a fifth of victims have returned ten times before they finally leave permanently (Anderson, 2003). Their reasons for returning range from lack of financial resources to continuing feelings of love for the abuser; from loneliness to fear of being killed by the abuser

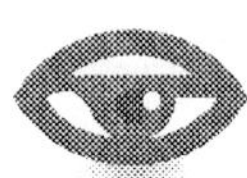

Self-Discovery

Your Criteria for a Healthy, Nonabusive Relationship

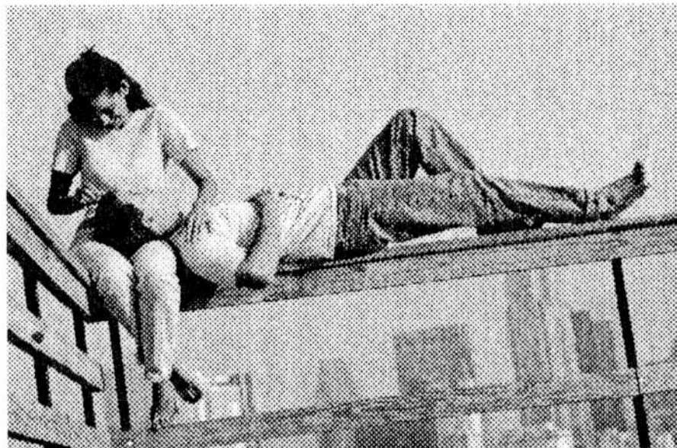

Survivors of abusive relationships can be more confident or finding a healthy relationship in the future if they are clear about their personal criteria for an intimate partner.

The ease with which a survivor of an abusive or violent relationship is able to complete this exercise offers an important clue about his or her readiness for a new relationship. Those who have survived such an unhealthy relationship should be clear about what they require and what is unacceptable in a partner *before* they begin a relationship with someone new.

A. List at least five qualities you will absolutely require in a new partner. These are nonnegotiable.

Qualities I will require:

1.
2.
3.
4.
5.

B. List at least five characteristics or behaviors you will avoid in a new partner. These you will not accept under any circumstances.

Characteristics I will not accept:

1.
2.
3.
4.
5.

Source: Adapted from Dugan and Hock (2006, p. 242).

(Anderson, 2003; Griffing et al., 2002). Reconstructing a life alone after an abusive relationship can be extremely difficult. Some survivors even say they were happier in the relationship than they are without it. Numerous new sources of stress may tend to eclipse the memory of the abuse. For many survivors, the horror of the abuse does not completely erase the positive aspects of the relationship (recall that the violence and abuse is cyclical, with good times as well as bad). However, survivors must guard against returning to a violent and potentially deadly relationship due to the stress of life alone and selective positive memories. When a victim returns to an abuser, the violence typically does not stop; instead, it tends to escalate with each successive episode (Anderson, 2003; Dugan & Hock, 2006).

Loving Again

Is someone who has survived a terribly abusive relationship ever able to risk an intimate relationship again? The answer is yes, but often the road back to love requires a great deal of careful thought and self-assessment. One common fear survivors face is becoming involved with another abusive or violent person. When victims look back on the violent relationship, they typically

Since You Asked...

10. Can someone who has been in an abusive relationship ever have a normal relationship again? Is it really possible to forgive and forget?

report that they never saw it coming; they simply fell in love with a person who showed no signs of the abusive nature that would later be revealed. However, signs that a person who *may* become a violent partner have been identified and are listed in Table 4.2. Knowing these signs is no guarantee that an abusive partner can be identified in advance, but they provide a backdrop against which to judge a potential partner early on in a relationship.

Finally, when survivors of violent relationships begin to consider a new relationship, they must apply what they have learned about themselves and about relation-

Table 4.2 WARNING SIGNS OF A POTENTIAL ABUSER

The following characteristics have been identified as more common in individuals who become abusive or violent partners. No one can know for sure if a relationship may turn violent, but an awareness of these features may help avoid a future tragedy.

CHARACTERISTIC OF POTENTIAL ABUSER	DESCRIPTION
Has a history of battering	May admit to hitting previous partners but will blame the partner for provoking the attacks; partner may learn about past abuse from relatives or ex-partners; battering behavior is independent of situation or partner.
Uses threats of violence	Makes threats of physical violence meant to control the partner; will attempt to excuse behavior by claiming "everybody talks like that."
Breaks or hits objects when angry	May break partner's favorite possessions or hit walls or furniture near partner to terrorize; action implies that "this could be you."
Uses force during an argument	May involve grabbing, pushing, physically restraining, blocking exit from situation, and so on.
Displays excessive jealousy	Is intensely jealous without reason or provocation, even in the very early stages of the relationship; will often claim jealousy is sign of deep caring.
Engages in controlling behavior	Attempts to take over all decision making; checks up on where partner is at all times; becomes angry at any lateness; takes charge of the money.
Becomes romantically involved very quickly	"Falls in love" very soon after meeting; pressures partner for commitment; desires to get married or live together after very short time (less than six months); comes on very strong with proclamations of undying and ultimate love.
Has unrealistic expectations	Expects relationship to fulfill both partners' every need and desire; assumes that partner automatically knows and will attend to all the abuser's physical and psychological needs.
Isolates partner from social contacts	Attempts to separate partners from all personal and social connections (work, friends, relatives) and establish sole and complete control.
Blames others for own problems	Any problem (job loss, car accident, etc.) is partner's or someone else's fault; never takes responsibility for any mistake or bad decision.
Blames others for own feelings	Blames partner for own anger and violence; believes partner is responsible for all negative actions or feelings.
Is hypersensitive to criticism	Is easily insulted and claims hurt feelings when partner is the one who is hurt and angry; interprets any small problem as a personal attack; sees world as basically unfair.
Displays cruelty to animals or children	May punish animals brutally or be insensitive to their pain; expects children to be capable of behaviors far beyond their abilities and is angered when they fail; may tease young children until they cry.
Uses "playful" force in sex	May desire to tie or hold partner down; demands sex regardless of partners' mood, desire, or willingness.
Engages in verbally abusive behaviors	Makes comments intended to be cruel and hurtful; verbally degrades partner; diminishes partners' accomplishments.
Subscribes to rigid male-female sex roles	Male batterer expects woman to serve him; may require that she stay at home; expects obedience in every way; sees women as inferior to men.
Displays "Jekyll and Hyde" mood swings	Has instantaneous mood swings; is pleasant one minute, but the next minute is explosive or "crazy."

Source: "Warning Signs of a Potential Abuser" adapted from The Project for Victims of Family Violence, Inc. Reprinted by permission of The Project for Victims of Family Violence, Inc.

ships. A reliable sign that survivors are ready to love and be loved in a happy, healthy relationship is that they are able to articulate what they want from that relationship and what they will never again tolerate from a partner. "Self-Discovery: Your Criteria for a Healthy, Nonabusive Relationship" provides a framework for survivors to test their level of clarity about potential future partners.

YOUR SEXUAL PHILOSOPHY

LOVE, INTIMACY, AND SEXUAL COMMUNICATION

Falling in love is one of the most emotionally charged events in our lives. Incorporating the issues discussed in this chapter into your working sexual philosophy *frees* you to enjoy love and intimacy to the fullest, because you know that you have the tools to avoid being swept away to a "destination" that is wrong for you. How might the information in this chapter fit into your developing sexual philosophy?

First, the more you know about your requirements for an intimate relationship, the better your ability to judge whether or not someone you meet and feel attracted to is likely to be right for you. This awareness does not *guarantee* that every potential relationship is going to work out and make you happy, but the more you develop a real sense of your needs and desires for a potential intimate partner, the better your chances of avoiding becoming involved with the wrong person, realizing too late that the person is totally wrong for you, and then enduring the pain of breaking up.

Second, effective communication can be difficult in love relationships, especially when the topics are about sensitive or sexual issues. Many if not most people enter into intimate relationships without understanding the basic strategies and barriers for intimate communication. This places them at a disadvantage from the start. If you have made an effort to familiarize yourself with at least a few proven techniques for successful communication, you will be better prepared and one step ahead when those first difficulties with your partner arise (and they always do).

Third, most of you will, unfortunately, experience at least one breakup of an intimate relationship, and many of you probably already have. The intense emotions that usually surround the ending of a relationship often leave people confused, bewildered, and asking, "What went wrong?" "How did something that seemed so great at the beginning end up causing so much pain?" Adding an understanding of why relationships end to your sexual philosophy will better prepare you to prevent a breakup of a good relationship; perhaps more important, you will "see the writing on the wall" sooner and reject potentially abusive relationships.

Your sexual philosophy will need to be crystal clear that you will not tolerate abuse or violence in your relationships. Most people who find themselves in a violent situation with a partner say they were completely shocked that their relationship transformed into such a nightmare. Knowing what these relationships are like and how they develop does not ensure completely that it can't happen to you, but it does allow you to be alert to warning signs and, ideally, escape at the earliest hint of violence or abuse before you become trapped by violence, danger, and fear.

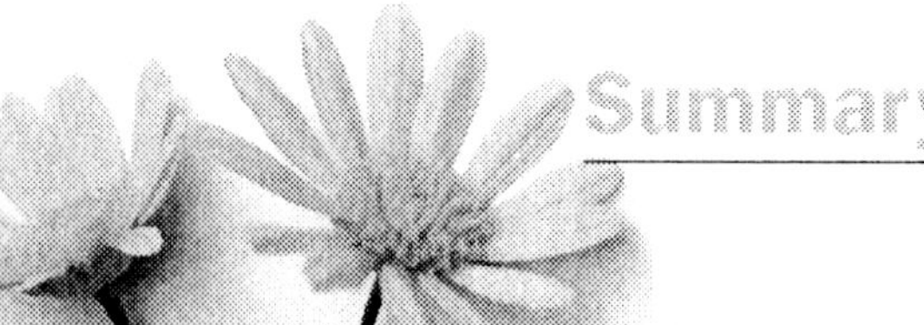

Summary

HISTORICAL PERSPECTIVES George and Martha in Love and Marriage

- In the 1700s, most marriages were undertaken for financial gain and social standing. Marriages were often arranged by the bride and groom's fathers to enhance the family's position in the community. Engagements, or courtships, tended to be relatively brief. The process of betrothed couples "getting acquainted" was speeded up through the practice of "bundling," or sleeping in same bed fully clothed, sometimes with a board between the young couple to prevent them from "losing control."

Establishing Early Intimacy

- Today courtship is more under the control of the couple themselves in most cultures. Many factors influence romance and intimacy and whether a couple make a lifelong commitment to each other. These factors include a person's field of eligibles, physical attractiveness, proximity, similarity, flirting, and reciprocity of attraction.

Love

- Individuals may be characterized by one or more of six "love styles" in intimate relationships: eros (intensely romantic love), ludus (game-playing love), storge (friendship love), mania (obsessive love), pragma (practical love), and agape (selfless love). Couples with differing love styles are less likely to sustain a relationship over time.
- Sternberg's triangular theory of love identifies the three primary components of love as intimacy, passion, and commitment. Relationships with all three components are called consummate love; when one or more of these components is lacking, the relationship may be characterized as empty love, mere infatuation, romantic yet short-lived love, friendship, companionate love, or fatuous love.

Communication in Love Relationships

- Self-disclosure tends to deepen as relationships intensify. Revealing personal information to a partner about your sexual preferences, fears, anxieties, desire, and values is all part of the challenge of sexual self-disclosure.
- Effective communication is fundamental in successful relationships. Researchers have identified three distinct communication styles in intimate relationships: validating, volatile, and conflict-avoiding. Poor communication patterns may signal that a relationship is weak and unstable. Warning signs of poor communication include criticism, contempt, defensiveness, and stonewalling. However, couples may improve their ability to communicate by learning new, more effective communication styles, such as holding regular "couple meetings," avoiding blame, and improving romantic communication.
- Communicating about sex is one of the most difficult challenges for couples because of embarrassment over sexual topics, lack of accurate information, cultural sexual taboos, and fear of being judged or rejected by the partner. Communicating about sex is a learning process that takes time as partners' comfort levels increase and their emotional intimacy deepens.

Losing Love: Why Relationships End

- Specific behaviors have been identified that contribute to the end of relationships. The most common factors include one or more of the following: lack of self-knowledge, acceptance of false relationship myths, poor communication, power imbalances between the partners, low self-esteem of one or both partners, social isolation of the couple from others, lying and cheating, excessive jealousy, controlling behaviors, and violence.

Abusive and Violent Relationships

- Abuse and violence are the dark side of love relationships. Relationship abuse includes physical violence, verbal abuse, and emotional abuse.
- Abusive patterns typically repeat in a cycle: the honeymoon phase, the tension-building phase, and the explosion of abuse or violence, followed by a return to the honeymoon phase. The pattern then repeats, with the abuse and violence typically escalating.
- The fear of this escalating violence, concern over children who may be part of the relationship, lack of money, loss of emotional support, and even the possibility of being murdered by the abusive partner are a few of the reasons abuse victims become trapped in these relationships and why, among those who do leave, most return to their abusers one or more times. Learning the signs of potential abusers may help prevent initial involvement or allow for earlier escape.

YOUR SEXUAL PHILOSOPHY: Love, Intimacy, and Sexual Communication

- Incorporating the issues discussed in this chapter into your working sexual philosophy frees you to enjoy love and intimacy to the fullest, because you will have the knowledge to avoid being swept into an intimate relationship that may be wrong for you. You will also have the tools to make a good relationship better or to help heal a relationship that may be having problems. Perhaps most important, you will be less likely to become trapped in unhealthy relationships that are abusive or violent.

Have You Considered?

1. Think of at least three people who are *not* in your field of eligibles. Briefly describe each one, and explain what characteristics cause you to exclude the person from any possibility of a romantic involvement.
2. Now think of a romantically involved couple, either people you know or celebrities, who violate the matching hypothesis. Explain why you think they are together and why their relationship is successful despite significant differences in level of attractiveness.
3. Imagine that you are in a romantic relationship that is lacking one of Sternberg's three basic components. If you had to accept less than a consummate relationship, which component would be the *least difficult* to live without? Which would be the *hardest* to live without? Explain your answers.
4. Complete the Styles of Love scale on page 107, and determine which style fits you best. Now go back and complete the scale as best you can for your "ideal partner" (not a current or past partner, necessarily, but the partner that you imagine would be perfect for you). Compare your love style with your ideal partner's style. How do they match up? Discuss what you learned about yourself from this exercise.
5. As discussed in the chapter, John Gottman believes that complaints can be positive in a relationship because they express an unmet need felt by one of the partners. Consider the following complaint in an intimate relationship: "I feel as if I'm doing all the yard work, and I wish we could share those responsibilities." Rewrite how that complaint would sound as a relationship begins to exhibit each of Gottman's four communication warning signs—(a) criticism, (b) contempt, (c) defensiveness, and (d) stonewalling.
6. Which of Notarius and Markman's six simple relationship truths do you think is the most important? Explain your answer.
7. Think about the unsuccessful relationships that you have had or observed in others. Discuss which of the ten relationship destroyers summarized in the chapter most likely caused those relationships to fail. Explain your answer.
8. Explain what you think are the three most common reasons survivors of abusive relationships return to their batterers, often many times, before they finally leave for good. Suggest possible interventions that might help survivors of an abusive relationship stay out of it once they are out.

Companion Website Resources

For further chapter resources go to **www.prenhall.com/hock.** This robust text website includes polling questions for you to vote on, regular news updates, quizzes, sample tests, suggested reading lists, and more.

SCENARIOS USA Also on the website are links to videos. *Scenarios USA*'s films portray real-life narratives that explore the non-biological aspects of relationships and sexual health. The films will help you consider how the themes of the text affect your own life and the lives of those around you.

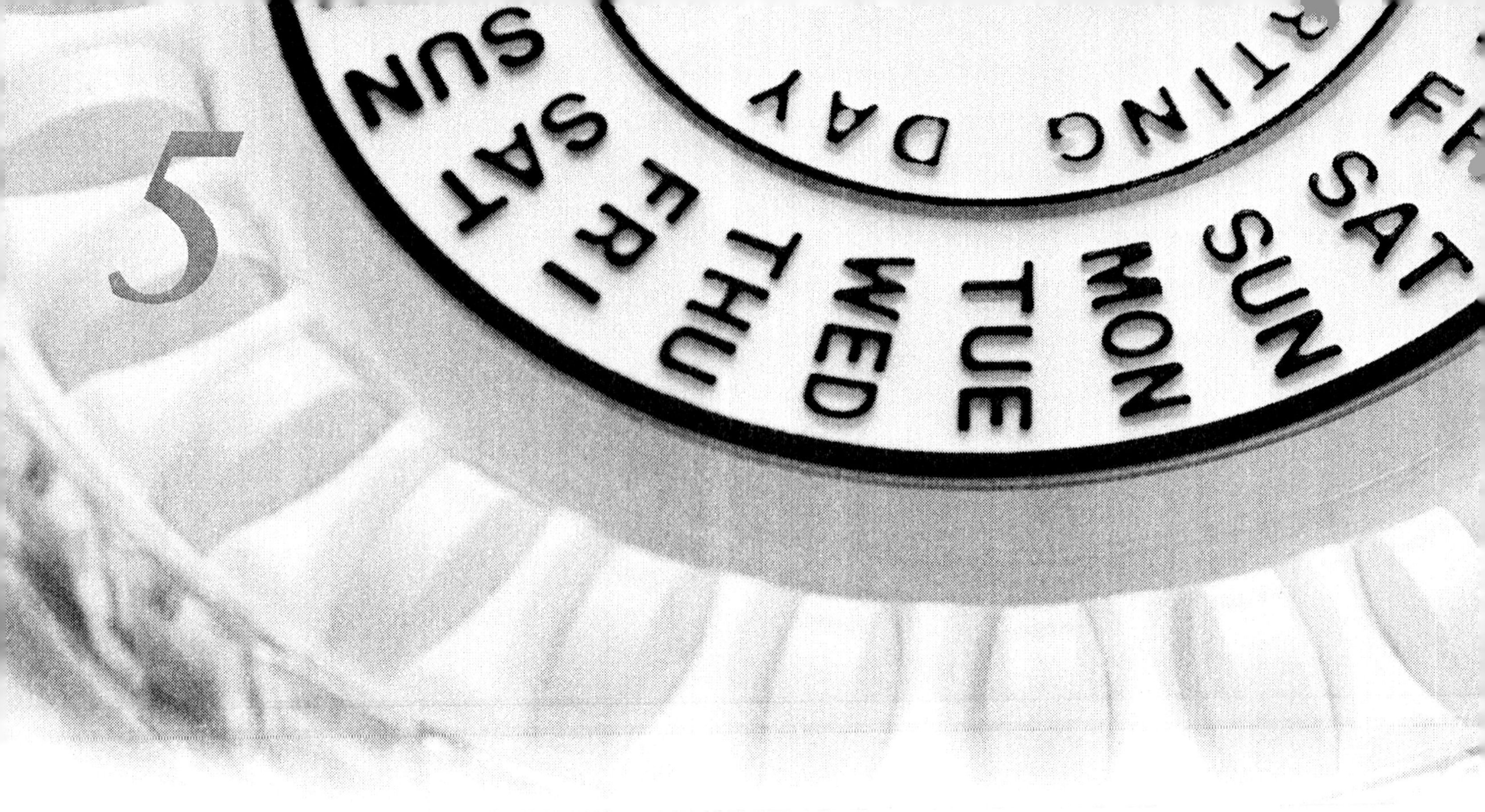

5

Contraception

Planning and Preventing Pregnancy

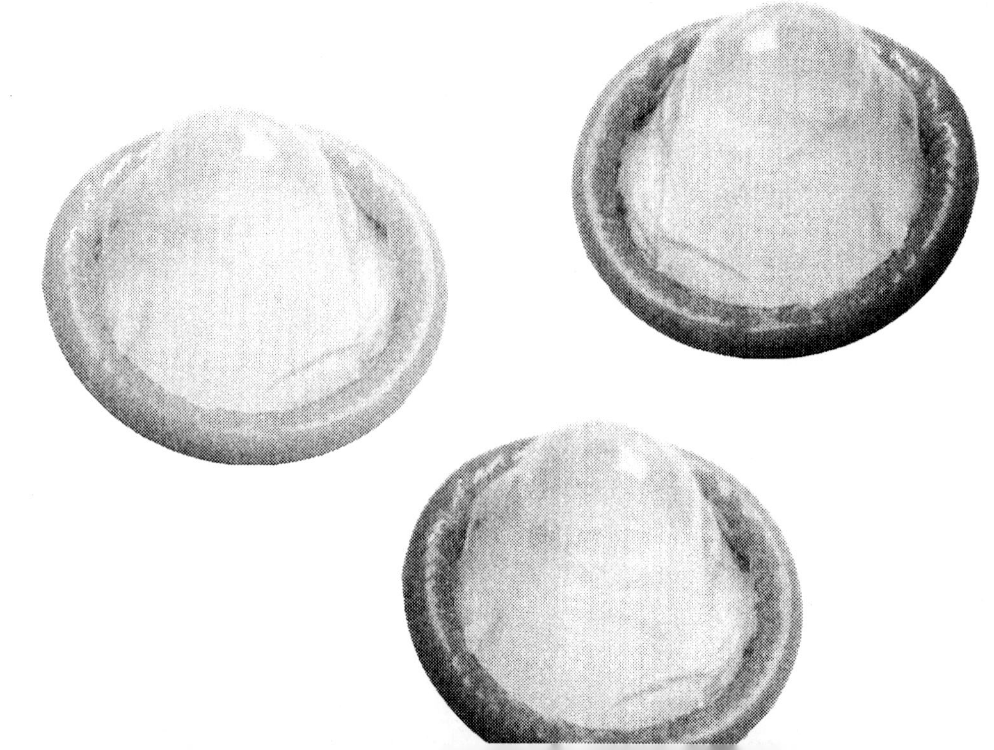

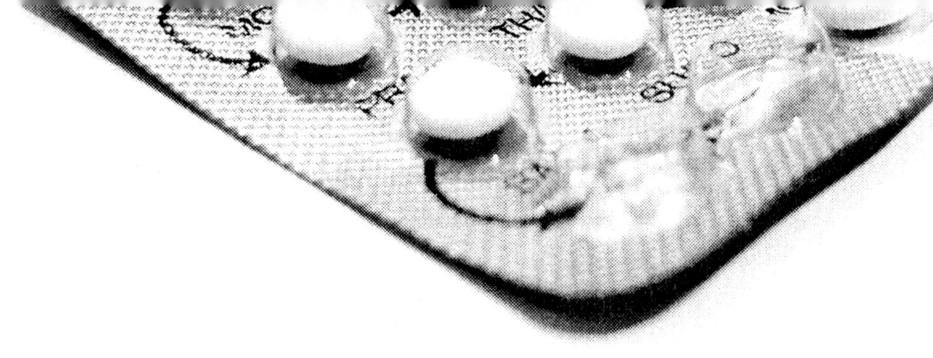

Since YOU Asked...

1. Which method of birth control is best? (see page 146)
2. When my girlfriend and I are having intercourse, I always pull out before I ejaculate. That means there's no chance of pregnancy, right? (see page 148)
3. Will the spermicidal lubrication on condoms protect against pregnancy if the condom breaks? (see page 155)
4. I don't like using condoms because they diminish sensation too much. Is there another safe method of birth control and STI prevention? (see page 157)
5. Does the female condom work as well as regular male condoms? (see page 158)
6. My girlfriend was on the pill, but she still got pregnant. How did that happen? (see page 162)
7. Is there really a "morning-after pill," and does it cancel the need for my boyfriend and me to use condoms? (see page 169)
8. What happened to the sponge method of birth control? I heard that the company went out of business. (see page 173)
9. When is it safe to have sex without contraception, before or after a woman has her period? (see page 175)
10. A friend told me that it is impossible for a woman to get pregnant when she is having her period. Is this true? (see page 175)
11. I've heard that the IUD is a painful and dangerous method of birth control. Is it still even available? (see page 178)
12. After a man has a vasectomy, does it feel different to have an orgasm without ejaculating sperm? (see page 180)

If you are having heterosexual intercourse, or planning to, and you do not want that activity to result in pregnancy or in the transmission of an STI, you must use birth control. A great deal of research has shown that most college students, men and women, are *not* using reliable contraception, and those who are tend to use it inconsistently (Desiderato & Crawford, 1995; R. Graham, 2001; Kusseling, Wenger & Shapiro, 1995). Even if you are not currently sexually active, and even if you do not plan to be in the foreseeable future, an accurate working knowledge of birth control is still important. Chances are that the day will come when you *will* want to be sexually intimate with someone. When that day comes, you will want to have thought about birth control in advance, rather than trying to make such decisions "in the heat of the moment." The point here is that even if you don't need contraception immediately, careful consideration now will help you make the best decisions about birth control later.

contraception Any process or means used to prevent the fertilization of the ovum by a sperm cell.

Simply put, **contraception** is about planning and preventing pregnancy. It is about your ability to plan when to conceive a child and your ability to prevent conception (the prefix *contra* means "against" or "opposing"). It is about *choice*. If you choose to have sexual intercourse with a member of the opposite sex and you choose not to use birth control, your choices will almost certainly eventually lead to pregnancy. For many couples, this may be exactly what they want. But for many others, especially couples of traditional college age, pregnancy is something they want to avoid, at least for now.

An unwanted pregnancy is a difficult and often traumatic experience for everyone involved. With very few exceptions, the *only* way for a couple to prevent conception (and pregnancy) is to make contraception a part of their sexual behavior. Acquiring the information you need to make the right choices about contraception may be one of the most important decisions in your sexual life.

You are probably aware of another important reason for using birth control other than to avoid unintended pregnancy: preventing sexually transmitted infections (STIs). As explored in detail in Chapter 8, "Sexually Transmitted Infections," an alarming number of potentially serious and even deadly infections can be contracted through unprotected sexual behavior. Some of these are painful and uncomfortable, some can have serious lifelong consequences if left untreated, others have no cure, and still others can kill you. The good news is that some contraceptive methods, while helping prevent pregnancy, also help protect you from these infections.

In this chapter, we will consider what an individual or couple must think about when choosing a personally comfortable and effective method of contraception. We will then examine in some detail the methods of birth control currently available, their degree of effectiveness in preventing pregnancy and STIs, and the advantages and disadvantages of each. We will also preview some future contraceptive options that may become available in the not-too-distant future. We will conclude, as always, by looking at how you can incorporate the information in this chapter into your sexual philosophy. First, however, let's take a brief look at the fascinating history of how contraception first became available in the United States. It is a shorter history than you might imagine.

Focus on Your Feelings

Contraception may not be one of the most emotionally charged topics in this book, but you might be surprised how often strong feelings can enter into the discussion of contraception methods, the choice of a method, and issues about using (or not using) contraception.

You may one day find yourself (if you haven't already done so) in an intimate relationship in which you and your partner disagree about using contraception or about the type of contraceptive method you want to choose. This can be very frustrating when you both desire an enjoyable sexual relationship but one of you may be more intent than the other on a contraception method that protects from pregnancy or STIs. Couples must work out these differences, no matter how emotional they become, if they are to make smart and healthy decisions about their sexual activities together. The more educated you both are about the methods that are available and how effective and safe they are, the more likely you will be able to come to a shared decision that is acceptable to both partners.

Emotions can also run high if contraception fails—that is, when a woman becomes pregnant or when an STI is transmitted. Incorrect or inconsistent use of the contraceptive method is usually the culprit, but even with perfect use, no method is 100 percent failure-proof (except total abstinence). If contraception has failed for anyone you know (or for you!), you know the range of emotions that are possible; you might feel frustration or anger, anxiety, or even panic about the eventual outcome of the situation.

You can see, then, that even though contraception seems on the surface to be a relatively straightforward, rational topic, it has its emotional side, which is important to keep in mind as you read this chapter.

Historical Perspectives

The Politics of Contraception

The early history of birth control in the United States is a story of radical politics. That's right, *politics*. In the early twentieth century, federal laws prohibited nearly everything related to birth control (D'Emilio & Freedman, 1988). These laws were contained in a bill referred to as the Comstock Act, named after its primary supporter, Anthony Comstock, an antiobscenity radical of the late 1800s and early 1900s who considered all contraceptive information and devices obscene and indecent. Under this act, it was illegal to sell or distribute birth control information or devices in any form. In addition, the act made it a crime for any mention of sexually transmitted diseases to appear in print. If that were not enough, doctors and nurses were prohibited from discussing these issues with their patients. Anyone found to be in violation of the provisions of the Comstock Act was subject to arrest and imprisonment (some unfortunates were arrested by Comstock himself).

Consequently, the only form of birth control available to most people in those years was the calendar-based rhythm method, a relatively unreliable method that will be discussed later in this chapter. At the time, even this method was largely misunderstood, and doctors often mistakenly advised couples who wanted to avoid pregnancy to engage in sexual activity at times when we now know they were *most* likely to become pregnant, not least!

Perhaps the most amazing fact about the history of birth control in the United States is that, essentially, one individual was single-handedly responsible for overcoming the Comstock Act and making contraception widely available. That person was Margaret Sanger (1883–1966), who is credited with coining the phrase "birth control."

Sanger was a nurse and mother of three children. In her 30s, she moved to New York City and became involved in socialist politics and active in the fledgling women's rights movement. Sanger believed that women's freedom to make choices about their personal and sexual lives depended on their ability to make choices about their reproductive lives. In 1912, she began to write and publish articles on female sexuality and on a woman's right to control her own reproductive body and to express herself sexually without the fear of pregnancy (D'Emilio & Freedman, 1988). She was proposing the separation of sex from reproduction. At the time, this was a very radical idea.

In the years that followed, Sanger fled to Europe to avoid arrest on obscenity charges (her writings about contraception were considered obscene and illegal at the time). While there, she visited a birth control clinic in the Netherlands, where women were being fitted by trained nurses with early versions of what we now know as the diaphragm. Convinced that this was the best and most effective form of birth control for women, Sanger returned to the United States and opened the first birth control clinic, located in Brooklyn, New York. After less than two weeks in operation, her clinic was raided by the police; Sanger was arrested on obscenity charges and spent 30 days in jail. Because of the publicity surround these events, Sanger became a celebrated and widely recognized leader of the birth control movement in the United States and in many countries throughout the world. By 1916, some 100,000 copies of her booklet, "Family Limitation," had been distributed, and birth control clinics had begun to open (Katz, 2002). This marked the start of a new sexual morality in the United States and of the modern age of contraception and family planning. Sanger's later work for contraceptive research funding resulted in the development of the first hormonal birth control pill in the late 1950s. She is considered one of the original founders of the organization known today as Planned Parenthood.

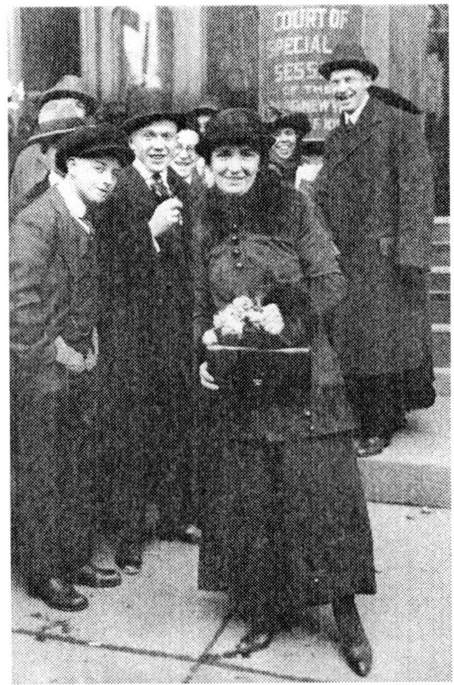

Margaret Sanger (1883–1966), crusader for the legalization and distribution of contraceptives in the United States.

As you will see in this chapter, in the decades since Sanger's early activism, the availability and variety of birth control methods has steadily grown. However, controversy and politics continue to complicate the contraception picture. Consider, for example, the debate over making condoms available in public high schools and whether doing so would promote an increase in sexual activity among teens or reduce disease and unintended pregnancy among sexually active teens (Francoeur, 1996). The goal in this chapter is not to attempt to resolve the controversies over birth control but rather to provide you with the information you need to make your own informed choices about this aspect of your sexuality.

Choosing a Method of Contraception

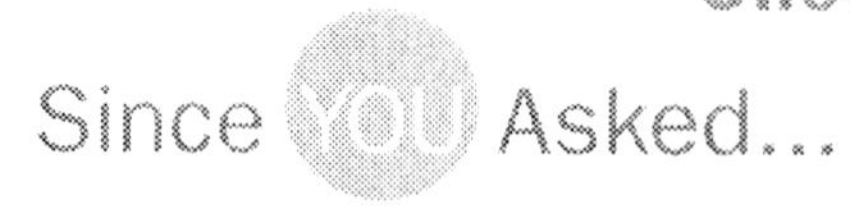

1. Which method of birth control is best?

Once you have made the decision to use contraception, you must determine what method is (or will be) best for you. To do so, you will need to do some homework. First, you must educate yourself about the many birth control methods. For each method, you need to understand its level of effectiveness, how to use it correctly, how well it is likely to fit with your sexual lifestyle, how comfortable you will be using it, and whether the method is one you can commit to using not only correctly but also consistently, *every time* you have intercourse.

An important part of this education will be to learn about the many common myths and erroneous beliefs about birth control so that you can avoid assuming you are safe when you are not. Research has shown that 53 percent of unplanned pregnancies occur in couples who are using contraceptives! Most of these contraceptive failures are due either to incorrect use of the contraceptive method or relying on false information about pregnancy and birth control (Henshaw, 1998).

An Individual or Shared Decision?

Both men and women have the option of making an individual choice about a method of birth control. However, if you are in an ongoing, intimate relationship for which birth control either is or will be necessary, it is probably best to discuss the options with your partner and decide on a method of contraception that will be effective and comfortable to both of you. If you cannot discuss and agree about birth control with a partner, deciding to have sexual intercourse with that person is probably a mistake. Moreover, research has demonstrated that couples who are able to communicate about contraception are more likely to use birth control consistently and are therefore at lower risk of unwanted pregnancy and contracting STIs (Edwards, 1994).

On the other hand, most college students who are sexually active are not in stable relationships, and some may even have more than one sexual partner at a given point in time (R. Graham, 2001; Sheer & Cline, 1994). Individuals may have little opportunity to make a joint decision about birth control with a prospective partner. In these situations, each person needs to be responsible for his or her own contraception choices and for using them correctly and consistently. To get an idea of whether your birth control method of choice is working for you, see "Self-Discovery: Contraceptive Method Comfort and Confidence Scale."

Lifestyle Considerations

Not all birth control methods are equally appropriate for all sexual lifestyles and life stages. To make a rational and informed decision about contraception, you need to do some serious self-appraisal about personal sexual life issues and activities, both now and in the future. For example, ask yourself the following questions:

1. Am I currently engaging in sexual activities that involve any risk of pregnancy or transmission of sexually transmitted infections?

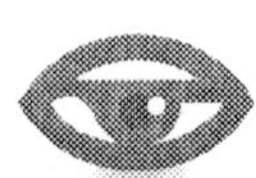

Self-Discovery

Contraceptive Method Comfort and Confidence Scale

To help you determine whether a contraceptive method suits your lifestyle and is a realistic choice for you, answer the following questions (yes or no) for each method you are considering.

_____ **1.** Have I had problems using this method before?

_____ **2.** Have I ever become pregnant while using this method?

_____ **3.** Am I afraid of using this method?

_____ **4.** Would I really rather not use this method?

_____ **5.** Will I have trouble remembering to use this method?

_____ **6.** Will I have trouble using this method correctly?

_____ **7.** Do I still have unanswered questions about this method?

_____ **8.** Does this method make menstrual periods longer or more painful?

_____ **9.** Does this method cost more than I can afford?

_____ **10.** Could this method cause me to have serious complications?

_____ **11.** Am I opposed to this method because of my religious or moral beliefs?

_____ **12.** Is my partner opposed to this method?

_____ **13.** Am I using this method without my partner's knowledge?

_____ **14.** Will using this method embarrass my partner?

_____ **15.** Will using this method embarrass me?

_____ **16.** Will I enjoy intercourse less because of this method?

_____ **17.** If this method interrupts lovemaking, will I avoid using it?

_____ **18.** Has a nurse or doctor ever told me NOT to use this method?

_____ **19.** Is there anything about my personality that could lead me to use this method incorrectly?

_____ **20.** Am I at any risk of being exposed to HIV (the AIDS virus) or other sexually transmitted infections if I use this method?

SCORING: How many total *yes* answers did you have?

A Few (0–3): Most people will have a few *yes* answers. *Yes* answers mean that potential problems may arise with that method. All methods have their strong points and their drawbacks. If you only have a few, chances are good that the method you've picked will work for you.

More than a Few (4 or more): If you have more than a few *yes* answers, you may want to talk with a physician, counselor, partner, or friend to help you decide whether to use this method or how to use it so that it will really be effective for you.

In general, the more *yes* answers you have, the less likely you are to use this method consistently and correctly each and every time you have sex. You might want to consider using another method.

Source: From *Contraceptive Technology* 18th edition by R. Hatcher, J. Trussel, F. Stewart, W. Cates, G. Stewart, F. Guest and D. Kowal (eds.).

2. Am I confident that I am in a one-on-one, exclusive relationship in which both of us are free of diseases that may be sexually transmitted?
3. How often do I engage in potentially risky sexual activities?
4. Do I have (or am I likely to have) more than one concurrent sexual partner?
5. How seriously would an accidental pregnancy disrupt my life?
6. Do I need to be in charge of contraception, or can I trust my partner to take care of it?
7. Do I feel comfortable overall with using this method of birth control?

How you answer these questions will help you determine exactly what features you need in the birth control method you choose. For example, if you answered yes to question 2, you may feel comfortable and safe selecting a method that is effective in preventing pregnancy, even though it may not provide protection from STIs. On the other hand, if your answer to question 4 is yes, prevention of pregnancy *and* STIs needs to be part of your decision process.

Unreliable Methods

Flawed information and beliefs about contraception often lead to poor decisions about birth control and safer sex. Here we focus on two commonly used yet very undependable methods of contraception: the withdrawal method, and douching.

The **withdrawal method**, in which the penis is withdrawn from the vagina prior to ejaculation (also called *coitus interruptus* or "pulling out") has been a widely practiced method of birth control for centuries. Theoretically speaking, it sounds as though this should be an effective way of preventing pregnancy, but it relies on too many ifs. *If* the man withdraws his penis from the woman's vagina before he ejaculates, and *if* he ejaculates well away from the vaginal opening, and *if* no semen enters her reproductive tract, and *if* no sperm are present in the pre-ejaculate, then pregnancy may be less likely to occur. All of these ifs combine to make the withdrawal method very risky (Kowal, 1998b). Also, as was discussed in Chapter 2, males secrete fluid from the Cowper's glands during the plateau stage *prior* to ejaculation. Under some circumstances this pre-ejaculate can contain live sperm cells capable of fertilization. Perhaps more important, the Cowper's gland secretions from the male and vaginal secretions from the female may contain HIV, hepatitis, or other sexually transmitted infectious agents; withdrawal prior to ejaculation provides no protection from these infections.

Since YOU Asked...

2. When my girlfriend and I are having intercourse, I always pull out before I ejaculate. That means there's no chance of pregnancy, right?

What all this means is that if withdrawal is the only method available to a couple who do not wish to become pregnant or transmit STIs, they would be safer waiting to have intercourse until such time as they can obtain a more reliable method of birth control. However, if sexually transmitted infections are not a risk, withdrawal, done correctly, will be more effective than using no method at all.

As recently as the late twentieth century, some individuals, couples, and even medical professionals believed that **douching** (the washing out of the vagina with a stream of water or some other liquid solution after intercourse) was an effective means of contraception. However, this is now known not to be the case at all. Sperm are already on their way into the uterus within 15 seconds of ejaculation, so any attempt at douching after unprotected intercourse will be too late. Furthermore, the stream of water can actually push the remaining sperm through the cervix even faster (they just surf right on through). Not only is douching not recommended for birth control, but most health professionals no longer recommend it at all as a routine hygiene practice for women because it may force bacteria higher into a woman's reproductive system and *increase* the risk of infections (Cornforth, 2001; Rosenberg & Phillips, 1992).

Over many centuries, people have tried and believed in numerous other unreliable, ineffective, and even foolish methods of birth control. One example is the belief that making love standing up will prevent conception because the sperm cannot swim uphill. This is *so* not true. Sperm are very skilled at swimming in any direction, with or against gravity! Another erroneous belief is that if a woman takes one or two of her friend's birth control pills prior to intercourse, she will be protected from pregnancy. Also not true. With specific exceptions (as you will see in our discussion of emergency contraceptive pills later in the chapter), oral

withdrawal method Removing the penis from the vagina just prior to ejaculation—an unreliable method of contraception; also called *coitus interruptus* and "pulling out."

douching Washing the internal vagina with a stream of water or any other liquid solution (not usually medically recommended).

question 2, you may feel comfortable and safe selecting a method that is effective in preventing pregnancy, even though it may not provide protection from STIs. On the other hand, if your answer to question 4 is yes, prevention of pregnancy *and* STIs needs to be part of your decision process.

Unreliable Methods

Flawed information and beliefs about contraception often lead to poor decisions about birth control and safer sex. Here we focus on two commonly used yet very undependable methods of contraception: the withdrawal method, and douching.

Since YOU Asked...

2. When my girlfriend and I are having intercourse, I always pull out before I ejaculate. That means there's no chance of pregnancy, right?

The **withdrawal method**, in which the penis is withdrawn from the vagina prior to ejaculation (also called *coitus interruptus* or "pulling out") has been a widely practiced method of birth control for centuries. Theoretically speaking, it sounds as though this should be an effective way of preventing pregnancy, but it relies on too many ifs. *If* the man withdraws his penis from the woman's vagina before he ejaculates, and *if* he ejaculates well away from the vaginal opening, and *if* no semen enters her reproductive tract, and *if* no sperm are present in the pre-ejaculate, then pregnancy may be less likely to occur. All of these ifs combine to make the withdrawal method very risky (Kowal, 1998b). Also, as was discussed in Chapter 2, males secrete fluid from the Cowper's glands during the plateau stage *prior* to ejaculation. Under some circumstances this pre-ejaculate can contain live sperm cells capable of fertilization. Perhaps more important, the Cowper's gland secretions from the male and vaginal secretions from the female may contain HIV, hepatitis, or other sexually transmitted infectious agents; withdrawal prior to ejaculation provides no protection from these infections.

What all this means is that if withdrawal is the only method available to a couple who do not wish to become pregnant or transmit STIs, they would be safer waiting to have intercourse until such time as they can obtain a more reliable method of birth control. However, if sexually transmitted infections are not a risk, withdrawal, done correctly, will be more effective than using no method at all.

As recently as the late twentieth century, some individuals, couples, and even medical professionals believed that **douching** (the washing out of the vagina with a stream of water or some other liquid solution after intercourse) was an effective means of contraception. However, this is now known not to be the case at all. Sperm are already on their way into the uterus within 15 seconds of ejaculation, so any attempt at douching after unprotected intercourse will be too late. Furthermore, the stream of water can actually push the remaining sperm through the cervix even faster (they just surf right on through). Not only is douching not recommended for birth control, but most health professionals no longer recommend it at all as a routine hygiene practice for women because it may force bacteria higher into a woman's reproductive system and *increase* the risk of infections (Cornforth, 2001; Rosenberg & Phillips, 1992).

Over many centuries, people have tried and believed in numerous other unreliable, ineffective, and even foolish methods of birth control. One example is the belief that making love standing up will prevent conception because the sperm cannot swim uphill. This is *so* not true. Sperm are very skilled at swimming in any direction, with or against gravity! Another erroneous belief is that if a woman takes one or two of her friend's birth control pills prior to intercourse, she will be protected from pregnancy. Also not true. With specific exceptions (as you will see in our discussion of emergency contraceptive pills later in the chapter), oral

withdrawal method Removing the penis from the vagina just prior to ejaculation—an unreliable method of contraception; also called *coitus interruptus* and "pulling out."

douching Washing the internal vagina with a stream of water or any other liquid solution (not usually medically recommended).

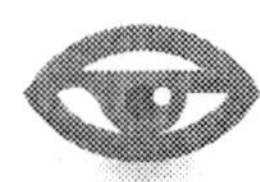

Self-Discovery

Contraceptive Method Comfort and Confidence Scale

To help you determine whether a contraceptive method suits your lifestyle and is a realistic choice for you, answer the following questions (yes or no) for each method you are considering.

____ 1. Have I had problems using this method before?

____ 2. Have I ever become pregnant while using this method?

____ 3. Am I afraid of using this method?

____ 4. Would I really rather not use this method?

____ 5. Will I have trouble remembering to use this method?

____ 6. Will I have trouble using this method correctly?

____ 7. Do I still have unanswered questions about this method?

____ 8. Does this method make menstrual periods longer or more painful?

____ 9. Does this method cost more than I can afford?

____ 10. Could this method cause me to have serious complications?

____ 11. Am I opposed to this method because of my religious or moral beliefs?

____ 12. Is my partner opposed to this method?

____ 13. Am I using this method without my partner's knowledge?

____ 14. Will using this method embarrass my partner?

____ 15. Will using this method embarrass me?

____ 16. Will I enjoy intercourse less because of this method?

____ 17. If this method interrupts lovemaking, will I avoid using it?

____ 18. Has a nurse or doctor ever told me NOT to use this method?

____ 19. Is there anything about my personality that could lead me to use this method incorrectly?

____ 20. Am I at any risk of being exposed to HIV (the AIDS virus) or other sexually transmitted infections if I use this method?

SCORING: How many total *yes* answers did you have?

A Few (0–3): Most people will have a few *yes* answers. *Yes* answers mean that potential problems may arise with that method. All methods have their strong points and their drawbacks. If you only have a few, chances are good that the method you've picked will work for you.

More than a Few (4 or more): If you have more than a few *yes* answers, you may want to talk with a physician, counselor, partner, or friend to help you decide whether to use this method or how to use it so that it will really be effective for you.

In general, the more *yes* answers you have, the less likely you are to use this method consistently and correctly each and every time you have sex. You might want to consider using another method.

Source: From *Contraceptive Technology* 18th edition by R. Hatcher, J. Trussel, F. Stewart, W. Cates, G. Stewart, F. Guest and D. Kowal (eds.). Copyright © 2004 by CTC, Inc. Reprinted by permission of the publisher, Ardent Media, Inc.

2. Am I confident that I am in a one-on-one, exclusive relationship in which both of us are free of diseases that may be sexually transmitted?
3. How often do I engage in potentially risky sexual activities?
4. Do I have (or am I likely to have) more than one concurrent sexual partner?
5. How seriously would an accidental pregnancy disrupt my life?
6. Do I need to be in charge of contraception, or can I trust my partner to take care of it?
7. Do I feel comfortable overall with using this method of birth control?

How you answer these questions will help you determine exactly what features you need in the birth control method you choose. For example, if you answered yes to contraceptives must be taken consistently over time to be effective in preventing pregnancy. And what about the good old plastic-wrap condom technique? Not even close. Plastic wrap might keep a penis fresh if it were in the fridge, but it will almost certainly slip off, leak, or break during intercourse and will not reliably protect anyone from pregnancy or STIs. Oh, and toothpaste is not a spermicide. Finally, the answer is a resounding "yes"—a woman *can* become pregnant the first time she has intercourse and regardless of whether she has an orgasm during sex.

Why have so many people believed in and used ineffective and even bizarre techniques for preventing pregnancy? The answer probably lies in the fact that most of the time when someone has intercourse using one of these methods, no pregnancy occurs, simply due to the law of averages. The couple may then *assume* that their method worked, when in reality the lack of pregnancy was simply a coincidence. Chances are, on that particular occasion of intercourse, no pregnancy would have occurred even if no attempt at birth control was made at all. Still, the myths persist that these are effective methods when in fact they are little better or even worse than no method at all. A fertile couple who use any of these methods will become pregnant sooner or later.

Many sexuality educators, medical professionals, and students are surprised at the persistence of the myths about birth control when so many effective choices of contraception exist and are readily obtained. As noted earlier, your choice of a successful method depends on your sexual lifestyle and your comfort and confidence in the method itself. If you trust that you and your partner are in a mutually exclusive, monogamous relationship, then you probably do not have to be concerned about STIs, unless one partner is already infected. Therefore, you may feel free to choose from *all* the methods discussed in this chapter for the prevention of pregnancy. However, most sexually active college students are in relationships that may not be monogamous, STI-free, and long-term. If that is or may be true for you, then you must consider *both* contraception and prevention of disease in your choice of birth control. We will turn now to methods that address both of these issues.

Reliable Contraception Methods

Choosing a method of birth control that is right for you requires knowledge of the different types available, including abstinence, hormonal methods, barrier methods, fertility awareness approaches, intrauterine devices, and surgical methods (sterilization). Table 5.1 summarizes the many different types according to the effectiveness, costs, STI prevention capabilities, advantages, and disadvantages of each. We explore all of the more accepted, more effective methods of birth control in the text. For our purposes, I have divided the various methods into two categories, those that serve to prevent pregnancy *and* STIs and those that help prevent pregnancy but offer little, if any, protection against STIs.

Methods for Preventing Pregnancy and STIs

Many individuals want contraception that accomplishes two important functions: preventing pregnancy and protecting against sexually transmitted infections. Contraception methods that do this include complete or selective abstinence ("outercourse") and two barrier methods—male and female condoms.

Table 5.1 SUMMARY OF CONTRACEPTIVE METHODS

CONTRACEPTIVE METHOD	TYPICAL FAILURE RATE (%)	PERFECT USE FAILURE RATE (%)	COST*	ADVANTAGES	DISADVANTAGES AND SIDE EFFECTS
No method (chance)	85	85	Average total cost of full-term pregnancy in the United States: $1,500–4,000	Provides best chance of pregnancy	No protection against pregnancy or sexually transmitted infections, high probability of "accidental" pregnancy or transmission of STIs
			METHODS THAT REDUCE RISK OF PREGNANCY *AND* STIs		
Abstinence, "outercourse"	Not known	0	Free but requires commitment and self-control by both partners	No cost, no risk of pregnancy, protection from STI transmission with committed and consistent use	Requires self-discipline, partner agreement, strong commitment; risk of unprotected intercourse if commitment wanes
Male condoms	12	3	$0.50–1.00 each	Accessible, portable, inexpensive; usable with many other methods; help protect against STIs and PID	Reduced male sensitivity reported by some, possible interruption of sexual "moment," latex may cause irritation (less likely with polyurethane condoms)
Female condoms	21	5	$2.50–$3.00 each*	Does not require male involvement in decision, may be inserted up to eight hours before intercourse	Potentially less interruption in sexual activity; some irritation and allergic reactions reported
			METHODS THAT REDUCE RISK OF PREGNANCY BUT *NOT* OF STIs		
Hormonal Methods					
Combination pills (estrogen and progestin)	2	0.1	$100–$300 per year	Very effective when taken consistently and correctly; eversible; safe for most healthy women under 35; decreases menstrual cramps and pain and regulates periods; may reduce premenstrual symptoms; acne improvement; may decrease risk of developing ovarian cancer, endometrial cancer, ectopic pregnancy, and PID	Must remember to take pills daily; some forms may be associated with missed periods; breakthrough bleeding or spotting between periods; weight gain, increased breast size; nausea; headaches; depression; possible rare complications of cardiovascular disease; most minor side effects decrease after first couple of months of use
Progestin-only pills (minipill)	2	0.5	$100–$300 per year	Fewer health risks overall than combination pills; reversible; decreased menstrual cramps or pain; less heavy bleeding; shorter periods; decreased PMS symptoms and breast tenderness	Must be taken same time every day, menstrual irregularities (breakthrough bleeding, cessation of periods), breast tenderness
90-day pills (Seasonale)	2	0.1	$300–400 per year	Four periods per year instead of 12; fewer menstruation-related problems including migraine headaches, cramping, mood swings, bloating; may reduce uterine fibroids and endometriosis symptoms	Greater chance of intermenstrual bleeding and spotting; breast tenderness; low but slightly increased risk of blood clots, heart attack, and stroke, especially in women over 35 who smoke
Implants	0.05	0.05	Approx. $190–$270 per year of protection	Long-term, effective contraception; reversible; light or no periods, decreased menstrual cramps and pain, decreased risk of developing endometrial cancer, ovarian cancer, and PID	Higher initial costs; headaches; menstrual irregularities (breakthrough bleeding or cessation of periods); breast tenderness; rare cases of prolonged periods

Table 5.1 (*Continued*)

CONTRACEPTIVE METHOD	TYPICAL FAILURE RATE (%)	PERFECT USE FAILURE RATE (%)	COST*	ADVANTAGES	DISADVANTAGES AND SIDE EFFECTS
Injectable (Depo-Provera)	0.3	0.3	Approx. $65 per injection (four needed per year)	Very high contraceptive efficacy; each injection provides three months of contraception; light or no periods; decreased menstrual cramps and pain; decreased risk of developing endometrial cancer, ovarian cancer, and PID	Return of fertility may take up to a year; discomfort of injections for some; return visits every three months, menstrual irregularities (breakthrough bleeding or cessation of periods); weight gain; breast tenderness; possible loss of bone mass (recovers when discontinued)
Contraceptive patch (Ortho Evra)	1.0–2.0	1.0	Approx. $60–$80 per three-pack (one pack needed per month)	Continuous, consistent dose of hormones; one patch per week eliminates need to remember daily pill; no interruption of sexual activity; helps regulate periods; less abdominal side effects than pill (hormones do not pass through digestive tract)	Breast tenderness and enlargement; headache; nausea; spotting or breakthrough bleeding; abdominal cramps and bloating; vaginal discharge; may expose women to level of hormones 60% higher than most oral contraceptives; serious risks include blood clots, stroke, or heart attack
Contraceptive Ring (NuvaRing)	1.5	0.7	Approx. $30 per ring (one per month)	Convenient once-a-month insertion; no medical fitting required; no interruption in spontaneous sexual activity; lowest dose of hormones due to release directly into mucous membranes	Headaches; vaginal irritation and discharge; may slip out during sexual intercourse (rare); weight gain; headache; nausea; serious risks include blood clots, stroke or heart attack
Emergency contraceptive pills (Plan B; Preven)	25–40[†]	25[†]	Approx. $25 per kit	Provides protection from pregnancy after unprotected intercourse or failure of primary method; highly effective in reducing risk of pregnancy; provides backup method for emergency situations; helps prevent	Should not be used if woman if already pregnant; nausea; vomiting; lower abdominal pain; fatigue; headache; dizziness; breast tenderness; and menstrual timing changes in month of use (side effects may last several days)
Barrier Methods					
Diaphragm with spermicide	20	6	$50–$150 including medical visit and fitting	Does not require male involvement in decision, need not interrupt intercourse (may be inserted up to six hours in advance); may protect against cervical abnormalities and cancer	Possible skin irritation from spermicide or latex; may cause increased risk of female urinary tract infections; additional spermicide must be used for repeated intercourse
Cervical cap with spermicide:			$50–$150 including medical visit and fitting	Does not require male involvement in decision; need not interrupt intercourse; protects for 48 hours	Low effectiveness, increased risk of urinary tract infections; should not be used during menstruation or left in place longer than 48 hours to avoid possible toxic shock syndrome; possible skin irritation from spermicide or latex; low effectiveness for women who have previously given birth
Women who have never given birth	18	9			
Women who have previously given birth	36	26			

Continued. . .

Table 5.1 (*Continued*)

CONTRACEPTIVE METHOD	TYPICAL FAILURE RATE (%)	PERFECT USE FAILURE RATE (%)	COST*	ADVANTAGES	DISADVANTAGES AND SIDE EFFECTS
Lea's Shield	20	6 with spermicide, 15 without	Approx. $65; no medical visit or fitting necessary	No fitting or prescription needed; one-size-fits-all; allows cervical secretions to escape through one-way valve; may be left in place for 48 hours; no interruption of sexual activities; silicone construction avoids latex reactions; additional spermicide not required for repeated intercourse	Must be used with spermicide for full protection; relatively expensive; must be replaced every six months; requires consistent use; not recommended for women with abnormal cervical cells in Pap test
Contraceptive sponges			$2.50–$3.00 each	Controlled by woman; can be inserted ahead of time; provides 24 hours of protection	Possible temporary skin irritation due to spermicide; low effectiveness for women who have previously given birth
Women who have previously given birth	40	20			
Women who have never given birth	20	9			
Vaginal spermicides	21	6	$0.50–$1.50 per use	Simple to use; available over the counter; provides increased effectiveness when used with other methods; provides extra lubrication for intercourse	Possible temporary skin irritation due to spermicide
Fertility Awareness Methods					
Calendar ("rhythm")	20	9	Either no cost or onetime thermometer purchase, $5–$80; ovulation prediction kit, $20–$50	Inexpensive; may be effective when used perfectly; no serious side effects; increases knowledge of reproductive physiology, enhances self-reliance	Requires careful record keeping; unforgiving of imperfect use; irregular menstrual cycles makes use more difficult
Cervical mucus	9	3			
Basal body temperature	20	9			
Postovulation	20	1			
Intrauterine Devices (IUDs)					
Progesterone T (Progestasert)	2.0	1.5	$300–$500 insertion cost;	Highly effective; safe; long-acting; hassle-free	Increased risk of PID; may cause menstrual problems; more risk for women who have never had children; requires trained personnel for insertion and withdrawal
Copper (Paragard T380A)	0.8	0.6	$40–$80 per month over five years continuous use		
Levonorgestrel (Mirena)	0.1	0.1			

Table 5.1 (*Continued*)

CONTRACEPTIVE METHOD	TYPICAL FAILURE RATE (%)	PERFECT USE FAILURE RATE (%)	COST*	ADVANTAGES	DISADVANTAGES AND SIDE EFFECTS
Surgical Methods					
Female sterilization (tubal ligation)	0.4	0.4	$1,500–$2,500	Highly effective; permanent; cost effective over time	Surgical procedure, expensive at time of surgery; permanent; reversibility difficult and expensive; usual risks that accompany surgery (anesthesia, hemorrhage, organ damage)
Male sterilization (vasectomy)	0.15	0.10	$500–$1,000	Highly effective; inexpensive in the long run; very safe; considered permanent, but successful reversals are common	Permanent; minor surgical procedure; expensive at time of surgery

* Many costs are significantly lower (or zero) at public health clinics and campus health services.

† Reduces chance of pregnancy by 75 percent in women who use ECP following unprotected intercourse during the two midcycle weeks.

Sources: American Health Consultants (2001); Best (2000); Hatcher et al. (1994, 1998, 2004); Kirn (2001); Napoli (2001); Roumen, Apter, & Mulders (2001); R. Rubin (2001).

Abstinence and "Outercourse"

The only 100 percent effective way to prevent pregnancy and avoid contracting STIs is to practice **abstinence** [from sex]. But what does abstinence from sex mean? Recall that sex is more than intercourse. Abstinence does *not* necessarily mean avoiding all sexual expression and activity—that's known as **celibacy**. In our current context, abstinence is the choice not to engage in sexual behaviors that involve any risk of pregnancy or spreading STIs. Some sexuality educators refer to this "selective" abstinence as **outercourse**, which means engaging only in sexual behaviors that are "safe" and avoiding those that are risky, such as vaginal or anal intercourse and oral sex (see Chapter 6, "Sexual Behaviors," for a detailed discussion of these activities). Many couples have freely chosen to abstain from such activities but want to express the sexual intimacy they may feel for one another. People who equate sexual behavior with intercourse have a rather limited view of the range and variety of sexual interactions that can provide intense feelings of intimacy and sexual satisfaction without the risk of pregnancy or STIs. Behaviors available to a couple practicing outercourse include holding hands, kissing, intimate touching, and exploring each other's bodies (Hatcher et al., 1994; Hatcher et al., 1998; Nelson et al., 2004). Contact of the hands and other parts of the body with the genitals, masturbation, mutual masturbation, and orgasm are all included in these activities, as long as the couple ensures that semen or vaginal fluids do not touch any mucous membranes or breaks in each other's skin (Reinisch, 1990).

Many couples who choose outercourse as their method of birth control find that their sexual interactions are especially satisfying precisely because they are free of the worry of pregnancy or STIs. However, everyone knows how easy it is for our judgment to be clouded in moments of great passion and sexual excitement. Therefore, deciding on abstinence or outercourse as your method of contraception takes a strong commitment combined with clear communication between partners.

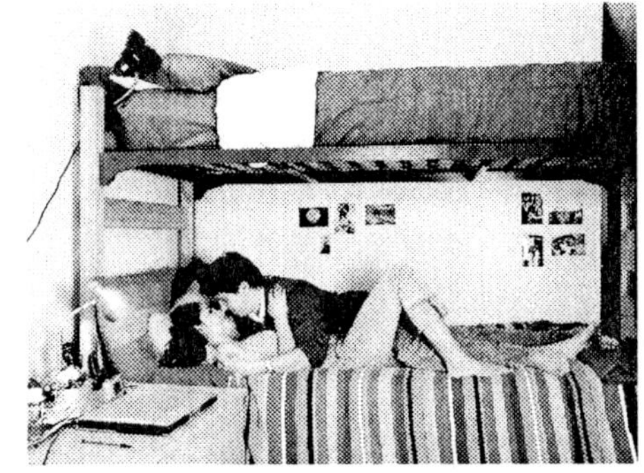

Outercourse, or "selective abstinence," implies that couples limit their intimate behaviors to those that carry little or no risk of pregnancy or STI transmission.

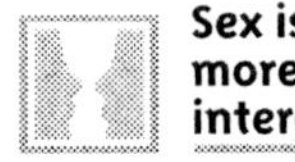

Sex is more than intercourse

sexual abstinence Avoiding sexual behaviors that involve any risk of pregnancy or the spread of STIs.

celibacy Abstinence from all sexual activities.

outercourse A form of abstinence in which a couple chooses to engage only in sexual behaviors that are unlikely to result in pregnancy or infection and to avoid all others, such as vaginal or anal intercourse and oral sex.

"In Touch with Your Sexual Health: Choosing Abstinence—Steps for Success" summarizes the steps that must be taken to ensure effective and successful reliance on outercourse.

Male Condoms

Today, virtually everybody knows about the **male condom**, a thin sheath of latex (rubber), polyurethane (plastic), or animal tissue that is placed over an erect penis prior to intercourse. Condoms are also sometimes referred to as "safes," "rubbers," or prophylactics. Condoms are a barrier method of birth control—the condom forms a barrier preventing sperm from entering the woman's reproductive tract.

Condom use has steadily increased over the past 25 years (Kaiser Family Foundation, 2001). Most people use condoms primarily for contraception, although some report using them strictly for prevention of STIs, either because they are relying on another highly effective method of contraception or because they are in a gay male relationship (Kaiser Family Foundation, 2001; Pilkinton, Kern, & Indest, 1994). Used correctly, condoms are an extremely effective method of contraception *and* of reducing the risk of virtually every sexually transmitted infection.

male condom A thin sheath of latex (rubber), polyurethane (plastic), or animal tissue that is placed over an erect penis prior to intercourse.

In the not-too-distant past, condoms were kept hidden and never mentioned openly. Now, at least in the United States, they are often discussed, incorporat-

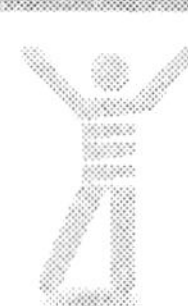

In Touch with Your Sexual Health

Choosing Abstinence—Steps for Success

When people or couples decide to make abstinence their method of choice for birth control, the effectiveness of the method depends on their ability to commit to the plan and maintain the necessary amount of self-restraint often required for success. Here are some ways to ensure that abstinence serves as an effective means of contraception.

1. Learn everything you can about sexual anatomy, response, what sexual behaviors are risky for pregnancy or STIs.
2. Decide about your specific sexual choices at a time when you feel clear-headed, confident, secure, and not under the influence of alcohol or other drugs that can cloud judgment and decision making.
3. If you have a regular current or potential sexual partner, make decisions together at a time when you feel close to each other and comfortable talking but *not* while you are being sexual. For example, talk as you take a walk holding hands or across the dinner table after a romantic dinner. Be sure you have plenty of time, so you won't need to rush the conversation.
4. Decide in advance what sexual activities you will engage in and those that you will not. Discuss these clearly and specifically with your partner in advance; don't wait until the last minute or when you are already engaging in intimate sexual behavior.
5. Avoid high-pressure sexual situations, and stay sober in all sexual settings.
6. Do not waver in your decisions. If you have decided a certain behavior is off limits, do not change your mind in the heat of passion. This will undermine your position on all of your decisions.
7. Be as informed as possible about safe sex and contraception, so you can be prepared if you change your mind about abstinence. Have condoms or another barrier method available, just in case.
8. Obviously, if you are using abstinence, you must use self-control to refrain from intercourse, especially if you do not have a ready means of contraception available.
9. Some people or couples, regardless of their intentions to practice abstinence, do "give in" and engage in intercourse, often without contraception (due to the fact that they were planning on being abstinent). If this happens, be informed about *emergency contraception pills*, which are quite effective in preventing pregnancy if taken within 72 hours of unprotected intercourse.

Source: Adapted from Kowall, 1998.

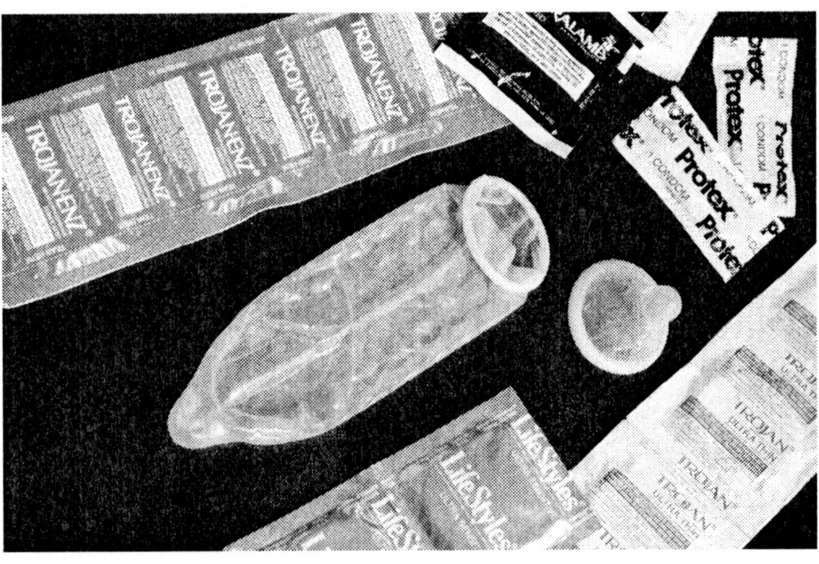

Today's condom market offers an amazingly wide selection to satisfy all tastes.

ed into plots on TV sitcoms and movies, and widely advertised. Twenty-five years ago, you could not find condoms on the shelves in your local drugstore; you had to request them (usually with some discomfort) from the person behind the counter. Today, drugstores and many supermarkets display racks full of condoms with more brands, styles, types, and packaging than anyone could ever have imagined. Types of condoms include those with and without lubrication, with or without spermicide (chemicals that kill sperm cells), with plain or reservoir tips, ultrathin, extra-strength, assorted colors, ribbed, textured, "snugger" or larger sizes, carrying case included, and yes, even flavored and glow-in-the-dark models. Entire stores such as Condom World in San Diego and Condomania in Boston are devoted exclusively to selling condoms and condom-related products. More than 100 different brands of condoms are available in the United States (Warner & Hatcher, 1998). And if it's variety you're after, look no further than the Internet. Web sites abound with every imaginable condom incarnation.

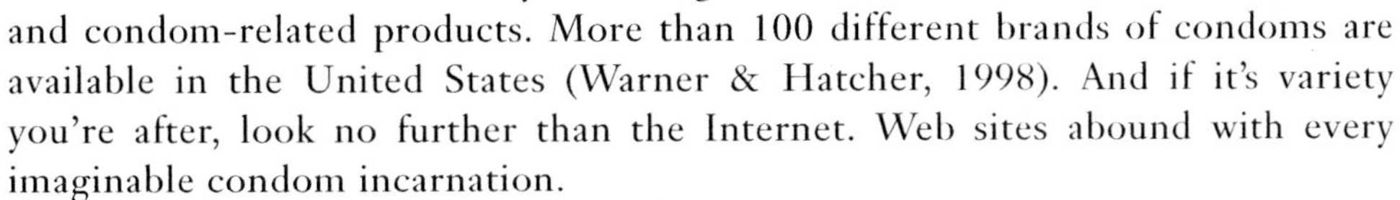

Such openness about this popular form of contraception and STI protection is far from universal. In China, for example, until recently, any advertising of contraception was illegal, and even discussion of related topics was taboo. As China has acknowledged and attempted to deal with its growing problem with sexually transmitted infections (including HIV), its repressive attitudes about contraception have undergone a revolution. As we first noted in Chapter 1, China's efforts to increase safer sex have even included the installation of condom vending machines in various locations throughout the country.

How Condoms Work

The way condoms work is not very mysterious. For contraception, they act as a barrier to prevent semen from entering the vagina. They also prevent contact of skin with mucous membranes and the exchange of genital fluids (semen, vaginal secretions) that can transmit sexually transmitted infections.

For the greatest protection against pregnancy and STIs, it is recommended that you follow these four rules:

1. *Use latex or polyurethane condoms only.* Natural membrane ("lambskin") condoms have small pores that may allow disease-causing viruses to pass through.
2. *Use lubricated condoms.* Inadequate lubrication during intercourse may cause a condom to break or tear. Using lubricated condoms greatly reduces this possibility. Condoms lubricated with a spermicide (usually nonoxynol-9) have sometimes been recommended because the spermicide may provide extra contraception protection in case the condom slips or breaks. However, recent evidence suggests that spermicides may cause irritation to the mucous membranes of the vagina and actually increase the possibility of HIV transmission. For that reason, nonspermicidal lubricated condoms may be the best all-around choice.
3. *Use condoms with a reservoir tip (or nipple).* This feature allows space at the end of the condom to catch the semen upon ejaculation so there is less chance of the condom breaking or leaking.

Since YOU Asked...

3. Will the spermicidal lubrication on condoms protect against pregnancy if the condom breaks?

4. *Use "unexpired" condoms.* Be sure the condoms you buy and use are not past the expiration date printed on the package.

Effectiveness of Condoms

As you can see in Table 5.1, the effectiveness of condoms depends a great deal on proper use. When condoms are used consistently and correctly for vaginal intercourse, they are very effective in preventing pregnancy. The 3 percent failure rate indicated in the table means that if 100 couples have intercourse an average of twice each week for a year and use condoms correctly each time, only three of the couples will become pregnant. This 3 percent failure rate is based on the couples using them, not condom failure itself. Think about it. If you do the math, this means that for that group of 100 couples, 10,400 condoms were used in a year and only three pregnancies occurred. That's an incredibly low *per-condom* failure rate of 0.028 percent (Warner & Hatcher, 1998).

However, looking further at Table 5.1 you can see that the pregnancy rate for condoms in the way couples *typically* use them is four times greater than for perfect use. The failures are not generally due to the product but to incorrect use. Why is typical use so poor? Here is a list of the most common mistakes people make when using condoms as their chosen method of contraception.

- Failing to use a condom every time they have intercourse (assuming it's a "safe" time of the month, not having them handy, making an exception "just this once," etc.)
- Putting the condom on too late, after the penis (and pre-ejaculate) has been in contact with the vulva or vagina
- Putting the condom on incorrectly (such as rolling it only partway down or failing to leave space at the tip)
- Withdrawing the penis from the vagina too late so that the man's erection has subsided and the condom can slip off
- Not holding the condom at the base when withdrawing
- Using old or damaged condoms
- Using the same condom more than once (jokingly referred to as "retreads")
- Inadequate lubrication during intercourse (increased friction can cause condom to tear)
- Using oil-based lubricants (such as Vaseline, baby oil, and most hand, body, and suntan lotions), which react with the latex and may cause the condom to break (these lubricants are not a problem with nonlatex polyurethane condoms)
- Storing condoms incorrectly (in wallet, in glove compartment, in direct sunlight, etc.)

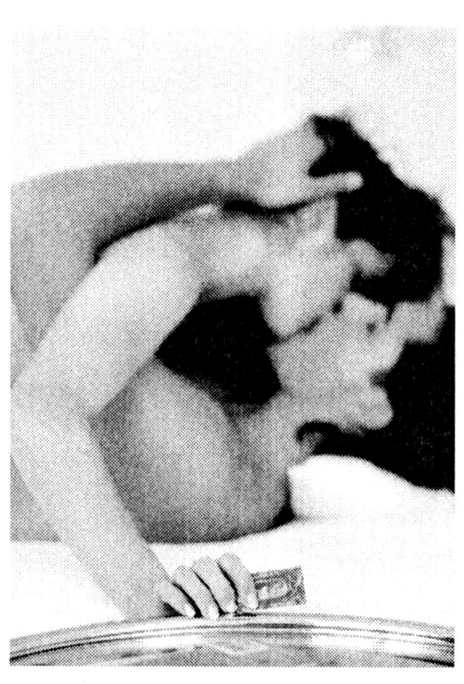

Incorporating condom use into lovemaking can enhance the couple's intimate experience.

Proper Use of Condoms

What is the *correct* way to use condoms? The procedures may sound somewhat complicated, but it's simple once a person becomes accustomed to them. The more a couple uses condoms, the easier and more natural-feeling they will become.

Many people argue that condoms interrupt or interfere with the flow and romance of making love. However, for many others, placing the condom on the man's penis (either by the man himself or by his partner) can be viewed as an enjoyable part of the sexual experience that can actually enhance rather than reduce intimacy and erotic feelings.

Using condoms correctly is the most important determinant of their effectiveness. Remember, failure of condoms themselves is rare, but failure due to incorrect use is all too common. "In Touch with Your Sexual Health: Using Condoms Correctly" summarizes the recommended steps for using condoms effectively.

Convincing Your Partner to Use Condoms

If you choose condoms as your preferred method of birth control, that does not automatically mean your partner will agree. Generally, men have less favorable attitudes

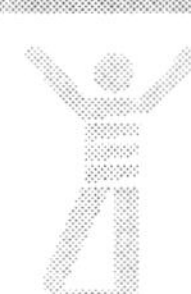

In Touch with Your Sexual Health

Using Male Condoms Correctly

1. Open the condom package carefully. Sharp fingernails or teeth can tear or puncture the condom.
2. Don't try to test the condom by filling it with air or water, as this will weaken the latex. Condoms are all pretested at the factory.
3. The condom should be placed on the erect penis before *any* contact between the penis and the partner's genital area.
4. To be sure which way the condom unrolls, place it over a finger and unroll it slightly. If the condom is placed upside down on the penis and then turned over, some pre-ejaculate fluid, and possibly sperm cells, may be left on the outside of the condom after it is unrolled.
5. Pinch the end of the condom as you unroll it to leave a small amount of empty space at the tip. This may help prevent breaking and may allow for more movement of the glans of the penis within the condom for increased sensitivity.
6. Unroll the condom all the way to the base of the penis.
7. Be sure there is adequate lubrication, either produced naturally from sexual arousal, from the lubricated condom, or from another source, prior to penetration.
8. If you are adding lubrication, do not use oil-based products such as hand creams, lotions, Vaseline, baby oil, cooking oil, massage oils, suntan lotions, or edible oils, as these will weaken the latex (they do not harm polyurethane condoms). Always use water-based lubricants such as K-Y jelly, spermicidal creams, or other lubricants made especially for sexual activity (available at most pharmacies).
9. If it feels as if the condom has broken or slipped off during intercourse, stop and check. If it has, replace it with a new one.
10. After ejaculation, hold the rim of the condom all the way around the base of the penis and withdraw the penis *before* loss of erection. This will help ensure that no semen comes in contact with the partner's genital area internally or externally. Accidentally leaving the condom inside your partner or spilling semen into or near the opening of the vagina greatly increases the risk of pregnancy and STIs. Sperm do *not* die immediately when exposed to the air as some people believe.

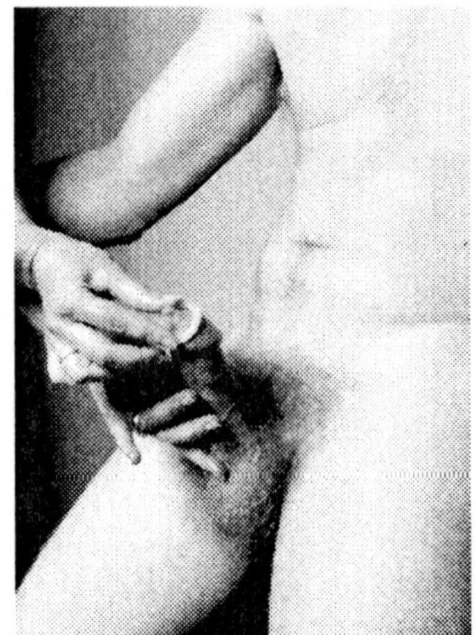

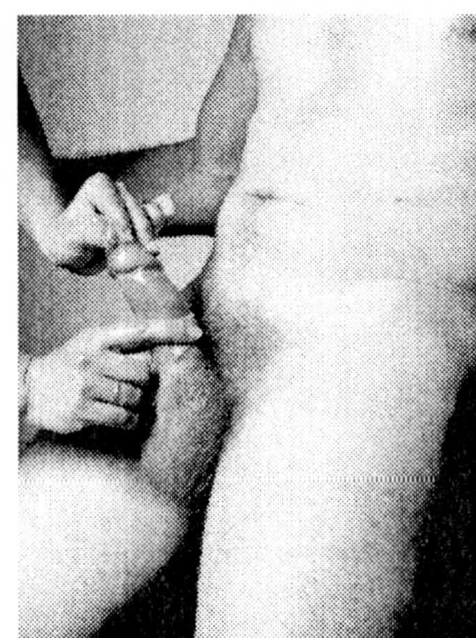

11. Holding the penis away from your partner, remove the condom and check it for signs of damage. Then wrap the used condom in tissue and throw it in the trash.
12. If you desire to have intercourse again, you must use a new condom. Condoms should never be reused.
13. If the condom breaks or slips off without your knowledge, consider using emergency contraception pills (discussed later in this chapter) to help prevent unwanted pregnancy.

All these steps might make condoms seem like a difficult method of birth control, but they're not. After a short time of using condoms as your chosen method of contraception, the process becomes easy, automatic, and even enjoyable.

Source: From *Contraceptive Technology* 18th edition by R. Hatcher, J. Trussel, F. Stewart, W. Cates, G. Stewart, F. Guest and D. Kowal (eds.).

toward condom use than women do (Conley & Collins, 2005; Franzini & Sideman, 1994). Many men are convinced that condoms will significantly reduce sensitivity during intercourse, interfere with erection, create an uncomfortable interruption in the lovemaking process, or make them seem "less macho." These and other objections, however, are not exclusive to males. In fact, when undergraduate students were surveyed, 30 percent of men and 41 percent of women reported that a partner had attempted to dissuade them from using a condom on at least one occasion (Oncale & King, 2001).

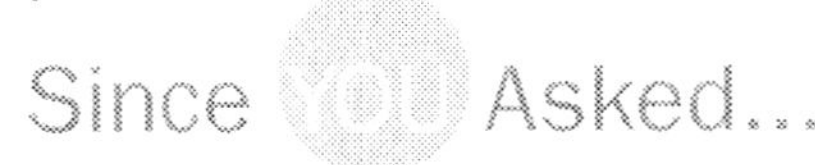

4. I don't like using condoms because they diminish sensation too much. Is there another safe method of birth control and STI prevention?

Table 5.2 STRATEGIES FOR INFLUENCING A RESISTANT PARTNER TO USE A CONDOM

College men and women were asked which strategies they had ever used to encourage condom use. The table summarizes the results.

STRATEGY	DEFINITION	SAMPLE STATEMENT
Reward	Promise of positive consequences if partner agrees	"Your respect for my feelings about using a condom would make our relationship even better."
Emotional coercion	Threat of negative emotional consequences if partner does not agree	"I'm upset and angry at you for not wanting to use a condom."
Risk information	Mention of the risk of STIs to persuade partner to agree	"It's risky to have sex without a condom. We'll both be safer from STIs if we use a condom."
Deception	False information or deception used to get partner to agree	"This is not a good time of the month, and I'm likely to get pregnant if we don't use a condom."
Seduction	Use of sexual arousal as distraction to get partner to agree	"I'll get you so turned on, you won't even know or care that we're using a condom."
Withholding sex	Decision to withhold sexual activity unless partner agrees	"Sorry, no condom, no intercourse."

Source: "Strategies for Influencing a Resistant Partner to Use a Condom" from "Influencing a Partner to Use a Condom" by S. DeBro, S. Campbell, and L. Peplau, *Psychology of Women Quarterly*, 18, (1994), p. 176. Copyright © 1994. Reprinted by permission of Blackwell Publishing.

Convincing a partner to use a condom remains a common problem, especially among college students. Often when a couple is in an ongoing relationship, concerns about using condoms can be overcome by experimenting with different brands and styles of condoms and incorporating their use into erotic touching and foreplay. If a partner steadfastly refuses to use a condom, various strategies have been reported that may be effective in overcoming the resistance and ensuring safer penetrative sexual activities (De Bro, Campbell, & Peplau, 1994). Table 5.2 details some of the strategies used successfully by college students to influence a partner to use a condom. Students were also asked to rate the effectiveness of the various strategies they used. All of the strategies were found to be moderately effective, but emotional coercion received the lowest ratings by both sexes. Women rated withholding sex, risk information, and deception as most effective (in that order), while men indicated deception as most effective, followed by withholding sex and seduction. Research such as this is important in helping increase our understanding of how condom use can be negotiated in college dating relationships. It may also be useful in developing or changing your personal sexual philosophy, which we'll discuss at the end of this chapter.

The Female Condom

Since YOU Asked...

5. Does the female condom work as well as regular male condoms?

The **female condom** (worn by the woman rather than the man) was approved for sale without a prescription in 1993 and does not need to be fitted by a health professional. It is marketed in the United States under the brand name Reality. Just as the male condom covers the penis to prevent genital contact or exchange of sexual fluids, the idea behind the female condom is to create a lining on the inside of the vagina and accomplish basically the same results. Female condoms consist of a tube (or pouch) of thin polyurethane, similar to the material in the polyurethane male condom, with a flexible ring at each end. One end is sealed and the other is open. The flexible ring at the closed end is squeezed in half and inserted into the vagina against the cervix, as shown in Figure 5.1. The internal ring holds the condom in place. The ring at the open end is positioned on the outside of the body, around the opening to the vagina. The condom is lubricated (though not with spermicide) and is sold with extra lubricant if needed for easier insertion or more comfortable movement. During intercourse, the female condom stays inside the vagina and the penis moves within it. After ejaculation, the condom must be removed by twisting the outside ring to trap the

female condom A tube or pouch of thin polyurethane with a flexible ring at each end. One end is sealed and the other is open. The condom is inserted into the vagina to protect against pregnancy and the transmission of STIs.

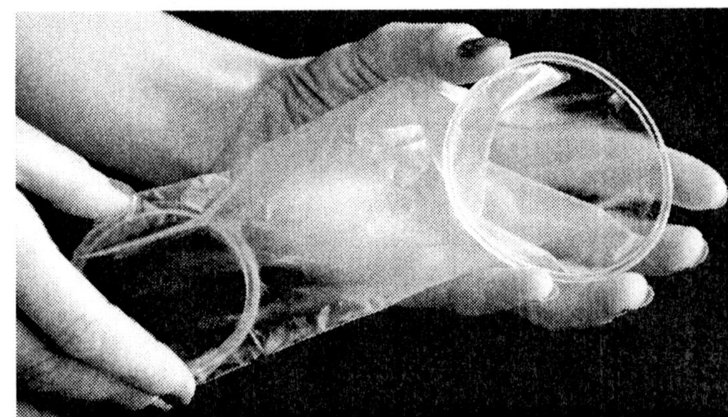

(a)

FIGURE 5.1 The Female Condom

The female condom consists of a tube of thin polyurethane, similar to the polyurethane male condom, but with a flexible ring at each end, as shown in the photo (a). The three-step procedure (b) illustrates how to insert a female condom. Care must be taken when removing the condom to prevent semen from spilling out.

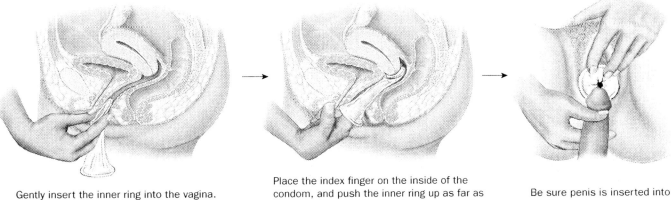

Gently insert the inner ring into the vagina. Feel the inner ring go up and move into place.

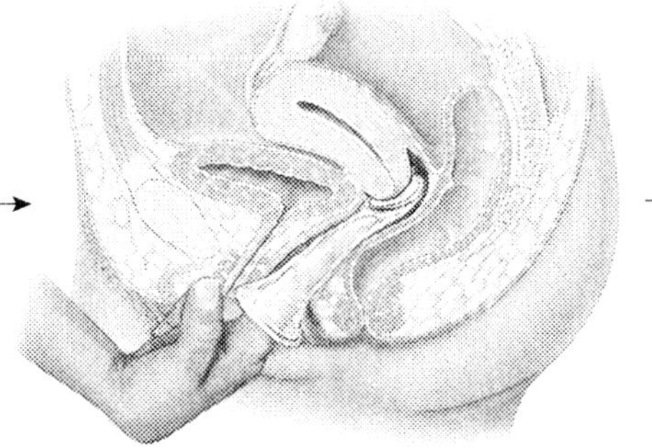

Place the index finger on the inside of the condom, and push the inner ring up as far as it will go. Be sure the sheath is not twisted. The outer ring should remain on the outside of the vagina.

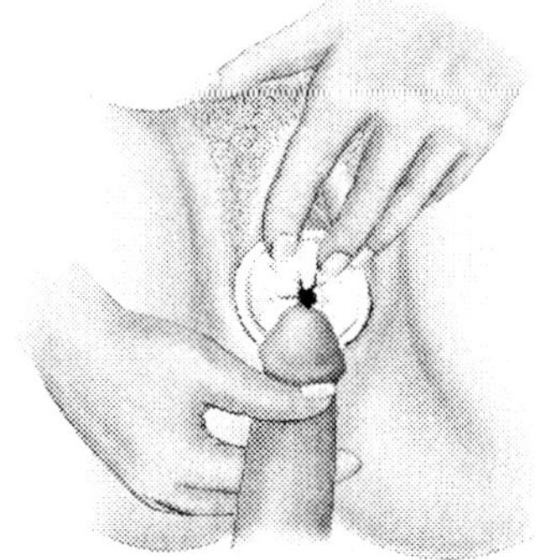

Be sure penis is inserted into condom, not next to it.

(b)

semen inside and gently pulling the condom out of the vagina. This should be done before the woman stands up to be sure none of the semen spills out of the condom into or around the vaginal area. As with male condoms, each female condom should be used only once. However, some studies have found that female condoms that have been carefully washed, dried, relubricated, and reused as many as seven times continued to meet FDA guidelines for effectiveness (Hollander, 2001).

The main disadvantage of the female condom is that typical-use failure rate is higher than for male condoms and is similar to other barrier methods, such as the diaphragm and cervical cap, discussed later. With incorrect or careless use, the female condom can be inserted or removed incorrectly, allowing semen to spill out in or near the vagina, or the penis may sometimes be inserted by mistake next to rather than inside of the condom. However, if used correctly and consistently, it is nearly as effective as the male condom. In fact, one study found that among such users in the United States, only 2.6 pregnancies occurred per 100 couples over a six-month period (Farr et al., 1994). The female condom has the advantage of allowing the woman to be in more control of contraception and preventing sexually transmitted infections. It also allows for greater spontaneity than the male condom because the female condom may be inserted up to eight hours before intercourse. For greater effectiveness, the female condom may be combined with hormonal contraceptives, but it should *not* be used at the same time as a male condom (this can create too much friction and cause the condoms to break). The female condom costs more than male condoms—approximately $3.00 each (although one online source offers them in wholesale lots of 100 for slightly over $200).

An additional advantage of the female condom is that, used correctly, it may provide slightly greater protection from STIs than a male condom. Because the polyurethane is stronger than latex, it is not degraded by the use of oil based lubricants; and the shape of the condom protects a wider area of skin between the base of the penis and the vulva or anus during intercourse (Nicolette, 1996). As mentioned, male and female condoms are not designed to be used simultaneously, as the effectiveness of each will be reduced. However, either the male or female condom may be combined with other contraceptive methods (such as hormonal or other barrier methods—see below) for increased protection against pregnancy and STIs.

Methods for Preventing Pregnancy (but *Not* STIs)

All of the remaining methods of birth control discussed in this chapter are designed only to help prevent pregnancy. Although a few of them may offer minimal protection against some STIs, they should not be used for that purpose. However, all of the methods discussed in this section may be combined with the condom for protection from STIs and added insurance against pregnancy.

Female Hormonal Methods

Female hormonal methods of contraception prevent pregnancy by altering certain characteristics of a woman's ovulation cycle or reproductive tract. Depending on the method, these hormonal alterations may prevent ovulation altogether, thicken the cervical mucus to create a barrier against sperm, or change the lining of the uterus so that even if an egg is fertilized, it will not implant and create a pregnancy. The various hormonal contraceptives on the market differ primarily in the specific hormonal formula and the method used to deliver the hormone to the body.

At this time, all hormonal methods of contraception are designed for women, but research is being conducted on possible male hormonal contraception methods, which we will discuss later in this chapter. As this book goes to press, five types of hormonal contraceptive delivery systems are on the market: oral, implant, injection, skin patch, and vaginal ring. All hormonal methods of contraception have both advantages and disadvantages—positive and negative side effects—so women and couples should strive to become as educated as possible about all the methods before selecting one.

Oral Contraceptives

In general, **oral contraceptives**, also referred to as birth control pills, are among the most popular reversible birth control methods used by women in the United States (Hatcher & Nelson, 2004). When used correctly, they provide a convenient and extremely effective method of preventing pregnancy. But they offer no protection against STIs. The two main categories of birth control pills are the **combination pill**, which contains a combination of estrogen and progestin, and the **minipill**, which contains progestin only.

How Oral Contraceptives Work. Combination oral contraceptives contain both estrogen and progestin. The contraceptive effect on a woman taking these hormones is that her body's normal hormonal cycle is altered, and ovulation (the release of an egg) is typically prevented. Different brands of combination pills have varying doses of hormones. In general, lower-dose pills are recommended because they are effective in preventing pregnancy and are less likely to produce negative side effects sometimes associated with oral contraceptives, such as spotting between periods, headaches, and breast tenderness. Although serious negative side effects are relatively rare, a woman's decision about com-

oral contraceptives Tablets containing female hormones that are ingested every day. They constitute the most popular reversible birth control method used by women in the United States; also known as birth control pills.

combination pill An oral contraceptive containing a combination of estrogen and progestin.

minipill An oral contraceptive containing progestin only.

bination oral contraceptives should be an informed one made in close consultation with her health care provider.

Birth control pills are sold in various types of packages that number and label each pill so that it is easier to keep track of the pills taken and whether a pill has been missed. Oral contraceptives must be taken for 21 consecutive days and then stopped for seven days, during which time the woman will usually have her period (for an exception to this rule, see the discussion on "90-day pills" next). Most popular brands of combined pills actually provide pills for all 28 days of the cycle, but the last seven pills in the pack contain no hormones and are supplied as "placeholders" so that the habit of taking a pill every day will not be interrupted.

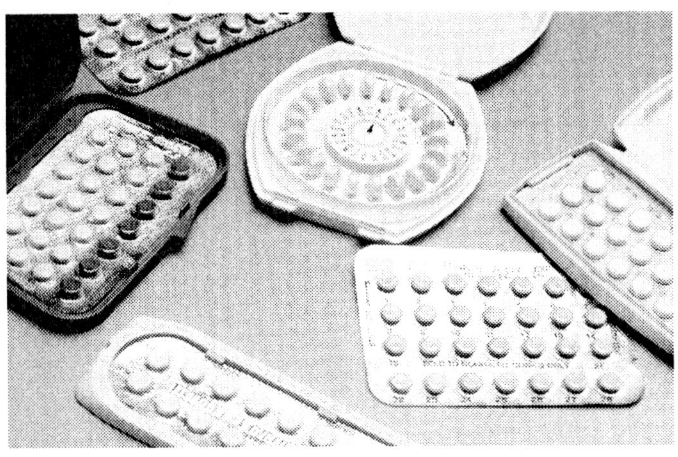

Numerous brands and formulations of oral contraceptives offer a great many options for women who choose this form of hormonal birth control.

The progestin-only minipill has a slightly, but only very slightly, higher failure rate compared to the combination pill (Hatcher & Nelson, 2004; World Health Organization, 1982). The main advantage of the progestin-only oral contraceptive pill is that it avoids some of the potential negative side effects associated with estrogen in the combination pill. However, many of the health benefits associated with the estrogen in the combined pill are also not present in the progestin-only pill. The pros and cons of oral contraceptives will be discussed shortly.

The contraceptive effect of progestin-only oral contraceptives (the minipill) not only interferes with ovulation but also causes a thickening of the mucus secreted by the cervix (Hatcher & Nelson, 2004). This thickening of the mucus sets up a barrier that is very difficult for sperm to penetrate. In addition, if some sperm were to get through this barrier, the lining of the uterus that develops to support a fertilized egg is thinner in a woman taking the minipill and is therefore less receptive to implantation and pregnancy.

Recently, a new way of taking oral contraceptives was approved by the Food and Drug Administration and introduced to the U.S. market under the brand name Seasonale. Instead of the traditional 21-day hormone regimen, Seasonale provides a daily dose of hormones for 84 consecutive days, during which a woman is protected against pregnancy and does not menstruate. She then takes the usual placebo pills for 7 days, during which she will typically have a period. The hormonal formulation in the "90-day pill" is basically the same as for standard 28-day oral contraceptives, but by taking the pills with hormones continuously for 84 days, a woman will have only 4 menstrual periods per year instead the average of 13 (Mangan, 2003).

Doctors and many women have been aware for decades that menstrual periods could be delayed or reduced in frequency if a woman skipped the placebo pills in the pack of oral contraceptives and went to a new pack immediately upon completing the 21-days of hormonal pills. This strategy has been recommended by doctors for women with menstruation-related health problems and used by women themselves to delay or skip a period due at an inconvenient or inopportune time (vacation, sports competition, honeymoon, etc.).

For many women, reducing the number of periods has various advantages beyond the convenience of less frequent menstruation. Women who experience especially painful periods, heavy bleeding, cycle-related migraine headaches, endometriosis, or other debilitating menstruation-related symptoms may benefit from reducing the annual number of periods. Moreover, many medical researchers contend that having fewer periods may actually be healthy (Kalb, 2003). In modern society, women have, on average, 450 periods during their lifetime. This is nearly three times as many as humans during the early hunter-gatherer era, when women spent far more time either pregnant or nursing their young. This has led some researchers to conclude that nature did not intend for women to have as many lifetime periods as they do today.

In studies of Seasonale, the most serious side effect was an increase in bleeding or spotting between periods. In one major study, 7.5 percent of women discontinued use of Seasonale due to breakthrough bleeding, compared to only 1.8 percent using standard 28-day birth control pills (Kalb, 2003). In addition, Seasonale, as a combination hormonal contraceptive, carries all the same health risks as other methods with similar formulations, as discussed earlier.

Some medical researchers are concerned about the potential negative side effects of the increased amount of hormones (nine additional weeks of hormones per year compared to conventional oral contraceptives) taken by women using the 90-day pill (Proust, 2004). Women considering Seasonale should be aware that because it is a relatively new hormone delivery system, additional studies will be needed over time to determine its long-term safety.

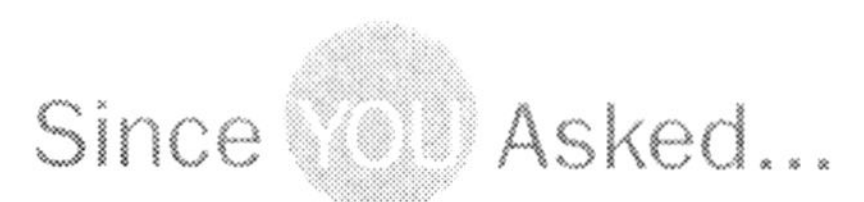

6. My girlfriend was on the pill, but she still got pregnant. How did that happen?

Effectiveness of Oral Contraceptives. Birth control pills offer one of the most effective methods of preventing pregnancy. Nevertheless, a very small percentage of women have become pregnant while taking oral contraceptives either because of the very unlikely event of inherent failure or due to incorrect use (such as skipping pills). However, when used correctly, as explained in the next section, only implants and sterilization have lower failure rates than oral contraceptives. With conscientious and careful use of the combination pill (meaning never accidentally forgetting to take a pill and being sure to take it at approximately the same time each day), only one woman in 1,000 should expect to experience an accidental pregnancy. For the progestin-only pill, that estimate increases to 5 in 1,000, still an impressive success rate.

Even with less than perfect use, such as the occasional missed pill, oral contraceptives have relatively high effectiveness rates. The combination pill's failure rate in the average user is about 3 percent. Depending on the study cited, estimated failure rates for the progestin-only pill range from 1 to 9 percent (Coustan, Haning, & Singer, 1995). As with nearly all forms of contraception, the most important factor in effectiveness is correct use.

Using Birth Control Pills Correctly. The most common incorrect use of oral contraceptives is forgetting to take them every day. Just how serious a problem is it to miss a pill or two? Potentially, very serious. Over the years since birth control pills first appeared on the market, the dose of hormones contained in them has been steadily reduced. This decrease has made the pill much safer in terms of negative side effects, but it has also increased the importance of regular doses. Women using combined oral contraceptives must take one pill every day of the 21-day course (in the 28-day pack, as noted earlier, the last 7 pills do not contain hormones and are there only to maintain the habit of taking one pill each day). Furthermore, women should try to take a pill at approximately the same time each day. This will maintain constant hormone levels in the bloodstream. Even the most conscientious of women may forget to take a pill. Because of this, and because the pill does not protect against STIs, most sexuality educators and health care professionals strongly recommended that women who choose oral contraception keep a backup method of birth control (such as condoms) readily available. If a woman misses a pill, she need not panic, but she should be aware of the steps to take to maintain maximum contracep-

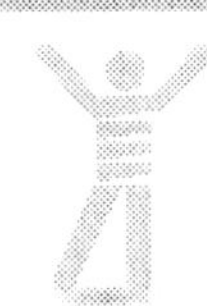

In Touch With Your Sexual Health

Missed Your Pill? Here's What You Should Do

Oral contraceptives are most effective when taken regularly, at about the same time each day. If you miss a pill, the effect on fertility depends on many factors such as when in your cycle the pill was missed, how many pills during a cycle were missed, and the timing of intercourse relative to the missed pill(s). Usually, pregnancy can be avoided even if pills have been missed through use of a backup barrier method or by taking emergency contraception pills, especially if intercourse has occurred in the past 5 days. The following chart offers recommendations about exactly what actions should be taken in the event of missed pills to maintain effective contraception.

# PILLS MISSED	WEEK PILLS MISSED	RECOMMENDATION	FINISH THIS PACK	EMERGENCY CONTRACEPTION	7-DAY BARRIER BACK-UP
1	1	Take 2 pills ASAP	Yes	Yes*	Yes
1	2–3	Take 2 pills ASAP	Yes	No	No
1	4	Skip placebo pills	Yes	No	No
2–4	1	Take 2 pills ASAP	Yes	Yes*	Yes
2–4	2	Take 2 pills ASAP	Yes	No	No
2–4	3	Start new pack	N/A	No	No
2–4	4	Skip placebo	Yes	No	No
5	Any	Take 2 pills; start new pack	N/A	Yes*	Yes

* Start emergency contraception as soon as possible. No need to double up on pills. Take the next pill on the next day.

Source: From *Contraceptive Technology* 18th edition by R. Hatcher, J. Trussel, F. Stewart, W. Cates, G. Stewart, F. Guest and D. Kowal (eds.).

tion protection. "In Touch with Your Sexual Health: Missed Your Pill? Here's What You Should Do" summarizes the steps a woman should take if she misses one or more pills during a cycle.

The start of protection from pregnancy depends on when in her cycle a woman begins taking oral contraception. The time after beginning birth control pills until she is safe from pregnancy is typically about a week. This, however, assumes that she begins taking combination pills during the first seven days after her menstrual period begins or, for progestin-only pills (the minipill), during the first five days. Although she is unlikely to be fertile during these days, a backup method of contraception, such as condoms, is recommended during the first week after beginning the pills. In addition she should consider emergency contraception pills (discussed later in this chapter) if she has had unprotected intercourse recently. However, if a woman begins taking birth control pills at any other time during her cycle, she should use a backup contraceptive during the first month of pills (Family Health International, 1996). Moreover, if a woman is at all concerned about exposure to sexually transmitted infections, she should continue to insist on condom use, even though she is protected from pregnancy by the birth control pills.

Advantages and Disadvantages of the Pill. When the first oral contraceptive pills came onto the U.S. market in the early 1960s, they were associated with some rare but potentially serious health dangers, such as blood clots and increased risk of stroke or heart attack. However, over the years, with changes in dose and type of hormones used in oral contraceptives, these dangers have been minimized or eliminated, and today oral contraceptives may even protect a woman from some serious diseases. One point is extremely clear: For nearly all women, the health risks associated with preg-

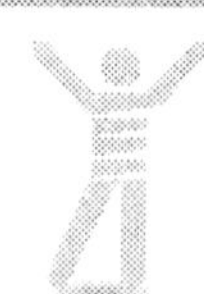

In Touch with Your Sexual Health

Pros, Cons, and Cautions of Using Oral Contraceptives

Here is a list of the major advantages and disadvantages of birth control pills. Also included is a list of warning signs of potentially serious side effects that may require immediate medical attention. Keep in mind that most of these pros and cons are also associated with other types of hormonal contraceptives discussed in this chapter.

Pros

- Very effective method of birth control
- No interruption of lovemaking
- Generally very safe
- Often makes menstrual cycle more regular and reduces or relieves symptoms of PMS and menstrual cramps
- May reduce length of period and amount of bleeding
- May protect against pelvic inflammatory disease, which can lead to infertility
- Appears to reduce risk of certain cancers, especially ovarian and endometrial cancers
- Does not interfere with future fertility
- May help clear up acne
- May reduce unwanted hair growth
- May reduce incidence and number of ovarian cysts

Cons

- Does not protect against any sexually transmitted infections
- Easy to miss doses
- Relatively expensive (depending on where purchased)
- Possible spotting (slight bleeding between periods)
- Possible nausea (infrequent and usually only during first cycle of use)
- Possible headaches and breast tenderness (usually solved by changing pill dose)
- Depression (rare)
- Cardiovascular disease (heart attack, stroke, blood clots; very rare and virtually always associated with women over 35 who smoke)

Cautions

- Oral contraceptives provide no protection against sexually transmitted infections. Many women choose to combine condoms with the pill for maximum prevention of both pregnancy and STIs.
- You should never begin taking oral contraceptives without a complete understanding of all the risks listed here and the correct use of the pills.
- You should be aware that the hormones in birth control pills may interact with other prescription medications (e.g. anti-seizure medications and certain antibiotics) and herbal remedies (e.g., Saint John's wort), causing a decrease in contraceptive effectiveness. Be sure to keep your health care provider informed of all medications and remedies you are taking.

Danger Symptoms

- When you are on the pill, you should be alert to all the side effects listed here. Furthermore, you should be alert to warning signs of serious problems that may be associated with the pill, especially if you smoke cigarettes. If you experience any of the following symptoms while on the pill, you should contact your doctor immediately. These danger signs are summarized by the acronym ACHES:

A—Abdominal pain (severe)
C—Chest pain (severe) with a cough or shortness of breath
H—Headache (severe), dizziness, weakness, numbness
E—Eye problems, vision loss, blurring, slurred speech
S—Severe leg pain

Source: Adapted from Hatcher & Nelson, 2004, pp. 427–442.

nancy are, overall, greater than those associated with oral contraceptives. It is impossible to address fully all of the advantages, disadvantages, health benefits, and dangers of birth control pills in this rather brief discussion. See "In Touch with Your Sexual Health: Pros, Cons, and Cautions of Using Oral Contraceptives" for a summary of considerations when choosing oral contraceptives as your birth control method. An excellent discussion of each specific type and brand of oral contraceptive may be found at *http://www.birthcontrol.com*.

Hormonal Implants

Hormonal implants are small tubes containing a progestin hormone that are surgically implanted under the skin of a woman's upper arm. These were marketed in the United States under the brand name Norplant. The matchstick-size tubes (called "rods") slowly released the progestin into the woman's system and were nearly 100 percent effective against pregnancy for approximately five years or until they were removed, whichever comes first. Like all other forms of hormonal contraception, implants do not not protect against STIs.

In 2000, the manufacturer of Norplant; Wyeth Pharmaceuticals, announced that some lots of the implants may have been defective and may not release adequate amounts of hormone to protect women from pregnancy. Wyeth advised doctors to stop inserting the implants and to provide Norplant patients with alternative forms of barrier contraceptives. Wyeth also announced that it was discontinuing distribution of Norplant. Consequently, as of early 2004, no contraceptive implant was available in the United States.

In 2005, Organon Pharmaceuticals, based in the Netherlands, received a positive review from the FDA for Implanon, a single-rod hormonal implant that releases a hormone similar to that found in many oral contraceptives. Implanon is easily inserted in about one minute, is continuosly effective for three years, and may be removed at any time to allow fertility to return. This new implant was expected to be available in the United States sometime in 2006 ("Bulletin," 2005).

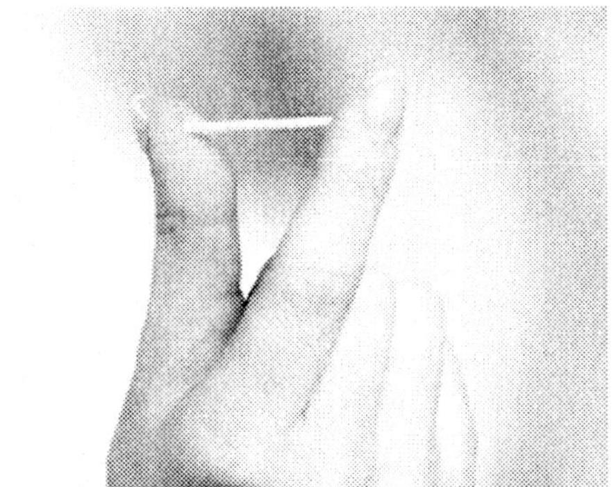

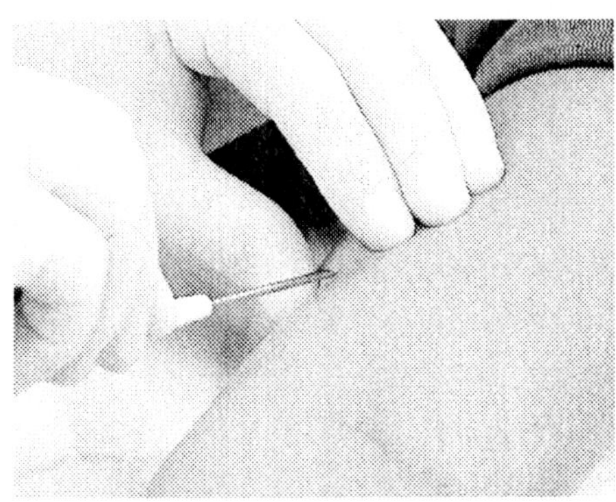

FIGURE 5.2 Hormonal Implants
Hormonal implants are small tubes that are surgically implanted under the skin of a woman's upper arm. Hormones contained in these tubes are slowly released into the woman's body over several years, thus preventing ovulation. Shown here is the single-tube Implanon implant device.

How Implants Work. The contraceptive action of implants is due to the slow release of hormones into the woman's body. The hormones prevent pregnancy by inhibiting ovulation, thickening the cervical mucus (similar to the minipill, described earlier), or both. Using a local anesthetic, a physician inserts the implant under the skin, usually on the underside of the upper arm (see Figure 5.2). The contraceptive effect is immediate (within 24 hours). Upon removal of the implant, fertility typically returns quickly.

Effectiveness of Implants. One of the greatest advantages of implant contraceptives is that once inserted, it is virtually impossible to use the method incorrectly. The contraceptive hormone is released over time so that protection is provided without any action at all on the woman's part. Therefore, as you can see in Table 5.1, no difference between typical and theoretical effectiveness exists. Perhaps more important is the extremely low failure rate of implants. Fewer than one woman in 2,000 became pregnant using Norplant in the first year, a 0.05 percent failure rate (Darney, 1994; Hatcher, 1998). The effectiveness of Implanon appears equally high. Among nearly 1,000 women participating in one large study of Implanon, not a single pregnancy was reported over a two-year period (Edwards & Moore, 1999; O'Connell, 2001).

Advantages and Disadvantages of Implants. The advantages of hormonal implants are their ease of use and near-perfect effectiveness. Still, hormonal implants are not without negative side effects. Overall, the majority of women who used Norplant when it was available in the United States were willing to overlook most of its problems and were satisfied with the method overall (Eilers & Swanson, 1994; Thomas & Le Melle, 1995). However, some women reported several negative experiences, including breast tenderness, complete cessation of menstrual flow, spotting or more frequent periods, higher initial cost, a slightly increased chance of benign ovarian cysts, and difficulty during the implant removal process (Eilers & Swanson, 1994; Frank et al., 1993; Hatcher, 1998). As new implants come onto the contraceptive market, their level of side effects and acceptability in the wake of Norplant remains to be seen. Studies of women using Implanon in Europe have found relatively high acceptance rates, with 80 percent of women continuing to use the implant method after two years or longer. In general, the side effects of Implanon are similar to those of Norplant (Edwards & Moore, 1999; O'Connell, 2001).

Injectable Hormonal Contraceptives

Another method of administering hormonal contraceptives is through an injection in the arm or hip. Injectable contraceptives offer convenience in that a woman does not need to remember to take a pill every day but instead must have a health care professional administer the shot. As of 2006, only one injectable contraceptive, Depo-Provera, was available.

Often referred to simply as "Depo," Depo-Provera has been in use throughout the world since the 1970s. It was approved in the United States in 1992. Each injection of the hormone gives a woman a minimum of three months of highly effective contraception. Like all other hormonal forms of birth control, Depo-Provera does not provide protection from STIs.

Another injectable contraception for women, developed in 2000, was a once-a-month combination hormone shot called Lunelle. Because Lunelle combined progestin-like and estrogen-like hormones, it avoided many of the negative side effects of Depo-Provera and offered many of the same benefits of combination birth control pills. However, due to errors in dosing and other marketing problems, the manufacturer of Lunelle recalled the product in late 2002 (Mechcatie, 2002a) and discontinued it in 2004. However, a demand clearly exists for such a product, and development is continuing (Mishell, 2004).

How Injection Methods Work. Depo-Provera consists of the hormone DPMA (medroxyprogesterone acetate), which is injected into the hip or arm. DPMA (a form of progestin) prevents pregnancy in the same manner as implants, by inhibiting ovulation, thickening the cervical mucus to prevent passage of sperm, and thinning the endometrial lining so that should fertilization occur, implantation (pregnancy) is unlikely. A single dose of DPMA provides contraceptive protection for at least three months, when another injection is required for continued effectiveness. This is a reversible method of birth control, although the return of fertility can take up to a year after discontinuing the method (Earl & David, 1994; Hatcher, 1998).

Effectiveness of Injectable Contraceptives. Depo-Provera is another extremely effective hormonal contraceptive with a failure rate of only 0.3 percent (about the same as for birth control pills). This rate assumes, of course, that the woman returns every three months for another injection. However, there is a buffer of effectiveness so that contraception is maintained for at least two weeks past the three-month recommended injection schedule (Earl & David, 1994; Hatcher,

1998). The contraceptive action of the method takes effect almost immediately following the first injection.

Side Effects of Injection Methods. Negative side effects associated with the use of Depo-Provera include menstrual changes, such as spotting and breakthrough bleeding (common), headaches (17 percent), nervousness (11 percent), decreased sex drive (5 percent), breast tenderness (3 percent), and depression (2 percent) (Hatcher, 1998). From those relatively low percentages you might assume that the majority of women using Depo are side-effect-free. However, when a reader poll conducted on the Women's Health Web site in 2002 asked women on Depo "Have you experienced side effects on Depo Provera?" only 20 percent said no.

Another side effect more common to Depo-Provera than other hormonal methods is **amenorrhea**, the cessation of a woman's period (Hatcher, 2004). The health risks of amenorrhea appear to be minimal and may even provide various benefits, such as the elimination of monthly symptoms of menstrual pain, bloating, and the emotional swings often associated with PMS (Huffman, 2002). Many women see this side effect as a plus. Furthermore, a woman's period typically returns soon after she stops using the method. Some evidence suggests that women on Depo-Provera experience decreases in HDL cholesterol levels (the "good" cholesterol), so blood lipids should be monitored in women with high overall cholesterol levels (Hatcher, 1998; 2004). Finally, one of the more serious side effects of DPMA is an increased loss of bone density (osteoporosis). To counter this side effect, most health care professionals counsel women who use Depo-Provers to make dietary alterations, use calcium supplements, exercise regularly, and have periodic bone scans (Kass-Wolf, 2001). In 2002, however, researchers found that any bone loss that occurs during the use of DPMA reverses within two to three years after discontinuation of the hormone ("Depo-Provera Bone Loss," 2002).

The Contraceptive Patch

No doubt you have heard about the nicotine patch. It delivers, through the skin, a continuous dose of nicotine that helps the smoker avoid withdrawal symptoms while trying to give up cigarettes. In a similar delivery process, the weekly hormonal **contraceptive patch** provides a precise dose of two hormones into a woman's body, through the skin, preventing ovulation. The contraceptive patch was introduced to the U.S. market in early 2002 under the name Ortho Evra. This hormonal contraceptive is a 1-inch-square patch that a woman wears like a Band-Aid on her abdomen, buttocks, upper body (front or back, but not on the breasts), or upper arm. Each patch is worn for one week, for three consecutive weeks, and then the fourth week is patch-free (the menstruation week). The adhesive in the patch allows it to stay on the skin throughout various activities including swimming, bathing, and exercising.

If this hormonal pattern sounds familiar, it is because the patch works exactly like oral contraceptives: three weeks of hormones and one week without, during which the menstrual period occurs. The primary difference here is the hormone delivery system. Side effects of the patch are generally the same as those discussed earlier for the combination pill: breakthrough bleeding between periods, weight gain or loss, breast tenderness, nausea, headaches, decrease or increase in sexual desire, and temporary symptoms of depression. However, recent studies have found that the patch may expose women to levels of hormones as much as 60 percent higher than most oral contraceptives. This may increase the risk of dangerous side effects including blood clots in the legs and lungs, and problems relating to clotting such as strokes and heart attacks. Although no increased incidence of

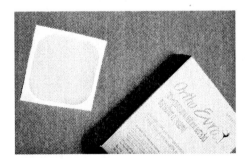

The contraceptive patch delivers hormones through the skin, preventing ovulation.

amenorrhea Cessation of a woman's period.

contraceptive patch A pad that delivers a precise dose of two hormones into a woman's body through the skin, preventing ovulation.

these side effects has been seen among women using the patch, the manufacturer has added a new label advising women of the possibility of increased hormonal exposure (Mechcatie, 2006).

The Contraceptive Ring

Another hormonal delivery system is the **contraceptive ring**. The first such ring, called NuvaRing, was released in the United States in 2002. No, it's not a ring worn on your finger (that would be a new twist on the engagement ring!). NuvaRing is a colorless, flexible, transparent silicone ring about 2 inches in diameter, similar to the ring in the female condom. When the ring is inserted into the vagina, it releases a continuous low dose of estrogenlike and progestinlike hormones into the bloodstream through the vaginal walls for three consecutive weeks. These are basically the same hormones found in other combination hormonal contraceptives. Are you beginning to see a pattern here? Researchers clearly believe they have found an effective, reasonably safe, and even beneficial combination of hormones to prevent pregnancy, and now various pharmaceutical companies are working to find the best method for delivering them to a woman's body.

Here's how the vaginal ring works. The woman inserts the ring into her vagina (in much the same way as inserting a diaphragm or sponge) and leaves it there for three weeks (see Figure 5.3). At the end of the three weeks, she removes it for a week, which will typically cause her to have her period, and then inserts a new one for the next three weeks (Chatfield, 2001). Because it is not a barrier device, such as a female condom or diaphragm, exact fit and position are not necessary for effectiveness (American Health Consultants, 2001). NuvaRing's effectiveness is excellent, with a failure rate of less than 1 percent when used according to the package instructions (Archer & Ballagh, 2003). Most couples are unaware of the ring during sexual activities, but it may be removed during intercourse as long as it is replaced within three hours. If the ring is removed for more than three hours, an additional form of barrier contraception should be used until the ring has been in the vagina for seven days (Archer & Ballagh, 2003).

The contraceptive ring offers the same pluses and minuses as other combined hormonal contraceptives—pill, implant, or patch. Some of the negative side effects, however, may be less severe for some women due to the ring's lower dose of hormones. The contraceptive ring is as effective as other combination hormonal methods but requires smaller amounts of hormones due to its location in the vagina, which targets the hormones exactly where they are needed for greatest effectiveness. On the down side, in addition to the overall negative side effects of combined hormonal contraceptives, a small number of women have experienced vaginal irritation and inflammation

FIGURE 5.3 The Vaginal Ring

The vaginal ring is a colorless, flexible silicone ring about 2 inches in diameter, as shown in the photo of a NuvaRing (a), that prevents ovulation by secreting hormones through the vaginal walls continuously for three weeks. The three-step procedure (b) illustrates how to insert a vaginal ring.

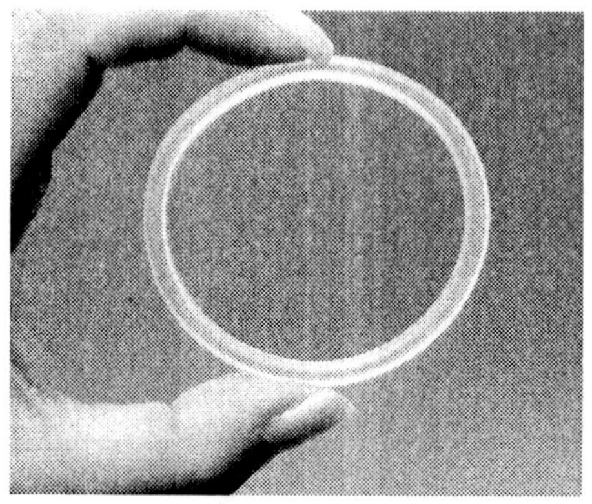

(a)

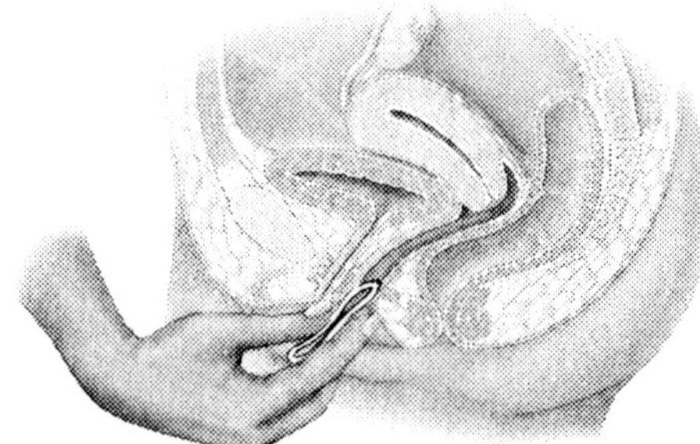

Squeeze the sides of the flexible ring together.

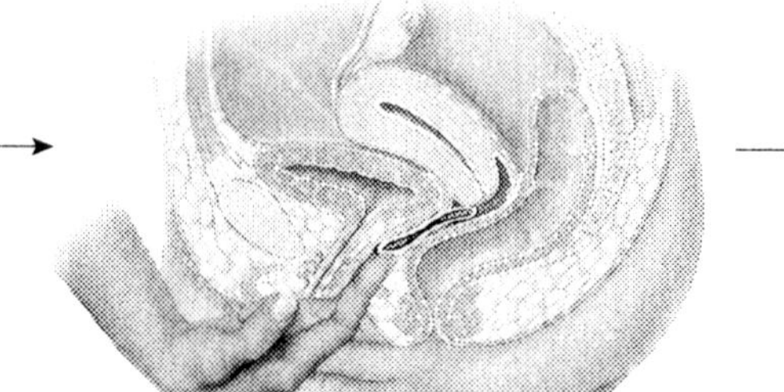

Insert the ring into the vagina.

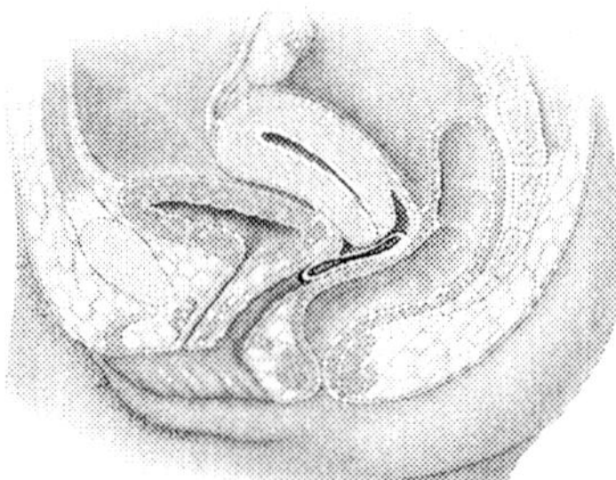

Position the ring deep in the vagina adjacent to the cervix.

(b)

also under local anesthesia, only a small puncture is made in the scrotum to allow access to the vas deferens, which is then snipped and blocked as in the scalpel method (see Figure 5.12). No sutures are required, and the punctures can hardly be seen following the procedure. Vasectomy complications are rare for either method but seem to be lower for the no-scalpel technique.

Still another method, approved by the FDA in 2003, requires no cutting of the vas deferens at all. Instead, tiny clips (shown in Figure 5.12) about the size of a grain of rice (brand name Vasclip) are passed into the scrotum through a small opening and placed around each vas deferens, clamping it shut and preventing the passage of sperm cells ("Vasclip," 2003). Early research findings have indicated that complications from the Vasclip procedure are fewer than for other vasectomy methods.

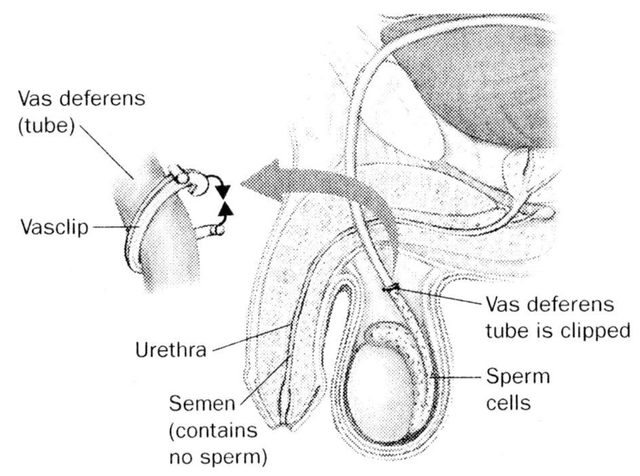

FIGURE 5.12 Vasectomy Procedures

A vasectomy severs or blocks each vas deferens tube so that no sperm can be ejaculated with the semen.

Effectiveness of Voluntary Surgical Contraception

Obviously, if you surgically prevent an ovum from ever encountering a sperm, you would have a 100 percent effective method of contraception. However, a very small failure rate (0.1 to 0.4 percent) is associated with this method. Why? Several reasons are possible, including poor surgical technique, spontaneous reconnection of a severed fallopian tube or vas deferens, and sperm cells that are left over in the male reproductive tract following surgery, which require as many as 20 ejaculations to clear (Stewart & Carignan, 1998). In rare instances, women have become pregnant before the male's reproductive structures were fully purged of sperm cells. Although this is not a failure of the method itself, these pregnancies have sometimes shown up in the effectiveness data (Stewart & Carignan, 1998). Excluding these infrequent errors in procedure, VSC is as near to a 100 percent effective method as exists today, other than true abstinence.

Advantages and Disadvantages of Sterilization

Interestingly, the main advantage of VSC is probably its main disadvantage: It is permanent (see the discussion in the next section regarding reversal). This means that a couple need no longer be concerned about using contraception. However, some people regret their decision and later wish that they were fertile. Some of the reasons for this regret include a change in desire for more children, loss of children through death, or divorce and remarriage. Regret is more common among individuals who choose VSC at earlier ages (Henshaw & Singh, 1986; Wilcox et al., 1991).

Other advantages of VSC include lack of long-term side effects and the low cost per year once the initial expense of the procedure is covered (about $2,000 for a tubal ligation and $600 for a vasectomy). An additional disadvantage is that both male and female sterilization requires surgery, which is accompanied by small but significant risks of medical complications.

Finally, some studies have demonstrated an increased risk of prostate and other cancers in men who have had a vasectomy, especially if the procedure was performed more than 20 years prior (Giovannucci et al., 1993). However, other studies have not found such a connection, and many health professionals believe that this risk factor has not been adequately demonstrated to warrant a widespread change in the current medical practice of vasectomy surgery (Howards, 1994; Stewart & Carignan, 1998).

The Reversibility of VSC

In some cases, reversal of a vasectomy or tubal sterilization is possible. For women who have reversal surgery, pregnancy rates following reversal range between 43 and 88 percent, depending on the type of blockage used in the sterilization and the techniques used in the reversal procedure. For men, pregnancy rates following reversal surgery range from 38 to 85 percent, depending primarily on the type of reversal surgery used, the length of time since the original vasectomy (the longer the time, the lower the success rates), and the presence or absence of sperm antibodies in the man's bloodstream (M. Fox, 1994; Pollack, Carignan, & Jacobstein, 2004; Stewart & Carignan, 1998). You may think that the new clip methods discussed earlier would be more reversible than other methods—simply "unclip"—however, a vasectomy using the Vasclip method is currently considered a permanent form of birth control, just like other surgical methods, and the reversibility of this new method has yet to be studied (Vasclip, 2005).

The most important point to consider is that reversal is a trickier and more extensive (also more expensive) surgery than the original procedure, and success is not guaranteed. Anyone considering voluntary surgical contraception should think of it as permanent.

Avoiding Abortion as Birth Control

You are undoubtedly aware that abortion is one of the most controversial topics in the United States today. The complexities of the abortion issue are discussed in detail in Chapter 9, "Conception, Pregnancy, and Birth." However, abortion must be mentioned here because it is most often the result of a couple's failure to use contraception correctly or at all. If these couples do not wish to conceive, they may turn to abortion as a birth control measure. Abortion is never an easy decision to reach and is usually a very trying and painful experience, both physically and emotionally. When people who do not wish to conceive, engage in unprotected intercourse, pregnancy is often the result. Many of these individuals will turn to abortion as a birth control measure. It is safe to say that virtually everyone on both sides of the abortion debate is opposed to the use of abortion as a birth control method. One of the best reasons for using contraceptives responsibly whenever you decide to have intercourse is never having to face the often painful and potentially life-changing decisions that accompany an unwanted pregnancy.

Experimental and Future Methods of Birth Control

New methods of birth control and contraception for women and men are continuously being researched in the United States and throughout the world. Ultimately, this research is likely to be beneficial in that the more choices we have to prevent unwanted pregnancies, the more likely it is that individuals will find and use a method that is best for them. Let us look at a few of the approaches to contraception that are under study and may reach the market in the not-too-distant future.

Future Methods for Men

You may be saying, "It's about time!" Well, it's true that nearly all of the many methods discussed in this chapter are for women. For men, there are just three: abstinence, condoms, and vasectomy. Many reasons may exist for this limited choice, ranging from systematic gender discrimination throughout the history of biomedical research (the "if men were the ones who got pregnant" position) to the very real fact that only one ovum is produced per month, whereas hundreds of millions of sperm cells are present in every ejaculation. The reasons, whatever they may be, are too complex for our discussion here. However, some promising new male contraceptive technologies are currently in various experimental stages (Schulman, 2000; Thompson, 2004). A brief list of what may be on the horizon follows.

Vas Injection Techniques

If you were to interfere with the sperm during ejaculation as they move from the epididymis up the vas deferens—perhaps block or change them in some way so they are unable to reach or fertilize an ovum—this would be a male contraceptive. A technique is currently under investigation to do just that. One is called RISUG, for *reversible inhibition of sperm under guidance*. Here a plastic-like compound is injected into each vas deferens using a very tiny needle and a local anesthetic (Guha, 2005; "RISUG", 2003.) The injected compound doesn't completely block the tubes, but as sperm pass through the material, it changes the acidity and electrical charge of the sperm cells, rendering them incapable of fertilization. The compound can later be dissolved with the injection of another agent that clears the vasa, allowing fertility to return. Preliminary research findings have demonstrated that this is a highly effective, reversible, nonhormonal contraceptive for men, and it was in clinical trials in India as of 2004 (Thompson, 2004).

Vas Occlusion Techniques

Studies are under way on several methods to occlude or plug the vasa deferentia. The plugs are made of polyurethane or silicone rubber and are either injected or inserted through small punctures in the scrotum. Again, the procedures are minimally invasive, performed under local anesthetic without an incision. (Schulman, 2000; Thompson, 2004). When and if the plugs are removed (an equally simple procedure), fertility should return.

Nifedipine

Nifedipine is one of a class of high blood pressure medications called calcium channel blockers. It is also widely prescribed for migraine headaches. By accident, an invitro fertilization (IVF) specialist noticed that among her couples, if the man happened to be taking nifedipine, none of the wives' eggs became fertilized during the IVF process. With further research of this curious finding, it appears that the drug may interfere with the calcium in the heads of sperm cells that enables them to dissolve the outer membrane of the ovum for fertilization (K. Johnson, 2000b; Travis, 2001). This research is in the early stages, but researchers are optimistic that a new direction in male contraception has been found. Nifedipine appears to have no negative side effects on men without hypertension. Reversal to fertility would simply require discontinuation of the medication.

A Male Hormonal Contraceptive?

A hormonal contraceptive for men is under investigation in many countries worldwide and began human clinical trials in late 2003. When such a contraceptive reaches the market, it will probably be in the form of an injection, an implant, a patch, or perhaps a combination of these delivery systems. As with the female hormonal methods, the goal is to alter male hormones so that sperm production decreases to the point of infertility. If a man has a sperm count of fewer than 20 million sperm per millimeter of semen, he's considered unlikely to be fertile (the average number is around 100 million per millimeter).

In early 2004, two pharmaceutical companies conducted clinical trials of a combination implant-injection in 14 research locales throughout Europe. The effectiveness and acceptability estimates of these trials appeared hopeful ("Large Clinical Trial," 2004). A great deal of study remains to be done, so you probably should not head to your corner pharmacy quite yet. But many researchers are predicting that a male hormonal method of birth control could become widely available by the end of this decade (Formichelli, 2001, Liu et al., 2006).

Immunocontraceptives

Imagine an injection that could vaccinate a man against fertility! Researchers are looking into once-a-year vaccines that may cause a man's immune system to develop antibodies against a specific hormone (FSH) necessary for sperm cells to mature. When the hormone molecules are destroyed, sperm are inactivated. The vaccine would eventually wear off, allowing fertility to return when and if desired (Schulman, 2000). Most of the immunocontraceptive research is being carried out for nonhuman animal population control (Fraker et al., 2002), but this method of birth control for humans is beginning to receive increased research and development attention (Anderson & Walton, 2005; "Human Immunocontraceptive Vaccine," 2000).

Future Methods for Women

As you have seen in this chapter, many advancements in contraception for women have occurred in the past decade. Women now have more choices of effective contraception than ever in history. The need today is for more methods that allow a woman to be in complete control of *both* her fertility and her degree of protection from STIs. Currently, only two methods offer her this level of control: the female condom and abstinence, neither of which is an overwhelmingly popular choice for most women. Clearly, a greater selection of nonhormonal, hassle-free methods would be welcome. To these ends, some exciting new female contraceptive research directions are emerging.

Antimicrobial Gels

A new gel that combines vaginal spermicide and microbicide (germ killer) began clinical trials in early 2002. It is designed to stop sperm dead in their tracks *and* block most of the pathogens that cause sexually transmitted infections such as HIV, genital herpes, gonorrhea, and syphilis. The effectiveness of BufferGel on both counts has been demonstrated in animals and was being tested on 1,000 human volunteers (Saltmarsh, 2001; "Two Trials," 2002). According to Dr. Richard Cone, professor of biophysics at John Hopkins University and director of the current research on BufferGel:

> "Not only must the compound kill both sperm and germs, it must do so without hurting the friendly bacteria in a healthy vagina, like the lactobacilli," he explains. "Also, it mustn't smell bad or taste bad. . . . And most importantly, it mustn't irritate sensitive vaginal tissues. BufferGel has met those standards both in animal trials and in extensive clinical safety trials." (Purdy, 2002).

Researchers are optimistic that microbicides such as BufferGel have the potential to provide a novel and effective method for reducing the risk of pregnancy and STIs. However, as for most new medications, the research and approval processes move slowly and the marketing of these products may be several years away (Dhawan & Mayer, 2006).

CatSper

In late 2001, researchers at Howard Hughes Medical Institute announced that they had discovered that something called an "ion channel protein," dubbed CatSper (short for "cation channel of sperm"), controls the flow of calcium to the tails of sperm cells (Quill, Sugden, Rossi, Doolittle, Hammer, & Garbers, 2003; Ren et al., 2001; Toma, 2001). This finding is similar to the news about nifedipine, mentioned earlier in our discussion of new male methods, but here a medication that blocks CatSper would render sperm unable to swim, leaving them incapable of reaching the ovum, thus preventing fertilization. Researchers suggest that the medication, in pill form, could be taken by a woman on a very short-term, as-needed basis, such as just before or even just after intercourse (Carlson et al., 2003). Moreover, early research suggests that drugs that block CatSper affect *only* sperm cells and appear to have virtually no negative effects on any other physiological systems, so virtually all the potential side effects associated with hormonal contraceptives might be avoided (Toma, 2001). Like the other new and experimental contraceptive developments mentioned here, CatSper blockers are not right around the corner. All the research so far has been on nonhuman animals.

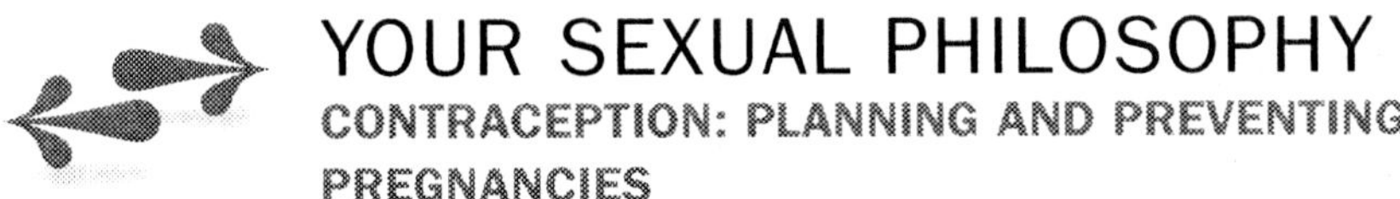

YOUR SEXUAL PHILOSOPHY

CONTRACEPTION: PLANNING AND PREVENTING PREGNANCIES

Over the past fifteen years, contraception research has exploded with innovative, simpler, and more effective methods of birth control. Never before have individuals and couples who wish to prevent pregnancy or engage in effective family planning had so many options. And we may be at the beginning of a rising research and development wave. If issues of birth control and contraception concern you, someone you care about, or someone who may rely on your counsel in such matters, consider it your personal goal to stay up-to-date and informed about existing, new, and upcoming methods of controlling fertility. Make use of the many online resources you can find at this book's Web site (*http://www.prenhall.com/hock*). This is a field of knowledge in which making informed, safe choices is crucial to everyone's sexual lives.

Deciding on a birth control method that is best and most comfortable for you is one of the fundamental components of your sexual philosophy. As mentioned at the outset of this chapter, if your choices about sexual behavior ever include heterosexual intercourse, that choice, by definition, includes the possibility of conception and pregnancy. If you carefully consider your contraception options now, based on all the available information from this chapter and other reliable sources, you will be able to make educated decisions about having a child or preventing an unwanted pregnancy. Regardless of your pregnancy plans, consider the importance of protecting yourself from sexually transmitted infections. This is equally important for men *and* women. If your decisions about birth control are based on a solid foundation of knowledge that is a part of your personal sexual philosophy, you can avoid the uncomfortable and risky position of trying to make the right choices about contraception and STI protection when you are unprepared or when your judgment may be clouded by the sexually charged events of an intimate sexual moment. Remember, your sexual philosophy is about knowing who you are, what you want or don't want, and planning ahead so that you can be in control of your sexuality rather than allowing it to control you.

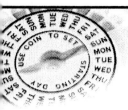

Summary

HISTORICAL PERSPECTIVES The Politics of Contraception

- Margaret Sanger led the birth control revolution in the early years of the twentieth century. It was largely through her efforts discussing birth control with health care providers that contraception for women became legal in the United States. Sanger believed that women could never achieve equal rights with men unless they were able to control their own reproductive bodies.

Choosing a Method of Contraception

- When choosing birth control, both sexual lifestyle and the various pros and cons of the available methods must be considered. This important decision may be made by an individual or is often a shared decision by a couple who are becoming involved in an intimate relationship.

Methods for Preventing Pregnancy and STIs

- Only two methods, abstinence (sometimes called "outercourse") and condoms (both male and female), are effective in helping prevent both pregnancy and STIs.

Methods for Preventing Pregnancy (but *Not* STIs)

- Hormonal methods for preventing pregnancy include the birth control pill, implants, the contraceptive patch, injections, and the vaginal ring. Differences among these methods are primarily in how the hormones are delivered to the woman's body. All hormonal contraceptives are highly effective in preventing pregnancy. However, they are not without some negative side effects. Having a clear understanding of the pros, cons, and cautions of hormonal contraceptives is important in deciding whether or not to use them.
- Vaginal barrier methods of contraception include the diaphragm, cervical caps, Lea's Shield, and spermicides; all are effective forms of contraception, but they have somewhat higher failure rates than some other methods.
- Fertility awareness methods of contraception may be effective for some couples. However, predicting ovulation accurately may be difficult for some women and requires very careful planning. Techniques for predicting ovulation include the calendar (rhythm) method, cervical mucus method, basal body temperature method, and symptothermal method. Ovulation prediction kits are now available that aid significantly in the timing of intercourse relative to ovulation so as to reduce (or enhance) the possibility of pregnancy.
- After early problems, the intrauterine device (IUD) is now back on the U.S. market. The IUD appears to be quite safe and offers an additional effective means of contraception for many women.
- Voluntary surgical contraception (VSC), commonly referred to as *sterilization*, is a popular permanent form of birth control. Methods include tubal ligation or tubectomy for women and vasectomy for men. Vasectomy is usually considered safer and less expensive than female tubal procedures and results in faster recovery time.
- Emergency contraception pills, now available over the counter in most states, allow a woman who has had unprotected intercourse within the past three to five days to significantly reduce her chances of conception.

Avoiding Abortion as Birth Control

- People on both sides of the abortion debate generally agree that relying on abortion as a method of birth control is inappropriate.
- Greater availability and proper use of contraception significantly reduces the need for and number of abortions.

Experimental and Future Methods of Birth Control

- Some of the new methods that may eventually reach the market include vas injections and blocking techniques, calcium channel blockers that disable sperm cells, combination vaginal spermicide-microbicides that help prevent pregnancy and STIs, immunocontraceptives that cause the immune system to destroy sperm cells, and a male hormonal contraceptive.

YOUR SEXUAL PHILOSOPHY: Contraception: Planning and Preventing Pregnancies

- Your decisions about birth control should be based on a foundation of accurate and complete information that are a part of your personal sexual philosophy. With this knowledge you will be prepared to make choices about contraception and safe sex practices with forethought and planning.

Have You Considered?

1. What would you do if contraception were illegal, as it was less than 100 years ago in this country and still is in others? Would you defy the law and obtain contraceptives on the black market? What other actions might you take?
2. Would you ever consider voluntary surgical sterilization as your birth control method of choice? Why or why not?
3. Imagine that you are the parent of a 19-year-old daughter who is home from college for a holiday weekend. You've always had a close relationship with her, so she comes to you explaining that she has met the man of her dreams and would like your advice about birth control. What would you want to be sure to tell her? What if your college student were a son? Would your advice to him be different? If so, in what ways? If not, why not?
4. Suppose that a heterosexual couple who have been in an intimate, loving relationship for nearly a year decide to go camping together. They're sitting by the fire under the stars feeling very romantic and sexually excited. Suddenly they realize they forgot to put the condoms in the backpack! Discuss how they might best deal with this situation.
5. Imagine a situation in which you truly want to make love, but it is extremely important to you to use condoms. However, your partner doesn't want to use them. Discuss at least three strategies you might employ to resolve this disagreement.

Companion Website Resources

For further chapter resources go to **www.prenhall.com/hock**. This robust text website includes polling questions for you to vote on, regular news updates, quizzes, sample tests, suggested reading lists, and more.

SCENARIOS USA Also on the website are links to videos. *Scenarios USA's* films portray real-life narratives that explore the non-biological aspects of relationships and sexual health. The films will help you consider how the themes of the text affect your own life and the lives of those around you.

6

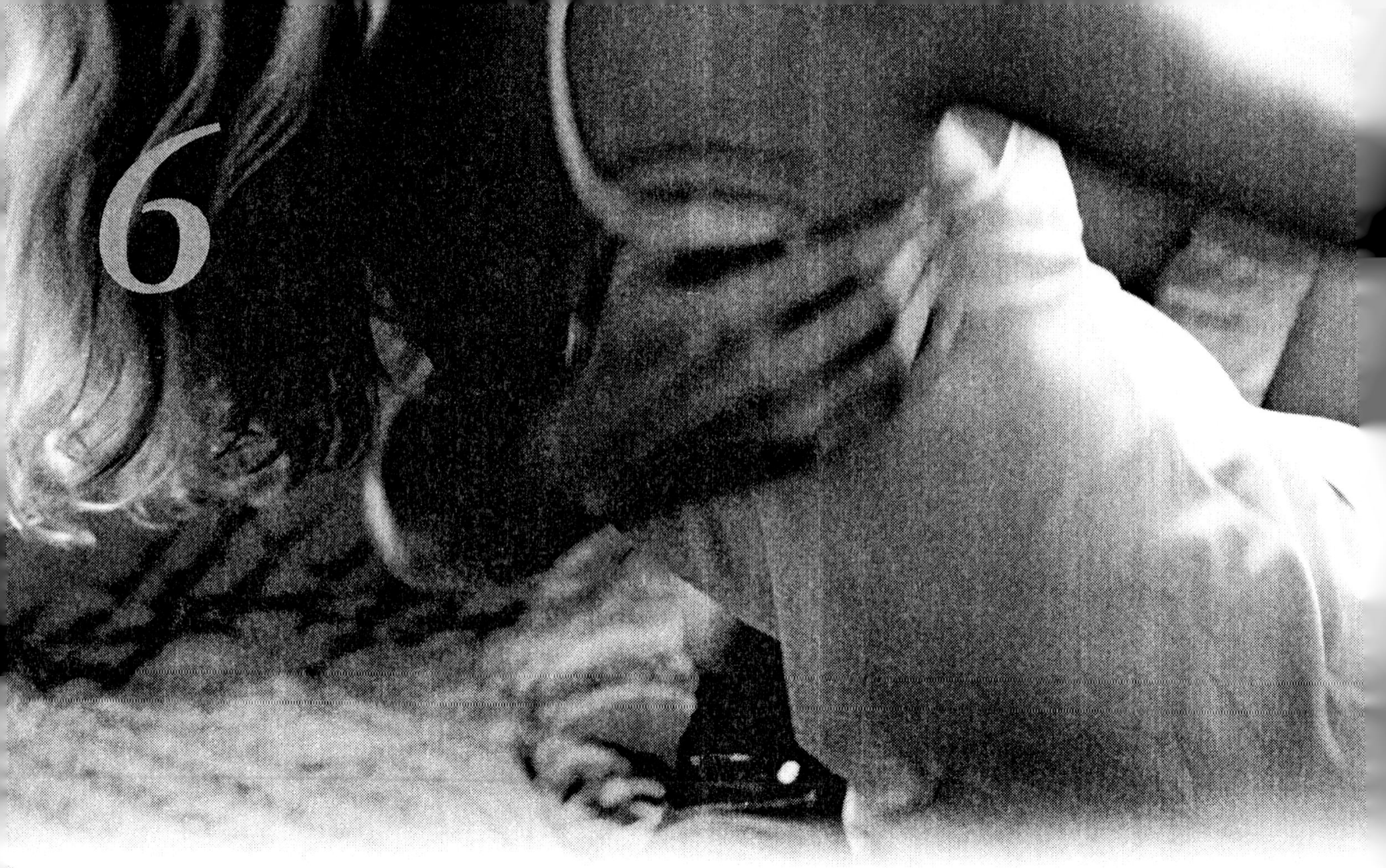

Sexual Behaviors

Experiencing Sexual Pleasure

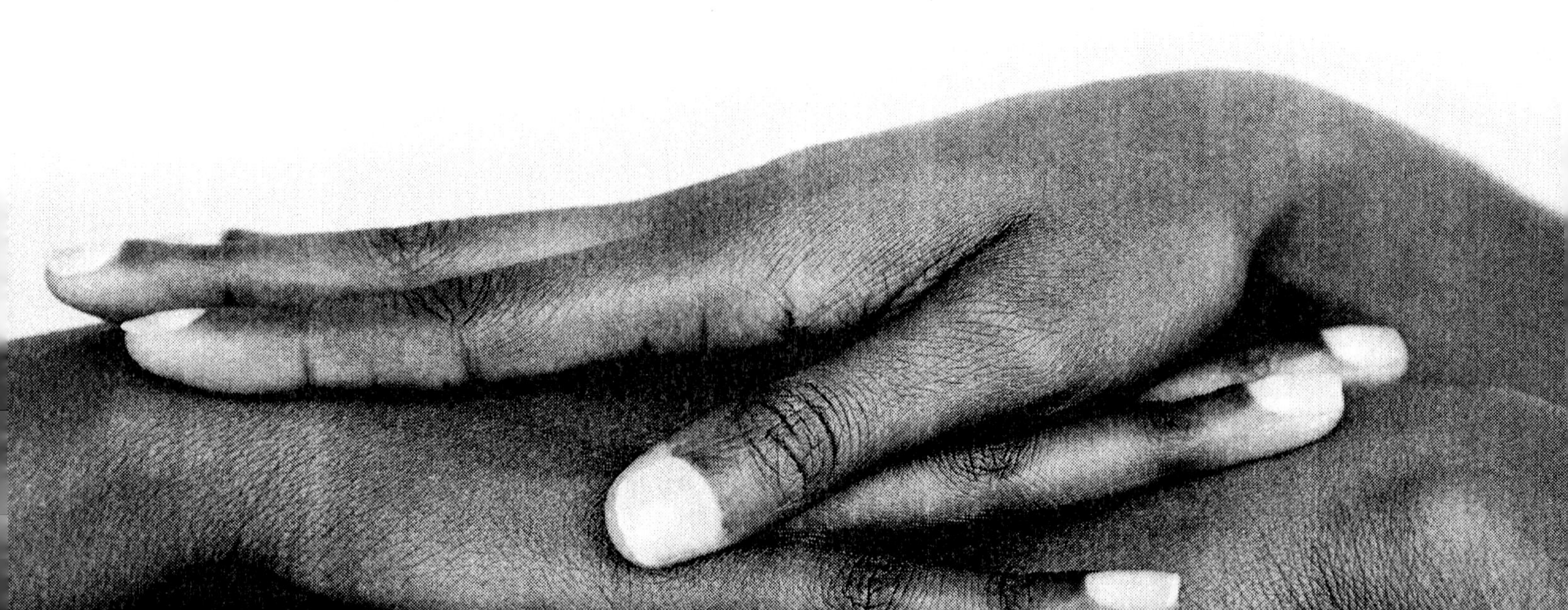

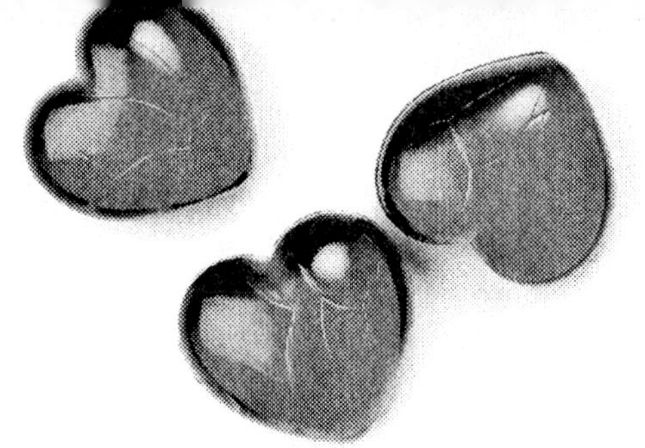

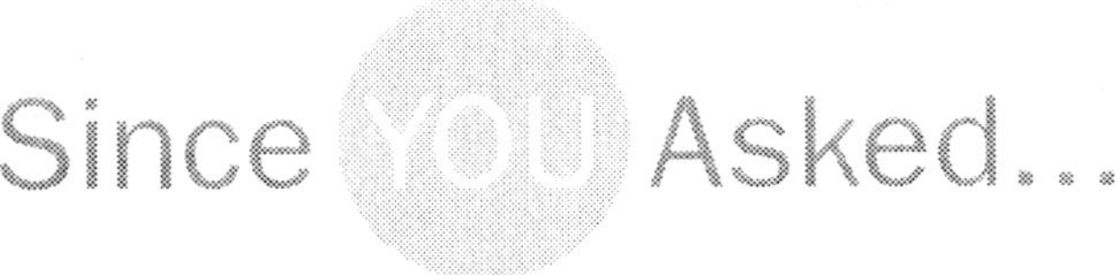

1. Why do people have sexual fantasies? (see page 196)

2. Some of my sexual fantasies involve things I would never really do, so why do I feel guilty just thinking about them? (see page 197)

3. If you are feeling sexually frustrated, how can you satisfy your sexual needs? (see page 204)

4. Does masturbation detract from one's sexual drive or pleasure? (see page 205)

5. I believe that foreplay is the best part of sex. Is that strange? (see page 212)

6. Do women get more pleasure from intercourse or oral sex? How and why? (see page 214)

7. My boyfriend says it's OK if we have oral sex because it doesn't spread sexual diseases. Is that true? (see page 215)

8. What is the best position for intercourse? (see page 217)

9. Is it abnormal to have intercourse four or five times a day with a partner whom you have been seeing for a long time? (see page 220)

10. Is there anything wrong with anal sex? (see page 222)

Being sexually intimate with the right person at the right time is one of the most physically and emotionally satisfying experiences in life. Approaching sexual activities responsibly—with accurate knowledge, mutual respect, and care—can enhance a person's self-esteem and happiness in general (McCabe & Cummins, 1998). Conversely, engaging in sexual acts irresponsibly—for example, at too young an age, when a person does not feel ready, or when care and respect between the partners are lacking—can lead to regret, guilt, and decreased self-esteem (Starks & Morrison, 1996; Wight et al., 2000).

That said, who decides when and with whom you are going to be sexual? You should, of course. You should be in charge of your body and what you do with it sexually. Unfortunately, some individuals have had sexually related experiences in the past, such as child sexual abuse or rape, that have taken that control over their body away from them through no fault of their own. This does not mean that they do not or cannot reclaim that control and take steps to prevent such painful events from ever happening again to them or to the people they care about.

In this chapter, we will explore what might be referred to as mainstream sexual behaviors: activities that are engaged in and enjoyed by a large percentage of couples and individuals. These include sexual fantasy, masturbation, touching and kissing, oral-genital sexual activities, sexual intercourse (coitus), and anal sexual activities. All of these activities (with the exception of coitus, which is, by definition a heterosexual behavior) can be engaged in by couples of all sexual orientations, whether straight, gay, lesbian, or bisexual. Although more research has been conducted pertaining to heterosexual sexual activities, most of our discussion here assumes that the readers may be of any sexual orientation. Furthermore, issues specifically pertaining to nonheterosexual orientations are the focus of Chapter 11, "Sexual Orientation." The goal of this chapter is to inform you about the variety of sexual activities so that you can make educated and responsible choices that are comfortable for you, whatever your sexual orientation, about your behavior now and in the future.

It's no accident that this chapter appears at this point in the book. Earlier chapters have discussed sexual anatomy, sexual responding, emotional intimacy in relationships, and contraception. These discussions have given you a foundation of knowledge for making your best personal choices about the behaviors you choose for yourself.

One last point for you to keep in mind as you begin this chapter: People's knowledge and experience of sexual activities varies greatly, due to our wide diversity of family background, cultural heritage, religion, past relationships, childhood events, sexual orientation, personal interest, and previous study or education. Although social norms in college often assume that everyone is

Focus on Your Feelings

The idea of sexual intimacy may produce a wide range of emotional responses. Usually, these emotions are positive and pleasurable; you may feel excitement or happiness, desire or contentment. Some of you, however, may experience negative emotions associated with sexual behavior; you may feel embarrassed, anxious, fearful, or even repulsed. These negative emotions can interfere with your enjoyment of intimacy and create barriers to fulfilling sexual experiences. However, when individuals and couples who are experiencing unpleasant feelings about sex come to understand the source of their emotions, they often discover ways of overcoming them. Your *emotional* responses to sex are primarily learned. They are the product of your sexual and relationship experiences throughout your life. If you have suffered from negative or traumatic sexual experiences in your past, current or future sexual behavior may become associated with those earlier events. Even though your *rational* self knows that this current situation, this partner, this current sexual experience may be far different from the negative events in your past, your *emotional* self may involuntarily react negatively. Psychologically speaking, present sexual cues tend to reactivate your emotional past.

Although no one can change the past, people can take steps to reduce the present emotional effects of a past negative sexual event. Often a caring, trusting relationship with a partner who is willing to be patient and understanding can allow a person to move beyond negative sexual associations from the past. Approaching sexual intimacy slowly, without demands or expectations, can help a partner feel safe, more in control, and less fearful. Sometimes, however, past events exert such a strong influence that the person may require more focused help through counseling with a trained professional therapist. Therapy for these kinds of emotional-sexual problems is extremely effective and nearly always successful in helping individuals overcome their sexual fears and find the intimacy they desire. If you feel that negative emotions are preventing you from enjoying a gratifying sexual life, counseling is usually available through your college or university health or counseling services, public and private counseling agencies, and therapists in private practice.

sexually knowledgeable, significant differences in that knowledge exist, and respecting those differences in each other is extremely important. As mentioned in the Preface of this book, whether you feel you know a little or a lot about sex, what you know will grow and change as you read and think about the issues in this chapter and throughout this book.

Although sexual activities themselves have not changed much throughout history, cultural attitudes toward them have undergone and are undergoing substantial social changes. Many sexual activities that were considered immoral, illegal, unhealthful, and evil less than a century ago are now commonly practiced, openly discussed, and even recommended by health professionals and therapists. Probably no better example exists of these social and cultural changes than the history of masturbation. Let's take a brief look back at how the act of "self-pleasuring" was regarded by some a mere 100 years ago.

Historical Perspectives

Masturbation Will Be the Death of You . . .

Few areas in Western cultural beliefs have changed as radically or as quickly as our attitudes about sexual behavior. Take one example, the M-word, *masturbation.* Although for many people, this is still an embarrassing and highly personal topic, consider the following excerpts from *Sexology*, a book by William H. Walling, published in 1904. The first quote is taken from the chapter titled "Masturbation, Male."

> Perhaps the most constant and invariable, as well as earliest signs of the masturbator are the downcast, averted glance, and the disposition of solitude. Prominent characteristics are loss of memory and intelligence, morose disposition, indifference to legitimate pleasures and sports, and stupid stolidity. The masturbator gradually loses his moral faculties; he becomes listless, incapable of all intellectual exertion; he is taken by surprise if required simply to reply to a child's question. (pp. 38–39)

You can see from this quote how extreme some professionals' views were in the early 1900s concerning the practice of masturbation among boys and men. However, their condemnation of the activity reached an even more fevered pitch when such behavior was suspected in women. Here's what Walling had to say in his chapter titled "Masturbation, Female":

> Alas that such a term is possible! O, that it were as infrequent as it is monstrous, and that no stern necessity compelled us to make the startling disclosures which this chapter must contain! We beseech, in advance, that every young creature, if she yet be pure and innocent, will at least pass over this chapter, that she may not know the depths of degradation into which it is possible to fall.
>
> The symptoms which enable you to recognize or suspect this crime [of masturbation] are the following: A general condition of weakness and loss of flesh; the absence of freshness and beauty; of color from the complexion; of the vermillion from the lips; and whiteness from the teeth; which are replaced by a pale, lean, puffy, flabby, livid physiognomy; . . . bluish circles around the eyes, dry cough, panting on the least exertion. (pp. 42, 46)

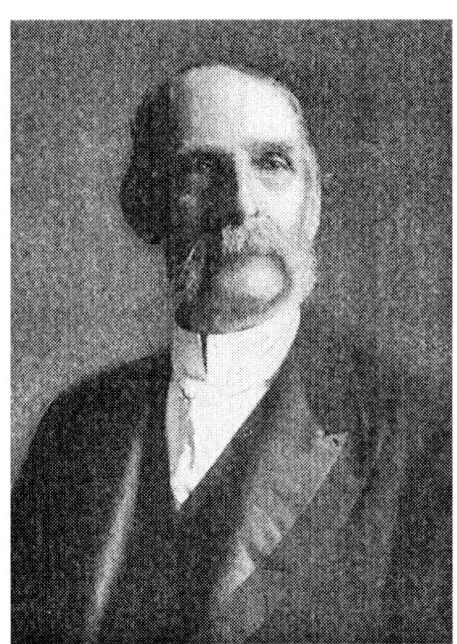
Dr. William H. Walling

For both male and female masturbation, Walling warned that left unchecked, masturbation would lead to sickness, wasting, and eventually death.

We will discuss today's prevailing views about masturbation in more detail in this chapter. The point of these quotes is to demonstrate the extent to which times have changed. Slightly more than a century after the publication of Walling's *Sexology*, masturbation has become a widely accepted sexual activity. As you will read, masturbation is today one of the key components of sex therapy and sexual satisfaction, and it has even been included in the plot lines of numerous television dramas and sitcoms. This does not imply that everyone masturbates or that everyone should. Masturbation, like all other sexual activities, is an individual choice. And for people to make those choices, they need to be as aware as possible of what sexual activities and sexual situations make them feel comfortable. Each person has his or her ideal "sexual comfort zone."

Your Sexual Comfort Zone

The extent to which you experience positive or negative reactions to sexual issues and behaviors determines what may be called your *sexual comfort zone*. People with wide sexual comfort zones are able to respond to various sexual topics and behaviors with relative ease and positive feelings. Those with narrower comfort zones are more likely to approach such issues with hesitation, negative emotions, and even fear.

Erotophobia-Erotophilia

How would you describe *your* sexual comfort zone? In the 1980s, a group of researchers developed the Sexual Opinion Survey (SOS) to measure and study people's reactions to sexual issues and behaviors (Fisher, 1988; Fisher et al., 1988). This scale measures people's place on a scale or continuum the researchers called **erotophobia-erotophilia**. *Erotophobic* individuals have narrow sexual comfort zones, respond negatively and uncomfortably to sexual cues, and may tend to avoid sexual information and activities. *Erotophilic* individuals feel more comfortable with sexual issues, seek out sexual information, enjoy sexual behavior, and respond with positive emotions to sexual cues. "Self-Discovery: Finding Your Sexual Comfort Zone" presents a modified version of the 21 items on the SOS, along with instructions for determining your sexual comfort zone. If you are curious, take a few minutes to answer all the questions and calculate your score. Be honest. There are no right or wrong answers, and no one will see your score but you. By the way, if you are in a relationship, you may want to write your answers on a separate sheet of paper so that your partner can take the survey, too, if he or she wishes.

Why Your SOS Score Is Important

Scores on the SOS have been linked to numerous sexual behaviors. Whether you score high (more erotophilic) or low (more erotophobic) or somewhere in the middle, you should understand what your score may predict about your sexual attitudes and choices. Table 6.1 summarizes some of the differences among people who score higher and lower on the SOS.

The measurement of erotophobia-erotophilia is not intended to place value judgments on people according to their score. Nevertheless, a high score on erotophilia may carry with it some potentially negative consequences. As you can see in Table 6.1, erotophobic individuals are uncomfortable about sexual issues and topics in general, so they are less likely to take precautions against sexually transmitted diseases, use birth control, or seek medical attention for sexual health problems. In addition, they tend to avoid opportunities to become more educated and thus less uneasy about sexuality. For these reasons, a person's score on the SOS can serve as a gauge of how emotionally and psychologically ready the person is to be involved in sexually intimate relationships.

erotophobia An attitude toward sexuality in which individuals are generally uncomfortable with sexual topics, respond negatively and uncomfortably to sexual issues, and tend to avoid sexual information and activities.

erotophilia An attitude toward sexuality in which individuals are comfortable with sexual issues, seek out sexual information, enjoy sexual behavior, and respond with positive reactions to sexual topics.

Sources of Your SOS Score

Your sexual feelings and attitudes develop throughout your life and are reflected, at least in part, in your SOS score. Humans are probably not born preprogrammed with any of these specific attitudes. Rather, you acquire them from your experiences and interactions with others (parents, mainly) as you move through childhood and adolescence into

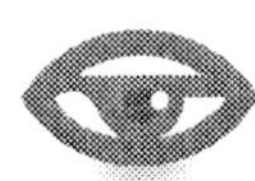

Self-Discovery

Finding Your Sexual Comfort Zone

Respond to each item as honestly as you can. There are no right or wrong answers, and no one but you need ever see your score. Use the following response key for your answers:

1 = I strongly agree 2 = I agree 3 = I somewhat agree 4 = I neither agree nor disagree
5 = I somewhat disagree 6 = I disagree 7 = I strongly disagree

(Note: This questionnaire was designed for individuals with a heterosexual orientation. Those with nonheterosexual orientations should make appropriate changes in the wording of some of the items.)

____ **1.** Erotica (sexually explicit books, movies, and other materials) is filthy, and people should not try to describe it as anything else.

____ **2.** If I found out that a close friend of mine was gay or lesbian, it would annoy me.

____ **3.** If people thought I was interested in oral sex, I would be embarrassed.

____ **4.** Almost all erotic (sexually explicit) material is nauseating.

____ **5.** It would be emotionally upsetting to me to see someone exposing his or her genitals in public.

____ **6.** Watching a stripper of the opposite sex would not be a turn-off.

____ **7.** I would not enjoy seeing an erotic (sexually explicit) movie.

____ **8.** When I think about seeing pictures showing someone of the same sex as myself masturbating, it nauseates me.

____ **9.** I do not enjoy daydreaming about sexual matters.

____ **10.** I am not curious about explicit erotica (sexually explicit books, movies, or other materials).

____ **11.** I think it would be very entertaining to look at erotica (sexually explicit books, movies, and other materials).

____ **12.** Swimming in the nude with a member of the opposite sex would be an exciting experience.

____ **13.** Masturbation can be an exciting experience.

____ **14.** Engaging in group sex is an appealing idea.

____ **15.** Thinking about engaging in sexual intercourse is arousing for me.

____ **16.** Seeing an erotic (sexually explicit) movie would be sexually arousing to me.

____ **17.** Thoughts that I may have homosexual tendencies would not worry me at all.

____ **18.** The idea of my being physically attracted to members of the same sex is not depressing.

____ **19.** The thought of engaging in unusual sex practices is highly arousing.

____ **20.** Touching and caressing my own genitals would probably be an arousing experience.

____ **21.** The thought of having long-term sexual relations with more than one sex partner (during the same time period) is not disgusting to me.

SCORING:

1. Total your ratings for items 1 – 10 = _______
2. Subtract from this number your ratings for items 11 – 21 (the result may be a negative number) minus = _______
3. Add 67 to this number plus 67 = _______
4. Your final score = _______

Your score will be somewhere between 0 (most erotophobic) to 126 (most erotophilic). To get an idea of what your score means, compare it to averages from other groups of heterosexual students from various parts of the world (Fisher, 1988).

Group Studied	Female Average	Male Average
U.S. students	54	72
Canadian students	72	78
Indian students (India)	64	70
Hong Kong students	48	59
Israeli students	59	71

Source: "The Modified Sexual Opinion Survey" from "Erotophobia-Erotophilia as a Dimension of Personality" by W. Fisher et al., in *Journal of Sex Research*, 25, (1988), pp. 123–151.

Table 6.1 EROTOPHOBIA-EROTOPHILIA: EFFECTS ON ATTITUDES AND BEHAVIORS

People who score high or low on the Sexual Opinion Survey (SOS) tend to differ in many ways relative to their sexual attitudes and behaviors. This table summarizes some of the most common differences researchers have found.

TOPIC	EROTOPHOBIC ATTITUDE	EROTOPHILIC ATTITUDE
Traditional sex-role behaviors	Accepting	Flexible
Sexual thoughts and behaviors	Source of guilt	Source of enjoyment
Masturbation	Negative	Positive
Sexual self-concept and attractiveness	Hesitant	Confident
Persons with nonheterosexual orientations	Negative, intolerant	Accepting, tolerant
Development of sexual problems	More likely	Less likely
Sexual health care (doctor visits, self-exams, etc.)	Less attentive	Attentive
Use of measures to prevent sexually transmitted infections	Less likely	More likely
Correct and consistent use of birth control	Less likely	More likely
Learning of sexually relevant materials	Reluctant	Enthusiastic
Sexual discussions between parents and children	Uncomfortable, avoidant	Open, comfortable
Sexual discussions with partner	Uncomfortable, avoidant	Open, comfortable
Engaging in sexual fantasy	Less likely	More likely
Enjoyment of sexual activities	Not great	Great
Breast-feeding in public	Uncomfortable	Comfortable
Accessing sexually explicit Internet sites	Less likely	More likely

Sources: Barak et al. (1999); Byers, Purdon, and Clark (1998); Fisher et al. (1988); Forbes et al. (2003); Garcia (1999).

adulthood. To demonstrate this, researchers asked subjects who had taken the SOS to fill out detailed questionnaires about their childhood and adolescent sexual influences.

Some of the factors found to influence partecipants' development of erotophobia include strict parental attitudes about sex play in childhood, religious training that inhibits free sexual expression, conservative family sexual attitudes, and guilt about masturbation in adolescence. Factors that lead to more erotophilic attitudes in adulthood include having parents who are good sexual educators and who are not embarassed to discuss sex, more frequent masturbation in childhood and adolescence, and a factual understanding of sexual topics in adolescence (Fischer et al., 1988).

If you think about these influences and compare them with your own memories of childhood and adolescence, you may gain some important insights into the sources of your sexual attitudes and feelings and how they relate to your current sexual philosophy. With that in mind, we turn to our discussion of sexual behaviors themselves.

Solitary and Shared Sexual Behaviors

As mentioned earlier, our discussion here is focused on "mainstream" sexual behaviors, relatively common behaviors that are engaged in by a majority or at least a large minority of people and couples. Moreover, these behaviors would not be considered particularly strange or deviant in most Western cultures (nonmainstream behaviors are discussed in Chapter 14, "Paraphilias"). Table 6.2 offers a glimpse of common sexual activities among college students at a major U.S. university. One sexual activity is conspicuously missing from the list in Table 6.2. It is one that many people fail to realize is the most common sexual activity of all and the one that we will discuss first: sexual fantasy.

Table 6.2 SEXUAL EXPERIENCES OF HETEROSEXUAL COLLEGE STUDENTS

Percentage of heterosexual U.S. university students who reported they had engaged in various sexual activities. (A percentage range represents the highest and lowest percentages reported in multiple studies.)

EVER EXPERIENCED	PERCENTAGE OF MALES	PERCENTAGE OF FEMALES	SIGNIFICANT DIFFERENCE
Masturbation	83	71	NO
Deep kissing	94–98	96–98	NO
Kissing sensitive areas (nongenital)	98	93	NO
Naked caressing and embracing	96	92	NO
Stroking or caressing partner's genitals	96–98	93–98	NO
Genitals caressed by partner	94	92	NO
Mutual touching of genitals to orgasm	89	82	NO
Having your genitals orally stimulated	94	89	NO
Oral stimulation of partner's genitals	89–91	89–91	NO
Mutual oral stimulation of genitals	78	83	NO
Sexual intercourse	80–91	80–91	NO
Intercourse, male on top	89	85	NO
Intercourse, female on top	87	84	NO
Intercourse, side by side	85	79	NO
Intercourse, rear-entry	77	79	NO
Having sex that lasts for hours	76	63	NO
Caressing partner's anal area*	61	37	YES
Having anal area caressed	61	50	NO
Anal intercourse	2–22	2–27	NO

* This is the only activity for which the difference between males' and females' responses was found to be statistically significant (greater than chance).

Sources: Hsu et al. (1994); Kelly (2001); von Sadovszky, Keller, & McKinney (2002).

We will follow sexual fantasy with a discussion of masturbation. Fantasy and masturbation are, for the most part, personal and solitary activities. When most people think of "sex," however, they think of interpersonal or *shared* behaviors; these will be the focus of our discussion in the balance of this chapter.

Most shared sexual activities carry some level of risk for contracting and transmitting sexually transmitted infections (STIs). See Table 6.3 for a summary of STI risks associated with different sexual behaviors (and see Chapter 8 for more in depth coverage of STIs). The importance of this point cannot be overemphasized: sexual intimacy can be one of life's most profound and enjoyable experiences if you are comfortable, confident, informed, and safe in the sexual choices you make. Doing everything possible to avoid the risks of STIs must be part of everyone's sexual decisions.

Sexual Fantasy

It has been said that the most sexual organ in the human body is the brain. Fantasizing about sex is generally considered the most common of all sexual activities (Ellis & Symons, 1990; Hicks & Leitenberg, 2001; Kinsey et al., 1953; Laumann et al., 1994; Person et al., 1989). In fact, it is so prevalent among college students that we would

Table 6.3 SEXUALLY TRANSMITTED INFECTION RISK FOR VARIOUS SEXUAL ACTIVITIES

ACTIVITY	RISK OF STI TRANSMISSION WHEN ONE PARTNER IS INFECTED
Sexual fantasy	Safe.
Masturbation (solo)	Safe.
Erotic touching	Safe (slight risk of transmitting herpes).
Genital touching to orgasm (mutual masturbation)	Safe, unless semen or vaginal secretions touch broken skin or mucous membranes. Possible, though unlikely, to transmit HPV (genital warts) or herpes simplex virus.
Cunnilingus (unprotected)*	*Giving partner*: risk of transmitting or contracting genital herpes in mouth area; genital warts in mouth and throat; gonorrhea; syphilis; hepatitis B; chlamydia; small risk of HIV. *Receiving partner*: risk of transmitting or contracting herpes from mouth to genitals; genital warts; gonorrhea; syphilis; hepatitis B; chlamydia; small risk of HIV transmission; may cause candidiasis infection (yeast from mouth to vagina) and possible nonspecific urinary tract infections.
Fellatio (unprotected)*	*Giving partner*: risk of transmitting or contracting genital herpes in mouth area; genital warts in mouth and throat; gonorrhea; syphilis; hepatitis B; chlamydia; very small risk of HIV. *Receiving partner*: risk of transmitting or contracting herpes from mouth to genitals; genital warts; gonorrhea; syphilis; hepatitis B; chlamydia; small risk of HIV transmission.
Coitus (unprotected)*	Risk of contracting and transmitting *all known STIs*. Risk generally greater for female than male.
Anal stimulation	Risk of vaginal, urinary, and reproductive tract infections if normal rectal bacteria are spread from anal area to vagina, vulva, or urethra (men and women). Risk of HIV, hepatitis B, HPV (from genital warts in anal area), chlamydia, and other bacterial risks from oral-anal contact (anilingus).
Anal intercourse (unprotected)*	Highest risk of transmission of HIV. Risk greatest to receiving partner due to semen contacting damaged rectal tissue. May also transmit genital warts, syphilis, chlamydia, and hepatitis B. Risk with condom higher than vaginal intercourse with condom.

* The use of protection such as a male or female condom or dental dam significantly reduces, but does not entirely eliminate, the risk of transmission.

not be surprised if you are doing it right now! One study found that, on average, college men reported having sexual fantasies approximately seven times a day and college women almost five times a day (Jones & Barlow, 1990). Another study found that teenage males report thinking about sex on an average of once every five minutes (Reinisch, 1990). Estimates of the percentage of male and females who have ever engaged in sexual fantasy ranges from 60 to 100 percent, depending on the study, the fantasy context, the subject sample, and the methods used to determine percentages (Cato & Leitenberg, 1990; Laumann et al., 1994; Leitenberg & Henning, 1995; Renaud & Byers, 1999). A review of numerous studies over 30 years places the percentage of people who report sexual fantasies in any context at about 95 percent (Leitenberg & Henning, 1995).

Since YOU Asked...

1. Why do people have sexual fantasies?

Sexual fantasies may arise virtually anytime, anywhere. They may begin spontaneously or through a conscious decision to fantasize about something sexual. They may or may not be accompanied by physiological sexual arousal, and emotionally they may be either positive or negative (Byers, Purdon, & Clark, 1998). Most people report using sexual fantasy as part of masturbation (S. Brody, 2003), and many people fantasize while engaging in sexual interaction with a partner, especially during intercourse (Davidson & Hoffman 1986; Lunde et al., 1991; Sue, 1979). Although some people may think these fantasies indicate a problem with the relationship (as indicated by statements such as "If you need to fantasize when we're together, you must not find me attractive"), research has shown that this is usually not the case. In fact, the vast majority of people (over 70 percent of men and women) have reported having sexual fantasies during sexual activities with a partner (Reinisch, 1990). Moreover, those who fantasize more tend to be better sexually adjusted overall, have fewer sexual problems, and report the greatest overall satisfaction in their sexual relationships (Leitenberg & Henning, 1995; Reinisch, 1990; Renaud & Byers, 2001).

Today, virtually all health professionals and sexuality educators consider sexual fantasy in all its contexts to be a normal and healthy part of a person's sexual life (Cato & Leitenberg, 1990; Janus & Janus, 1993; Leitenberg & Henning, 1995). In fact, as shown in Table 6.4, sexual fantasy has been shown to enhance sexual enjoyment and satisfaction in many different ways, whether with a partner or by oneself.

When Sexual Fantasies May Cause Problems

Sexual fantasies are usually harmless, enjoyable activities; however, under some circumstances, they can be a source of discomfort. Sexual fantasies may cause a problem in the following four ways.

- *The person having the fantasies is psychologically and emotionally troubled by them.* Some people feel that their fantasies are somehow wrong, sinful, or immoral, and this can create a great deal of guilt and worry (Renaud & Byers, 2001). One study found that 25 percent of male and female college students reported feeling guilty about having sexual fantasies during intercourse (Cato & Leitenberg, 1990). Other research has revealed that 84 percent of college students report experiencing intrusive or unpleasant sexual fantasies (Byers et al., 1998). This is not surprising, considering that Western religions typically teach that a sinful *thought* is morally equivalent to actually carrying out the behavior or at least feeling the temptation to do so. Indeed, when conservative Christian

Since YOU Asked...

2. Some of my sexual fantasies involve things I would never really do, so why do I feel guilty just thinking about them?

Table 6.4 POSITIVE FUNCTIONS OF SEXUAL FANTASY

FUNCTION	POSITIVE EFFECTS
Provide a safe sexual outlet	By definition, a fantasy does not involve any physical contact, so there is no danger of pregnancy or STIs. By itself or combined with masturbation, fantasy can provide a completely safe sexual experience.
Enhance arousal	Probably the most common reason people fantasize is to increase and enhance their feelings of sexual excitement. Fantasy in a nonsexual setting has the potential to enhance future sexual encounters, and fantasy during masturbation or lovemaking can strengthen physical and psychological responses.
Relieve boredom	Sex therapists often recommend fantasy to spice up a couple's sex life that has become routine and predictable.
Treat sexual problems	Fantasy (usually combined with masturbation) is a cornerstone of sex therapy. It has been shown to increase sexual desire, arousability, orgasm, and sexual satisfaction in general.
Relieve sexual anxiety, guilt, and doubt	Nearly everyone at one time or another feels anxiety, guilt, or self-doubt about sexual issues. Fantasy offers an opportunity to think about sexual values, to replay sexual scenes, and to learn about one's sexual identity.

Sources: Alfonso, Allison, and Dunn (1992); Byers, Purdon, and Clark (1998); Cato and Leitenberg (1990); Davidson and Hoffman (1986); Leitenberg and Henning (1995); Masters, Johnson, and Kolodny (1995); Reinisch (1990); Renaud and Byers (1999); Striar and Bartlik (1999).

college students were studied, a significantly higher proportion (95 percent) reported substantial guilt related to their sexual fantasies. Interestingly, the same study found that those who felt the greatest guilt about their sexual fantasies also reported higher levels of sexual dissatisfaction and sexual problems in their relationships (Cato & Leitenberg, 1990).

People who feel guilty about having sexual fantasies are less likely to discuss their fantasies with others or to seek information about them. Often when these people discover that fantasizing about sex is a common and healthy activity, their own guilt and uneasiness falls away, and it ceases to be a source of worry.

- *The fantasies become compulsive or addictive.* For a small percentage of people, fantasies can become so dominant in their thinking that they interfere with the activities of daily life. Others may find that they are unable to function sexually or respond to their partner without constant use of a specific sexual fantasy (Janus & Janus, 1993; Reinisch, 1990). An example of this might be the person who must fantasize about a previous lover in order to become aroused with the current partner. Although these are relatively rare occurrences, they can be very disturbing to the person experiencing them. Fortunately, counseling is usually successful in helping these individuals redirect their sexual thoughts in directions that are more acceptable and comfortable for them (Reinisch, 1990).
- *The sexual fantasies are indiscriminately shared with a partner.* Sometimes sharing fantasies (such as thinking of a previous lover) may cause a partner to feel embarrassed, uncomfortable, pressured, or threatened in some way; this can in turn have a negative impact on the relationship (Masters, Johnson, & Kolodny, 1995). Therefore, if sharing of fantasies is to occur in a relationship, couples should do so with great care and sensitivity to each partner's feelings and sexual attitudes. Under some circumstances, sharing fantasies can enhance intimacy and trust between two people and open up new areas for a couple to explore sexually. This positive aspect of fantasy sharing will be discussed shortly.
- *Rarely, sexual fantasies may be associated with antisocial or criminal sexual behavior.* Many people have fantasies of "forbidden" or even illegal sexual acts but would never consider acting on them in real life (Byers et al., 1998). Evidence does exist, however, that some criminal sex offenders (such as child molesters, rapists, and exhibitionists) fantasize about these illegal behaviors and activities more often than nonoffenders (Leitenberg & Henning, 1995), and this is especially true of predatory sex offenders (Deu & Edelmann, 1997). We cannot know for sure if the fantasy led to the criminal behavior or if the behavioral tendencies caused the fantasies, but it is important to be aware that the association exists in this population of sexual offenders.

Sex Differences in the Experience and Content of Sexual Fantasy

If you were to ask around, most people would probably say that men and women differ a lot in how much they think about sex and in the content of their sexual fantasies. But is this common view supported by the available research? Several studies on sexual fantasy have focused on male-female differences, and the results have been mixed. As mentioned earlier, men report having more frequent sexual fantasies overall during the day than women do, and men are more likely than women to fantasize about someone other than their current partner (Hicks & Leitenberg, 2001; Laumann et al., 1994). Most studies have also found that men are more likely than women to have sexual fantasies during masturbation. However, research has not found significant overall differences between the number of men and women who engage in sexual fantasy during intercourse or experience sexual daydreams.

Another area in which male and female differences have been found is in the content of some of their sexual fantasies. For example, while the vast majority of people engage in sexual fantasies about someone other than their current relationship partner, men are more likely to do so (98 percent) than women (80 percent) (Hicks & Leitenberg, 2001). Many sexual fantasy topics appear to be common for women and men. Within very broad and general categories of sexual fantasy (such as "traditional sexual behaviors" or "exploratory sexual behaviors"), research finds little difference between the number of men and women who have experienced fantasies (Rokach, 1990). However, some sex differences do emerge when more specific fantasy content is studied. When students at a large university in the western United States were asked whether they had ever experienced certain specific sexual fantasies, a more precise picture of these differences unfolded (Hsu et al., 1994). Table 6.5 lists some of the *specific* fantasies found to be experienced more often by one sex or the other (usually more often by men) and some that were equally common for men and women.

Looking at specific fantasies in greater detail, several categories emerge that differ significantly between men and women. In an extensive review of the research on sex differences in the content of heterosexuals' fantasies, Leitenberg and Henning (1995) reached the following conclusions:

> Men's fantasies are more active and focus more on the woman's body and on what he wants to do with it, whereas women's fantasies are more passive and focus more on men's interest in their [own] bodies. Men's sexual fantasies also focus on explicit sexual acts, nude bodies, and physical gratification, whereas women use more emotional context and romance in their sexual fantasies. Men are more likely to fantasize about multiple partners and group sex than are women. Finally, women are more likely to have submission

Table 6.5 COMPARING THE CONTENT OF MEN'S AND WOMEN'S SEXUAL FANTASIES

SEXUAL FANTASY CONTENT	MEN EXPERIENCING (%)	WOMEN EXPERIENCING (%)
FANTASIES WITH NO SIGNIFICANT SEX DIFFERENCES		
Touching or kissing sensuously	98	97
Naked caressing	93	92
Sex in unusual locations	89	82
Intercourse in unusual positions	87	82
Masturbating your partner	83	75
Performing sexual acts in a mirror	61	61
Having your partner watch you masturbate	56	53
Being tied up during sex	41	43
FANTASIES WITH STATISTICALLY SIGNIFICANT SEX DIFFERENCES		
Watching your partner undress	98	81
Oral sex	96	84
Sex with a virgin	85	32
Two or more lovers at the same time	76	45
Sex with a mysterious stranger	70	47
Getting married	52	71
Being rescued by a future lover	26	46
Homosexual fantasies if heterosexual or heterosexual fantasies if homosexual	19	33

Source: Adapted from Hsu et al. (1994)

> fantasies, whereas men are more likely to have dominance fantasies, although both types of force fantasies may serve the same purpose: affirming sexual power and irresistibility. Each of these gender differences in fantasy content is consistent with sex role stereotypes and with the different sexual scripts taught to men and women. (p. 484)

Bear in mind that these differences are based on averages and that many people who have sexual fantasies contradict these stereotypes. Furthermore, although we see these differences in sexual *fantasy*, we do not find similar differences in *real-life* sexual experiences (see Table 6.3). The real-life sexual experiences of male and female college students have been found to be essentially the same (Hsu et al., 1994; Person et al., 1989). This brings us to the important discussion of the relationship between fantasy and reality.

Fantasy versus Reality

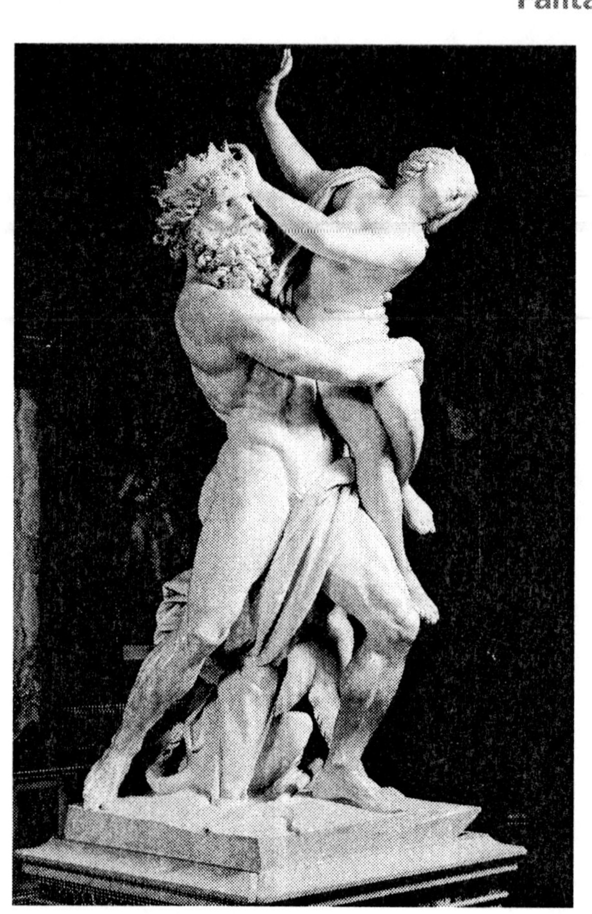

Women's fantasies of forced sex are completely *different from real-life rape.*

Sometimes sexual fantasies are about a sexual situation or activity that the fantasizer has experienced or would like to experience in real life. Some couples will even share their fantasies with each other as a way of expanding their sexual repertoire and enhancing their relationship. However, many people report having sexual fantasies that they would never truly want to experience in real life (Byers et al., 1998; Renaud & Byers, 1999). These fantasies may involve famous people; unusual, "forbidden," or "taboo" sexual activities; or even situations that in reality might be frightening or dangerous. Two-thirds of women and about a third of men who have these fantasies have no desire to act them out (Masters et al., 1995).

One important example of such a fantasy is the forced-sex or "rape fantasy." Some analysts have suggested that a woman who has fantasies of being sexually overpowered has a secret desire to be raped. Nothing could be further from the truth. Although many women do have fantasies of forced sex, the women who have these fantasies are very clear that they have no wish whatsoever to be raped in reality (Kanin, 1982; Reinisch, 1990; Strassberg & Lockerd, 1998). A fantasy of being forced to engage in a sexual act bears no resemblance to the terror, violation, and violence of real sexual aggression. In a woman's fantasy, the woman is completely in charge of the situation; it plays out as more of a seduction than a rape; the "lover" is imagined as a desirable male; she experiences no pain; she suffers no real violence; and she has no reason to fear being injured or killed (Strassberg & Lockerd, 1998). Often in fantasy rapes, the woman actually sees *herself* as the powerful one, so irresistible that the man cannot control himself, and she allows his *illusion* of his dominance to give *her* pleasure (Hariton, 1973; Strassberg & Lockerd, 1998). Obviously, in a real rape, none of this is true. For the victim, real-life rape is entirely about violence, dominance, and humiliation (we will discuss this topic in greater detail in Chapter 13, "Sexual Aggression and Violence: Rape, Child Sexual Abuse, and Harassment").

Clearly, it would be a serious mistake to assume that simply because people have certain sexual fantasies, they want to act them out in real life. On the other hand, are there ways in which sexual fantasies may be shared or be acted out to enhance a couple's sexual life? The answer for most couples is maybe and sometimes yes.

Using Sexual Fantasy to Enhance Your Relationship

One of the most common problems in long-term relationships is boredom and loss of sexual desire. A technique frequently suggested by relationship counselors and sex therapists (and often discovered by couples themselves) is for the couple to share and experiment with each other's sexual fantasies (Striar & Bartlik, 1999). However, many couples are hesitant to share their fantasies out of fear of embarrassment or rejection. In addition, many people have not taken the time to think about exactly which of their sexual fantasies might be exciting to actually try out with their partner. The "Self-Discovery: What Turns *You* On?" offers you the opportunity to analyze your own fantasies and, if you are in a close, trusting relationship, discover whether some of them might add some variety and spice to your sexual life with your partner. This exercise requires a great deal of mutual trust and respect, so approach it carefully, and be sure to read *all* the instructions!

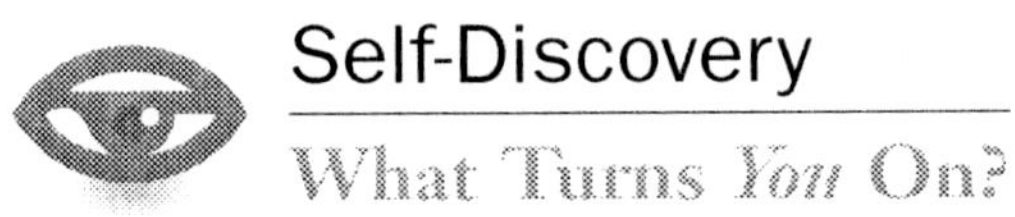

Self-Discovery

What Turns *You* On?

Below is a list of various intimate activities that are the focus of some people's sexual fantasies. To get an idea of your own fantasies, rate each activity, and if you so choose, share your answers with your partner, now or in the future. If you are in a trusting, caring relationship, you may want your partner to complete this exercise as well.

Use the following ratings key to respond to each item on the scale. Be honest with yourself; no one ever has to see your answers but you.

Key

1 = I think I would like this a lot.
2 = I think I would probably like this.
3 = I'm not sure, but I might be willing to try it.
4 = I'm sure I would not like this at all.

Note: this is an intensely personal exercise, so you might want to use a separate sheet of paper for your answers.

Intimate Activity	Your Rating			
	1	2	3	4
1. New or unusual positions for intercourse				
2. For me to initiate lovemaking more often				
3. For my partner to initiate lovemaking more often				
4. A "quickie" once in a while or more often				
5. More touching before intercourse				
6. Lovemaking to last longer				
7. To watch my partner undress				
8. For my partner to watch me undress				
9. More oral stimulation of me				
10. More oral stimulation of my partner				
11. To watch my partner masturbate				
12. For my partner to watch me masturbate				
13. To take showers or baths together				
14. To be touched to orgasm				
15. To touch my partner to orgasm				
16. Some anal stimulation				
17. Anal intercourse				
18. To experiment with sex toys together				
19. To explore erotic materials together (videos, etc.)				

Continued. . .

Intimate Activity	Your Rating			
	1	2	3	4
20. To make love in new and different locations				
21. To make love while bouncing up and down on a trampoline while eating ice cream				
22. To make love in front of a mirror				
23. More sex talk during lovemaking				
24. To make love blindfolded				
25. To wear sexy clothes for lovemaking				
26. To have my partner wear sexy clothes for lovemaking				
27. To make love outdoors				
28. To share sexual fantasies				
Add a few of your own, if you wish:				
29.				
30.				
31.				
32.				

How to evaluate your ratings: There is no overall score on this exercise. The point is to consider how you rate each item individually. You will begin to discover for yourself what fantasies turn you on, which ones you are willing to share with your partner, and which ones you might want to try.

Sharing your answers with your partner: If you are currently in an intimate relationship and both you and your partner have taken the test, you can decide together if you want to share your answers. If you do, remember to be open and nonjudgmental of each other's answers. Some of your answers will match and some probably won't. But you will learn something about each other that may add to your enjoyment of your relationship and shared sexual intimacy.

Masturbation

You may have heard the Woody Allen quote, "Don't knock masturbation. It's sex with someone I love!" A more recent twist on the same theme, though not so catchy, goes something like this: "Masturbation is safe sex with someone whose sexual history I know completely!" ("Politics of Masturbation," 1994).

Masturbation refers to sexual activities performed on oneself, typically focusing on manipulation of the genitals to orgasm. Most people masturbate, yet it remains one of the most secretive, embarrassing, and taboo of all sexual topics of discussion (Halpern et al., 2000; Laqueur, 2004). Why? Because most Western cultures are still feeling the effects of hundreds of years of extremely negative attitudes about masturbation. We will address this history in a moment, but first let's look at a few statistics. Ever since Kinsey's 1940s and 1950s survey data on men and women, researchers have been trying to determine just how many people masturbate. Percentages vary a great deal from study to study, depending on who the subjects were and how they were surveyed. Kinsey's early work found that 92 percent of men and 58 percent of women reported that they had masturbated to orgasm (Kinsey, Pomeroy, & Martin, 1948; Kinsey et al., 1953). A large survey in the 1970s found similar percentages, with 86 percent of men and 60 percent of women reporting masturbating within the past year (Hunt, 1974). The much publicized study on sex in America, the National Health and Social Life Survey, published in the mid-1990s, found that about 60 percent of men and 40 percent of women between the ages of 18 and 60 reported masturbating during the previous year (Laumann et al., 1994).

masturbation Any sexual activity performed on oneself by oneself, typically focusing on manipulation of the genitals to orgasm.

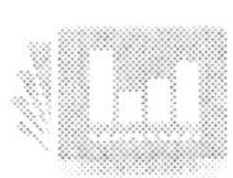

Evaluating Sexual Research

Self-Reporting of Personal Information

Imagine that you've been asked to be part of a sex survey and a researcher comes to your house to interview you and ask you a lot of questions. One line of questioning goes something like this: "Have you ever masturbated to orgasm? When was the last time you masturbated? How often do you masturbate?" How likely is it that you would be completely honest in your answers? What if the same questions were asked in an anonymous, written questionnaire? Might your answers be different? Many people are embarrassed talking about (or even thinking about) sexual topics, and many are especially uncomfortable discussing masturbation (Catania, 1999; Halpern et al., 2000). Their discomfort, guilt, or shame about this or other behaviors may cause them to withhold information or to be less than truthful in their answers, creating bias in the survey's results.

This bias may help explain some of the differences seen in the statistics about masturbation or other behaviors reported in the various studies cited in this chapter. Perhaps students in the Midwest really do masturbate less than students in California or New York, and maybe people in general are masturbating less today than in past decades. But some of these differences across studies could also be due to higher levels of guilt or embarrassment among midwestern or New England students, leading to a greater hesitancy to report that they have masturbated or to underreport how often they do so. In the case of a well-known 1990s survey, *The Social Organization of Sexuality: Sexual Practices in the United States* (Laumann et al., 1994), researchers actually went to people's homes for interviews, and in some cases it was reported that spouses and children of the respondents were also present at the time. You can see how this situation might lead to less than truthful responses given to the interviewers to sensitive questions about behaviors such as masturbation (Catania, 1999; Reiss, 1995). This is not to say that the researcher's findings in this survey or in any survey are wrong. The point is that the statistics reported in this survey and in all surveys of sexual behavior do not tell us how many people masturbate or engage in any other sexual activity but only how many are *willing to report* that they do.

Several recent surveys of college students have found conflicting results. One survey of students at a university in New York City found that 85 percent of females and 95 percent of males reported masturbating (Person et al., 1989). Another survey conducted at a Southern California university found rates of 71 percent for women and 83 percent for men (Hsu et al., 1994). Moving away from coastal and urban settings, however, a survey of students at the University of Kansas found that only 42 percent of women and 73 percent of men reported masturbating (Reinholtz & Muehlenhard, 1995), and another survey at a university in Vermont found the percentages to be 45 percent for women and 81 percent for men (Leitenberg, Detzer, & Srebnik, 1993). How would you account for the discrepancies in all these findings? Think about this for a moment and then read "Evaluating Sexual Research: Self-Reporting of Personal Information."

Centuries ago, people believed that masturbation would lead to various forms of mental illness, including a condition known as "masturbatory hysteria."

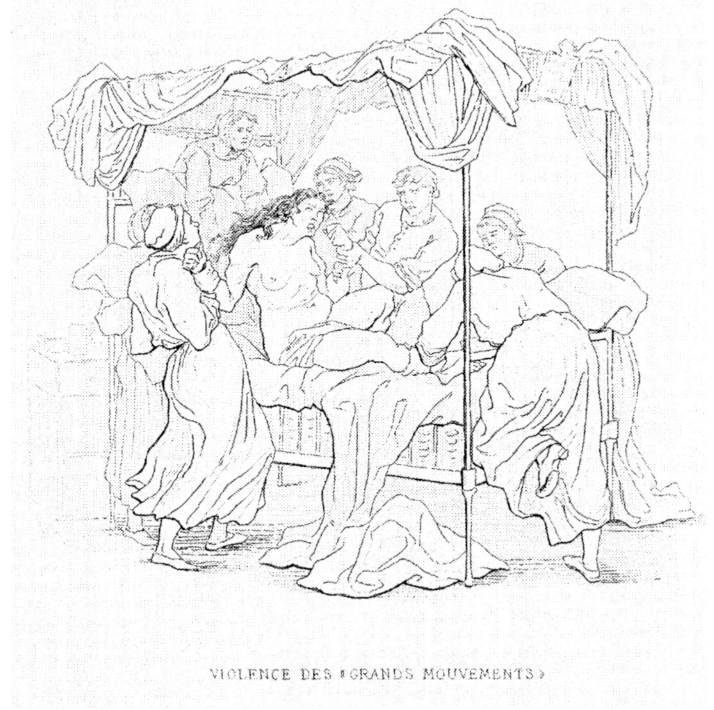

Changing Attitudes about Masturbation

Few, if any, human sexual behaviors have a history of such terrible press as masturbation has had, as demonstrated by the quotes from William Walling at the beginning of this chapter. But times have changed, right? When discussing masturbation, the answer to that question is yes and no. Few people believe today, as many did a century ago, that masturbation will lead to hairy palms, genital cancer, blindness, insanity, hysteria, sterility, impotence, asthma, reduction or increase in penis size, loss of future enjoyment of sex with a partner, or instant death from too much sexual excitement (Flanagan, 1990; "The 'M' Word," 1995). And fewer people still would buy the notion suggested by J. H. Kellogg in 1888 that masturbation can be prevented by eating plain, whole-grain foods such as cornflakes (Michael et al., 1994).

Nevertheless, negative views and taboos concerning masturbation can still be found in far more recent events. It was not until 1972 that the American Medical Association declared masturbation to be a normal sexual behavior. Furthermore, even though most people consider masturbation to be a natural part of life (Dodson, 2002; Janus & Janus, 1993), a significant percentage of adults (14 to 47 percent) feel guilty about masturbating (Dodson, 2002; Michael et al., 1994). As recently as 2003, a "Doonesbury" cartoon strip that made reference to the medical news that masturbation may have a preventive effect on prostate cancer was pulled from 300 newspapers in the United States because it was considered offensive and in poor taste (Evans, 2003).

Perhaps the most telling example in recent history of ongoing negative attitudes about masturbation occurred in 1994 when U.S. Surgeon General Joycelyn Elders was addressing a UN delegation on the spread of sexually transmitted diseases. Following her talk, a member of the audience asked if she would consider promoting masturbation as a way of discouraging children from trying riskier forms of sexual behavior. Elders replied, "With regard to masturbation, I think that is something that is part of human sexuality and part of something that should perhaps be taught" (Popkin, 1994). The storm of controversy that her comment set off was so intense that President Bill Clinton, who had appointed her 15 months earlier, reluctantly had to dismiss her from her position. Apparently, the notion of teaching young people about masturbation was still too radical to receive "official" support in American society. Since that time, no U.S. surgeon general has discussed the topic of masturbation. Elders went on to write her autobiography and is coauthor of a book about the value of a comprehensive sex education, including information about masturbation, titled *Harmful to Minors: The Perils of Protecting Children from Sex* (Levine & Elders, 2002).

In spite of all the negative attitudes and news about masturbation, an increasing amount of evidence suggests that America and many other countries are beginning to recognize its many beneficial aspects, and acceptance of the practice is growing. In 1999, even the Catholic church, while continuing to declare masturbation wrong, no longer deemed it a sin (Sked, 1999). These cultural changes can also be seen in writings from some of the more liberal popular press publications, such as the following example:

> Recent signals point toward a veritable Age of Masturbation. In the shadow of AIDS, and in the spirit of self-exploration, many people are choosing to [masturbate] as a means of sexual expression. Despite the fact that conservatives are equating sex with everything bad—including, but not limited to, death—a new sexual vanguard is touting fresh and exciting ways to enjoy your body. Masturbation could turn out to be the disco of the 90s. (Brooks, 1992, p. 24)

Indeed, considering the masturbation statistics given earlier in this discussion, this quote appears to have been remarkably prophetic. Furthermore, beyond these changing popular beliefs and attitudes, sexuality researchers, therapists, and educators, recognizing that no evidence exists that masturbation is harmful in any way for most people, have begun to recognize the physical and psychological health *benefits* of masturbation. These are detailed in Table 6.6.

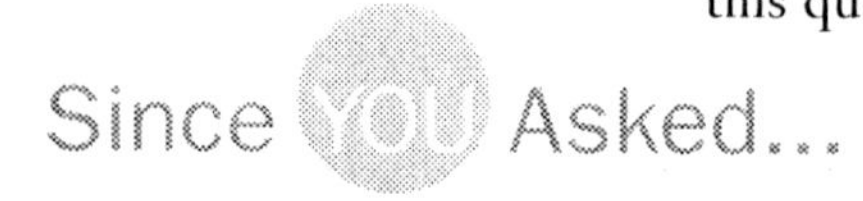

3. If you are feeling sexually frustrated, how can you satisfy your sexual needs?

Table 6.6 THE BENEFITS OF MASTURBATION

BENEFIT	FUNCTION
Sexual self-discovery	Masturbation provides a "laboratory" for exploring and experimenting with one's own sexual feelings and sensations. This learning process is important for achieving sexual satisfaction with a partner and in life in general.
Release of sexual tension or frustration	Masturbation may be used to alleviate feelings of sexual frustration resulting from romantic and sexual activities with a partner that do not lead to orgasm or general sexual tensions that may build up over time.
Enhancement of sexual interactions with a partner	Masturbation appears to be related to a person's sexual satisfaction with a partner now and in the future. Research has shown that people in relationships who masturbate are more sexually satisfied with their partner and their relationship.
Resolution of sexual problems, including inhibited sexual desire, premature ejaculation, difficulty with orgasm, erectile problems, general arousal difficulties, and delayed orgasm (these are discussed in Chapter 7, "Sexual Problems and Solutions")	Many common sexual problems are treated with the help of masturbation. The therapeutic benefits of masturbation exercises may be part of a treatment program prescribed by a professional counselor or a self-help strategy individuals or couples may discover on their own.
Orgasm	Masturbation has been reported, especially by women, as providing the most reliable and most intense orgasms.
Relief from stress	Many people who masturbate find it helpful in relieving stress, tension, and sleeplessness that are not necessarily related to sex per se.
Relief from menstrual pain	For some women, masturbating before or during their period reduces or even eliminates menstrual cramps.
Compensation for a disparity in a couple's levels of sexual desire	A common problem couples face is that one wants more frequent sexual contact than the other. While couples may solve this problem using various strategies, masturbation can often help reduce the guilt, demand, and frustration often felt by couples in this situation.
Safe sex	Solo masturbation poses zero risk of STIs or pregnancy. You cannot give yourself an STI or make yourself pregnant. Even when masturbation activities are shared by a couple, it is one of the lowest-risk sexual behaviors.

Sources: Davidson and Moore (1994); Kay (1992); Kelly, Strassberg, and Kircher (1990); Masters and Johnson (1974); "The Politics of Masturbation" (1994); Tiefer (1998).

Masturbation's Role with Other Sexual Behaviors

A common belief about masturbation is that it serves as a substitute for sexual activities with a partner. This belief then leads to other assumptions—that masturbation must be a sign of dissatisfaction with one's partner, that people masturbate only when they don't have a sexual partner, that people who masturbate are sexually deprived, or that masturbation is simply an outlet for people who do not have any other form of sexual release. The truth is that all of these beliefs and assumptions are wrong. Instead of substituting for sex with a partner, masturbation is typically a normal component of a sexually healthy life (Michael et al., 1994).

Research clearly demonstrates that many people do not stop masturbating when they enter a sexual relationship. In fact, most people continue to masturbate after marriage (Janus & Janus, 1993). Moreover, those who are having the most sexual intercourse with their partner are the most likely to masturbate (Michael et al., 1994). Finally, people who masturbate are more likely than those who don't to be both physically and emotionally satisfied with their overall sex lives (Davisdon & Moore, 1994). Taken together, the evidence is quite strong that masturbation is far more than an activity people simply do in place of other sexual activities or a sign of a sexual problem; rather it is an integral part of the diverse repertoire of normal human sexual activities.

Since YOU Asked...

4. Does masturbation detract from one's sexual drive or pleasure?

Techniques of Masturbation

One important point should be made before discussing techniques of masturbation: It is perfectly OK *not* to masturbate. Although masturbation is discussed more openly in society and its benefits are more widely known, no one should interpret this as evidence that something is wrong or abnormal with choosing not to masturbate. As for all sexual behaviors, this is each person's individual choice. If you are not comfortable with the idea of masturbation and you have chosen to refrain from that activity for any reason (or for no reason at all), that is a completely legitimate decision, and you should never feel pressured to do anything sexual that feels wrong or uncomfortable to you. If you already masturbate regularly, you probably know what feels best and how you prefer to do it, so the techniques discussed here may be of less value to you than to others who have never masturbated or are in the early stages of experimentation. When people masturbate, their bodies typically progress through the same pattern of sexual responses as would happen if they were with a partner. For a better understanding of the bodily changes that usually accompany masturbation, you may want to review Chapter 3, "The Physiology of Human Sexual Responding."

Following are the aspects often reported as part of many people's most pleasurable masturbation experiences.

- **Privacy.** First, be sure you have a comfortable place to be by yourself where you are sure you will not be interrupted or intruded upon.
- **Time.** Allow plenty of time so that you do not need to feel rushed or pressured in any way.
- **Sexual Self-Awareness.** To allow yourself pleasurable masturbation experiences, become familiar with your own sexual anatomy. Take a few minutes and examine your own body (see Figure 6.1). You may find that a small hand mirror is helpful for seeing everything. As you do this exam, touch parts of your sexual anatomy gently and allow yourself to become familiar with them. If you find this

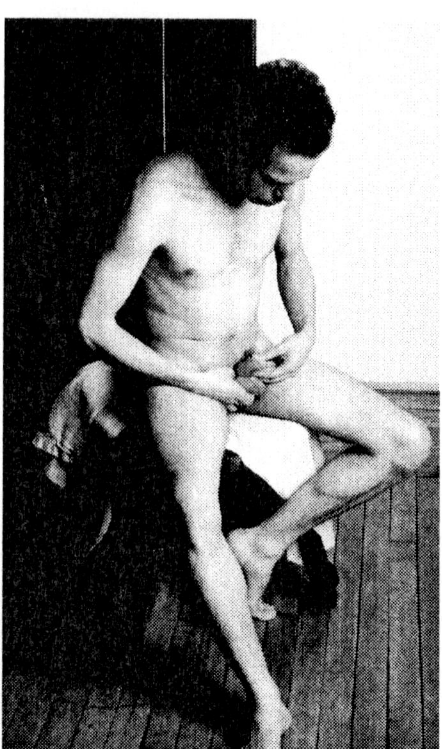

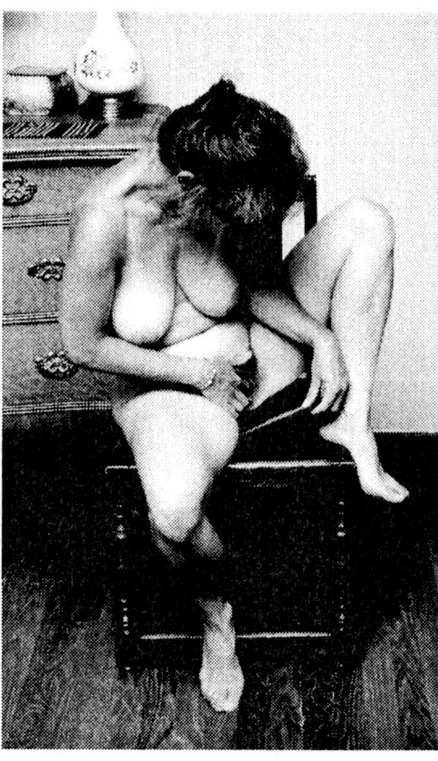

FIGURE 6.1 Sexual Self-Awareness Sexual self-examination allows for enhanced knowledge of sexual anatomy and greater pleasure from masturbation.

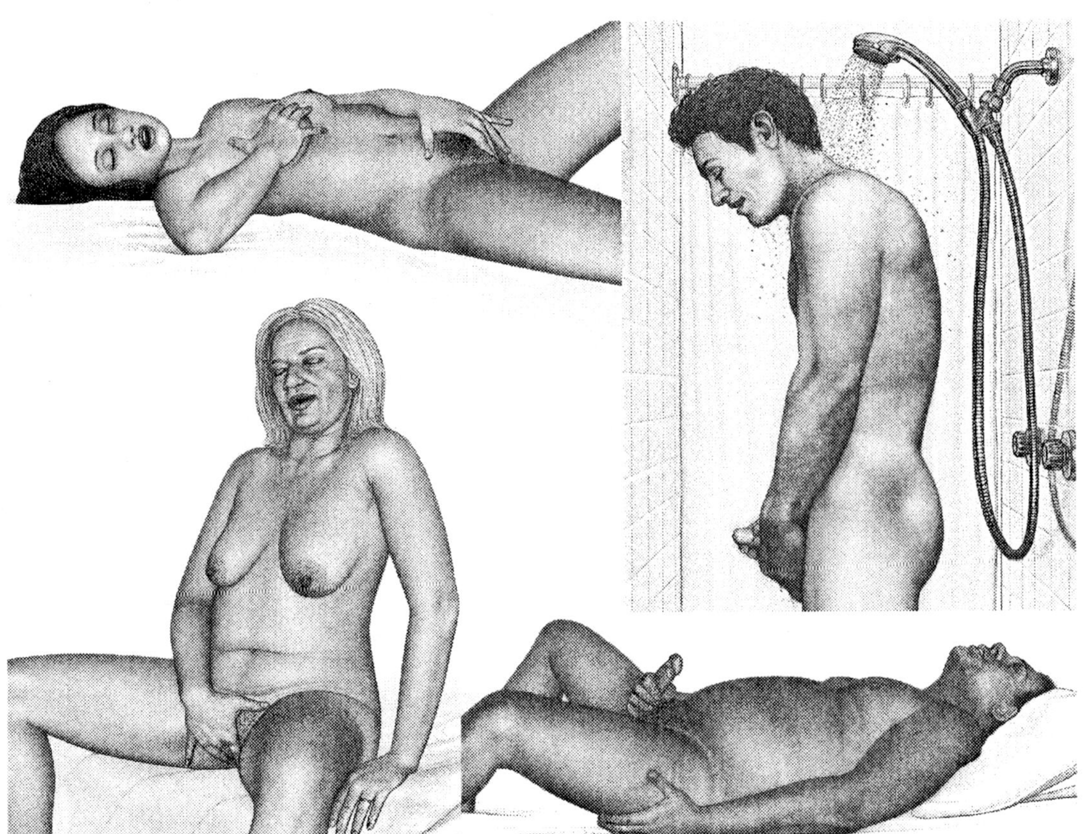

FIGURE 6.2 Masturbation
A variety of positions can be used while masturbating.

exercise difficult and embarrassing, as many of you will, just proceed slowly and do as much self examination as feels comfortable for now. As time passes and you continue this activity, you will become increasingly at ease with your body.

- **Arousal.** As you examine and touch yourself, you may begin to become sexually aroused. The physical changes accompanying masturbation parallel those during sex with a partner. A woman may notice her clitoris becoming enlarged or an increase in vaginal lubrication. A man's penis becomes erect, and he may be aware of changes in the skin of his scrotum and the position of his testicles.
- **Techniques of Stimulation.** Of course, each individual has unique preferences, but some similarities may be found in typical styles of masturbation among men and women relating to position, touch, and orgasm.
  - *Position.* Most men and women masturbate while lying face up. However, variations may include sitting in a chair or on the edge of a bed, kneeling, or standing (see Figure 6.2). Some people masturbate lying face down and rubbing against the bed or an object.
  - *Touch (Men).* In general, men grasp the penis with the whole hand or between the thumb and one or more fingers. They usually stroke the shaft and glans of the penis in an up-and-down motion. Men who are uncircumcised will often use the foreskin as a "sleeve" for movement over the glans. The pressure and speed of stroking varies among men, but usually these will both increase as the man becomes increasingly aroused and closer to orgasm. A man should be aware that as he becomes aroused, the Cowper's gland will secrete a clear, slick fluid that may appear at the urethral opening before he ejaculates. This pre-ejaculate is completely normal. Some men will stimulate their testicles, anus, or nipples while masturbating, though this is the exception rather than the rule.

- *Touch (Women).* Techniques women use for masturbation are often significantly more varied. Most women touch, stroke, rub, massage, or otherwise stimulate the outer and inner labia and the area of the clitoris. Some women enjoy direct clitoral stimulation; others find this uncomfortable due to the extreme sensitivity of the clitoral glans. Contrary to popular belief, very few women ever insert anything into the vagina while masturbating. Also, only a small percentage of women stimulate their breasts and nipples during masturbation. A minority of women masturbate by rubbing the vulva area against an object such as a pillow, using the friction of pressing their thighs together to achieve desired stimulation, or incorporating some form of water massage. As a woman becomes aroused, she will notice an increase in vaginal secretions. This fluid may be used by the woman to lubricate the rubbing or massaging of the vulva.

- **Orgasm.** Some people may not experience orgasm the first few times they try masturbating. Eventually, however, nearly everyone who masturbates on a regular basis has an orgasm every time, and most people feel that orgasm is the goal, if not the main point, of masturbating (for most men, this will invariably include ejaculation of semen). For someone who has never experienced an orgasm, the strength of the physical and psychological sensations during masturbation as orgasm approaches can sometimes feel too intense and even a little frightening. Remember, masturbation is about self-pleasuring. If at any time you feel uncomfortable, just stop. As you experiment over time, the sensations will become increasingly predictable and enjoyable.
- **Artificial Lubrication.** Many men and women will often add some lubrication while masturbating to allow for easier movement of the hand against the genitals, which often intensifies sensations. Water-based lubricants specifically designed for sexual use are probably best for this purpose because they have excellent lubricating properties and will usually not cause irritation to sensitive body areas. However, many people have found that hand creams, lotions, or body oils work just as well.
- **Vibrators.** Electric and battery-operated vibrators have become increasingly popular and more readily available in recent years. They can be purchased at various retail outlets, through mail order catalogs, and on the Internet. They come in a variety of shapes and sizes, some of which are shown in Figure 6.3. In addition, entire books have been written describing vibrators and their uses (Venning & Cavanah, 2003; Winks & Semans, 2002). Many people enjoy the sensations produced by incorporating a vibrator into their masturbation experiences. In addition, some women who have had difficulty reaching orgasm report that using a vibrator (usually on the clitoral area, not inserted into the vagina) has allowed them to have orgasms more easily, which in turn helps them to experience orgasms more readily without the vibrator.

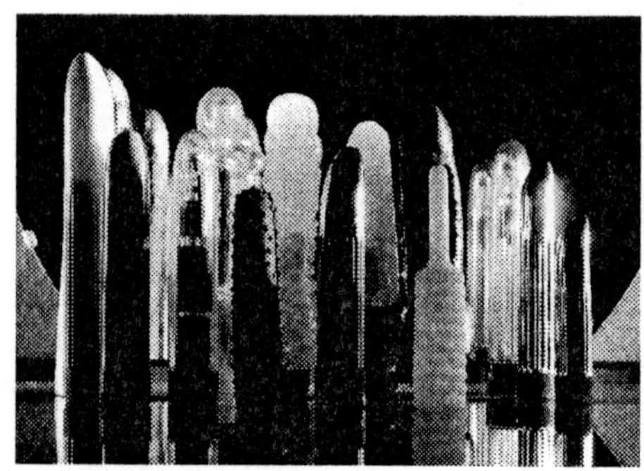

FIGURE 6.3 Sexual Vibrators
Many people find that sexual vibrators enhance their masturbation experiences.

Erotic Touch

Sex is more than intercourse

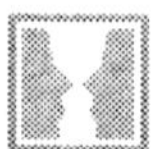

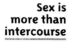

erotic touch Intimate or sexual touching between partners, usually with the hands, for the purpose of sexual arousal and sharing sexual or sensual pleasure.

Erotic touch refers to intimate or sexual touching between partners, usually with the hands, for the purpose of sexual arousal and sharing sexual or sensual pleasure. Specifically, the activities discussed in this section include kissing, sensual massage, caressing of the breasts and nipples, and genital touching. Keep in mind, however, that any type of touch in any location on the body may be sexy and arousing to couples, depending on their personal preferences.

Many people view erotic touching as "foreplay," a routine step on the path to intercourse, as expressed in this statement: "We kiss for a while, then we touch each other for a while, and then after we touch each other's genitals for a while, it's time for 'real sex.'" However, touch is far more than that. Research has clearly demonstrated that human infants need close physical contact with others in order to thrive or even to survive. Throughout life, touching continues to be an important means of communicating closeness, affection, and sexual intimacy. The famous sexuality researchers Masters and Johnson, in their book *The Pleasure Bond* (1974), are very clear on this point:

> For the man and woman who value each other as individuals and who want the satisfactions of a sustained relationship, it is important to avoid the fundamental error of believing that touch is a means to an end. It is not. *Touch is an end in itself.* It is a primary form of communication, a silent voice that avoids the pitfall of words while expressing the feelings of the moment . . . establishing a sense of solidarity between two people. Touching is a sensual pleasure, exploring the texture of the skin, the suppleness of the muscle, the contours of the body, with no further goal than the enjoyment of tactile perceptions. (p. 238)

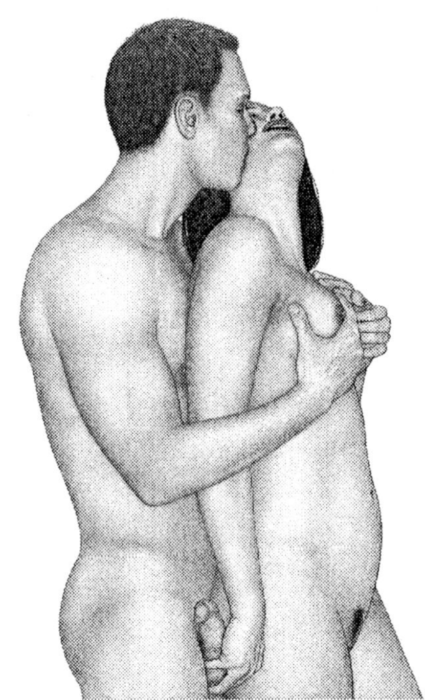

FIGURE 6.4 Erotic Touch

Erotic touch is a pleasurable, intimate behavior by itself and need not necessarily lead to other sexual activities.

This does not mean that touch cannot lead to other sexual activities, such as intercourse, and for many couples it often does. But when touching is seen as *only* a prelude to intercourse, it often loses much of its pleasurable value and becomes no more than a way signaling a desire or demand for something else. Many couples report that early in their relationship, touching was central to their physical intimacy together. Touch was extremely erotic, almost electrically charged. Then, as intercourse became a more common part of the sexual relationship, touching began to take a back seat, so to speak, and became a much more perfunctory or superficial part of their lovemaking. This shift in focus from a whole body sensuality to genitally focused intercourse sometimes leads to the sexual problems we discuss in the next chapter. Interestingly, one of the exercises recommended for helping couples who are experiencing sexual problems is to return to a focus on touch, rather than on intercourse.

How to Touch Your Partner

How should you touch your partner sexually? The answer to that question is obvious. You should touch your partner in the way your partner likes to be touched! (see Figure 6.4). But how do you know exactly what your partner likes? Sometimes you can tell by changes in movements, facial expressions, breathing, and vocalizations of pleasure. However, unless you are a mind reader (and you're not), these nonverbal clues can often be misleading. Consider the following common scenario of a couple's sexual interaction. He enjoys a firm, rapid style of touching, similar to a massage, but she prefers a lighter, slower, stroking touch. In an attempt to communicate to each other what they like, he will touch her more and more firmly and she will touch him increasingly lightly. Each has the feeling that the other just isn't getting it. So they try harder to demonstrate what they like. He touches harder still, she lightens up even more until both become disappointed and frustrated (this is called "mirroring" and is discussed further in Chapter 7). What's the solution? The best way to discover your partners preferences for being touched (or for any intimate activity) is to *ask*.

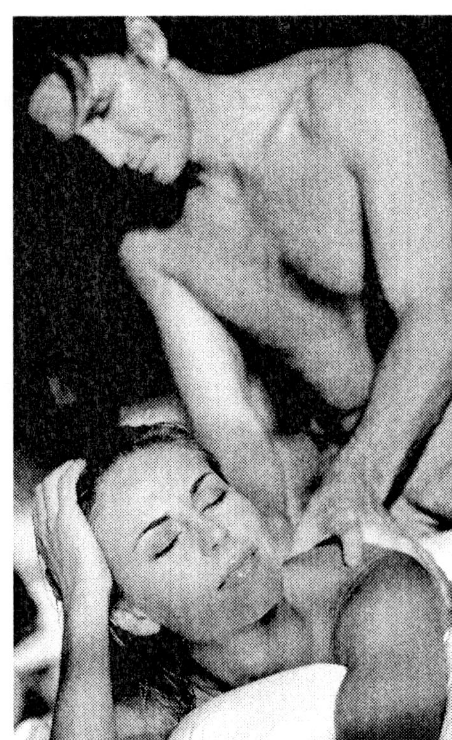

Mutual sensual massage often enhances sexual feelings between partners.

One way to communicate what you like is to reinforce your partner when he or she does something that feels especially good. Saying "That feels really good" or "What you were just doing is exactly how I like it" helps your partner learn the behaviors that most satisfy you. Another strategy is to bring up the issue at a time when you are feeling close and comfortable but not being sexual. Be positive and talk about your feelings. Say, "I really like it when you touch me slowly and lightly," *not* "You really don't touch me the way I like." Hopefully, then, the next time you are involved in erotic touching with your partner, your discussion will be put into practice. Finally, another way to let your partner know what you like is to demonstrate. An exercise devised by Masters and Johnson (1970) and often suggested by sex therapists is for you to guide your partner's hand over your body to illustrate how and where you most enjoy being touched. Many people are embarrassed by this at first, but slowly it will become more comfortable and will actually open up new lines of sexual communication (see Chapter 4, "Love, Intimacy, and Sexual Communication," and Chapter 7, "Sexual Problems and Solutions," for more discussion of these issues).

Kissing

In most Western cultures, kissing is a very common and popular form of erotic touching (see "Sexuality and Culture: Cultural Variations in Kissing Behavior"). Many forms of kissing are popular, from a friendly or familial peck on the cheek to more arousing and romantic kissing known as French, deep, or soul kissing (see Figure 6.5). Interestingly, research on kissing in the human sexuality literature is conspicuously lacking. Kinsey's work in the 1940s and 1950s found that nearly all couples (87 percent) in the United States include deep kissing as part of lovemaking (Kinsey et al., 1948).

Since then, however, kissing has been overlooked in most studies and surveys of sexual behavior. Why do you think this is the case? A possible explanation may be that kissing in Western culture does not "count" as a sexual behavior (see Irving, 1995). The 1994 national survey of sexual behavior (Michael et al., 1994) does not mention kissing at all. Even the famous *Hite Report* on female sexuality, which covered a wide range of sexual behaviors, only addressed kissing in the last page-and-a-half of the book (Hite, 1976). This is an unfortunate and misguided omission, because the mouth, lips, and tongue are very sensitive structures capable of producing pleasure and sexual arousal when stimulated by another person's mouth, lips, and tongue. Kissing continues to be one of the most popular sexual activities among college students. One recent study of college students that did include this behavior found that 88 percent reported deep kissing within the past month and over 93 percent said they fantasized about it, making deep kissing the most common fantasy (Hsu et al., 1994). Kissing is a very safe behavior in terms of STI transmission; however, the herpes virus may be transmitted if one person has active sores on the lips or mouth.

FIGURE 6.5 Kissing

Kissing is one of the most common intimate activities in most Western cultures.

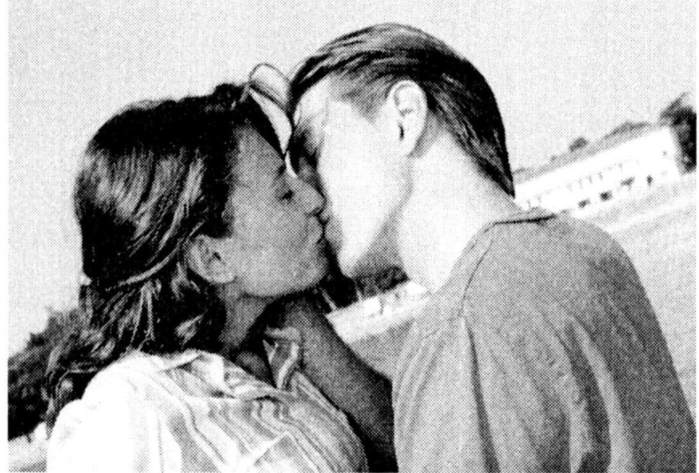

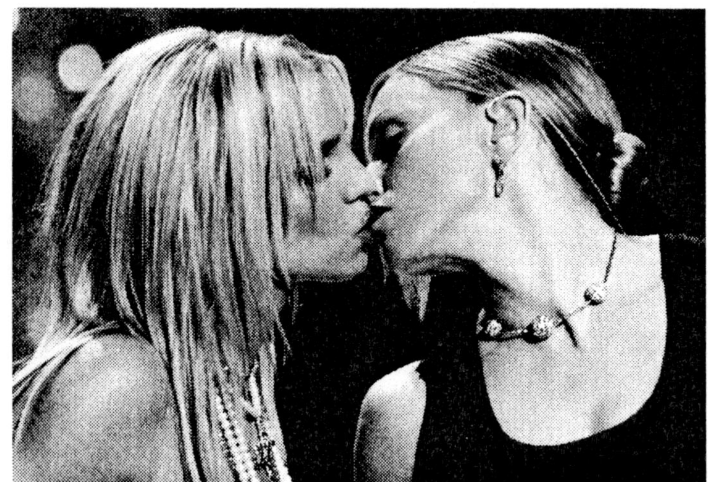

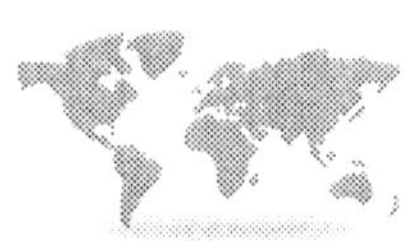

Sexuality and Culture

Cultural Variations in Kissing Behavior

Leonore Tiefer is a clinical psychologist with a remarkably broad background in all aspects of human sexuality. The following is an excerpt from "The Kiss," in her latest collection of essays, *Sex Is Not a Natural Act*.

I became fascinated by the remarkable cultural and historical variations in styles and purposes of kissing, given how "natural" it seems to pursue whatever customs each of us has grown accustomed to. Clellan Ford and Frank Beach (1951) compared the sexual customs of the many tribal societies that were recorded in the Human Relations Area Files at Yale. Few field studies mentioned kissing customs at all. Of the twenty-one that did, some sort of kissing accompanied intercourse in thirteen tribes—the Chiricahua, Cree, Crow, Gros Ventre, Hopi, Huichol, Kwakiutl, and Tarahumara of North America; the Alorese, Keraki, Trobrianders, and Trukese of Oceania; and the Lapps in Eurasia. There were some interesting variations: the Kwakiutl, Trobrianders, Alorese, and Trukese kiss by sucking the lips and tongue of their partners; the Lapps like to kiss the mouth and nose at the same time.

But sexual kissing is unknown in many societies, including the Balinese, Chamorro, Manus, and Tinguian of Oceania; the Chewa and Thonga of Africa; the Siriono of South America; and the Lepcha of Eurasia. In such cultures, the mouth-to-mouth kiss is considered dangerous, unhealthy, or disgusting, the way Westerners might regard a custom of sticking one's tongue into a lover's nose. Ford and Beach reported that when the Thonga first saw Europeans kissing, they laughed, remarking, "Look at them—they eat each other's saliva and dirt."

Deep kissing apparently has nothing to do with degree of sexual inhibition or repression in a culture. On certain Polynesian islands, women are orgasmic and sexually active, yet kissing was unknown until Westerners and their popular films arrived. Research in parts of Ireland, by contrast, where sex was considered dirty and sinful, and, for women, a duty, shows that the Irish also were oblivious to tongue kissing until recent decades.

Many tribes across Africa and elsewhere believe that the soul enters and leaves through the mouth and that a person's bodily products can be collected and saved by an enemy for harmful purposes. In these societies, the possible loss of saliva would cause a kiss to be regarded as a dangerous gesture. There, the "soul kiss" is taken literally. (It was taken figuratively in Western societies; recall Christopher Marlowe's "Sweet Helen, make me immortal with a kiss! Her lips suck forth my soul.")

Although the deep kiss is relatively rare around the world as a part of sexual intimacy, other forms of mouth or nose contact are common—particularly the "oceanic kiss," named for its prevalence among cultures in Oceania but not limited to them. The Tinguians place their lips near the partner's face and suddenly inhale. Balinese lovers bring their faces close enough to catch each other's perfume and to feel the warmth of the skin, making contact as they move their heads slightly. Another kiss, as practiced by Chinese Yakuts and Mongolians at the turn of the century, has one person's nose pressed to the other's cheek, followed by a nasal inhalation and finally a smacking of lips.

The oceanic kiss may be varied by the placement of the nose and cheek, the vigor of the inhalation, the nature of the accompanying sounds, the action of the arms, and so on; it is used for affectionate greeting as well as for sexual play. Some observers think that the so-called Eskimo or Malay kiss of rubbing noses is actually a mislabeled oceanic kiss; the kisser is simply moving his or her nose rapidly from one cheek to the other of the partner, bumping noses on route.

Small tribes and obscure Irish islanders are not the only groups to eschew tongue kissing. The advanced civilizations of China and Japan, which regarded sexual proficiency as high art, apparently cared little about it. In their voluminous display of erotica—graphic depictions of every possible sexual position, angle of intercourse, and variation of partner and setting—mouth-to-mouth kissing is conspicuous by its absence. Japanese poets have rhapsodized for centuries about the allure of the nape of the neck, but they have been silent on the mouth; indeed, kissing is acceptable only between mother and child. (The Japanese have no word for kissing—though they recently borrowed from English to create *kissu*.) In Japan, intercourse is "natural"; a kiss, pornographic. When Rodin's famous sculpture *The Kiss* came to Tokyo in the 1920s as part of a show of European art, it was concealed from public view behind a bamboo curtain.

Among cultures of the West, the number of nonsexual uses of the kiss is staggering: greeting and farewell, affection, religious or ceremonial symbolism, deference to a person of high status. (People also kiss icons, dice, and other objects, of course, in prayer, for luck, or as part of a ritual.) Kisses make the hurt go away, bless the sacred vestments, seal a bargain. In story and legend a kiss has started wars and ended them, awakened Sleeping Beauty and put Brunnhilde to sleep.

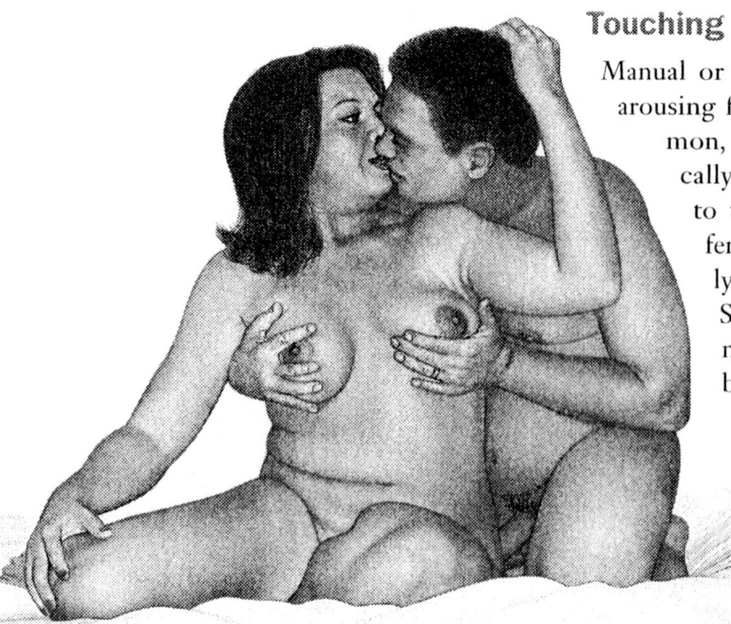

FIGURE 6.6 The Breasts and Sexual Behavior

Most women and many men find breast and nipple stimulation very sexually exciting.

Touching the Breasts and Nipples

Manual or oral stimulation of the breasts and nipples can be very sexually arousing for both men and women (see Figure 6.6). It is much more common, however, for women to have their breasts touched or kissed erotically than it is for men (Hsu et al., 1994). This may be due in large part to the importance placed on (some would say obsession with) the female breast in U.S. culture. Women also report being more sexually aroused by having their breasts and nipples touched than men do. Some women are even able to have an orgasm through breast and nipple stimulation alone (Masters & Johnson, 1966). A commonly believed myth is that larger breasts are more sexually sensitive to touch, but no relationship has been shown in the scientific literature between breast size and sensitivity to erotic touching.

Exactly how people prefer to have their breasts touched is probably as individual as fingerprints. Some prefer a firmer touch, some a softer stroking, while others may like the nipples pinched or sucked. Like all shared sexual activity, the best way to learn about your partner's preferences is through open, honest communication.

Genital Touching

Some people choose to limit their sexual interactions with a partner to touching. They may have any number of reasons for this, such as religious or moral beliefs about intercourse, reducing their risk for STIs or unwanted pregnancy, or a desire to wait until a later time in life (closer relationship, marriage, etc.) to engage in other sexual behaviors. Many couples find touching of the genitals, often referred to as shared or **mutual masturbation**, a very exciting, intimate, and satisfying activity. Among college students, 82 percent of females and 89 percent of males report experiencing mutual genital touching to orgasm (Hsu et al., 1994), and some men and women say that it is their preferred method of having an orgasm (Janus & Janus, 1993). In addition, some couples find watching each other masturbate very sexually exciting (Benedict, 1997). One online survey found that approximately half of the respondents masturbate occasionally or regularly while being watched by a partner ("Polls and Surveys," 2004).

Since YOU Asked...

5. I believe that foreplay is the best part of sex. Is that strange?

Again, as with all sexual behavior with a partner, everyone has specific preferences for genital touching. As mentioned earlier, you should avoid assuming that your partner likes the same style of genital touching as you, because you'll probably be wrong. The best way for a couple to learn about their preferences is to talk about them and, if the relationship is open and comfortable, to show and tell. This said, here are some general guidelines for genital touching.

Both men and women usually prefer a gentle, slower touch at first, with increasingly firmer pressure and faster stroking as excitement builds. Most men like to have the erect penis encircled by their partner's hand and stroked up and down. Usually, there will be some contact with the glans, but some men find the tip of the penis too sensitive for focused stimulation. Some men enjoy gentle touching and massaging of the scrotum, testicles, and anal area as well. Most women enjoy having the outer and inner labia gently massaged or stroked and the area of the clitoris stimulated. Some women like more focused touching of the clitoris, while others prefer more general, overall massaging of the vulva. The glans of the clitoris is extremely sensitive for some women, making direct stimulation uncomfortable or

mutual masturbation Partners' touching of each other's genitals, often to orgasm and enjoyed as a sexually intimate and satisfying activity.

even painful. Many women also enjoy some stimulation of the outer part of the vagina and anus (the vulva and vagina should not be touched by the same part of the hand that has stimulated the anus, because bacteria that exist normally in the rectum may be transferred from the anal area, creating a risk of vaginal or urinary tract infections). Most women do not prefer a finger or fingers inserted deeply into the vagina during mutual masturbation, and some even find it uncomfortable or distracting ("Female Masturbation," 2001; Hite, 1976; Masters & Johnson, 1979).

Often, but not always, genital touching leads to orgasm. Many couples find this to be a very pleasurable and satisfying form of sexual intimacy and release. It allows those who are in relationships but do not feel ready for other activities such as oral sex or intercourse to enjoy the intense pleasure and closeness that sexual intimacy can provide (see Figure 6.7).

Finally, genital touching, even to orgasm, is relatively free from the risks of sexually transmitted infections. To be confident of this, however, couples must make sure that semen and vaginal fluids come into contact only with skin that is healthy and unbroken (Reinisch, 1990).

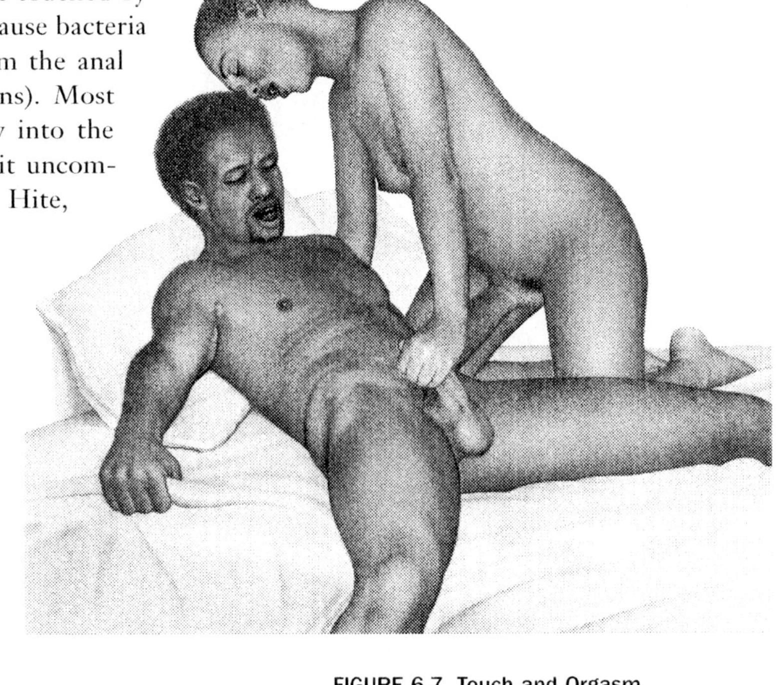

FIGURE 6.7 Touch and Orgasm

A couple can experience intense pleasure, including orgasm, from mutual erotic touching.

Oral Sex

Sometimes referred to as "going down," "giving head," "eating out," "blow job," and many other slang terms; oral sex, like masturbation, is something most people have experienced but few are comfortable admitting or talking about it openly. Recent surveys have found that nearly 80 percent of people have engaged in oral sex and almost 90 percent feel that it is a normal and acceptable sexual activity (Billy et al., 1993; Janus & Janus, 1993; Laumann et al., 1994). Among college students, the percentages are even higher, with over 90 percent of men and women reporting experience with oral sex (Hsu et al., 1994; von Sadovszky, Keller, & McKinney, 2002). For younger populations in general, 55 percent of never-married individuals between 15 and 24 reported having experienced oral sex (Hoff, Greene, & Davis, 2003). In another study of over 1600 young adults (18 to 24 years old), 78 percent reported receiving oral sex and 57 percent reported performing oral sex (Ompad et al., 2006).

Sex is more than intercourse

Oral sex involves two distinct behaviors, depending on the recipient of the activity. **Cunnilingus** is oral sex performed on a female, and **fellatio** is oral sex performed on a male. Each of these behaviors also involves two components: giving oral sex and receiving it. Slightly more college men and women report receiving oral sex than report giving it (Hsu et al., 1994).

Cunnilingus

The word *cunnilingus* is derived from the latin *cunnus*, meaning "vulva," and *lingere*, "lick." The behavior itself, however, often involves many other activities besides licking. Techniques of cunnilingus are extremely varied, and each woman is different in her preferences for receiving oral sex. In general, the vulva is stimulated by the mouth, lips, and tongue of the woman's partner (see Figure 6.8). This may include kissing, licking, sucking, and sometimes light biting of the outer and inner labia, the clitoral hood, and the shaft and glans of the clitoris. Some women also enjoy the tongue

cunnilingus Oral sex performed on a female.

fellatio Oral sex performed on a male.

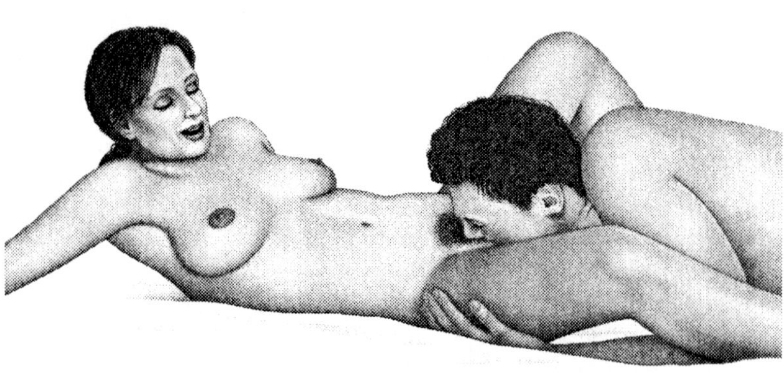

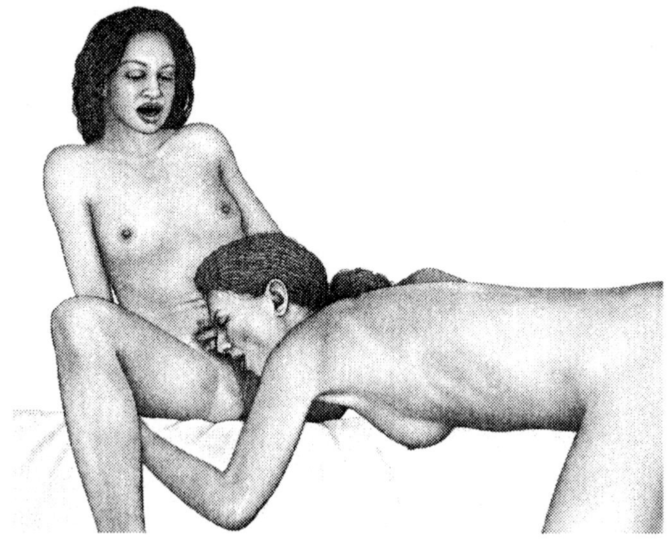

FIGURE 6.8 Cunnilingus

Cunnilingus is the stimulation of the vulva with the mouth, lips, and tongue.

inserted into the outer part of the vagina. The contact of the mouth with the vulva may range from very light, slow stroking with the lips and tongue to faster, firmer movements of the tongue and strong sucking of the labia and clitoris. Many women enjoy simultaneous manual stimulation of the woman's outer vagina, G-spot area, anus, or breasts and nipples during oral sex.

Fellatio

The word *fellatio* originates from the Latin *fellare*, meaning "suck." This is actually something of a misnomer because sucking is usually not a major component of this activity and vigorous sucking may even become uncomfortable or painful to the man. Like women, men vary a great deal in exactly how they like oral sex to be performed on them. In fellatio, a man's genitals are stimulated by his partner's mouth, lips, and tongue (see Figure 6.9). This may include kissing and licking of the penis including the shaft, glans, and frenulum. Often the entire penis is taken into the mouth and stimulated by moving the penis in and out of the mouth, caressing it with the tongue, and perhaps sucking lightly. Some men also enjoy oral stimulation of the scrotum and testicles, including gentle sucking of the testicles through the scrotum. Some men enjoy simultaneous stimulation of other parts of the body during oral sex, including the testicles, anus, or breasts and nipples.

Why Some People Like Oral Sex

Since YOU Asked...

6. Do women get more pleasure from intercourse or oral sex? How and why?

Most people who engage in oral sex, whether giving or receiving, find it to be an extremely intimate, pleasurable, and exciting activity. In the National Health and Social Life Survey conducted in the mid-1990s, a clear majority of men and women rated giving and receiving oral sex as somewhat or very appealing (Laumann et al., 1994). In studies of sexual fantasy, oral sex is one of the most common fantasies reported by college students, with 96 percent of men and 84 percent of women reporting fantasizing about oral activities (Hsu et al., 1994).

People report a wide variety of reasons that they enjoy oral sex. Some couples feel that giving and receiving oral sex creates more intense feelings of intimacy than any other sexual behavior, even intercourse. Others enjoy the feeling of the mutual enjoyment and acceptance of their partner's entire body that oral sex represents. Most people who engage in oral sex find it a highly physically arousing behavior in which stimulation can be focused exactly where and how it feels the best. Some find that orgasms through oral sex feel different or better than masturbation, touching, or even intercourse. Many women and some men report that the best or only way they have orgasms with a partner is through oral sex. Shere Hite, in her reports on female and male sexuality, quotes women as saying:

> "A tongue offers gentleness and precision and wetness and is the perfect organ for contact. And besides, it produces sensational orgasms!"
>
> "It really puts me in orbit, and I always have an orgasm!" (Hite, 1976, p. 234)

Hite also offers the following quotes about oral sex from men:

> "This is by far my favorite sexual activity. I always orgasm and it is more intense for me than an intercourse orgasm."
>
> "Fellatio is the best. Besides the physical sensations, I feel the woman really loves and appreciates my body." (Hite, 1981, p. 539)

Another reason that many couples enjoy oral sex is that it can serve as a substitute for intercourse. Some couples who have made a decision to avoid intercourse either due to personal moral beliefs, the choice to be safe from unwanted pregnancy, or a desire to wait until a later point in time for intercourse will engage in oral sex as a way of exploring sexual intimacy without intercourse. However, contrary to the belief held by many people, especially adolescents, oral sex is *not* safe sex and can transmit most sexually transmitted infections (see "In Touch with Your Sexual Health: Oral Sex and STIs").

Why Some People Object to Oral Sex

In contrast to people who enjoy oral sex, others are uneasy with oral sex or averse to it. No one should ever be coerced into any sexual behavior that is not freely chosen. If you do not feel comfortable about giving or receiving oral sex, that is your choice, and you do not need a justification for refusing. About 10 to 30 percent of people surveyed considered oral sex unusual, kinky, or unappealing (Janus & Janus, 1993; Michael et al., 1994). In addition, some people who agree to engage in oral sex may not actually

Since YOU Asked...

7. My boyfriend says it's OK if we have oral sex because it doesn't spread sexual diseases. Is that true?

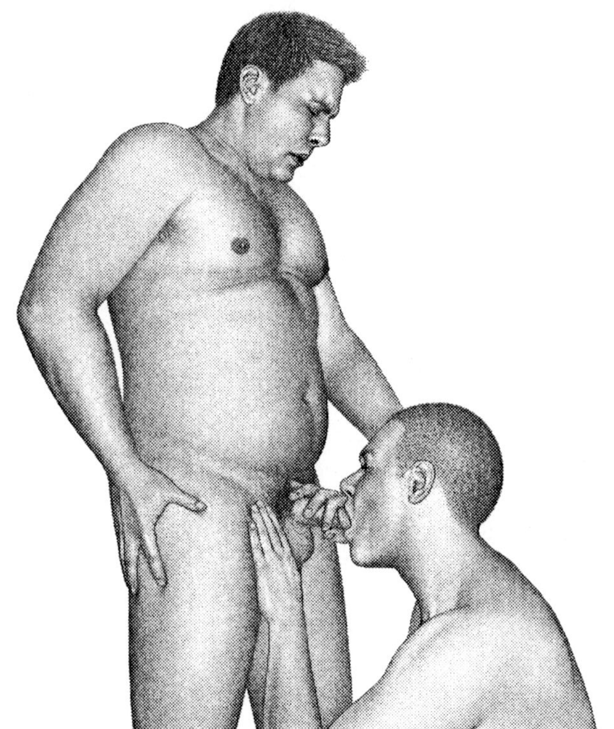

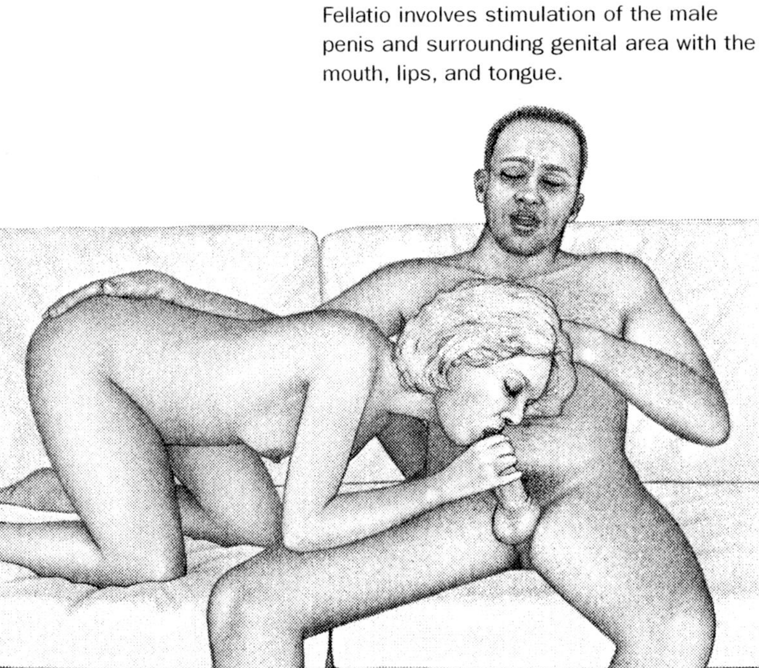

FIGURE 6.9 Fellatio

Fellatio involves stimulation of the male penis and surrounding genital area with the mouth, lips, and tongue.

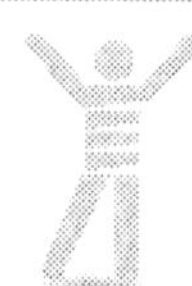

In Touch with Your Sexual Health

Oral Sex and STIs

Oral sex carries a clear risk of transmission of various STIs, including human papilloma virus (genital warts, which may lead to oral cancer), herpes simplex virus, hepatitis B, gonorrhea, syphilis, chlamydia, chancroid, and HIV (see Chapter 8, "Sexually Transmitted Infections," for more information on all STIs) (Centers for Disease Control and Prevention, 2000b; "Oral Sex Linked," 2004; Remez, 2000). In addition, research has found that oral sex may be a major cause of recurring vaginal yeast infections because the mouths of one-third to one-half of all adults normally contain yeast bacteria that can overwhelm the normal balance of yeast and other organisms in the vagina (Geiger & Foxman, 1996; "Oral Sex, Masturbating," 2004).

On a related note, a worrisome recent trend points to a significant upturn in the number of adolescents engaging in oral sex (Remez, 2000). The primary reason for this may be the erroneous belief among these teens that oral sex poses little or no risk of STI transmission and allows them to be sexually active while maintaining their *perception* of virginity. Some protection from transmission of STIs during oral sex is provided by using condoms during fellatio (nonlubricated condoms are usually preferred for this) and dental dams (thin sheets of latex placed over the vulva) for cunnilingus. Also, a condom may be cut lengthwise, opened up, and placed over the vulva for STI protection during cunnilingus. While the risk for transmission of HIV through oral-genital contact appears to be relatively low, unprotected oral sex should never be thought of as safer than vaginal or anal intercourse in terms of the risk for STIs overall.

enjoy it (Hite, 1976). At times, oral sex can become a problem in a relationship if one person desires to give or receive it and the other doesn't. There also appear to be differences in oral sex preferences by groups (Laumann et al., 1994). Individuals with more years of education are more likely to engage in oral sex than those with fewer years of schooling. Another consistent finding is that oral sex is significantly more common among whites than blacks in the United States (Billy et al., 1993). In addition, differences with age have been found as well, with older adults (over 50) reporting less experience with oral sex than younger individuals (Laumann et al., 1994).

Many reasons have been suggested as to why someone may feel uncomfortable with oral sex and wish to avoid it. One of the most obvious relates to an individual's morals and attitudes about sex. Some believe that oral sex is simply wrong and conflicts with their personal code of acceptable behavior. Other reasons concern the mechanics of the behavior itself. Some partners are often concerned that the penis will be pushed too deep into the mouth and throat or the inserting partner will ejaculate in the mouth, causing a gag reflex or other unpleasant reactions. Although swallowing semen is not harmful or dangerous in itself (assuming no STIs), many people are uncomfortable or repulsed by the idea (by the way, since many students ask, semen is a "low-cal food," containing only about 5 calories in the average ejaculate). Both men and women worry that the smell or taste of the female genitals will be unpleasant or offensive in some way. Western society has encouraged this view with the numerous "feminine hygiene" products on the market that send the message that a woman's natural genital odor is bad and should be covered up. In reality, female genitals that are washed with normal regularity have a natural fragrance that most people find attractive and enjoyable. A strong or unpleasant odor from a woman's vagina may be a sign of an infection that may require treatment.

The bottom line is that if two people desire oral sex, all of their concerns can usually be overcome through sensitivity, respect, and open communication.

Coitus

All of the sexual activities we have discussed so far—sexual fantasy, masturbation, erotic touching, and oral sex—are practiced and enjoyed by people who are straight, gay, lesbian, or bisexual. An exception is **coitus**, which refers to penis-vagina intercourse and is therefore by definition a *heterosexual* behavior. In most cultures around the world, coitus, commonly referred to as *sexual intercourse* (a more general term), is the shared sexual behavior that is considered most appealing, most acceptable, and most common among heterosexuals. One large survey in the 1990s found that 95 percent of heterosexual men and women of all ages rated vaginal intercourse as either very or somewhat appealing (Michael et al., 1994). Studies of college students reveal that a greater number have experienced intercourse than masturbation or oral sex. Depending on the particular study, 73 to 93 percent of college women and 87 to 97 percent of college men say they have had sexual intercourse (Davidson & Moore, 1994; Hsu et al., 1994; Kelly, 2001; Reinholtz & Muehlenhard, 1995). Among all young adults between age 15 and 24, some 60 percent report having had intercourse (Hoff et al., 2003).

When discussing coitus, three issues appear to be of greatest interest to researchers and people in general. The first involves the various positions for intercourse and the pros and cons of each. The second relates to duration and frequency of intercourse (probably so that people can compare averages with their own duration and frequency). And the third focuses on intercourse and female orgasm.

Positions for Coitus

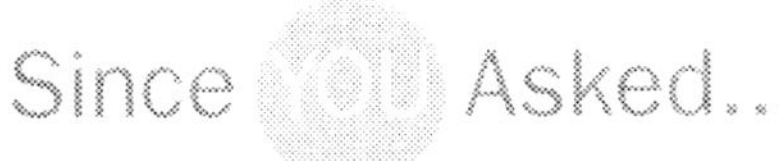

8. What is the best position for intercourse?

How many positions for coitus are there? The easy answer is, as many as people can imagine: man on top, woman on top, side by side, facing each other, facing away from each other, sitting, standing, hanging from the chandelier, and numerous variations on each of these themes. Which position is best? This depends completely on the couple engaging in the activity. Each person and each couple are different in their preferences for coital positions. It would be impossible here to even try to discuss or picture all the possible variations. Instead, I will sketch some of the basic positions and offer a brief description of some of the advantages and disadvantages of each. As we discuss some of these, remember: Coitus in *any* position without a condom is a high-risk behavior for the transmission of STIs if one or both partners are infected.

coitus Penis-vagina intercourse.

Man on Top, Face to Face

This is the most common position in Western cultures. It is often referred to as the "missionary position," so named after the Christian missionaries who introduced the position to the people of the Polynesian Islands (see Figure 6.10). Prior to the missionaries' arrival, these island cultures traditionally practiced woman-on-top coital positions.

Pros

- Ease of insertion of penis into vagina
- Either partner can guide penis into vagina
- Good for kissing and eye contact
- Woman can touch and stroke man's body, buttocks, scrotum
- Wide variation of leg positions for woman
- Man feels dominant (often an expectation in Western cultures)

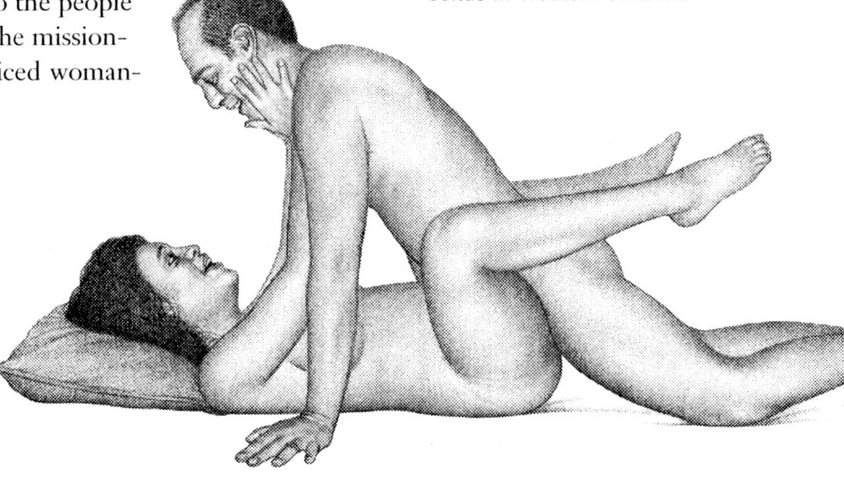

FIGURE 6.10 Man-on-Top Coital Position

The man-on-top position requires somewhat more physical effort on the part of the male; it is the most common position for coitus in Western cultures.

Cons

- Difficult for man to caress woman's body
- Difficult for clitoral stimulation by man
- Only moderate clitoral stimulation from thrusting
- Highly stimulating for man, less control over ejaculation
- May be tiring for man to support weight on arms and legs
- May be too much weight on woman
- Woman may feel too passive and submissive

Woman on Top, Face to Face

Most people are surprised to learn that the woman-on-top or **female-superior position** is the most common position for coitus throughout the world (see Figure 6.11). People use many variations of the female-superior position; usually the woman is kneeling or squatting over the man, but she may also lie down on him. By the way, the expression "female-superior" does not imply anything about power or sex roles; it simply means "woman above." The man-on-top position is preferred primarily in Western cultures.

Pros

- Woman has more control over angle of penetration, movement, and angle and speed of thrusting
- Usually considered best position for woman's orgasm
- Partners may caress each other's body
- Either partner may stimulate clitoris during intercourse
- Man can stimulate woman's breasts manually or orally
- Less physically stimulating for male; easier to control ejaculation
- Woman feels more active and in charge both physically and psychologically (which may be desirable for some women and men)

female-superior position A position for heterosexual intercourse in which the woman is sitting on or crouching over the male; this is the most common intercourse position throughout the world.

Cons

- Difficult for man to thrust with hips
- Some men (and some women) feel man is too passive in this position
- Less stimulation for man if he has difficulty reaching orgasm

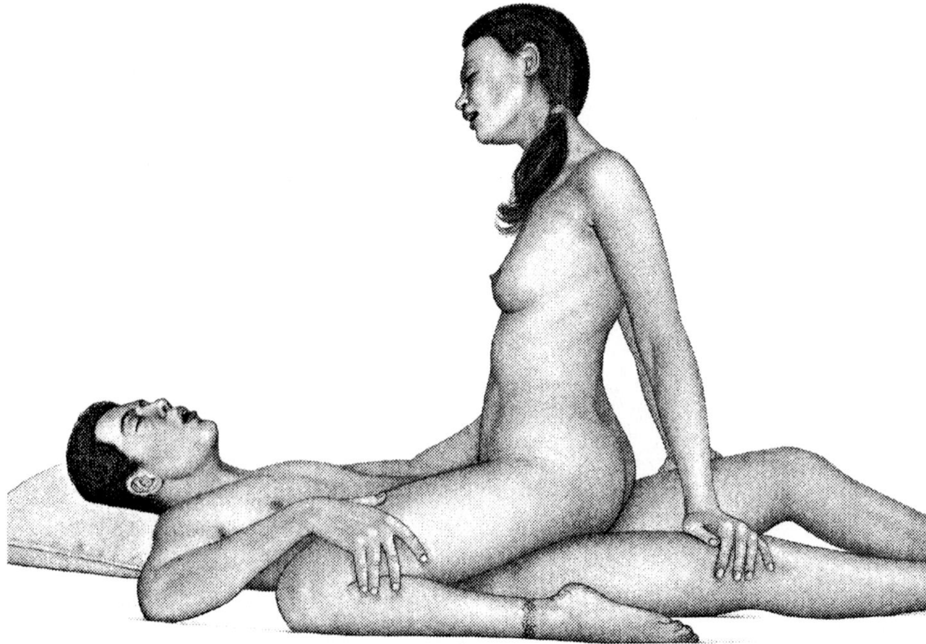

FIGURE 6.11 Woman-on-Top Coital Position

The female-superior position allows the woman more control over angle and depth of penetration and the man greater control over his orgasm.

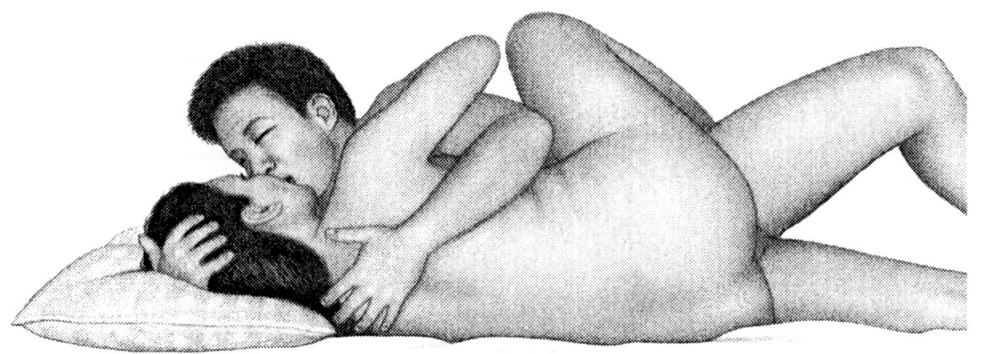

FIGURE 6.12 Side-by-Side Coital Position

The side-by-side position requires less physical effort for both partners and allows more freedom of movement for mutual caressing during intercourse.

Side by Side, Face to Face

In this position, both partners lie on their side, facing each other with their legs intertwined (see Figure 6.12). Insertion of the penis into the vagina can sometimes be difficult in this position, so some couples will begin intercourse in another position and roll into a side-by-side posture.

Pros

- Neither partner is supporting own or other's weight
- Not physically demanding
- Good for extended coitus
- Shallower penetration
- Caressing is easy with free (top) arm
- Easy to control movements; good for controlling ejaculation
- Less hot and sweaty in warm temperatures

Cons

- Difficult to insert penis into vagina
- Shallower penetration
- Difficult clitoral stimulation
- Chance of penis slipping out of vagina during thrusting
- More difficult position for exuberant thrusting
- Arms underneath may fall asleep

rear-entry position: A position for heterosexual intercourse in which the penis is inserted into the vagina while the man is behind the woman.

Rear Entry

In the **rear-entry position**, the penis is inserted into the vagina from behind the woman (see Figure 6.13). Regardless of similarities in appearance, this coital position should not be confused with anal intercourse. Several variations on the position may be used, including lying side by side, front to rear ("like spoons"); sitting with the woman in the man's lap, facing away; or the woman kneeling and the man behind her (often called "doggy style").

Pros

- Deeper penetration of penis in vagina possible
- Man may reach around woman for breast or clitoral stimulation
- Woman may reach back to stimulate man's scrotum
- Some men and women report different and enjoyable feelings of stimulation
- Good position during pregnancy

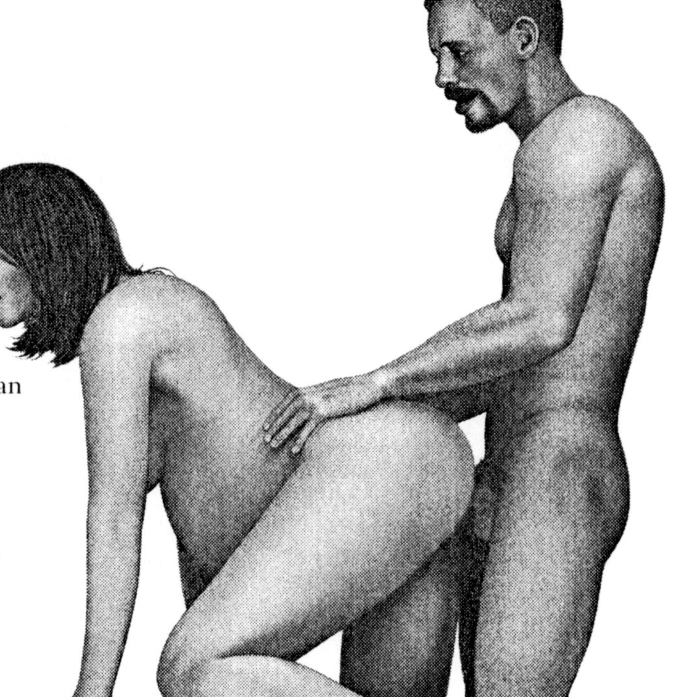

FIGURE 6.13 Rear-Entry Coital Position

Some people enjoy the sensations provided by the rear-entry position; it may also be more comfortable if the woman is pregnant.

Cons

- Penetration may be uncomfortably deep
- Kissing and eye contact difficult
- Lack of face-to-face contact may feel too impersonal
- For some, association with animals may be a turnoff
- For some, association with anal intercourse may be a turnoff

Frequency and Duration of Coitus

Since YOU Asked...

9. Is it abnormal to have intercourse four or five times a day with a partner whom you have been seeing for a long time?

In the 1940s and 1950s, Alfred Kinsey's surveys (see Chapter 1) revealed that the average number of times married couples reported having intercourse (coitus) was 2.8 times per week (for those in their 20s). Suddenly, nearly everybody in the country had a "yardstick" with which to compare their own sex lives. And since 2.8 was an *average*, most people saw themselves as "abnormal": "Oh, no! We're sex fiends, honey! We do it twice a day!" or "Something must be wrong with our marriage, dear. We only do it once a week." The National Health and Social Life Survey (Laumann et al., 1994; Michael et al., 1994) and an annual survey conducted by the Durex condom company (2003), provided people in countries around the world with some newer averages to ponder, such as an annual intercourse frequency average of 118 in the United States compared to 152 in Hungary (see Tables 6.7 and 6.8).

Such statistics are interesting to know, but they really should not be taken too seriously by most couples. The *ideal* frequency of sexual intercourse (or any sexual activity) is as often as feels good and comfortable to each individual and couple. One couple might have intercourse twice a day or more and another once a month or less; as long as they are happy with their sexual life together, that is their "normal" frequency. Furthermore, a couple's frequency of sexual encounters is unlikely to be very stable over time. Depending on stress, fatigue, illness, presence or absence of kids, vacations, and so on, some days, weeks, months, or years are likely to be more sexually active than others, and sometimes this variation can be large.

What about duration of coitus? How long should intercourse last? This is another question that each couple must answer for themselves. For some couples, a fast, super-

Table 6.7 FREQUENCY OF COITUS IN THE UNITED STATES

AGE	NOT AT ALL IN THE PAST YEAR (%)	A FEW TIMES IN THE PAST YEAR (%)	A FEW TIMES A MONTH (%)	TWO OR THREE TIMES A WEEK (%)	FOUR OR MORE TIMES A WEEK (%)
MEN					
18–24	15	21	24	28	12
25–29	7	15	31	36	11
30–39	8	15	37	33	6
40–49	9	18	40	27	6
50–59	11	22	43	20	3
WOMEN					
18–24	11	16	32	29	12
25–29	5	10	38	37	10
30–39	9	16	36	33	6
40–49	15	16	44	20	5
50–59	30	22	35	12	2

Source: Table 8, p. 116 from *Sex in America* by R. Michael, J. Gagnon, E. Laumann, & G. Kolata.

Table 6.8 ESTIMATE OF AVERAGE ANNUAL FREQUENCY OF COITUS IN SELECTED COUNTRIES, 2003

Total	127	Austria	123
Hungary	152	South Africa	123
Bulgaria	151	Spain	123
Russian Federation	150	Germany	120
Serbia/Montenegro	147	Netherlands	120
Croatia	144	Canada	119
Czech Republic	144	Italy	119
France	144	United States	118
India	138	Denmark	114
Belgium	136	Finland	114
Iceland	136	Taiwan	113
United Kingdom	135	Thailand	105
China	132	Vietnam	104
Slovakia	131	Hong Kong	103
New Zealand	130	Sweden	102
Poland	126	Malaysia	100
Australia	125	Singapore	96
Norway	124		

Source: Durex Corp. (2003).

ficial, lovemaking session (commonly known as a "quickie) is perfectly fine with both of them, while another couple might feel cheated if sex is less than a half-day production. Most couples who are comfortable and happy with their sexual life find that duration of lovemaking varies from one time to the next, depending on many of the same issues that influence frequency. Of course, lovemaking usually includes behaviors other than coitus itself, and the entirety of the experience is important to most people. Laumann and colleagues (1994) found that about 70 percent of men and women reported that their last lovemaking (referred to in the survey as a "sexual event," meaning the entire lovemaking session, not just coitus) lasted from 15 minutes to an hour, and 20 percent of men and 15 percent of women said it lasted an hour or more. Only 11 percent of men and 15 percent of women said that their most recent sexual event was less than 15 minutes. In terms of intercourse itself, researchers have found that the length of time of actual penile-vagina thrusting varies from approximately 2 to 7 minutes (Patrick et al., 2005).

Coitus and Orgasm

As was discussed in Chapter 3, virtually all men will routinely experience orgasm through the act of coitus itself. However, most women do not. This is due primarily to the stimulation that is produced by the thrusting of the penis in the vagina. The glans of the penis is surrounded by the vaginal walls and usually receives more than adequate stimulation for orgasm. In fact, many men report that intercourse provides *too much* stimulation, causing them to reach orgasm and ejaculate sooner than they would like (see Chapter 7, "Sexual Problems and Solutions," for a discussion of this). However, for the woman, this thrusting by itself may not provide much stimulation to the clitoris, especially as the clitoris retracts during the plateau phase (see Chapter 3). For most women, this makes

anal intercourse A sexual position in which the penis is inserted through the partner's anus into the rectum.

anilingus Oral stimulation of the anus.

orgasm difficult if not impossible to achieve from intercourse alone. Although the duration of intercourse is related to reaching orgasm for some women, at least half of all women (some research reports the number is as high as 75 percent) do not experience orgasm from coitus *regardless of the duration of thrusting* (Hite, 1976; Laumann et al., 1994; Reinisch, 1990; Singh et al., 1998; Slob, van Berkel, & vander Werff ten Bosch, 2000).

Although the majority of women do not routinely reach orgasm during coitus, many men and women believe that a woman *should* achieve orgasm with penile thrusting alone, and this perception can lead to problems in the relationship. Once a couple understands the facts about female orgasm and intercourse, the "problem" is easily solved. For women who do not receive the stimulation during coitus that they need and want for orgasm, additional stimulation to the clitoral area can be provided through touching or oral sex before or after coitus or with manual stimulation during intercourse. Using these techniques, virtually all women are able to experience orgasm as part of lovemaking if they so desire.

Anal Stimulation

Anal stimulation, which includes **anal intercourse**, manual stimulation of the anal area, and oral-anal stimulation (**anilingus**), is the least common of the sexual activities discussed in this chapter. A widespread belief among heterosexuals is that anal sex is practiced primarily by gay men and that all gay men engage in anal intercourse. However, the incidence of anal sexual behavior among heterosexual couples is significantly higher than most people would expect. Between 15 and 30 percent of heterosexual men and women report experience with anal intercourse (Billy et al., 1993; Flannery et al., 2003; Laumann et al., 1994; Reinisch, 1990). Among college students, 15 to 20 percent report experiencing anal intercourse, and over 50 percent have engaged in caressing of the anus (Hsu et al., 1994; Flannery & Ellingson, 2003). To further debunk the myths about anal sex, not all gay men engage in anal intercourse with their partners. Studies have shown that between 10 and 40 percent of gay men do not include anal intercourse in their lovemaking activities, and that percentage increased dramatically during the 1980s and early 1990s due the gay community's awareness of the high risk of HIV transmission from anal intercourse (Goldbaum, Yu, & Wood, 1996; Voeller, 1991). However, during the late 1990s and early 2000s, public health officials were reporting a troubling increase in the number of gay men in the United States who were returning to the highly risky practice of unprotected anal intercourse (Halkitis, Parsons, & Wilton, 2003).

Some people feel that the anus is dirty or unappealing, and to include it in sexual behavior seems to them unpleasant or simply wrong. However, the tissues of the anus and rectum are very sensitive, and many people find stimulation of these areas pleasurable (see Figure 6.14). Anal erotic activities may include touching or massaging the outer anal area, insertion of a finger into the anus, kissing or licking the anus (anilingus), or anal intercourse. For some people, anal stimulation, especially when accompanied by stimulation of the penis or clitoris, may lead to intense orgasms. However, anal sexual activities involve some unique health risks that must not be overlooked.

Cautions Regarding Anal Intercourse

Unprotected anal intercourse is the *highest-risk sexual behavior* for the transmission of virtually all STIs, including HIV, hepatitis B, and human papilloma virus (which may cause anal cancer) if the inserting partner is infected. This is due to the fact that the lining of the rectum is thin and fragile, without the elastic qualities of the vagina. Also unlike the vagina, the anus and rectum do not produce any natural lubrication upon sexual arousal. Therefore, a high likelihood exists of damage to rectal walls (small tears, abrasions, or fissures), allowing direct

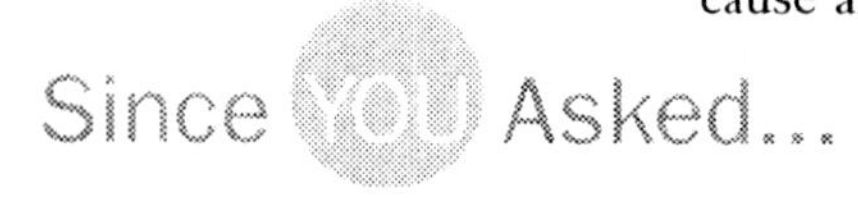

10. Is there anything wrong with anal sex?

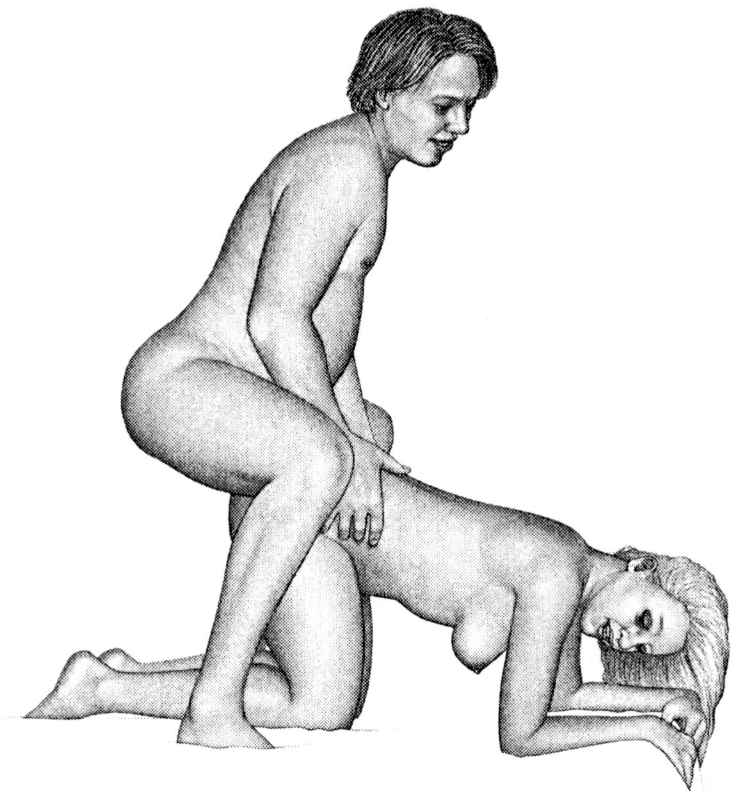

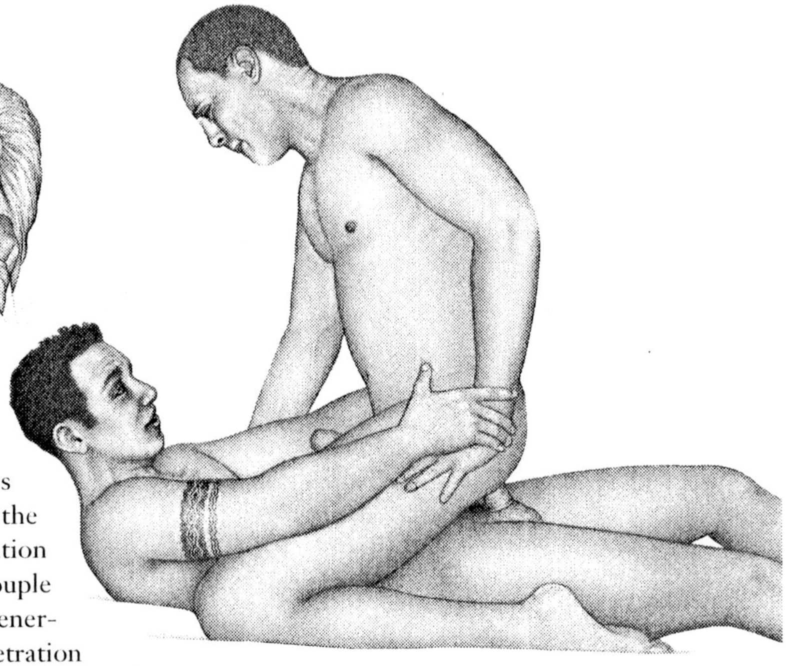

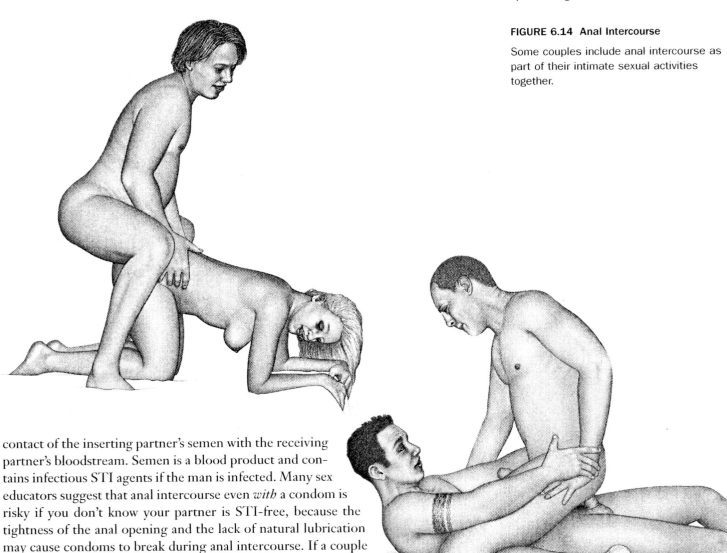

FIGURE 6.14 Anal Intercourse

Some couples include anal intercourse as part of their intimate sexual activities together.

contact of the inserting partner's semen with the receiving partner's bloodstream. Semen is a blood product and contains infectious STI agents if the man is infected. Many sex educators suggest that anal intercourse even *with* a condom is risky if you don't know your partner is STI-free, because the tightness of the anal opening and the lack of natural lubrication may cause condoms to break during anal intercourse. If a couple who are free of STIs wishes to engage in anal intercourse, generous amounts of artificial lubricant should be used and penetration should be done very slowly and carefully. Some evidence suggests that frequent anal intercourse over time may lead to large and painful anal fissures, hemorrhoids, and potential weakening of the anal sphincter muscles.

Finally, if the normally harmless bacteria in the anus and rectum are somehow transferred to the urethra (in men or women), the vagina, or the vulva, they can cause vaginal, reproductive, and urinary tract infections. Therefore, it is extremely important that if a couple have engaged in anal stimulation or anal intercourse, they should carefully avoid any vaginal stimulation or intercourse until the hand, mouth, or penis has been washed or the condom has been changed.

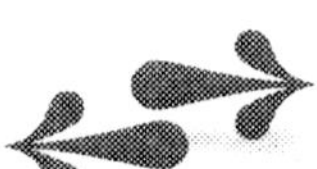

YOUR SEXUAL PHILOSOPHY

SEXUAL BEHAVIORS: EXPERIENCING SEXUAL PLEASURE

The information in this chapter has offered you the knowledge you need for an enhanced appreciation for the range of behaviors available for experiencing and sharing sexual pleasure, expressing your sexual desires, and conveying feelings of closeness, intimacy, and love between two people. A clear understanding of these activities is crucial when faced with sexual choices and decisions people must make throughout their lives.

Without a foundation for making sound choices that are right for you, these usually pleasurable activities can sometimes become uncomfortable, frightening, and even dangerous.

This might be a good time to stop again and consider how all this information might fit into your sexual philosophy. Think for a moment about the sexual choices you have made up to this point in your life. Do you feel comfortable with your sexual decisions? Have you made mistakes? Do you have regrets? Do you feel guilty or ashamed? Would you change anything if you could? Next, consider the sexual choices you are making now and may make in the future.

The decisions you make about sex (or anything else, for that matter) throughout your life should be based on applying the sum of your experience, knowledge, and past and present feelings. Exploring who you are sexually and what path you want your sexual life to take allows you to make clear choices that feel right to you when the time to act on those decisions arrives. To clarify your personal feelings about the behaviors discussed in this chapter, ask yourself the following questions:

1. Is this behavior something I want to do and would feel comfortable and positive about doing?
2. What sort of relationship with a partner do I need in order to feel comfortable sharing this activity (casual, monogamous, marriage)?
3. What if my partner wants to do something that makes me uncomfortable? Will I agree anyway? If so, why? If not, how will I handle the situation if my partner continues to pressure me?
4. If the behavior involves the risk of STIs or unwanted pregnancy, how will I be sure I am protected?
5. Will I be able to discuss my feelings about this activity with my partner?

This kind of self-exploration provides you with opportunities to place the many aspects of human sexual behavior into the context of your personal life and gain valuable insights into yourself as a sexual being now and in the future. Remember, your sexual philosophy is about discovering who you are, knowing what you want and don't want, and planning ahead. The information in this chapter, perhaps more than any other in this book, plays a crucial role in the development of your personal sexual philosophy so that you can take charge of your sexual life, rather than having it take charge of you.

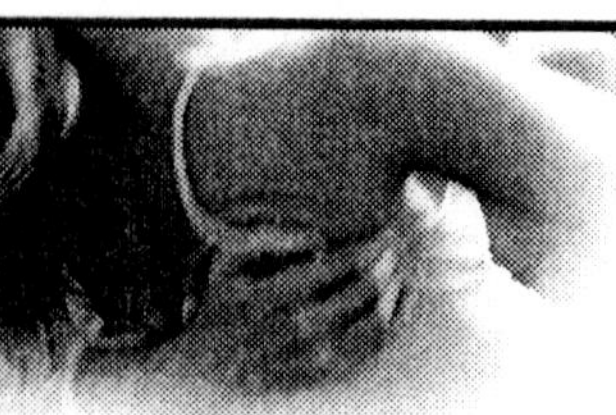

Summary

HISTORICAL PERSPECTIVES Masturbation Will Be the Death of You . . .

- Historically, masturbation was regarded as an unhealthy, immoral activity that could lead to serious health consequences and even death. Today, most health professionals and sexuality educators view masturbation as a normal, healthy sexual activity; it is sometimes incorporated into therapy for certain sexual problems.

Your Sexual Comfort Zone

- The erotophobia-erotophilia scale predicts one's sexual comfort zone. It measures a person's level of ease in learning and talking about sexual issues.
- The erotophobia-erotophilia scale may also predict how likely people are to use contraceptives and to engage in risky sexual behaviors.

Solitary and Shared Sexual Behaviors

- The sexual activities covered in this chapter are engaged in by a majority or large minority of people. These behaviors would not be considered strange or deviant by most people in our culture.

Sexual Fantasy

- Sexual fantasy is by far the most common sexual "behavior." Estimates are that 95 percent of people have engaged in

sexual fantasy. Sexual fantasies may occur as daydreams, while masturbating, or during sex with a partner. Although sexual fantasy has many useful functions, it can create guilt in some people and in a small percentage of people become obsessive.
- Some sexual fantasies, such as sex in unusual locations and positions, are equally common among men and women; others, such as having sex with two partners at once or with a mysterious stranger, show significant differences between the sexes. For some couples, sharing sexual fantasies may enhance their intimate relationship.

Masturbation

- Masturbation, contrary to old beliefs, is a common behavior. It does not cause hairy palms, genital cancer, sterility, blindness, or a decrease in enjoyment of sex with a partner.
- Masturbation has been found to have many health benefits. For example, research has found that people who masturbate while in an intimate relationship have more active and more satisfying sex lives with their partner.

Erotic Touch

- Erotic touching is an enjoyable sexual behavior in itself and need not always lead to intercourse.
- Individual preferences for where and how to be touched vary greatly. In general, the breasts and nipples are sexually sensitive areas for women *and* men. Genital touching can be a safe source of great pleasure, intimacy, and sexual satisfaction and does not necessarily lead to other less safe sexual activities.

Oral Sex

- While most people find oral sex to be an appealing, intimate behavior, some find the activities involved to be morally wrong or physically offensive.
- Oral contact may spread most sexually transmitted infections.

Coitus

- Coitus, defined as penile-vaginal intercourse, is the only strictly heterosexual sexual behavior. All other sexual activities may be engaged in by straight, gay, lesbian, or bisexual individuals. The man-on-top coital position is most common in Western cultures, but the woman-on-top position is the most common elsewhere in the world. Various coital positions have specific advantages and disadvantages.
- The movements of coitus typically do not, in themselves, provide adequate stimulation for most women to reach orgasm routinely through intercourse without additional stimulation, usually of the clitoral area.

Anal Stimulation

- Anal sex among heterosexual couples is more frequent than is commonly believed. Among gay male couples, it is less frequent than is commonly believed.
- Unprotected anal intercourse has the highest risk of transmission of HIV and other sexually transmitted infections of all sexual behaviors.

YOUR SEXUAL PHILOSOPHY: Sexual Behaviors: Experiencing Sexual Pleasure

- Understanding the full range of sexual activities available to humans in intimate relationships enhances one's ability to experience and share sexual pleasure, express sexual desires, and convey feelings of closeness, intimacy, and love with another individual.

Have You Considered?

1. Assume for a moment you are in a sexually active relationship with someone you love deeply and with whom you are hoping to spend the rest of your life. One evening, your partner expresses a desire to engage in a sexual activity that you are not interested in and that you find somewhat offensive (you pick the activity). How would you react? Explain what you think would be the best way to handle this situation in your relationship.
2. Suppose that a heterosexual couple are feeling a strong mutual desire to be sexually intimate, but they've agreed that intercourse (coitus) should be saved for marriage. Explain how they might balance their desire for sexual intimacy with their moral convictions regarding sex and marriage.
3. Imagine for a moment that you have a 14-year-old daughter and you are discussing sexual issues with her. What would you want her to know and understand about the behaviors discussed in this chapter? Explain your answer.
4. Now imagine for a moment that you have a 14-year-old son and you are discussing sexual issues with him. What would you want him to know and understand about the behaviors discussed in this chapter? Explain your answer. Were your answers different for a daughter and a son? Why or why not?
5. Consider a situation in which sexual partners are discussing experimenting with various sexual positions. Explain why some couples might find the various positions appealing while others might reject some of them.
6. Discuss the influences or experiences from childhood or teen years that you feel often shape people's adult feelings and attitudes toward sexual activities.

Companion Website Resources

For further chapter resources go to **www.prenhall.com/hock.** This robust text website includes polling questions for you to vote on, regular news updates, quizzes, sample tests, suggested reading lists, and more.

SCENARIOS USA Also on the website are links to videos. *Scenarios USA*'s films portray real-life narratives that explore the non-biological aspects of relationships and sexual health. The films will help you consider how the themes of the text affect your own life and the lives of those around you.

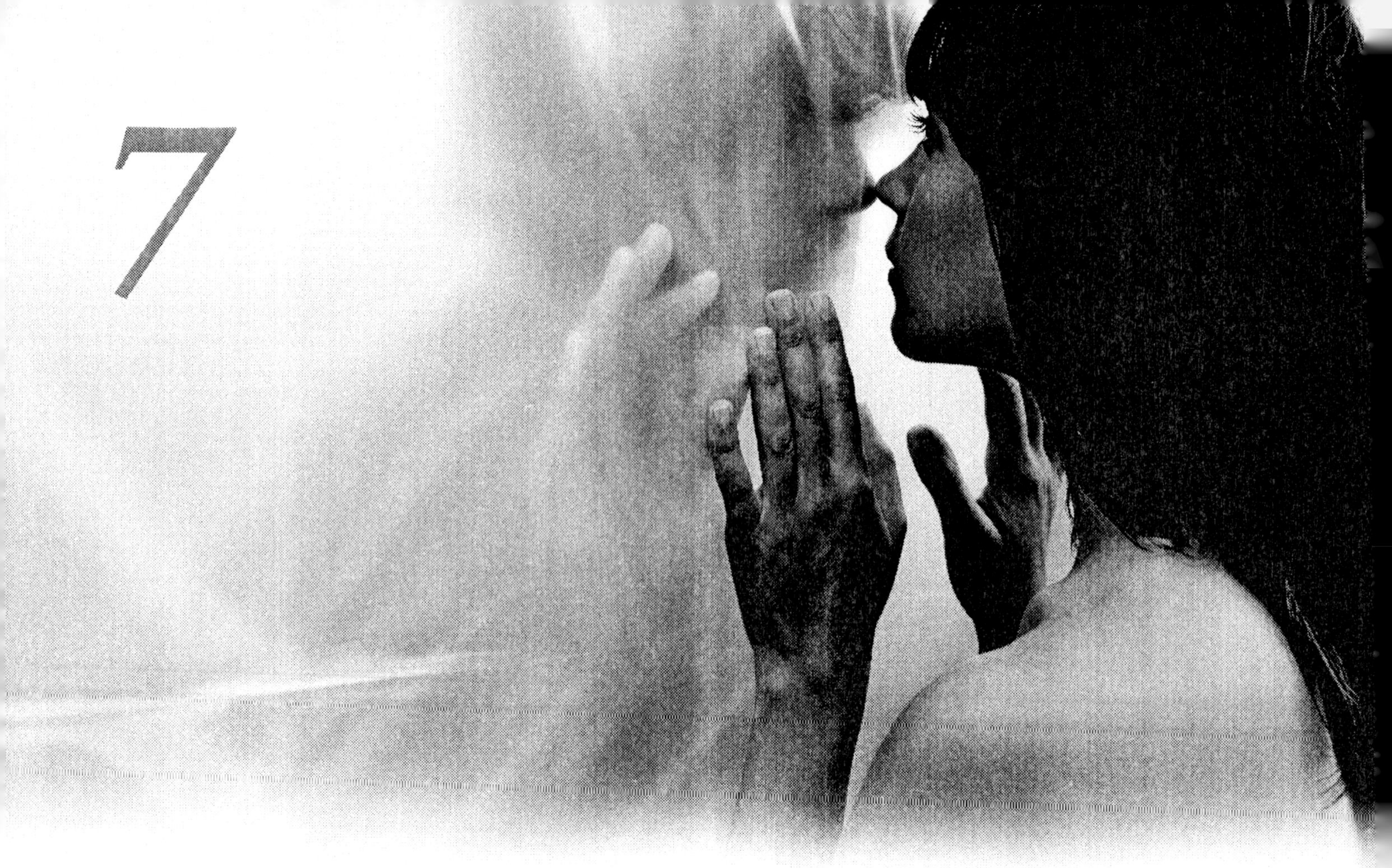

7

Sexual Problems and Solutions

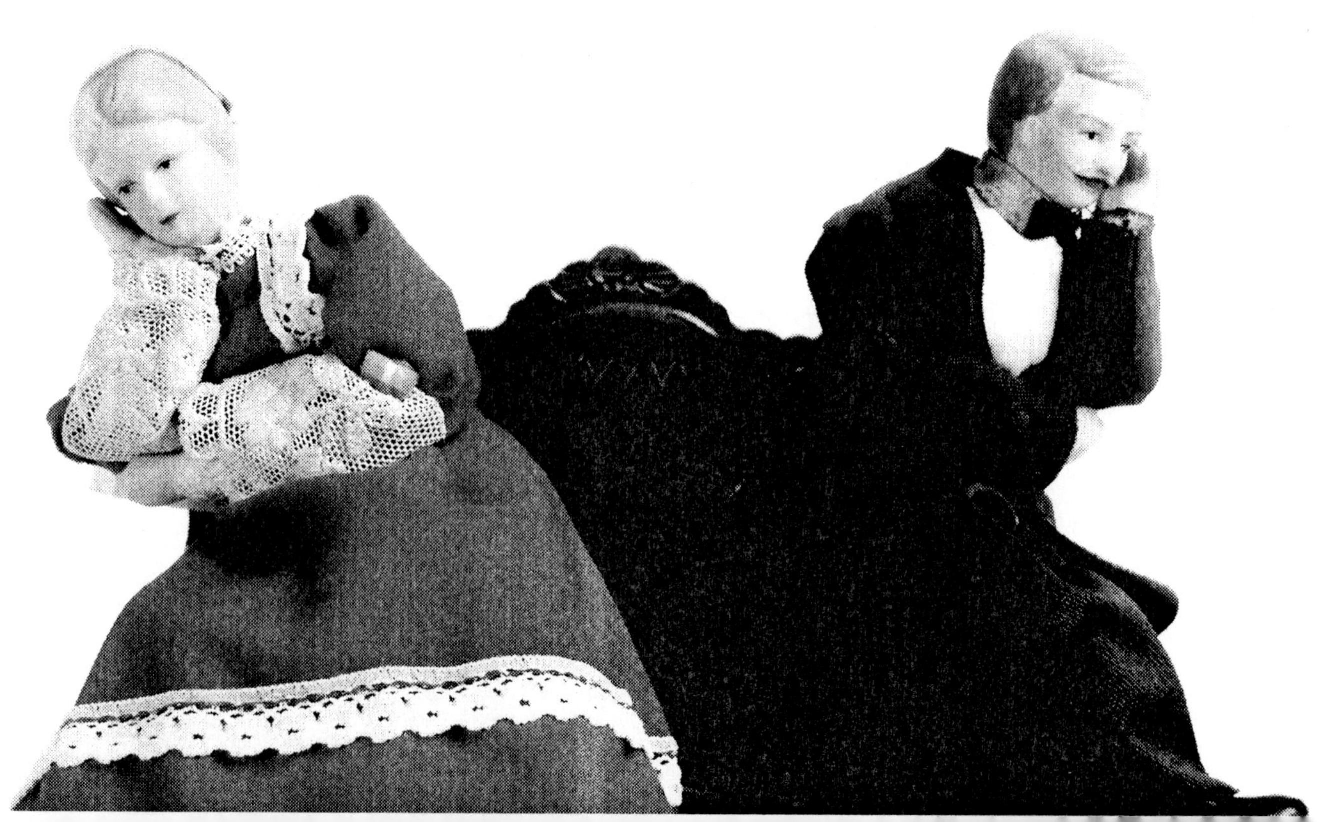

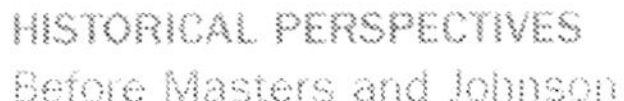

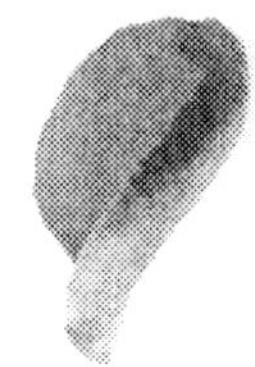

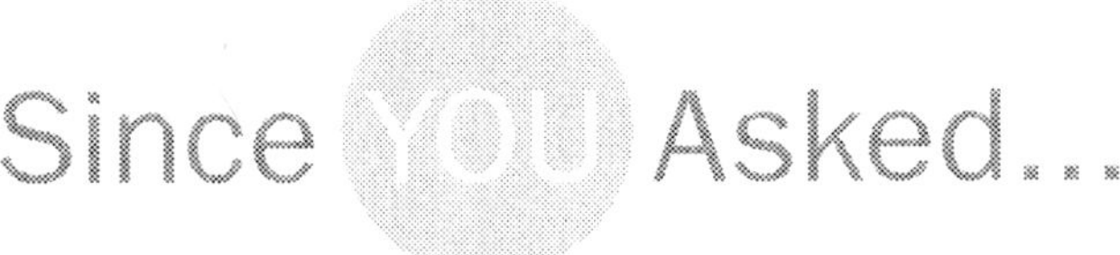

Since YOU Asked...

1. What is "bad" sex? How do you know if you are doing it right? (see page 230)

2. My girlfriend is from India. We've been together for nearly a year, but she doesn't seem interested in sex at all. Could this be due to growing up in a different culture, or is it something in our relationship? (see page 240)

3. How can a couple who have been together for a long time (married three years) get their sexual feelings back? We have a good relationship, but we hardly ever make love anymore. (see page 241)

4. I'm a male and I'm curious if it is odd that I have never masturbated. Is masturbation healthy? (see page 243)

5. I can't tell if my partner is satisfied or not when we make love. What are the signs that a person is sexually satisfied? (see page 244)

6. I want to have sex four or five times a week, but my boyfriend would be happy with once a week or less. What can I do to get him more interested in sex? (see page 246)

7. Is impotence always psychological? Does Viagra work for everyone? (see page 250)

8. What causes a woman to be unable to experience orgasm during sexual intercourse even though she can have an orgasm during oral sex? Is it a physical thing or mental? Maybe both? (see page 258)

9. Are there ways for a guy to control orgasm and last longer? (see page 260)

10. How can a woman get past the step of intercourse hurting her even when she's doing it with someone she loves? What can she do to help relieve the pain? (see page 264)

Most people assume that sex is a *natural* act, and it follows from this assumption that sexual behaviors and responses should occur *naturally*—that the mind and body should do what they are programmed "by nature" to do whenever they are supposed to do it. After all, that is how sex works for nonhuman animals, right? Well, yes, more or less; however, for humans, sex is *not* a natural act, at least, not entirely (Tiefer, 2004).

Our abilities to think and feel add layer upon layer to the human sexual experience until it resembles that of nonhuman animals hardly at all. In other words, humans have an intellectual and emotional investment in virtually everything sexual. This investment, on the one hand, infuses people's sexual interactions with immense joy and passion, while on the other, it can create psychological insecurities, doubts, or other negative perceptions that may lead to sexual problems. As you will see in this chapter, such problems, and the emotions surrounding them, are more common than most people think.

You may have noticed that this chapter focuses on "sexual problems" rather than "sexual disorders" or "sexual dysfunctions." The reason for this word choice is that nearly all sexual problems are readily treatable, and with very few exceptions, no one should have to endure chronic, long-term sexual difficulties. Words such as *disorder* and *dysfunction* imply that these conditions are more serious and much less likely to respond to treatment. Sometimes the words themselves can discourage individuals from seeking the help they need to solve whatever problems they are facing. Nevertheless, you might see words such as *disorder* or *dysfunction* used occasionally in this chapter because they may be incorporated into formal psychological or medical diagnoses for specific sexual problems. However, they are just words, and you should not be put off by them. As the title of this chapter suggests, sexual problems are no different from most other difficulties in life, and although they may be emotionally or physically painful, they all have solutions.

That said, sexual problems seldom confine themselves to the bedroom. They have a persistent tendency to intertwine with other aspects of the relationship and with each partner's contentment with life in general. Determining which came first, the sexual problem that led to the relationship issues or other nonsexual conflicts that affected the couple's sexual connection, is important and often difficult. Regardless, the bottom line is that sexual and relationship problems nearly always go together. This, then, often causes the couple to feel an increased sense of concern and urgency to solve the problem.

This chapter will examine many facets of sexual problems and their solutions, starting with how common sexual difficulties are and how to know whether you have a sexual problem. We will then move on to how sexual problems can be evaluated and classified in ways that allow them to be understood as clearly as possible. Once we have a clear understanding of a particular sexual problem, we can better pinpoint the possible causes that led up to the condition. Then, with a clear understanding of the problem and its possible causes, we will be in the best position to discuss treatments and solutions to specific sexual problems and methods to enhance sexual enjoyment and satisfaction in general.

Focus on Your Feelings

For some people, the topics covered in this chapter evoke intense emotions. Sexual feelings and responses are closely linked to our expectations about sex. Most people *expect* sex to work correctly and feel good. They *expect* their bodies to do what they are supposed to do during sexual activities. They *expect* that they and their partners will be sexually satisfied and content. When expectations are not met, people have a tendency to react with stronger than usual emotions. When your sexual expectations are not met, when your body or your partner's body does not "behave" the way it "should," you are likely to become emotional about it in one way or another.

What emotions are you likely to feel? Almost anything except happiness. You might be disappointed in yourself or worried that you have disappointed your partner. You might feel embarrassed because, well, sexual problems are embarrassing! You might feel afraid because you are unsure what is wrong with you and how long it's likely to last. You might be frustrated because you really want to enjoy sexual intimacy with your partner and this is getting in the way of that. You might feel guilt over the frustration you perceive in your partner. You might experience anger—at yourself, at your body, at your partner, or at the world in general for the unfairness of it all.

Becoming educated about sexual problems and their solutions *before* they occur (or before the next one occurs) is the key to minimizing the intensity and duration of your potential negative feelings. When they do occur, with your emotions in check, you will be able to think rationally about your problem and take the necessary steps to find a satisfying solution. Moreover, worrying less about these problems goes a long way toward helping you resolve them.

Before we begin our journey through the field of sexual problems and solutions, let's place them into a historical frame by looking back to a time when sexual problems were, for the most part, invisible. It wasn't that these problems did not exist or that people did not suffer from them. The difference was that people typically did not talk about or acknowledge them to their partners or even to themselves, much less to anyone else, such as their doctor or a therapist. Furthermore, people saw little point in discussing such private matters because nobody really knew very much about how to treat them. If this sounds like ancient history to you, it isn't; we only have to go back about 40 years.

Historical Perspectives

Before Masters and Johnson

A careful examination of the history of sexual dysfunction prior to the 1960s reveals little published literature and a quagmire of myths and faulty information. Prior to Masters and Johnson's pioneering research into the physiology of sexual response (discussed in greater detail in Chapter 3, "The Physiology of Human Sexual Responding"), most sexual difficulties were attributed, depending on how far into the past we want to go, to anything from demonic possession to the Freudian notion of unresolved, unconscious childhood conflicts stemming from poor parenting practices (Weiderman, 1998). Based on these old models of sexual problems, most attempts at helping people overcome them generally met with poor success, due in large measure to the difficulty of understanding and treating sexual problems without the benefit of a road map of human sexual anatomy, physiology, and response.

The work of William Masters and Virginia Johnson in the early 1960s revolutionized our understanding of human sexual anatomy and sexual responding. They revealed, for example, how erection of the penis and clitoris prepare the body for sexual interactions and what types of stimulation produce (or fail to produce) sexual excitement and orgasm. But the goals of their careful laboratory observations of human sexual response, far beyond simply describing sexual structures and their functions during sexual activity, were to help couples and therapists apply that knowledge to solve sexual problems and to enhance people's sexual lives (Masters & Johnson, 1970). Although some flaws and errors in Masters and Johnson's early work have been pointed out over the decades since they first published their findings, they clearly accomplished the goal of bringing sexual problems and solutions into the open, offering people solutions and hope.

The insights from the sex laboratories of Masters and Johnson awakened a new era of treatment methods for sexual dysfunctions (Annon, 1974; Kaplan, 1974). As you will see in this chapter, today's successful treatments of sexual difficulties rely heavily on an *interaction* of psychological and physical factors. Prior to the work of Masters and Johnson, the overall ineffectiveness of the approaches to treating sexual difficulties led to a widespread belief that such problems and conditions must be endured in silence. Today, thanks to the work of Masters and Johnson and the many advances in psychological and biomedical sciences that have followed their work, most sexual problems are relatively easy to treat and cure.

What Is a Sexual Problem?

Probably the best response to the question "Do I have a sexual problem?" is another question: "Do *you* think you do?" Although this may seem like a frivolous response, it is not, because most sexual problems are self-diagnosed. This means that sexual problems are to a large degree a matter of the extent to which individuals or

Table 7.1 CATEGORIES OF SEXUAL PROBLEMS

CATEGORY	PROBLEM	PERSISTENT OR RECURRENT SYMPTOMS
		MALE
Desire	Hypoactive sexual desire	Few or no sexual fantasies and little or no desire for sexual activity
Arousal	Erectile problems (erectile disorder)	Inability to attain or maintain an adequate erection during sexual activity
Orgasm	Rapid (premature) ejaculation	Ejaculation with minimal sexual stimulation before, upon, or shortly after penetration
	Delayed ejaculation (uncommon)	Delay or lack of orgasm and ejaculation regardless of amount or degree of sexual stimulation
Sexual pain	Dyspareunia (rare)	Genital pain associated with sexual intercourse
		FEMALE
Desire	Hypoactive sexual desire	Few or no sexual fantasies and little or no desire for sexual activity
	Sexual aversion	Extreme dislike and avoidance of genital contact with a partner
Arousal	Inhibited sexual arousal	Inability to attain or maintain adequate sexual excitement (i.e., lubrication, engorgement of genitals) during sexual activity
Orgasm	Inhibited orgasm	Delay or lack of orgasm regardless of amount or degree of sexual stimulation
Sexual pain	Dyspareunia	Genital pain associated with sexual intercourse
	Vaginismus (uncommon)	Painful, involuntary spasm of the musculature of the outer third of the vagina that interferes with vaginal penetration

couples perceive that a problem exists. That said, sexuality educators and clinicians usually divide sexual problems into four categories: sexual desire disorders, sexual arousal disorders, orgasm disorders, and sexual pain disorders (see Table 7.1). Each of these will be discussed in turn later in this chapter. However, the existence of any of these problems depends largely on each individual's or couple's subjective analysis of their sexual experience. In other words, one person's sexual problem may be another's perfectly satisfactory sexual life. For example, imagine a couple who have been happily married for several years and make love once every couple of months. Would you assume that they have a sexual problem? Or consider a man who makes love with his partner several times a week but is able to achieve an erection only once or twice a month. Does he have a sexual problem? How about the couple in which one partner always experiences an orgasm during their lovemaking but the other never does. Is this a sexual problem?

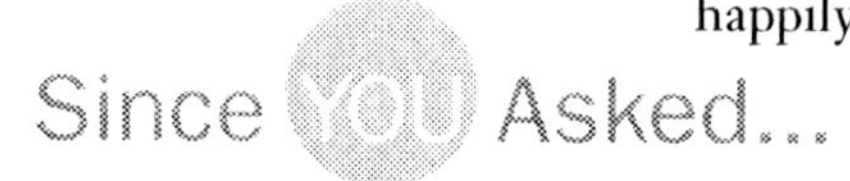

1. What is "bad" sex? How do you know if you are doing it right?

You get the idea. If you are like most people, you may have found yourself surprised by these couples' situations, but you stopped short of assuming that they were experiencing sexual problems. You probably thought something along the lines of "It depends. If they feel happy and satisfied with their sexual lives, then these are probably not sexual problems *for them*." But if infrequent lovemaking, problems with erections, lack of orgasm, or any other sexual difficulties are causing frustration, emotional pain, or relationship discord, they can probably be diagnosed as sexual problems.

Remember, however, that not everyone knows for sure if he or she is experiencing a sexual problem. It is quite common for someone to feel sexually unfulfilled but not understand why or lack an awareness of what constitutes a satisfying sexual life. For this reason, becoming knowledgeable about sexual activities and about problems that may arise in one's sexual life is important for living a healthy and satisfying sexual life.

How Common Are Sexual Problems?

Sexual problems are more common than people think. Why? Because people typically do not discuss their sexual lives, and especially their sexual difficulties, with others. When people are experiencing a sexual problem, they often assume that they are the only ones suffering from that particular difficulty. They assume that "everybody else's sex life must be just fine, but ours is in trouble!" Therefore, they keep the problem to themselves, acting as if everything is normal and suffering in silence. In the meantime, however, numerous others experiencing sexual problems are thinking the very same thing, hiding their problem, and also pretending everything is OK! Consequently, when people with a particular sexual problem observe others, everyone else does indeed appear fine, which in turn reinforces their false assumptions. This is a psychological phenomenon called *pluralistic ignorance.* In reality, if people were more open about sexual difficulties, they would find they have plenty of company, and they all would feel less isolated and anxious. Fortunately, the Internet now offers individuals and couples a safe and reasonably private mode of communication about sexual problems.

Masters and Johnson (1970) estimated that half of all married couples experience a "diagnosable" sexual problem at some point in their marriage. Other studies have found rates for various sexual problems to range from 10 to 52 percent for men and 24 to 63 percent for women (Bancroft, Loftus, & Long, 2003; Heiman, 2002; Rosen et al., 1993; Spector & Carey, 1990). A U.S. national survey conducted in the 1990s found that over the previous 12 months, the percentage of individuals who reported at least one sexual problem lasting at least one month ranged from 3 to 33 percent, depending on the particular problem and the person's sex (Laumann, Gagnon, Michael, & Michaels, 1994). Table 7.2 summarizes these findings.

Other studies have shown significant variations in the prevalence of certain sexual problems among some groups. For example, one survey of women who had recently received routine gynecological care reported the remarkable finding that nearly all (98.8 percent) of the respondents reported at least one sexual problem when the following categories were included: loss of desire, arousal difficulties, orgasm problems,

Table 7.2 PREVALENCE OF SEXUAL PROBLEMS IN THE UNITED STATES

PROBLEM	INDIVIDUALS REPORTING THE PROBLEM DURING THE PREVIOUS 12 MONTHS, ALL AGES (%)	
	Men	**Women**
Hypoactive (low) sexual desire	15.8	33.4
Erectile disorder	10.4	N.A.
Premature ejaculation	28.5	N.A.
Difficulty lubricating	N.A.	18.8
Inability to reach orgasm	8.3	24.1
Pain during sex	3.0	14.4
Performance anxiety*	17.0	11.5
No pleasure in sex*	8.1	21.2

N.A. = not applicable.

*May be the cause or the result of a sexual problem.

Source: Table, "Prevalence of Sexual Problems in the US" from *The Social Organization of Sexuality* by E. Laumann, J. Gagnon, R. Michael, and S. Michaels. Copyright © 1994. Reprinted by permission of The University of Chicago Press.

painful sex, and poor body image (Nusbaum et al., 2000). Another study found that just over 24 percent of women reported experiencing distress about their sexual relationship or their own sexual abilities (Bancroft et al., 2003). The point here is simply to demonstrate that sexual problems are very common. This is an important piece of information because when people suffering from sexual problems and understand that many others experience similar difficulties, they are more likely to seek help, find solutions, and live happier, more satisfied lives (Rosen & Laumann, 2003).

Evaluating a Sexual Problem: A Three-Dimensional Model

To understand and treat a specific sexual problem effectively, it can be helpful to consider three dimensions of the problem: its duration, its context (the settings in which the problem occurs), and its frequency in that context. These three distinct dimensions, taken together, clarify the nature of any specific sexual difficulty in what can be viewed as a **three-dimensional model of sexual problems**. We'll briefly explore each dimension.

Duration: Primary or Secondary

This first dimension helps clarify how long a person has been experiencing the problem. A *primary* sexual problem is one that has always existed in the person's sexual life; a *secondary* problem is one that is occurring now but was not present at some point in the person's past sexual experiences. For example, if a man is having difficulties achieving and maintaining an erection, it is important to determine if his problem is primary or secondary. If it is primary, this implies that he has always had difficulty with erections; if it is secondary, this would indicate that his erections have been fine in the past, say, in a previous relationship or at a younger age, but are not so fine now. Likewise, if a woman is unable to experience an orgasm and this problem is primary, it means she has never been able to experience one. However, if in the past she was orgasmic and now is not, her problem is secondary.

Context: Global or Situational

Saying that a sexual problem is "global" does not mean it occurs everywhere throughout the world! Rather, a *global* problem is one that occurs for an individual or couple in virtually *all* settings. On the other hand, a *situational* problem is experienced in specific settings but is absent in other contexts. For example, if a man has a global erectile problem, he is unable to achieve an erection in all situations including, say, during masturbation, spontaneously during sleep, and with a partner. If, however if his erection problem is situational, we can assume he is capable of having erections in some settings, such as masturbation, but not others, such as while making love with his partner. Likewise, if a woman is orgasmic, say, when she masturbates or during oral sex but not with her partner, this would be a situational problem. Alternately, if she is unable to reach orgasm regardless of the setting or activity, her problem would be classified as global.

Frequency: Total or Partial

A *total* sexual problem is one that occurs invariably, that is, every time, *in a given setting*. A problem defined as *partial* occurs often enough to cause distress but not on every occasion in that particular setting. For instance, a man who is able to have an erection *sometimes* when he and his partner make love (but not as often as he or they would like) is experiencing a partial erectile problem (not a partial erection, a partial *problem*). However, if he is *never* able to achieve an erection during lovemaking with his partner, regardless of his erections elsewhere, that would be classified as total. If a woman is able to achieve an orgasm with her partner when they go on vacation but not during their regular home life, this would be considered a partial problem with orgasm.

three-dimensional model of sexual problems A method of classifying or diagnosing sexual problems according to their duration, context, and frequency.

Table 7.3 APPLYING THE THREE-DIMENSIONAL MODEL TO SOME SPECIFIC SEXUAL PROBLEMS

EXAMPLE OF PROBLEM	DURATION		CONTEXT		FREQUENCY		SUSPECTED CAUSES
	Primary	**Secondary**	**Global**	**Situational**	**Total**	**Partial**	
A 30-year-old woman has never experienced an orgasm with or without a partner in any setting.	√		√		√		Physical, organic, or hormonal disorder; psychological issues from past sexual abuse and trauma; repressive family environment
A 40-year-old man who has had erections in the past is now completely unable to achieve an erection in any setting.		√	√		√		Advanced circulatory (vascular) illness; complications from prostate surgery; physical injury; nicotine, drug, or alcohol abuse; severe psychological trauma; depression
A 45-year-old woman finds that she rarely achieves orgasm regardless of the sexual setting. This has not been a problem for her in the past.		√	√			√	Serious relationship difficulties; hormonal imbalances; drug or alcohol abuse; depression
A 25-year-old man is never able to achieve or maintain an erection with his current partner but has no such difficulty when he masturbates.		√		√	√		Relationship problems such as anger, resentment, or guilt; sexual orientation issues; performance anxiety; fear of pregnancy or STI transmission; drug or alcohol abuse in settings with partner
A 25-year-old woman finds that she often, but not always, fails to reach orgasm during lovemaking with her partner. This has not been a problem for her with past partners, and she is fully capable of orgasm through masturbation.		√		√		√	Relationship problems such as anger, resentment, guilt, or abuse; sexual orientation issues; pregnancy or STI concerns; lack of adequate stimulation during sexual encounter; fatigue, stress, or anxiety in settings with partner; unrealistic expectations of intercourse and female orgasm

Think for a moment how much better everyone's understanding of a particular sexual problem will be once these dimensions have been considered and, consequently, how much more effective any potential solution is likely to be. If you think about it, you will see how, for example, a primary, global, and total problem would suggest very different potential causes and treatments than one that is secondary, situational, and partial. Table 7.3 can help you visualize how these three dimensions might be used in determining the suspected causes of specific sexual problems.

Sources of Sexual Problems

Now that you have some idea of how sexual problems may be defined, classified, and understood, the next step in resolving them may lie in determining where or how the problem may have originated. Although many treatments for sexual problems are often effective regardless of the cause, finding the *best* treatment for a specific difficulty will usually require some clarification of the source of the problem. The source of most sexual problems usually fall into one or more of the following four categories: biological or physiological causes, psychological causes, relationship issues, and cultural expectations. If the reasons for a sexual problem are not immediately evident (as is often the case), a skilled sex therapist can usually help clients uncover the true causes through careful questioning and discussion. Here is a brief discussion of each of the potential causes of sexual problems.

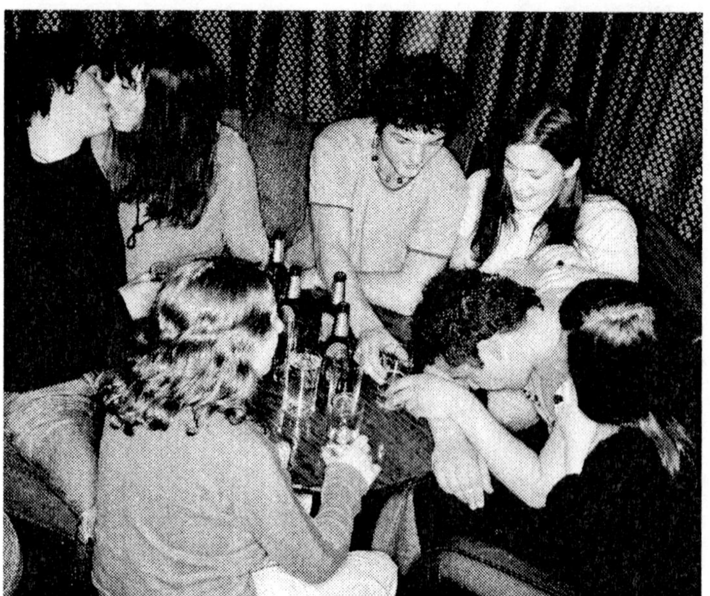

Although alcohol may reduce inhibitions against sexual behavior, it may also interfere with sexual responding.

Biological or Physiological Causes

Sexual problems stemming from biological or physiological sources typically occur when the physical body is *incapable* (usually temporarily) of responding appropriately, regardless of the partner, the setting, or the sexual activities that may be occurring. These causes can be neurological, such as spinal cord or other nerve damage; hormonal, involving imbalances in the hormones that control and activate sexual responding; or vascular, meaning that the circulatory system is malfunctioning so that blood is not circulating as it should for sexual arousal. Such circulatory deficiencies may be due to disorders such as heart disease, diabetes, or atherosclerosis (hardening of the arteries) arising from cigarette smoking or poor diet. Physiological causes may also arise from physical injuries or trauma to the genitals or to the brain and nervous system.

Included in this category of sources of sexual problems is the use and abuse of alcohol and other recreational drugs. Use of alcohol and other drugs often accompanies sexual interactions because many people believe that drugs enhance the sexual experience. Such enhancement may be true for some people some of the time, usually in very small doses. In general, however, most recreational drugs *interfere* with normal, desirable sexual functioning. Probably the most common "antisex drug" is alcohol.

Calling alcohol an antisex drug may surprise you, because many people believe that drinking alcohol makes people feel *more* sexual, not less. Indirectly, this may be true in some ways. Alcohol acts on the brain to reduce inhibitions of all kinds, including sexual ones. Small to moderate amounts of alcohol might cause some people to become less sexually inhibited and to engage in various sexual behaviors more readily than they would if sober. However, as a drug, alcohol is a general nervous system *depressant*, and if your nervous system becomes too depressed, normal sexual responding is inhibited. Beyond this depressant effect, alcohol also causes blood vessels throughout the body to dilate, which can reduce blood flow to the genitals and inhibit such responses as penile erection, clitoral engorgement, and vaginal lubrication (Graber, 1993; Norris, 1994). Chronic alcohol abuse may also alter the balance of sex hormones, reducing those that are directly responsible for sexual arousal and response in both men and women (Kreslin, 1993).

Alcohol is not the only culprit in drug-related causes of sexual problems. Most so-called recreational drugs, including amphetamines, heroine, cocaine, and marijuana, produce negative sexual side effects, especially with heavy or long-term abuse. The nicotine in heavy cigarette use has been found to interfere with erections in men (and possibly arousal in women) by causing plaque to build up in the arteries and reducing blood flow to the genitals. In fact, sometimes a male patient's complaint of erection difficulties is a physician's first hint of possible heart disease (Sadovsky, 2003). Table 7.4 summarizes some of these recreational drugs and their effects on sexual response.

In addition to the "recreational" drugs summarized in Table 7.4, many prescription medications have negative sexual side effects. Certain blood pressure medications are known to cause sexual problems, especially erectile difficulties in men. Other drugs, including some antihistamines, antipsychotic medications, and prescription tranquilizers, may interfere with sexual desire or orgasm.

Table 7.4 EFFECTS OF DRUG ABUSE ON SEXUAL FUNCTIONING

SUBSTANCE	SEXUAL DISORDER	FREQUENCY OF OCCURRENCE
Alcohol		
Immediate effects	Erectile disorder	· · ·
	Desire disorder	· · ·
	Delayed orgasm	· · ·
Long-term effects	Erectile disorder	· · ·
	Desire disorder	· · ·
Amphetamines		
Low doses	Increased desire	·
	Delayed orgasm	·
High doses or chronic use	Delayed or no ejaculation (men)	· · ·
	Erectile disorder	· ·
	Inhibition of orgasm	·
Amyl nitrite (poppers)	Decreased arousal and lubrication	·
	Erectile disorder	·
	Delayed orgasm or ejaculation	·
Barbiturates	Decreased desire	· · ·
	Erectile disorder	· · ·
	Inhibited ejaculation	· · ·
Cocaine	Erectile disorder	· · ·
	Spontaneous or delayed ejaculation	·
	Priapism	·
Marijuana	Decreased desire	·
	Hormonal alteration	·
MDMA (Ecstasy)	Erectile disorder	· · · ·
	Inhibited ejaculation	· · · ·
	Delayed orgasm	· · · ·
	Decreased desire	· ·
Methaqualone (Quaaludes)	Erectile disorder	·
	Inhibited ejaculation	·
	Decreased desire	·
Morphine (heroin)	Decreased desire	·
	Erectile disorder	·
	Hormonal alterations	·
Tobacco		
Short-term effects	Erectile problems	·
Long-term effects	Erectile disorder	· · ·

Key: · rare; · · infrequent; · · · common; · · · · very common.

Source: Table, "Effects of Drug Abuse on Sexual Functioning" from "Medications That May Contribute to Sexual Disorders" by W. Finger, M. Lund and M. Slagle, *Journal of Family Practice*, 44, (1997), pp. 33–43. Copyright © 1997. Reprinted by permission of The Journal of Family Practice.

Probably the most common sexual side effects from prescriptions medications today relates to the widespread use of drugs that have revolutionized the treatment of depression over the past 20 years: the **SSRIs** (which stands for *selective serotonin reuptake inhibitors*). These drugs, known by the various trade names of Prozac, Zoloft, Paxil, Luvox, Lexipro, and Celexa, are highly effective in treating depression, usually without most of the negative side effects associated with earlier antidepressants. Unfortunately, however, for some patients taking these medications, one common side effect involves sexual problems, usually relating to inhibition of orgasm. A more complete discussion of these drugs and their effect on sexual functioning appears later in this chapter.

SSRIs Selective serotonin reuptake inhibitors, drugs administered to treat depression that may cause various sexual side effects, especially inhibited or delayed arousal or orgasm.

Psychological Causes

Although sexual problems may stem from various or multiple causes, it is safe to say that most are either *psychogenic* (having primarily a psychological cause) or involve one or more psychological components. While the cause of a sexual difficulty may be psychological, the effect is usually physically manifested in the form of no erection, no arousal, no orgasm, reaching orgasm too rapidly or too slowly, and so on. This is not surprising in light of the many recent discoveries in psychology and biomedical research demonstrating a link between mind and body.

We know that strong emotions such as stress, fear, guilt, anxiety, and depression trigger responses in your nervous and endocrine systems that are incompatible with sexual arousal. If you stop to think about it, there's a very good reason for this. When your brain senses that you are feeling threatened in some way, it activates some systems such as heart rate, blood pressure, and adrenalin secretion to prepare you to meet the challenge of the perceived danger. This is called the "fight or flight response." At the same time, however, your brain shuts down networks in your body that are unnecessary for fighting or fleeing, such as digestion, salivation, and, yes, sexual responding. These built-in responses have helped humans to survive as a species for millions of years of evolution; we probably wouldn't be here without them. After all, if you are being chased across the plains by a wooly mammoth, wasting energy on sexual responding will do you no good at all!

However, for most of you in today's world, the threats you face over life's issues, such as relationships, money, jobs, family problems, school, grades, deadlines, and computer crashes, are not the sort of dangers that require you to fight or run away (physically, that is). Rather, the difficulties and challenges in your life cause you to worry, experience anxiety, become overly stressed, feel fearful, feel guilty, or become depressed. Nevertheless, when your responses to those threats become strong enough, your brain senses the danger you are perceiving and orders your nervous system to react much as it would to that wooly mammoth. Your body becomes ready to fight or run away (whether you need to or not), and it also becomes very unready to respond sexually. Table 7.5 lists some of the most common psychological causes of sexual problems. Many of these will be touched on again in later discussions of the various specific sexual problems.

Table 7.5 COMMON PSYCHOLOGICAL CAUSES OF SEXUAL PROBLEMS

FEAR OF . . .	ANXIETY ABOUT . . .	GUILT OVER . . .	STRESS DUE TO . . .	OTHER CAUSES
Pregnancy	Relationship issues	Lack of feelings for partner	Job or work	Feelings of powerlessness
Infertility	Money	Unfaithfulness	Money	Feeling trapped
Abuse	Ability to respond	Masturbation	Nonsexual relationship problems	Past or current abuse
Partner violence	Ability to please partner	Sexual fantasies	Family problems	Posttraumatic stress
Transmitting or contracting STIs	Lack of sexual experience or knowledge	Past behaviors	Illness	Poor self-image
Pain	Infertility	Betrayal of partner	Loss or grief	Low self-esteem
Being walked in on during sex	Pregnancy	Lying	Children and child rearing	Loss or grief
	Past sexual trauma	Cheating	Other family responsibilities	Serious illness (self or loved ones)
	Childhood sexual abuse	Other deception		Infertility
		Repressive family environment in childhood		Physical or sexual abuse by partner

Relationship Issues

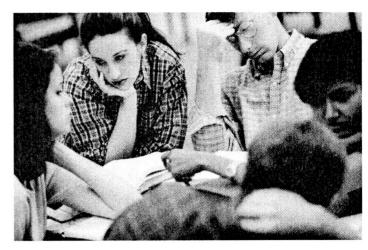

One of the most common causes of sexual problems today is the stress of modern life.

Because nearly all sexual problems occur in the context of a relationship between two people, it is logical to suspect that the causes may lie in issues within the relationship. Sometimes problems will arise that neither partner has ever experienced before, or some people may see a pattern of similar difficulties in past relationships. Whatever the case, determining if specific relationship factors are contributing to the couple's sexual problem and then defining and resolving the issues may be key in solving their sexual troubles. Although individual couples experience a wide variety of specific relationship problems, those that are most likely to affect the sexual side of a relationship are trust, communication, anger or resentment, sexual expectations, respect, and love.

Loss of Trust

Successful intimate relationships rely on trust, and the same is true of healthy, satisfying sexual interactions (Besharat, 2003; Kaplan, 1974). Most couples need to trust that their partner is faithful, is honest in expressing feelings, will not inflict emotional or physical pain, and is not withholding important information that might negatively affect the relationship. Sexual problems such as desire disorders, arousal difficulties, erectile problems, and orgasm difficulties may sometimes be linked to the lack or loss of trust in a relationship. When this basic trust is lost, it stands to reason that the overall relationship will suffer, and the sexual side especially may begin to deteriorate (Smyth, 2002).

Poor Communication

How often have you heard someone who is experiencing relationship problems say something like "We just don't communicate!" Effective communication is a cornerstone of a good relationship, and good sexual communication is usually the foundation of a good sexual relationship (Weeks & Gambescia, 2000). Unfortunately, many couples, even those who enjoy excellent communication about most topics, find communicating about sex difficult. As discussed at the beginning of this chapter, people tend to expect that good sexual interactions simply happen "naturally," that we should be able to "sense" our partner's needs, wishes, and desires, and that something must be amiss if we have to *talk* about it. In reality, just the opposite is true. Sure, sex just "clicks" for some couples, but for most, the truth is that *words enhance sex*. The ability to express sexual feelings, sexual desires, insecurities about sex, specific behavior and stimulation preferences, and other concerns is crucial in establishing and maintaining a sexually satisfying relationship. Counselors, therapists, and physicians who work with couples with sexual problems should encourage the couples to discuss openly their sexual likes and dislikes, desires, and priorities. Often simply setting aside time or increasing the amount of time a couple allow for talking to each other about intimate issues and sharing feelings can go a long way toward increasing physical and emotional intimacy. Many couples complain of a gradual loss of intimacy over time; making the romantic side of the relationship a greater priority can help rekindle feelings of pleasure and intimacy (Leiblum & Rosen, 2000).

Anger and Resentment

Strong negative emotional reactions, especially anger and resentment, work directly against sexual responding. If you are feeling angry or resentful toward your partner, regardless of the reasons, responding sexually is going to be difficult (Bélanger,

Laughrea, & Lafontaine, 2001; Kaplan, 1974). In anger, two barriers to sexual intimacy are functioning simultaneously. One is specific physiological responses of the autonomic nervous system, which are incompatible with sexual arousal; the other is the psychological distance and loss of desire for intimacy with the partner that accompanies the anger. Anger and conflict occur in all relationships, but couples who are unable to resolve their conflicts and manage anger effectively often find levels of resentment building and sexual problems developing (see the discussion on defining and resolving anger later in this chapter). One of the most difficult tasks in sex therapy is helping angry and resentful couples find strategies for resolving their conflicts and moving past the hostility. If they refuse to do so, the therapy they are seeking for their sexual difficulties is likely to fail (Weeks & Gambescia, 2000).

Conflicting Sexual Expectations

Everyone grows up with expectations about sex, and no two people's expectations are the same. When two people enter into a sexually intimate relationship, they are sure to have some differing expectations about sex that will need to be negotiated and reconciled. For example, one of the most common differing expectations about sex is how often they "should" make love. If one partner desires and expects that having sex is a daily event while the other feels that once a week is ideal, they are likely to experience some very difficult conflicts if they fail to work out a compromise. Or if one partner expects to be the initiator of sex but the other often enjoys making the first move, these differing expectations, if not reconciled, can lead to a serious imbalance in the relationship and potential sexual problems. When both partners are willing and able to communicate and discuss differences in expectations, chances are good they can work them out. However, sometimes partners have expectations of each other or about the relationship that they keep hidden, each assuming that the other should "just know what I want" and behave accordingly. This has been called the *myth of the lover as mind reader*. These hidden expectations are often extremely problematic and can lead to difficult conflicts, sexual and otherwise (Weeks & Gambescia, 2000).

Lack of Respect

Lack of respect in an intimate relationship will invariably undermine sexual feelings, desire, and responses. Two distinct yet related types of respect are fundamental to successful and satisfying relationships: *self-respect* and *mutual respect*. A lack of self-respect, and the low self-esteem that invariably accompanies it, usually causes one or both partners to feel unworthy of experiencing sexual pleasure and undeserving of sexual pleasure that may be offered by the other. In fact, a person lacking self-respect may actually lose respect for a partner who attempts to initiate sexual intimacy (Leiblum & Rosen, 2000).

Mutual respect is equally important in that each partner needs to feel that his or her wishes, ideas, attitudes, desires, abilities, and unique characteristics as a person are honored and valued by the other. When this mutual respect is absent, the foundation for successful and satisfying sexual interactions crumbles away, and along with it go other keys to intimacy such as trust, communication, and love.

Loss of Love

Everyone knows that sexual interactions sometimes occur outside a context of love. However, in an intimate relationship, sexual satisfaction and functioning often falter when feelings of love between the partners decrease. Love is probably the most difficult to define of all the factors in intimate relationships that can influence sexual functioning. It is at least as important as the others, possibly the most important of all (Sprecher, 2002). Perhaps love is a blend of the various aspects of relationships we have been discussing. Or maybe it doesn't really matter how we define love here. It proba-

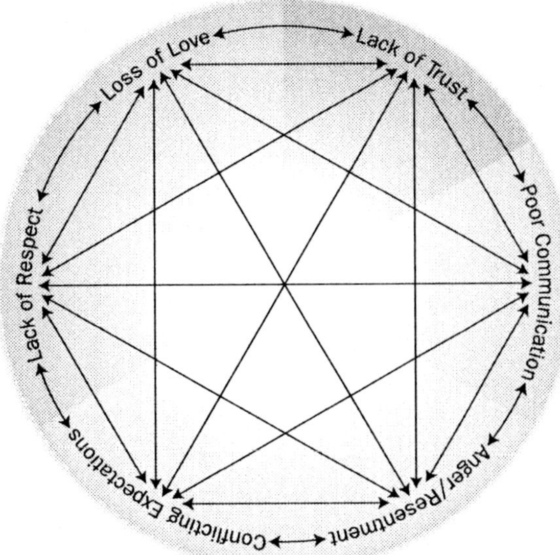

FIGURE 7.1 The Circle of Relationship Issues and Sexual Problems

Any single relationship factor on the circle may lead to, or be caused by, any other factor, which may in turn cause another relationship problem, and so on, until sexual intimacy is lost.

bly suffices to say that love is an emotional, psychological, and physical condition about which most people are able to say, "I know it when I'm in love." What does matter here—most people would agree—is that sex combined with love is very different from sex without love. People generally make very clear distinctions between "making love" and "having sex" (Faulkner, 2003). Even sex therapists are careful about helping couples not focus too much on the sexual component lest lovemaking be reduced to "sexmaking" (Weeks & Gambescia, 2000). The main point here is that for most people, when they feel that love is fading or is absent, the likelihood of sexual problems grows.

Interactions among the Six Factors

Trust, communication, anger and resentment, sexual expectations, respect, and love are so closely intertwined that it is virtually impossible for a couple to be experiencing a problem with one factor without also feeling the effects on at least some of the others. For example, if a couple lack effective communication skills, they will likely have difficulty reconciling conflicting sexual expectations. Their conflicting expectations could in turn lead to feelings of anger and resentment, a loss of respect for each other, and the eventual loss of feelings of love. You can start from any one of the relationship problems we have been discussing and logically trace a chain of escalating barriers to sexual intimacy to all or most of the other five. Figure 7.1 visually depicts this interdependent circle of relationship issues that may lead to sexual problems.

Cultural Expectations

In general, behavioral scientists are realizing with increasing clarity that if we are to have any hope of studying and correctly interpreting all human behavior, including human sexuality, it must be considered within its cultural context (Bancroft, 2002; Triandis, 1989; Triandis et al., 1988). Moreover, few complex human interactions are influenced by culture more than sexuality.

As we become more global in our human interactions through freer economic trade, the internet, and the ease of travel, intimate relationships are forming across cultural and national boundaries. Consequently, the sexual problems sometimes experienced by partners from diverse ethnic, social, and religious backgrounds have come into sharper focus (see "Sexuality and Culture: Forbidden Love").

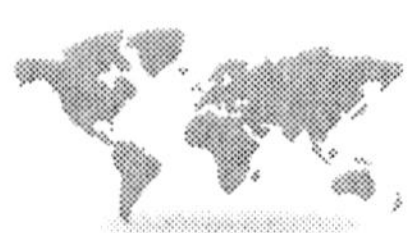

Sexuality and Culture

Forbidden Love

In June 2001, former U.S. Marine Jason Johnson married Bahraini princess Meriam Al-Khalifa in Las Vegas. In her home country, where they met, she was forbidden to marry a non-Muslim (he is Mormon) and was expected to marry someone of similar royal standing in her country. In Bahrain, young women are not even allowed to be alone with men, so she had to sneak out to meet him at a mall and eventually secretly ran away from her country to marry Johnson. Their romance inspired the 2001 television movie *Forbidden Love*. Unfortunately, the couple were unable to resolve their cultural differences, and the princess returned to Bahrain alone less than a year after the marriage.

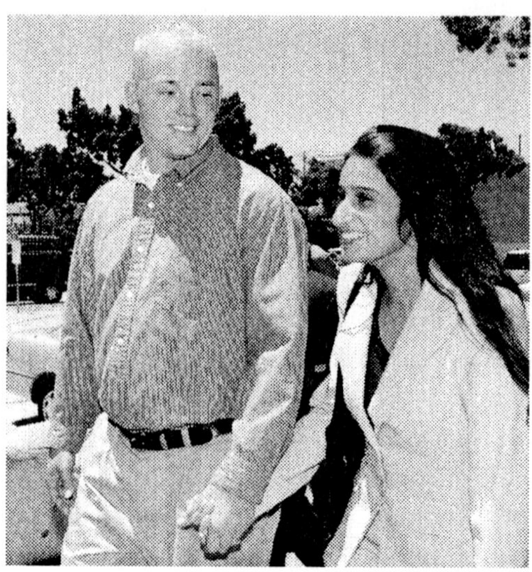

American Jason Johnson with his wife, Bahraini princess Meriam Al-Khalifa.

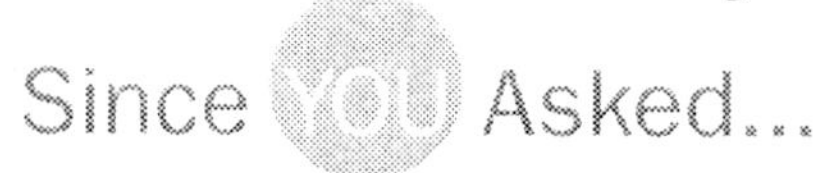

Since You Asked...

2. My girlfriend is from India. We've been together for nearly a year, but she doesn't seem interested in sex at all. Could this be due to growing up in a different culture, or is it something in our relationship?

When people from different cultures become involved in a romantic relationship, their deeply ingrained attitudes and expectations about sex may clash dramatically, causing sexual problems. For example, cultures differ greatly in attitudes and expectations about nudity, modesty, acceptable sexual behaviors, sexual roles and responsibilities of men and women, privacy, parts of the body that are considered sexual and nonsexual, religious teachings about sex, and even expectations about sexual responding. These often profound differences were recognized and written about over half a century ago when the famous sociologist Margaret Mead suggested that the prevalence of orgasm in women may be culturally determined: "There seems to be a reasonable basis for assuming that the human female's capacity for orgasm is to be viewed much more as a potentiality that may or may not be developed by a given culture" (Mead, 1949, p. 217).

This is not to say that cross-cultural unions are doomed. On the contrary, the recognition of cultural sexual diversity has led today's sex therapists and researchers to pay significantly more attention and sensitivity to cultural differences and conflicts in their study and treatment of sexual problems (Osman & Al-Sawaf, 1995; Ribner, 2003; Sunger, 1999). Beyond the professionals, however, this cultural awareness is growing throughout the general population. As our globe continues to shrink, cultural barriers to intimate relationships are increasingly likely to fade with time and interpersonal contacts across cultural boundaries.

In the next section, we begin discussing some general principles for helping individuals and couples resolve sexual problems. You may be wondering why a discussion of treatments appears before considering the specific problems themselves. The answer will become clear as you read on.

General Treatment Principles

The solutions or treatments for most sexual problems typically incorporate one or more basic strategies, combined with some specific methods designed for each individual difficulty. We will refer to these general treatment principles later as we review the various sexual problems and the specific solutions for each. Therefore, a basic understanding of these approaches now is helpful in appreciating how they can be effective for such a wide variety of problems. The most prominent of these general principles are sensate focus, therapeutic masturbation, and enhanced communication.

Sensate Focus

In their groundbreaking book *Human Sexual Inadequacy*, Masters and Johnson (1970) described a comprehensive sex therapy program for couples dealing with various sexual problems. Mutual "pleasuring exercises" were a central feature of their program. They referred to this approach as **sensate focus**. Sensate focus, in various interpretations, forms, and applications, continues to play an important role in sex therapy practices today (Albaugh & Kellogg-Spadt, 2002).

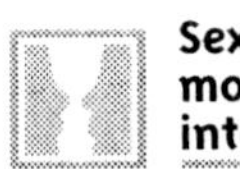

Sex is more than intercourse

Sensate focus is an interesting and paradoxical treatment for sexual problems because it assumes, in essence, that the sex will be better if a couple *stop doing it*! The idea behind this strange-sounding notion relates to Western cultures' insistence on equating sex with intercourse. For most couples, especially among heterosexual partners, "having sex" means engaging in sexual intercourse. However, most sexual problems occur in the context of either having or leading up to having intercourse. Erectile difficulties, lack of arousal, rapid ejaculation, lack of orgasm, inhibited orgasm, and painful sex usually occur while a couple is having or trying to have intercourse. In other words, the focus is on the goal of intercourse. Sensate focus exercises require that the partners redirect their emphasis away from intercourse and focus on their capacity for *sensuality*.

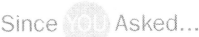

Since You Asked...

3. How can a couple who have been together for a long time (married three years) get their sexual feelings back? We have a good relationship, but we hardly ever make love anymore.

Here is one way you may be able to relate to this idea. Most couples can remember times in their lives when they were being sexual with a partner, perhaps early in the relationship, but there was an agreement, spoken or unspoken, that their sexual behavior would not lead to intercourse for any number of reason. Usually, people recall those sexual encounters as intensely arousing; the possibility that the body might not respond "correctly" was the farthest thing from their minds because their bodies were responding powerfully and effortlessly. Often, however, when a relationship progresses to having intercourse, much of that sensual, intensely sexy behavior disappears and becomes simply "foreplay," behaviors leading up to intercourse. If later on, either person begins to experience a sexual problem, the couple begin to feel anxious about sex, worried that the problem, whatever it is, will happen again when they have intercourse. This anxiety may in turn lead to other sexual problems or even the avoidance of sex altogether because any sexual activity triggers the awareness that intercourse is approaching. Therefore, the first rule of sensate focus is "no intercourse."

Here's how sensate focus typically works. Assuming any underlying physical causes have been ruled out or corrected, a couple who are experiencing a sexual problem are instructed to find quiet, private time together one or more times each week. The length of time may vary, depending on the individual couple's needs. During these sessions, they are to remove their clothing and spend the time taking turns touching and caressing each other, focusing on the pleasure they feel in touching and being touched. However, they must not touch each other's breasts or genital areas. "Self-Discovery: A Sex Therapist's Instructions for Sensate Focus Exercises" provides clear instructions for sensate focus from one of the most famous sex therapists of the twentieth century, Helen Singer Kaplan.

As the therapeutic process proceeds, usually over several weeks, the caressing is allowed to expand to include nipples and genitals, but the goal continues to be sensual and pleasurable sensations, *not orgasm*. Genital touching that may lead to orgasm is

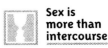

sensate focus A sex therapy technique that requires a couple to redirect emphasis away from intercourse and focus on their capacity for mutual *sensuality*.

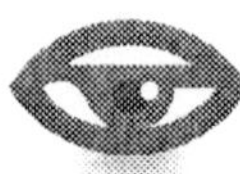

Self-Discovery

A Sex Therapist's Instructions for Sensate Focus Exercises

I'd like you both to get ready for bed—to take off your clothes, shower, and relax. I want you [the woman] to lie on your belly. Then you [the man] caress her back as gently and sensitively as you can. Move your hands very slowly. Begin at the base of her neck, caress her ears, and work your way down to her buttocks, legs, and feet. Use your hands or your lips (or both). Concentrate only on how it feels to touch her body and her skin.

In the meantime, I want you [the woman] to focus your attention on the sensations you feel when he caresses you. Try not to let your mind wander. Don't think about anything else; don't worry about whether he's getting tired or whether he's enjoying it or anything else. Just concentrate on your sensations; let yourself feel everything. Communicate with him. Don't talk too much . . . but remember that he can't possibility know what you are feeling unless you tell him. Let him know where you want to be touched and how, and where his caresses feel especially good; and let him know if his touch is too light or too heavy or if he is going too fast. If the experience is unpleasant, tell him so. Try to identify those areas of your body that are especially sensitive or responsive.

When you have both had enough of this, I want you [the woman] to turn over on your back so that you [the man] can caress the front of her body. Start with her face and neck and go down to her toes. But this first time don't caress her sexual organs. Skip her nipples, vagina, and clitoris. Again, both of you are to concentrate only on what it feels like to caress and be caressed. Stop when this becomes tedious to either of you. Now it's your [the man's] turn to receive. I want you [the woman] to do the same to him.

Source: Adapted from Kaplan (1974), p. 209.

prohibited. The idea is for the couple to experience pleasure for pleasure's sake, not as a preliminary to intercourse (Figure 7.2).

Masters and Johnson (1970, p. 68) reported that for most couples in treatment,

> the sensate focus exercises represent the first opportunity they have ever had to "think and feel" sensuously and at leisure without intrusion upon the experience by the demand for [orgasm] (own or partner's), without the need to explain their sensate preferences, without the demand for personal reassurance, or without a sense of need to rush to "return the favor."

Typically, within a few weeks (and sometimes sooner), with the pressures and expectations of intercourse removed, couples find that sexual, sensual, and romantic feelings and responses are reawakening in them. As the therapeutic process continues, they are allowed to begin to touch each other to orgasm and eventually to engage in intercourse once again. Couples feel emotionally closer, men with erectile dysfunction are having good erections, women who were experiencing arousal difficulties become fully aroused, sexual desire increases for couples whose desire had been waning, and orgasm problems are often resolved.

This is not to say that sensate focus is a sexual cure-all. Many couples with deep emotional or psychological problems in their relationship have a great deal of difficulty agreeing to and beginning the exercises. Other couples may find the intimacy and arousal of the exercises too threatening to continue. Still others, as they find themselves becoming aroused during the sessions, will depart from the instructions and have intercourse. As Kaplan (1974) notes, it is not unusual for a therapist to hear the following comment: "He started to touch me and we got so excited that we thought we shouldn't waste it, so we had intercourse" (p. 213). This demonstrates the power of sensate focus to enhance sexual feelings, but "breaking the rules" can lead to less successful long-term outcomes.

As sensate focus strategies have been researched, adapted, and refined over the years, various findings have brought the method into sharper focus. For example,

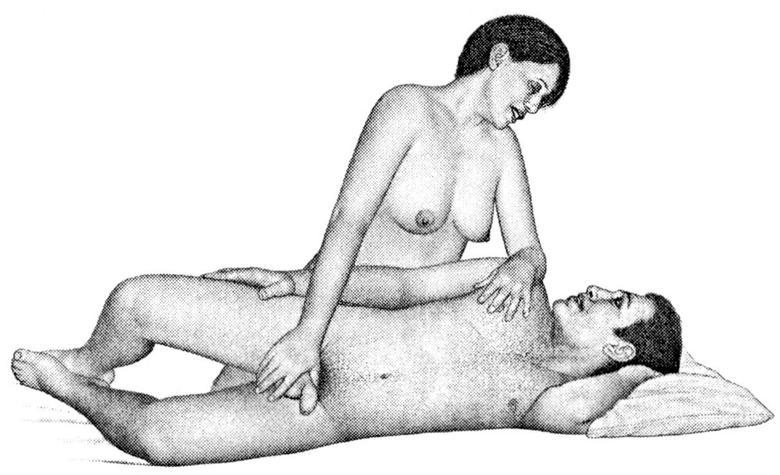

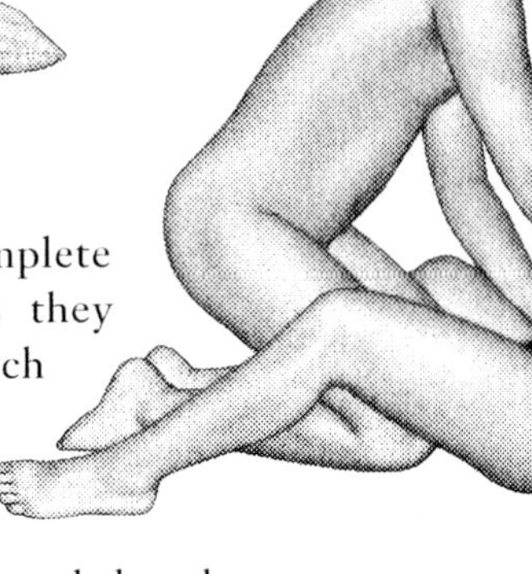

FIGURE 7.2 Sensate Focus Exercises

Sensate focus exercises are designed to help a couple reconnect on a sensual, rather than sexual, level, without expectations or demands. After a while, the couple may begin to include touching of genitals and breasts, but without orgasm.

studies have suggested that nearly half of all couples who complete sex therapy programs fail to maintain the improvements they accomplished (Hawton, Catalan, & Fagg, 1992). To combat such relapse rates, other researchers have suggested that couples plan "booster sessions" of nonintercourse sensate focus exercises from time to time or following disappointing sexual interactions (McCarthy, 1993). Finally, research has suggested that the experience and effectiveness of traditional sensate focus exercises may not be equivalent for men and women (Wiederman, 2001).

Nevertheless, sensate focus continues to be a mainstay of sexual therapy. You will see how it is applied to specific sexual problems later in this chapter.

Masturbation as Treatment

As noted in Chapter 6, secular attitudes toward masturbation have undergone a complete turnaround compared to 100 years ago. Back then, masturbation was regarded by most people as an unhealthy and even perverted behavior that would lead to various unpleasant outcomes, including loss of energy, blindness, genital cancer, and sexual dysfunction. Today, medical and psychological professionals, and most Western cultures in general, consider masturbation a normal and healthy sexual activity. Indeed, far from its past reputation as leading to a loss of sexual performance and enjoyment, masturbation today is a central component in the treatment of various sexual problems. Why? Several reasons have been suggested: (1) It allows individuals to become more aware of their own bodily sensations during sexual arousal and orgasm, which in turn (2) helps partners explain to each other what kinds of stimulation feels best; (3) it serves as a sexual release while couples are working on solving their sexual problems; and (4) it helps individuals work on specific sexual difficulties without a partner or issues they are not comfortable exploring with a partner.

Since YOU Asked...

4. I'm a male and I'm curious if it is odd that I have never masturbated. Is masturbation healthy?

This does not imply that a person or couple can simply "masturbate their way out of a sexual problem." The use of masturbation in sex therapy is usually referred to as **directed masturbation** (this does *not* mean that the therapist offers suggestions *while* you do it!). The idea is for the therapist to advise the client on how masturbation activities might effectively be used to help overcome a sexual problem (Kaplan, 1974).

directed masturbation A sex therapy strategy in which the therapist advises the client on how to use masturbation activities to help overcome a sexual problem.

Directed masturbation has been demonstrated to be an effective therapeutic component in the treatment of most common sexual problems, such as premature ejaculation, erectile dysfunction, arousal disorder, and especially inhibited or lack of orgasm, (Leiblum & Rosen, 2000; O'Donohue & Geer, 1993). Specific applications of masturbation in treating these problems will be discussed shortly in the context of each specific problem. For now, here is the key to understanding why masturbation is such a powerful tool in treating sexual disorders: People who are experiencing a sexual problem with their partner rarely encounter the same problem when masturbating. For example, among the 510 couples who participated in Masters and Johnson's early studies of their therapy method, only 11 women and no men were unable to achieve orgasm through masturbation. When a sexual problem exists with a partner and is present during masturbation as well, this is often a sign that the problem is global and may stem from either physical or deep-seated psychological causes.

Note that the use of masturbation in therapy is not always appropriate for all people, even if their sexual problem might be helped by it. Not everyone feels comfortable with masturbation no matter what the reasons. Furthermore, in some relationships, one or both partners' attitudes about masturbation may create a situation in which the therapy serves to compound their sexual and relationship problems rather than solve them. To avoid this, therapists must be aware of when and with whom recommendations of masturbation as therapy are appropriate (Christensen, 1995).

Communication

The importance of effective communication in intimate relationships is discussed in detail in Chapter 4 and was also touched upon in relation to the causes of sexual problems earlier in this chapter. "Communication issues" between intimate partners comes up so often, it seems almost a cliché, but this only demonstrates communication's significant role in the success or failure of these relationships. A common misconception is that if a couple have to *talk* about their sexual interactions, they must be doing something wrong. Nothing could be further from the truth. If you don't communicate your sexual desires, likes, dislikes, preferences, and feelings to your partner, how is he or she supposed to know them? Mind reading? No scientific evidence exists that people are telepathic about sex (or anything else, for that matter).

What about nonverbal communication? Certainly, nonverbal forms of communicating, such as moans and groans and body language, play a part in sexual interactions, but these signals are often vague and easily misread. What you might hear as a moan of pleasure from your partner might actually be a sign of encouragement to do something more intensely because it feels so good or a request to stop whatever it is you are doing because it has become overly stimulating or even painful! Sometimes you simply cannot be sure without using *words*. The "Self-Discovery: Mirroring" demonstrates how relying on nonverbal communication can backfire. It may sound familiar to you.

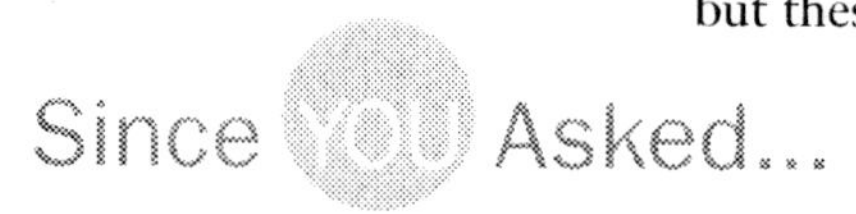

5. I can't tell if my partner is satisfied or not when we make love. What are the signs that a person is sexually satisfied?

Virtually all sex therapy strategies involve an element of enhancing communication between partners (Carey, 1998; Everaerd, 1993; Kaplan, 1974; Masters & Johnson, 1970; Striar & Bartlik, 1999). Poor communication is an important factor in the development, escalation, and persistence of many sexual problems. Helen Singer Kaplan's words in her 1970 book *The New Sex Therapy* continue to ring true:

> Trying to be an effective lover for oneself and for one's partner without communicating is like trying to learn target shooting blindfolded. One needs reciprocal feedback to develop a good sexual interaction and to secure and give effective erotic stimulation. . . . Open and genuine communication is a wonderful tool for correcting and remedying problems between two people. . . . When real needs and desires are expressed without fear or shame, they are often met eagerly by the partner. When fears of failure and humiliation are disclosed, they lose a good deal of their power to hurt. (p. 134)

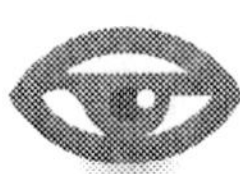

Self-Discovery

Mirroring: A Potential Problem with Nonverbal Communication

Here is an example of how a lack of verbal communication about the seemingly simple act of sexual touching can lead to frustration and dissatisfaction; it is called *mirroring*. A couple are beginning to make love. She prefers to be touched in soft, slow strokes, but he likes to be touched in a firm and more rapid rubbing motion. As they explore each other's bodies, she attempts to signal her touch preferences to him by demonstrating, touching him as she wants to be touched, softly and slowly, so that he can "mirror" the behavior back to her. But this gentle touching is not what feels best to him, so he begins to touch her more firmly and rapidly, hoping that she will mirror his behavior in how she is touching him. She then perceives that her message is not getting through, so she touches him even more lightly and slowly, to which he responds with even firmer and faster rubbing. This continues to escalate until the pleasure evaporates in a cloud of frustration and neither feels much like touching at all anymore. What's the solution to this problem? Communication using *words*.

In the next section, you will see how these basic treatment principles—sensate focus, therapeutic masturbation, and communication enhancement—combine in the treatment of specific sexual problems.

Specific Problems and Solutions

As mentioned earlier in this chapter, sexual problems are usually divided into four categories: problems with desire, arousal, orgasm, and pain. We will discuss each category in turn and focus on the most common problems for men and women in each group. For each specific sexual problem, you will find a description of the problem, an overview of possible causes of the difficulty, and a brief discussion of treatment methods that have been shown to be most effective. Because this is a textbook and not a self-help book, we won't discuss the treatments in great depth or detail. We will, however, touch on a suggestion or two for each problem, in addition to referring to the general treatment principles discussed earlier. If you are concerned about a sexual problem in your life, many resources are available to you in self-help books, on the Internet (see the suggestions at the end of this chapter), and from qualified sex therapists.

Problems with Sexual Desire

These are problems couples typically experience before any physical sexual responses begin. Very low or lack of desire for sex with a partner is referred to as **hypoactive sexual desire (HSD)**.

Description. *Hypo-* means "under," "low," or "not enough" (as opposed to *hyper-*, which indicates "over," "high," or "too much"). Hypoactive sexual desire, also referred to as *inhibited sexual desire*, is formally defined as "persistently or recurrently deficient or absent sexual fantasies and desire for sexual activity" (American Psychiatric Association [APA], 2000, p. 539). In other words, individuals or couples who do not think about sex very much, who do not feel desirous of sexual activities very often, *and* who find this to be a problem in their life and relationship may be diagnosed with HSD.

Typically, a person with HSD is sexually functional—that is, able to respond, become aroused, and reach orgasm—but feels little or no desire for sex. In some cases, this lack of desire exists for sexual interactions with the partner only, but often desire fades for all forms of sexual activity, including masturbation. Low sexual desire has

hypoactive sexual desire (HSD) A persistently low level or lack of sexual fantasies or desire for sexual activity; also known as *inhibited sexual desire*.

historically been assumed to afflict women more commonly than men, and a greater amount of research on HSD has focused on women than on men. However, this difference may be due to cultural expectations and stereotypes and not on actual numbers. Many therapists report approximately equal numbers of men and women who are treated for desire difficulties (Leiblum & Rosen, 2000).

Since YOU Asked...

6. I want to have sex four or five times a week, but my boyfriend would be happy with once a week or less. What can I do to get him more interested in sex?

Problems with desire are the most common sexual problems presented in therapy and are generally considered the most difficult to treat (Pridal & Lo Piccolo, 1993; H. S. Singer, 1979; Trudel et al., 2001; Weeks & Gambescia, 2002). As you will see later, most sexual problems can be addressed with specific behavioral interventions that, if the quality of the relationship allows, provide relatively rapid and effective solutions. This is generally not true of HSD. The underlying reasons for the loss or lack of sexual desire may be complex and difficult to uncover and reverse. Moreover, reigniting passion between two people for whom it has been lost is rarely a simple or straightforward endeavor.

Further complicating this disorder is the fact that HSD may occur in different ways for different couples. In some cases, both partners may have lost their sexual desire for each other. In others, however, sexual desire may have become a "one-way street," in that one partner's desire for sex with the other is not returned, or any sexual desire may be unbalanced, with one partner consistently feeling higher levels of desire than the other. Each of these situations carries its own set of issues that must be addressed in treatment. What could be going on here? Why are so many couples lacking desire for what most people consider one of the most pleasurable, intimate, enjoyable, and even necessary activities of human existence? The causes may be even more complex than the problem itself.

Causes. In attempting to determine the possible causes of HSD, the three-dimensional classification system described earlier in this chapter and demonstrated in Table 7.3 becomes extremely important. In cases involving low desire that is primary (lifelong), global (occurs in all settings), and total (occurs consistently), underlying biological causes such as hormonal imbalances or neurological pathology must be considered. However, for desire difficulties that are secondary (current but not in the past), situational (desire is present in some settings), and partial (desire occasionally increases), nonphysical factors such as psychological, relationship, or cultural issues are more likely to be in play. And virtually *any* of the factors listed in Table 7.5, alone or in combination, may play a role in a person's or a couple's loss of sexual desire. Among the most commonly suggested nonphysical causes are anxiety over relationship and other sexual issues, depression, fear (of pregnancy, STIs, or pain), and past sexual victimization (Kaplan, 1979; Leiblum & Rosen, 2000; Letourneau & O'Donohue, 1993). "In Touch with Your Sexual Health: Uncovering a Possible Cause of Hypoactive Sexual Desire" uses a dialogue between a therapist and her client to show one way the loss of sexual desire might develop.

Solutions. Due to the complexity of HSD in terms of both diagnosis and causal factors, the most important piece of the treatment puzzle may be uncovering the reasons for the low desire. Often a therapist will ask to talk with each partner individually before resuming joint sessions. This allows the therapist to discuss relevant issues that each partner may be unwilling to reveal to the other; issues that could facilitate or hinder the treatment process. Examples of such issues might be sexual orientation confusion, current or past affairs, masturbation issues, current relationship abuse, past sexual trauma, or a combination of these. In addition, the therapist must determine that both partners independently perceive that a problem exists and that they both truly wish to work toward a solution.

Depending on a couple's specific set of circumstances, a therapist may suggest various therapeutic interventions. All three general treatment principles discussed earli-

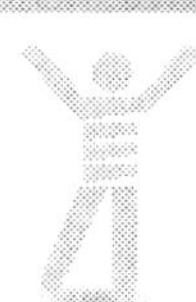

In Touch with Your Sexual Health

Uncovering Possible Causes of Hypoactive Sexual Desire

Client: My biggest concerns is that I just don't seem to desire sex with my husband.

Therapist: Are you and your husband having sex at all?

Client: Well, yes, but not very often.

Therapist: When was the last time?

Client: Maybe a month ago. I feel bad. And guilty. I love him and I know he wants to . . . But I'm just not interested.

Therapist: Did you and your husband have sex more often in the past?

Client: Oh, yeah! At the beginning we made love every day, at least. And even after two or three years, we still had sex a few times a week.

Therapist: So do you have a sense of when that changed?

Client: Around the time our third child was born, a year ago. After the first two, we got back to making love as soon as we could. But not this time. I'm pretty exhausted all the time with three kids.

Therapist: So, you dont't want more children?

Client: No! We're clear about that. In fact, the third one wasn't planned. We love her dearly, but she was definitely a surprise. I'm totally at my limit with three.

Therapist: What form of birth control are you using?

Client: (*pausing, sheepish*) We, uh, don't.

Therapist: No birth control at all?

Client: We try to time it right, you know.

Therapist: Have you ever used birth control in your marriage?

Client: Actually, . . . no.

Therapist: What do you anticipate will happen now if you have sex with your husband?

Client: Well, I guess I'll probably get pregnant, but I just can't handle another child!

Therapist: Do you think these concerns could have any bearing on your lack of sexual desire?

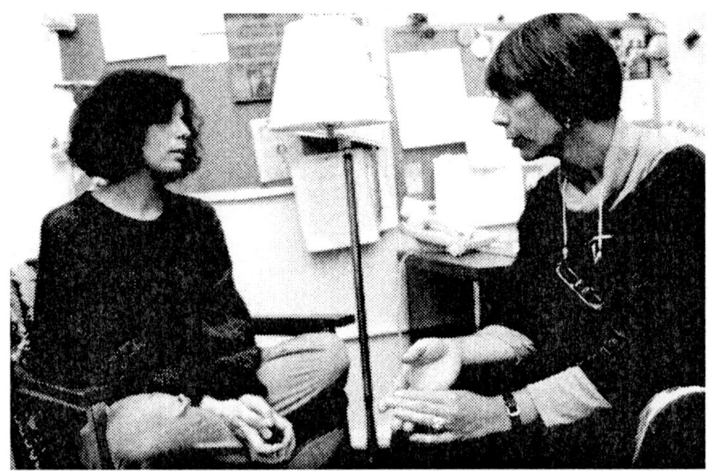

er offer potential benefits for HSD. Sensate focus, in reducing anxiety about intercourse and fears about performance, may reawaken sensuality for the couple and spark new sexual feelings. Masturbation exercises may assist in reacquainting each partner with the pleasurable personal sensations of sexual response and in turn increase desire. Of course, enhanced communication between partners is crucial if they are to rediscover their desire for each other. By the time a couple seek professional treatment for HSD, they are often at their wit's end and even close to divorce. Sometimes they have stopped communicating about sex completely because it has become too uncomfortable and painful a topic. Typically, when a couple are suffering from low or nonexistent sexual desire, they avoid *all* forms of affection because touching, kissing, and even holding hands triggers negative feelings about sexual activities. And when affection and sexual desire fade, the communication that comes from sexual intimacy deteriorates as well (Leiblum & Rosen, 2000).

Some researchers and therapists have suggested varied yet similar versions of **cognitive-behavioral therapy** in treating HSD (Bass, 1996; Klein, 1997; Trudel et al., 2001). As the name implies, cognitive-behavioral therapy for sexual desire problems is designed to (1) assist an individual or a couple in identifying and exploring

cognitive-behavioral therapy A therapeutic approach designed to gradually eliminate specific thoughts and associated behaviors that may be contributing to sexual problems.

irrational, faulty, and self-defeating beliefs and attitudes (*cognitions*) that underlie sexual difficulties; (2) develop strategies to discard those ineffective cognitions and replace them with new, more accurate, and more constructive thought processes; and (3) gradually eliminate undesirable *behaviors* that were based on the old ways of thinking and replace them with new and effective actions stemming from the new belief systems. These approaches to overcoming low-desire problems have been shown to result in relatively high rates of success for both increasing sexual desire and enhancing overall relationship satisfaction. To help you grasp a sense of how cognitive-behavioral techniques help with sexual desire problems, Table 7.6 summarizes one such program (McCarthy, 1995).

Table 7.6 A COGNITIVE-BEHAVIORAL APPROACH TO HYPOACTIVE SEXUAL DESIRE

Barry W. McCarthy at the American University/Washington Psychological Center developed a cognitive-behavioral approach for treating couples dealing with low sexual desire. He introduced his method as follows:

> The optimal sexual process involves positive anticipation [of sex], an emotionally stable relationship, non-demand pleasuring [such as sensate focus], multiple stimulation, sharing orgasm, emotional satisfaction, and a regular rhythm of sexual activity. The dysfunctional pattern is negative anticipation, blaming and alienation, performance anxiety, goal-oriented stimulation, intercourse focus, failure, and sexual avoidance. (1995, p. 133)

McCarthy described a five-component model of treatment that focused on sexual anticipation, owning your own sexuality, deserving sexual pleasure, arousal and orgasm problems, and valuing emotional intimacy. Here is a brief description of each component.

COMPONENT	DESCRIPTION
Sexual anticipation	It's tough to desire sex if you are not looking forward to it. When one or both members of a couple feel pressured to desire sex, the result is usually the opposite: loss of desire and even avoidance of sex. Couples can build greater positive anticipation of sexual interactions in two ways. First, a couple should set specific "sexual dates" that they can plan for and look forward to. These should be when both partners are at their best in terms of mood, energy, and time. Second, couples should avoid falling into predictive or boring lovemaking routines by communicating their sexual desires and planning special sexual turn-ons.
Owning your own sexuality	You are the one who is in charge of your own sexuality. It's your responsibility, not your partner's, to be sexually satisfied; to develop a respectful, trusting, and intimate relationship; and to insist on your sexual rights, such as not fearing unwanted pregnancy, being safe from STIs, and rejecting abusive behaviors. You must accept your sexual history, including any negative sexual experiences you may have suffered in your past, and work to resolve any lingering guilt. You must be willing to communicate to your partner your sexual feelings, desires, and needs, as well as activities that turn you on.
Deserving sexual pleasure	Not all people feel that they deserve to experience sexual pleasure. This may be due to such issues as family upbringing, past negative sexual experiences, low self-esteem, or negative body image. If you don't feel you deserve sexual pleasure, how are you going to desire sexual interactions? The answer is, you're not. All people deserve sexual pleasure because they are human beings, and that pleasure should not depend on the presence or absence of any particular personal characteristic or experience.
Arousal and orgasm problems	Problems with arousal or orgasm go hand in hand with HSD. "For males, dysfunction problems almost always precede desire problems. The male apologizes or tries to cover up his erection, early ejaculation, or [delayed ejaculation] problem. He feels he is failing sexually, avoids [sex], and this inhibits his desire. . . . For females, the mistaken assumption was if the woman could only learn to have orgasms, or better orgasms, or more orgasms, then the desire problem would take care of itself—a seductive, but false assumption" (pp. 138–139).
Valuing emotional *and* sexual intimacy	Emotional intimacy in a relationship is not the same as sexual intimacy. When emotional intimacy is *combined* with sexual intimacy, a couple usually do not have a problem. Emotional intimacy problems tend to be more of a male problem, contends McCarthy, and men must alter their cognitions about emotional involvement if desire problems are to be avoided or overcome. "Both the male and his partner need to value intimate, interactive sex. . . . The major psychological aphrodisiac is an involved, aroused partner" (p. 140).

Source: Table, "Cognitive-Behavioral Approach to Hypoactive Sexual Desire" by B. McCarthy in *Journal of Sex Education & Therapy*, 21, (1995), pp. 132–141.

McCarthy (1995) also reminds us that hypoactive sexual desire is usually a problem for the couple as a unit:

> Conceptualization, assessment, and treatment of [HSD] needs to focus on this as a couple issue and broadly examine cognitions, knowledge, scripts, family of origin, sexual socialization, systems issues, comfort, skills, and flexible variable sexual scenarios and techniques. [HSD] is a changeable pattern as the couple identify and confront inhibitions and build bridges to desire. (p. 140)

Problems with Sexual Arousal

Both men and women may suffer from arousal problems; for some reason, they don't seem to be able to become sexually excited, even though they want to. In other words, it is not a lack of desire, as is the case with HSD, but rather the body seems to fall short of the desire a person feels. Of course, many psychological and physiological factors combine to produce sexual arousal in humans, but an arousal problem is defined specifically for a man by his difficulty achieving or maintaining erections (called **erectile disorder**, or **ED**) and for a woman by her lack of vaginal lubrication and swelling of the genital structures during sexual stimulation, usually with a partner (called **female sexual arousal disorder**).

Male Erectile Disorder

A common sexual myth is that the penis should be ready for sexual intercourse at any moment; it should become hard and erect whenever a man (or his partner!) wants it to; and it should stay that way until he (or his partner) is done with it. This expectation has been linked historically to a man's overall strength and masculinity as a person. Male erectile disorder used to be called "impotence," which implied that the potency or vitality of a man somehow vanishes if his penis doesn't become erect well enough, fast enough, and for a long enough period of time. Over the past decade, sex therapists, physicians, and educators have phased out "impotence" as a label for this sexual problem, even though it is still quite common to hear it in nonprofessional settings.

Difficulties with erections at some point in a man's life are extremely common. Over half of all men responding to surveys say they have experienced problems with erections during intercourse at least on occasion (Feldman et al., 1994), and one study estimates that by age 40, fully 90 percent of men have experienced erectile difficulties at least once (McCarthy, 1992).

Description. The clinical definition of erectile disorder is a "persistent or recurrent inability to attain or maintain an adequate erection until completion of sexual activity" (APA, 2000, p. 545). In addition, such an inability must be perceived as a problem by the man or the couple to be diagnosed as a disorder. As discussed early in this chapter, the mere fact that a man is having trouble with his erections does not automatically imply that he has a sexual problem.

As you may have noticed, this definition of ED leaves a great deal of room for interpretation. What is meant by "persistent" and "recurrent"? How would you describe an "adequate" erection? And just what "sexual activity" is implied, and how does one know when it is "complete"? In real life, erectile problems usually mean that the man is having difficulty achieving an erection and maintaining it for the penetration, thrusting, and orgasm (his and maybe hers) involved in sexual intercourse. In fact, vaginal and anal intercourse are really the only sexual activity for which an erect penis is absolutely necessary. Some couples do not find the occasional or even the frequent lack of penile erection to be an important problem in their sexual life together and have developed ways of "working around it" without

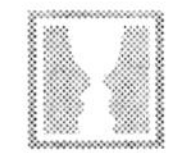

Sex is more than intercourse

erectile disorder (ED) Recurring or persistent difficulty in achieving or maintaining an erection.

female sexual arousal disorder A woman's frequent or persistent inability to attain or maintain sexual arousal.

feeling deprived of sexual satisfaction or intimacy. Remember, intercourse is not the only path to sexual fulfillment.

That said, however, erectile problems are typically quite upsetting to most men and most couples. A complex set of psychological and emotional reactions typically accompany erectile disorder—embarrassment, rejection, shame, frustration, anger, fear, and anxiety, just to name a few. Such reactions may lead to withdrawal from all intimacy in the relationship in order to avoid the possibility of further failure. Erectile problems are rarely only a physical malfunction of a penis; they are usually either a result or a cause of psychological, relationship, or intimacy problems.

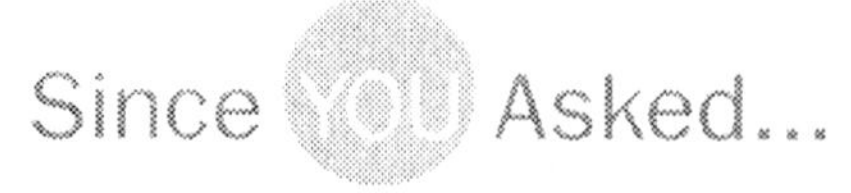

7. Is impotence always psychological? Does Viagra work for everyone?

Causes. The current consensus among sex researchers and therapists is that erectile problems usually stem from some combination of physical, psychological, and social factors, and rarely is only one of those three categories of causes at work (Chillot, 2002; Weeks & Gambescia, 2000). If you look back to the section on "sources of sexual problems" earlier in this chapter, it is not difficult to see how a biological factor such as blocked coronary arteries (preventing adequate blood flow to the penis), a psychological factor such as anxiety or depression, and a social factor such as relationship problems or cultural issues could combine to produce recurring erectile problems.

Due in part to societal expectations placed on the penis's assumed boundless ability for erections, many men (and often their partners) are concerned over *any* loss of erection during lovemaking. The irony of this concern is that it is quite normal for penile erection to vary, sometimes a lot, during a sexual encounter. Nevertheless, when it subsides, a common reaction is, "Ohmygod! What is wrong with me!" Consequently, one or more instances of erectile difficulty, regardless of the initial reason, frequently leads to a new cause: *performance anxiety*, the fear of not being able to perform "as expected." The development of performance anxiety was first described in a therapeutic setting by Masters and Johnson (1970) and has been seen in numerous studies over the years since their early work (Vares et al., 2003; Weeks & Gambescia, 2000). Masters and Johnson (1970) described it as follows:

> With each opportunity for sexual connection, [the impotent male's] immediate and overpowering concern is whether or not he will be able to achieve an erection. Will he be able of "performing" as a "normal" man? He is constantly concerned not only with achieving but also with maintaining an erection of quality sufficient for [penetration]. . . . The impotent man is gravely concerned about the functional failure of a physical response which is not only naturally occurring, but in many phases, involuntary. . . . It is his *concern* which discourages the natural occurrence of erection. Attainment of an erection is something over which he has absolutely no voluntary control. . . . No man can will, wish, or demand an erection. . . . Many men, contending with fears for sexual function, have [so] distorted this basic natural response . . . that they literally break out in a cold sweat as they approach sexual opportunity. (pp. 11–12)

You can see how this process may produce a vicious cycle: Perceived sexual failure leads to fear and anxiety, which leads to more failure, which increases the fear and anxiety, which produces more failures, and so on.

Performance anxiety may also play a role in producing another common factor in ED and other sexual problems referred to as **spectatoring**. Spectatoring is not about watching your partner during sex or your partner watching you. It is about you "watching" yourself mentally. When a person feels sexually insecure, a common and perhaps natural reaction is to become very self-aware during sexual inter-

spectatoring Mentally observing and judging oneself during sexual activities with a partner; may cause sexual problems.

actions. If a man becomes anxious about his sexual performance and fearful about achieving or maintaining an erection, he begins to second-guess everything he does during sex. Instead of allowing himself to be spontaneous and enjoy the feelings and responses of sexual interaction, he's watching and judging himself: "Am I becoming turned on fast enough?" "How's my erection doing?" "Oh, am I losing it?" Spectatoring serves to increase his anxiety, create an emotional and psychological distance from the pleasure of lovemaking, and turn his erectile fears into self-fulfilling prophecies.

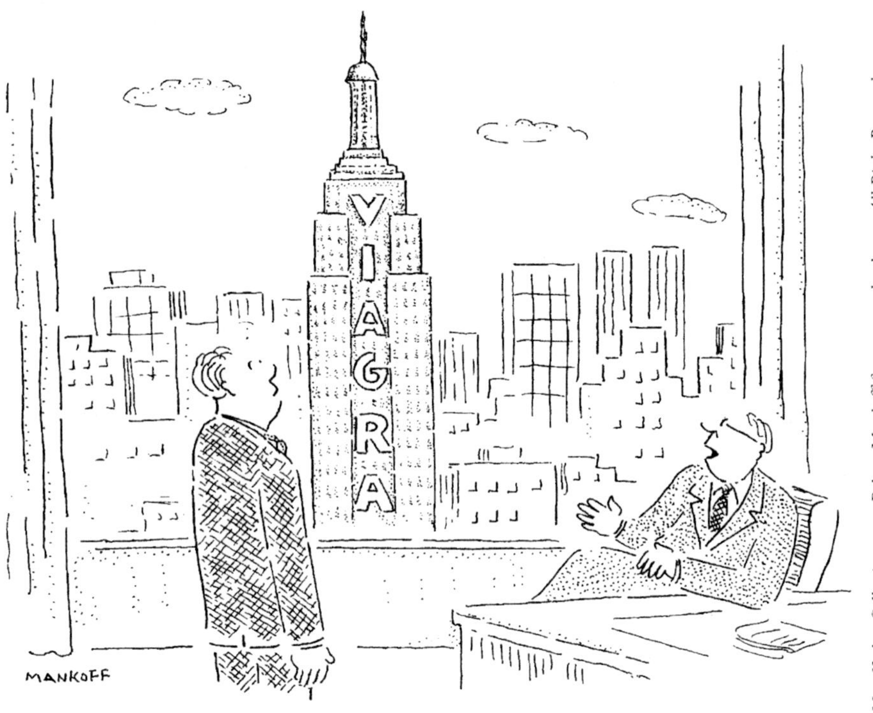

"Now, that's product placement!"

Solutions. I know what you're thinking—"Viagra!" True, the treatment of ED has undergone a major revolution in recent years, in the form of a little blue pill called Viagra (sildenafil citrate), approved by the FDA in 1998 as the first pill for the treatment of erectile problems. In the early 2000s, second-generation erectile medications—including Cialis (tadalifil), and Levitra (vardenifil)—began appearing on the market; they produce similar effects but stayed in the man's body longer, allowing him to increase the level of spontaneity for sexual activity. These drugs are helping millions of men overcome problems with erection, but it would be a mistake to assume that they are a cure for every case of erectile disorder. These medications enhance the body's ability to *respond* to sexual stimulation with increased blood flow to the penis. These drugs are not "erection pills"; they do not *induce* an erection or increase desire in and of themselves (Weeks & Gambescia, 2000). If a man were to take one of these medications before a final exam in his class, he would probably *not* be taking the exam with an erection.

Many men with ED who have been prescribed Viagra, Cialis, or Levitra, especially those with nonphysical causes of erection problems, report using it once or twice and then returning to satisfying sexual activity with perfectly fine erections without it. Simply knowing that the drug is handy, sort of an "erection good luck charm," is enough to alleviate their fears and return them to satisfactory functioning. It is important to remember, however, that although these medications offer treatment from a biological perspective, they cannot treat psychological, relationship, or desire problems that often contribute to sexual difficulties (Leiblum & Rosen, 2000). If you or someone you know is wondering whether he may have ED and might need a medication such as Viagra, "Self-Discovery: Self-Screening for Erectile Dysfunction" can provide a rough idea of the seriousness of the problem.

It is very important for a man who is experiencing problems with erections to see a physician for a physical exam to rule out potential physical causes. Such an exam goes beyond simply determining if the "sexual plumbing" is functioning properly. Loss of erections may be a sign of a larger health problem such as arterial blockages, heart disease, or diabetes. Often the man himself knows whether his difficulty is mainly physical or psychological. How does he know? Because he has erections in some settings, such as when he masturbates, when he awakens in the morning, or when he is with different partners.

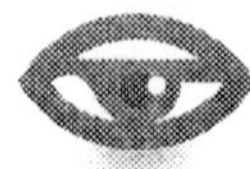

Self-Discovery

Self-Screening for Erectile Dysfunction

This quiz can help you figure out if you may have erectile dysfunction (ED). It is designed for men who are, or have been, sexually active, including vaginal or anal intercourse. If you think you may be having a problem with ED, be sure to take your results to your doctor. Only your doctor can decide if you have ED and if medication is right for you.

Pick the answer for each question that fits you best. Then add up the point values for your answer choices as indicated at the end of the scale.

1. How do you rate your confidence that you could get and keep an erection?
   a. Nonexistent
   b. Very Low
   c. Low
   d. Moderate
   e. High
   f. Very high

2. When you have had erections with sexual stimulation, how often were your erections hard enough for penetration (entering your partner)?
   a. Avoided sexual intercourse
   b. Almost never or never
   c. A few times (much less than half the time)
   d. Sometimes (about half the time)
   e. Most times (much more than half the time)
   f. Almost always or always

3. During sexual intercourse, *how often* were you able to maintain your erection after you had penetrated (entered) your partner?
   a. Avoided sexual intercourse
   b. Almost never or never
   c. A few times (much less than half the time)
   d. Sometimes (about half the time)
   e. Most times (much more than half the time)
   f. Almost always or always

4. During sexual intercourse, *how difficult* was it to maintain your erection to *completion* of intercourse?
   a. Avoided sexual intercourse
   b. Extremely difficult
   c. Very difficult
   d. Difficult
   e. Slightly difficult
   f. Not difficult

5. When you attempted sexual intercourse, *how often* was it satisfactory *for you*?
   a. Avoided sexual intercourse
   b. Almost never or never
   c. A few times (much less than half the time)
   d. Sometimes (about half the time)
   e. Most times (much more than half the time)
   f. Almost always or always

6. When you attempted sexual intercourse, *how often* was it satisfactory *for your partner*?
   a. Avoided sexual intercourse
   b. Almost never or never
   c. A few times (much less than half the time)
   d. Sometimes (about half the time)
   e. Most times (much more than half the time)
   f. Almost always or always

Scoring: For each letter you circled, give yourself the following number of points.
a. = 0 b. = 1 c. = 2 d. = 3 e. = 4 f. = 5 Total = ______

Interpreting your score:
This quiz can help a man, along with discussion with his doctor, figure out if he may have erectile dysfunction (ED). According to the pharmaceutical company that makes and markets Viagra, a score below 24 *may* indicate some degree of ED. However, this is only an estimate, and if any man's sexual response is troubling him, he should discuss it with his doctor, regardless of his score on this scale.

Source: Adapted from Pfizer (2005).

A common test for the underlying cause of ED is to monitor **nocturnal penile tumescence (NPT)**—nighttime erections. Typically, men experience three to six erections per night as a normal part of rapid-eye-movement or dreaming sleep. These erections are a normal, routine physiological response during REM sleep and do not imply that the man is dreaming about sex. However, if a man's penis is becoming erect during REM sleep, his body is probably functioning adequately, and his problems with erections likely stem from nonphysical sources. How can he know if he is having erections at night if he's asleep? If he has a bed partner (or very close friend), he could ask this person to watch his penis during the night, but for most people, that's probably asking a lot. Today, inexpensive devices called penile tumescence monitors are available that are worn on the penis during the night and indicate whether the man has had an erection (see Figure 7.3).

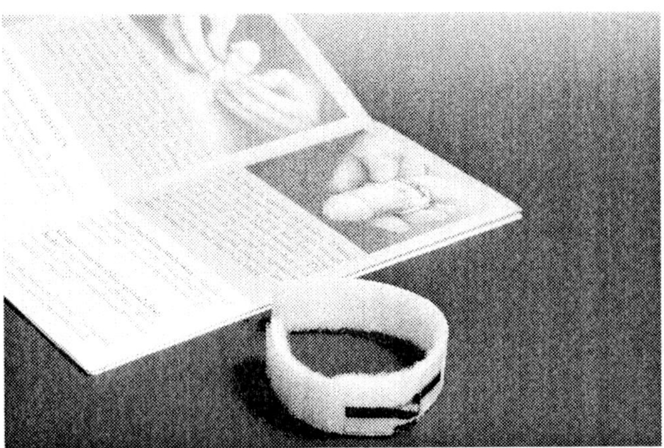

FIGURE 7.3 Home Screening for Erectile Disorder

Devices such as these allow men to determine if they are having normal erections during sleep.

Many, if not most, erectile problems, especially if they are primarily psychological and not physical, can be treated effectively without drugs. In fact, ED is a perfect example of a sexual problem that may be helped by some form of sensate focus exercises such as those discussed earlier in this chapter. When the pressure to perform—to achieve and maintain an erection for intercourse—is removed, many men find that erections cease to be a problem. When the agreement has been made between partners to engage in "nondemand pleasuring," such as kissing, touching, and caressing, for the sake of pleasure itself, and not as a prelude to intercourse, many men who have been dealing with erectile disorder find themselves very aroused and very erect throughout the entire session.

Of course, other factors that may be contributing to the erection difficulties should be resolved so that the overall quality of relationship that may have deteriorated either prior to or during the period of the specific erectile disorder may be improved. As mentioned earlier, these issues may be psychological, such as depression, fear of pregnancy or STIs, or the effects of past sexual traumas. They may be social problems relating to the current relationship, such as anger, resentment, guilt, loss of trust, and so on. Table 7.7 provides some important information relating to male arousal and erections that can help couples in understanding and overcoming ED.

The important point here is that psychological and medical science have advanced to the point where no man need resign himself to life without erections. Virtually any and every case of erectile difficulty can now be solved.

Female Sexual Arousal Disorder

Female arousal problems are defined in physiological terms as they are for men, although, as is also true for men, the underlying causes are likely to be more a combination of biological, psychological, and interpersonal factors. In the past, women suffering from female sexual arousal disorder were often referred to as "frigid," but this negative, judgmental term has disappeared from the professional literature, as has "impotence" when discussing ED.

Description. The formal, clinical definition of female sexual arousal disorder (or FSAD) is "a persistent or recurrent inability to attain, or to maintain until completion of the sexual activity, an adequate lubrication-swelling response of sexual excitement" (APA, 2000, p. 543). Also, as with virtually all sexual problems, this

nocturnal penile tumescence (NPT)
Erection of the penis while a man is asleep.

Table 7.7 UNDERSTANDING MALE AROUSAL AND ERECTIONS

ISSUE	INTERPRETATION
It's common.	By age 40, fully 90 percent of all men experience at least one instance of erectile difficulty. This, then, is normal and does not indicate the presence of an erectile disorder.
Don't overreact.	The key to overcoming an erection problem is to avoid overreacting and labeling yourself "impotent" or some sort of sexual failure.
Men are people, too.	Reject the myth of the "male machine" who should be ready, willing, and able to have and use an erection at any moment, with any partner, and in any situation. A man and his penis are human, not performance machines.
Erections come and go.	Remember, during sexual activity of, say, 45 minutes, it is completely normal for an erection to come and go several times. You cannot *will* it to return, and trying too hard will backfire. Simply relax and enjoy the moment, and chances are your erection will return.
Sex is far more than intercourse.	It is not necessary to have an erect penis to be a good lover and to satisfy your partner. Even if you are having difficulty achieving and maintaining an erection during lovemaking, pleasure and satisfaction may be realized through a multitude of sexual behaviors such as manual or oral stimulation or with the use of "sex toys."
Stop thinking about an erection.	Instead of focusing on your erection, try to involve yourself physically and mentally in giving and receiving sexual pleasure. Remember, lovemaking is a participatory, shared activity, not a "spectator sport." Through participation and involvement, an erection will often follow in the natural course of events.
Communicate, communicate, communicate.	Try to become comfortable communicating your desires and needs to your partner. Tell your partner if you feel pressured, if things are moving too fast, or if you need more or different stimulation. Your partner will probably appreciate the feedback, and overall intimacy will be the result.
Try it by yourself.	Masturbation alone is a good method for overcoming ED. You can practice having an erection, losing it, and gaining it again through masturbation exercises. Through these exercises, you can become more familiar with your body's responses and more confident during lovemaking.
Erection is separate from ejaculation.	Although they usually occur together, it is not necessary to have an erection in order to ejaculate. They are separate physiological functions.
Not all erections are for sex.	Avoid assuming that a morning erection means you should immediately have sex. An erection upon awakening is a result of routine physiological arousal during the sleep cycle, and a "use it or lose it" attitude often leads to loss of the erection.
Think of sex as pleasure, not sex as performance.	Rather than focusing stimulation on a totally flaccid penis, engage in "nondemanding" sensate focus exercises instead. Become involved in the sensual feelings, and the sexual responses will often follow. The heart of good sex is pleasure, not performance.
Not all sexual encounters are perfect.	"Feelings about a sexual experience are best measured by your sense of pleasure and satisfaction rather than whether you got an erection. Accept that some sexual experiences will be great for both of you, some will be better for one than the other, some will be mediocre, and there will be others that are poor or downright failures. Do not put your self-esteem on the line for each sexual encounter" (McCarthy, 1992, p. 31).

Source: Table, "Understanding Male Arousal and Erections" from "Erectile Dysfunction and Inhibited Sexual Desire: Cognitive-Behavioral Strategies" by B. McCarthy in *Journal of Sex Education and Therapy*, 18, (1992), pp. 22–34. Copyright © 1992. Reprinted by permission of American Association of Sex Educators, Counselors & Therapists.

"inability" must be causing personal or relationship distress to be diagnosed formally as a disorder.

If you think this sounds even more subjective and vague than the definition of ED, you are correct. Arousal problems in men can be assessed by the couple and by the therapist fairly easily by "measuring" the quality of his erections. Engorgement of the genitals in women is not as easily observed, and a lack of natural lubrication may be difficult to determine if the couple is using sexual lubricants in their lovemaking (Rosen & Leiblum, 1995). Furthermore, engorgement and lubrication from arousal are not technically required for sexual intercourse, but an erection is. Because, historically, sexual problems revolved around whether or not a *couple* were able to complete the act of intercourse, arousal problems in women received relatively little attention by researchers and therapists in past decades (except in terms of suspected hormonal imbalances). In contrast, erection problems have been a primary research and treatment focus (Bartlik & Goldberg, 2000). This discrepancy, however, has begun to change, and as ED has entered the public spotlight with the introduction of Viagra, greater research and therapeutic attention is being placed on female arousal and pleasure issues as well.

Female sexual arousal disorder may be considerably more common than most people believe. One large survey found that nearly a fifth of women under the age of 60 reported difficulty with lubrication, and the percentages are considerably higher for women past the age of menopause (Laumann, Paik, & Rosen, 1999; Rosen et al., 1993). Although for men, ED may be a distinct and separate problem, women typically experience arousal problems in combination with other sexual disorders such as hypoactive sexual desire (discussed earlier) and orgasm difficulties (to be discussed shortly). It stands to reason that a lack of desire or past difficulties reaching orgasm might contribute to a woman's lack of sexual arousal with a partner. Because of the frequency of multiple diagnoses in women, some researchers are suggesting that future therapeutic guidelines (such as the DSM-V, currently in development and due in 2010) differentiate between *genital* arousal disorder (primarily the lack of lubrication) and a more general "sexual excitement disorder" that would take into account a wider range of criteria and, ideally, enhance treatment strategies for women dealing with FSAD (Leiblum, & Rosen, 2000). Moreover, many leading researchers and sexuality educators are contending that female sexual problems, such as arousal difficulties, are fundamentally different, physically and psychologically, from those of men and may require a separate diagnostic scheme if they are to be understood fully (Bancroft et al., 2003). Consequently, you may notice that some of the issues discussed for the causes and treatments for female problems do not necessarily correspond to those discussed for men.

Causes. FSAD may stem from biological, psychological, relationship, or cultural causes or any combination of these. The most common biological issues relate to hormones.

Arousal in women appears to be more closely tied to hormonal balance and imbalance than it is in men. A woman's hormonal levels are cyclical and may vary considerably during her fertility cycle, with pregnancy, during breast-feeding, with certain medications, and with menopause. For example, low levels of estrogen are a common cause of vaginal dryness. This is a problem especially among women who are postmenopausal or whose ovaries are not functioning properly or have been removed for health reasons (Morokoff, 1993). Hormones may also be associated with sexual responses in women. One in particular that has been receiving increased attention is testosterone. You're probably thinking, "Testosterone? That's a male hormone, isn't it?" Yes it is, but women have some too, although about one-twentieth as much as men. In women, testosterone is produced by the ovaries along with estrogen. And it appears to be an important factor in female sexuality. Abnormally low levels of testosterone in women seems to be linked to low levels of desire, arousal, and even low sexual sensitivity in the nipples, vagina, and clitoris (Bartlik & Goldberg, 2000).

As discussed earlier in this chapter, various prescription medications, especially the class of antidepressants known as the SSRIs (selective serotonin reuptake inhibitors), such as Prozac, Zoloft, and Effexor, have been found to produce negative sexual side effects, including arousal problems in both men and women. This all-too-common side effect of the SSRIs will be discussed in greater detail shortly in the section on problems with orgasm. Other less common physiological considerations in the source of FSAD include substance abuse, thyroid problems, diabetes, and multiple sclerosis.

Many women experiencing FSAD may have no physiological problems at all, and their difficulties in becoming sexually aroused stem from psychological or relationship issues. The usual list of psychological difficulties involved in various sexual disorders may play a role in FSAD (see Table 7.5). The most common of these include depression, anxiety, fear, and guilt (Bancroft et al., 2003). Loss of sexual desire is one of the hallmarks of clinical depression. Depressed people typically withdraw from human contact altogether and from sexual intimacy especially. Other psychological obstacles to arousal include anxiety and fear from past sexual abuse or rape, concern about one's ability to reach orgasm with a partner, fear of pregnancy or STIs, or other sources of personal or sexual distress. Women who have grown up in a sexually restrictive cultural or religious family setting often find it difficult to enjoy what they were taught was wrong, bad, and sinful, and instead they feel guilty. To be able to relax and enjoy the pleasure of lovemaking is the key to becoming aroused for women and for men. Just as a man cannot "will, wish, or demand an erection," neither can a woman command herself to become aroused.

Most sexuality educators agree that the quality of the relationship is key to the enjoyment of sexual interactions. Relationship difficulties are a common reason that a woman may have difficulty becoming aroused with her partner. Suppressed anger, fear of rejection, imbalances of power, poor sexual communication, lack of trust, infidelity, specific deep conflicts between the partners, and conflicting expectations may interfere with a woman's ability to respond sexually with her partner. Beyond these relationship problems, however, it is important to note that when a woman ceases to become aroused with a partner who is abusive or who employs coercive or violent tactics to obtain sex from her, she does *not* have a sexual disorder. The discussion of sexual problems and solutions assumes an appropriate, mutual, and noncoercive relationship (Morokoff, 1993). This issue of relationship abuse in discussed in detail in Chapter 4, "Love, Intimacy, and Sexual Communication," and Chapter 13, "Sexual Aggression and Violence."

Solutions. Therapy for FSAD typically includes a combination of the general treatment guidelines discussed throughout this chapter: enhanced communication, specific sensate focus exercises (see Table 7.8), and directed masturbation. These treatment strategies are all designed to help a woman understand her body's responses to sexual stimulation, acquire a sense of mastery over her ability to become aroused, and enhance intimacy between her and her partner.

New medical treatments are finding some success as well. Interestingly, although several of the newer antidepressants on the market have the negative side effect of causing sexual problems, one of these antidepressants, bupropion (Wellbutrin, Zyban), which affects brain chemicals other than serotonin, is showing promise as a *treatment* for low sexual desire and arousal (Clayton, Warnock, & Kornstein, 2004). Some women prescribed bupropion show marked increases in sexual desire, sexual thoughts, and sexual pleasure.

If a lack of normal levels of testosterone in women contributes to FSAD, then shouldn't medically prescribed small doses of testosterone help return women to normal levels of desire? Current research indicates that the answer to that question may be yes. Although negative side effects must be carefully monitored and avoided, testosterone replacement therapy in pill, sublingual (under the tongue), patch, or cream form has been shown to increase sexual desire and genital responsiveness in women with FSAD (Bartlik & Goldberg, 2000; Chu & Lobo, 2004; K. Johnson, 2004).

Research continues on the effectiveness of Viagra and similar drugs for women. Most of the current evidence for Viagra use in women is anecdotal, but some small studies have found increases in sexual fantasy, desire, and function in women using Viagra (K. Johnson, 2002; Salerian et al., 2000). However, the makers of Viagra and

Table 7.8 FIVE-STEP SENSATE FOCUS FOR FEMALE SEXUAL AROUSAL DISORDER

Helen Singer Kaplan, one of the pioneers in applying Masters and Johnson's theory of sensate focus to solving sexual problems, suggested the following five-step sensate focus process for addressing FSAD specifically. These steps should take place over several weeks, not in one or two intimate sessions.

> The aim of treatment . . . is to reduce the anxiety which is evoked during the excitement phase, and which inhibits its expression. The original Masters and Johnson method is effective, although there are advantages to employing some flexibility to accommodate to the patients' individual dynamic needs. (Kaplan, 1979, p. 4)

STEP	INSTRUCTIONS TO COUPLE
1. Sensate focus I	The couple should take turns pleasuring each other; caressing each other's bodies while avoiding genital stimulation, as with the standard sensate focus exercises.
2. Sensate focus II	The couple now begin to stimulate each other's body sexually, using gentle, nondemanding genital stimulation, but not to the point of orgasm.
3. Slow teasing genital touch—no orgasm	The couple now turn to slow, teasing caressing involving the vulva, clitoris, vaginal opening, and nipples. This should proceed until the woman senses that orgasm may be nearing and then interrupted for a short time until her arousal level decreases somewhat. This process is then repeated several times.
4. Withhold intercourse or other corresponding activities	For heterosexual couples, vaginal intercourse (or other corresponding activities for same-sex couples) should be withheld until the woman is very aroused and well lubricated. To avoid frustration of her partner and pressure on herself, the partner may have orgasms through other means that do not involve intercourse.
5. Slow, teasing return to intercourse or other corresponding activities	Finally, slow, teasing entering of the vagina with the woman on top, so that she is in control of the process and may better focus her genital sensations. For lesbian couples, their preferred sexual activity may now resume, also in a slow and teasing fashion, with the woman who has been having arousal difficulties in control.

Source: Adapted from Kaplan, 1974.

its offshoots seem unconvinced and are unlikely to market the drug for women (Mayor, 2004). More likely are efforts among major drug companies to develop medication targeted specifically for female sexual problems.

Problems with Orgasm

When a woman is experiencing a problem with orgasm, it usually means she is not having orgasms often enough or "quickly" enough. This is known as **female orgasmic disorder**. By contrast, the most common orgasm problem for men is reaching orgasm *too* quickly, known as **premature ejaculation**. Sexual difficulties such as these are very common and, like most sexual problems, typically quite easily treated. A less common condition is retarded ejaculation in men, or **male orgasmic disorder**, which will be covered briefly in this discussion.

female orgasmic disorder A sexual problem in which a woman rarely or never reaches orgasm or whose orgasms are delayed; also known as *inhibited female orgasm* or *anorgasmia*.

premature ejaculation (PE) A man's tendency to have an orgasm suddenly with little penile stimulation, typically just before, upon, or shortly after penetration of the penis into the vagina; also referred to as *rapid* or *early ejaculation*.

male orgasmic disorder A frequent or recurring delay or inhibition of orgasm and ejaculation; a relatively rare disorder.

Female Orgasmic Disorder

Women who rarely or never reach orgasm or whose orgasms are delayed in one or more settings may be experiencing *female orgasmic disorder* also referred to as *inhibited female orgasm*, or *anorgasmia* (lack of orgasm). Regardless of the orgasm difficulty being experienced, it must be causing personal or relationship distress to be diagnosed

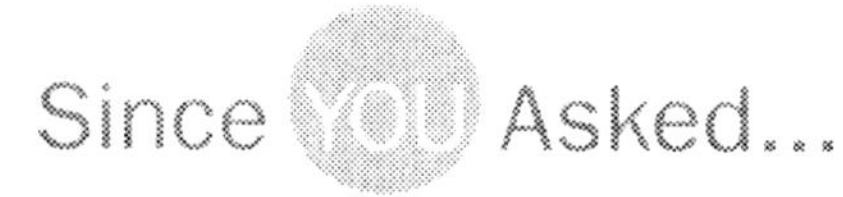

8. What causes a woman to be unable to experience orgasm during sexual intercourse even though she can have an orgasm during oral sex? It is a physical thing or mental? Maybe both?

as a clinical problem. Difficulties with orgasm are among the most common sexual complaints of female college students.

Description. The circumstances surrounding a woman's orgasm difficulties are especially important. A woman who has never experienced an orgasm under any conditions is often referred to as "preorgasmic," implying that all women have the capacity for orgasm, even if they have never had one. This type of problem would be classified as *primary anorgasmia*.

Primary anorgasmia is relatively rare and accounts for only 5 to 15 percent of all cases of FOD (Comer, 1998; Hite, 1976; Spector & Carey, 1990). Most instances of female orgasmic disorder are secondary and situational (and may be either total or partial). Many women who are capable of achieving orgasms through masturbation, oral sex, manual stimulation by partner, or use of a vibrator rarely or never do so during penis-vagina intercourse. Other women reporting orgasm difficulties may be orgasmic through masturbation but never or rarely with a partner, regardless of the type of stimulation. Still others may experience orgasm with a partner on rare occasions but far less often than they desire.

Causes. Again, a wide variety of potential causes for female orgasmic disorder must be considered, including organic, psychological, and relationship-based issues. When attempting to determine the source of this problem, its classification on the dimensions of primary-secondary, global-situational, and total-partial is crucial.

Organic or physiological causes may include hormonal imbalances as discussed previously, use or abuse of alcohol or other recreational drugs, or side effects of prescription medications. As noted in Chapter 3, "The Physiology of Human Sexual Responding," alcohol is notorious for suppressing orgasm in both men and women. As a central nervous system depressant, moderate to heavy amounts of alcohol interfere with the body's ability to respond to sexual stimuli. Under alcohol's influence, arousal slows significantly and orgasm becomes less intense or often disappears altogether (Geller, 1991; Rosen & Ashton, 1993).

As alluded to earlier, one of the most significant recent developments relating to physiological causes of orgasm problems involve side effects of the new class of prescription antidepressant medications known as the selective serotonin reuptake inhibitors. These medications are widely prescribed for depression and various other psychological difficulties such as obsessive-compulsive disorder, premenstrual distress, and even smoking cessation. Virtually all of these medications have been shown to produce sexual side effects in some users, the most common of which is delayed or suppressed orgasm in both men and women (Clayton et al., 2004; Rosen, Lane, & Menza, 1999). Usually, this side effect can be reversed by changing the specific medication, altering the dose, or combining other medications with the SSRI (Keltner, McAfee, & Taylor, 2002).

Turning to the nonphysical causes of female orgasmic disorder, the most common is simply lack of adequate or desired sexual stimulation. You'll recall from Chapter 3 that stimulation of the clitoris is necessary for orgasm in most women. You may also remember from earlier discussions that during intercourse, the thrusting of the penis in the vagina may not provide much contact with the clitoris. Consequently, it is quite common for women not to experience orgasm during intercourse alone without additional simultaneous clitoral stimulation (Kaplan, 1974). One study found that women reported experiencing an orgasm during sexual activity with a male partner between 11 and 34 percent of the time over the previous month (Bancroft et al., 2003).

The problem is that there continues to be widespread misunderstanding of this basic physiological concept, and many women (and men) incorrectly believe that both *should* experience orgasm during intercourse. An all-too-common expectation is that if the man can "last long enough," that is, can hold off his own orgasm and continue thrusting, the woman *should* reach orgasm. When this does not happen, she may feel distressed that she has failed to please *him* (Nicholson & Burr, 2003). In reality, lack of orgasm in women during intercourse is *normal*. Most women do not routinely experience an orgasm through intercourse, regardless of how long their male partner "lasts." However, 90 percent of all women are orgasmic through activities other than or in addition to intercourse, such as masturbation or manual or oral stimulation (Stock, 1993). Today, women who do not have orgasms during intercourse are *not* considered to have a sexual problem based on that symptom alone.

Finally, as for all sexual problems, various additional causes must be considered (Stock, 1993). For example, research has found that age, marital status, and education level appear to be linked to orgasm. Women who are younger, are not married, and have less education report greater problems with orgasm (Laumann et al., 1999). Past sexual traumas including sexual harassment, childhood sexual abuse, sexual assault, and rape have also been shown to relate to orgasm difficulties. And of course, as has been mentioned for all sexual problems discussed here, psychological issues, such as depression, anxiety, and fear; relationship factors, such as infidelity, anger, and resentment; and cultural factors, including religion, values, and role expectations, may all play a role in sexual responding and orgasms.

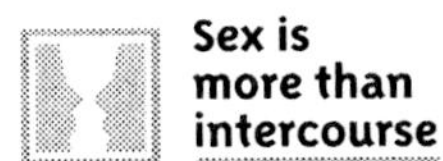
Sex is more than intercourse

Solutions. Treatment strategies for female orgasmic disorder generally incorporate a combination of the treatment guidelines discussed earlier in this chapter, especially masturbation and sensate focus exercises. Historically, in Western cultures, women have been given significantly less "permission" than men to think and act in sexual ways. The effects of this double standard are still felt today. Consequently, many women are insufficiently familiar with their own bodies and with their individual sensations when responding sexually. Sexual self-exploration through masturbation can be a powerful tool for a woman to discover that she is capable of achieving orgasms and where and how she needs to be touched to achieve them. Sometimes the incorporation of a vibrator into her masturbatory repertoire can assist a woman who has never or rarely experienced orgasm by providing maximal stimulation leading to more predictable orgasms and thereby enhancing self-awareness (Davis et al., 1996).

Once a woman is reasonably comfortable with her own body and her ability to have orgasms, nondemanding sexual exercises, such as sensate focus, can begin to include her partner. In some cases, she may masturbate in her partner's presence as a way of demonstrating, educating, and involving both as a team. As part of their sensate focus program, a specific position was developed by Masters and Johnson to allow the woman to guide her partner in ways of touching and pleasuring that provide the sensations and stimulation that is most effective for her (see Figure 7.4). Not only does

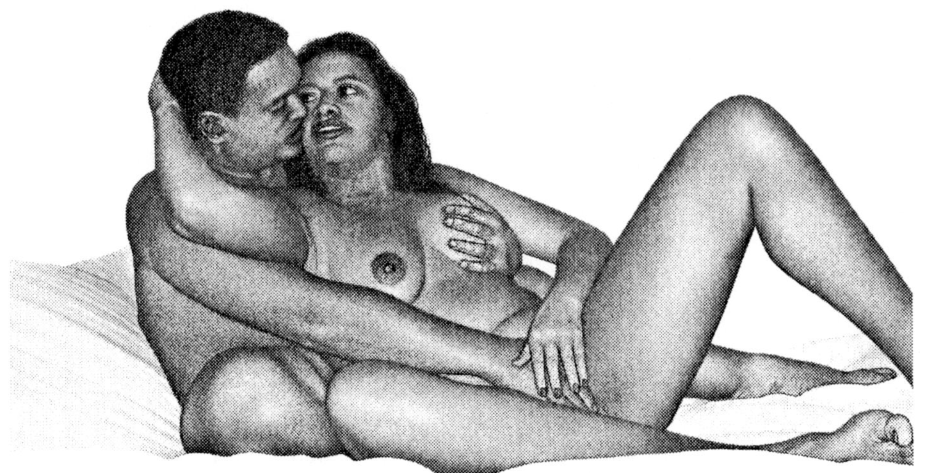

FIGURE 7.4 Back-to-Front Sensate Focus Position

The back-to-front position allows the woman to guide the man's touching movements—to help him understand what feels best to her.

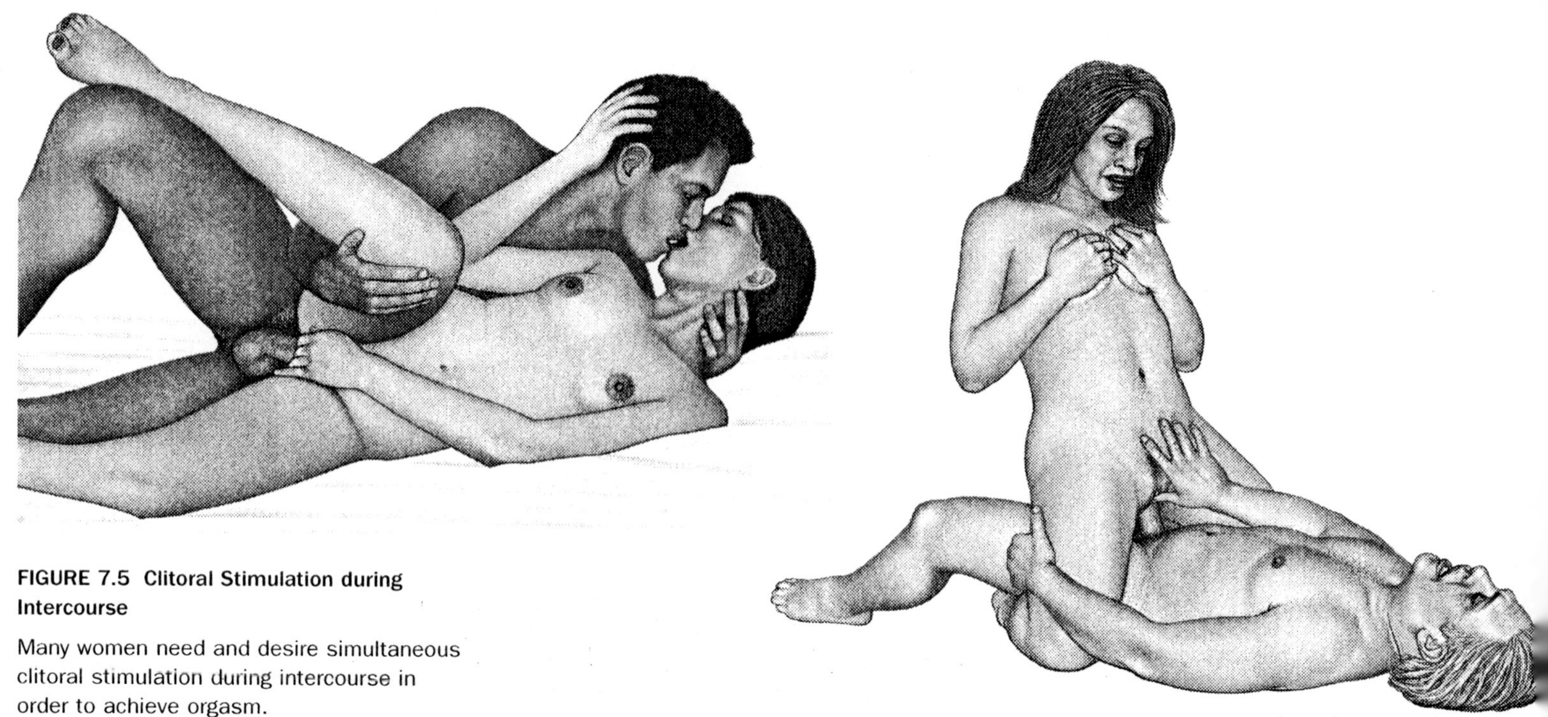

FIGURE 7.5 Clitoral Stimulation during Intercourse

Many women need and desire simultaneous clitoral stimulation during intercourse in order to achieve orgasm.

this exercise help inform her partner about what feels best to her, but it also tends to enhance closeness and communication in general (Masters & Johnson, 1970).

For heterosexual couples, these exercises are usually carried out during a period of time when intercourse is banned, as discussed earlier, so the pressure of performing according to old expectations is removed. When the woman is comfortable with her ability to have orgasms through these exercises, intercourse may be resumed. If the goal for the couple is for both to reach orgasm during intercourse, this is now usually accomplished through the addition of manual stimulation by either partner to the clitoral area during penetration (see Figure 7.5). These methods, and various adaptations of them, appear to be quite successful in helping most women with female orgasmic disorder—as many as 90 percent—become orgasmic alone, with a partner, and sometimes during intercourse (Segraves & Althof, 1998).

Premature Ejaculation

Reaching orgasm and ejaculating "too soon" with a partner is the most common sexual complaint of men (especially younger men) and may be the most frequently encountered sexual problem (other than low desire) in sex therapy. Estimates are that 25 to 35 percent of men are affected by this sexual problem (Byers & Grenier, 2003).

Since YOU Asked...

9. Are there ways for a guy to control orgasm and last longer?

Description. Premature ejaculation (PE), also often referred to as *rapid* or *early ejaculation*, has always been difficult to define. Masters and Johnson (1970) diagnosed PE for heterosexual relationships when the man reaches orgasm before his partner more than 50 percent of the time during intercourse. But you already know that is way off the mark, because half or more of all women do not have orgasms routinely during intercourse *regardless* of how long intercourse takes. Some have attempted to define PE as the man's subjective experience of having an orgasm sooner than he wants to. This definition is problematic as well due to the fact that many men define their own ability to control orgasm based on the same myth of lasting long enough for their partner to have one. Other definitions have included ejaculatory latency (how long until ejaculation occurs), perceived ejaculatory control (how much control the man feels he has over when he ejaculated during sexual stimulation), concern over ejaculating more rapidly than desired, satisfaction with ejaculatory control, and the frequency of antiportal (prior to penile insertion) ejaculation.

Clinically, the definition of PE has focused on the man's tendency to have an orgasm suddenly and without much stimulation, just before, immediately upon, or shortly after penetration of the penis into the vagina (APA, 2000, p. 552). Most men who suffer from PE report that ejaculation often "takes him by surprise . . . and the ability to decide when to ejaculate is missed" (Polonsky, 2000, p. 310).

Like most sexual problems discussed in this chapter, PE revolves around sexual activities with a partner, usually vaginal or anal sex. Rarely is a man concerned with reaching orgasm too fast during masturbation, oral sex, or other activities with a partner. The reason that PE is such a common problem is in part due to the emphasis placed on intercourse as the singular goal of lovemaking, as has been discussed throughout this book. Obviously, if a man ejaculates before intercourse can even get under way, both he and his partner may see this as a serious problem in their sexual lives. In heterosexual couples, the man's inability to delay his orgasm may be interpreted (often erroneously) as the cause of whatever orgasm problems she may be experiencing. Consequently, he feels inadequate as a lover, ashamed of his perceived lack of control, and filled with anxiety and even dread as each new sexual encounter approaches. These reactions may in turn lead to erectile difficulties, loss of sexual desire, and potentially avoidance of sex with a partner altogether. Fortunately, PE is one of the easiest sexual problems to treat, as you will see shortly.

Causes. Many causes for rapid ejaculation have been hypothesized, but none has been clearly demonstrated by scientific research. With this lack of solid evidence for any specific cause in mind, here is a brief list of some of the suggested origins of PE. Each item is followed by a brief summary of overall research findings (Grenier & Byers, 1995; Hong, 1984; Masters & Johnson, 1970; O'Donohue, Letourneau, & Geer, 1993; Polonsky, 2000). Research suggests the following about men who experience premature ejaculation:

1. They may be more sensitive physically to sexual stimulation, which causes them to become aroused more quickly (some research support, some refutation; more research needed).
2. They may have faster-acting reflexes in the pelvic and genital muscles that control orgasm and ejaculation, so that ejaculation may occur prior to full arousal (some research support; further study needed).
3. They may be less able to perceive the moment in their arousal sequence that signals the onset of orgasm and ejaculation ("the point of no return") (some clinical support, some refutation; findings unclear).
4. They may be angry with or dislike women in general or their partners specifically and unconsciously wish to deprive them of their pleasure (little to no support).
5. They may tend to have longer periods of abstinence between sexual encounters, leading to faster arousal and ejaculation (some research support; findings unclear).
6. They may be conditioned over time to ejaculate quickly due to rushed masturbation and sexual encounters during their developmental years when the threat of getting caught placed a premium on finishing quickly (some anecdotal and clinical support; little scientific evidence).
7. They may be normal. This theory contends that as humans evolved, ejaculating quickly had survival value in that males who were able to mate quickly could impregnate more females and were in a condition of increased vulnerability (that is, easy to attack while mating) for shorter periods of time (generally refuted).
8. They may have higher levels of testosterone (convincingly refuted).

What's the bottom line on the cause of premature ejaculation? No one really knows for sure. Perhaps a more important question, then, is, how can a man acquire better ejaculatory control? Fortunately, treatment strategies and outcomes for PE are much more definitive than its origins.

Solutions. Men who consistently ejaculate very quickly typically strive to delay their orgasm during intercourse using strategies that, unfortunately, have been shown to be generally ineffective. The most common of these strategies involves attempts to distract themselves from the sexual act in which they are engaged (Grenier & Byers, 1997), usually by focusing on anti-arousing thoughts such as an ugly teacher, STIs, counting backward from 100, dead animals on the side of the road, or parents walking in, to name just a few. Other common behavioral strategies include drinking alcohol before intercourse, withdrawing for a few minutes during intercourse, and applying anesthetic (numbing) cream to the penis. These are usually unproductive tactics for two reasons. One, they are rarely effective in delaying orgasm, and two, they detract from the pleasure of the sexual encounter. Think about it: Who would want to be thinking of road kill or have a numb penis while making love? (Slob, van Berkel, & van der Werff ten Bosch, 2000, for one study suggesting sexual enhancement for some rapid ejaculating men using a penile anesthesia technique.)

What are some more effective solutions for PE? Once again, if you remove *intercourse* from the sexual equation, most men do not have a rapid ejaculation problem. Sensate focus exercises in which intercourse is banned often help the man with PE feel more in control and allow for greater intimacy between partners by extending each overall lovemaking session. It is important for couples to remember that pleasure, closeness, intimacy, and sexual satisfaction can be achieved through various sexual behaviors and not through intercourse alone.

Sex is more than intercourse 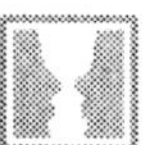

Beyond sensate focus, however, most treatments for PE approach the problem from exactly the opposite direction than most men attempt. The solution is found not in *distraction* from sexual sensations, but greater focus on them. Most treatments employ one of many variations on a treatment developed by Masters and Johnson (1970) called the "squeeze technique." This method requires the man's partner (remember that all of Masters and Johnson's original clients were heterosexual couples) to stimulate the man's penis manually until he feels he is close to orgasm and ejaculation. She then stops the stimulation and squeezes the glans area (tip) of the penis firmly between her thumb and fingertips. The pressure she exerts should be fairly strong but not to the point of causing pain. The typical effect of this is that "he will immediately lose his urge to ejaculate" and "may also lose 10 to 30 percent of his full erection" (Masters & Johnson, 1970, p. 104). She should then wait about 30 seconds and resume penile stimulation until his orgasm is once again looming and repeat the same squeeze maneuver. Using this technique, men who ejaculated very quickly in the past can learn to delay orgasm for more than 15 minutes (see Figure 7.6).

After several sessions using the squeeze technique, the next step is for the couple to have slow, nondemanding intercourse in the woman-on-top position. When the man feels he is nearing orgasm, he lets her know this verbally, and "she then can elevate from the penile shaft, apply the squeeze technique . . . for 3 or 4 seconds, and reinsert the penis . . . without the added stimulus of pelvic thrusting" (Masters & Johnson, 1970, p. 107). The couple then practices this process until the man gains increased conscious control over his body's progression toward ejaculation. Masters and Johnson reported this treatment method to be highly successful, with only two failures out of 186 men with PE. The same technique with some obvious modifications would be effective for gay male couples as well.

Today, variations of the squeeze technique remain the treatment of choice for PE. However, most sex therapists and researchers agree that the actual squeezing of the

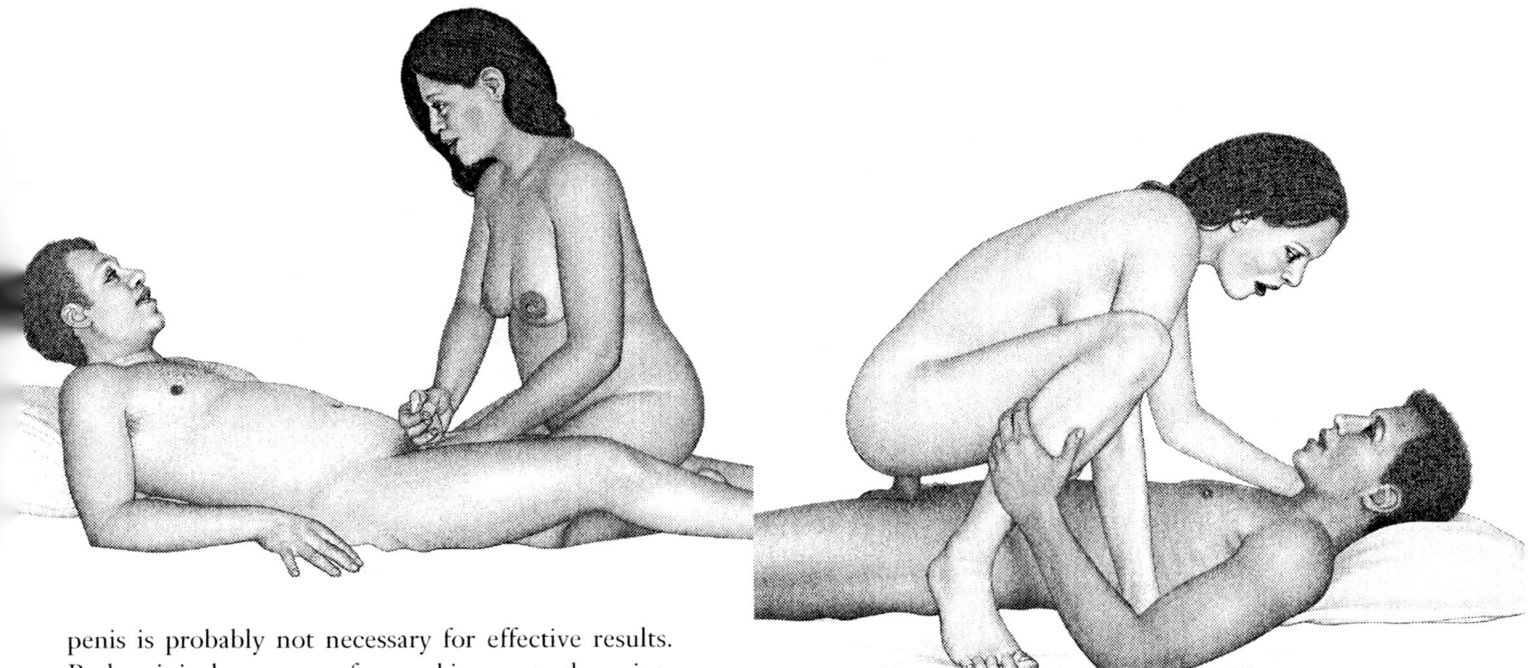

penis is probably not necessary for effective results. Rather, it is the process of arousal just up to the point of no return, followed by a retreat from that point, over and over, that allows the man to focus on his physical sensations and develop conscious control of what was formerly purely reflexive. Furthermore, it is not absolutely necessary for a man to do this with a partner. He can begin to learn about his responses and acquire some conscious control over his orgasms by engaging in "squeeze" or "start-stop" techniques while masturbating by himself (Polonsky, 2000).

FIGURE 7.6 Treatment for Premature Ejaculation

Masters and Johnson's "squeeze technique" (a) and newer versions called "start-stop techniques" (b) help some men overcome a problem with rapid ejaculation.

These treatment strategies for PE are effective because the man is learning to recognize his *moment of ejaculatory inevitability*, as discussed in Chapter 3. This is the moment in his response cycle when the physiological mechanisms of ejaculation kick in, after which the event is reflexive and out of his conscious control. To acquire *conscious* control over ejaculation, he must learn to identify with some precision the sensations immediately preceding that moment. That is why focusing on his arousal, rather than distracting himself from it, is the key to overcoming premature ejaculation.

One last note on treatment of PE returns us to the SSRIs medications discussed earlier. These medications frequently produce the side effect of delaying orgasm in both men and women. When that side effect was discovered, doctors began to prescribe the medications (especially Prozac, Zoloft, and Paxil) to *treat* PE (Stone, Viera, & Parman, 2003). Many men have found that taking Prozac or some other SSRI effectively allows them to engage in intercourse longer and feel more in control of their orgasms (Rosen et al., 1999; Waldinger & Olivier, 1998). However, some sex therapists and physicians believe that taking such a powerful psychotherapeutic medication for PE is akin to using a sledgehammer to swat a fly. What this colorful analogy implies is that PE is typically treated quite easily and successfully using the behavioral techniques just described, and resorting to a pill that alters the balance of brain chemicals, though convenient, may be unnecessary and may risk other unwanted side effects.

Male Orgasmic Disorder

Although relatively rare, some men experience delayed or inhibited ejaculation, referred to as *male orgasmic disorder* (APA, 2000; Apfelbaum, 2000). As with female orgasmic disorder, delayed ejaculation in men is characterized by an inability to reach orgasm after long periods of stimulation that should in most cases be adequate in terms of focus, intensity, and duration (APA, 2000). Although this "problem" may sound advantageous to some men (and to some women), the real effect of the problem is extreme frustration, usually in both partners, which may lead to other relationship problems and avoidance of lovemaking. Most of the time, this difficulty is secondary and situational, in that the problem has not been present in the past or with other partners. Men who experience inhibited ejaculation typically have no difficulty obtaining or, indeed, maintaining an erection, and their erections typically last throughout the extended period of time they are attempting to reach orgasm.

The causes of inhibited ejaculation are unclear but may include many of the psychological and relationship issues discussed earlier in this chapter, such an anger, fear of pregnancy, or guilt. Treatment usually consists of identifying and resolving such psychological and relationship issues and then applying behavioral treatments to the problem itself. For heterosexuals, this includes masturbation exercises with a partner in which the man masturbates or is masturbated by his partner until the moment of ejaculatory inevitability, at which time he quickly inserts his penis into her vagina. This process is repeated over time, with penetration occurring at increasing intervals in advance of orgasm. In this way, the man becomes accustomed to and confident in having intravaginal orgasms with his partner.

Painful Sex

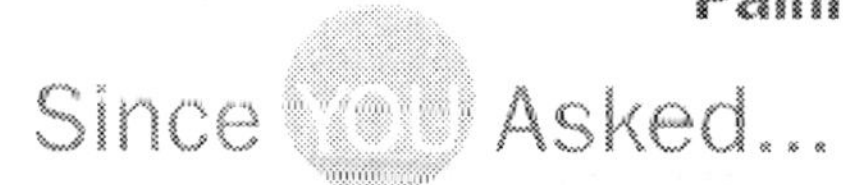

10. How can a woman get past the step of intercourse hurting her even when she's doing it with someone she loves? What can she do to help relieve the pain?

If sex hurts, something is probably wrong. That may sound overly simple, but it is very difficult to think of an exception (except, of course, the consensual, voluntary inflicting or receiving of pain for sexual pleasure, called *sadomasochism*, which will be discussed in Chapter 14, "Paraphilias"). What we are discussing here is physical pain experienced during sexual activities. Such pain can occur with a variety of sexual activities, including oral sex, manual stimulation by a partner, or anal intercourse, but it is most commonly reported with penile-vaginal sexual intercourse.

The human body is designed for the act of heterosexual intercourse to work smoothly and to feel good. After all, this is how we survive as a species! If we were designed so that sex hurt, the human race would probably have become extinct long ago. That is why pain associated with intercourse, especially if the pain occurs on a regular basis, is not normal. Both men and women may experience pain with sexual intercourse, but it is four to five times more common in women (Laumann et al., 1994). The two most common sexual problems involving painful sex are dyspareunia and vaginismus.

Dyspareunia

Dyspareunia (dis-puh-ROO-nee-uh) means painful sexual intercourse. In women, it refers to physical pain experienced in the vagina, the vaginal opening, or deeper in the abdominal cavity during or just after intercourse. Although dyspareunia is relatively rare in men, it involves external or internal pain relating to the penis, testicles, or other deeper areas in the reproductive tract. Dyspareunia is one of the most common sexual problems in women, with as many as 23 percent of women reporting that such pain occurs at least a few times per year and approximately 15 percent experiencing the problem over a period of at least several months (Butcher, 2003; Laumann et al., 1994; Spector & Carey, 1990). Many causes of dyspareunia have been identified, and most are physical in nature, prompting some researchers to suggest that dyspareunia should be classified as a pain disorder that interferes with sexual activity rather than as a sexual disorder (Binik et al., 2002).

Regardless of the specific classification, the most common cause for vaginal dyspareunia is lack of adequate vaginal lubrication prior to and during intercourse. As you know from Chapter 3, sexual arousal causes the vagina to secrete a fluid that lubricates and protects the walls of the vagina during intercourse. If penetration is attempted before the woman is fully aroused or if she is not feeling sexually excited for any reason, lubrication will be minimal, and the thrusting of the penis can irritate the vagina, resulting

dyspareunia Painful sexual intercourse, usually experienced as pain in the vagina, the vaginal opening, or deeper in the abdominal cavity during or just after intercourse.

in itching, burning, and stinging both during intercourse and sometimes for hours after. Usually, this cause of dyspareunia can be readily overcome through increased arousal or the use of a topical water-based vaginal lubricant. However, it is important to note that lack of lubrication may be a sign of unresolved psychological or relationship problems that are preventing the woman from becoming aroused with her partner.

Other sources of vaginal irritation include infections (Stewart, 2003) such as yeast infections, bacterial vaginosis, trichomoniasis, or herpes simplex virus (refer to Chapter 8, "Sexually Transmitted Infections," for a more detailed discussion). In addition, various medications may contribute to dyspareunia due to their effect on vaginal lubrication (Stewart, 2003). Some women have a sensitivity or allergy to the latex or spermicides used in condoms and other forms of contraceptives. This allergy may cause an inflammation in the vagina that can be further irritated by intercourse (Stewart, 2003).

A second type of pain in women during and after intercourse is called *deep dyspareunia*. The pain is not experienced as localized external or vaginal irritation but as a deeper *ache* in the lower abdominal area. Usually, this is the result of deep thrusting during intercourse, when the erect penis makes forceful contact with the cervix. This contact creates pressure on the uterus, which in turn affects the ovaries. The ovaries are very sensitive to trauma, much like the testicles in men. Altering sexual positions and decreasing the intensity of thrusting usually reduces or eliminates this problem. Deep dyspareunia may also be a sign of *endometriosis* (discussed in Chapter 2) or *pelvic inflammatory disease*, typically a result of various untreated sexually transmitted infections. The most important point to keep in mind here is that pain during sex is *not normal.* If you experience either form of dyspareunia, even over a short period of time, you should consult your doctor for appropriate consultation, diagnosis, and treatment.

For men, dyspareunia is usually due to a localized infection either on the penis or in the reproductive tract, including the scrotum, testicles, and anus, or in some cases headache following sexual activity (Partner Therapy Group, 2003). If the skin of the penis is inflamed or irritated due to vigorous masturbation without adequate lubrication, a sensitivity to contraceptive chemicals or latex condoms, or infections such as herpes or HPV, intercourse is likely to exacerbate these conditions, resulting in pain. Other causes of dyspareunia in men involve infections (usually bacterial) of the male sexual anatomy, including the urethra, the prostate gland, the testicles, and the epididymis on one or both sides.

Treatment of dyspareunia in men must address the underlying physical causes to reduce inflamation, enhance proper hygiene, and where indicated, alleviate infections through antibiotics or other medications.

Vaginismus

Vaginismus refers to a condition in women that causes pain *prior* to intercourse, due to involuntary contractions and spasms of the muscles controlling the opening to and outer third of the vagina. These contractions occur in the moments just before intercourse as penetration is anticipated. Typically, women diagnosed with vaginismus are unable to engage in sexual intercourse or tolerate vaginal penetration of any kind (Leiblum, 2000). The percentage of women experiencing this problem is unclear, with estimates ranging anywhere from 1 to 30 percent, depending on the definition and degree of severity of the disorder (Comer, 1998; Leiblum, 2000; Read, King, & Watson, 1997). The symptoms of vaginismus often generalize to nonsexual vaginal penetration situations, such as gynecological examinations, Pap tests, and the use of tampons (Reissing et al., 2004; Sadovsky, 2000). Consequently, beyond a difficult sexual problem, vaginismus may interfere with a woman's reproductive health and create a frustrating obstacle to becoming pregnant.

The underlying causes of vaginismus demonstrate the powerful link between mind and body. Research is in general agreement that this sexual problem is primarily psychological

vaginismus Pain in a woman just prior to intercourse, due to involuntary contractions and spasms of the muscles controlling the opening to and outer third of the vagina.

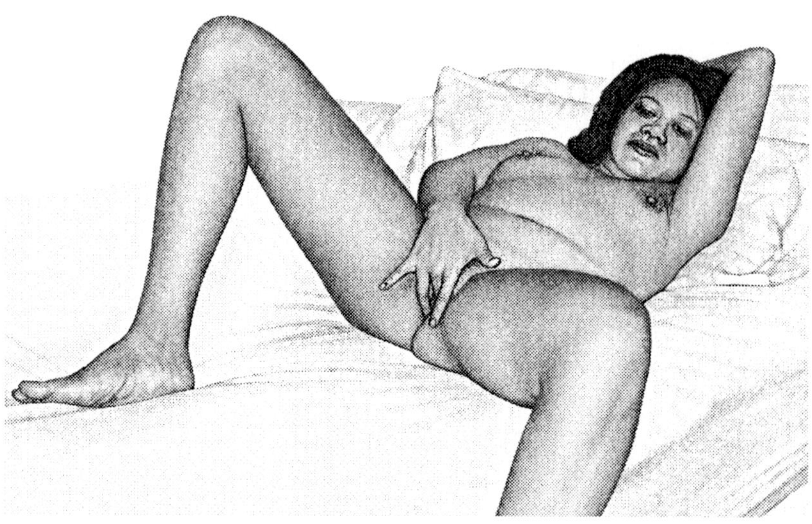

FIGURE 7.7 Treatment for Vaginismus

Treatment exercises for vaginismus typically involve gradual, smaller-to-larger vaginal penetration using special dilators or finger insertion in a relaxed, fear-free setting, sometimes in conjunction with therapy to deal with the source of the fear.

and probably based on a deeply conditioned fear that penetration will be painful or traumatic in some way, which may indicate a potential link between dyspareunia and vaginismus (Butcher, 1999; Reissing et al., 2004). The origins of that fear can vary widely from one woman to another and may include childhood sexual abuse, painful past intercourse experiences, rape and sexual assault trauma, belief in myths about painful and bloody first intercourse, or extreme fears about unwanted pregnancy or STIs. Most physicians and sex therapists who treat vaginismus agree that it is rare to see a case that lacks at least one serious past sexual trauma.

Vaginismus is generally treated using a combination of psychological and physical strategies. Usually, treatment includes sensate focus exercises to enhance intimacy between the partners and help the woman feel more relaxed and familiar with her sexual arousal without worrying about approaching penetration. Next, the woman practices exercises to learn voluntary control of the muscles that surround the vagina. Finally, a gradual process of nonthreatening vaginal insertion allows her to become less sensitive to penetration.

Traditionally, this step-by-step therapy has been accomplished using a set of *dilators*, smooth, round-ended cylinders in graduated sizes from very small (the width of a pencil) to the approximate size of an erect penis. In conjunction with self-exploration, relaxation, and masturbation exercises, the woman inserts these dilators sequentially, beginning with the smallest, to become accustomed to penetration. Currently, the use of dilators is decreasing, and women are often instructed simply to use the tip of a little finger at first, and slowly increasing finger insertion up to two or three fingers at once (see Figure 7.7). When she feels ready, her partner may join the process and continue to proceed slowly until eventually penetration becomes possible. Using these techniques, success rates of 80 to 100 percent have been reported (Segraves & Althof, 1998).

A "New View" of Female Sexual Problems

In Chapter 3, we introduced a recent model for understanding sexual problems, called "A New View of Women's Sexual Responding." This model has been suggested as an alternative to classifying male and female sexual problems based on a single model such as Masters and Johnson's traditional categories of excitement, plateau, orgasm, and resolution. The underlying assumption of this New View is that men's and women's sexual problems cannot be explained using the same classification scheme because sexuality and sexual functioning are fundamentally different for each sex. The researchers who proposed the New View (12 women scientists, researchers, and clinicians) developed a classification system that they contend more accurately reflects the complexities of female sexual problems that may not always be present in male sexual problems. This model, published as a "manifesto," is a response to the trend to "medicalize" sexual problems and attempt to find "cures" in the form of drugs, symbolized by the huge success of male erectile dysfunction medications such as Viagra. Proponents of the New View contend that although a medical model of sexual problems may be effective for men, women's sexual problems often involve nuances and complexities that cannot be treated successfully with a simple pill. Instead they suggest an approach that goes well beyond Masters and Johnson's four phases of sexual response, including various sexual, cultural, political, and economic considerations. These are described in greater detail in Table 7.9.

Table 7.9 SUMMARY OF THE MANIFESTO "A NEW VIEW OF WOMEN'S SEXUAL PROBLEMS"

The following classification system was designed by the Working Group on a New View of Women's Sexual Problems as an alternative to the traditional model of assigning problems to such categories as desire, excitement, and orgasm. The group's "manifesto" defines sexual difficulties for women as "discontent or dissatisfaction with any emotional, physical, or relational aspect of sexual experience [that] may arise in one or more of the following interrelated aspects of women's sexual lives."

CLASSIFICATION CATEGORY	DEFINITIONS
Sexual problems due to sociocultural, political, or economic factors	• Ignorance and anxiety due to inadequate sex education, lack of access to health services, or other social constraints. • Sexual avoidance or distress due to perceived inability to meet cultural norms regarding correct or ideal sexuality. • Inhibitions due to conflict between the sexual norms of one's subculture or culture of origin and those of the dominant culture • Lack of interest, fatigue, or lack of time due to family and work obligations
Sexual problems relating to partner and relationship	• Inhibition, avoidance, or distress arising from betrayal, dislike, or fear of partner, partner's abuse or couple's unequal power or arising from partner's negative patterns of communication • Discrepancies in desire for sexual activity or in preferences for various sexual activities • Ignorance or inhibition about communicating preferences or initiating, pacing, or shaping sexual activities • Loss of sexual interest and reciprocity as a result of conflicts over commonplace issues such as money, schedules, or relatives or resulting from traumatic experiences such as infertility or the death of a child • Inhibitions in arousal or spontaneity due to partner's health status or sexual problems
Sexual problems due to psychological factors	• Sexual aversion, mistrust, or inhibition of sexual pleasure due to past experiences of physical, sexual, or emotional abuse; general personality problems with attachment, rejection, cooperation, or entitlement; depression or anxiety • Sexual inhibition due to fear of sexual acts or of their possible consequences, such as pain during intercourse, pregnancy, sexually transmitted disease, loss of partner, or loss of reputation
Sexual problems due to medical factors	• Local or systemic medical conditions affecting neurological, neurovascular, circulatory, endocrine or other systems of the body • Pregnancy, sexually transmitted infections, or other sex-related conditions • Side effects of drugs, medications, or medical treatments

Sources: FSD Alert (2000); Kaschak and Tiefer (2002).

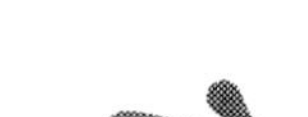

YOUR SEXUAL PHILOSOPHY

SEXUAL PROBLEMS AND SOLUTIONS

By now you know that sexual problems are quite common and usually are not particularly serious or difficult to overcome. The biggest obstacles to solving sexual problems are ignorance, embarrassment, and acceptance of the many myths and misconceptions that usually accompany sexual difficulties and poor communication. After reading this chapter, you now have the tools to overcome those hurdles and are better prepared to deal rationally and effectively with sexual difficulties when and if they arise.

Most people never give sexual problems even a passing thought until one happens to them or their partner. This is a bad idea. Although you may never experience a diagnosable sexual disorder, most people do at some point in their lives. An awareness and understanding of sexual problems and their solutions is a vital component of your sexual philosophy. Why? Here are just a few good reasons.

First, knowledge is prevention. If you realize that sexual problems are both common and easily treated, your anxiety level at the first potential sign of one will be much lower than if you lacked this knowledge. That reduction in anxiety may help you head off the problem before it worsens or leads to relationship complications.

Second, knowledge is treatment. After reading this chapter, you now know many strategies to help you or your partner deal with sexual problems as soon as they appear. You will be less likely to feel embarrassment, confusion, frustration, or various other emotions that often lead to denial of a problem, discomfort with intimacy, loss of desire, and avoidance of lovemaking altogether. You will be better able to communicate about the problem with your partner and help your partner through it too. You will likely feel more comfortable discussing the problem with your doctor, and you will be more open to the possibility of seeking the help of a counselor or sex therapist. In other words, should you ever need to confront sexual difficulties, you will be better equipped to handle the situation in rational, mature, and effective ways.

Finally, knowledge is support. With this base of knowledge added to your sexual philosophy, you may be able to help others who might seek your advice and reassurance at a time when they are experiencing sexual difficulties. Who knows? The person in need of your assistance might be a close friend, a brother or sister, a son or daughter, or even a parent (I know that's difficult to imagine, but it's not impossible!). Even if you never need all your new information about sexual problems, someone else just might.

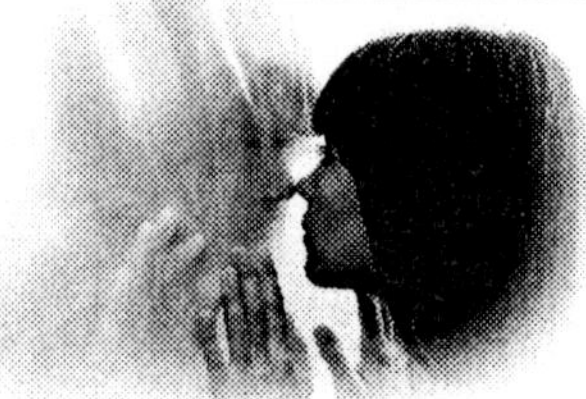

Summary

HISTORICAL PERSPECTIVES Before Masters and Johnson

- Masters and Johnson's research during the 1960s led the way into modern sex therapy. Their research was the first to examine and explore the typical physical responses of the human body to sexual stimulation. Their goal was to achieve greater understanding of these responses in order to improve couples' and therapists' ability to solve sexual problems.

What Is a Sexual Problem?

- Most sexual problems are self-diagnosed. This means that generally, if individuals or couples perceive that they have a sexual problem, they probably do. However, feeling that a sexual problem exists is very different from knowing what it is and how to treat it successfully. Fortunately, most sexual problems are quite common and usually easily treated.
- Sexual problems may be classified into three dimensions for more accurate diagnosis: duration of the problem (primary versus secondary), the context in which the problem occurs (global versus situational), and the intensity or frequency of the problem (total versus partial). Classifying the problem into these three ways assists in discovering the origins of the problem and how best to treat it.

Sources of Sexual Problems

- The origins and causes of sexual problems vary widely. They may include physical, psychological, relationship-based, or cultural issues or a combination of these factors.

General Treatment Principles

- Sexual problems may be reduced by temporarily banning the sexual behavior during which the problems occur. Using the sensate focus technique, the sexual activity, such as intercourse or oral sex, that is at the center of a particular sexual problem may be regarded as "off limits" while the couple focus on exploring other sensual activities to assist them in overcoming their anxiety.
- Today, masturbation is not only regarded as normal but also as a key ingredient in sex therapy.
- Effective communication is the most basic key to successful relationships and satisfying sex. Successful sexual communication must rely primarily on words. Nonverbal communi-

cation may often be misinterpreted and has been found to be an unreliable and even harmful strategy for attaining sexual compatibility.

Specific Problems and Solutions

- Loss of sexual desire (*hypoactive sexual desire*) is the most commonly reported sexual problem. The treatment of low sexual desire is often more complex and difficult than for other sexual problems, but most couples who are motivated to do so can find a solution.
- Both men and women may experience difficulties with arousal. Among men, this is usually referred to as *erectile disorder,* while for women is typically called *female sexual arousal disorder.* Treatments for arousal disorder include sensate focus exercises, directed masturbation, and sometimes (mainly for men) medications such as Viagra, Cialis, or Levitra.
- Lack of orgasm for women during intercourse has been found to be the norm, not a disorder. Most women (50 to 80 percent) do not achieve orgasm through heterosexual intercourse but need additional stimulation to clitoral area before, during, or after intercourse to reach orgasm. Therefore, contrary to popular belief, lack of orgasm during intercourse is common and normal for women.
- SSRI antidepressant medications (such as Prozac, Effexor, and Paxil) have been found to inhibit and delay or even prevent arousal and orgasm in some men and women.
- Premature or rapid ejaculation is the most common sexual problem among younger men. Treatment techniques, often called "start-stop methods," are generally quite effective for premature ejaculation. Mental distraction strategies attempted by many men (thinking about sports or car accidents during intercourse) often fail to provide dependable help with the problem.
- Sex should *never* be painful. Painful sexual experiences are more common for women than men and include *dyspareunia* (pain after sex) and *vaginismus* (pain and muscle cramping just prior to insertive sex). Vaginismus is often the body's reaction to past sexual trauma. Sexual pain difficulties can usually be treated successfully.
- Overall, sexual problems are common and usually easy to treat and cure. No one should suffer unnecessarily or for long periods of time with sexual problems.

YOUR SEXUAL PHILOSOPHY: Sexual Problems and Solutions

- Knowledge and understanding of the characteristics, causes, and treatments are the most important keys to solving sexual problems if and when they arise in a person or couple's life. Therefore, the information in this chapter plays an important role in the development of your comprehensive sexual philosophy.

Have You Considered?

1. Imagine that you begin to experience one of the sexual problems discussed in this chapter (your choice). Explain how you would probably feel. Assuming that the problem does not have a physical cause, what strategies would you use to understand and resolve the problem?
2. Now imagine that your partner (who has not read this book) begins to experience one of the sexual problems discussed in this chapter (your choice). Again, explain how you would probably feel. Also, assuming no physical cause, how would you help your partner understand and resolve the problem?
3. Suppose that a man is having trouble with premature ejaculation. Describe how his problem might manifest itself if it was classified in each of the following ways: (a) primary, global, total; (b) secondary, situational, partial; (c) secondary, global, partial; (d) primary, situational, total.
4. A couple who have been in an intimate relationship for two years are not feeling much sexual desire for each other any more. Discuss at least three ways in which improved communication between them might help them overcome their HSD.
5. Explain why a man with erection problems and a woman with arousal difficulties are both able to become very excited (he has firm long-lasting erections and she easily becomes aroused and lubricated) during sensate focus exercises but not during lovemaking.
6. Do you think a couple could have a satisfying sexual relationship without ever having sexual intercourse? Explain your answer.
7. Other than hypoactive sexual desire, which sexual problem do you think would be most difficult to solve? Explain your answer.

Companion Website Resources

For further chapter resources go to **www.prenhall.com/hock**. This robust text website includes polling questions for you to vote on, regular news updates, quizzes, sample tests, suggested reading lists, and more.

SCENARIOS USA Also on the website are links to videos. *Scenarios USA's* films portray real-life narratives that explore the non-biological aspects of relationships and sexual health. The films will help you consider how the themes of the text affect your own life and the lives of those around you.

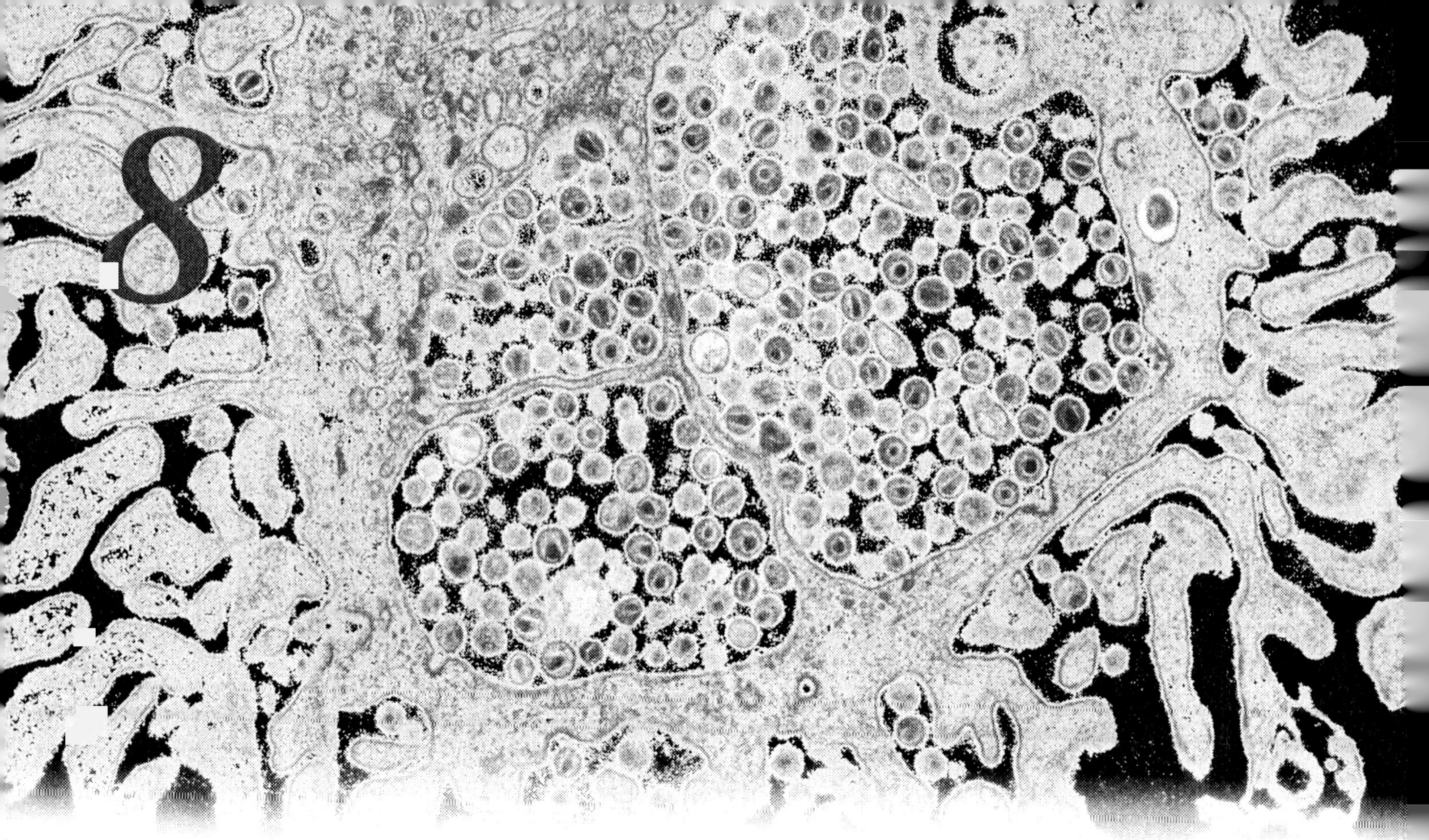

8

Sexually Transmitted Infections

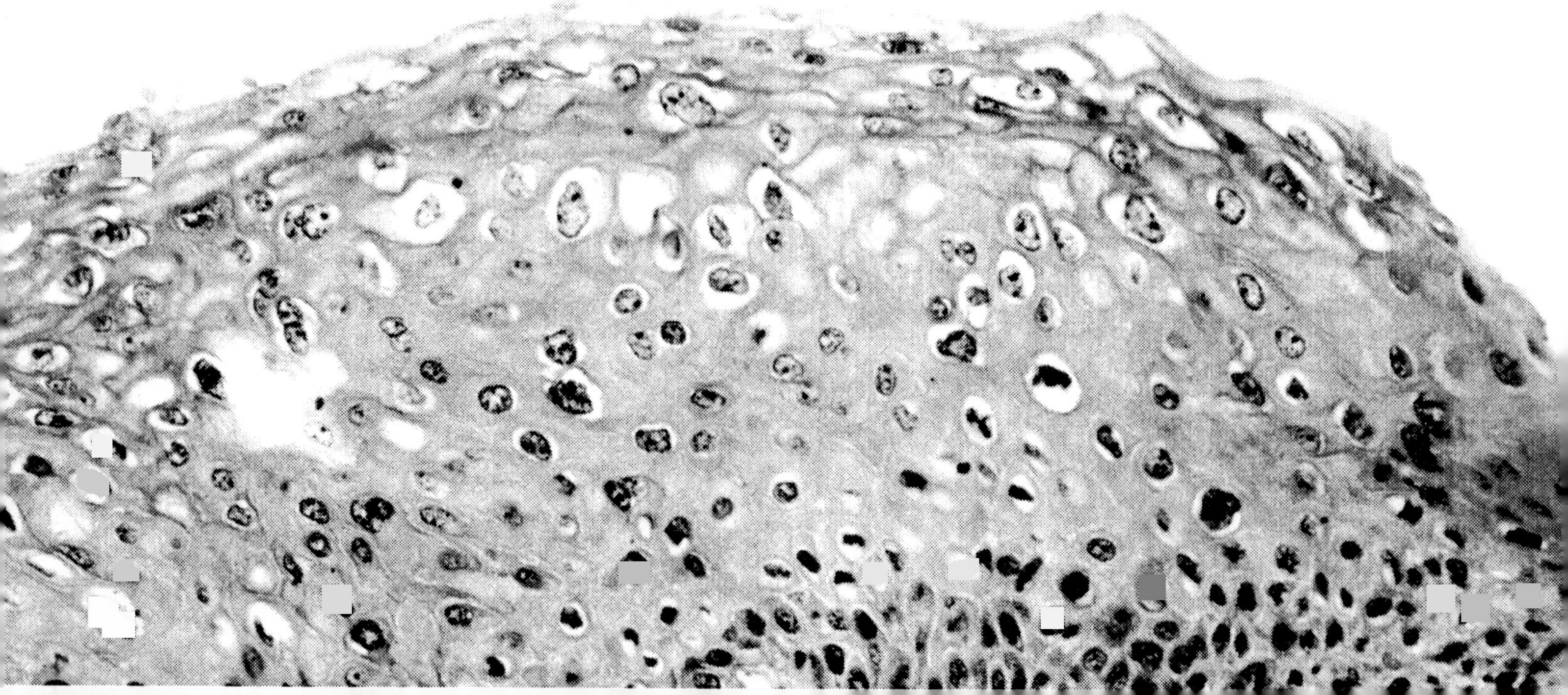

Since YOU Asked...

1. How would I know if I had a sexually transmitted disease? (see page 275)
2. Other than AIDS, what is the worst sexually transmitted infection? (see page 282)
3. My boyfriend told me he had an outbreak of herpes two years ago. Could I still catch it from him? (see page 286)
4. I have an uncle who says he had hepatitis B, but he is now cured. I thought viruses could not be cured, so how is this possible? (see page 288)
5. Is it true that genital warts can cause cancer? (see page 289)
6. I heard that AIDS has been nearly eliminated in the United States. Is this true? (see page 296)
7. Can people get an STI from having oral sex? (see page 297)
8. There is a rumor that people with AIDS are swimming in the community pool in my neighborhood. Should I be concerned about letting my kids swim there? (see page 298)
9. Are the STIs caused by viruses and bacteria basically the same? (see page 303)
10. If I had sores on my genitals but the sores went away, does that mean I'm cured? (see page 308)
11. What are crabs, and how can I tell if someone has them? (see page 312)
12. Once I start having sex, how can I be sure to never catch an STI? (see page 313)

sexually transmitted infections (STIs) A group of viral, bacterial, and other infections that are spread primarily by sexual behaviors.

Throughout this book, you have read about many issues related to your sexual health. In this chapter, the primary focus is on sexual health—in particular, on a group of viral, bacterial, and other infections that are directly caused and spread by sexual behaviors. Most people know these as *sexually transmitted diseases* (STDs), but the terminology among health professionals and sexuality educators today is **sexually transmitted infections (STIs).** The name change is meant to emphasize an important message—that these are *infectious* conditions (unlike many diseases such as heart disease or diabetes, for example) that are spread from one person to another through certain behaviors and also that these infections are treatable or curable.

Paradoxically, the same activities that can bring us so much pleasure and allow us to express our most intimate feelings toward another person can also spread infections that may be uncomfortable or embarrassing at best and deadly at worst. By the time you finish reading about all of the many sexually transmitted infections, you may feel as though you never want to touch another person again, at least not sexually. Of course, that's far from the goal of this chapter. No one has to give up being sexual or sharing sexual pleasure to avoid sexually transmitted infections. However, your ability to protect yourself from contracting an STI or to keep from infecting others if you happen to become infected depends on becoming as educated as possible about STIs. *That* is the purpose of this chapter. Even though you may be troubled by the sheer number of these infections and the disturbing symptoms that may accompany them, ignoring them won't make them go away. Knowing all you can about them can help you avoid them and reduce their spread overall.

The worldwide STI epidemic is showing few, if any, signs of slowing. Consequently, everyone, whether sexually active currently or not, must acquire the information needed to make informed, healthy sexual choices. In this chapter, we will review each of the most common STIs: the infection's symptoms and diagnosis, how it is spread, how to know if you have it, and how it can be treated or cured. We will also focus on prevention, which is always more desirable than treatment for any health problem. Before we begin our discussion of STIs today, let's take a look back at how one common sexual infection, syphilis, was at the center of a shameful, racist event in the medical history of sex.

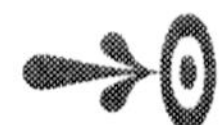

Focus on Your Feelings

STIs tend to stir up a variety of negative emotions. One, of course, is fear of contracting an STI. This fear is real—*if* you don't know how to prevent an STI. As you will see in this chapter, everyone has the ability to avoid STIs by understanding how they are spread and how contracting them can be avoided.

It is not unusual for people to react with disgust to any disease that produces symptoms such as ulcerations of the skin or bodily discharges. With STIs, the disgust is often extended beyond the disease to the infected person, which increases the stigma that already surrounds these infections and in turn contributes to people's hesitation to be tested or seek treatment. STIs are a fact of life (albeit a preventable one) and should be seen in the same light as any other curable or treatable illness.

Anxiety over STIs typically peaks *after* people have engaged in risky sexual behavior. The distress over the possibility that they may have contracted an STI can be overwhelming. If you find yourself in this situation, the best way to alleviate your anxiety is to be tested. The relief of receiving a negative result (which is the most likely outcome) may motivate you to avoid unsafe behaviors in the future. If, however, you do discover that you have contracted an STI, you may feel angry at the person who transmitted the infection to you. Although this hostility is understandable, remember that most STIs have no symptoms, and the person who spread the infection may have had no idea he or she was infected.

For most STIs, the physical pain is minor and subsides fairly quickly once treatment begins. However, the emotional pain of dealing with the stigma attached to having an STI and, in the case of viral infections, the prospect of living with an STI for the rest of one's life may be devastating. This pain may be lessened through education about exactly what to expect from the disease, obtaining the best treatments and care available, and joining support groups with others who are in the same situation. Sometimes a person who has been diagnosed may experience severe depressive symptoms or even thoughts of suicide. Anyone experiencing such extreme emotional reactions should seek professional help immediately. All STIs can be treated and managed effectively to allow the infected person to live a happy and fulfilling life in spite of the infection.

Historical Perspectives

The Tuskegee Syphilis Study

One of the darkest episodes in the history of medical research was the Tuskegee Syphilis Study, the details of which only came to light publicly in the late 1990s. In the early 1930s, the U.S. Public Health Service set about studying the short- and long-term effects of the sexually transmitted infection caused by the syphilis bacterium (which we will discuss in detail later in this chapter). The methodology employed by the researchers at that time was to *deny treatment* to 400 low-income African American men who tested positive for the disease. In fact, the researchers decided not to tell the men that they even had syphilis and conspired to prevent them from obtaining treatment elsewhere. Finally, when it was discovered that penicillin could cure the illness, they did not inform the patients of this because, the researchers decided, to treat them would destroy the potential findings of their long-term study of untreated syphilis.

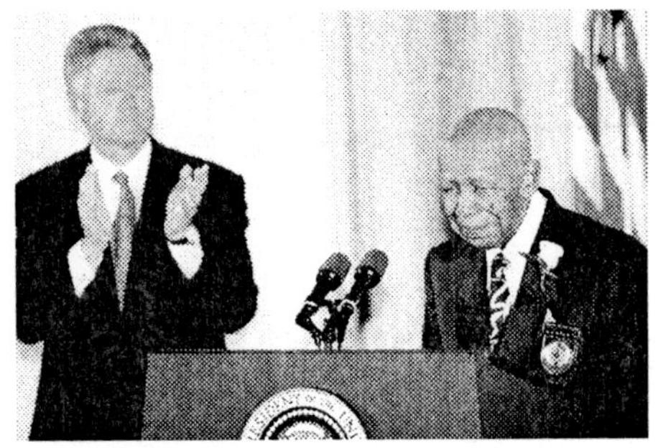

The Tuskegee syphilis study was one of the most unethical studies in the history of modern medicine. In 1997, President Bill Clinton offered the victims and their families an official apology and compensation for the injustice done to them.

As you will see later in this chapter, without treatment, syphilis is a particularly insidious infection that slowly, over years and decades, invades various systems of the body, causing tumors of the skin, bones, or liver; aneurisms of the heart valves and arteries; and major disorders of the central nervous system leading to symptoms of severe mental illness (referred to historically as "syphilitic insanity"). Most of the men in this group faced shortened lives, full of illness and pain for themselves and their families. In addition, some of these men undoubtedly passed the disease on to their sexual partners.

Today, everyone agrees that this was a horribly inhumane abuse of science and research, clearly reflective of the state of bigotry and discrimination at that time. Although evidence of the study began to come to light in the 1970s, it was not until 1997 that President Bill Clinton made an official apology to the victims and their families and made funds available to compensate them for their suffering. However, no amount of money or regret can change the legacy of mistrust the Tuskegee study created between the African American community and the medical establishment in the United States (Fairchild & Bayer, 1999).

The STI Epidemic

Sexually transmitted infections are among the most common causes of illness and disease worldwide. On any given day, more people are suffering from STI-related symptoms, discomfort, or illness than the total number of people with the common cold. Every year, according to the Division of STD Prevention (DSTDP) of the Centers for Disease Control and Prevention (CDC), approximately 15 million new cases are diagnosed in the United States alone, and over 65 million Americans are living with an *incurable* STI (DSTDP, 2004b). Before discussing the various infections in detail, I will summarize some statistics for the more common STIs so you can get a feel for the sheer size of this epidemic.

At least one person in four will contract an STI at some point in life, and an estimated 15 million people are infected with an STI each year (CDC, 2000b). People between the ages of 15 and 30 are at greatest risk for becoming infected with an STI. The most common STIs in this age group are *gonorrhea*, *chlamydia*, and the *human papillomavirus* (HPV), which is the cause of genital warts. However, this age group is vulnerable to all the STIs discussed in this chapter. Among teens, the estimated rate of chlamydia in the United States is between 5 and 10 percent (CDC, 2003c) and is higher overall among women than men (this sex difference is true for most STIs, for reasons we will discuss later in this chapter). A study of STIs in juvenile detention centers found infection rates of 5.1 percent for gonorrhea and 14.7 percent for chlamydia among youths 18 years and younger. Female adolescents in the study were three times more likely to have contracted gonorrhea or chlamydia than males of the same age (Broussard, Leichliter, & Evans, 2002). Figure 8.1 illustrates these infection rates for two common STIs.

Rates of STIs such as herpes and HPV also appear to affect young people disproportionately. Accurate estimates are difficult to make because, as you will see shortly, many STIs, such as genital warts and chlamydia, may not present obvious symptoms. Among women under 25, studies have found HPV (genital wart) prevalence rates ranging from 28 to 46 percent. By the time young people reach adulthood, 15 to 20 percent will have

FIGURE 8.1 Chlamydia and Gonorrhea Rates by Age and Sex

Source: DSTDP (2001), pp. 12, 20, and 32.

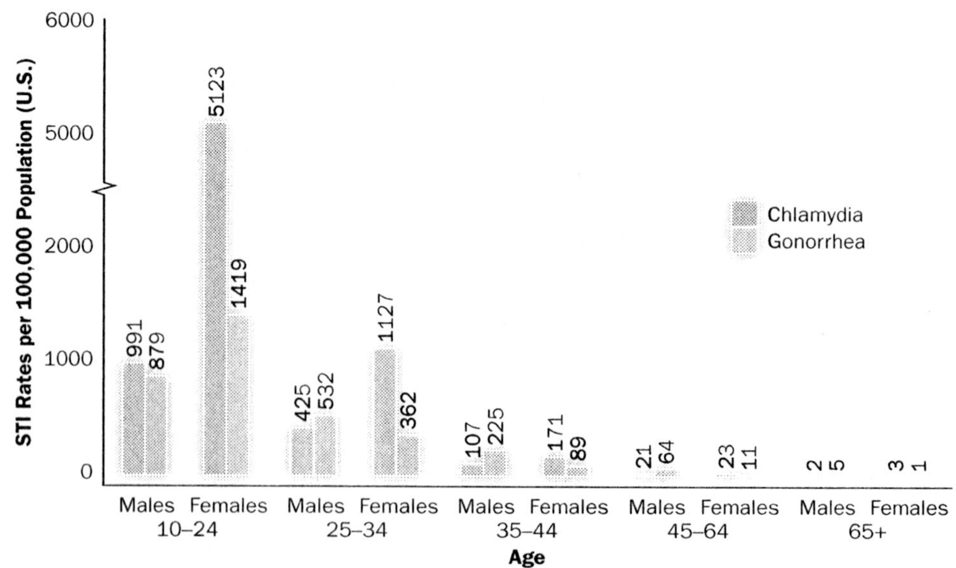

become infected with the herpes virus (DSTDP, 2000). HIV and AIDS are major worldwide epidemics. According to statistics presented at the 2005 National HIV Prevention Conference in Atlanta, in the United States alone, over 1 million people are living with HIV and AIDS, and the number of new cases per year is estimated at between 40,000 and 60,000. The cumulative number of U.S. deaths from AIDS-related illnesses as of 2003 was approximately 525,000 (CDC, 2004b). Worldwide, the numbers are staggering: Over 40 million people are infected with HIV, 3 to 5 million new HIV infections occur each year, and approximately 20 million people have died from AIDS-related illnesses since the epidemic began officially in 1981 (Avert.com, 2004).

The estimated comprehensive financial costs of STIs are in the tens of billions of dollars per year in the United States alone and over $100 billion worldwide. Moreover, the human and financial costs of STIs increase dramatically when STIs are not identified and treated early. In addition to the life-threatening nature of some STIs, two of the most dangerous additional long-term consequences of untreated STIs are *pelvic inflammatory disease* (PID) and *infertility*. Both can have a significant impact on a person's quality of life and future plans. The more immediate personal consequence of STI infections is that they increase a person's the risk of becoming infected with other STIs including HIV, further fueling the overall epidemic.

Risk Factors for STIs

If you ask people why the transmission of STIs is so common, they will probably say something such as "unsafe sex, of course!" and they would be right. However, that is only a small part of the story. For a full understanding of STI risks, we must examine the medical, educational, psychological, and emotional factors behind people's decisions to engage in risky sexual activities. Later in the chapter, we will discuss how you can avoid contracting STIs altogether.

Lack of STI Symptoms

A common misconception about STIs is the assumption that if you become infected, the signs will be obvious: a rash, a discharge, a sore, an odor, urination pain, and so on. The specific symptoms, when present, for each STI will be covered in our discussion in this chapter. However, clear symptoms of certain sexually transmitted infections are often absent.

Since You Asked ...

1. How would I know if I had a sexually transmitted disease?

Many STIs are **asymptomatic**, meaning they may produce no noticeable symptoms at all, especially in women. But no symptoms does not imply no disease. Infected people who are asymptomatic are capable of unknowingly transmitting the infection to their sexual partners. In addition, these infected individuals are unlikely to seek testing or treatment because they show no signs of the illness. If you have an STI that is asymptomatic or have risky sexual contact with someone with an asymptomatic STI, you may not even be aware of your risks of transmission.

Most doctors and sexuality educators recommend periodic, routine screening for various STIs for people who are sexually active, especially if they are not in faithful, monogamous relationships. We will discuss the tests available for specific STIs throughout this chapter. Knowing the risks of contracting STIs and preventing them altogether is a far better health strategy than diagnosing and subsequently treating them.

Lack of Accurate Information

In Western societies, the age at which people first become sexually active has been steadily decreasing. Currently, in the United States, the average age of first intercourse is approximately 16 years for both boys and girls (CDC, 2001a; Kahn et al., 2002). Researchers have observed a significant increase in early teen oral sex during the early 2000s, based on a widespread misconception that oral sexual activities do not pose significant risks of STI transmission (M. O'Brien, 2003; Prinstein, Meade, & Cohen, 2003). These two trends, combined with inconsistent or nonexistent sex education programs in schools—for example, those that teach only abstinence and provide no information about sexual behaviors and their consequences—create an environment that not only fails to prevent but actually *increases* the spread of STIs when teens, in order to avoid intercourse, substitute other risky behaviors such as oral sex (Schaalma et al., 2004). In Chapter 12, "Sexual Development throughout Life," you can find a more detailed discussion of these teen sexual issues. However, this lack of accurate STI information is not limited to teens. Individuals and couples in all age groups may place themselves at risk of STIs due to misconceptions, ignorance, or gaps in their knowledge about how these infections are spread (Shelby, 2003).

When people, for whatever reason, are poorly educated about sexuality and STIs, they are likely to make decisions about sexual behavior based on false or distorted beliefs. Table 8.1 summarizes some of the common and persistent myths about STIs. You can see that faulty beliefs such as those listed in the table may lead individuals and couples to engage in risky behaviors without even being aware of the dangers.

"Unhealthy" Sexual Emotions

In addition to faulty beliefs and misinformation, negative emotions surrounding sexual behavior, such as guilt, shame, fear of stigma, and embarrassment, may create a risky environment for the spread of STIs. Often these unpleasant emotions about sex stem from life experiences such as traumatic past events, restrictive parental attitudes toward sex, cultural expectations, or religious teachings about sex. When people with these feelings become sexually active, the emotional distress they experience may decrease their ability to make choices and take appropriate actions that will protect them from contracting or transmitting STIs (Fortenberry et al., 2002). For example, people who feel shame, guilt, embarrassment, or fear of being stigmatized over sexual activities or contracting an STI are more likely to avoid discussing sexual risks with a partner, resist STI testing, delay or avoid seeking medical care for suspected STI infection, and shy away from sexuality information and STI education (Barth et al., 2002; Nzoom.com, 2003). In addition, those who hold negative attitudes and emotions about sexual issues often

asymptomatic Having no noticeable symptoms despite the presence of an infectious agent.

Table 8.1 COMMON MYTHS ABOUT STIs

The following statements about STIs are widely believed; however, they are all false.

MYTH	TRUTH
Only people who have sex with many partners get STIs.	A single sexual encounter can transmit an STI; someone's only partner may have other partners.
Condoms prevent STIs.	Condoms, used correctly, greatly reduce the chances of STI transmission, but condoms alone are not a 100 percent effective form of prevention.
A lack of any symptoms of an STI probably means no infection.	Many STIs "hide" in the body and do not show any obvious or visible symptoms.
I don't know anyone who has an STI; it must not be a problem in my town.	Unfortunately, STIs are everywhere.
You can get an STI only from vaginal or anal sex.	Vaginal and anal sex are common routes of transmission, but other activities such as oral sex, intravenous drug use, and do-it-yourself tattooing may transmit STIs as well.
I'm on the pill, so I'm pretty well protected from STIs.	Hormonal forms of contraception offer no protection from STIs.
People cannot get an STI the first time they have sex.	Yes, they can.
STIs only transmit if the man ejaculates inside his partner.	STIs may be transmitted through oral, vaginal, or anal sex without ejaculation of semen; vaginal secretions and preejaculate fluid may contain STI microbes.
Getting an STI is no big deal; the infections are easy to treat and then you're immune from them in the future.	Some STIs, if untreated, may infect other areas of the reproductive tract and cause problems with fertility later in life; other STIs have no cure, and some may be deadly.
A person who is clean, well-dressed, and neatly groomed is at low risk of STIs.	Bacteria, viruses, and parasites do not discriminate based on a person's appearance.
The risk of STIs is very low except in certain geographical or low-income areas.	STIs are common in all socioeconomic groups.

resist availing themselves of authoritative education and information about risks and prevention. This resistance, in turn, typically leads to a reliance on often inaccurate sources of information about STIs, such as common myths, peers, or the popular media.

Poor Sexual Communication

As discussed in detail in Chapter 4, "Love, Intimacy, and Sexual Communication," talking about sexual issues in meaningful and effective ways is one of the most difficult areas of communication for many intimate couples, even in well-established, long-term relationships. You can imagine, then, how uncomfortable many people would feel talking openly about sex, negotiating safer sex agreements, insisting on condom use, or avoiding certain high-risk behaviors in new or more casual relationships. Nevertheless, such communication is crucial in preventing STIs. Research has consistently demonstrated that communication between partners is one of the most important factors predicting safer sex practices, including condom use (Feeney et al., 1999; Palmer, 2004; Sheeran, Abraham, & Orbell, 1999). Interestingly, your parents' communication styles and openness about discussing sexuality with *you* may have molded your ability to engage in safe-sex discussions with potential or current sexual partners. A study by Troth and Peterson (2000) found the following links between parents' communication styles and their children's ability to talk about safe sex and use of condoms in their early sexual relationships:

1. Children of parents who openly discussed sexual matters are more willing to discuss safe sex with their dating partners.

2. Children whose parents were less involved in their sexual education are less willing to discuss safer sex with their partners.
3. Parents who use avoidance as their primary strategy for resolving conflicts have children who are less willing to discuss condom use and negotiate safer sex practices with their partners.
4. In general, most parents did not provide meaningful sex education or communicate effectively with their children about safe sex. Children in the study who held more positive attitudes about discussing safer sex were more likely to have talked to their partners about HIV/AIDS and to have used condoms upon becoming sexually active.

As an indication of your personal attitudes toward safer sex practices and condom use, "Self-Discovery: STI Risk Scale" provides on opportunity to measure your own sexual risk, based on your specific attitudes about sexual activities and STIs.

Substance Abuse

Another behavior inextricably linked to the spread of STIs is substance abuse. The nature of this link involves the use of psychoactive drugs, especially alcohol, that cause the user to take sexual risks that he or she would be unlikely to take when sober, such as unsafe sexual activities and lack of condom use (Dunn, Bartee, & Perko, 2003; Knight, 2004). One in five teens reports engaging in unprotected intercourse after drinking alcohol or using other drugs ("Teens Cite," 2003). A study of alcohol consumption and STIs between 1983 and 1998 in all 50 states found a clear association between the two (Chesson, Harrison & Stall, 2003). For every 1 percent rise in alcohol consumption, the researchers found about 0.5 percent increase in gonorrhea incidence rates and about a 2.5 percent increase in the rate of syphilis infection.

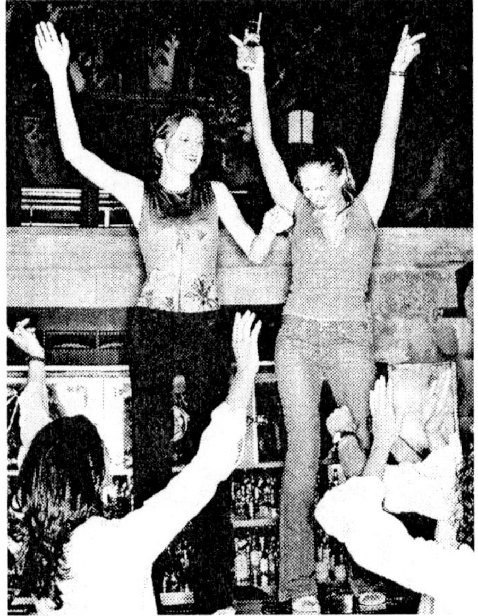

One explanation for why alcohol use leads to poor sexual decision making is called the alcohol myopia theory.

Why does alcohol have these effects on sexual behavior and the spread of STIs? A hypothesis frequently proposed to explain this phenomenon is known as **alcohol myopia theory** (Steele & Josephs, 1990). This theory suggests that under the influence of alcohol, people are more likely to focus on immediate, "feel-good" behaviors (such as sexual arousal) and discount the more distant, long-term consequences of the activity (such as the possibility of contracting an STI). In other words, when it comes to making good decisions about sexual activity, alcohol causes your brain to be myopic or nearsighted, able to see up close but not at a distance (Cooper, 2002; George & Stoner, 2000).

Beyond this decreased ability to make clearheaded decisions, recreational drug use also facilitates the spread of STIs by creating enhanced routes of transmission. You are aware that bloodborne STIs, such as HIV and hepatitis, are often transmitted through the sharing of needles by intravenous drug users. Beyond this, however, drug use is commonly associated with a greater number of sexual partners. These partners are more likely to be drug users themselves and therefore more likely to be infected with one or more STIs (Ramisetty-Mikler et al., 2004). The bottom line to all this is that in terms of STIs, drug use and sexual behavior do not mix. Together, they create a complex environment conducive to many negative sexual experiences and outcomes, including poor sexual decision making and the spread of STIs.

High-Risk Sexual Behaviors

Nearly all sexual behaviors with a partner (except phone and Internet sex) carry some risk of transmitting STIs, and some activities are far riskier than others. As you read through the discussion of specific STIs in this chapter, you will see in greater detail how

alcohol myopia theory The belief that under the influence of alcohol, people are more likely to focus on immediate, "feel-good" behaviors (such as sexual arousal) and ignore future negative consequences.

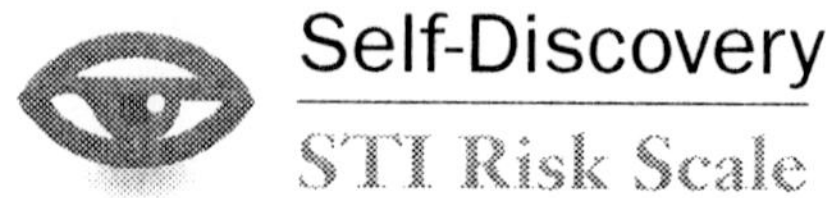

Self-Discovery

STI Risk Scale

This brief scale will help you assess you personal risk profile relative to your chances of contracting an STI. After completing the scale, use the scoring and score interpretation to get an idea of your STI risk level. Be honest in your answers; only you will know the outcome of the scale.

Rate each statement using the following scale: 5 = strongly agree; 4 = agree; 3 = not sure; 2 = disagree; 1 = strongly disagree.

____ 1. Sexual behavior choice plays a major role in your risk of contracting STIs.

____ 2. Obtaining and using methods of STI prevention are really pretty simple.

____ 3. Being tested for STIs is a good idea for most young, sexually active people.

____ 4. Getting to know your sexual partner's history before becoming sexually intimate is a good STI prevention strategy.

____ 5. Insisting on testing for a potential sexual partner makes a lot of sense.

____ 6. If you found out you had an STI, you would get treated as fully and as quickly as possible.

____ 7. You believe condoms are a good way to reduce a person's risk of contracting or transmitting an STI.

____ 8. You are comfortable talking to your sexual partner about sex and STIs.

____ 9. If you had physical symptoms that you thought might be an STI, you would see the doctor immediately.

____10. You would be likely to use "selective abstinence" (avoiding specific sexual behaviors) to avoid STIs.

____11. If you were having sex with more than one partner, you would get tested for STIs more often.

____12. You are comfortable examining your sexual anatomy for signs of an STI.

____13. If you were at all unsure of a potential sexual partner's STI status, you would not have sex with that person.

____14. You feel that everyone should become educated about the risks and prevention of STIs.

____15. You believe that anyone may possibly be infected with an STI.

____16. You know that even when no symptoms are present, a person may still be infected.

____17. You would tell your sexual partner if you are or were diagnosed with an STI.

____18. You are careful to avoid excess alcohol or other drugs when in a potential sexual situation.

____19. You are reasonably comfortable discussing STIs with your doctor or other health professional.

____20. If your partner will not agree to your requirements for safe sex, you will not have sex.

Add up your score, which will range between 20 and 100. *The higher your score, the safer you are from contracting an STI.*

Here is what your score means:

Scores below 40 indicate that you may be at a very high risk for contracting one or more STIs.

Scores between 41 and 60 indicate a moderate to high risk.

Scores between 61 and 80 indicate a moderate to low risk.

Scores over 80 indicate that you are at a fairly low risk for STIs.

Regardless of your score on this scale, everyone must be educated about STIs to minimize risks of transmission.

Table 8.2 SEXUAL BEHAVIORS: RISK LEVELS FOR SPECIFIC INFECTIONS

BEHAVIOR	INFECTION	LEVEL OF RISK
Fantasy, solo masturbation, phone or Internet sex	None	None.
Kissing	Herpes	Very low (no sores present); high (sores present or recently healed). Deep, intense kissing with blood in saliva may pose risk of HIV or hepatitis transmission.
Mutual masturbation	HIV, syphilis, hepatitis	Very low, unless sores, cuts, or abrasions are present on hands.
Fellatio, with condom	Herpes, genital warts	Low to moderate, depending on presence of sores or warts. Virus may transmit skin-to-skin around condom.
Fellatio, without condom	Chlamydia, herpes, genital warts, gonorrhea, hepatitis, syphilis, HIV	Low to high, depending on infection and presence of lesions. Risk is *not* reduced by avoiding ejaculation in mouth.
Cunnilingus	Chlamydia, herpes, genital warts, gonorrhea, hepatitis, syphilis, HIV	Low to high, depending on infection and presence of lesions. Risk may be higher during menstruation. Risk may be reduced significantly by use of dental dam.
Vaginal intercourse with condom	Herpes, genital warts, pubic lice	Moderate to high, depending on presence of sores or warts and extent of lice infection.
Vaginal intercourse without condom	All	Moderate to high.
Oral-anal contact	All	Moderate to high, depending on presence of infection and routes of transmission through skin.
Anal intercourse (insertive or receptive) with condom	All	Moderate to high.
Anal intercourse (insertive or receptive) without condom	All	High.

certain sexual behaviors pose risks for contracting or transmitting that particular infection. However, we can discuss some general guidelines here.

Overall, the more intimate and genitally oriented the activity, the more risk it carries. However, abstaining from vaginal or anal intercourse does not ensure that you are safe from infection. Skin-to-skin contact involving the lips and the genital areas may transmit some STIs regardless of any exchange of bodily fluids. Furthermore, the use of condoms, while greatly reducing the risk of contracting or transmitting all STIs, is not a 100 percent effective strategy. Table 8.2 summarizes the specific STI risks of various mainstream sexual behaviors.

Your ultimate defense against STI infection and transmission is education, knowledge, awareness of unsafe behaviors, and *planning ahead* to ensure your sexual health. This is discussed further near the end of this chapter in "Your Sexual Philosophy: STIs."

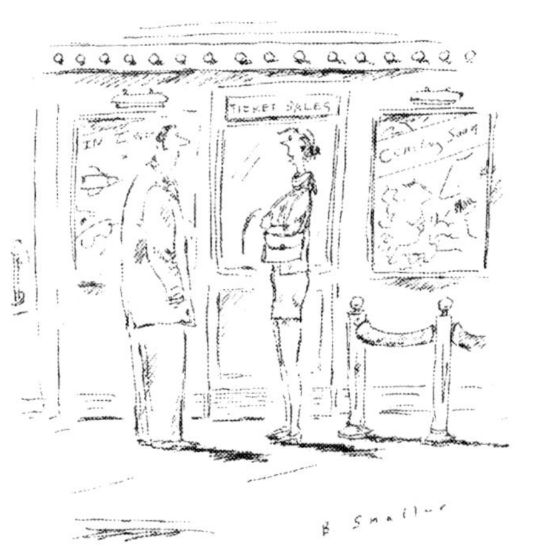

Yes, I realize that we are free agents, but I have to take on the additional risk of pregnancy and am more susceptible to certain sexually transmitted diseases, so I think you should pay for the movie.

Specific Sexually Transmitted Infections

Now we are ready to begin our discussion of the STIs themselves. The various infections may be divided into categories based on the type of pathogen (germ) that causes the infection: viral, bacterial, and parasitic. For each category, we will discuss the characteristics and symptoms of specific infections, the typical modes of transmission, the tests available for diagnosing the infection, and the cures or treatments available now and newer treatments that may become available in the near future. These are summarized in Table 8.3.

Table 8.3 SEXUALLY TRANSMITTED INFECTIONS

INFECTION	TYPICAL SYMPTOMS	MODE OF TRANSMISSION	TREATMENT	VACCINE AVAILABLE?	POTENTIAL COMPLICATIONS
		VIRAL STIs			
Herpes simplex virus (HSV), type 1 and type 2	Often asymptomatic. Clusters of small, painful blisters in genital and anal areas or around mouth. General flu-like symptoms: mild fever, fatigue, and tenderness in lymph nodes, perhaps urinary pain.	Oral, vaginal, or anal sexual activities; kissing	No cure. Treated with antiherpetic drugs (acyclovir, famciclovir, valacyclovir)	No vaccine available as of 2006. Research is under way.	Sores create route of transmission for other STIs. May be passed from pregnant mother to child during birth.
Hepatitis B (HBV)	Usually no symptoms unless virus becomes active. Jaundice, a deep yellowing of the skin and eyes. Loss of appetite, fatigue, abdominal pain, nausea, vomiting, darkening of the urine, rash, and joint pain.	Contact with blood, serum, semen, vaginal fluids, and in rare instances saliva. Routes of transmission are sharing needles, sexual contact, and sometimes tattooing and body piercing.	No cure. Acute infection: bed rest, increased fluid intake, good nutrition, and avoiding alcohol (which may exacerbate liver inflammation). Chronic infection: Alpha interferon boosts the body's immune system; lamivudine, antiviral medication, slows liver infection.	Yes. Series of three injections over 6 months. Prevents infection for life.	In small percentage of chronic cases: serious liver disease, including cirrhosis and liver cancer, which may lead to liver failure and either a liver transplant or death.
Human papilloma virus (HPV): Genital warts	Visible warts on the penis, opening to the vagina, cervix, labia minora, or anal area. Warts may also appear inside the vagina or anus and may not be noticed at all. Warts are flat or lumpy; they may be single or in groups and vary in size. Sometimes the warts may be too small or flat to be seen or felt.	Skin-to-skin contact; vaginal, oral, or anal sexual activities. Transmission possible with or without visible warts.	No cure. Removal of warts through cryosurgery (freezing), laser therapy, surgery, and topical medications applied by the patient. Removing warts does not cure infection.	Vaccine in human trials appears to be effective in preventing transmission; vaccine to prevent infection approved by FDA in 2006.	Major cause of cervical and anal cancers.
HIV/AIDS	HIV: Initially no symptoms or mild fever, headache, fatigue, and rash. As virus progresses: loss of energy; unexplained weight loss; frequent fevers and night sweats; frequent yeast infections; enlarged lymph glands; persistent skin rashes; short-term memory loss; mouth, genital, or anal sores; and blurred vision. AIDS diagnosed when CD4+ T-cell count dips to below 200 or when the person becomes infected with one or more opportunistic infections.	Transmission requires that semen, vaginal fluids, or blood from an infected person enters the bloodstream of an uninfected person. The most common routes of HIV are through sexual contact, primarily vaginal and anal intercourse and, less commonly, oral sex.	No cure. More than 20 specific medications for fighting HIV are currently on the market, including protease inhibitors, nucleoside-nucleotide reverse transcriptase inhibitors, nonnucleoside reverse transcriptase inhibitors, and fusion inhibitors. Also available are immune system enhancers and specific treatments for AIDS-related infections.	No. Research is continuing.	With proper treatment, life span of HIV infected individuals is rapidly increasing (approaching 25 years in the United States). Survival following diagnosis with AIDS is approaching 10 years.

Continued. . .

Table 8.3 (*Continued*)

INFECTION	TYPICAL SYMPTOMS	MODE OF TRANSMISSION	TREATMENT	VACCINE AVAILABLE?	POTENTIAL COMPLICATIONS
		BACTERIAL STIS			
Chlamydia	Thick, cloudy discharge from the vagina or penis occurring 1 to 3 weeks after exposure; less common: pelvic pain, irregular periods, increased pain during menstrual periods, discomfort during urination, or irritation of the vaginal and/or anal area; often asymptomatic.	Oral, vaginal, and anal sex. Extremely contagious bacterium; may be transmitted during a single sexual encounter with an infected partner.	Oral antibiotics will cure most cases. All sexual partners must be treated concurrently to prevent reinfection.	No. Research is ongoing.	Untreated may lead to infections of reproductive system and pelvic inflammatory disease in women and epididymitis in men, a major cause of infertility.
Gonorrhea	Men: painful, burning sensation during urination or bowel movement, and/or a cloudy discharge from the penis or anus. Women: often no noticeable symptoms. Cloudy vaginal discharge, irritation during urination, or vaginal bleeding between periods. Rare symptoms: lower abdominal pain or pain during intercourse.	Vaginal, anal, or oral sexual contact. Transmission to newborns can occur at delivery and cause eye infections.	Oral antibiotics will cure most cases. Some strains are becoming antibiotic-resistant. All sexual partners must be treated concurrently to prevent reinfection.	No. Research is ongoing.	Untreated may lead to infections of reproductive system and pelvic inflammatory disease and possible infertility in women and epididymitis or prostatitis in men.
Nongonococcal urethritis (NGU)	Similar to gonorrhea infection: discharge from the urethra; burning and itching at the end of the urethra or upon urination.	Vaginal, anal, or oral sexual contact.	Oral antibiotics will cure most cases. All sexual partners must be treated concurrently to prevent reinfection.	No.	Untreated may lead to infections of reproductive system and pelvic inflammatory disease and possible infertility in women and epididymitis or prostatitis in men.
Chancroid	A soft, painful chancre sore, or cluster of sores, similar in appearance to a syphilis chancre, on the penis, vaginal entrance, internal vagina, or perineum. Pain when urinating, defecating, or having sex; rectal bleeding. Swelling and pain of the lymph nodes located in the groin area.	Sexual contact, including vaginal, anal, and oral sexual practices.	Oral antibiotics will cure most cases. All sexual partners must be treated concurrently to prevent reinfection.	No.	Pain of ulcers may require hospitalization. Ulcers may return following treatment.

Continued. . .

Table 8.3 (*Continued*)

INFECTION	TYPICAL SYMPTOMS	MODE OF TRANSMISSION	TREATMENT	VACCINE AVAILABLE?	POTENTIAL COMPLICATIONS
Syphilis	Primary stage: characterized by a sore called a *chancre* that appears at the point of infection. Usually heals completely within a few weeks. Secondary stage: occurs within weeks or months; symptoms include low grade fever, sore throat, fatigue, headache, alopecia (hair loss), and skin rashes, typically on the hands or feet. Late stage: extensive spread of the bacterium leading to organ damage, neurological damage, paralysis, mental illness, and death.	Sexual contact, including vaginal, anal, and oral sexual practices.	Antibiotics, primarily penicillin, typically cure the infection. All sexual partners must be treated concurrently to prevent reinfection.	No. Research is ongoing.	Untreated, bacterium spreads to all bodily systems, causing new symptoms and eventual destruction of organs and brain tissue and death.
Pelvic inflammatory disease (PID)	Not an STI but a condition resulting from several STIs. Lower abdominal sensitivity and pain, pain during intercourse, irregular periods, cervical discharge and tenderness, fever, nausea, and vomiting.	Direct result of various STIs transmitted through sexual contact.	Various oral or injected antibiotics.	No. Vaccines that will prevent STIs such as chlamydia and gonorrhea will have the effect of preventing millions of cases of PID.	PID can affect the uterus, ovaries, fallopian tubes, or other related structures. Untreated, PID causes scarring and can lead to infertility, tubal pregnancy, chronic pelvic pain, and other serious consequences.

Continued. . .

Viral STIs

All STIs are serious to varying degrees, and no one would willingly choose to contract one. Nevertheless, some STIs are more serious than others. Among various criteria we might use to judge the seriousness of a particular infection, perhaps the most important is our ability to cure someone who is diagnosed with it. Using this as a bright-line test, many researchers would argue that the most serious STIs are those caused by viruses. Why? Because medical science has not yet discovered how to cure viruses. Viruses, one-hundredth the size of bacteria, invade the body's cells and essentially transform those cells into virus factories that produce still more viruses that invade still more cells. Any agent that will destroy the virus will likely have to destroy the cell as well, leading to highly undesirable side effects, including the death of the host (the

2. Other than AIDS, what is the worst sexually transmitted infection?

Table 8.3 (*Continued*)

INFECTION	TYPICAL SYMPTOMS	MODE OF TRANSMISSION	TREATMENT	VACCINE AVAILABLE?	POTENTIAL COMPLICATIONS
PARASITIC STIs					
Trichomoniasis	Men: usually asymptomatic. Possibly: irritation of the urethra, slight discharge, pain after urination or ejaculation. Women: yellow or greenish vaginal discharge accompanied by an unpleasant odor, genital irritation, and pain upon urination.	Sexual contact, including vaginal, anal, and oral sexual practices.	Oral antibiotics will cure most cases. All sexual partners must be treated concurrently to prevent reinfection.	No.	Without proper treatment, may cause PID among women and NGU among men.
Pubic lice	Genital irritation and extreme itching, often said to be the most intense itching imaginable, caused by lice biting the skin to feed on blood.	Sexual contact, sharing bedding, sharing clothing.	Prescription shampoos, creams, and ointments containing chemicals that are toxic to the lice. Washing of all bedding and clothes in hot water.	No.	No serious complications. Difficult to cure completely and easily spread.
Scabies	Irritation and rash in genital or anal area or on hands or feet.	Sexual activities as well as nonsexual skin-to-skin contact.	Prescription lotions (permethrin, lindane, crotamiton) applied to all areas of the body from the neck down and washed off after 8 to 14 hours. Decontamination of all clothing and bedding.	No.	No serious complications. Difficult to cure completely and easily spread.

patient). This is why we do not have a cure for the common cold (which is caused by various strains of the *rhinovirus*), the flu (caused by various *influenza viruses*), or viral STIs. Consequently, if you contract a viral STI, no pill, injection, or other treatment can cure it. As you will see, however, this does not mean that viral STIs are not preventable or treatable, and the symptoms of these infections may be controlled and limited to varying degrees. The most common viral STIs that we will focus on here are herpes, genital warts, hepatitis, and HIV, which causes AIDS. Because viral STIs are not curable, "In Touch with Your Sexual Health: Living with an Incurable STI" discusses important considerations for those who have contracted viral STIs.

Herpes Simplex Virus (HSV)

Researchers have identified at least eight strains of the human herpes virus. One of these causes chickenpox, another causes shingles, and a third causes mononucleosis. Two viruses in the herpes family are STIs: *herpes simplex virus type 1* (HSV 1) and *type 2* (HSV 2) (Corey & Wald, 1999). HSV-1, the more common of the two, is most often the cause of oral herpes: cold sores or fever blisters on the lips, on the tongue, or in the mouth.

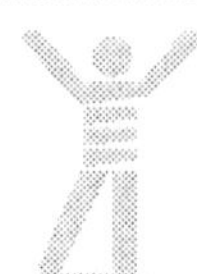

In Touch with Your Sexual Health

Living with an Incurable STI

Although STIs caused by viruses are treatable, they are not curable at this time. Consequently, anyone who contracts a viral STI must become educated about the best strategies for living a healthy life with the virus. Here we present information for living with herpes simplex, hepatitis B, and the human papilloma virus, which causes genital warts. Our discussion of the unique challenges of living with HIV and AIDS is included in the body of the chapter.

Emotional distress is a common reaction when a person discovers that he or she has been infected with an incurable STI. However, stressing out does little good and may in fact exacerbate outbreaks of the infection. Stress, anxiety, attitudes about being infected, and lack of social and information support have all been linked to outbreaks (Longo & Koehn, 1993). The reverse has also been found to be true. People living with STIs have been shown to have lower self-esteem, experience greater daily challenges, and demonstrate greater psychological problems (Swanson, Dibble, & Chenitz, 1995).

Disclosing an infection to potential sexual partners is another issue in the lives of people with STIs. Studies have found that these STIs can spread even in the absence of sores or other symptoms (Wald, 1998; Wald et al., 2000). Despite such evidence, many people continue to believe that they are contagious only during obvious symptoms or an active outbreak of lesions. A key question in the minds of most people is when and to whom they should disclose their STI status. This is a question with no easy, one-size-fits-all answer. Some argue that in casual sexual encounters, when condoms are used consistently, disclosure may not be necessary. Others contend, however, that disclosure should be automatic with all potential sexual partners, regardless of the nature of the relationship. Ultimately, this becomes an ethical and philosophical decision each person living with these viruses must make.

People who discover they are infected often find counseling to be helpful in developing effective coping strategies for living with the infection. Feelings such as depression, fear of being "found out," anxiety about being seen as "damaged goods," social rejection, and anger can be debilitating, even for those who have lived with the virus for many years. Due to the chronic nature of these viruses, patients may need one on one therapy during the first few months to the first year after the initial diagnosis. Social support, particularly support groups made up of people living with viral STIs, can be found in most parts of the country, and there is a national STI hotline, set up by the CDC, to help people find the resources they may need: (800) 227-8922. Such support groups can be very helpful for people who need reassurance that they are not alone and who may need the help of others in the same situation. Support groups can also help with issues of disclosure, including when to disclose to partners. Last but not least, support groups provide a safe environment for socializing with understanding others and the possibility for new intimate relationships.

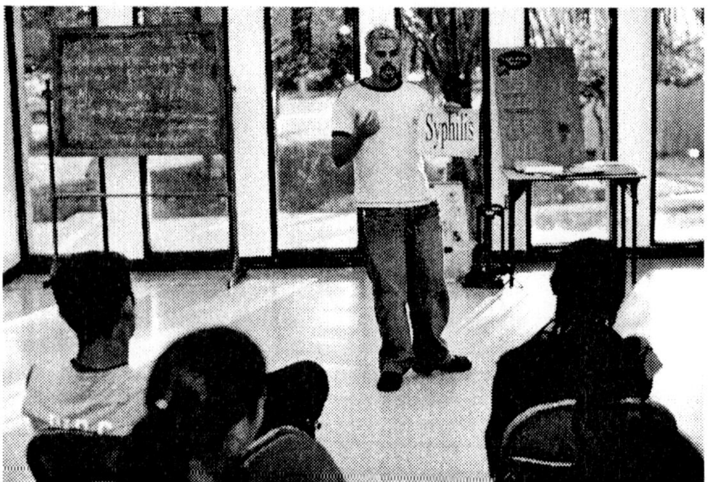

A diagnosis of an incurable STI is never easy. However, health care, information, resources, and support all work together to create and sustain a quality of life that can be rich and satisfying despite the infection.

HSV-2 is the primary cause of **genital herpes**, which is characterized by painful sores and blisters (much like cold sores) that occur in the genital or anal area. However, HSV-1 and HSV-2 are extremely similar and often interchangeable; that is, either or both may produce infection in either the oral and genital areas, or both (Xu et al., 2002).

genital herpes An STI caused by the herpes simplex virus (type 2) and characterized by painful sores and blisters, usually in the genital or anal area.

Herpes infections are extremely common. Approximately 45 million people over age 12 are infected with genital herpes in the United States alone (DSTDP, 2004b). That means that approximately one in every five Americans has had genital herpes.

From the late 1970s to the early 1990s, herpes prevalence increased by 30 percent, with the greatest increases occurring among teens and young adults (Mark, Hanahan, & Stender, 2003; Wald, 1999). Most of the people currently infected have never noticed any signs of the virus and are unaware of their infection. In one study, over 25 percent of subjects tested positive for HSV-2, but only 4 percent reported being aware of any history of the infection ("New Study," 2003). Because HSV may transmit, in some cases, without active lesions, this lack of awareness of infection contributes significantly to its spread.

Herpes is more common among women than men. Approximately 25 percent of women are infected, compared to approximately 20 percent of men. The increased risk for women is due mostly to the fact that transmission of most STIs is more likely from males to females than vice versa (DSTDP, 2004a).

Symptoms

Symptoms of HSV occur 2 to 10 days after exposure to the virus. Many people may experience general flu-like symptoms, including a mild fever, fatigue, tenderness in lymph nodes in the groin or neck, and perhaps urinary pain or discomfort (DSTDP, 2004a). The primary symptom of genital herpes infection is the appearance of clusters, or *crops*, of small, painful blisters in the genital area—labia, vaginal opening, vagina, anal area, penis, or scrotum. Less commonly, the sores may appear in other parts of the body, such as the thighs or buttocks, and tend to be less painful than the genital outbreaks. Other symptoms sometimes include itching, pain during intercourse, vaginal or urethral discharge, and sensitivity in the abdominal area. Typically, the first episode of a genital herpes outbreak is the most severe, in terms of both symptoms and duration of the outbreak (see Figure 8.2).

Within a few days, the blisters rupture and ooze fluid. This fluid is full of millions of herpes virus particles, and the risk of transmission is highest at this point. Over the next week or two, the blisters scab over and heal without leaving a scar. If the lesions are inside the vagina, anus, or mouth, healing may take longer. We should mention that these sores are sometimes confused with other STIs such as chancroid and syphilis (to be discussed later), so diagnosis by a qualified health care professional is important for proper treatment and management of the infection.

After the blisters heal, HSV typically enters a latency period when the person is free of outbreaks. However, this does not mean that the virus is gone. Latency simply implies that the infection is suppressed, usually temporarily. Recurrent outbreaks of herpes are common, but the severity of the symptoms tends to become less

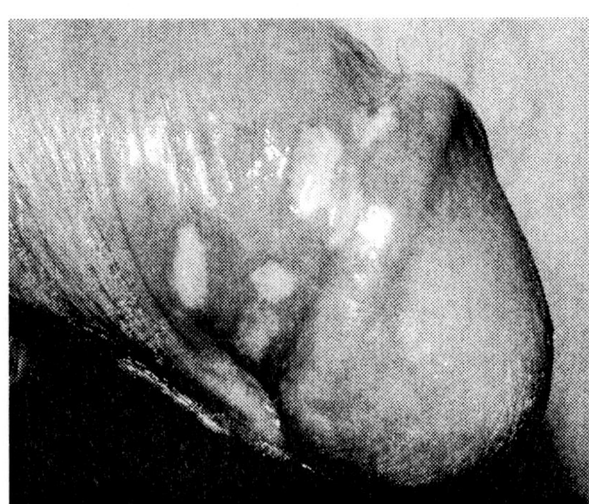

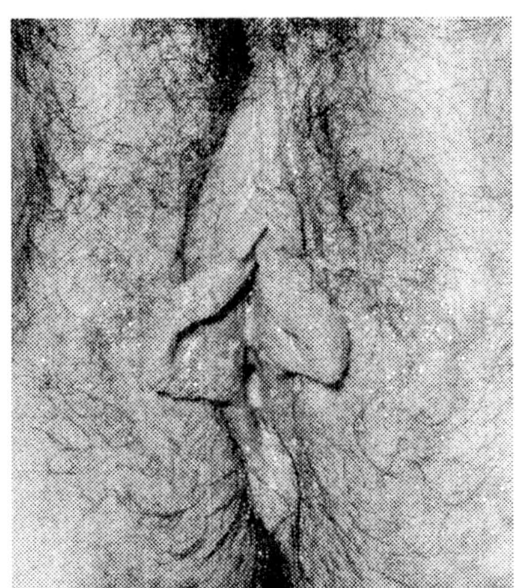

FIGURE 8.2 Herpes Simplex Virus

Shown here are male and female examples of active genital herpes lesions.

pronounced over time and is often limited to blisters, without the accompanying bodily discomforts. Many people with herpes learn to recognize the early warning signs of an impending attack. These **prodromal symptoms** include itching, burning, pain, and sensitivity, often in the same areas where the initial outbreak occurred.

Most people infected with HSV-2 will experience recurring outbreaks ranging from once a year or less to twice a month, with an average of five new outbreaks in the first year (Murphy & Risser, 1999). The number of recurring episodes tends to decrease over time and may be significantly limited or even eliminated with medications (to be discussed shortly). The exact cause of these recurrences remains somewhat unclear. Some of the factors in herpes outbreaks that have received research support to varying degrees include hormonal changes associated with a woman's menstrual cycle; emotional stress; physical stress; vigorous sexual intercourse; exposure to ultraviolet light, especially sunlight; another illness (especially with fever); steroidal medications; or poor nutrition.

Transmission

Herpes is nearly always transmitted through oral, vaginal, or anal sexual activities. It is the only STI that may be transmitted through kissing. Herpes is readily transmitted via oral sex, which is largely responsible for the high number of cross-infections of oral and genital herpes. People who become sexually active at younger ages, who have had numerous sexual partners, or who have been diagnosed with other STIs are at increased risk of becoming infected with HSV (Corey & Wald, 1999; DSTDP, 2004a).

Some anecdotal evidence has suggested that the herpes simplex virus may be transmissible in nonsexual ways, through toilet seats, shared towels, contaminated surfaces, hot tubs, and so on. However, the herpes virus can survive outside the body for only about 10 seconds. In hot, moist environments, survival time may be somewhat increased, but the likelihood of nonsexual transmission of HSV is virtually nonexistent, and no case of transmission from towels or toilet seats has ever been documented. Therefore, medical professionals assume that *all* cases of genital herpes have been transmitted the "old-fashioned way," through sexual contact.

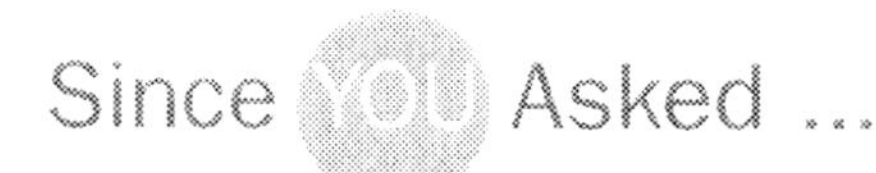

3. My boyfriend told me he had an outbreak of herpes two years ago. Could I still catch it from him?

In the past, most people believed that if no herpes sores were visible, the virus was not contagious. However, more recent research has found that many people who are infected with HSV may release virus particles, referred to as **viral shedding**, when they have no symptoms of the infection. This is called **asymptomatic shedding** and is far more common than most people believe. Studies have found that among people diagnosed with genital herpes, and among many who have not, the virus is shed on days when no clinical signs (blisters or sores) of infection are present (Corey & Wald, 1999; Wald et al., 2002). Moreover, because most people (75 to 90 percent) who are infected with genital herpes are unaware of having been infected with HSV, transmission of the virus to a sexual partner is *most* likely to occur on days when no herpes lesions are present.

Diagnosis and Treatment

Herpes is typically diagnosed visually by the person who has the infection or by a health care provider. Diagnostic tests may be done directly on the fluid from the sores if the infection is active.

As was pointed out earlier, herpes is not curable, but it is treatable with medications. Several antiviral drugs, known as **antiherpetics**, are currently available that are

prodromal symptoms Warning signs, such as itching, burning, or pain, that an outbreak of an infection such as herpes may be impending.

viral shedding The release of virus particles that can potentially spread the infection to others.

asymptomatic shedding Release of infectious virus particles when no symptoms of infection are present.

antiherpetics Medications developed to treat (reduce or prevent but not cure) outbreaks of the herpes virus.

quite effective in suppressing the action of the herpes virus and preventing outbreaks. The most common medication is *acyclovir* (trade name, Zovirax; also available in generic form). Others include *famcyclovir* (trade name, Famvir) and *valacyclovir* (trade name, Valtrex). All of these drugs are taken orally and appear to be equally effective. The newer drugs, famcyclovir and valacyclovir, differ from acyclovir in the convenience of the dosing schedule (fewer doses each day). These medications may be taken at the first preinfection sensations or at the earliest sign of an outbreak of genital herpes. They are generally taken for 7 to 10 days during the first outbreak or for 5 days during subsequent episodes.

All of these antiherpetic medications, when taken on a continuous daily basis, are effective in suppressing outbreaks of herpes altogether. In general, suppressive therapy is recommended for individuals who suffer six or more outbreaks per year (Woodward & Fisher, 1999), but it is often prescribed for people who experience less frequent recurrences. One 2002 study found that daily doses of Valtrex limited outbreaks to an average of 1.6 per year, compared to more than 7 episodes for those using the same medication only "as needed," when outbreaks occurred ("Suppressive Drug Therapy," 2002). Moreover, the length of time between outbreaks for the suppressive therapy group was 180 days, compared to 57 days for the groups receiving the drug at each flare-up. When episodes of blisters do occur, various nondrug treatments, including warm baths, loose-fitting clothing, and avoiding activities that might further irritate the affected area, such as some sports or sexual activities, may be helpful in managing the pain and discomfort that often accompany an outbreak.

Research has also found that suppressive, or continuous, dosing of valacyclovir also appears to significantly reduce the rate of transmission of HSV from an infected to an uninfected partner (W. Elliot, 2004). Finally, research is under way to develop a vaccine to prevent HSV, and results of early tests look promising (Randerson, 2003). However, vaccine research and FDA approval typically move very slowly, and a widely available and effective vaccine is unlikely to be available until around 2010.

Hepatitis B Virus (HBV)

Hepatitis, meaning inflammation of the liver, is a disease marked by an impairment of liver functioning caused by a viral infection. Although six strains of hepatitis are found in humans, you are probably most familiar with those designated A, B, and C. Currently, the only type of hepatitis officially designated as a *sexually* transmitted infection is **hepatitis B (HBV)**, which accounts for about a third of all cases of hepatitis in the United States (Lemon & Alter, 1999). Although theoretically, *hepatitis C* may be transmitted sexually, actual transmission through sexual activities has been shown to be virtually nonexistent (Marincovich et al., 2003).

It is estimated that around 5 percent of the U.S. population is infected with HBV (DSTDP, 2000). Over 45,000 new cases of hepatitis are reported each year, but public health officials suspect that the actual number of new cases *not* reported to public health authorities could be as many as five to ten times that number (Lemon & Alter, 1999).

Symptoms

People infected with hepatitis B typically show no symptoms until the virus becomes active and begins to affect the liver. When this occurs, symptoms usually appear between 1 and 6 months after exposure. The most noticeable symptom is **jaundice**, a

hepatitis B virus (HBV) A virus that may be sexually transmitted and may lead to inflammation and impaired functioning of the liver.

jaundice A symptom of hepatitis characterized by a deep yellowing of the skin and eyes.

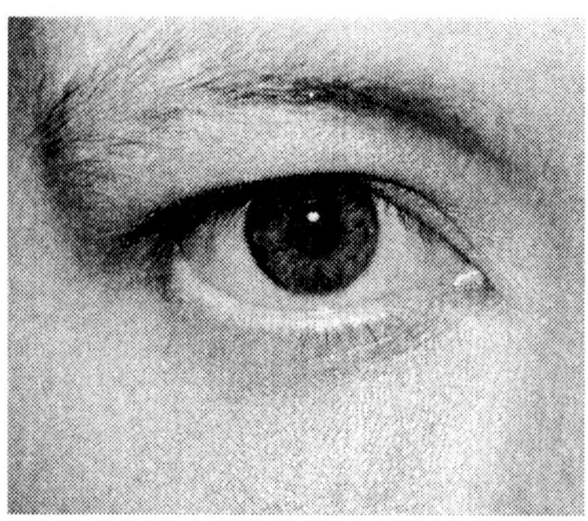

FIGURE 8.3 Jaundice Caused by Hepatitis
One of the most obvious signs of an active hepatitis infection is a yellowing of the skin and eyes.

deep yellowing of the skin and eyes (see Figure 8.3). Other symptoms include loss of appetite, fatigue, abdominal pain, nausea, vomiting, darkening of the urine, rash, and joint pain.

HBV infection may be acute or chronic. An *acute* hepatitis infection is essentially a new infection that may or may not involve the symptoms just described. In approximately 90 percent of cases, the illness runs its courses and the person recovers fully, is no longer contagious, and may not even test positive for antibodies to the virus. However, the remaining 10 percent of those infected as adults become chronically infected and are lifelong carriers of the virus (for infants and young children, infection leads to *chronic carrier* status in 50 to 90 percent of cases). Approximately 10 to 15 percent of chronic carriers of hepatitis B will develop serious liver disease, including **cirrhosis of the liver** and liver cancer, which may lead to liver failure and, without a liver transplant, death.

Transmission

HBV is spread by contact with blood products, semen, vaginal fluids, and in rare instances, saliva. These bodily fluids of an infected person must enter the bloodstream of another person for the virus to transmit. The most common routes of transmission are sharing needles, sexual contact and, occasionally, tattooing and body piercing. HBV is not spread by casual contact or by respiratory droplets (sneezing or coughing). HBV may also be transmitted from an infected woman to her infant during pregnancy or birth.

Any sexual activity that allows the blood or blood product of an infected partner to enter the bloodstream of an uninfected partner may transmit HBV. The riskiest behaviors are unprotected vaginal and oral sex, intercourse without a condom, anal intercourse with or without a condom, and oral-anal activities (refer to Table 8.2).

Diagnosis and Treatment

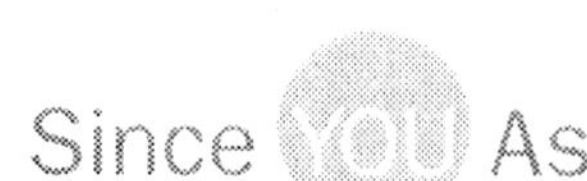

4. I have an uncle who says he had hepatitis B, but he is now cured. I thought viruses could not be cured, so how is this possible?

Jaundice, in combination with reports of other symptoms, is the most common indicator of HBV infection. The diagnosis is usually then confirmed by a blood test that detects antibodies to the hepatitis virus. After a person is initially exposed to the virus, 1 to 4 months is required for the body to produce antibodies. During this **incubation period**, the virus may not be detectable (although the person may transmit the virus), so an initial blood test is often followed by a confirmatory test 3 to 6 months later. A home test may already be available in the United States for hepatitis B (such a test has been available for hepatitis C, and a home test for HBV was introduced in some European countries in 2004).

Once a person has been diagnosed with acute HBV, treatment options are limited. As mentioned earlier, the body's immune system usually resolves an acute infection on its own. For those with symptoms of acute infection, most doctors recommend bed rest, increased fluid intake, good nutrition, and avoiding alcohol (alcohol may exacerbate liver inflammation). The symptoms of acute hepatitis usually last 4 to 12 weeks, and the body usually eliminates the virus entirely within 6 months (Lin & Kirchner, 2004).

In cases of chronic infection, two medications are currently prescribed when and if a person shows signs of liver infection. *Alpha interferon*, a protein that boosts the body's immune system response to the virus, and two antiviral medications (trade names, Lamivudine and Hepsera) slow the rate at which the hepatitis B virus multiplies, which helps prevent inflammation that can lead to liver damage. Beyond

cirrhosis of the liver A potentially serious liver disease that may lead to liver cancer.

incubation period The time between infection and the appearance of physical symptoms of illness.

these approved medications, various new antiviral agents that show promise in the treatment of HBV are currently in human trials and should be available within a few years (Zepf, 2003a).

Of course, preventing any illness is preferable to treating it. To that end, an HBV vaccine that will prevent infection with near certainty has been available since the early 1980s. The vaccine is recommended for *everyone* by most medical organizations in the United States, and it is now part of the routine vaccination schedule recommended for infants. Moreover, the HBV vaccine is required routinely for public school admission in most states. The vaccine is given in a series of three injections over a 6-month period and imparts lifetime immunity to the virus. Over a 20-year period, the vaccine has reduced the annual number of new cases of hepatitis B in the United States from 300,000 to under 80,000 (Lin & Kirchner, 2004). The vaccine does not contain live HBV viruses, so it cannot "accidentally" cause hepatitis. Studies have shown the vaccine to be safe, with no serious negative side effects (Kimmel, 2002).

Human Papilloma Virus (Genital Warts)

Genital warts, caused by certain strains of the **human papilloma virus (HPV)**, may be the most common STI in the United States today among young, sexually active individuals (DSTDP, 2004b). Some researchers estimate that 50 to 75 percent of Americans of reproductive age may be infected with HPV (Cates, 1999b). In addition, approximately 5 million Americans become infected with HPV every year (Cates, 1999b; DSTDP, 2004b). Moreover, *most* people infected with HPV have never noticed an active outbreak of warts and are unaware they are infected with the virus (CDC, 2002).

Symptoms

Over 100 types of HPV, the virus that causes warts, are present in humans, and about 30 of them are transmitted through sexual contact and appear primarily in the genital or anal area. Although most of these strains of the virus are relatively harmless, a few types have been shown to increase the risk of other potentially serious and even deadly diseases such as cervical dysplasia (abnormal cells of the cervix), cervical cancer, or other cancers of the reproductive tract, mouth, and anus (Jancin, 2004; Koutsky & Kiviat, 1999; Stoler, 2000). Two strains of HPV (types 16 and 18) in particular have been shown to be implicated in virtually all cases of cervical cancer (McNamara, 2004; Pinto et al., 2003). Women infected with other types of genital HPV may still develop genital warts but are unlikely to be at increased risk for cervical cancer. Based on this clear connection between HPV and cancerous cellular abnormalities, the American Cancer Society has issued new guidelines for the detection and prevention of cervical cancer. These are explained in "In Touch with Your Sexual Health: HPV, Cervical Cancer, and the Pap Test: Advances in Cervical Cancer Screening."

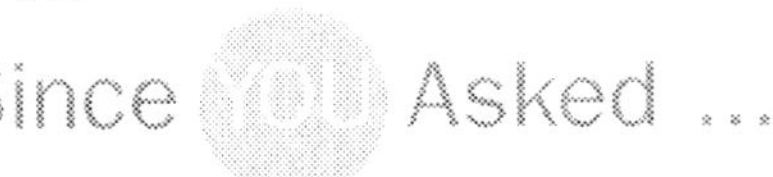

5. Is it true that genital warts can cause cancer?

HPV infection is typically discovered by noticing the presence of visible warts or clusters of warts in the genital area. The warts may be on the penis, opening to the vagina, cervix, labia minora, or anal area. However, warts may also be inside the vagina or anus and may not be noticed at all. In such cases, the person may be unaware of the infection.

Warts typically appear 4 to12 weeks after exposure. Usually the warts are painless, but in some sensitive areas such as the urethra, they may be uncomfortable or cause pain. The warts can have a flat, lumpy, or cauliflower appearance; they may occur

human papilloma virus (HPV) A sexually transmitted virus typically characterized by warts in the genital or anal area and that may lead to some forms of cancer; also known as *genital warts*.

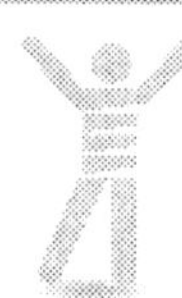

In Touch with Your Sexual Health

HPV, Cervical Cancer, and the Pap Test: Advances in Cervical Cancer Screening

Over the past 50 years, use of the Pap test to screen for cervical cancer has reduced the incidence of the disease by 70 percent in the United States. Yet despite this enormous success, each year thousands of American women develop cervical cancer and die unnecessarily.

In 2002, the American Cancer Society published new guidelines for cervical cancer screening, and the following year, the American College of Obstetricians and Gynecologists (ACOG) released new recommendations for screening. Both sets of guidelines recognize new cervical cancer screening and detection techniques and contain important information concerning the prevention and early detection of cervical cancer, including the following:

- Cervical cancer screening should begin approximately 3 years after a woman begins having vaginal intercourse, but no later than 21 years of age.
- Cervical screening should be done every year with regular Pap tests or every 2 years using liquid-based Pap tests. Women up to age 30 should undergo annual cervical cytology (microscopic) screening.
- Starting at age 30, women who have had three consecutive normal Pap tests may continue screening every 2 to 3 years. However, it is recommended that women continue to see their health care providers on an annual basis for health checkups and to learn good prevention practices.
- Women 70 years of age and older who have had three or more normal Pap test results and no abnormal results in the last 10 years may choose to stop cervical cancer screening. ACOG notes that due to limited studies of older women, it is difficult to set an across-the-board upper age limit for cervical cancer screening and therefore recommends that testing continue in non-high-risk women over the age of 70.

Recently, the Food and Drug Administration also approved a new approach to cervical cancer screening for women 30 years of age and older: the use of the HPV test in conjunction with the Pap test. This new test can accurately determine which women are at risk of developing cervical cancer and which women have little or no risk of developing cervical disease or cervical cancer in the near future. If both test results are negative (normal), neither test will need to be repeated more often than every 3 years. If the Pap test is negative (normal) and the HPV test is positive, the HPV test should be repeated in 6 to 12 months. If both tests are positive, a woman's physician will discuss the next steps with her.

In 2006, the FDA approved a vaccine that prevents HPV in women. The vaccine is approved for women between the ages of 9 and 26 and is likely to be expanded in the future to include men and older women. Keep in mind that the vaccine must be given *prior* to HPV infection.

Source: Adapted from National Cervical Cancer Public Education Campaign (2006).

singly or in groups; and they may vary in size. Sometimes the warts may be so small or flat that they cannot be seen or felt (see Figure 8.4).

Transmission

Although HPV in humans has existed for decades and perhaps even centuries, only recently has it been elevated to "high-threat" status. Three reasons account for this new danger. First, as mentioned earlier, HPV cannot be cured. When the warts are visible, they can be removed using chemical or laser treatments (to be discussed next), but the virus remains in the body for at least a year until, in most cases, the immune system is able to fight and eradicate it (if no reinfection has occurred). While the virus is in the body, it can express itself with a new outbreak at any time. The second and more important issue is the discovery that certain types of HPV are the major cause of cancer of the cervix, as we have already discussed. The third factor generating increased concern is that HPV is relatively easy to transmit *despite the use of condoms*

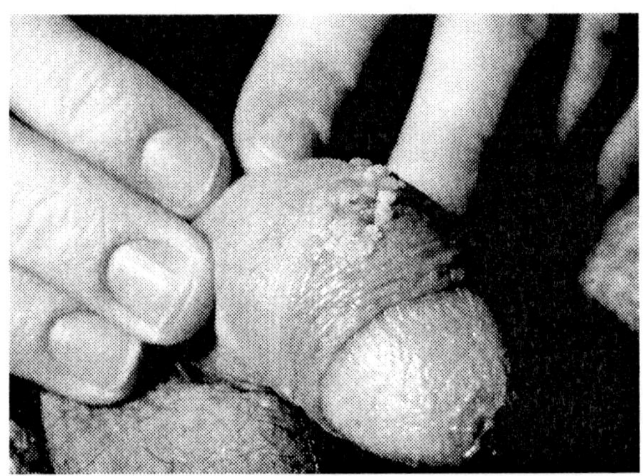

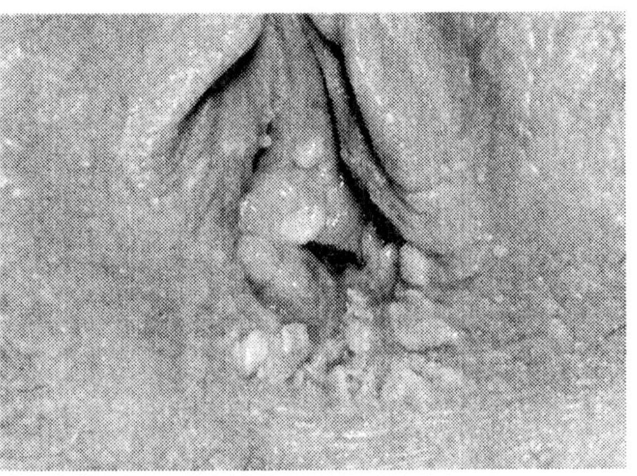

FIGURE 8.4 Genital Warts
Shown here are typical, observable cases of male and female genital warts.

because the virus can shed from the infected person to his or her partner during sexual acts, through skin-to-skin contact in genital areas that are not well protected by a condom (Groopman, 1999; Rothenberger, 2001).

That said, HPV is *most* likely to transmit when warts are visible (Koutsky & Kiviat, 1999). The virus usually transmits from genitals to genitals, but may also be spread through oral and anal sexual activities. It can be spread to the mouth and throat through oral sex with an infected partner. Genital warts are *not* caused by contact with other types of warts on the skin (such as the hands, feet, or face). HPV transmission is, as for all STIs, also linked to the number of sexual partners. One study that examined the rates of HPV among college women found that of the 604 women in the study, 7 percent of women who reported one male lifetime sex partner were infected with HPV, compared to 33 percent with two to four lifetime male sex partners, and 53 percent who had five or more lifetime male sex partners (Burk et al., 1996). Similar patterns of infection increasing with the number of partners have been found among men.

Diagnosis and Treatment

Genital warts are typically diagnosed visually by a health care professional. However, given that HPV infection is often asymptomatic, infection is often not suspected by the infected person or by a health care provider. Tests are now available to detect HPV and to reveal the exact strain of the virus. However, testing for HPV beyond visual inspection is usually not part of standard medical care for women or men.

As this text went to press, new guidelines for HPV screening were under consideration by various medical organizations in the United States. Past practices have recommended an HPV test for women who received Pap test results indicating abnormal cervical cells (referred to as ASCUS, for *atypical squamous changes of unknown source*). Approximately 5 percent of all Pap smear tests find such abnormalities, and only a small percentage of these women are eventually diagnosed with cervical cancer upon follow-up testing. Currently, however, HPV testing is becoming increasingly common for women as part of the routine annual gynecological exam (as noted in "In Touch with Your Sexual Health: HPV, Cervical Cancer, and the Pap Test").

A new Pap test method called the *thin-prep Pap* collects enough cervical cells to allow for an HPV test to be done immediately if abnormal cells are found. If strains of HPV associated with cancer are discovered, the woman can be monitored more closely and more often for signs of cervical cancer and receive early, effective treatment (Friedman, 2002). Beyond this use of HPV testing, however, some medical researchers are suggesting that the Pap test be *replaced* by HPV screening for all women, because a positive test for specific HPV strains is significantly more sensitive than the Pap smear in identifying women at risk of cervical cancer ("Can HPV Testing," 2003). However, such testing is not yet routine, so women need to be aware of these new findings and request the appropriate tests from their doctors. One more point must be made about HPV and cancer: In addition to HPV's link to cervical cancer, evidence exists that the virus may also play a role in anal and oral cancer in men and women. Consequently, tests for these cancers are recommended for anyone, male or female, infected with cancer-related strains of HPV (Kubetin, 2002).

Many visible outbreaks of genital warts resolve on their own. In cases where this does not happen, various methods are available for removal of the warts, including cryosurgery (freezing with liquid nitrogen), laser surgery, and several topical medications that are designed to be applied by the patient (CDC, 2002). In pregnant women with genital warts, surgical removal is recommended. Perhaps most important, HPV may be spread without any obvious signs of infection. Typically, after 1 to 2 years without a recurrence of warts or reinfection by a partner, the body's immune system will often suppress or eliminate the virus from the body (CDC, 2002)

Although no medical cure exists for HPV, and prospects for one in the foreseeable future are not bright, two vaccines against the virus appear close to reality (Bloom, 2005; Walsh, 2003b). As of 2005, vaccines were in large-scale human trials, and results indicate near 100 percent effectiveness in preventing infection with the strains of HPV that cause genital warts and are most closely linked to cancer (Russell, 2005). In 2006, the FDA approved a vaccine for HPV.

HIV and AIDS

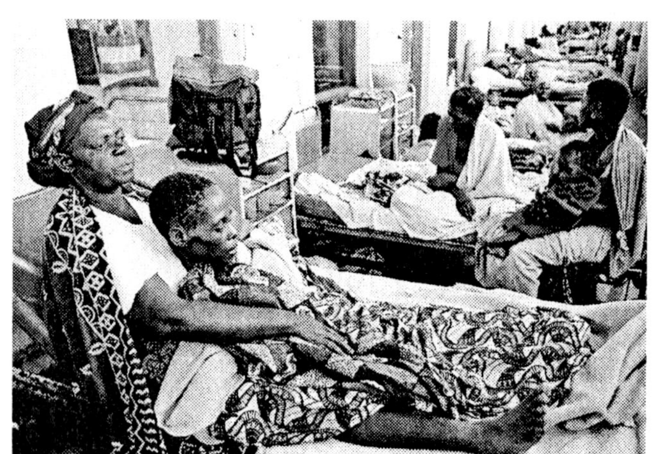

HIV continues to outpace efforts to slow its spread worldwide.

One of the most profound and frightening public health crises of the last century is the HIV/AIDS worldwide **pandemic**. It is safe to say that HIV/AIDS has changed forever how the world views sexuality and sexual behavior. The staggering numbers of people who have died (and continue to die) as a result of AIDS; the vast numbers who are infected with HIV, the virus that causes AIDS; and the effect of HIV on human sexuality necessitate a somewhat deeper and wider discussion than we have provided for the other STIs in this chapter. Therefore, in this section we will focus on the background and origins of HIV/AIDS, the prevalence and incidence of the infection, symptoms and progression of HIV/AIDS, the proven routes of transmission, myths and misconceptions, diagnosis and testing for HIV, current treatment options, and the challenges of living with HIV. We will focus our attention on HIV and AIDS in the United States, but the devastating toll AIDS is taking around the world is discussed in "Sexuality and Culture: The HIV/AIDS Pandemic." Indeed, in 2004, the United Nations announced that new cases of HIV infection worldwide reached a record high in 2003, of 5 million new infections, and only one out of every ten infected individuals was receiving the treatment needed to combat the virus. As one UN official summed it up, "The virus is running faster than all of us" (Intelihealth, 2004b; UNAIDS, 2004).

pandemic A widespread epidemic.

human immunodeficiency virus (HIV) The virus that causes AIDS.

acquired immune deficiency syndrome (AIDS) A gradual failure of the immune system, leading to serious infections and death.

Background and Origins of HIV and AIDS

Most likely, everyone reading this is familiar, to some extent, with **HIV**, the **human immunodeficiency virus**, and **AIDS**, **acquired immune deficiency syndrome**, that is caused by HIV. What may surprise many people is that HIV in its current forms has been present in humans since the 1930s, and perhaps earlier. Most scientists today

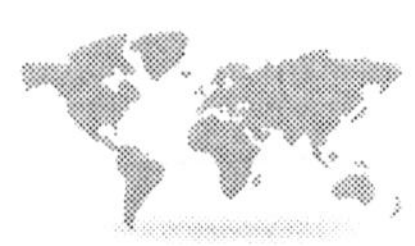

Sexuality and Culture

The HIV/AIDS Pandemic

HIV and AIDS have become a global pandemic and one of the greatest health threats of our time. Over 3 million deaths are attributed to HIV infection every year around the world, and it is estimated that over 40 million people throughout the world are currently living with HIV infection (UNAIDS/WHO, 2005a).

The United States and European countries were among the first to report AIDS cases, but less economically developed countries in regions such as sub-Saharan Africa are the most severely affected and were among the first to report *epidemic* levels of HIV infection and AIDS-related deaths. Over 25 million people in sub-Saharan Africa are HIV-positive; most are between 15 and 49 years old (UNAIDS/WHO, 2005a). The affected countries are losing entire generations of people, and HIV is a threat to entire cultures.

Recently, some African countries such as Uganda, Kenya, and Zimbabwe have seen slight drops in the rate of HIV and AIDS infection. One of the first, and most important steps taken in these countries was acknowledging their high rates of HIV, and then instituting government-sponsored prevention and intervention efforts, including condom promotion and distribution, mass HIV testing, screening and treatment for STIs, and community mobilization. Nevertheless, these countries remain among the most severely affected countries in the world (UNAIDS/WHO, 2005b). In some Zimbabwe communities, as many as 40 percent of adults are infected with HIV. In South Africa, nearly 30% of pregnant women are HIV positive and the death rate of those aged 15 or older increased 62 percent between 1997 and 2002.

As the maps show, rates of HIV infection and AIDS are becoming major problems in Asia, Europe, and Latin America as well. World health organizations are focusing intensively on the extreme danger of an even larger and more widespread increase of HIV throughout China and Southeast Asia.

Worldwide spending on HIV/AIDS is approximately $5 billion annually, which is estimated to be less than half the amount needed to fight the epidemic effectively. Another problem is a shortage of trained medical personnel to treat and care for HIV and AIDS patients. This further adds to the costs of this illness.

If a bright side to these overwhelming statistics exists at all, it lies in the fact that the world is finally being shocked into coming to grips with this worldwide pandemic. The 2003 report from the Joint United Nations Program on HIV and AIDS found something of a silver lining in the following quote:

> Globally, the AIDS response is moving into a new phase. Political commitment has grown stronger, grass-roots mobilization is becoming more dynamic, funding is increasing, treatment programs are shifting into gear, and prevention efforts are being expanded." (UNAIDS, 2003, p. 5)

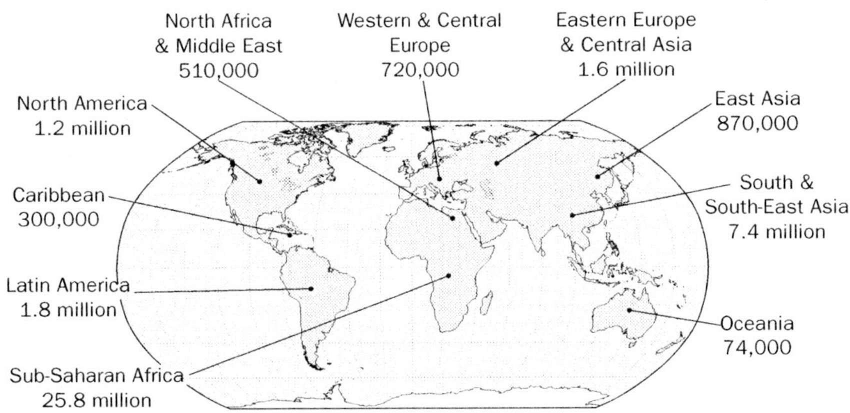

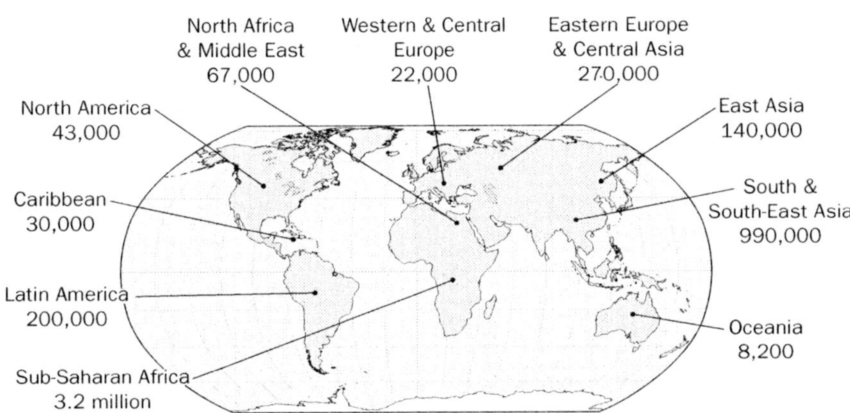

These maps show the total number of people estimated to be living with HIV/AIDS worldwide as of the end of 2005 and the number of new HIV infections around the world recorded in 2005.

Source: World Health Organization, (2005).

agree that the virus probably crossed from chimpanzees and other nonhuman primates infected with a simian form of HIV (called SIV) to humans between 1930 and 1945. Although SIV was harmless to the nonhuman population, in humans it leads to the immune system destroying disease known as AIDS. The cause of this animal-to-human crossover is thought to be the practice in some parts of Africa of capturing, killing, and eating nonhuman primate meat, leading to an exchange of blood products from simians to humans and thus the transfer of the virus ("HIV Puzzle Cracked," 2003; Watanabe, 2004).

Awareness of HIV and AIDS in the United States, dates back only to the early 1980s. On June 5, 1981, the Centers for Disease Control and Prevention released their first report that a few cases of a rare form of pneumonia (*pneumocystis carinii pneumonia*, or PCP), had been diagnosed among gay men in New York, Los Angeles, and San Francisco. Soon other mysterious diseases including a rare form of skin cancer (*Kaposi's sarcoma*, or KS) and other infections, normally thwarted entirely by the human immune system, were being diagnosed among more and more men in the gay community. Because these diseases only establish themselves in the human body through the opportunity of a weakened immune system, they are referred to as **opportunistic infections**. Doctors and medical researchers were bewildered at that time by the array of symptoms and diseases exhibited by the patients who had first contracted the infection that would become known as AIDS; they were helpless to stop the disease's progression. These symptoms included unexplained weight loss, rare forms of pneumonia, rare cancers, and various infections caused by microbes not normally found in normally healthy human populations. Within one year, over 1,500 cases of this new illness had been diagnosed, and over 600 of the infected men had died.

In the early years after the discovery of AIDS in the United States, the illnesses and deaths were occurring primarily within the gay male community. On the street and among the population in general, the disease was regarded as a "gay plague," adding fuel to the already hot fire of prejudice and discrimination against nonheterosexual individuals. However, even to the professional health community, AIDS did indeed appear, at first, to be limited to gay men. Consequently, the first official, medical designation for AIDS was GRID, for *gay-related immune deficiency*. Soon, however, AIDS was discovered in populations beyond gay males, including women, intravenous drug users, and large groups of people in other countries, especially, at that time, Haiti and Africa. Consequently, in 1982, the CDC officially changed the name of the disease to *acquired immune deficiency syndrome*, or AIDS.

By the middle of 1983, scientists had not yet discovered the cause of AIDS. In May of that year, the following quote appeared in the *New York Times:*

> In many parts of the world there is anxiety, bafflement, a sense that something has to be done—although no one knows what—about this fatal disease whose full name is Acquired Immune Deficiency Syndrome and whose cause is still unknown. The World Health Organization (WHO) plans to convene a meeting of experts in Geneva from November 22 to 25. ("Concern over AIDS," 1983)

In late 1983 and early 1984, American and French researchers discovered that the causal organism for AIDS was a virus, or more specifically, a **retrovirus**. Retroviruses are especially insidious because they survive by using their RNA to invade and destroy the DNA of normal body cells and then copy the virus's DNA into the hosts cells' chromosomes. This process replicates over and over, manufacturing more viruses, which in turn migrate into additional cells. Only a handful of human retroviruses have been discovered, including ones that cause certain cancers and two that cause HIV.

opportunistic infections Diseases that establish themselves in the human body when the immune system is weakened and incapable of fighting them off.

retrovirus A type of virus, such as HIV, that survives by invading and destroying the DNA of normal body cells and then replicating its own DNA into the host cell's chromosomes.

Prevalence and Incidence of HIV/AIDS

As of 2004, the cumulative number of diagnosed AIDS cases (the **prevalence**) in the United States grew to 930,000. Of these, over 520,000 have died from AIDS-related illnesses (CDC, 2004b). In addition, 1.3 million people are estimated to be infected with HIV, and as many as a third of those are unaware of their HIV status. Approximately 40,000 new cases of HIV infection (the **incidence**) have been reported each year in the United States alone. This incidence rate had been relatively stable until early in the new century, when the CDC reported an upturn in new cases of HIV, from approximately 14,000 per year to 43,000 in 2003 (CDC, 2004b). This increase will be discussed in more detail shortly. The number of AIDS-related deaths in the United States was just over 18,000 in 2003 (CDC, 2004b).

Although HIV infection crosses all ethnic, age, and economic boundaries, it is diagnosed disproportionately in certain populations. Nearly 40 percent of AIDS cases and 50 percent of new HIV infections are among African Americans. In comparison, white Americans account for 42 percent of AIDS cases and 35 percent of new HIV infections. Table 8.4 details the number of new HIV infections by ethnicity and sex. The rate of AIDS is four times higher among men than women; however, the number of new HIV infections is growing alarmingly fast among women, particularly African American and Hispanic women.

In 2003, public health officials reported a disturbing increase in HIV infections in the United States. Between 1999 and 2002, new cases of HIV infection among men rose 7.3 percent, 17 percent among men who have sex with men, and 26.2 percent among the Latino population (CDC, 2003a). Researchers attributed these increases to two primary shifts in attitudes among the public about prevention. One of these shifts is the growing *erroneous* belief that the new, more effective drugs now available to treat HIV infection can actually cure the disease or render it harmless and noninfectious (which they cannot). Combined with this growing confidence that HIV is no longer a serious health threat—a "death sentence"—is a phenomenon that has been termed **safe-sex fatigue**, the feeling of being fed up with always practicing safer sex behaviors. These changing attitudes are causing some people, especially within the gay male and college communities, to abandon safer sex practices and return to more

prevalence The total cumulative number of cases of a disease in a given population.

incidence The number of new cases of a disease in a given population over a specific time period.

safe-sex fatigue A loss of tolerance for the necessity of always practicing safer sex behaviors.

Table 8.4 ESTIMATED NEW HIV/AIDS CASES BY RACE/ETHNICITY AND SEX (2004)

RACE/ETHNICITY	NEW HIV/AIDS CASES
Caucasian	11,806
African-American	19,206
Hispanic	6,970
Asian/Pacific Islander	394
American Indian/Alaska Native	208
Other	146
SEX	**NEW HIV/AIDS CASES**
Females	28,273 (73%)
Males	10,457 (27%)
Total	38,730

Source: CDC, (2004c). Cases of HIV infection and AIDS in the United States 2004. HIV/AIDS Surveillance Report, 16, 1–46.

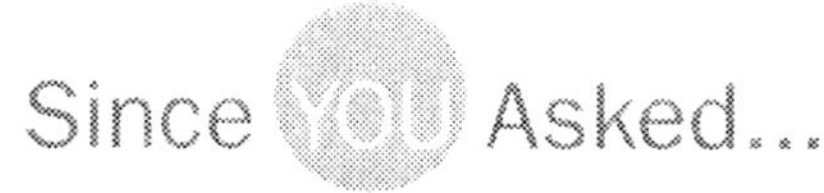

6. I heard that AIDS has been nearly eliminated in the United States. Is this true?

risky sexual behaviors (Kellogg, 2002; Tun et al., 2003). Furthermore, many young adults in the United States today have not experienced at first hand the staggering numbers of deaths from AIDS that occurred in the earlier years of the disease and seem to fear the virus far less. Paradoxically, advances in the treatment and management of HIV and AIDS seem to be undermining public health efforts to promote safer sex behaviors.

Symptoms

Most people who become infected with HIV at first experience no symptoms at all. If symptoms do occur, they may resemble those of the common cold or flu, including fever, headache, fatigue, and rash—all the usual signs that the immune system is responding to a foreign microorganism. These signs of infection typically occur within a few days to several weeks after exposure and usually resolve within 1 to 3 weeks; however, these symptoms are too general to serve as reliable indicators of HIV infection. The only accurate diagnosis of HIV is an HIV antibodies test (to be discussed in the next section).

Once the initial symptoms of infection, if any, subside, the infected person feels normal and in typically good health. However, he or she now carries the virus, and the immune system is busy manufacturing antibodies in an attempt to fight the infection. More important, the person is now capable of transmitting the virus to others, primarily through the exchange of blood or blood products during sexual contact or injectable drug use. Over time, HIV continues to multiply in the body, attacking and killing immune system cells, especially CD4+ T-cells, the body's first line of defense against most infections. As the immune system weakens, new and more severe symptoms begin to appear. These include loss of energy; unexplained weight loss; frequent fevers and night sweats; frequent yeast infections; enlarged lymph glands; persistent skin rashes or flaky skin; short-term memory loss; mouth, genital, or anal sores; and blurred vision (Aggarwal & Rein, 2003; Davis, 2004; Engender Health, 2003).

In the United States, the time between initial HIV infection and the diagnosis of AIDS is 8 to 10 years on average but varies greatly from person to person. Until recently, individuals diagnosed with HIV progressed to full-blown AIDS and died from AIDS-related diseases within 8 to 12 years following initial infection. This time interval has been steadily increasing as treatments for HIV have improved. Today, there are people who have been infected with HIV for over 20 years who continue to live healthy lives.

A diagnosis of AIDS is made in a person who tests positive for HIV when two criteria are met: the person's immune system CD4+ T-cell count dips to below 200, which is less than half the normal lower limit, and when the person becomes infected with one or more of over 20 opportunistic infections. In the United States, the most common AIDS-defining opportunistic infection is the *Pneumocystis carinii pneumonia* virus (PCP). The interval between a diagnosis of AIDS and death due to various opportunistic infections has also been increasing. The current interval range is 1 to 10 years (CDC, 2003b).

Transmission

The human immunodeficiency virus in transmissible amounts is found in the semen, vaginal fluids, and blood of infected persons. Transmission of HIV requires that one of those virus-containing bodily fluids from an infected person enters the bloodstream of an uninfected person. The most common sexual routes of HIV transmission are through unprotected vaginal and anal intercourse. The act of vaginal intercourse itself does not *automatically* ensure the transmission of HIV if one partner is infected. The probability of transmission of HIV from a single instance of unprotected vaginal intercourse between monogamous couples, where one is infected, is approximately 1 in 1,000 (Gray et al., 2001). However, the probability increases greatly as the number of viruses in the blood, called *viral load*, increases, especially in the early or *acute stage* of HIV. The acute stage of HIV infection (also called *primary HIV*) is the first few months following a person's initial infection, when the virus is multiplying fastest and the individual is most likely to be unaware of his or her HIV-positive status. During the first 5 months of infection, sexual transmission is 8 to 10 times more likely compared to later stages of infection (Pilcher, 2003). Odds of infection also increase dramatically with the presence of genital lesions, such as herpes sores or genital warts, on either partner. Regardless of these statistics, the consequences of contracting HIV are far too great to "play the odds," because transmission *can* occur during *any* instance of vaginal intercourse, including the first one.

Overall, women are at greater risk of contracting HIV through heterosexual intercourse than men are during any given sexual encounter. This difference is primarily due to biological and anatomical factors, including the larger surface area of mucous membrane exposed during sex in women than in men, the greater volume of bodily fluids transferred from men to women during vaginal or anal intercourse, the higher total number of viruses in male sexual fluids, and the small tears or other lesions that may occur in vaginal (or rectal) tissue during sexual penetration (World Health Organization [WHO], 2000). In addition, research has demonstrated that the viral load required to transmit HIV is considerably lower for male-to-female transmission than for female-to-male transmission (WHO, 2003). Findings have indicated that women who transmit HIV to men have a 4 times greater viral load than women who are HIV-positive and do not transmit the virus. In contrast, men who transmit HIV to women have only a 1.5 times greater viral load than HIV-positive men who do not transmit the virus ("Gender Makes a Difference," 2001).

Anal intercourse presents a significantly different picture relative to HIV transmission risk. The overall risk of transmitting HIV through *protected anal* intercourse (with a condom) is 10 times greater than through *unprotected vaginal* intercourse, or 1 in 100 (Levin, 2002). The probability of transmission through *unprotected anal* intercourse is 10 times greater than that, or nearly 1 in 10 (Vittinghoff et al., 1999). This holds true for both straight and gay couples who engage in anal intercourse.

Various reasons account for the high risk of transmission through anal sex. The mucous membrane lining the rectum is only one cell layer thick and does not lubricate during sexual activity as the vagina does. This means that rectal tissues can be damaged easily. Slight tears or abrasions in the rectal walls allow an easy route of transmission from the semen of an HIV-positive insertive partner to the receptive partner. The reverse may also be true: If the receptive partner is HIV-positive, the virus may enter through damaged mucous membranes at the opening to the urethra or through a sore or abrasion on the penis. Moreover, condoms offer less protection during anal intercourse than during vaginal intercourse because the lack of natural lubrication and the tightness of the anal opening may cause condoms to tear or break.

Evidence suggests that the risk of oral transmission of HIV is real but significantly lower than vaginal or anal sexual contact (Gottleib, 2003). Oral transmission is difficult to demonstrate because so few sexually intimate couples limit their sexual activities to oral sex exclusively. However, new and faster HIV testing methods have allowed researchers to zero in more accurately on how HIV is transmitted. Although some studies have suggested that the risk of HIV through oral sex is close to zero, other studies have disputed this claim (Gottleib, 2003; D. Hawkins, 2001). One study found that nearly 8 percent of men who had oral sex with other men had contracted HIV through those oral sex activities ("Oral Sex

Since YOU Asked ...

7. Can people get an STI from having oral sex?

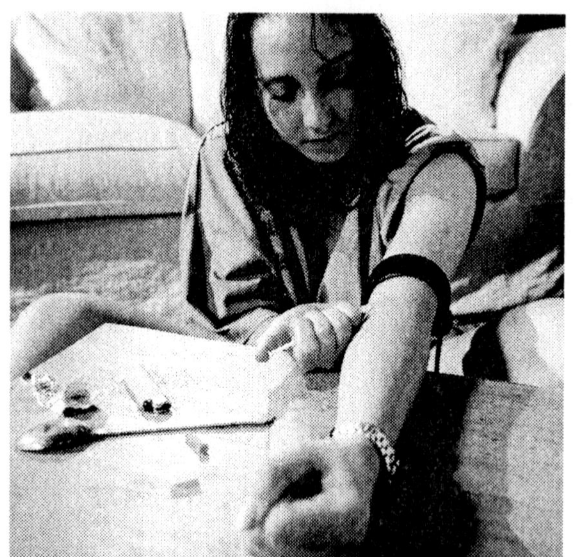

Sharing needles used to inject drugs remains a major route for HIV infection.

Transmission," 2000). This is an extremely important finding because many people, regardless of sexual orientation, hold the mistaken belief that oral sex is safe sex, a falsehood that leads to further spread of HIV (as well as most other STIs). Finally, some research suggests that the risk of HIV infection through oral sex is increased by the practice of genital piercing ("Genital Piercing," 2002).

HIV may also be spread through various nonsexual routes, including the sharing of needles by intravenous drug use, accidental needle sticks among health care workers, blood transfusions, tattooing, and body piercing. When an HIV positive person injects a drug, some of his or her blood is likely to be drawn into the syringe. If another person then uses the same needle, a highly infectious route of transmission is established. Health care professionals have contracted the virus when caring for an HIV patient by accidentally sticking themselves through gloves or other protective clothing with a needle that has been used to give an injection or draw blood. This mode of transmission has decreased over time as greater precautions have been taken and better protective materials have been developed. Early in the HIV epidemic (prior to 1985), one of the most common routes of transmission was through transfusions of blood donated by people who were unaware of their positive HIV status. Today, in most industrialized countries, the blood supply is routinely screened for HIV and numerous other diseases and is very safe. The current risk of an HIV-infected donated blood sample is less than 1 in 500,000 (CDC, 2003e; Intelihealth, 2004a).

Tattooing or body piercing is theoretically a risky activity in terms of potential for HIV transmission. If nonsterile or unsanitary utensils are used for piercing or tattooing, HIV may be spread among customers, especially if the time interval between procedures is short. Most tattoo and piercing businesses are required by law to use universal sanitary precautions to prevent infections of all kinds, and these precautions, if followed, are generally effective in preventing HIV transmission (Brown, Perlmutter, & McDermott, 2000). More worrisome are do-it-yourself piercing and tattooing, because groups of individuals may share whatever sharp tools they may be using, creating a route of HIV transmission if one of them is infected with the virus.

If there is any good news in this discussion, it is that many of the ways people worry about the transmission of HIV are simple myths and misconceptions. For example, no evidence exists that HIV can be transmitted through bites by insects (such as mosquitoes or flies); the sharing of dishes, food, or even toothbrushes; donating blood; sharing hot tubs or swimming pools; contact with pets or other animals; or nonsexual contact with HIV-positive people. Contact with saliva, tears, or sweat does not transmit HIV. Using the same toilet, restroom, towels, or washcloths as an HIV-positive person will not cause transmission. HIV is not airborne, so coughing and sneezing are not risk factors. And probably most important, caring for a person with AIDS is not a risk factor for transmission, especially if no needles are involved.

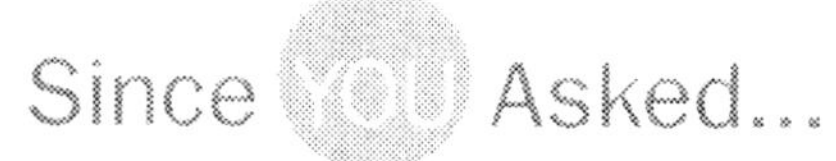

8 There is a rumor that people with AIDS are swimming in the community pool in my neighborhood. Should I be concerned about letting my kids swim there?

HIV Testing

Simple, accurate, and minimally invasive tests for HIV are widely available throughout most of the developed world. The tests are designed to detect antibodies that the body's immune system has manufactured in response to HIV infection, not the virus itself (which is very difficult to detect). After a person is exposed to HIV, the immune system goes to work attempting to fight off the newly introduced virus by manufacturing antibodies designed to attack and kill the viral invader. However, because HIV is so skilled at hiding in the body's cells, the human immune system is usually unsuccessful in destroying it. Nevertheless, the antibodies remain in the blood indefinitely and are detectable by an HIV antibodies test. The number of antibodies needed to be detected by HIV tests may not build up in the blood for as long as 6 months after infection. Therefore, a *conclusive* negative result usually cannot be obtained until 6 months after the time of possible infection. Therefore, a person planning on being tested for HIV should refrain from *all* risky activities for 6 months prior to obtaining the test. When an HIV antibody test produces a positive result, it is always followed up by at least one additional confirmatory test using an alternate method, to confirm the results.

Testing methods for HIV have changed considerably in recent years. Formerly, a person had to provide a blood sample in a doctor's office or clinic and then wait anxiously for 1 to 2 weeks for the result. Although many HIV testing facilities still follow this procedure, a newer testing method called Orasure, developed in the late 1990s, uses a sample of the mucus from the mouth rather than blood. HIV antibodies are present in saliva, but the virus itself is not reproduced in sufficient quantities to be transmissible in saliva. The saliva-mucus test requires the patient to hold a specially treated cotton pad between the cheek and lower gum for 2 minutes. The sample is then sent to a lab, where it is tested for the presence of HIV antibodies. If the test is positive, the person will undergo a confirmatory blood test. The saliva-mucus test is growing rapidly in popularity because it does not involve blood or needles. However, saliva-mucus tests are more expensive than the standard blood test and do not allow for simultaneous testing for other STIs, such as syphilis, which still requires a blood test.

Another important breakthrough in HIV testing is the OraQuick Rapid HIV-1 Antibody Test ("Oral Fluid Based," 2004; Silverman & Peters, 2003). Using saliva or less than a drop of blood, OraQuick is able to detect antibodies to HIV in about 20 minutes with 99.6 percent accuracy. In addition to the rapid results, this test does not require refrigeration or specialized equipment and may be used in situations outside of the standard medical office or clinic setting, such as schools, bars, social service agencies, counseling centers, detention centers, and jail. Another new HIV test that promises results in only 3 minutes, the *Reveal Rapid HIV-1 Antibody Test*, was also approved by the FDA in 2003 (Kaye, 2003). Tests that provide nearly immediate results are important in the fight against the spread of HIV and AIDS because thousands of people who are tested for HIV each year using conventional tests never follow up or check their results. Expanded use of new rapid-results testing technologies that provide while-you-wait findings greatly increases the effectiveness of screening, counseling, and prevention.

Usually, the HIV testing process includes counseling. Counseling individuals who are concerned about their HIV risk is important for public health programs because it enhances their ability to reduce future risky sexual and drug behaviors (regardless of the test results), determine the most common risk behaviors for various populations, provide timely and effective treatments for those with positive test results, help patients cope with the emotional and psychological stresses of a positive test, and reduce the probability of spread of the virus. Unlike other STIs, for which testing is usually carried out in a doctor's office or clinic, many venues offer HIV testing. Table 8.5 lists the testing options, all or some of which may be found in virtually all cities and towns in the United States.

Making the decision to be tested for HIV (or any STI) is an important part of taking responsibility for one's own health and health care. Test sites usually use either **confidential testing** (in which the patient's name and other identifying information is obtained for statistical purposes but kept confidential) or **anonymous testing** (in which the patient is assigned a number and provides no identifying information at all). Anyone who has any concern about HIV status should be tested—the sooner, the better. A negative result, which is very likely for most people, provides a deep sense of

confidential testing Medical test results that are kept confidential by the testing agency and not shared with anyone other than the patient and certain state record-keeping offices.

anonymous testing Tests administered without collecting any personal information about clients, who are identified only by an assigned code number.

Table 8.5 LOCATIONS FOR HIV COUNSELING, TESTING, AND REFERRAL

- Adolescent health clinics, school-based health centers, university health centers
- AIDS services organizations
- Clinics serving men who have sex with men
- Community-based organizations
- Community health centers
- Correctional facilities
- Drug or alcohol prevention and treatment programs
- Family planning clinics
- Freestanding HIV test sites
- Hospital emergency departments
- Hospitals/other urgent care centers
- Managed care organizations
- Men's health clinics
- Migrant health centers
- Occupational/employee health clinics
- Outreach programs (e.g., syringe exchange programs)
- Prenatal clinics
- Private-sector service providers
- Publicly funded counseling and testing sites
- Sexually transmitted disease clinics
- Tuberculosis clinics
- Women's health clinics

Source: CDC (2001a).

relief and allows for a fresh start in avoiding risks and *staying* negative. A positive result, while psychologically and emotionally difficult, allows for early medical intervention and emotional support to help the person develop and sustain a healthy and satisfying quality of life while living with HIV (more on this issue shortly).

Treatment

As of 2006, no cure or vaccine for HIV or AIDS had been found, and the prospects for either were not optimistic. However, treatments for HIV, focusing on preventing the development of AIDS symptoms, have improved greatly since the virus was discovered. Treatment consists of a three-pronged approach: attacking the virus itself, strengthening the immune system, and preventing and controlling opportunistic infections and diseases. The treatment for each HIV-positive individual depends on the person's specific health status and involves working with doctors to tailor a program to the patient's needs. The typical treatment for HIV involves combinations of various medications in conjunction with healthy lifestyle changes.

highly active antiretroviral therapy (HAART) A combination of several medications prescribed for people who are HIV-positive to delay the onset of AIDS.

entry inhibitors A relatively new class of HIV medications that prevent the virus from entering immune system cells.

immune-based therapies Medications that are designed to help an infected person's immune system fight a virus, such as HIV, more effectively.

More than 25 specific medications for fighting the HIV/AIDS virus are currently on the market (Grossman, 2004a). The most effective treatment at present involves a combination of several medications. When HIV-positive individuals have access to this "drug cocktail," referred to as **highly active antiretroviral therapy, or HAART**, management of HIV is optimized for most: The HIV viral load is significantly reduced, survival is extended, and quality of life is enhanced (R. Johnson, 2002; A. D.

Walling, 2004). Figure 8.5 shows the improvement in 10-year survival rates before and after the introduction of the HAART treatment protocol. Perhaps even more striking is the fact that the average number of years of survival from HIV infection to an AIDS diagnosis increases significantly with the number of medications combined in HAART treatment, as shown in Figure 8.6. One of the current global health challenges is making these drugs affordable and accessible to the millions of HIV-positive people worldwide who currently go untreated for this devastating illness.

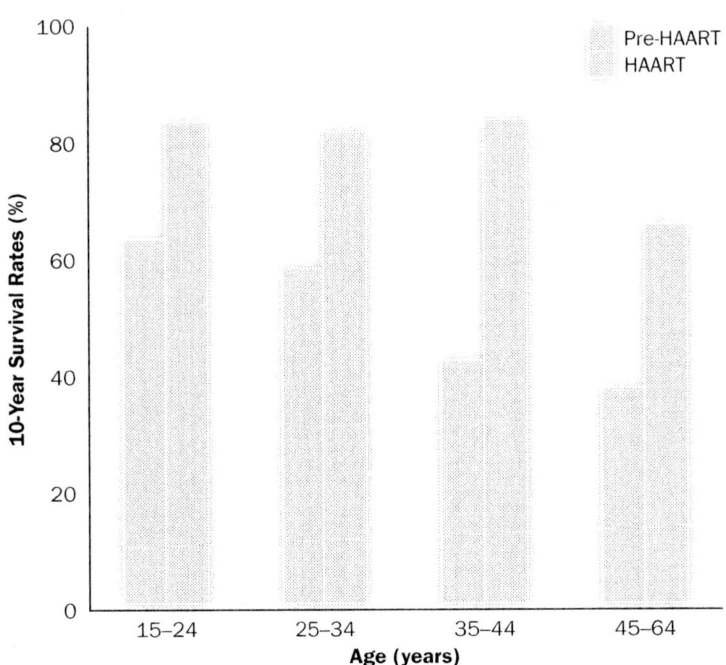

FIGURE 8.5 Ten-Year Survival Rates Before and After Introduction of Highly Active Antiretroviral Therapy (HAART)

Source: Graph, "The Changing Face of AIDS" by R. Johnson from *Aids Read*, Vol. 12, No. 9, (2002), pp. 373–375.Copyright © 2002, THE AIDS READER, Cliggott Publishing Group. All rights reserved.

Although HAART appears to be effective in slowing and even reversing the progression of HIV, it is not without negative side effects. Research has indicated that long-term use of HAART therapy for HIV may increase a person's chances of developing coronary heart disease. Researchers have reported a 26 percent increase in heart attack risk among HIV-positive individuals who had been taking HAART for 4 to 6 years (Friis-Moller et al., 2003). However, the study's authors also pointed out that even this increased rate represented a small absolute risk and must be weighed against the significant survival and quality-of-life benefits of HAART. Another downside to HAART treatment regimens concerns the development of resistance to the medications over time. HIV is a very adaptable virus and can sometimes develop resistance to the drugs that are being used to combat it ("Most Resistance," 2003). In the face of such drug resistance, a different combination of antiretroviral drugs is often substituted, with varying success (Griffin, 2004). HAART, as beneficial as it has been for many of those infected with HIV, is not a *cure* for HIV or AIDS. Increasingly effective treatments for HIV should not be seen as a reason or excuse for abandoning safe sex and other health-related practices (A. D. Walling, 2004).

A newer class of anti-HIV drugs, called **entry inhibitors**, actually prevent the virus from entering immune system cells altogether, rather than preventing replication of the virus within the cell. Entry inhibitors attach to receptors on the outside of immune cells, essentially blocking HIV from binding to the cells prior to entry. As of early 2005, only one of these drugs, *enfuvirtide* (trade name, *Fuzeon*), had been approved by the FDA. It is intended for use among HIV-positive individuals for whom other therapies have been ineffective. This is an important addition to the anti-HIV arsenal because those HIV-positive people who eventually become resistant to the other classes of drugs may still be helped by entry inhibitors.

In a separate but parallel approach to HIV treatment, researchers are working on a different type of drugs referred to as **immune-based therapies**. Instead of attacking HIV itself, these medications are designed to enhance or "train" the infected person's immune system to fight the virus more effectively. These drugs are still in early trials and are unlikely to be available for several years ("Lab Technique," 2003).

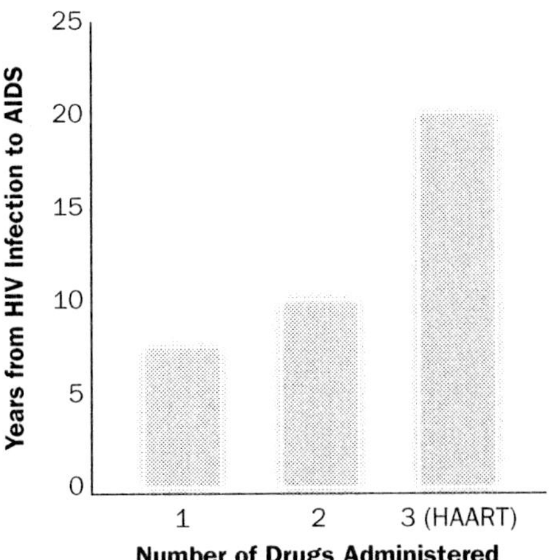

FIGURE 8.6 The Impact of HAART on Time from HIV Infection to AIDS

Source: Graph, "The Impact of HAART on Time from HIV Infection to AIDS" by R. Johnson from *Aids Read*, Vol. 12, No. 9, (2002), pp. 373–375. Copyright © 2002, The Aids Reader, Cliggott Publishing Group. All rights reserved.

As noted earlier, HIV weakens a person's immune system, allowing various opportunistic infections to invade the body. Part of a comprehensive treatment program for people with HIV must include specific treatments for these infections if and when they arise. They fall into six main categories: malignancies (cancers) and bacterial, viral, fungal, protozoal, and neurological infections. Although only some of these opportunistic infections are curable, all are treatable to varying degrees of effectiveness. Choice of treatment will depend on the nature and seriousness of the infection (Grossman, 2004b, for a summary of these infections and their treatments).

Living with HIV

For about the first 10 years of the HIV epidemic in the United States, most people thought of HIV as a death sentence, and with good reason. Until the availability of more effective medications, people diagnosed with HIV commonly died of AIDS-related infections within a year or two. Today, as you can see in Figures 8.5 and 8.6, combinations of treatments are allowing people with HIV to live longer with a greatly improved quality of life. This is evidenced by the fact that HIV infections are remaining stable or slowly increasing but deaths from AIDS are dropping. Today, a diagnosis of HIV is no longer considered a death sentence in the United States (R. Johnson, 2002; Schmitt & Stucky, 2004). New and better medications and effective combinations of drugs, such as HAART, have extended the life expectancy of many of those diagnosed with HIV to 20 years and beyond, with the prospect of a relatively normal life during this time.

Psychologists and other health professionals have made extensive efforts to change negative attitudes about HIV and AIDS. Many people now understand that HIV is an infection that one can live with but, like all serious health issues, something that must be treated and carefully monitored. This reframing of HIV has served to begin to destigmatize those who are infected and to focus attention on prevention, treatment, and cure. Improvements in treatment and survival have also had another very important effect: to give people living with HIV and their loved ones *hope*. The mind-body connection can be a powerful healer in itself, and hope is a key element in that healing process. That said, the impact of a diagnosis of HIV should not be minimized. It is a serious illness with potentially fatal consequences, but it is an illness that can be managed, and a full, productive life can be sustained in the face of an HIV diagnosis.

HIV, Lifestyle, and Health

Obviously, adopting safer sexual behaviors is particularly important for people living with HIV to prevent the spread of the virus to others. Unfortunately, studies indicate that as many as 55 percent of people who know they are HIV-positive continue to engage in unsafe sexual activities and fail to inform their partners of their HIV status (Josephson, 2003). In addition to the danger this poses to their sexual partners, unsafe sex is also a serious health threat to HIV-positive individuals themselves (Clottey & Dallabetta, 1993). At one time, people believed that a couple who both were HIV-positive (called *HIV-seroconcordant couples*) had little reason to worry about unprotected sexual activities; after all, what could possibly happen that was worse than HIV? Researchers, however, have strongly refuted that idea. People who have been diagnosed for HIV continue to be at risk for all other STIs, and for many, the risk and seriousness of infection is much greater than for those whose immune systems are not compromised by HIV. Furthermore, more than one strain of HIV exists; infection with multiple strains of HIV may be much more serious and deadly than infection with only one and may cause the progression to AIDS to accelerate (Goulder & Walker, 2002). Many seroconcordant couples appear to be aware of these risks. A study conducted with HIV-concordant couples found that the primary reasons these couples used condoms was to reduce their risk of other viral STIs such as herpes, HPV, and hepatitis (S. P. Williams, 2001). The point here is that the importance of safer sex does not end with a couple's HIV-positive test results; instead, safer sex practices become even *more* essential.

The Future of HIV/AIDS

More than two decades have passed since the first cases of AIDS were identified in the United States. In that time, enormous effort and resources have been poured into HIV education and prevention. However, far more resources are needed to fight this disease. For every new case of HIV that is diagnosed and treated, many more have yet to be discovered. Clearly, defeating HIV is one of the single greatest challenges the world has ever faced. Worldwide, factors such as poverty, drug use, poor health care, violence, famine, and hopelessness all contribute to a lack of adequate HIV education, which in turn perpetuates an epidemic that is far from being controlled.

Fortunately, we can find *some* cause for optimism amid this terrible epidemic as newer and more effective treatments are developed and made available, driving the sickness and death rate from HIV/AIDS downward. A pill form of an existing HIV treatment drug (*tenofovir*) is currently in the testing stages to see if it might actually prevent HIV infection altogether (Dotinga, 2004), and research on a vaccine to immunize people against HIV infection is proceeding worldwide ("G-8," 2004; "Initial Results," 2003). As is true of all disease, prevention is the best hope for a future without HIV and AIDS.

That said, it is important to keep in mind as you read this that treatment for HIV and AIDS is significantly more available and effective in Western and First World countries than in developing nations, especially Africa, where the disease is having the most devastating impact (as discussed in "Sexuality and Culture: The HIV/AIDS Pandemic" earlier in this chapter). This discrepancy in resources and treatment must be addressed globally if we are to save millions of lives and, it is hoped, one day rid the world of this deadly virus.

Bacterial STIs

Although the various viral infections we just finished discussing are quite common, *most* sexually transmitted infections in the United States are bacterial. Bacterial STIs are infections caused by single-celled organisms called *bacteria* that are spread primarily by sexual contact. These organisms are harbored in bodily fluids (saliva, mucous membranes, vaginal secretions, semen, blood, etc.) and may be transmitted during oral, vaginal, or anal sex, when contact with these fluids occurs.

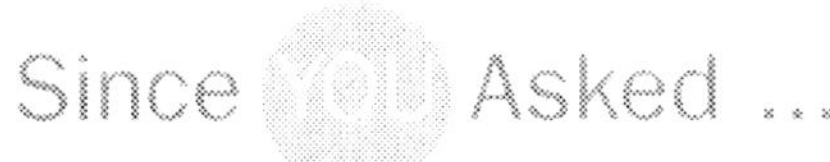

9. Are the STIs caused by viruses and bacteria basically the same?

Medical science is far more capable of curing bacterial infections than viral ones. Think about it: When you have a common cold, which is caused by a virus, no cure exists—you must let the illness run its course. However, if your upper respiratory symptoms are caused by a bacterial infection, a week or two of treatment with an *antibiotic* readily cures you. So it is with bacterial STIs—for the most part, they are curable and fairly easy to treat, provided that they are diagnosed early and have not mutated and become resistant to common antibiotics. However, even in the most difficult cases requiring repeated treatment, a cure is highly likely. The most important factor in treating bacterial STIs is medical attention at the first signs of infection.

For each bacterial STI, we will follow the format used for viral infections: description, signs and symptoms, routes of transmission, and available tests. However, because treatments for all bacterial STIs are similar, we will examine treatment issues in a single section toward the end of our discussion.

Chlamydia

Chlamydia is an infection caused by the *Chlamydia trachomatis* bacterium, which survives in the cells of bodily fluids such as vaginal secretions and semen. The bacterium is transmitted primarily through sexual contact between an infected person and an uninfected partner. Chlamydia is the most commonly diagnosed and reported STI in the United States, where an estimated 3 million new infections occur each year (DSTDP, 2004b). Anyone can be infected with chlamydia, but the highest rates of

chlamydia A sexually transmitted bacterium, often causing a thick, cloudy discharge from the vagina or penis; may be asymptomatic, especially in women.

pelvic inflammatory disease (PID) A painful condition in women marked by inflammation of the uterus, fallopian tubes, and ovaries; typically caused by one or more untreated STIs.

urethritis A painful inflammation of the urethra; often caused by one or more untreated STIs.

epididymitis A painful swelling and inflammation of the epididymis, the structure at the back of each testicle that stores maturing sperm; often caused by one or more untreated STIs.

infection are among women under the age of 25 (DSTDP, 2004b). One reason for these troubling high numbers is that chlamydia is one of several STIs that often produce no noticeable symptoms, so many people are unaware they are infected. However, the bacterium is highly contagious whether it produces symptoms or not.

Symptoms

Seventy-five percent of women and 50 percent of men infected with chlamydia experience no noticeable symptoms and may have no idea that they have been exposed to an STI (DSTDP, 2004b). Often a diagnosis is made during a routine medical examination or while obtaining care for an unrelated medical issue.

When signs are present, the most common symptom of chlamydia infection is a thick, cloudy discharge from the vagina or penis occurring 1 to 3 weeks after exposure to the bacterium. This discharge is typically less noticeable in women than in men. Most women experience some normal fluid discharge from the vagina associated with hormonal changes of the menstrual cycle. However, the fluid associated with chlamydia is typically greater in quantity and cloudier in appearance. Other symptoms women may experience include pelvic pain, irregular periods, increased pain during menstrual periods, discomfort during urination, or irritation of the vaginal or anal area (see Figure 8.7).

Men who become infected may experience a discharge from the penis and a burning sensation upon urination. Men may also notice irritation or inflammation at the opening to the urethra, and in the morning the urethra may be red and sealed together with dried secretions (Beers, 2004).

If left untreated, any symptoms that may be present for either sex usually diminish and disappear within about a month. However, the infection itself is not cured, remains highly transmissible, and may lead to more serious health problems.

Untreated chlamydia may lead to serious illness damage to the reproductive system of both men and women. As the infection moves up the reproductive tract, women may develop **pelvic inflammatory disease (PID)**, a painful condition in women marked by inflammation of the uterus, fallopian tubes, and ovaries. PID has the potential to cause infertility, chronic pelvic pain, and ectopic (tubal) pregnancy (see Chapter 9, "Conception, Pregnancy, and Birth"). We will discuss PID in greater detail later in this chapter. Among men, untreated chlamydia infection may lead to **urethritis**, an uncomfortable condition that is marked by the inflammation of the urethra, or **epididymitis**, a painful swelling and inflammation of the epididymis, the

FIGURE 8.7 Chlamydia Infection
Examples of male and female chlamydia symptoms. Most people who contract chlamydia, however, exhibit no symptoms at all.

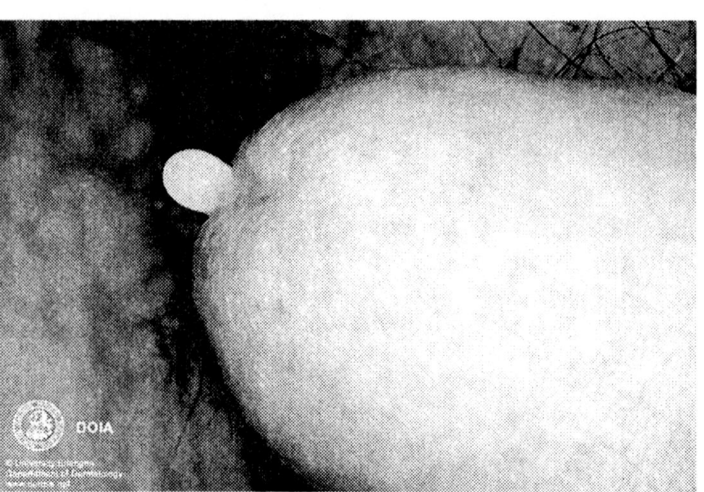

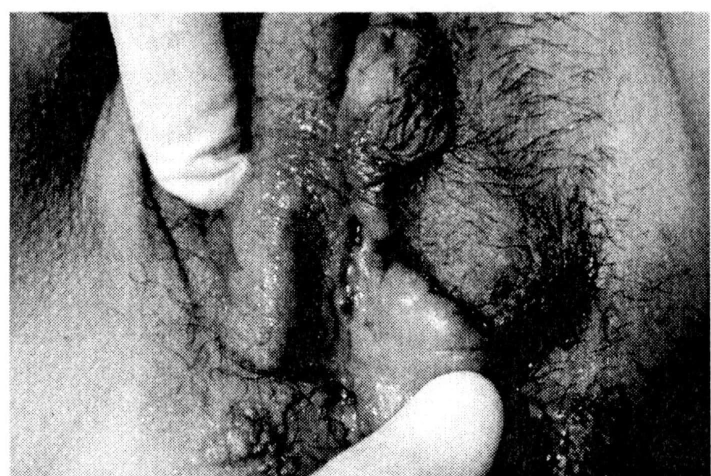

structure at the back of each testicle that stores maturing sperm. Chlamydial infection may play a role in altering the formation of sperm cells or blocking the transport of sperm cells, leading to infertility in men ("Previous Chlamydia," 2004).

Chlamydia is becoming a major public health issue, and public health agencies such as the Centers for Disease Control and Prevention are working to prevent the spread of chlamydia through increased awareness, testing, and screening. The number of new annual cases declined by 25 percent during the 1990s (Cates, 1999b). This decrease was most likely due to the increased screening efforts, particularly among adolescents and young women under the age of 20, who are at greatest risk of infection (Burstein et al., 2001; Marrazzo et al., 1997).

Transmission

Chlamydia, like most STIs, is transmitted through sexual contact, primarily oral, vaginal, and anal sex. The bacterium is extremely contagious and can easily be transmitted during a single sexual encounter. Vaginal or anal intercourse is the most common route by which chlamydia is transmitted between sexual partners. Chlamydia infection of the throat may result from oral sex, although this type of transmission occurs less frequently than transmission through vaginal or anal sexual contact. Chlamydial infection can also be spread to the eyes if a person touches an infected area on themselves or a partner and then touches the eyes. Chlamydia may also be passed from a pregnant mother to her infant with potentially serious health consequences for her baby.

Diagnosis

Several types of tests may be used to detect *Chlamydia trachomatis*. Testing for chlamydia, as for most STIs, must be done by a health care professional at a doctor's office or clinic. A home test for chlamydia is not currently available, but research for such a test is under way. Tests typically use a sample of cells from the infected area—genitals, anus, or throat. The sample is then examined microscopically for the presence of the *Chlamydia trachomatis* bacterium (bacteria are 10 to 20 times larger than viruses and are far easier to see under a microscope). A newer method for chlamydia screening is *urine-based testing*. Instead of collecting fluid from the vagina, cervix, urethra, or anus, a sample of urine is collected and analyzed for chlamydia. This testing method is allowing for greater chlamydia screening because it is noninvasive and can be carried out in a larger variety of locations—virtually anywhere there is a bathroom. This is important due to chlamydia's asymptomatic nature and the need for and acceptance of widespread screening regardless of people's awareness of infection (Gunn et al., 1998; Pimenta et al., 2000).

Given the high prevalence of asymptomatic chlamydia infections, yearly screening is recommended for sexually active adolescents, especially young women, and all women who have new or multiple sexual partners, even if they don't have any symptoms (DSTDP, 1998). Screening is also recommended for women during pregnancy due to complications that may be caused by the bacterium to both the infant and the mother (DSTDP, 2004a; Jacobson et al., 2001).

Finally, chlamydia infection is found to coexist in many people diagnosed with gonorrhea. Because of this link, a new test has been developed that can detect both STIs in a single sample of genital fluids or urine.

Gonorrhea

Gonorrhea is a sexually transmitted infection caused by the bacterium *Neisseria gonorrhoeae*. Vernacular names for gonorrhea include *clap*, *drip*, and *burn*. Gonorrhea has been infecting humans for centuries; it is even mentioned in the Bible (Leviticus 15:1–15).

gonorrhea A sexually transmitted bacterium typically producing pain upon urination and a thick cloudy discharge from the penis or vagina; often asymptomatic, especially in women.

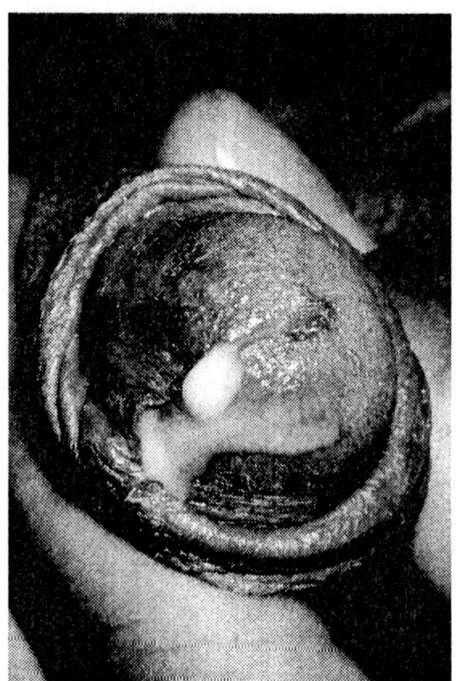

FIGURE 8.8 Gonorrhea Symptoms in the Male
The most common symptoms of gonorrhea in the male are a cloudy discharge from the penis and painful urination. In women, the infection usually has no obvious symptoms, but when symptoms do appear, a similar discharge from the vagina may be observed accompanied by painful urination.

In the 1970s, gonorrhea was one of the most frequently reported STIs. During the 1980s and 1990s, due in part to an increase in public awareness campaigns to prevent all STIs, gonorrhea rates declined at a rate of 10 percent per year (DSTDP, 2000). According to the CDC, rates stabilized around 1996 and then began to increase again. An estimated 650,000 new cases are reported each year in the United States, but this figure is believed to understate the true number of infections by about half (DSTDP, 2004b). Gonorrhea rates are highest among young people, particularly among those between the ages of 15 and 24. At one time, rates were substantially higher among men than women, but the gender gap is closing due primarily to increased screening programs for women that are revealing infections that formerly went undetected.

Symptoms

As with chlamydia, symptoms tend to be more obvious among men than among women. In men, symptoms are likely to occur within 2 to 5 days of exposure to gonorrhea (DSTDP, 2004a; Hook & Handsfield, 1999), although the incubation period can range from 1 to 14 days.

Infection in men may occur in the urethra, anus and rectum, or mouth and throat (see Figure 8.8). Symptoms typically include a painful, burning sensation during urination or bowel movement and a cloudy discharge from the penis or anus. In the case of oral infection, the main symptom is a severe sore throat. Untreated, gonorrhea may spread to other regions of the reproductive tract and can cause epididymitis (discussed in conjunction with chlamydia), acute or chronic prostatitis (inflammation of the prostate gland), and eventual scarring of the urethra, leading to restricted urine flow and urinary tract infections (Parsons, 2002; Hook & Handsfield, 1999).

Among women, the vagina and cervix are the primary sites of infection for the gonorrhea bacterium, and most women have no observable symptoms. The asymptomatic nature of the infection in women contributes to delayed diagnosis and treatment, increased chance of transmission to others, and more complicated and more serious medical conditions.

When symptoms are present, women may notice a cloudy vaginal discharge, irritation during urination, or vaginal bleeding between periods. Other symptoms, such as lower abdominal pain or pain during intercourse, may be indicative of a more complicated infection (Hook & Handsfield, 1999). Unlike men, who have a shorter and more defined incubation period, symptoms in women may not appear until months after initial exposure to the microorganism (DSTDP, 2004a). The longer period between exposure and detection in women contributes to increased complications in women and to long-term consequences such as pelvic inflammatory disease, scarring of the uterus and fallopian tubes, and potential infertility (DSTDP, 2004a; Miller et al., 1999).

Sometimes a woman may confuse gonorrhea with non-STIs that may produce a vaginal discharge. The most common of these is *candidiasis*, better known as a yeast infection, which is an inflammation of the vagina due to microorganisms that may be present in women regardless of sexual activity. This is discussed in greater detail in Chapter 2, "Sexual Anatomy."

Pharyngeal gonorrhea (infection of the throat) can occur as a result of oral sex. Fellatio is a more efficient means of transmission than cunnilingus, which explains the greater prevalence of pharyngeal infection among individuals who have oral sex with men (Hook & Handsfield, 1999).

A less common systemic complication of gonorrhea that may afflict both men and women is *disseminated gonococcal infection* (DGI). The most common clinical manifestations of DGI are skin rashes and joint pain, usually in only one joint in the hands or wrists (Angulo & Espinoza, 1999; Hook & Handsfield, 1999).

nongonococcal urethritis (NGU) A sexually transmitted bacterial infection of the urethra characterized by urethral inflammation and discharge, but not caused by the gonorrhea bacterium.

syphilis A sexually transmitted bacterium characterized by a sore, or chancre, at the point of infection; untreated, it may progress to more serious stages and even death.

Transmission

Gonorrhea thrives in the moist mucous membrane of the throat, genitals, and anus and is easily transmitted through vaginal, anal, or oral sexual contact. Transmission to newborns can occur during delivery and cause infection of the infant's eyes that may lead to blindness or life-threatening blood infections (DSTDP, 2004a). These risks may be minimized with appropriate treatment of the infant soon after birth. The risk of transmission from infected mother to infant is between 30 and 47 percent (Brocklehurst, 1999). Additional complications of gonorrhea infection during pregnancy include low birth weight, preterm delivery, and postpregnancy maternal infection (Brocklehurst, 1999; Ramus et al., 2001).

Diagnosis

Routine screening for gonorrhea is recommended for adolescents during their annual medical exams, and yearly tests are also recommended for anyone with new or multiple sexual partners (DSTDP, 1998). Gonorrhea infection is diagnosed by examining fluid from the urethra, vagina, cervix, rectum, or throat. A swab that looks like a long Q-Tip is used to collect a sample of the fluid from the infected areas. The specimen is then either cultured or stained to reveal the presence of the gonorrhea bacterium. The results are usually known in 1 to 2 weeks and are 90 to 95 percent accurate. Another test now in widespread use is a urine-based screening ("Chlamydia, Gonorrhea Test," 2000). As for chlamydia, urine-based tests are easier to perform, patients appreciate their less invasive nature, and results may be known in as little as 20 minutes. Urine-based tests tend to be more expensive than traditional forms of testing, but they may lead to wider testing, better treatments, and reduced spread of infection.

Nongonococcal Urethritis (NGU)

As the name implies **nongonococcal urethritis (NGU)** is inflammation of the urethra *not* caused by the gonorrhea bacterium. It is caused by various other bacteria (including *chlamydia*), but the symptoms often mimic those of gonorrhea. NGU is typically characterized by a discharge from the urethra as well as burning and itching at the end of the urethra or upon urination. It is far more common in men than in women. Approximately 4 million cases of NGU occur annually in the United States (Terris, 2003). NGU is usually transmitted through insertive sexual activity, primarily vaginal and anal intercourse. NGU can be diagnosed with a microscopic examination of cells from the urethra or with a urine test.

Syphilis

Syphilis is one of the earliest recorded and most infamous of the STIs. The list of famous people who purportedly died of untreated syphilis includes King Henry VIII, Napoleon, John Keats, Paul Gauguin, Vincent van Gogh, and Al Capone. Today, virtually no one dies of syphilis; in fact, it is a relatively uncommon STI in the United States, with fewer than 7,000 cases reported in 2002 (CDC, 2003g). Syphilis is caused by the bacterium *Treponema pallidum* or *T. pallidum*. First identified in 1905, the bacterium is also sometimes referred to as a *spirochete* because of its spiral or corkscrew shape (see Figure 8.9).

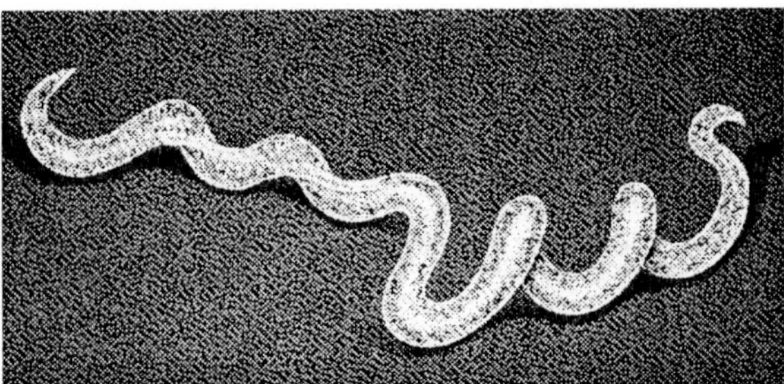

FIGURE 8.9 Syphilis Bacterium
The syphilis bacterium, magnified here over 1000 times, is called a spirochete due to its spiral or corkscrew shape.

Prior to the discovery and widespread use of penicillin during the 1940s, more than 50,000 people became infected with syphilis each year, and thousands of those died from the infection. When penicillin was found to be an effective treatment, rates dropped drastically. In the early 1990s, a resurgence of syphilis occurred in the United States, especially in the South and

chancre A sore that typically appears at the site of infection with syphilis.

large urban areas. At that time, the CDC increased attention on syphilis prevention in the affected areas, including more efficient partner notification and better testing and treatment. In response to these stepped-up efforts, syphilis rates began to drop. By the late 1990s, syphilis had decreased to a historic low of less than 8,000 cases. The CDC saw an opportunity to eliminate syphilis entirely from the United States. In September 1999, a national plan was initiated to reduce the U.S. annual syphilis rates to less than 1,000 cases per year (DSTDP, 1999a). Initially, the plan appeared to be working. As of late 2000, syphilis rates were decreasing, but then a new increase was once again observed by mid-2001. This time, the increases were in large western cities such as San Francisco and Seattle, where syphilis had not been a major problem previously. The increases have been seen primarily among gay and bisexual men (Tuller, 2003). This increase is disturbing for many reasons, not the least of which is that infection with syphilis and the unprotected sexual behaviors that cause it also increase the incidence of more serious, incurable STIs, including HIV and hepatitis. In response to these new statistics, the CDC is targeting those geographical areas for new efforts in education and prevention.

Symptoms

Symptoms of syphilis occur in four distinct stages. The *primary stage* is characterized by a sore called a **chancre** (pronounced "shank-er") that appears at the point of infection within 10 days to 3 months (with an average of 3 weeks) after exposure to the virus (see Figure 8.10). Chancres have hard edges with a watery center and vary in size. The center of the chancre is teeming with syphilis bacteria, making transmission highly probable. Often the chancre may go unnoticed, because it is painless and may be hidden inside the mouth, vagina, or anus. After a few weeks without treatment, the chancre heals and disappears on its own. However, without treatment, the bacterium stays in the body, continuing to multiply, and is highly transmissible to others through sexual contact.

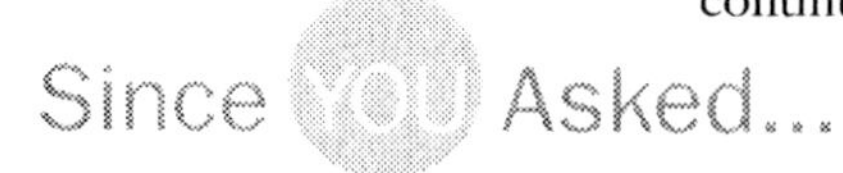

10. If I had sore on my genitals but the sores went away, does that mean I'm cured?

The *secondary stage* of syphilis occurs within a few weeks to up to 6 months of the initial infection. Secondary symptoms include low-grade fever, sore throat, fatigue, headache, alopecia (hair loss), and skin rashes, typically on the hands or feet (see Figure 8.11). Secondary indications are more apparent and more uncomfortable than primary symptoms, but they are likely to be misdiagnosed as various other health problems. Untreated, secondary symptoms also resolve on their own, but the person is still infected and can transmit the organism to others.

FIGURE 8.10 Syphilis Chancre
The first sign of syphilis infection for males and females is a chancre, or sore, at the point of initial infection.

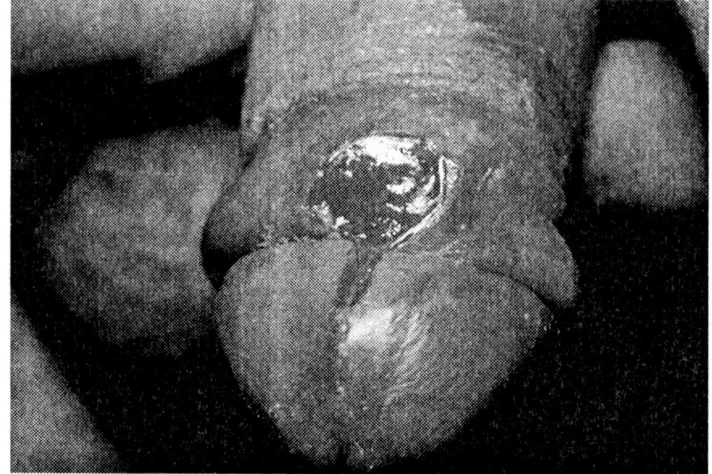

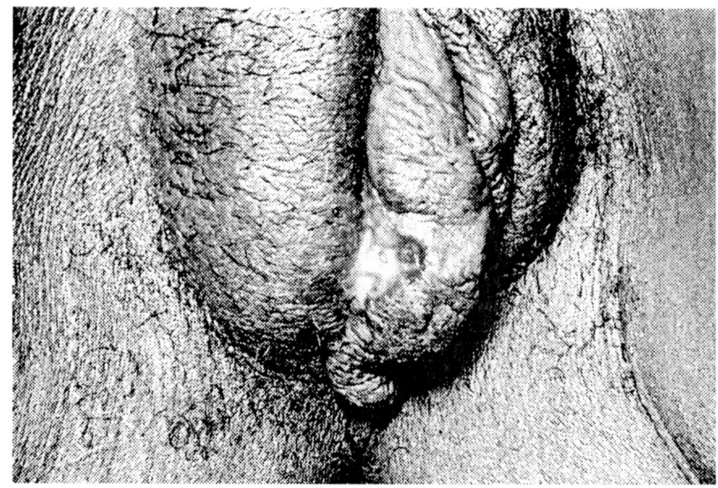

Following the disappearance of secondary-stage symptoms, the infected person enters the *latent stage* of syphilis. This stage has no symptoms, but blood testing would indicate the presence of *T. pallidum.* This stage can last for years or even decades. Although the person is no longer contagious during the late latent stage, the bacteria are continuing to spread throughout the entire body, attacking the heart, muscles, lungs, liver, brain, skin, and nervous system. Ten to 20 years after initial infection, the disease enters the *tertiary stage* or *late stage* of syphilis. In this stage, extensive damage has occurred, often leading to organ failure and neurological injury resulting in paralysis, mental illness, and death. The long-term neurological damage caused by the syphilis bacterium was once known as "syphilitic insanity" but is now called *neurosyphilis.* Today, with antibiotic treatment for syphilis, the infection rarely moves beyond the primary or in rare cases the secondary stage before being treated and cured.

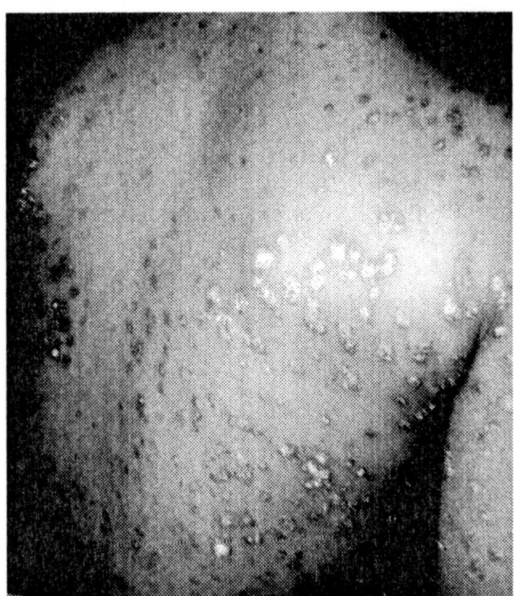

FIGURE 8.11 Secondary Syphilis Rash
If untreated, syphilis progresses to more serious symptoms, including a pronounced skin rash that may appear anywhere on the body.

Transmission

All bacterial STIs are transmitted in basically the same ways: through sexual contact, especially vaginal, anal, and oral sexual practices. Syphilis may be transmitted between heterosexual, gay, or lesbian couples (Campos-Outcalt & Hurwitz, 2002). As noted earlier, the sore that typically appears soon after infection is located at the point of bacterium entry, so it may be found on or in the genitals, the anus, or the mouth.

Diagnosis

During the primary and secondary stages, diagnosis can be made with visual inspection, if symptoms are present. Fluid from the chancre can be sampled and examined microscopically for bacteria. In the absence of symptoms, a blood sample can be taken and tested for the presence of *T. pallidum* antibodies. Although the microscope test indicates infection with the organism, a laboratory blood test can reveal infection *and* how much of the organism is present in the blood. This may be important, because even after people infected with syphilis are cured, they will always have small amounts of antibodies in their blood. If the amount of antibodies is very low, a past, inactive infection is indicated.

Chancroid

Chancroid is a genital ulceration infection that is caused by the bacterium *Haemophilus ducreyi. H. ducreyi* is found in some areas of the United States, but it is far more prevalent in developing countries, especially in tropical or subtropical locales such as Africa, Asia, and the Caribbean. Worldwide, over 7 million cases of chancroid occur yearly (Steen, 2001). In the late 1980s, over 5,000 annual cases were reported in the United States, primarily in urban areas with high rates of prostitution and substance use (Alien, 2001; Tucker, 2001). By 2000, the rate in the United States had dropped below 200 cases, which were confined to specific urban areas such as New York City and Memphis (Tucker, 2001).

Symptoms

Unlike many other STIs, chancroid nearly always presents noticeable symptoms. The primary symptom is a soft chancre sore, similar in appearance to a syphilis chancre, on the penis, vaginal entrance, internal vagina, or perineum (see Figure 8.12). Unlike syphilis chancres, chancroid chancres are often painful and typically occur in groups at the point of infection. Men are more likely to present with genital ulcerations, while women are more likely to have pain when urinating, defecating, or having sex or to experience rectal bleeding. Infected persons are also likely to notice swelling and pain

chancroid A sexually transmitted bacterial infection causing one or more painful soft chancre sores in the genital or anal area.

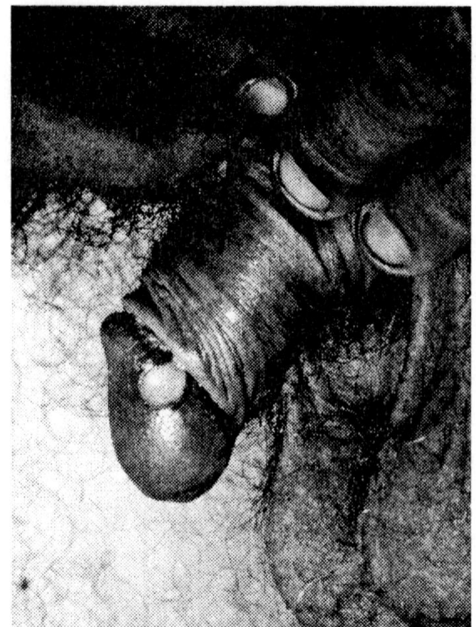

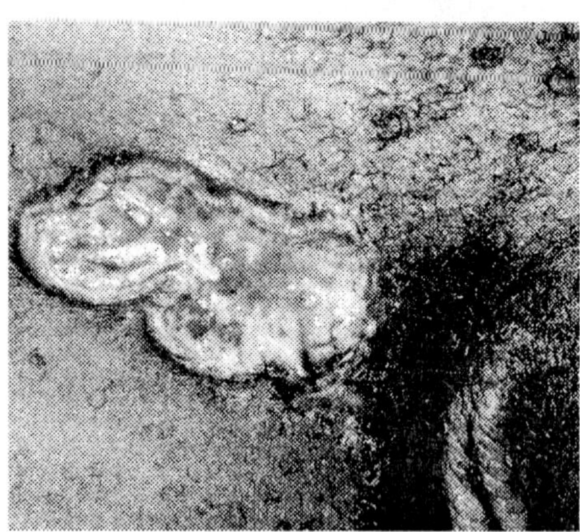

FIGURE 8.12 Chancroid
Symptoms of chancroid for males and females include chancre sores in the genital region and swollen lymph nodes in the groin.

in the lymph nodes in the groin area. The incubation period is 4 to 7 days after exposure. The chancres usually do *not* heal on their own and become increasingly serious until the infected person seeks treatment. In some cases, ulcerations and pain can be so severe that hospitalization is necessary. Once treatment begins, complete healing may take 30 days or more. Ulcers may reappear at any time after healing, usually in the same location.

Transmission

Haemophylus ducreyi is transmitted through oral, vaginal, or anal sexual contact, but infection can occur in areas other than the genitals, such as the fingers or the eyes. Risk behaviors including substance abuse and prostitution are most often associated with the disease. Although chancroid bacterial infections themselves are typically treated and cured relatively easily in most settings, the presence of chancroid lesions can increase the chances of contracting other STIs, including HIV, gonorrhea, and herpes, by as much as 400 percent (CDC, 2002).

Diagnosis

Chancroid is usually diagnosed by inspecting the affected area. However, given the similarities between chancroid ulcerations and those of other STIs, such as herpes or genital warts, visual diagnosis requires that the health care provider be familiar with the distinct differences between various STIs that may cause genital ulcerations. Infection is confirmed by testing the fluid from a sore by culturing or microscopic examination. Even if a chancroid diagnosis seems obvious, testing for syphilis should be conducted to avoid misdiagnosis and ensure appropriate treatment.

Pelvic Inflammatory Disease (PID)

Aside from AIDS, the most common and most serious complication of sexually transmitted infections among women is *pelvic inflammatory disease*, an infection of the upper genital tract. PID can affect the uterus, ovaries, fallopian tubes, or other related structures. Untreated, PID causes scarring and can lead to infertility, tubal pregnancy, chronic pelvic pain, and other serious consequences (Bortot, Risser, & Cromwell, 2004; U.S. Department of Health and Human Services, 2003).

Each year in the United States, over 1 million women are diagnosed with PID, and the highest incidence is among teenage girls. However, the number of cases among young women may be decreasing, due in part to the increase in STI screening in settings other than STI clinics, such as during regular doctor visits. PID is a major cause of infertility; at least 100,000 women become infertile each year as a result of the condition (Bortot et al., 2004). The risk of infertility as a result of PID is approximately 10 percent following the first episode of PID and rises to more than 50 percent after three or more episodes. PID is also an important causal factor in ectopic (tubal) pregnancies.

PID results when bacteria from the vagina, cervix, or urethra migrate up into the deeper regions of the woman's reproductive tract. Most cases of PID are caused by either chlamydia or gonorrhea bacteria. These bacteria then settle into the uterus, fallopian tubes, and ovaries and continue to multiply, causing inflammation and scarring and sometimes leading to fallopian tube blockage and hence infertility.

Common symptoms include lower abdominal sensitivity and pain, pain during intercourse, irregular periods, cervical discharge and tenderness, fever, nausea, and vomiting. Often these symptoms are not felt until the infection has progressed to a dangerous stage. PID is difficult to diagnose because the symptoms are so similar to those of various other health problems.

Recommended treatment typically consists of the combined administration of two or more antibiotic medications (Bortot et al., 2004). In the past, hospitalization was recommended for all PID cases so that bed rest and intravenous medications could be initiated (DSTDP, 1998). Today, however, hospitalization for PID is rare, indicated only when treatment regimens appear to be failing to treat the symptoms adequately or when intravenous antibiotic treatment is deemed necessary. Follow-up is necessary within 3 days of treatment and then again 4 to 6 weeks after treatment is complete to be sure the infection has been cured. It is also recommended that sexual partners of the diagnosed woman be treated if they had sexual contact with the patient within 60 days of the onset of symptoms (CDC, 2002).

Treatment for Bacterial STIs

Nearly all bacterial STIs are effectively treated with a single course of antibiotic medication. The most commonly used antibiotics for uncomplicated cases of bacterial STIs are *azithromycin* and *doxycycline*, both of which can be taken orally. Other oral antibiotic treatments include *cefixime*, *ceftriaxone*, *ciprofloxacin*, *erythromycin*, *levofloxacin*, *ofloxacin*, and *penicillin*. With the exception of penicillin, which continues to be primarily used to treat syphilis, almost all these medications can be used to treat gonorrhea, chlamydia, and chancroid. Prescribing considerations that should be taken into account by the patient and medical professional include the severity of the infection, the age of the patient, coinfection with other diseases, and pregnancy. All of these antibiotics may be taken orally, over a course of 1 day to 2 weeks. In most cases, the antibiotic will cure the infection, but little may be done to reverse any physical damage to the infected area or scarring due to ulcerations.

Follow-up examination is very important when treating bacterial STIs to ensure that the infection has been cured and that no reinfection has occurred. Women are at risk of becoming reinfected with an STI that was previously treated. A recent study examined the rates of repeat infections among women who tested positive and were treated for chlamydia. Among the women who had a repeat infection, the average time between first infection and repeat infection was a little over 7 months (Burstein et al., 2001). The results of this study and others indicate that a considerable number of patients' sexual partners are not being properly treated, or treated at all, for STIs. Therefore, treatment of all sexual partners of an infected person is of paramount importance, to prevent both reinfection and further spread of the bacterium. What this implies is that taking an antibiotic for a bacterial STI is only part of a complete treatment. Effective treatment also requires notification and treatment of the person's sexual partner or partners and a conscious decision to avoid anonymous or unprotected sexual encounters.

antibiotic-resistant strain A strain of bacteria that has mutated and is no longer treatable with the current antibiotic therapy.

To ensure effective management or cure of STIs, treatment of all sexual partners of an infected person is necessary.

Moreover, some **antibiotic-resistant strains** of bacterial STIs have been diagnosed in recent years. For example, in the early 2000s, 14 percent of all cases of gonorrhea in Hawaii and 0.4 percent on the West Coast of the United States were found to be resistant to usual antibiotic treatment ("Ciprofloxacin-Resistant Gonorrhea," 2002). Moreover, these numbers and locations of resistant gonorrhea are increasing, and cases of other resistant bacterial STIs are beginning to appear. So far, the development of newer antibiotic medications is keeping pace with these new strains of diseases, but researchers fear that one or more STIs may eventually mutate so fast that it becomes extremely difficult or impossible to treat (S. Smith, 2004). Furthermore, as new strains of resistant bacteria appear, doctors may treat the infection using the usual antibiotics, and the patients, assuming the drugs will cure the disease, will instead continue to be infected and potentially increase the rate of spread.

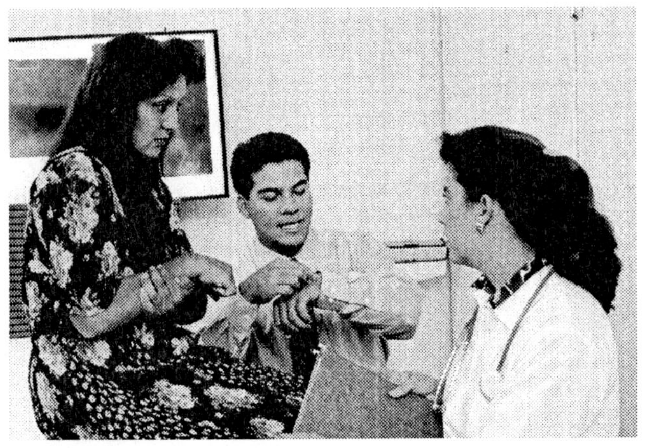

Parasitic STIs: Sexually Transmitted Bugs?

A *parasite* is an organism that attaches itself to a host and uses the host's resources to survive. A common example of a parasite in botany is mistletoe, which spreads through various species of trees and if left unchecked may eventually kill the host. In animals, an all-too-familiar parasite is the common flea. You are aware that some parasites found in food can cause serious illnesses in humans. In the same fashion, some sexually transmitted infections are caused by parasites. Three of these are trichomoniasis, pubic lice, and scabies.

Trichomoniasis

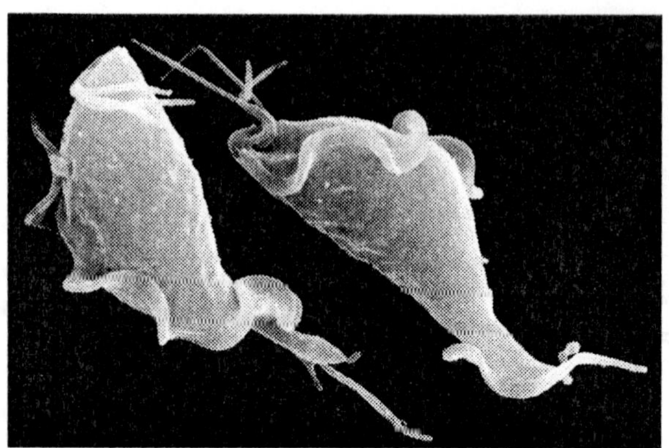

FIGURE 8.13 Trichomoniasis Parasite Trichomoniasis is caused by this microscopic protozoan parasite, *Trichomonas vaginalis*.

Trichomoniasis, also known as "trich," is caused by a protozoan parasitic organism called *Trichomonas vaginalis* or *T. vaginalis* (see Figure 8.13). *T. vaginalis* is the most common nonbacterial, nonviral STI, and it accounts for one-third of all STI diagnoses in the United States each year, or about 5 million cases ("Treatment Options," 2004). Estimates are that approximately 170 million people worldwide are infected with the *T. vaginalis* parasite and that one in four will be infected at some point in their lifetime (Tucker, 2003). Most men who contract trichomoniasis have no symptoms, but they are contagious and can pass the infection on to their sexual partners. If men do experience symptoms, they are usually irritation of the urethra, a slight discharge, and pain after urination or ejaculation. Among women, common symptoms include a yellow or greenish vaginal discharge accompanied by an unpleasant odor, genital irritation, and pain upon urination. Some women may have very mild symptoms or no symptoms at all. Transmission of *T. vaginalis* is almost exclusively through sexual contact. Without proper treatment, trichomoniasis may cause PID among women and NGU among men.

Trichomoniasis can usually be treated effectively with a single dose of *metronidazole* (brand name, Flagyl), an antibacterial, antibiotic-like drug taken orally. Due to a significant risk of reinfection, all sexual partners of an infected person should be treated for the infection (DSTDP, 1998). Metronidazole is not recommended for pregnant or nursing women. A follow-up visit is not typically necessary; however, if symptoms persist, a higher dose of the same medication is usually prescribed.

Pubic Lice

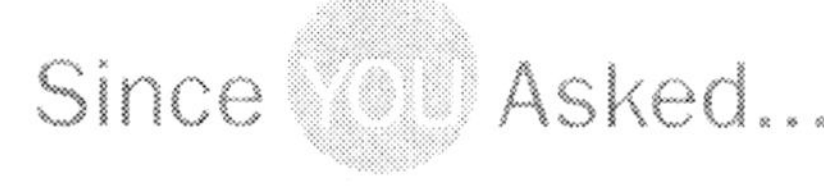

11. What are crabs, and how can I tell if someone has them?

This is an STI that almost no one really wants to hear about. **Pubic lice** are tiny buglike parasites that are visible to the unaided eye, often referred to as "crabs" because they look somewhat like the crustaceans. Pubic lice are *not* the same as head lice, which commonly occur among children of school age.

Estimates of how many people are affected by public lice are difficult because treatments are readily available without a prescription. However, sales of those treatments indicate more than 3 million cases a year in the United States (Billstein, 1999).

Pubic lice live on the blood of their host in the moist, warm areas of the genitals, anus, and abdomen (see Figure 8.14). They invade the pubic area and live among the pubic hair. They can survive up to 30 days on a host or 24 hours without a host. Adult pubic lice are about the size of a sesame seed and can be seen with the naked eye. Lice's only goal in life appears to be to procreate, because once they reach adulthood, they mate until they die. The female louse lays about four eggs a day, attaching them with a sticky fluid to the base of the pubic hairs. These eggs hatch in 5 to 10 days. Even away from the host, public lice can survive on clothing, sheets, or towels and continue to multiply.

trichomoniasis A common sexually transmitted protozoan parasite causing symptoms in women, including genital irritation, painful urination, and a foul-smelling vaginal discharge; infected men are typically asymptomatic, yet contagious.

pubic lice Small buglike parasites, usually sexually transmitted, that infest the genital area causing extreme itching; often referred to as "crabs," because of their resemblance to a sea crab.

The most obvious symptom of lice infestation is irritation and extreme itching, often said to be the most intense itching imaginable. The itching is a result of the lice biting the skin to feed on the host's blood and attaching themselves to the shaft of the pubic hairs. When an infested person scratches, it irritates the skin and creates further opportunities for the lice to feed and spread.

Pubic lice are diagnosed by visual inspection. A skilled examiner will be able to see the adult lice and maybe even the eggs. The lice may also look like scabs from scratching, but when they are removed and placed under a microscope, the "scabs" may actually scamper away!

Pubic lice and their eggs are difficult to remove completely. Pubic lice are typically treated with prescription and nonprescription shampoos, creams, and ointments (with brand names such as Elimite or Kwell) containing chemicals that are toxic to the lice. Following treatment, the pubic hair should be combed with a special fine-mesh comb to remove any remaining eggs, or the pubic hair may be completely shaved. Typically, one treatment is insufficient to rid the body of all lice, and a follow-up treatment a week later is recommended to be sure any newly hatched lice are killed. In addition, all clothing, towels, bedding, and other materials that may have come in contact with the lice should be washed in hot water or sprayed with special medicated spray and sealed in plastic bags for 2 weeks (AllRefer.com, 2003b).

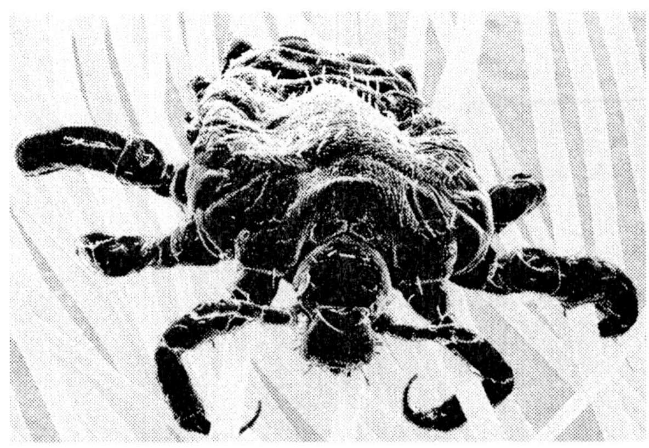

FIGURE 8.14 Pubic Lice Infestation
Pubic lice infest the genital area and lay eggs at the base of the pubic hairs. This is a highly magnified photograph of a pubic louse attached to pubic hairs.

Scabies

Scabies, also known as *Sarcoptes scabiei* or "itch mites," are tiny parasitic mites. Scabies mites are not visible to the naked eye. They infest the host by attaching themselves to the hair shaft and burrowing under the skin on the hands, feet, and genitals, where females lay approximately three eggs daily (see Figure 8.15). Scabies are transmitted through direct skin-to-skin contact, including, but not limited to, sexual activity (Wendel & Rompalo, 2002). Scabies mites have a body structure that enables them to burrow easily into the skin and makes them difficult to remove without medical assistance. They belong to the same class of insects as spiders, ticks, and chiggers, but they most closely resemble the dust mite (Platts-Mills & Rein, 1999).

Scabies infestation is diagnosed visually by examining the burrows underneath the skin or by examining the infested skin, lesions, or sores. Scabies are successfully treated with prescription lotions (*permethrin*, *lindane*, or *crotamiton*) applied to all the areas of the body from the neck down and washed off after 8 hours (CDC, 2002). As with pubic lice, all bedding and clothing must be decontaminated, washed, and dried at high temperatures. Symptoms may take several weeks to resolve fully, and some experts suggest retreatment within a week of the initial treatment. Treatment is suggested for all persons who came in close contact, sexual or otherwise, with the infested person within 30 days of the infection.

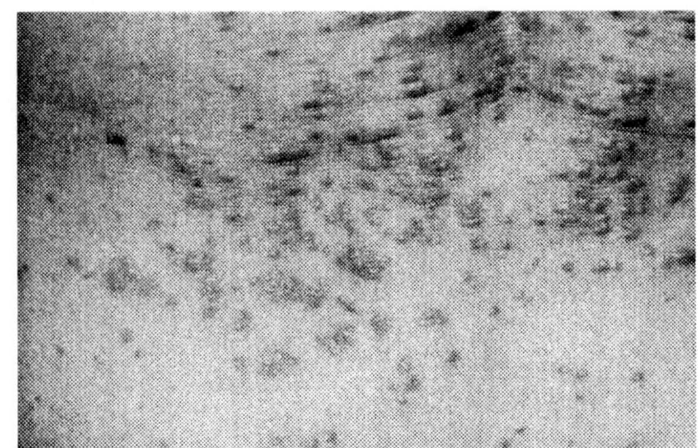

FIGURE 8.15 Scabies Infestation
Scabies are parasites that burrow under the skin anywhere on the body. The lice themselves cannot be seen without magnification, but their burrows and the irritation from scratching is shown here.

Preventing STIs

Throughout this chapter, we have talked about the various behaviors that transmit STIs. With the exception of coercive situations, such as rape, your STI risks are determined by your individual *choices* of behaviors. To sum up prevention strategies, we must return to the five major risk categories discussed at the beginning of this chapter and examine how you can reduce or eliminate each of them. As you may recall, the five risk categories are lack of accurate information, negative emotions and faulty beliefs, poor sexual communication, substance abuse, and risky sexual activities.

Since YOU Asked ...

12. Once I start having sex, how can I be sure to never catch an STI?

scabies Microscopic parasitic mites, often sexually transmitted, that burrow under the skin on the hands, feet, and genitals and cause extreme itching.

Obtaining Accurate Information about STIs

As we noted at the beginning of our discussion of STIs, the research evidence is clear: People who are effectively and appropriately educated and informed about the causes, symptoms, routes of transmission, and treatment options for all STIs are *far* more likely to make healthy sexual decisions (Ross & Williams, 2002).

As Table 8.2 makes abundantly clear, most sexual behaviors that involve physical contact with a partner carry at least some risk of STI transmission. Therefore, each person must make an educated and thoughtful assessment of the amount of risk he or she is willing to take when choosing to be sexually active. This is referred to as a person's level of **acceptable risk**. In this sense, sexual behavior is no different from other health-related behaviors that we all make choices about, based on what we perceive to be an acceptable risk. For example, some people smoke cigarettes, eat a high-fat diet, or fail to wear a seat belt, even though they know these behaviors are clear risks to their health. For them, however, these are acceptable risks; otherwise, in theory, they would not take those actions. Sexual behavior should be based on a similar principle. Like it or not, sex is a *health behavior*, and each person's level of acceptable risk should determine what sexual activities the person chooses or chooses not to engage in relative to STIs (this concept also relates to other sexual decisions such as birth control and pregnancy).

Here is the most important point about acceptable risk: No one can intelligently determine one's acceptable risk without knowing what all the risks are! Now that you have read this chapter, you are better equipped to make decisions about your sexual behaviors, based on your level of acceptable risk, but it doesn't end here. You have a responsibility to *stay* informed and educated about sexual risks throughout your life.

A thorough understanding of the symptoms, modes of transmission, diagnosis, and treatment of all STIs is crucial for individuals and couples to determine their acceptable risk levels and make effective choices about their sexual behavior. The key here is that the knowledge be as accurate as possible and not based on myths, such as those exposed in Table 8.1. Some individuals and couples are able to obtain solid factual information about STIs on their own, through reading, researching, and talking to knowledgeable professionals such as counselors, sexuality educators, and physicians. A perhaps more far-reaching source for this information is high-quality, effective sex education in school and college classes.

The solution does not lie in merely *offering* sex education to young people, however. Research has shown that even among teens who receive STI education in school or from parents, their *working knowledge* of sexual risks remains poor (Clark, Jackson, & Allen-Taylor, 2002). When teens were asked about their sex education history, 97 percent said they had received specific education about STIs. Most of the participants knew that HIV is a serious STI, but only 2 percent could name all eight major STIs (HIV, gonorrhea, syphilis, herpes, chlamydia, hepatitis B, trichomoniasis, and genital warts), 9 percent could name the four curable bacterial infections, and 3 percent could name the four viral incurable infections. The study suggested that STI education efforts may be spending a disproportionate amount of time and resources on HIV education at the expense of other STIs that are much more common among young people.

Overcoming Unhealthy Emotions about Sex

As people become educated and knowledgeable about human sexuality in general and about STIs specifically, the negative STI emotions discussed earlier in this chapter (shame, guilt, fear of stigma, embarrassment) all tend to decrease. The reduction in these emotions opens the door for better communication between partners, greater comfort with their own and each other's bodies, greater awareness of the symptoms of

acceptable risk The level of risk one is willing to accept when making behavioral choices about one's health and well-being.

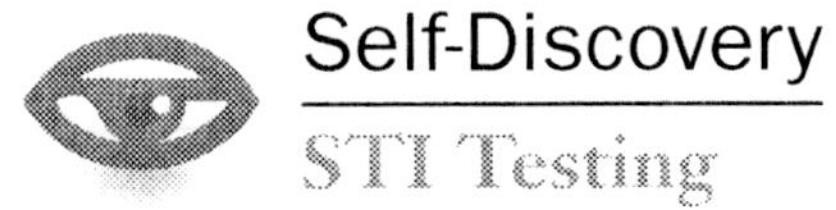

Self-Discovery

STI Testing

No one likes to think that he or she will be at risk for an STI. The reality is, however, that most sexually active people will at some time in their lives come in contact with a sexual partner who is or was infected with an STI. For this reason, it is important to practice safer sex, such as consistent condom use, as well as to consider STI testing part of your preventive health care.

Currently, STI testing is usually not a standard preventive medical practice. In fact, most physicians do not routinely test for STIs during annual or biannual health visits. If you want to be tested for STIs, you usually have to ask, which in itself can be an uncomfortable experience. However, the stigma of being tested for STIs is disappearing, and doing so is now often seen as a smart move.

When STIs are diagnosed and treated early, their transmission and potential negative side effects can usually be reduced or prevented. You may feel uncomfortable requesting STI testing, but it's your health, and unless you take charge, you may not get this important health care service. You can be your own best health advocate, so consider the following the next time you're scheduling a health exam.

1. ____**Am I comfortable talking about my sexual health with my health care provider?** The experience of STI testing can be easier when your health care provider is someone with whom you feel comfortable discussing your sexual history and activities. This is particularly important if one is diagnosed with an STI such as herpes or HIV that requires long-term management.
2. ____**Have I requested STI testing?** Because STI testing is usually not a standard health care practice, you must request it. Avoid assuming you are not infected with an STI if your health care provider does not identify an infection or recommend STI testing.
3. ____**Should I consider being tested for STIs routinely during my annual health exams?** Because STIs can have few or no observable symptoms, if you are sexually active, routine testing during annual health exams may identify an unknown infection. Annual testing is not considered an STI *prevention* method but may allow an STI to be identified and treated in its earliest stages.
4. ____**Has my partner been tested? Can we both be tested at the same time?** It is often not enough for one person in the relationship to be tested for STIs. The results of one partner do not necessarily apply to the other partner. Being tested with your partner and being sexually faithful are signs of mutual caring and among the safest sexual practices of all.

STIs, greater willingness to seek medical attention for possible infection, less discomfort with STI testing (see "Self-Discovery: STI Testing"), and an enhanced ability to make intelligent choices about living a healthy sexual life. We all have the responsibility to take charge of our sexual lives and assert our needs, desires, and rights as sexual people. The negative emotions discussed here undermine that goal. Those who are unable, for whatever reason, to face and overcome negative sexual feelings may end up—literally—risking their lives.

Communicating Effectively about Sex

Many people fail to realize that effective sexual communication is an important *safe sex behavior*. The ability to communicate openly and honestly is key to avoiding contracting or transmitting all of the STIs we have discussed in this chapter. The topics of communication that relate directly to STI prevention include issues such as number of previous sexual partners, past or current STI infections, and agreements to use condoms or to avoid specific risky sexual behaviors. Disclosing infection with an incurable STI to a partner can be the most difficult communication challenge of all. "In Touch with Your Sexual Health: Disclosing an STI Infection to a Sexual Partner" discusses the importance of disclosure and offers some tips for feeling less uncomfortable.

Discussing these issues does not come easily to most people, and many avoid it out of embarrassment, fear of rejection, or assumptions about their risks of contracting or transmitting STIs. One study of college students found that although 99 percent felt knowledgeable about safe sex practices, only 77 percent considered disclosure of past

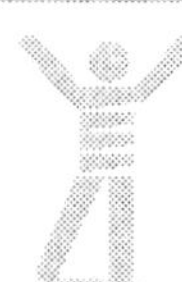

In Touch with Your Sexual Health

Disclosing an STI to a Sexual Partner

Discovering you are infected with an STI, especially one that has no cure, can be devastating. It can shake your trust in others and in yourself. However, in addition to obtaining as much information as possible on the infection and seeking out the best treatments available, you also have to prepare yourself for disclosing your status to current or potential sexual partners. Informing a sexual partner of your STI status is an ethical and potentially a legal responsibility.

If you have a steady partner at the time of your diagnosis, you should not assume that he or she intentionally infected you with the STI. As you know from your reading of this chapter, many people who are infected are unaware of it because they have never had symptoms or they mistakenly assume they have been cured. Moreover, you may have been infected *prior* to your current relationship. If so, you may have transmitted it to your partner, rather than the other way around. From a personal health perspective, the issue of who infected whom is secondary to the immediate need for screening and treatment for your sexual partner or partners.

So what is the best way to break the news to your partner? This is so individual, it's difficult to make one overall recommendation. However, here are a few suggestions that may help.

Be Honest with Yourself

It's easy to get treated for an STI, especially one that is curable, and forget that it ever happened or to have genital warts removed or wait until herpes blisters heal and hope (mistakenly) that you then have no chance of spreading the infection. However, once you accept that you have or have had an STI, breaking the news to your partner will be easier.

Say It, Don't "Show It"

Often people are too scared or embarrassed to tell their partner about the infection, so they attempt to make the partner figure it out. Some indirect strategies people use to disclose STI status include leaving STI pamphlets around, testing the partner's reaction by telling stories about "other people," or suggesting that they both be tested together (that way someone else can tell the partner). However, using a direct, honest approach, talking or perhaps writing a personal note (and then following up with a discussion; an e-mail would probably be too impersonal!), is likely to be a more effective way of initiating a discussion about these health issues, ensuring effective treatment for both partners, and preserving the closeness and trust of the relationship.

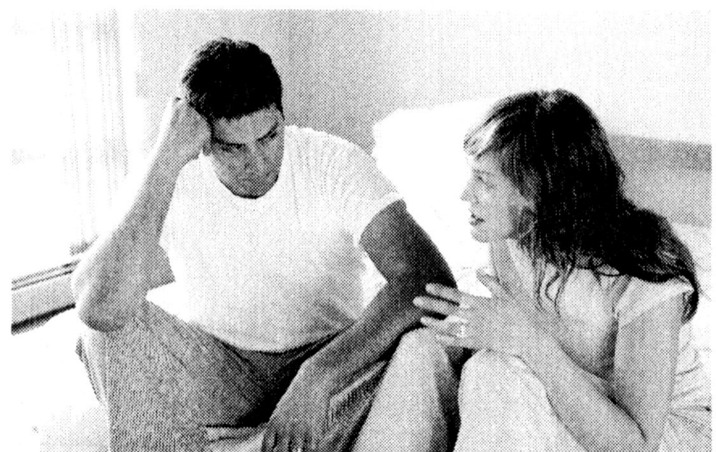

Avoid the Blame Game

As mentioned earlier, wasting energy on determining who gave the STI to whom can be destructive and may not be in the best interest of your relationship. When people are blamed for something that they may or may not be responsible for, they become defensive. Most people would never intentionally set out to infect another with an STI. When transmission does occur, it is often because the infected person is unaware of having been infected or did not fully understand the risk of transmitting the infection to others.

Telling a partner that you have an STI is never easy. The goal of sharing positive (or negative) STI test results leads to a responsible course of action that will include treatment and prevention strategies for the future. By being honest with yourself, talking directly about your infection status, and encouraging your partner to get immediate testing and treatment, you and your partner can move past the diagnosis and focus on developing the positive aspects of your relationship.

or current STI infections a safe sex practice, only 58 percent regarded disclosure of the number of previous sex partners as a safe sex practice, and 37 percent did not feel that disclosure of the number of partners should be a requirement prior to becoming sexual with a new partner (Lucchetti, 1999). Moreover, the same study found that over 30 percent of students had *actively avoided* such discussion with at least one sexual partner, and over 20 percent admitted to misrepresenting their prior sexual history to their new sexual partners.

Your ability to communicate and make agreements with a sexual partner or potential partner about the risks of STIs relies in part on successfully navigating the two skills discussed previously: becoming knowledgeable about STIs and overcoming negative emotions about them. Both of these skills allow you to obtain clarity in your own mind, which in turn smooths the way for communicating about these issues with a potential partner. Here are some general tips that often help people add communication to their arsenal of STI prevention strategies (Office of Health Education and Wellness, 2003):

- Become as educated and knowledgeable as you can about the symptoms, causes, and treatments of all STIs.
- Do not allow embarrassment, guilt, shame, or fear stop you from protecting your health and your life. If you need to, practice with a friend, make notes, rehearse.
- Do *not* wait until you are sexually intimate to start communicating.
- Think about what you want to say, and how you will say it, ahead of time.
- Be clear about your limits, and decide what you are comfortable doing sexually.
- Keep your sense of humor, and avoid becoming overly serious, but don't avoid saying what you need to say.
- Be flexible about when you will talk. Find a private, quiet, nonsexual setting when you have plenty of time so you won't feel rushed.
- Communicate with your partner honestly, so that you can both make clear, informed choices.
- Give your partner time to think about what you have said, and listen carefully to his or her responses.
- Decide *in advance* what you both feel comfortable doing sexually, based on all the information you have communicated, and stick to your agreements.
- Never allow yourself to be seduced, cajoled, persuaded, or coerced into agreeing to behaviors that you feel are too risky or make you uncomfortable.
- If you and your partner cannot agree to respect each other's level of acceptable sexual risk, you may need to reevaluate your relationship.

Avoiding Mixing Sex and Substance Abuse

The best-laid plans for sexual communication, however, often go away when people's ability to communicate and make rational decisions is compromised by alcohol or other drug use. Research has left little doubt that in terms of STIs, drugs and sex simply do not mix. Drugs, especially alcohol and marijuana, often accompany sexual interactions. In college and university settings, they nearly *always* occur together. However, as noted early in this chapter, this is a dangerous and potentially deadly mix. No matter how educated and informed a person may be, regardless of that person's level of comfort with sexual issues, and notwithstanding that person's ability when sober to communicate about sex with a partner, alcohol or other drug use may lead to poor sexual choices and the spread of STIs. It is interesting to note that efforts in the United States to

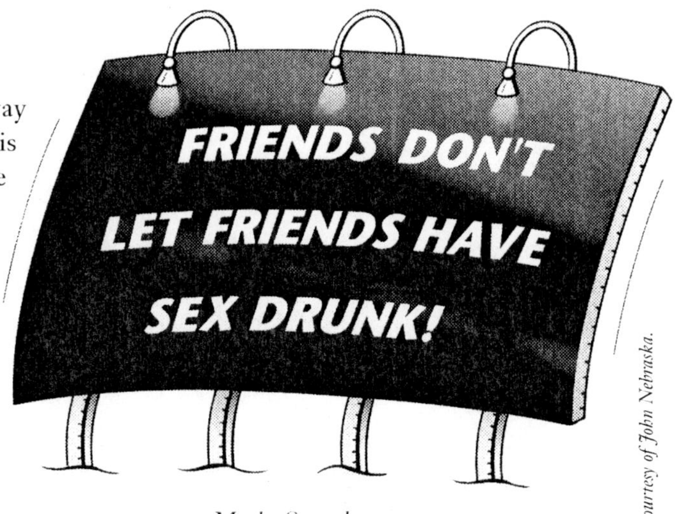

Maybe Someday . . .

Courtesy of John Nebraska.

stop people from drinking and driving ("Friends don't let friends drive drunk") have found significantly greater support than similar campaigns to reduce the dangers of mixing alcohol and sex. Yet the connection is equally strong. Perhaps one day, billboards and TV ads will read, "Friends don't let friends have sex drunk." Of course, a "designated sex partner" program is unrealistic, but perhaps, people will get the message nevertheless.

Refraining from Risky Sexual Behaviors

You already know that the absolute best method for avoiding STIs is abstinence. However, the reaction of most college students to the suggestion of abstinence is along the lines of "Yeah, right." Indeed, as you can see in Chapter 6, "Sexual Behaviors," the vast majority of college students choose to be sexually active, and a great deal of research shows that teaching "abstinence only" is a *very ineffective* way of reducing unsafe sexual practices (J. Brody, 2004; Sparks, 2005). However, abstinence must be part of any STI prevention discussion, if for no other reason that it is, obviously, the *most* effective means of avoiding STIs.

Sex is more than intercourse 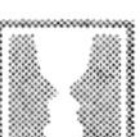

Having said that, however, not everyone interprets abstinence in the same way. To some people, it implies no sex of any sort, a concept closer to **celibacy**. To others, abstinence is the process of picking and choosing which sexual behaviors a person is willing to engage in, either alone or with a partner, in order to enjoy sexual feelings and activities while avoiding exposure to infections or pregnancy. From your reading of this chapter and looking at Table 8.2, you may be thinking, "That's great, but what safe sexual behaviors are left?" Well, there are many; you just have to be smart and, sometimes, *creative*! Here are some suggestions from various sexuality educators on how to have sexually intimate relationships while minimizing your risks for STIs.

First, limit your *number* of sexual partners. The more sexual partners a person has, the greater the chances of contracting an STI no matter how careful the person may be in practicing safer sex practices.

Second, get to know a potential sexual partner before initiating a sexual relationship. If more couples would do this, many STI risks could be avoided. This point relates to our earlier discussion about sexual communication. As difficult as clear, honest sexual communication may be, it becomes increasingly easier as two people become emotionally closer. Making psychological intimacy a higher priority than sexual intimacy is a very effective safer sex strategy.

Third, ensure that you and your potential sexual partner are free of STIs. This means agreeing to be tested *prior* to engaging in any risky sexual behavior together. For many people, that means waiting 6 months from their last sexual encounter before being tested so that the presence of all STIs, including HIV, is reasonably sure to be detected. Six months is a long time for many couples to postpone their sexual involvement, especially at the beginning of a new relationship when excitement is running high. However, the sexual side of the relationship does not have to be put completely on hold, as will be explained next.

Fourth, practice safe sexual behaviors, often referred to as **selective abstinence** or "outercourse" (detailed in Chapter 6). If a couple are clear about their intentions to be safe and wait until they can both be tested, they may still engage in intimate, low- or no-risk *noninsertive* sexual activities such as kissing, hugging, massaging, body exploration through touch, rubbing genitals together clothed, mutual genital touching, and mutual masturbation. These activities can be extremely exciting and allow the couple to get to know each other's bodies and responses. Then, when their tests come

celibacy Engaging in no sexual activities whatsoever.

selective abstinence Choosing to engage in or avoid certain sexual behaviors on the basis of their risks of STIs or pregnancy.

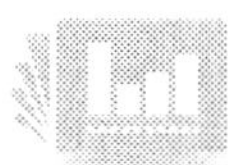

Evaluating Sexual Research

The Condom Effectiveness Controversy

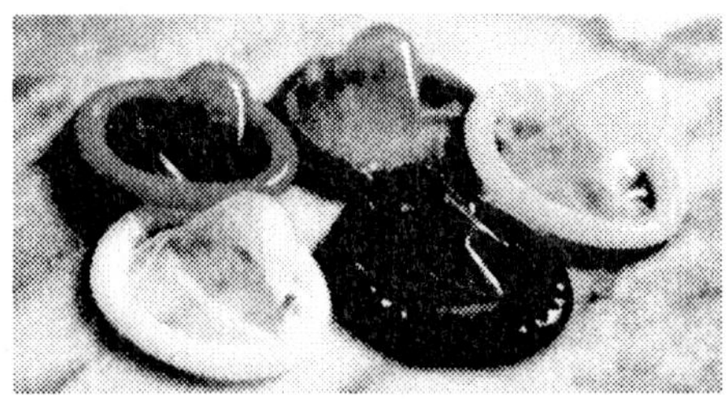

Condoms have been available for over a century, with the first condom dating back to the late 1800s. Condoms were initially marketed for people who were having sex with prostitutes. It was not until much later that condoms were considered a viable pregnancy prevention method. Over the decades, condoms have continued to be an effective contraceptive method, and STI prevention was secondary. However, the rise of HIV in the early 1980s changed the way we perceived the utility of condoms, and their use became the single most effective method of preventing STI and HIV transmission among sexually active people.

The increasing rates of HIV, combined with evidence that condoms are an effective means of preventing the exchange of bodily fluids, influenced the prevention messages given to populations at high risk of contracting STIs. HIV also fueled the safer sex approach to prevention that encouraged condom use as the most viable prevention method, second only to abstinence.

Throughout the HIV epidemic, individuals and groups opposed to the safer sex message (preferring the teaching of abstinence only) pointed to the limitations of condom use in preventing HIV, such as, breakage, slippage, and punctures. However, such limitations were and continue to be due primarily to *human error*, not faulty condoms. And the minuscule number of condom failures represent a *much* smaller risk than the failure to use condoms at all.

Today, many groups who support abstinence-only prevention programs, including the Catholic church, are spreading erroneous information that condoms do not prevent STIs and that promoting condoms for safer sex encourages unsafe sex practices and gives people a false sense of security. It is true that some STIs, such as genital warts or syphilis, may be transmitted even when a condom is used correctly, depending on where the warts or chancre is located. Thus the condom's effectiveness in preventing infection sometimes depends on which STI is being prevented and the physical location of the symptoms. However, the effectiveness of condoms in reducing the risk of STI transmission is indisputable based on all the scientific evidence. Claims that HIV and other viruses may pass through the latex in the condom are absolutely false. Some groups have even gone so far as to claim that condoms are the *cause* of people dying from HIV (Kruger, 2003). This is simply and blatantly untrue.

Although no one has ever claimed that condoms are 100 percent effective at preventing HIV or other STIs, they are *far* more effective than unprotected sexual activities. Therefore, unless a strategy can be found to stop all unsafe sexual activity worldwide, referred to as "universal abstinence" (a goal that is clearly impossible), the importance of condom use must continue to be stressed as a crucial part of STI prevention.

back negative (which is likely), they will be (very!) ready for further sexual exploration together. If one or both test positive for one or more STIs, they will then probably feel close and intimate enough to make rational decisions about further sexual activity and their acceptable levels of risk.

Finally, use safer sex practices. If a couple choose to engage in insertive sexual behavior without waiting and testing, they must try to be as safe as possible. This includes all of the issues we have discussed in this section: education, emotions, communication, substance abuse, and testing. However, the first line of defense against most STIs, in most real-world settings, is the use of male condoms for vaginal, anal, and oral sexual activities. You will notice that I use the word *safer*, not *safe*. As discussed in "Evaluating Sexual Research: The Condom Effectiveness Controversy," condoms are not 100 percent effective in preventing any STI, but the risks are significantly lower with consistent and correct condom use.

Remember, when you look at your sexual choices from the perspective that sex is a *health behavior*, you will find it easier to understand the cause-and-effect relationships between your sexual decisions and their potential consequences.

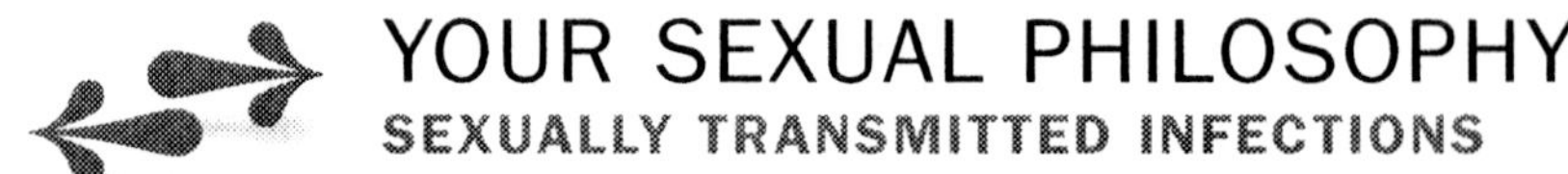

YOUR SEXUAL PHILOSOPHY
SEXUALLY TRANSMITTED INFECTIONS

From our earliest stirrings of sexual feelings in puberty, we often make the misguided and potentially dangerous assumption that sex will just "take care of itself." We plan for college, we plan a major, we plan a career, we may even plan ahead for marriage, but too often we fail to plan for life as a sexual being. Then, when we are faced with sexual decisions, sexual situations, sexual pressures, or the heat of sexual moments, instead of being in control of those situations, we allow them to take control of us. The result: poor sexual choices, including an increased likelihood of exposure to STIs.

The information in this chapter is essential to an effective sexual philosophy. Combining accurate information and education with carefully considered attitudes and goals will help you know who you are, know what you want and don't want, and *plan ahead.* Although it is true that sometimes the best-laid plans go awry, a strong personal sexual philosophy serves as the best foundation for a healthy, disease-free sexual life.

The goal of this chapter was not to frighten you away from sexual intimacy altogether. On the contrary, the objective has been to provide you with a solid base of knowledge about sexually transmitted infections: what they are, their symptoms (or lack thereof), how they are transmitted, how they are diagnosed, and available treatment options. When you incorporate the information in this chapter into your sexual philosophy, you will help to *enhance* sex and intimacy in your life by making decisions and choices that provide a satisfying and healthy sexual life. With this knowledge, you will be able to be part of the solution to stopping the spread of STIs, rather than another STI statistic.

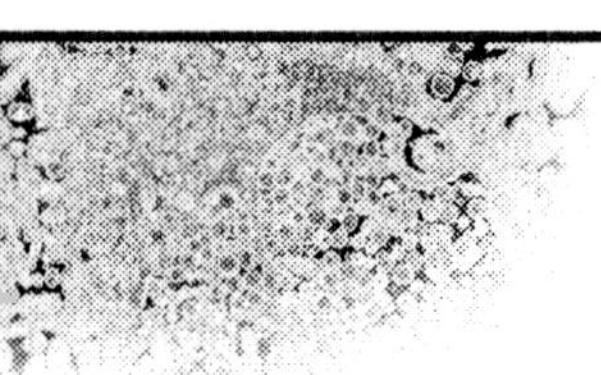

Summary

HISTORICAL PERSPECTIVES The Tuskegee Syphilis Study

- In the 1930s, in Tuskegee, Mississippi, doctors hid the diagnosis and denied treatment to a group of black men with syphilis in order to study the long-term effects of the disease. The study was publicly revealed in the 1970s, and President Clinton in 1997 issued a national apology to the victims and their families.
- The racist aspects of the Tuskegee syphilis study still have repercussions today, as many minorities continue to mistrust the U.S. medical system.

The STI Epidemic

- Approximately 25 percent of the population of the United States will contract an STI at some point in life, and an estimated 15 million people are infected with an STI each year. Sexually active people between the ages of 15 and 30 are at greatest risk of contracting STIs.
- Gonorrhea, chlamydia, and the human papillomavirus (HPV), which causes genital warts, are the most common agents causing STIs among teens and young adults.

Risk Factors for STIs

- STIs are among the most common illnesses throughout the world. Many STIs may have no obvious symptoms and may go undiagnosed and untreated, allowing them to spread more widely.
- Lack of education, negative emotions about sex, poor communication, substance abuse, and risky sexual activities all contribute to the current worldwide STI epidemic.

Specific Sexually Transmitted Infections

- STIs may be categorized according to the type of microbe causing the infection.

Viral STIs

- STIs that are caused by viruses currently have no cure. (This is true of virtually all viruses.)
- Millions of people in the United States are infected with viral STIs. The most common of these are herpes, hepatitis B, and the human papilloma virus.

- HIV, the virus that causes AIDS, has caused a global pandemic, with an estimated 40 million individuals infected worldwide. In the United States, at least 40,000 new cases are reported each year.
- No cure for HIV or AIDS exists. A recent increase in new HIV cases may reflect "safe sex fatigue" stemming from the mistaken belief that new HIV treatments and medications, which are often effective in treating symptoms, actually cure AIDS.
- A simple oral saliva test is now available for HIV, and researchers are working around the clock to find an effective HIV vaccine, which still appears many years away from becoming a reality.

Bacterial STIs

- Although most bacterial STIs are readily cured with antibiotics, when they are asymptomatic and untreated, they can lead to more serious conditions of the reproductive tract, including infertility.
- Virtually all bacterial STIs are spread primarily through unprotected oral, vaginal, or anal sexual activities. Bacterial STIs include chlamydia, gonorrhea, syphilis, and chancroid.

Parasitic STIs: Sexually Transmitted Bugs?

- Parasitic STIs are caused by organisms that attach to and feed off of the human body. The most common of these are trichomoniasis, pubic lice, and scabies. The main symptom of sexually transmitted parasites is usually intense itching. These infections are relatively easy to treat and cure.

Preventing STIs

- Prevention is always preferable to curing STIs. This is true of any infection or disease.
- Strategies for preventing STIs include education about their causes, symptoms, and treatments; overcoming negative sexual feelings that often interfere with treatment; effective communication between partners to help avoid transmission; resisting the use of mind-altering substances that cloud judgment and may lead to unsafe sexual practices; and engaging in safer sexual activities.

YOUR SEXUAL PHILOSOPHY: Sexually Transmitted Infections

- Incorporating an accurate and working knowledge of STIs into your sexual philosophy is the very best way for you to stay safe and help others to avoid contracting or transmitting one of these infections. In terms of sexual health, this may be the most important area for accurate information in a person's sexual philosophy of life.

Have You Considered?

1. Imagine that you are the public health director of a major city. You have been hired to stem the STI epidemic in the city. Explain three strategies you feel would be most effective in reaching your goal (and keeping your job) and how you might go about implementing them.
2. Do you think sex education should be part of the curriculum in junior high and high schools? Why or why not? If a school system decided to add sex education to its standard curriculum for high schools, how would such a program be implemented in light of many parents' objections to such teaching?
3. Suppose for a moment that you are a parent of a 14-year-old daughter. She has a boyfriend, and although she hasn't said anything specific to you, you suspect she may be on the verge of becoming sexually active. What would be the three most important pieces of advice and information you would want to be sure to communicate to her about STIs? Discuss how you might approach the subject with her.
4. Summarize the link between HPV and cervical cancer and what women should do to prevent cervical cancer.
5. Discuss why a diagnosis of HIV is no longer considered a death sentence in the United States.
6. Imagine that you meet someone you really like and you begin to date. As the relationship progresses, you become closer and more intimate, but the relationship still has not progressed beyond the kissing and touching stage. Your feelings for each other are deepening, and you know you are falling in love. Then one night, this person sits you down for a serious talk and discloses to you, very gently and lovingly, that he or she is HIV-positive. What do you think your reaction would be? Would you continue seeing the person? Why or why not?
7. Discuss three reasons sexually active people should be tested for STIs regardless of any obvious symptoms.
8. For most college and university students, alcohol and sexual activity are usually connected. This is a often a dangerous mix. Explain why alcohol increases the risk of STI transmission and how colleges and universities might reduce alcohol use in potential sexual situations.

Companion Website Resources

For further chapter resources go to **www.prenhall.com/hock**. This robust text website includes polling questions for you to vote on, regular news updates, quizzes, sample tests, suggested reading lists, and more.

SCENARIOS USA Also on the website are links to videos. *Scenarios USA*'s films portray real-life narratives that explore the non-biological aspects of relationships and sexual health. The films will help you consider how the themes of the text affect your own life and the lives of those around you.

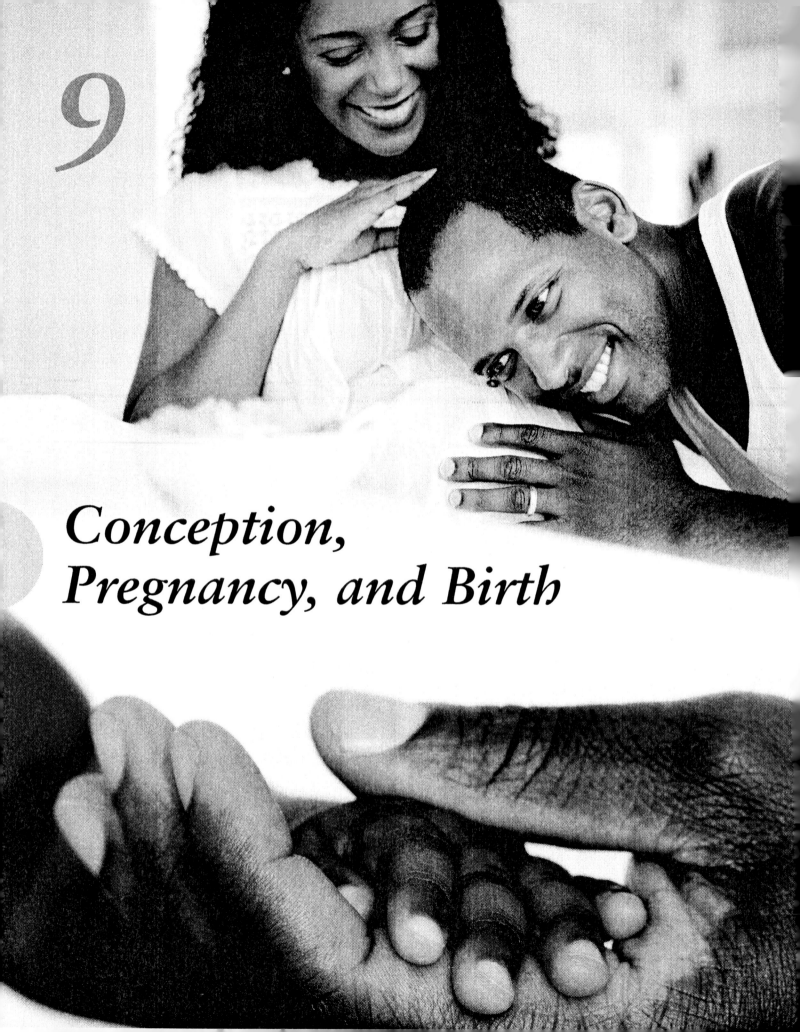

9

Conception, Pregnancy, and Birth

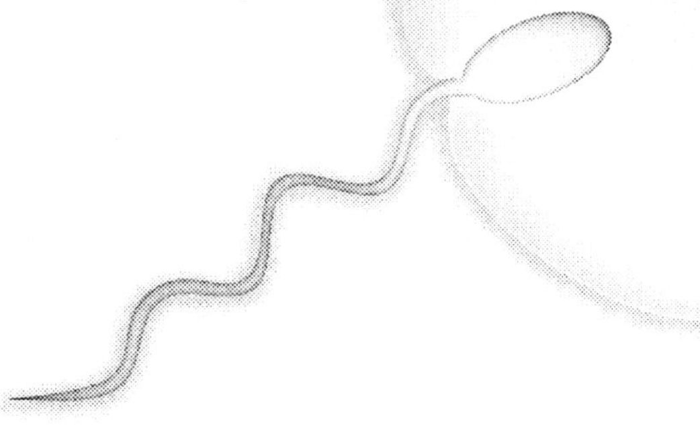

HISTORICAL PERSPECTIVES
The Pain of Giving Birth

DECIDING WHETHER OR NOT TO HAVE A CHILD
Choosing *Not* to Have a Child

Self-Discovery: Are You Ready to Be a Parent?

Influence of the Child's Sex

Sexuality, Ethics, and the Law: Sex Preselection Technology

CONCEPTION
Ovulation: The Ovum's Journey
The Sperm's Journey
The Ovum-Sperm Rendezvous

PREGNANCY
First Trimester
Second Trimester
Third Trimester

POTENTIAL PROBLEMS IN PREGNANCY
Ectopic Pregnancy
Miscarriage
Preterm Birth
Fetal Abnormalities (Birth Defects)
Teratogens
Embryonic and Fetal Testing

ABORTION
Abortion Procedures

Sexuality, Ethics, and the Law: The Abortion Controversy

The Psychological and Emotional Experience of Abortion
Reducing the Number of Abortions

Sexuality and Culture: Russia's Legacy of Abortion

BIRTH
Labor
Choices and Decisions in Childbirth

POSTPARTUM ISSUES
Postpartum Depression

Self-Discovery: A Postpartum Depression Checklist

Sexual Activities after Childbirth
Return of the Fertility Cycle

IMPAIRED FERTILITY
Scope of the Infertility Problem
Causes of Impaired Fertility
Fertility Testing
Solutions to Impaired Fertility

ADOPTION

YOUR SEXUAL PHILOSOPHY

Since YOU Asked...

1. My older sister (she's 28) really wants to get pregnant, but her husband is saying he's not ready. Is there any way she can convince him to agree? (see page 326)

2. I feel that I really do not want to have children ever! Does that make me totally weird? (see page 326)

3. After a woman's period, how soon is the next egg released, and when is she most fertile? (see page 331)

4. Last week, I took two pregnancy tests that were both negative. But I still haven't started my period. Could I be pregnant? (see page 334)

5. A few months ago, I started my period very late and had a lot of blood and very bad cramps (worse than usual). My friend said it was probably a miscarriage. Is that possible? (see page 338)

6. My aunt's baby was born after only 25 weeks of her being pregnant. The baby is probably going to be OK, but will the baby have any problems later on? (see page 340)

7. I heard that there's a pill a woman can take to have an abortion. What's that about? (see page 346)

8. My sister wants to have a midwife deliver her baby. Is this dangerous compared to having a doctor handle the birth? (see page 354)

9. Why do some women get so depressed after giving birth? That seems so opposite of how a new mother should be feeling, if she really wanted the baby. (see page 357)

10. What is sterility, and what causes it in both males and females? (see page 360)

Most college students are typically more concerned about *preventing* pregnancy than about conception, pregnancy, and birth. And it's probably safe to say that most young adults probably see the processes of conception, pregnancy, and birth as far simpler than they are. The reality is that reproduction is one of the most intricate and elegant of all human biological functions. It is also one of the most important reasons we are sexual beings—without it, the human species would have ceased to exist a long time ago. Biological science has progressed to the point that we now understand most of the human reproductive processes; yet still today, we do not understand them completely. As you will see throughout this chapter, conception, pregnancy, and birth remain, in very real ways, mysterious and miraculous.

It is very likely that you already have or will have children one day. Sometimes pregnancy and the birth of a baby happen when the parents plan for it to happen. You may be surprised to learn, however, that in the United States, nearly half of all pregnancies are unplanned (J. O'Brien, 2004; Santelli et al., 2003). This is not to say that all unplanned pregnancies are *unwanted*. On the contrary, many unplanned pregnancies are greeted with acceptance, pleasure, and even joy, once the initial surprise wears off. However, the fact that over 2 million unplanned pregnancies occur in the United States each year makes a strong case for a generally poor understanding among the general public of the realities of exactly how, when, and why conception occurs. This lack of understanding, perhaps combined with poor decision making about sexual behavior, is probably linked to incomplete education regarding conception, pregnancy, and birth. This very important and very basic information has traditionally been referred to as "the birds and the bees"—clearly indicating a desire to sidestep the straightforward details of *human* reproduction.

Although you may know more about human reproduction than the average person who has received the "birds and bees" talk, let's put an end to the cycle of incomplete information right here. After you read this chapter, you'll know a lot more, and one day you may be in a position to pass your knowledge on to others, perhaps to your own children.

For perspective, we'll begin with a look back at some early and rather crude-sounding childbirth practices. Then, returning to the present, we will cover the sometimes complex issues people face in life as they make decisions relating to whether and when to have a child. Whether such a conscious decision is made or not, pregnancies happen. And they all begin with the fascinating series of events leading to conception, the meeting and joining of the male sperm with the female egg, or ovum. If the fertilized ovum survives, the next step in under-

Focus on Your Feelings

Becoming pregnant, being pregnant, and giving birth are times of great emotion. For those who want to get pregnant, the emotions experienced upon learning the news are typically joy and excitement, perhaps mixed with nervousness about what's to come. As the pregnancy progresses, many women acquire a kind of glow that accompanies the happiness of being pregnant, but they may also grow weary of the inescapable discomforts of pregnancy. Pregnancy is also the time when most women and couples are preparing emotionally, sometimes with some trepidation, for parenthood. They may also feel concern that the fetus is developing properly and no complications are arising.

When a woman or couple who want to have children have difficulty conceiving, they usually experience intense feelings of disappointment and frustration as time passes without a pregnancy. They often feel that for some reason they are being denied one of their most cherished and anticipated life goals, and many couples feel a deep emotional loss of a child who has not yet been conceived. Luckily, nearly always, the couple will find a solution to their infertility issues that is right for them.

Another example of the emotional topics covered in this chapter relates to the loss of an unborn child. When a couple must endure the early, spontaneous loss of their unborn baby, it is rarely "just a miscarriage." To most couples, it is the profound loss of a future child whom they had already grown to love and cherish; the emotions they feel are similar to those felt upon losing any loved one through death. If you focus on what your feelings might be if you ever have to deal with a miscarriage (although chances are good that you won't), you will be much better prepared to offer the kind of understanding and support close friends or relatives may need should they ever have to face this difficult event.

Few people are ambivalent about the topic of abortion. Many fiercely stake out and defend ideological territories about the morality of choosing to terminate a pregnancy. Whatever your personal attitudes about abortion, you probably feel strongly about them. When or how this contentious issue will be resolved is anybody's guess, but if we can work together to reduce the number of unwanted pregnancies, that will be one step in a direction on which everyone can agree.

standing reproduction is taking a close look at the many changes in the growing embryo and fetus, as well as in the mother, during approximately nine months of pregnancy. It is also important to be aware of some of the problems and decisions that sometimes accompany pregnancy, including miscarriage (also called *spontaneous abortion*) and voluntary, or induced, abortion. Next we will turn to the final stage in pregnancy: childbirth, and the issues accompanying the birthing process, both during and after. Finally, we will examine infertility issues some couples face and solutions available today to assist them in becoming pregnant or, if they so choose, to adopt. Many of the issues discussed in this chapter (such as abortion or infertility) may trigger some strong emotional responses in you. This is normal and to be expected.

Historical Perspectives

The Pain of Giving Birth

Everyone knows that physical pain is usually a part of childbirth. Today, medical science in most developed nations has advanced to the point that a woman has the option of giving birth with minimal or tolerable levels of pain while remaining awake and fully aware of the profound moment her baby enters the outside world. These modern pain-reducing techniques, however, are relatively new to the history of human birthing practices. In fact, the use of medical pain control for childbirth did not come into common practice until the mid to late nineteenth century. The earliest methods required the mother to be deeply sedated under *general anesthesia*.

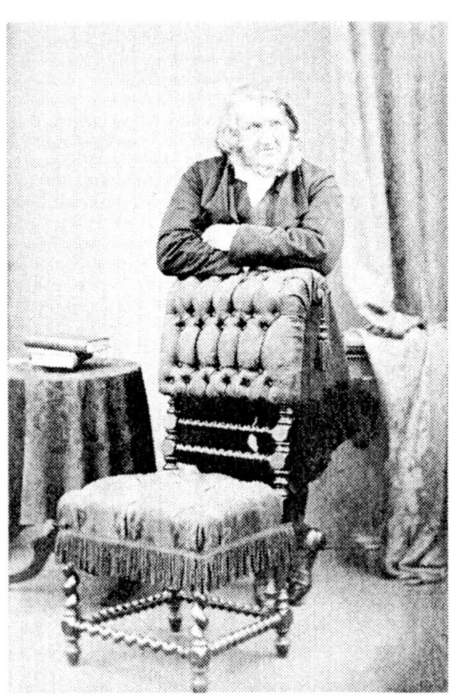

The earliest form of childbirth pain medication was deep sedation using a handkerchief saturated with a few drops of chloroform, a chemical discovered by Sir James Simpson (shown here) in the mid–1800s.

In the early 1800s, the pain-reducing qualities of ether, a mildly sedating and pain-reducing gas, had been discovered, and it was beginning to be used during childbirth. Although ether was often effective for pain, large amounts were required for full pain relief, and many medical professionals feared that such high levels of the drug might lengthen the birth process and potentially harm the fetus.

In 1847, an obstetrician and professor of **midwifery** (the practice of assisting women in pregnancy and childbirth) at Edinburgh University, Dr. James Young Simpson, invited two of his medical colleagues to dinner. After dinner, he asked them to try a new anesthetic he had been working on. A couple of hours later, the story goes, Dr. Simpson awoke underneath his dining room table and observed his fellow physicians still asleep and snoring peacefully next to him (Fissell, 1999b). This was exactly the medical result he had hoped for (although the dinner party itself may have fallen short of expectations) and within a month, he had used his new discovery, *chloroform*, on more than 50 women during the birth process (Gazeteer, 1995). The method of administering the drug was primitive: A handkerchief with a few drops of the liquid was held over the woman's nose and mouth (today we tend to see this in movies when someone is kidnapped). Sedation was quick and deep and did not have many of the negative side effects associated with ether.

A few years after Simpson's discovery, acceptance of the use of chloroform for childbirth grew rapidly when Queen Victoria demanded and received chloroform during the birth of her eighth child in 1853. For the next 50 years, chloroform became widely accepted for the pain of childbirth and for other painful medical procedures. The drug however popular at the time, was not entirely free of potentially serious side effects. The handkerchief method of delivery was imprecise, and overdose was not uncommon. In addition, around 1900, the drug was found to cause liver damage in some patients, and its use decreased drastically. Chloroform is still available today, but it is used primarily as a solvent in paint thinner and not at all in modern medicine.

midwifery The practice of assisting women through normal pregnancy and childbirth.

About the time chloroform was losing favor, a new method of childbirth pain control, called *twilight sleep*, was being developed. Pioneered by Dr. Bertha Van Hoosen, a gynecology professor at the University of Illinois Medical School, twilight sleep used a combination of two injectable drugs: morphine and scopolamine (Fissell, 1999a). These two drugs combined have the advantage of pain relief (morphine) and amnesia (scopolamine), so the woman awoke without any memories of labor or delivery (which most back then considered a positive side effect). Furthermore, if the morphine administered was kept to a minimum, the mother was capable of hearing, speaking, and participating emotionally in the birthing process, although, due to the effects of the scopolamine, she would have no memory of it. Even though the mother's memories of childbirth, if any, were vague, many women at the time saw twilight sleep as the most natural method of childbirth available. Because in twilight sleep the pelvic and uterine muscles are not paralyzed, as they are with ether and chloroform, the woman was able to assist in the birthing process and help push the baby out. Overall, twilight sleep made the entire birth process easier on the mother and the newborn, and women began to demand this method of childbirth as part of the growing women's rights and suffrage movement of the early 1900s.

Over the past several decades, childbirth has undergone nothing short of a total revolution as the emphasis has turned to natural or other methods of childbirth that reduce pain while allowing the woman to be awake, actively participate in, and have a full recollection of the delivery of her baby. Current childbirth methods and pain reduction techniques will be discussed in detail later in this chapter.

Deciding Whether or Not to Have a Child

Most people see having children as an important and necessary part of their lives. Most realize as well that becoming a parent is not a decision to be taken lightly. Having and raising a child carries with it challenges and responsibilities that are, arguably, the greatest that we humans face in a lifetime. However, most parents will tell you without hesitation that along with those challenges and responsibilities, parenting is also their greatest source of joy, love, pride, and meaning, especially in terms of their sense of a lasting contribution to the future of humankind.

How can you know if and when you are ready to have a child? The truth is, most people probably can't, at least not for sure. Indeed, as mentioned at the beginning of this chapter, many prospective parents are not even planning on becoming parents, at least not at that particular point in their lives, when they discover that a baby is on the way. Nevertheless, adults can ask themselves some important questions as they consider their future as parents. Some of these questions are discussed in "Self-Discovery: Are You Ready to Be a Parent?" You may find the questions and your answers to them quite revealing, whether you already have children or if parenthood still seems far in the future.

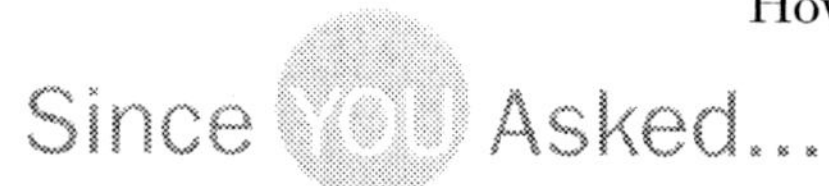

1. My older sister (she's 28) really wants to get pregnant, but her husband is saying he's not ready. Is there any way she can convince him to agree?

2. I feel that I really do not want to have children ever! Does that make me totally weird?

Choosing *Not* to Have a Child

Not everyone feels destined to be a parent. In fact, a small but increasing percentage of Americans are choosing *not* to have children. These individuals and couples are often fertile and biologically capable of conceiving, but they feel more comfortable and content to live lives that do not include parenting. They often prefer to be called "childless by choice" or "child-free." Some people react to this decision with disbelief, assuming that a life without kids is incomplete or lacking in some way. Those who choose to be child-free see it very differently.

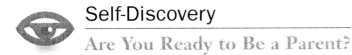

Self-Discovery

Are You Ready to Be a Parent?

If you are wondering if and when you might be ready to become a parent, here is a list of questions and considerations that may be helpful. Even if you already have children or if you know for sure you are *not* ready now, a little self-analysis never hurts. If you are in a relationship that you see as potentially long-term, you might want to go through these items with your partner.

Your Expectations about Yourself as a Parent

- **Do you currently spend time with children and teens? Do you enjoy it?** Whether you answer yes or no doesn't predict how you'll feel about your own children, but giving some thought to the issue can highlight some of your assumptions and attitudes about life with children.
- **What are your thoughts on the responsibilities and commitment of parenthood?** This question is just a way to help you reflect on the demands of parenting and whether you're comfortable with them. Parenthood is permanent; you can't just raise your kids during the "fun" years.
- **How do you cope with stress? Is your stressed-out self something you would want your child to witness?** Research shows that your level of stress can affect your children and your ability to parent effectively. If you feel you don't have a good handle on managing your stress, now is a great time to start learning some new coping mechanisms.
- **What are your hopes and fears about parenthood?** Being a parent isn't all shared hugs and fits of giggling. You will have tough times and disappointments, and your children will not always meet your expectations. Some aspects of parenting can be frightening—it's a big responsibility. But voicing your fears and examining them now can help. Our own parents are the strongest models we have for raising children. Some of their lessons are positive and others negative. Examine your life with your parents, and think about what you can learn from their successes and shortcomings. Think about what you'd like to emulate from your own childhood and what you'd like to change or avoid altogether.

Your Values and Expectations about Life

These questions will help you pinpoint the personal attitudes and values you'll bring to the role of parent. They will also help identify differences that may exist between you and your current or future partner.

- **What values and morals would you like to pass on to your children? What attitudes would you want to be sure your child avoids?** This question helps you verbalize what you think is important to bring to the role of parent. If you're having trouble deciding whether you want children, it may have something to do with unresolved issues from your own childhood.
- **What are your priorities for your children? For example, do you want them all to have a college education? What are your expectations about their social lives, relationships, marriage, and careers?** We all come to parenthood with a set of expectations, often unspoken. This question helps you clarify your hopes and dreams for your children.
- **What are your thoughts about disciplining children? How strict or permissive do you think you would be as a parent? Why?** This is an area where many new parents are unprepared and partners often disagree. Thinking about these issues now will help you in planning strategies for setting limits, establishing acceptable and unacceptable behaviors, and developing consistent consequences for your child's actions.

Your Lifestyle and How It Will Change

Answering these questions will give you insight into the practical realities of your situation, which you should consider before taking on parenthood.

- **Talk to people you know who've decided not to have children; talk to others who've decided to have children. How does what they tell you make you feel?** This is not to suggest that you base your decision on what others say, but hearing friends and relatives talk about their own parenthood choices can raise new issues for you to consider.
- **What does your support system look like?** You don't need a *whole* village to raise your child, but a few people to lean on can really help. Child rearing is difficult to do on your own. Do you have a partner or family and friends nearby to whom you can look for assistance? A circle of support isn't a prerequisite for parenthood, but it's a wonderful addition.
- **What do you do when you have free time? What will you do when you don't have any?** This is one of the practical realities of parenthood. Your needs, goals, and activities will become secondary to those of your child most of the time. He or she will become your number one priority almost all the time—are you ready for that?
- **How do you think your life will change?** It will. Big time. Most parents say it's for the better, but the effect on your time and energy can be enormous. Take a moment now to think seriously about the new life you are considering.

Source: Adapted from Evaluate Your Parenting Readiness (2005).

Is it OK to decide not to have children? Of course it is. But the decision may not be as easy as it sounds. Most societies place strong expectations on their members to become parents, and those expectations are not particularly subtle. Just think for a moment how history has treated childless marriages. Women without children were called "barren," and men and their families would often reject, punish, or even murder wives who did not produce children, regardless of where the fault for the infertility lay. Today, most world cultures are seemingly more civilized and understanding about a lack of offspring, but couples often still experience great turmoil and emotional pain when they have difficulty conceiving, and some couples are unable to sustain their marriage after the discovery that they are infertile. A major biotechnological industry has grown to assist infertile couples to conceive, usually at great expense to the couple (to be discussed later in this chapter). Additionally, many couples turn to adoption (also discussed later) to create a family.

What about those who choose not to have children regardless of their biological ability to do so? Among women of childbearing age in the United States, 6.6 percent define themselves as "voluntarily childless" ("Childless by Choice," 2001). That's over 4 million women. Nevertheless, such a decision is often seen as a violation of expectations in a child-oriented society, and such women and couples are viewed negatively (Gillespie, 2003; Mueller & Yoder, 1999). Many child-free couples (sometimes called DINKs, for "dual income, no kids") face subtle and sometimes not-so-subtle forms of discrimination, disapproval, and even punishment from various groups in their lives (Cannold, 2003).

In Western cultures, we are beginning to see a decrease in the social stigma attached to couples who make the decision to be childless by choice, and they cite many advantages of their decision. Consider for yourself some of the pros and cons of a child-free life in Table 9.1.

Table 9.1 ADVANTAGES AND DISADVANTAGES OF CHOOSING A CHILD-FREE LIFE

ADVANTAGES	DISADVANTAGES
Greater discretionary income	Potential feelings of loneliness and missing an important part of life
More free time	Possible lifelong conflict or regret over decision to be child-free
Greater education opportunities	Lack of child's unconditional love
Greater freedom to have second job	Lack of feeling needed by child
More time for hobbies and passions	Negative judgment by others (selfish, immature, unhappy)
No interference with career path	Disappointment of potential grandparents
More satisfying marriage*	Discrimination at work (being expected to do more than others due to "no kid" status)
Sense of not contributing to world overpopulation	Less ability to enjoy more flexible hours and possible shorter workweeks
Not subjecting children to dangers and perils of modern life	Lack of support when ill or elderly
Fewer worries in general	Difficulty finding other adults and couples for socializing
Calm and uncluttered home life	Lack of child tax credits
More time and energy for spouse	Tendency to become more rigid, less flexible
Better sex life	Risk of becoming overly independent and isolated from society at large
Opportunities for travel	More difficult search for self-knowledge without the "education" of having children
More time for charitable volunteer work	Greater chance of divorce*
Energy for spiritual and stress-relieving activities	
More time to explore personal goals and values	

*Child-free couples who stay together consistently report great marital satisfaction compared to traditional married couples, but divorce rates are higher among child-free couples, probably due to the greater financial independence of both partners and lack of perceived obligation to stay together "for the sake of the children."

Sources: Arenofsky, 1996; "Childless by Choice," 2001; Connidis and McMullen, 1999; Kopper and Smith, 2001; La Mastro, 2001; Morell, 2000; and Salzman, 1998.

Influence of the Child's Sex

If you were deciding whether or when to have children, do you think you might be influenced by being able to choose the sex of the child? Just one girl? A boy first and then a girl? How about two girls and then a boy? What if you could take your pick? Just drink the blue medicine to make a boy baby and the pink medicine for a girl. Of course, this is just a fantasy. Prospective parents can't actually choose the sex of their children; they just have to take what they get. Or do they? Although a 100 percent accurate method of sex selection as simple as a pink or blue drink does not exist (yet!), researchers have developed laboratory techniques that allow parents to choose, with a high degree of success, the sex of their child *prior to pregnancy* (Fackelmann, 1998; Lockwood, 2000; Meadows, 2004).

The theory behind such a choice is simple. The egg released from a woman's ovary contains only female (X) sex chromosomes. The man's sperm cells, however, may contain either X or Y chromosomes. An egg that is fertilized by an X-bearing sperm cell will be a girl, and one fertilized by a Y-bearing sperm cell will be a boy. Consequently, if only X, or only Y, sperm cells are allowed to reach the ovum in the fallopian tube, the sex of the resulting child is a sure thing.

Because of inherent DNA differences, X-bearing sperm cells are slightly larger than Y-bearing cells. Based on this difference, medical techniques have been developed to separate X- and Y-bearing sperm cells in the lab. Once the sperm cells have been sorted, samples rich in the cells that will determine the desired sex of the future child (X or Y) are used to inseminate the woman, or incorporated in other assisted reproductive techniques (discussed later in this chapter). Methods of sperm sorting are not perfect, but they are achieving approximately 90 percent success rates in producing male babies and 80 percent for girls, and these success rates are improving rapidly (Westphal, 2004). In another sex-selection method that is becoming more common, couples use in-vitro fertilization to create embryos. Using DNA testing, the embryos are then sorted into male and female and only the ones of the desired sex are implanted in the uterus.

As you probably guessed, sex preselection technology is quite controversial and provides much material for debate (Dickens, 2002; Lockwood, 2002; *New Scientist*, 2004). In purely medical terms, however, some very serious and even deadly inherited diseases are linked to the X and Y chromosomes, and these risks may be reduced through sex selection technologies. Beyond medical considerations, many parents feel that the procedures provide them with the opportunity to achieve the desired gender makeup of their family: to have all of one sex, to create a balance between the sexes of their children, or whatever combination they prefer. But what are the ethical and social considerations of this technology? These are discussed in "Sexuality, Ethics, and the Law: Sex Preselection Technology."

Conception

Conception requires a single sperm cell from a man to penetrate and fertilize an ovum (egg) from a woman. Sounds pretty basic, doesn't it? And in many ways it is; after all, it may be the single most important event in the survival of the human species. However, as you will see, the journey of that sperm and that ovum prior to reaching the moment of conception is amazing and complex. Our story begins with the woman, before she is born.

Ovulation: The Ovum's Journey

When a female fetus is born, her ovaries already contain approximately 2 million immature eggs (called *oocytes*). As the girl develops through childhood, the number of oocytes in her ovaries decreases until puberty, when the first mature ovum is released, at which point her ovaries contain approximately 400,000 oocytes

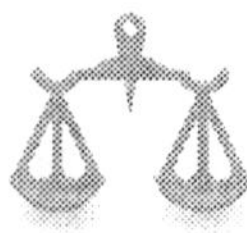

Sexuality, Ethics, and the Law

Sex Preselection Technology

The worldwide social and ethical considerations in the face of increasingly available methods for allowing prospective parents to select the sex of their children are deeply disturbing. What, for example, might these procedures mean for male-female sex ratios in countries such as China, India, or the Middle East, where boy babies are highly prized and preferred over girls? The effect of China's one-child policy is that boys are so highly prized that an estimated 500,000 to 2 million baby girls are secretly abandoned to orphanages or murdered every year so that the parents may try again for a boy (K. Johnson, 1996; Lubman, 2000).

Recognizing the future sociological implications of infant sex selection, China and India have passed laws prohibiting abortions based on parental sex preferences (Mudur, 2002). In addition, China has begun to restrict assisted fertility clinics that may be engaged in prepregnancy sex selection technologies and to reward families monetarily who have only one son or who have no son but have and keep two daughters ("China Rewards," 2005; Glenn, 2004; Kalb, Nadeau, & Schafer, 2004; Reproductive Health Technologies Project, 2000). Although the technology allowing for the *preselection* of the sex of children (prior to conception) may help reduce sex-based abortions, the consequences of such a choice to the population of countries that place a high value on male offspring could be devastating to the gender balance in those countries in future decades.

These concerns notwithstanding, infant sex selection is here to stay. Individuals, couples, cultures, and countries will approach the issues in their own way and from their own legal, moral, and ethical perspectives. As with so many new and emerging technologies, scientific advances in human sexuality may be used for positive or negative ends, and the choices we make must therefore be as informed and accurate as possible.

(Frishman, 1995b). This turns out to be hundreds of thousands more than a woman will release in her lifetime, but nature is taking no chances: Most women will have approximately 35 to 40 fertile years between the onset of puberty and menopause. Releasing one ovum each month, this amounts to a lifetime total of 400 to 500 ova released from a woman's ovaries.

During puberty, a set of preprogrammed hormonal changes occur in a girl's body, triggering menarche, her first menstrual period and, soon thereafter, the beginning of ovulation, the release of one ovum each month (puberty and menarche are discussed in greater detail in Chapter 12, "Sexual Development thoughout Life").

Following the onset of a woman's menstrual period each month, a combination of hormones released over the next two weeks promotes the growth of *ovarian follicles*, small sacs on the surface of the ovaries, each of which contains a developing ovum (a more thorough explanation of menstruation and the menstrual cycle may be found in Chapter 2, "Sexual Anatomy," and Chapter 5, "Contraception." As this **follicular phase** of her fertility cycle begins, the pituitary gland at the base of the brain begins to secrete *follicle-stimulating hormone* (FSH), which further enhances follicle growth and ovum development. The many ovum-containing follicles that have been growing now release their own hormone, *estradiol*, a powerful form of estrogen (see Table 9.2 for a summary of hormone production during a woman's fertility cycle). At this point, the follicles are in a kind of competition, because only one follicle will eventually rupture and release the ovum into the fallopian tube for possible fertilization (more than one ovum may be released in relatively rare cases, resulting, if fertilized, in fraternal twins or multiple births).

follicular phase The early period during a woman's monthly fertility cycle when the pituitary gland secretes *follicle-stimulating hormone* to enhance ovum development.

By about a week after the first day of a woman's period, the follicle producing the most estrogen receives an extra dose of FSH, causing it to become the "dominant

Table 9.2 HORMONAL CHANGES IN WOMEN DURING A TYPICAL FERTILITY (MENSTRUAL) CYCLE

MENSTRUAL PHASES	DAYS IN PHASE	HORMONAL ACTIONS
Follicular (proliferative) phase	Days 1–6: Beginning of menstruation to end of blood flow	Estrogen and progesterone start out at their lowest levels. Follicle-stimulating hormone (FSH) levels rise. Ovaries start producing estrogen and levels rise, while progesterone remains low.
	Days 7–13: Endometrium (inner lining of the uterus) thickens to prepare for egg implantation	
Ovulation	Day 14	Level of luteinizing hormone (LH) surges. Largest follicle on ovary bursts and releases egg into fallopian tube.
Luteal (secretory) phase, also known as the premenstrual phase	Days 15–28	Ruptured follicle develops into corpus luteum, which produces progesterone. Progesterone and estrogen stimulate a blanket of blood vessels to prepare for egg implantation.
If fertilization occurs:		Human chorionic gonadotropin (hCG) hormone begins to increase in the woman's body. Fertilized egg attaches to blanket of blood vessels and becomes placenta. Corpus luteum continues to produce estrogen and progesterone.
If fertilization does not occur:		Corpus luteum deteriorates. Estrogen and progesterone levels drop. Blood vessel lining sloughs off, and menstruation begins.

follicle," while the others will deteriorate (Hatcher et al., 1998). This dominant follicle then continues to grow, produces increasing amounts of estrogen, and forms a pouch, looking somewhat like a water-filled blister, on the ovarian wall and will grow to nearly 0.75 inch in diameter just prior to rupturing and releasing the ovum (see Figure 9.1).

The continuing rise in estrogen levels signals a further increase in secretion of FSH, along with the release of *luteinizing hormone* (LH). These two hormones now combine to cause the wall of the follicle at the edge of the ovary to break down, and about a day later, the follicle ruptures, releasing the ovum into the abdominal cavity. This is the precise moment of ovulation. A human ovum is a very large cell, relatively speaking, one of the largest in the human body: It measures 0.004 inch across (about the size of a sharp pencil point) and is visible to the naked eye (see Figure 9.2).

The fallopian tubes are not actually connected to the ovaries; rather the threadlike structures (the *fimbriae*) at the upper end of the tubes rest adjacent to and against the ovaries. The back-and-forth motion of these fimbriae set up a current in the abdominal fluid that draws the newly released ovum into the fallopian tube (see Figure 9.2). Once the ovum has entered the fallopian tube, the woman is "officially" fertile. For a natural pregnancy to occur, sperm cells and ovum must meet, and one sperm must penetrate the ovum's outer membrane during its brief journey along the upper region of the fallopian tube (more on this shortly).

After the ovum is released, estrogen production decreases and progesterone and LH secretions begin to rise. Over the next 14 days of a woman's cycle, called the **luteal phase**, the growth of new follicles in the ovaries is suppressed, and the lining of the uterus (the *endometrium*) thickens in preparation to receive a fertilized ovum.

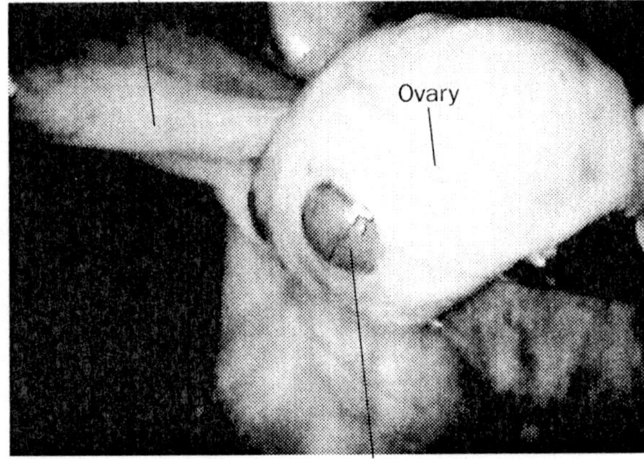

FIGURE 9.1 A Mature Ovarian Follicle

As an ovum matures, its follicle on the wall of the ovary grows nearly three-quarters of an inch in diameter.

3. After a woman's period, how soon is the next egg released, and when is she most fertile?

luteal phase The later period of a woman's monthly fertility when the lining of the uterus thickens in preparation for receiving a fertilized ovum if conception has occurred.

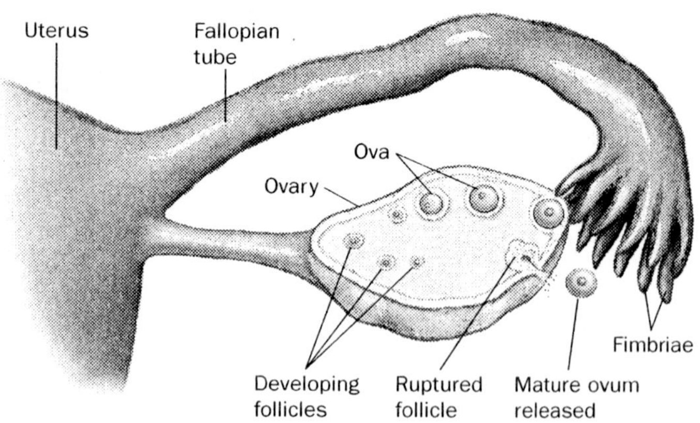

FIGURE 9.2 Ovulation

Ovulation occurs when the ovarian follicle containing a mature ovum ruptures and releases the ovum toward the opening of the fallopian tube.

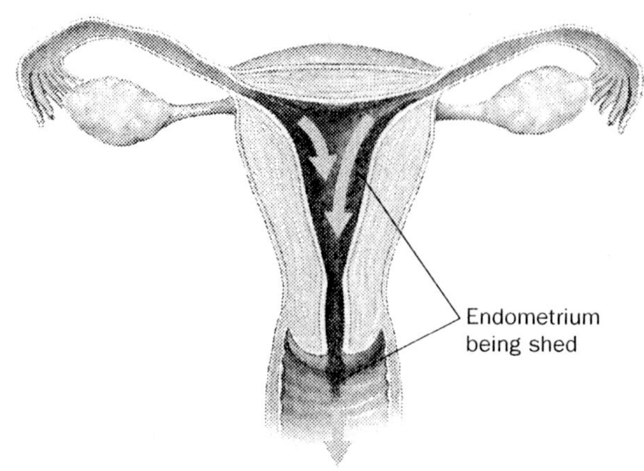

FIGURE 9.3 Menstruation

If fertilization of the ovum does not occur, the lining of the uterus is shed as menstrual fluid during a woman's period.

seminiferous tubules Tightly packed tubes in the testicles in which sperm cells are produced.

If no fertilization occurs, changes in hormone secretions cause a breakdown in the lining of the endometrium, which then drains, typically over several days, through the cervix and out the vagina (see Figure 9.3). This draining of the uterine lining and fluid (menstruation) is what is commonly known as a woman's period.

The Sperm's Journey

Unlike girls, boys are not born with a lifetime supply of reproductive cells. However, upon reaching puberty, boys normally begin to produce sperm cells in astonishingly large numbers and continue to produce them throughout their life. Sperm cells are produced in the testicles. The testicles are made of up of tightly packed **seminiferous tubules**, literally "seed-bearing tubes" (see Figure 9.4). When these tubules are stimulated by male secretions of follicle-stimulating hormone (FSH, which is produced by the male system just as by the female) and testosterone, millions of primitive cells that line the tubules begin to develop into sperm cells. These cells then migrate from the testicles to the epididymis, the structure attached to the back side of each testicle (see Figure 9.5). Once in the epididymis, the sperm cells mature and develop their ability to swim.

The length of time needed for the sperm cells to develop from migration from the tubules to the epididymis to ejaculation is approximately 68–72 days. In other words, the sperm cells that are beginning to develop in a man's testicles today will not be ready to be ejaculated and fertilize an ovum for ten weeks (Frishman, 1995b).

Sperm cells are minuscule, especially compared with the ovum. What sperm lack in size, however, they make up for in sheer numbers. In normal adult men, the number of sperm cells in a single ejaculate ranges from approximately 20 million to 200 million per milliliter (cubic centimeter) of semen, with an average of about 60 to 70 million (see Figure 9.6). The normal volume of semen ejaculated ranges from 2 to 6 milliliters (a teaspoon holds about 5 milliliters). This means that somewhere between 40 million and 1 *billion* sperm cells may be contained in a single ejaculation (Frishman, 1995b; Male Infertility Specialists, 2002; Zepf, 2001).

"Why so many?" you may ask. This is a very good question, especially when you consider that an ovum is fertilized by only a single sperm. Probably the most important reason is that although sperm are numerous, they are not particularly hardy. Some may be abnormally formed, some may become trapped among other body cells, some

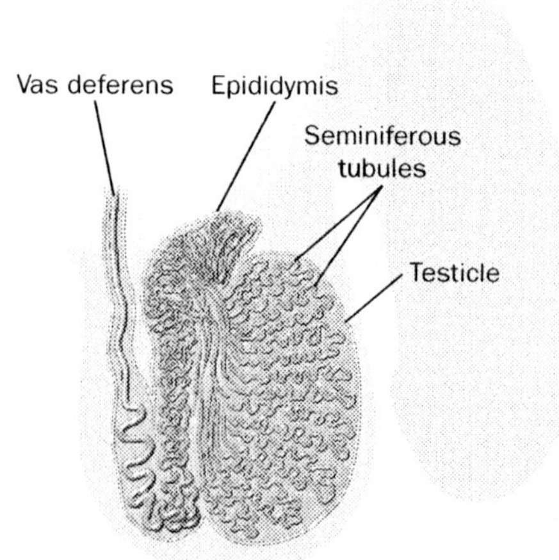

FIGURE 9.4 Tubules in the Testicle

Each testicle contains hundreds of feet of tightly coiled seminiferous ("seed-bearing") tubules.

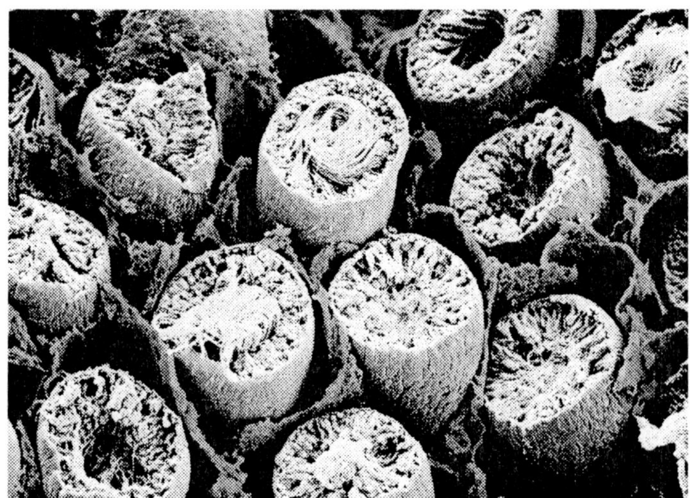

FIGURE 9.5 Sperm Cells in the Epididymis

Sperm are transported from the testicle to the epididymis, where they continue to mature at varying rates in preparation for ejaculation and potential fertilization of an ovum.

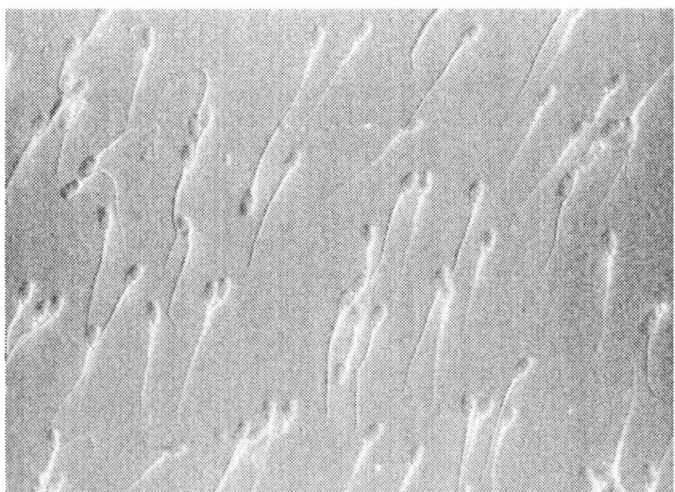

FIGURE 9.6 Sperm Cells in the Ejaculate

The typical male ejaculate contains an average of around 400 million sperm cells.

may be attacked by antibodies in the woman's body, many will die in the normal acidic environment of the vagina, and many just don't have the necessary stamina to make the 3-inch trip (a long way for a microscopic sperm) from the vagina through cervix into the uterus and on into the fallopian tube. Therefore, to help ensure the survival of the human species, nature has provided plenty of reinforcements (Bainbridge, 2003).

The Ovum-Sperm Rendezvous

Assume that the ovum is in the fallopian tube and the sperm cells have recently been ejaculated into the vagina. The ovum is gently whisked along the tube by *cilia*, tiny hairlike structures that create a current in the intrafallopian fluid. The ovum is capable of being fertilized for only 12 to 18 hours, so the best chance for fertilization is if sperm cells are already high up in the fallopian tube when the ovum arrives. Because sperm cells may survive in the female reproductive tract for about two to four days, the average couple is fertile for approximately five to six days each month. In other words, if ejaculation occurs in the vagina from four days before to approximately one day after ovulation, live sperm cells may have an opportunity to encounter the ovum in the fallopian tube. This in itself, however, does not guarantee pregnancy. In fact, the odds of pregnancy are only about 1 in 5 from a single act of intercourse and only 1 in 2 or 1 in 3 when a couple is trying to become pregnant and the timing of intercourse is right (Dunson, Colombo, & Baird, 2002).

Only about 100 to 1000 of all those hundreds of millions of sperm manage to make it all the way to the upper portion of the fallopian tubes where fertilization occurs. On their way there, the sperm cells have undergone physical and chemical changes that make them capable of penetrating the outer membrane of the ovum by releasing an enzyme that literally digests the ovum's inner wall (Frishman, 1995b). These survivor sperm then surround the ovum in a sort of competition to be the first to penetrate and fuse their chromosomes with those of the ovum (see Figure 9.7). Immediately after the first sperm successfully penetrates the ovum's outer membrane, biochemical changes triggered in the ovum create a barrier that effectively

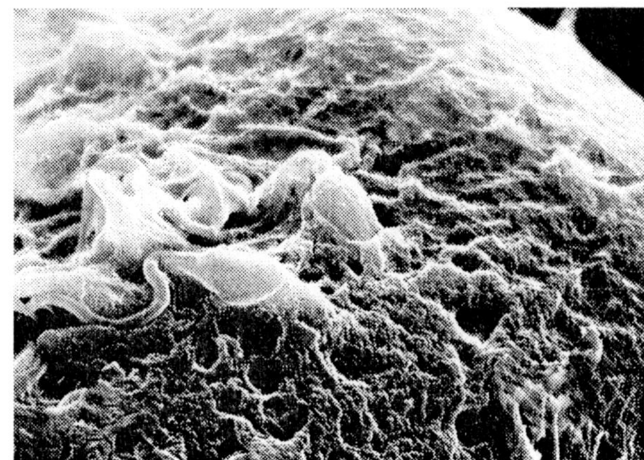

FIGURE 9.7 Sperm Cells on the Surface of the Ovum

Only one sperm cell will be allowed to penetrate the ovum's membrane.

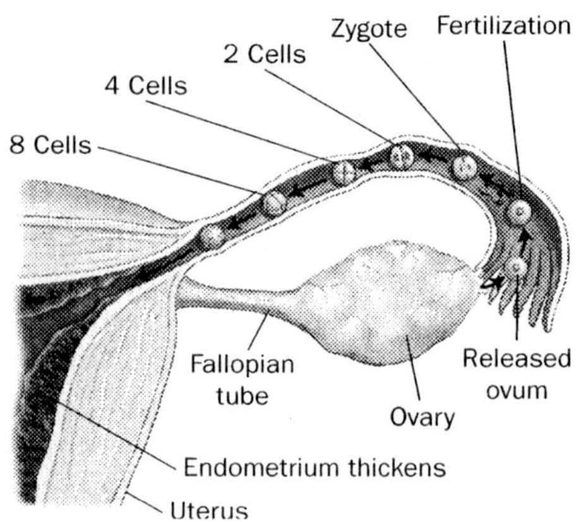

FIGURE 9.8 Zygote Moving through the Fallopian Tube

The fertilized egg, now known as a *zygote*, begins to divide as it travels along the fallopian tube.

blocks any other sperm cells from entering because the DNA of only one sperm cell is required for conception.

Upon successful fertilization, the DNA of the man's sperm and the woman's ovum join together, and a new organism, combining the genetic material of both, is created. Within hours, this organism, now called the **zygote** (see Figure 9.8), divides into two cells, then four, and eight, and so on as it continues its two- to four-day journey along the remainder of the fallopian tube to the uterus (Frishman, 1995b; Namnoum & Hatcher, 1998). Immediately upon fertilization, a hormone called *human chorionic gonadotropin* (hCG) begins to increase in the woman's body. Within about two weeks after conception, this hormone has reached high enough levels that conception can usually be determined using a standard home pregnancy test that measures the level of the hormone in the woman's urine. The level of hCG continues to increase day by day, so the test becomes more reliable each day following the initial two weeks.

Pregnancy itself has not been established until about two weeks after conception because the zygote has not yet implanted into the lining of the uterus (this will be discussed in the next section). Therefore, what we call a "pregnancy" test is often, in reality, a *conception* test. If a woman has a positive test result, she should assume that she has conceived until proved otherwise through a doctor visit or additional tests. She should not use alcohol or other drugs, be sure to take a multivitamin containing folic acid (an important B-vitamin for normal fetal development), and stop smoking. If a woman is planning on conceiving or is not taking steps to prevent an unwanted pregnancy, she should engage in a healthy lifestyle and avoid activities that are dangerous to a fetus (such as ingesting alcohol and all other drugs) *before* conception occurs.

4. Last week, I took two pregnancy tests that were both negative. But I still haven't started my period. Could I be pregnant?

zygote A fertilized ovum (or egg) moving down the fallopian tube.

blastocyst The developing zygote, with cells surrounding a fluid-filled core, upon entering the uterus and before implanting in the uterine wall.

embryo A blastocyst that has implanted in the uterine wall.

pregnancy The period of growth of the embryo and fetus in the uterus.

Pregnancy

During nearly all of the 400 to 500 fertility cycles in an average woman's lifetime, pregnancy will not occur. As mentioned earlier, if the ovum is not fertilized by a sperm cell, progesterone and estrogen levels diminish during the second half of a woman's cycle, blood flow to the uterus decreases, and the lining of the uterus is shed during the woman's period.

If fertilization has occurred, however, the lining of the uterus, signaled by hormones, continues to thicken in preparation for the arrival of the zygote. About four days after fertilization, the zygote enters the uterus. It has already divided many times and consists of approximately 90 cells surrounding a fluid-filled core. It is now called a **blastocyst**. On the sixth or seventh day after fertilization, assuming that the endometrium lining has formed properly, the blastocyst, containing over 100 cells, may implant into the wall of the uterus. Once implantation occurs, the blastocyst is referred to as an **embryo**. The blastocyst's successful attachment to the uterine lining is the beginning of **pregnancy** (see Figure 9.9).

As pregnancy is established, an organ, called the **placenta** begins to develop on the uterine wall adjacent to the embryo. The placenta contains a rich supply of blood vessels and is, in essence, the life-support system that biologically unites the developing embryo to the mother. As it grows along with the embryo, the placenta serves as a "transfer station" for nourishment and oxygen from the mother's body to the fetus, and for waste products from the fetus back to the mother's blood stream for disposal. During childbirth, the placenta, often referred to as the *afterbirth*, is typically expelled from the uterus following the newborn and examined for any abnormalities that could signal problems for the infant.

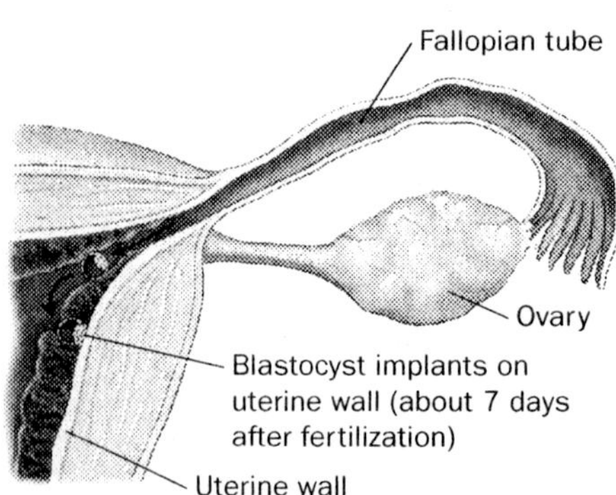

FIGURE 9.9 Blastocyst Implanting on Uterine Wall

Pregnancy begins when the developing zygote has left the fallopian tube, grown to become a blastocyst, and embedded itself in the uterine wall. At this point, the blastocyst is now referred to as an embryo.

Throughout pregnancy, the placenta is attached to the abdominal wall of the fetus by the **umbilical cord**, which reaches an average length of approximately 22 inches during pregnancy and consists of one large vein and two arteries. Its function is to transport nutrients, oxygen, and fetal waste products back and forth between the fetus and the placenta. When a baby is born, the umbilical cord is tied off and severed. The small portion still attached to the infant shrinks and detaches within about 2 weeks, leaving a scar we all know as the navel.

Assuming a normal, healthy pregnancy, the embryo will now begin to grow in predictable stages over the next nine months (Bainbridge, 2003; Fetal Development, 2005; D. Singer, 1995; Sutter Health Network, 2002). The following photographs and brief explanations highlight the remarkable process of the transformation from a cluster of cells to the birth of a new life. For the sake of discussion, the 40 weeks of a full-term pregnancy are often divided into phases of about three months each, called **trimesters**.

placenta An organ that develops on the uterine wall during pregnancy joining the developing embryo to the mother's biological systems, transferring nourishment, oxygen, and waste products between the fetus and the mother.

umbilical cord A structure of approximately 22 inches in length, consisting of one large vein and two arteries, that transport nutrients, oxygen, and fetal waste products back and forth between the fetus and the placenta.

trimester One of three periods of about three months each that make up the phases of a full-term pregnancy.

embryonic period The initial eight weeks of pregnancy following fertilization.

fetus An embryo after eight weeks of pregnancy.

quickening The first movement of the fetus that is felt by the mother.

First Trimester

The first three months of pregnancy begin with the **embryonic period**, usually considered to be the initial eight weeks following fertilization. At the end of this period, the embryo becomes known as a **fetus**. This first trimester is a critical time for the developing embryo. During this time, it is at highest risk of *miscarriage* (also referred to as *spontaneous abortion*) due to various genetic, structural, hormonal, or environmental causes. Approximately 10 to 20 percent of *confirmed* pregnancies (in women who know they are pregnant) end in miscarriage (D. Singer, 1995; Tong et al., 2004). You will find a more complete discussion of miscarriages a bit later in this chapter. Barring early termination of pregnancy, here are some of the milestones reached during this first trimester.

- *Month 1* The embryo resembles a tadpole or tiny shrimp; buds of arms and legs begin to appear; the heart begins to beat; the embryo is about the size of the eraser on a pencil and weighs less than 1 ounce.
- *Month 2* The embryo grows to about 1 inch long; distinct fingers and toes appear; the heart muscle has divided into chambers; facial features are visible; the placenta is functioning, bringing nutrients to the embryo and carrying wastes away; the embryo takes on more human appearance.
- *Month 3* The embryo, now called a fetus, grows to about 3 inches in length; fingers and toes have nails; the fetus begins to move in the uterus, but movements cannot usually be felt by the mother; all vital organs and muscles are formed and functioning by the tenth week. The fetus now weighs about 1.2 ounces (the equivalent of a dozen U.S. pennies).

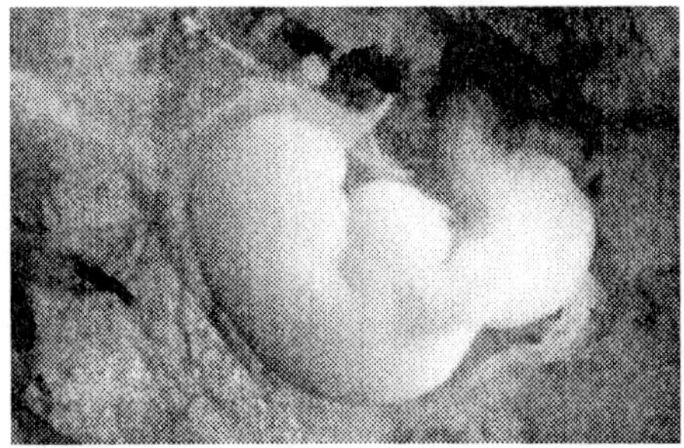

Embryo at one month.

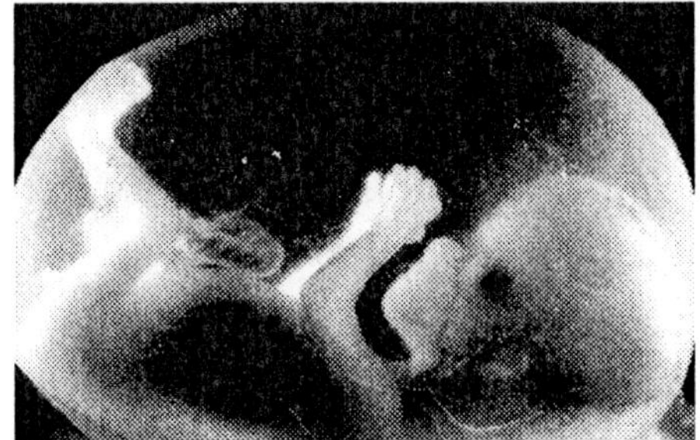

Fetus at three months.

Second Trimester

Usually by the fourth month, the pregnancy is firmly established and the risk of miscarriage decreases significantly. It is early in this second trimester that the mother will begin to feel the fetus move, which is called **quickening**. During these months, the growth of the fetus accelerates greatly. Here are some of the developmental changes during this phase.

- *Month 4* Fetal movement increases and includes kicking, sucking, and swallowing; about 20 tooth buds develop; fingers and toes are more clearly defined; the sex of the fetus may now be determined by observing the growth of the genitals with ultrasound. The fetus grows to 6 or 7 inches long and now weighs around 6 or 7 ounces.

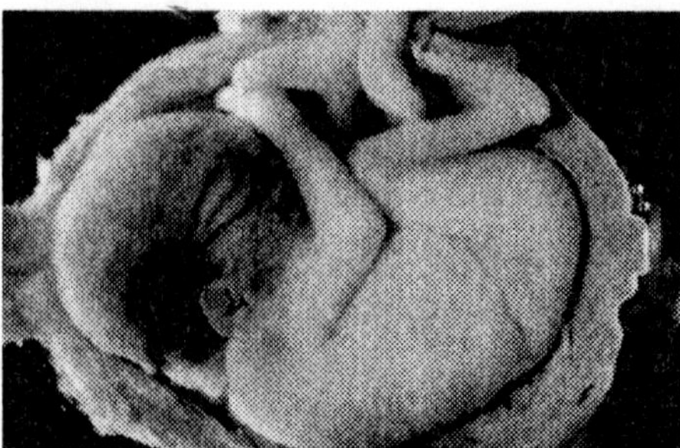

Fetus at five months.

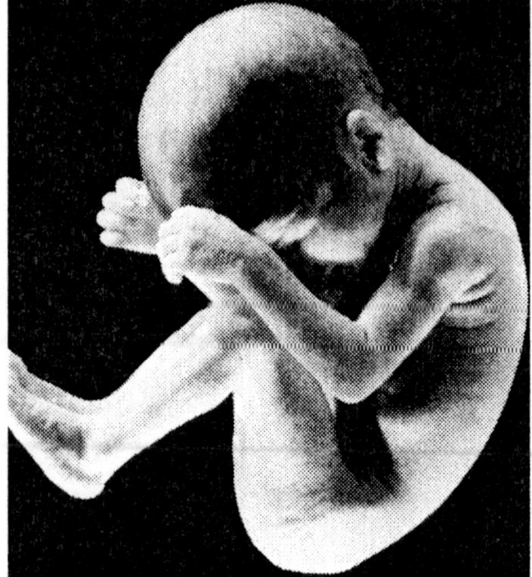

Fetus at seven months.

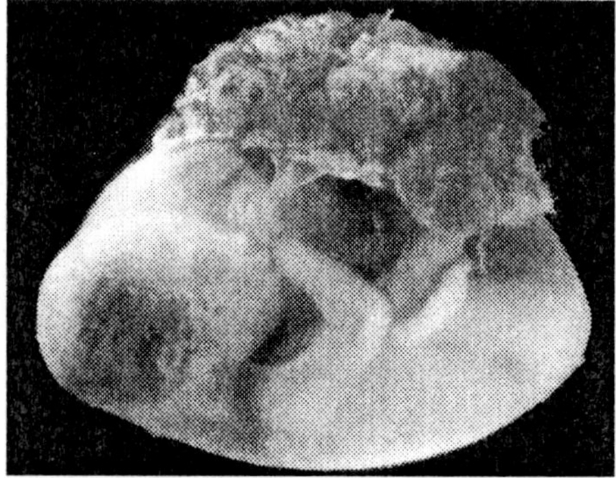

Nearly full-term fetus (eight to nine months).

- *Month 5* Fetal activity increases further and may even include rolls, flips, and somersaults; the fetus enters a predictable waking-sleeping cycle; the mother will feel frequent unmistakable movements of the fetus; fetal eyelashes and eyelids appear; growth accelerates to 8 to 10 inches long, and weight increases to nearly a pound by the end of the fifth month.
- *Month 6* Fetal skin is red and wrinkled and covered with a protective coating called the *vernix*; the eyes open and close; the fetus's lungs are "breathing" the amniotic fluid in and out; the fetus is capable of hearing sounds from the outside world; rapid growth continues as the fetus reaches 11 to14 inches in length and 1.5 to 2 pounds. If born in this month, the baby, although very premature, will have a good chance of survival with specialized intensive care (see the discussion of premature births later in the chapter).

Third Trimester

The last three months of pregnancy are marked by a dazzling increase in the rate of growth of the fetus. During the third trimester, the fetus will typically add up to a foot in length and at least 7 more pounds. Also, changes will accelerate that prepare the baby for birth, including internal organ maturation, layers of fat, muscle tone, and rotation into a head-down position in the womb. Here are the major events as birth approaches.

- *Month 7* The fetus's taste buds have developed, and it may be observed sucking its thumb; muscle tone develops through kicking and stretching; clear responses to external sounds may be observed; layers of fat are forming beneath the skin; internal organs are maturing quickly. If born prematurely at this time, the baby has high chance of survival and a normal life with proper medical care. The fetus reaches 14 to 16 inches long and about 3 pounds by the end of the seventh month.
- *Month 8* Fetus rotates to head-down position; brain grows quickly; overall growth now at a rate of a half pound per week; fetus's kicks and elbow thrusts now become visible from the outside surface of the mother's abdomen; the fetus's internal organs, except for the lungs, are nearly fully developed; the skull bones are flexible and not yet connected to allow them to compress for passage through the birth canal; size is approximately 18 inches long, and weight is 4 to 6 pounds at the end of this month.
- *Month 9* The fetal lungs develop fully and are ready to breathe air; the skin typically becomes pink and smooth; the fetus now turns and settles head down, low in the mother's uterus, in preparation for birth; activity decreases, producing fewer noticeable movements; on average the fetus reaches 18 to 22 inches in length and 6 to 9 pounds as the onset of labor approaches (labor and birth will be discussed shortly).

Potential Problems in Pregnancy

The vast majority of pregnancies proceed virtually trouble-free from conception to birth, except for some common discomforts for the expectant mother, such as nausea and vomiting, backache, swollen feet and ankles, and hemorrhoids. Nonetheless, these "normal" discomforts can make for a difficult eight to nine months for many women, and the burdens on her body and overall well-being should not be ignored. Table 9.3 summarizes some of these effects on the expectant mother, along with some causes and possible remedies. As you can see from the table, these typical problems that may occur during pregnancy usually do not threaten the eventual well-being or survival of mother or fetus. Much less frequently, serious and even life-threatening difficulties may arise during pregnancy. Here we will examine some of the more serious problems of pregnancy and then look at some of the prenatal tests that can be used to screen for genetic or physical defects.

Table 9.3 COMMON DISCOMFORTS OF PREGNANCY AND SOME REMEDIES

Many women proceed through pregnancy with very little distress and few problems. However, as the body changes to accommodate a new human life growing within it, certain discomforts are bound to occur. Here is a list of the more common discomforts associated with pregnancy for the woman, along with some possible causes and suggested remedies.

SYMPTOM	CAUSE	REMEDIES	SITUATIONS TO AVOID
Nausea and vomiting	Common discomforts of early pregnancy, affecting between 50 and 80 percent of all pregnant women. Although often referred to as *morning sickness*, nausea and vomiting can occur at any time and may persist throughout the day.	Increase amount of sleep. Avoid triggering odors. Exercise more. Eat smaller amounts of food more often. Eat whatever sounds good at the moment, even if it is junk food. Take more vitamin B_6 or ginger (which combats nausea).	Some women may need medical support to avoid severe dehydration. They should contact their doctor if they experience persistent vomiting and are unable to keep any fluids down for more than 24 hours.
Leg cramps	Caused by poor circulation, not enough calcium, pressure on nerves.	Increase calcium in the diet. Try a calcium supplement like Tums. Stretch the calf muscles by flexing the foot to relieve cramps. Apply a warm cloth or heating pad to leg muscles. Put feet up.	Avoid too much phosphorus in foods (phosphorus is linked to the depletion of calcium).
Backache	Caused by strain of increased uterine weight on back muscles and ligaments, made worse by poor posture.	Stand straight. Wear flat shoes with arches. Sleep on a firm mattress. Try pelvic-rocking exercises while on hands and knees. A maternity belt or sling might help as well.	Avoid high heels; avoid becoming overly fatigued or overexertion using the back muscles.
Shortness of breath	Pressure of the growing uterus on the diaphragm; anemia can exacerbate.	Stand up straight. Sleep with extra pillows to prop upper body up.	Quit smoking. Do not exercise to the point of fatigue.
Varicose leg veins	Progesterone, one of the pregnancy hormones, causes the veins to dilate or relax and not return blood to the heart as efficiently.	Elevate legs frequently. Walk daily. Put on support hose immediately upon wakening.	Avoid standing for long periods, sitting with crossed legs, and knee socks with tight tops.
Sleeplessness	Usually in the last months, caused by difficulty getting comfortable, frequent trips to the bathroom, worries, and the baby's movements.	Take a warm bath. Drink warm milk or chamomile tea at bedtime. Increase B vitamins by eating whole grains. Ask someone for a relaxing back rub. Lavender aroma may help with sleep.	Do not take sleeping pills or tranquilizers; avoid caffeinated drinks such as coffee, tea, and colas.
Numbness in fingers or arms	Usually due to fluid retention putting pressure on nerves.	Sit and stand up straight. Do shoulder circling exercises. Sleep with wrists slightly bent up on a pillow.	Avoid lying for prolonged periods on either arm; avoid sleeping with wrists curled up under the body.

Source: Adapted from Obstetrics-Gynecology and Infertility Group (2001).

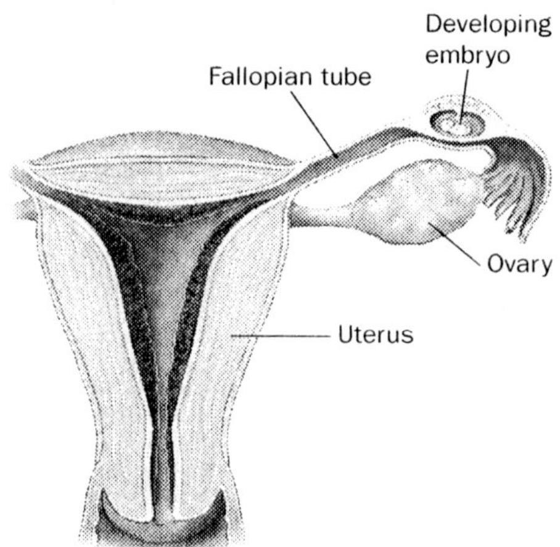

FIGURE 9.10 Ectopic Pregnancy

An ectopic pregnancy occurs when the zygote implants outside the uterus, usually in the fallopian tube.

Ectopic Pregnancy

An **ectopic pregnancy** (*ectopic* means "out of place") occurs when a zygote implants somewhere in the woman's body other than the uterus, most often in one of the fallopian tubes. Ninety-seven percent of ectopic pregnancies occur on the wall of the fallopian tube where fertilization has just taken place (Frishman, 1995a) and are often referred to as *tubal pregnancies*. Invariably, ectopic pregnancies are short-lived because, as you might imagine, the fallopian tube, while ideal for conception, is far too small for the developing embryo (see Figure 9.10).

Tubal pregnancies carry a high risk of rupture of the fallopian tube, causing internal bleeding, hemorrhaging, and even death of the pregnant woman if not diagnosed and treated quickly. Ectopic pregnancies occur in approximately 2 percent of all pregnancies and account for between 9 and 13 percent of all pregnancy-related deaths, or about 40 to 50 deaths per year in the United States (Advanced Fertility Center, 2005; Shima, 2002).

Over the past several decades, the number of ectopic pregnancies in the United States and Europe has been increasing ("Ectopic Pregnancy," 1995; Shima, 2002; Tay & Walker, 2000). The reasons for this increase are unclear, but a likely cause may relate to a similar climb in rates of certain sexually transmitted diseases, especially chlamydia and gonorrhea. As discussed in Chapter 8, "Sexually Transmitted Infections," these bacteria, if not properly treated, may lead to pelvic inflammatory disease, which may damage a woman's fallopian tubes and increase the risk of ectopic pregnancy (Sadovsky, 2001; Shima, 2002).

In the early stages, an ectopic pregnancy often produces all the signs and symptoms of a normal pregnancy, including absence of the menstrual period, nausea, and positive results on a pregnancy test. Six to eight weeks after the missed period, however, as the zygote grows in the fallopian tube, symptoms begin to appear, most commonly vaginal bleeding and abdominal pain (Sadovsky, 2001). Usually, a physician will be able to diagnose a tubal pregnancy using a combination of physical examination, hormonal blood tests, and ultrasound imaging techniques (Frishman, 1995a).

Treatments for ectopic pregnancies range from a single injection of a medication called *methotrexate*, which inhibits cell growth in the zygote and allows it to be expelled, or laparoscopic surgery to remove the cell mass and part or all of the fallopian tube (Advanced Fertility Center, 2005; K. Johnson, 2000a; Sadovsky, 2001). In the past, ectopic pregnancies usually caused the loss of the fallopian tube and the potential for reduced future fertility. Today, the use of tube-preserving treatment techniques has increased the rate of normal future pregnancy and delivery among women who have had one ectopic pregnancy to approximately 50 to 60 percent (Advanced Fertility Center, 2005). Moreover, as medical treatments for ectopic pregnancy and assisted fertility techniques continue to develop, the most negative effects of ectopic pregnancies are likely to decrease significantly.

ectopic pregnancy Implantation of a zygote somewhere in the woman's body other than the uterus, most often in one of the fallopian tubes, in which case it is also called a *tubal pregnancy*.

miscarriage The loss, (without any purposeful intervention) of an embryo or fetus during the first 20 weeks of pregnancy; also called *spontaneous abortion*.

Miscarriage

Miscarriage, or spontaneous abortion, is the loss (without any purposeful intervention) of an embryo or fetus during the first 20 weeks of pregnancy (Frishman, 1995a; McBride, 1991). You may be surprised to learn that at least 40 percent of all pregnancies end in miscarriage, with some estimates ranging up to 80 percent (Frishman, 1995a; Lockwood, 2000; McBride, 1991). Many of these are called *silent miscarriages* because they occur before the woman is aware that she is pregnant, and the spontaneous abortion mainfests itself as a somewhat late and often unusually heavy menstrual period. Of pregnancies that have been confirmed, about 10 to 20 percent end in miscarriage (D. Singer, 1995; Tong et al., 2004).

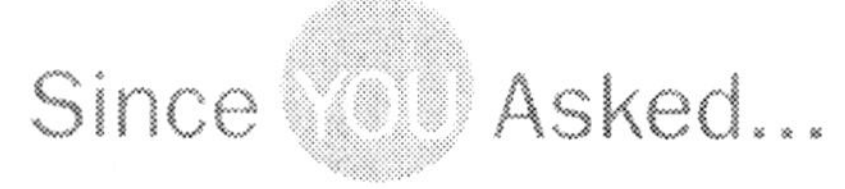

5. A few months ago, I started my period very late and had a lot of blood and very bad cramps (worse than usual). My friend said it was probably a miscarriage. Is that possible?

Most commonly, miscarriage is the result of one or more serious genetic fetal abnormalities. In these cases, the aborted embryo would probably not have survived beyond the first trimester, no matter what. Other possible causes for spontaneous abortions include the mother's or father's age (the chances of miscarriage increase as parental age increases), maternal illness or infection (such as rubella, or "German measles"), sexually transmitted infections, abnormalities of the uterus, hormonal imbalances, environmental toxins such as recreational drug use by the mother (especially alcohol and cocaine), radiation, heavy caffeine intake, and medical procedures such as amniocentesis (Frishman, 1995a; Lockwood, 2000; Slama et al., 2003).

Those who have never experienced the loss of a pregnancy often find it difficult to understand the deep sadness experienced by the prospective parents. Indeed, most miscarriages happen very early in pregnancy, well before the embryo would have any chance of survival outside the womb. Moreover, the vast majority of miscarriages happen for important biological reasons that would probably have rendered the fetus nonviable under any circumstances. Usually, however, these seemingly rational "justifications" for the miscarriage provide little comfort for the parents, who must deal with the loss of a future child whom they had already incorporated into their psychological and emotional lives (Hock, 2003; Lasker & Toedter, 2003; J. Rodriguez, 1990). When a miscarriage occurs, the parents may have already selected names for the baby, told friends and relatives the happy news of the pregnancy, and even begun decorating the baby's room.

Often doctors, nurses, and friends of the parents try, with all the best intentions, to offer condolences such as "Don't worry; you'll be able to become pregnant again. You'll still be able to have a child" or "But you were hardly even pregnant at all!" These attempts at comfort, however, frequently occur too soon after the loss, sometimes even while the woman is still in the hospital recovering from the miscarriage. She and her partner at that point may not have had even a moment for the grieving process, a process that is very real, very painful, and very personal (Lasker & Toedter, 2003). To consider, even for a moment, the idea of "replacing" the baby they have just lost is usually the last thing on their minds.

Preterm Birth

Preterm birth, also known as *premature birth*, is the birth of a fetus well before the nine-month, 280-day pregnancy period is complete. More specifically, preterm birth is defined as any delivery of a normally formed infant that occurs less than 37 weeks (259 days) after conception, which is three weeks less than a full-term pregnancy (Morantz & Torrey, 2004). The reasons for premature births are unclear, but it is the leading cause of fetal death in the United States and occurs in approximately 10 percent of births each year. Moreover, the rate of premature births has increased by over 20 percent since 1980 ("Predicting Preterm Births," 2002).

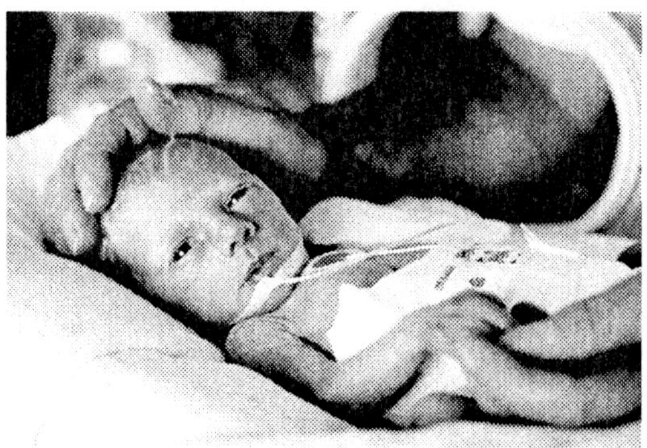

The rate of premature births has been increasing in the United States, but survival rates of preterm babies is on the rise as well.

On the other hand, significant medical advances now allow many more preterm infants not only to survive but also to live relatively normal, healthy lives. Today, even infants born as early as 22 weeks have a fighting chance of survival (Draper et al., 2003). That's 18 weeks or more than *four months* before full term! Figure 9.11 illustrates the rates of survival of premature infants, by weeks of gestational (developmental) time in the womb.

Nevertheless, giving birth to a very early-term infant is a difficult and stressful challenge for any parent (Preyde & Ardal, 2003; Singer et al., 1999). Typically, premature infants require special and often highly intensive care in a hospital setting before they

preterm birth Birth of an infant less than 37 weeks after conception.

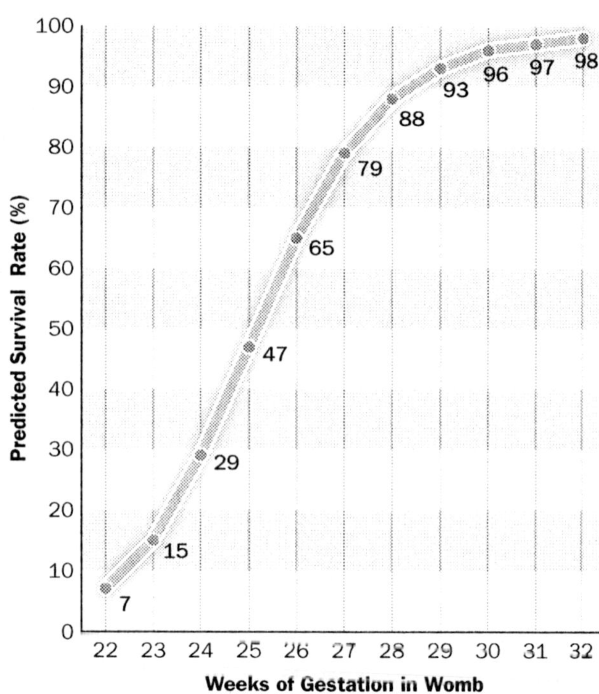

FIGURE 9.11 Predicted Survival Rates for Preterm Infants

Note: Full term is 40 weeks.

Source: Adapted from Draper et al. (2003).

are strong and healthy enough to be taken home. Premature births are often associated with a wide range of developmental difficulties for the child and consequently for the parents (Feldman et al., 2002). Preterm infants often exhibit early deficits in cognitive, attention, and motor skills, some of which may continue into later childhood. Moreover, preterm infants tend to be less alert and slower to acquire early visual skills compared to full-term babies. These cognitive and perceptual difficulties may interfere with the interactions between the mother and the infant, which may in turn disrupt the normal mother-child bonding process. This lack of social interaction and bonding between the preterm infant and the mother may further intensify the developmental delays for the child (Feldman et al., 2002).

Predicting if or when a pregnancy is likely to end in a preterm delivery has been generally unsuccessful (Colombo, 2002; "Predicting Preterm Births," 2002). Research has attempted to define the factors most often associated with preterm birth. However, as with all correlational research, researchers often have a difficult time determining with confidence whether certain factors, such as drug use, cigarette smoking, or various infectious agents, actually cause preterm births or may coexist with other risk factors, such as poor nutrition, that lead to early labor and birth. Approximately half of all preterm births occur for unknown reasons.

One often-mentioned "cause" of premature births relates to intercourse during pregnancy. Contrary to popular belief, however, no scientific research has demonstrated that sexual activity during the later stages of pregnancy increases the risk of preterm labor (Sayle et al., 2001). A common misconception (pun not really intended) is that couples should avoid having intercourse during pregnancy, especially as the pregnancy progresses into the later months. However, research shows that sexual activity, including intercourse, throughout the duration of a normal pregnancy poses no risk to the developing fetus or to the mother. Sexual activity does not normally increase the chances of premature birth or birth defects, does not affect birth weight or birth length, and won't cause the uterine membranes to rupture (Bing, 2001; Gerszberg, 1998). In fact, sexual intercourse and orgasm for the woman late in pregnancy, even during the last two weeks, appear to be associated with *lower* rates of preterm deliveries (Brown, 2001). This does not hold true, however, if the woman has or contracts a sexually transmitted infection such as syphilis or chlamydia during pregnancy. These have been shown to relate to increased preterm labor and birth (Jancin, 2000).

Since YOU Asked...

6. My aunt's baby was born after only 25 weeks of her being pregnant. The baby is probably going to be OK, but will the baby have any problems later on?

None of this implies that the woman or the couple will necessarily feel like having intercourse in the later stages of pregnancy. Sexual desire varies a great deal among pregnant women and their partners. Some feel more sexual and more sexually desirous of their partners, while others feel that sex is the last thing on their mind. Clearly, some of the normal side effects of pregnancy, such as nausea, fatigue, and body changes, may interfere with sexual feelings for some pregnant women. Moreover, sometimes it is the woman's partner who is hesitant to engage in intercourse for fear of harming her or the baby, even though those risks are virtually nonexistent.

Couples who choose to have intercourse during pregnancy may need to experiment with various positions to accommodate the changes in the woman's body as the fetus and the woman's abdomen grow (see Chapter 6, "Sexual Behaviors," for more about various sexual positions). Finally, as you read so often throughout this book, sexual intimacy and satisfaction need not involve sexual intercourse, at least not all the time. Many pregnant women and couples find that they are able to fulfill their sexual needs through other intimate and satisfying activities such as oral sex and mutual masturbation if they choose to avoid vaginal penetration during pregnancy but still desire sexual closeness and sexual release.

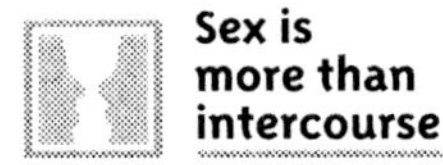
Sex is more than intercourse

Fetal Abnormalities (Birth Defects)

One of the worst fears prospective parents face is that their baby will be born with a condition commonly referred to as a **birth defect** (Cunniff, 2004). A birth defect is a physical abnormality or a dysfunction of metabolism (body chemistry) that is present at birth and results in physical or mental disability. Some birth defects may be serious enough to cause the death of the infant. Over 4,500 specific birth defects have been identified, and they are the second leading cause of infant mortality, after preterm birth ("March of Dimes Update," 2003). Fortunately, the actual odds of any these problems occurring are low, as you can see in Table 9.4. Moreover, testing of the fetus while in the uterus for various abnormalities is becoming ever safer and more accurate (Marcus, 2000). Early embryonic testing for genetic abnormalities will be discussed in greater detail later in this chapter.

birth defect A physical abnormality or metabolic dysfunction that is present at birth and may result in physical or mental deficits.

Table 9.4 INCIDENCE OF BIRTH DEFECTS

BIRTH DEFECT	ESTIMATED INCIDENCE
STRUCTURAL AND METABOLIC PROBLEMS	
Heart and circulation defects	1 in 115 births
Muscle and skeleton defects	1 in 130 births
Genital and urinary tract defects	1 in 135 births
Nervous system and eye defects	1 in 235 births
Chromosomal syndromes	1 in 600 births
Club foot	1 in 735 births
Down syndrome (mental retardation; physical abnormalities)	1 in 900 births
Respiratory tract defects	1 in 900 births
Cleft lip or palate	1 in 930 births
Rh disease (mismatched mother-fetus Rh factor)	1 in 1,400 births
Spina bifida (defect in spinal vertebrae)	1 in 2,000 births
Metabolic disorders	1 in 3,500 births
Anencephaly (lack of brain matter)	1 in 8,000 births
PKU (absence of a digestive enzyme)	1 in 12,000 births
CONGENITAL (PRESENT AT BIRTH) PROBLEMS	
Fetal alcohol syndrome	1 in 1,000 births
Congenital syphilis	1 in 2,000 births
Congenital HIV infection	1 in 2,700 births
Congenital rubella ("German measles") syndrome	1 in 100,000 births

Source: Adapted from March of Dimes Perinatal Data Center (2004).

Teratogens

The developing fetus needs a safe, natural, toxin-free environment in the uterus to have the best chance of developing into a normal, healthy baby. To accomplish this, the pregnant woman must be careful to avoid putting or allowing any substance into her body that may cross through the placenta into the fetus and cause complications in its physical development. Any outside agent, whether it is a drug, a microbe, a chemical, or radiation, that has the potential to cause a fetal abnormality is called a **teratogen**. Teratogens can be ingested by a pregnant woman by any means, including eating, smoking, or injecting. The Food and Drug Administration (FDA) has developed a coding system for over-the-counter and prescription drugs to rate their safety during pregnancy. It uses the codes A (safest), B, C, D, and X (most harmful) to indicate the danger of a substance to a fetus. Various teratogens are more or less harmful, depending on the timing of exposure during the nine months of pregnancy. As a rule, a woman who is pregnant should not take any drug or medication without first consulting her doctor.

Embryonic and Fetal Testing

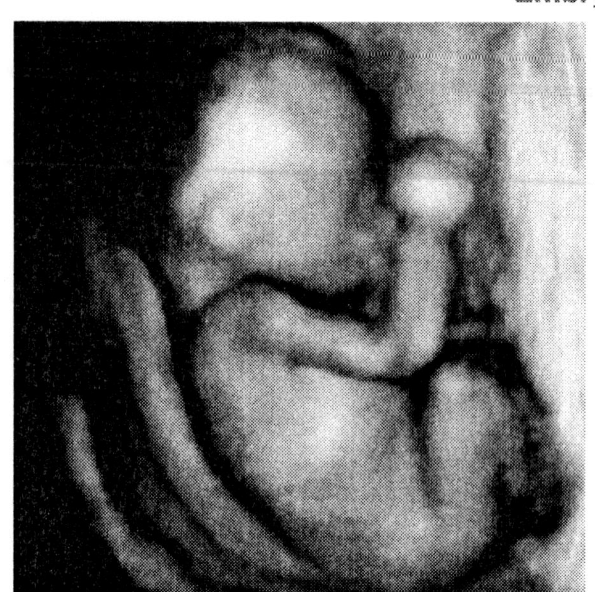

FIGURE 9.12 Three-Dimensional Sonogram of a Fetus in the Uterus

Ultrasonic visualization of the fetus inside the uterus lets doctors and parents monitor the progression of pregnancy and can alert them to the presence of any birth defects.

Several prenatal tests for some birth defects are used fairly widely, and medical science's ability to screen for genetic or physical defects of the embryo or fetus has been growing rapidly (Cunniff, 2004; Harmon, 2004). Moreover, many of these tests can now be carried out far earlier in pregnancy than was previously possible, often within the first 8 to 12 weeks. Blood tests performed on the expectant mother measure levels of proteins and hormones that can predict an increased risk of some disorders such as *spina bifida* (a neural tube defect in which the spinal column fails to close completely during fetal development), and *Down syndrome* (a chromosomal condition characterized by some degree of mental retardation, often combined with specific physical and medical problems such as small stature, lowered resistance to infection, vision and hearing difficulties, and in some, heart defects that are usually correctable). However, blood tests can have a high false-positive rate that often adds unnecessarily to stress and worry for the parents. Today, ultrasound, three-dimensional ultrasound, and magnetic resonance imaging (MRI) exams allow parents and health professionals actually to see the fetus in the uterus (as shown in Figure 9.12) and assist greatly in diagnosing fetal abnormalities earlier and with greater accuracy (Finn, 2004). These safe, noninvasive exams may be performed as early as the twelfth week of pregnancy and can assist greatly in diagnosing or ruling out various fetal abnormalities with far fewer errors than blood tests.

Amniocentesis and *chorionic villus sampling* (CVS) are invasive tests that require the extraction of a small amount of fluid from the sac surrounding the fetus (in amniocentesis) or a sample of placental tissue (in CVS). The cells in these substances contain the full genetic code for the fetus and can be used to diagnose many genetic abnormalities such as Down syndrome, cystic fibrosis, hydrocephalus (fluid pressure in the skull), sickle cell anemia, and hemophilia (O'Shea, 1995).

Amniocentesis requires that a long needle guided by ultrasound be inserted into the uterus through the abdomen (see Figure 9.13), and CVS uses a small tube inserted through the cervix or a thin needle passed through the abdominal skin. Although most women report only minor discomfort from these procedures, the disruption to the uterine balance carries a slight increased risk of miscarriage.

teratogen Any agent that has the potential to cause a fetal abnormality.

Therefore, these tests are usually reserved for women at higher risk of pregnancy complications and must be considered carefully in consultation with their doctor. Typically, one of these tests will be recommended for pregnant women over 30 because the risk of all birth defects, and especially Down syndrome, increases with maternal age. In addition, if other risk factors are present, such as a family history of abnormalities or exposure to environmental toxins, these genetic tests are more likely to be prescribed.

All of these prenatal tests allow parents to better prepare and plan for an infant that may be born with a serious abnormality or to make an informed decision to terminate the pregnancy, if they so choose. The most frequent outcome of prenatal testing, however, is the relief and peace of mind that come with knowing that the development of their baby will be normal and healthy (Marcus, 2000).

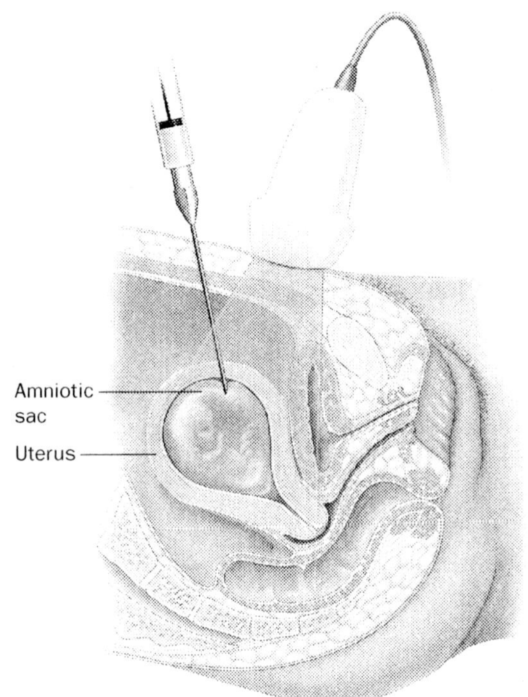

FIGURE 9.13 Amniocentesis Procedure

During amniocentesis, fluid from the sac surrounding the fetus is extracted and tested for genetic abnormalities.

Abortion

We discuss abortion at this point in the text because it is one of the many problems that may occur for some women or couples during pregnancy. As you learned earlier in the chapter, termination of a pregnancy from natural causes prior to the twentieth week of pregnancy is referred to as a *spontaneous abortion* or *miscarriage*; after twenty weeks, it is referred to as a *preterm birth*. However, spontaneous abortions are clearly distinguished from our everyday understanding of the meaning of **abortion**, which is the *voluntary* termination of a pregnancy, or an *induced abortion*. Although induced abortions are often unrelated to physical health problems of the embryo or the mother, it is an important and common event that must be included in our examination of conception and pregnancy. Over 850,000 legal abortions are performed in the United States each year, and one pregnancy in every five ends in voluntary abortion (Finer & Henshaw, 2003).

The debate over induced abortion is, and has been for decades, one of the most polarizing controversies in the United States and elsewhere in the world. The two sides of this controversy in the United States are summarized in "Sexuality, Ethics, and the Law: The Abortion Controversy." Beyond this impassioned debate, however, various issues relating to abortion are important to discuss briefly here. These topics include how abortions are performed; the possible psychological and emotional effects on the woman, and often on the father as well; how and when the choice is made to end a pregnancy; and suggested strategies to reduce the number of abortions, a goal on which people on both sides of the controversy can agree.

Abortion Procedures

The options available to a woman for choosing to terminate her pregnancy decrease as the time since conception increases. In general, a decision to abort in the first 8 weeks of pregnancy offers the woman the greatest number of choices of methods and carries the lowest risk of complications. That said, however, termination of a pregnancy may also be performed after 8 weeks and at any time during the first two trimesters (the first 24 weeks of pregnancy) with relatively little risk of serious complications for the woman (Cates & Ellertson, 1998). The two types of procedures for terminating a pregnancy are surgical abortions and medical abortions.

abortion Termination of a pregnancy before week 37; in common usage, assumed to be the result of an intentional act as opposed to a miscarriage.

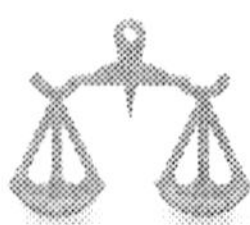

Sexuality, Ethics, and the Law

The Abortion Controversy

In the United States and elsewhere, intense debate and even violence surround the issue of abortion. Some people are ambivalent, unsure, or stake out some middle ground about abortion. But most fall fairly clearly into one of two camps, commonly referred to as **pro-choice** (those who believe that a woman has the moral and legal right to chose to abort her pregnancy) and **pro-life** (those who are morally opposed to abortion, believe it is akin to murder, and hold that it should be made illegal). Here is a summary of the central ideological points of these two sides of the abortion issue.

The Pro-Life Position

- Pro-life ideology is based on the belief that human life begins at the moment of conception and that the embryo or fetus, from conception to full gestational term, has the same inalienable right to survival as any other human.
- The pro-life position tends to encompass more than an antiabortion position; many of those who believe in basic pro-life principles also tend to oppose assisted suicide and stem cell research but, paradoxically, tend to favor capital punishment.
- While those adhering to a pro-life position may do so for many reasons, most pro-life individuals have a strongly Christian religious orientation (they are sometimes referred to as "fundamentalist" or "evangelical" Christians); many claim that the basic assumptions of the pro-life movement are based on Christian ideology.
- Some people within the pro-life movement allow for little, if any, gray area in the debate. They hold that any and all abortions are wrong, immoral, and tantamount to murder. This often includes the abortion of pregnancies caused by rape or incest and pregnancies that may have medical complications that threaten the life of the mother. Others, however, who consider themselves to believe strongly in pro-life principles are willing to make exceptions in some of these cases.

The Pro-Choice Position

- Pro-choice ideology is centered on the belief that a woman has the right to control her own body and reproductive life.
- Pro-choice individuals are not proabortion per se; that is, they do not *want* pregnant women to have abortions. Rather, they believe in the right of every woman to make an educated decision about her reproductive rights and responsibilities and to do so in consultation with her partner, family, or doctor, if she so chooses.
- Some of the gray area within the pro-choice movement relates to the father's degree of responsibility for the decision to abort a pregnancy and his moral and legal duty to support a child born of a pregnancy he would have chosen to abort. Pro-choice advocates tend to be more liberal politically in general and may also support assisted suicide legislation and stem cell research. They also tend to oppose the death penalty.
- Another controversial aspect of the pro-choice movement is the topic of late-term abortions (referred to by the pro-life movement as "partial-birth abortions"). Some disagreement exists within the pro-choice movement regarding the ethics of these late-term abortions unless the health or life of the mother is at stake.

Note: Research assistance: La Sara W. Firefox, New College, Santa Rosa, California.

pro-life The belief that voluntary abortion is akin to murder, and that it should be illegal.

pro-choice The belief that a woman has the moral and legal right to choose freely to abort her pregnancy.

Surgical Abortions

Until the late 1990s, virtually all abortions performed in the United States used surgical procedures, and nearly all of those used a technique called **vacuum aspiration** (see Figure 9.14). Today, most early surgical abortions (usually defined as within the first 12 weeks of pregnancy) use a process called *manual vacuum aspiration* (MVA). This technique incorporates a syringe device that is operated by hand or a small hand-

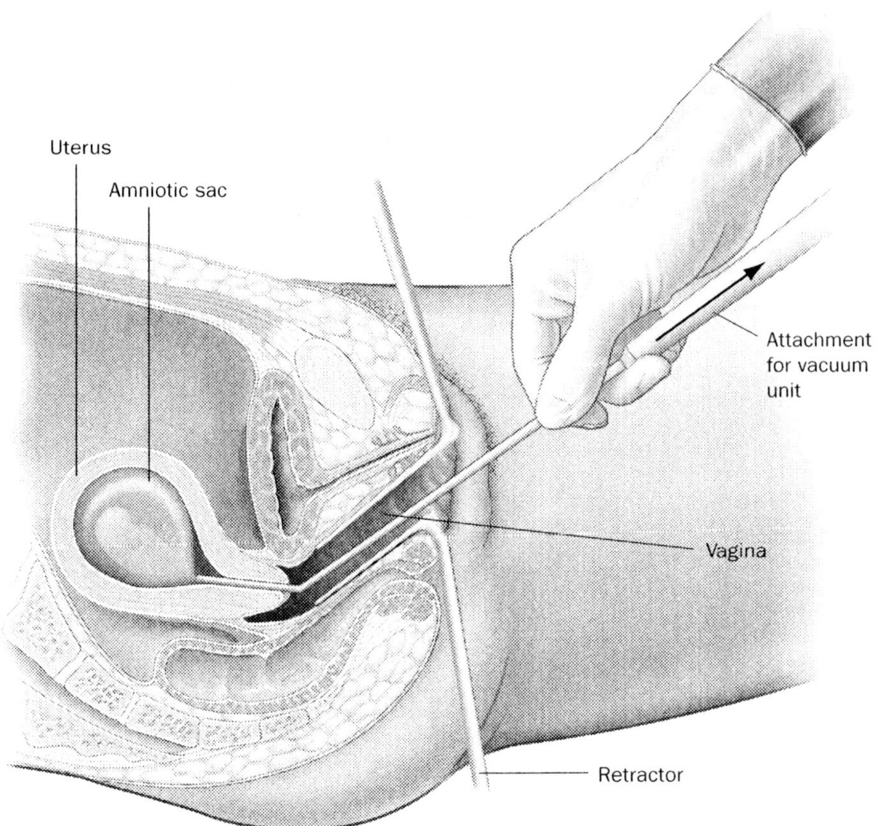

FIGURE 9.14 Vacuum Aspiration Procedure

In vacuum aspiration, the most common abortion technique for early pregnancies, a small tube is inserted through the cervix. Suction is then applied to the tube, creating a slight vacuum effect that draws out the contents of the uterus, including the uterine lining and the embryo.

held electrical vacuum device. Both vacuum methods have been shown to be equally safe and effective (Todd et al., 2003). Vacuum aspiration, as the term implies, incorporates a small tube that is inserted through the cervix to which suction is applied, creating a slight vacuum that draws out the contents of the uterus, including the endometrium lining and the embedded embryo. The procedure takes 5 to 15 minutes and, where abortion is legal, is typically performed in a doctor's office or medical clinic under local anesthetic. Usually, over-the-counter pain relievers (such as ibuprofen) are adequate for postsurgical pain and cramping. Normal side effects of the procedure include abdominal cramping and usually some bleeding. Serious complications are rare and may include perforation of the uterine wall or infection (Cates & Ellertson, 1998; Hollander, 2003; Reproductive Health Technologies Project, 2005).

If pregnancy has progressed beyond the first trimester, the usual termination procedure is **dilation and evacuation**, commonly called **D&E** (see Cates & Ellertson, 1998; Reproductive Health Technologies Project, 2005; WebMD, 2002). D&E is a more invasive and extensive procedure than MVA, largely because by the second trimester (13 to 26 weeks), the pregnancy is more firmly established and the developing fetus in the uterus is larger. The procedure therefore typically requires greater dilation of the cervix than a first-trimester abortion. Prior to the procedure, the woman is usually given sedatives and a local or general anesthetic. Then the cervix is dilated so that a vacuum tube may be inserted to remove the fetus and most of the remaining contents of the uterus. Next, a curved surgical instrument called a *curette* is inserted to scrape the lining of the uterus to free any additional tissue. Finally, suction may be applied to be sure the uterus has been fully emptied.

A D&E is typically performed as "day surgery" in a hospital setting. A woman should expect to experience cramping for several hours to several days and bleeding

vacuum aspiration A method of abortion in which a small tube is inserted through the cervix to extract the contents of the uterus, including the endometrium lining and embedded embryo.

dilation and evacuation (D&E) A method of abortion commonly used when a pregnancy has progressed beyond the first trimester, involving scraping of the uterine walls and suctioning out of the contents.

for about two weeks following the procedure. Postsurgical pain is usually relieved with over-the-counter medication such as acetaminophen or ibuprofen. Rare but serious complications of this procedure may include damage to the uterine wall, severe bleeding (hemorrhaging), and infection.

Surgical abortion, since becoming legal in the United States in 1973, is considered quite safe (Cates, Grimes, & Schulz, 2003), with risks to the health and life of the mother significantly lower than the risks of pregnancy and giving birth. However, in countries where abortion is illegal, abortion is often one of the the leading causes of maternal deaths (Berer, 2002). This was also true in the United States before the legalization of abortion.

Both MVA and D&E are highly effective methods of terminating pregnancy. Studies have shown that the long-term effects on the mother's fertility from a single abortion performed during the first trimester of pregnancy has little effect on the woman's future ability to become pregnant and give birth (Cates & Ellertson, 1998). However, the effects of later-term abortions or of multiple abortions on future fertility and pregnancy have yet to be evaluated in scientific studies. One study of 96 women who had undergone D&E procedures during their second trimesters of a past pregnancy found future preterm births or future first-term miscarriages among these women to be no more frequent than the average for pregnant women overall (Chasen et al., 2003).

Medical Abortions

Today, a clear trend can be seen away from surgical abortions for early pregnancies and toward medical methods of terminating pregnancy. A **medical abortion** relies on specifically targeted drugs to terminate a pregnancy rather than surgical procedures. As this text goes to press, the frontline medications used in abortions are either *mifepristone* (brand name, Mifeprex; formerly referred to as RU-486) or *methotrexate* combined with *misoprostol* (a synthetic form of the hormone *prostaglandin*). Here's how a medical abortion works (Creinin et al., 2003; Foubister, 2000; Schaff & Mawson, 2001).

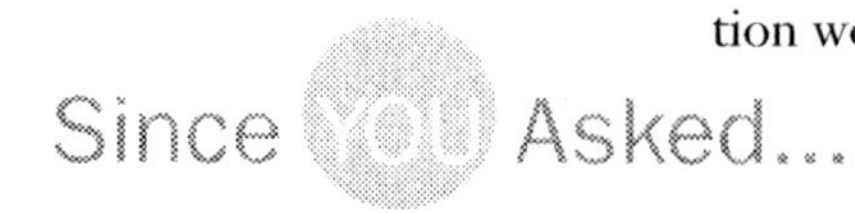

7. I heard that there's a pill a woman can take to have an abortion. What's that about?

When a woman chooses to have a medical abortion, the doctor administers either mifepristone or methotrexate to the pregnant woman during an office visit. Mifepristone is administered as one to three pills; methotrexate is usually delivered by injection into the muscle of the upper arm. After two or three days, the woman returns to the doctor for a single dose of misoprostol in pill form that can either be swallowed or inserted into the vagina. This combination of medications causes the uterus to contract, the embryo to detach from the uterine wall, and the cervix to soften somewhat to allow the contents of the uterus to be expelled (Creinin et al., 2003; Foubister, 2000; Knowles & Dimitrov, 2002; Schaff & Mawson, 2001). The woman must then return to the doctor at least once more to confirm that the abortion process has been completed. Both combinations of medications appear to be equally effective and have about the same rate and profile of typical side effects (Hollander, 2002). About 5 percent of medical abortions will either fail to abort or will partially abort. In those cases, a surgical abortion must then be performed.

The most common negative side effects of medical abortions are cramping and bleeding. Usually, more vaginal bleeding will occur following a medical abortion than a surgical one, as the uterus contracts and passes the embryo and other uterine contents through the cervix. Typically, blood clots will be passed during the abortive process, but at the time these abortions are carried out, the embryo is usually still too small to be seen. Most women will be unaware exactly when it has been expelled. A smaller percentage of women report additional side effects, including headache, nausea, and diarrhea (Knowles & Dimitrov, 2002).

medical abortion A method of abortion using drugs rather than surgery to terminate a pregnancy.

Surgical or Medical Abortion: Pros and Cons

If a woman has chosen to have an abortion, she will need to decide which method she prefers. This decision should be made in consultation with her partner (if appropriate) and with her health care provider. Her choice may be based on many factors, such as the time since conception, possible side effects of the procedure, and her own emotional and psychological preferences. Table 9.5 summarizes the pros and cons for surgical versus medical abortions.

The Psychological and Emotional Experience of Abortion

Some people mistakenly believe that a woman's decision to terminate her pregnancy is a relatively easy, uncaring, or detached decision. Yet most women who have chosen to have an abortion rarely describe the experience in such terms. Most are conflicted about the decision and may experience complex, painful, and confusing emotional reactions about the unwanted pregnancy and their decision to terminate it (Kero et al., 2001).

That said, fewer than 1 percent of all women who choose to have an abortion suffer from severe short- or long-term negative psychological outcomes afterward. The

Table 9.5 PROS AND CONS OF MEDICAL AND SURGICAL ABORTION METHODS

MEDICAL ABORTION	SURGICAL ABORTION
PROS	
High success rate (greater than 95%)	High success rate (99%)
Allows woman more control over abortion process	Available early and later in pregnancy
Seems more natural to some women, similar to a heavy period	Usually requires only one visit to doctor, hospital, or clinic
May be less emotionally painful than surgery for some women	Does not necessarily require follow-up doctor visits (although usually recommended)
Avoids invasive procedure and anesthesia	Requires less involvement by woman; may choose general anesthesia
Affords more privacy; much of process occurs at home	More certainty and less doubt about abortion outcome
Little to no risk of physical injury	Typically shorter duration of cramping following procedure
	Procedure typically completed in a single day (usually less than 15 minutes)
CONS	
Available only during first trimester of pregnancy	Allows for less sense of control by woman over the abortion process
Requires at least two or possibly more doctor visits	Involves an invasive procedure, sedation, or general anesthesia
Requires follow-up to ensure abortion is complete	Less natural-feeling, similar to any surgical procedure
Requires woman's active involvement and participation in abortion process (may be seen as a plus by some women)	Sometimes greater sense of grief and loss follows the procedure
Can take days to weeks to complete the abortion process	Slight risk of injury or infection during or following the procedure
Less certainty that abortion is occurring properly and fully	Possible distress caused by the noise of the electrical vacuum aspirator (manual aspirators are quiet)
Typically more cramping during and following procedure	May be inappropriate for women with allergies to anesthesia or serious anemia
Usually more bleeding following procedure	
Possible sight of blood clots and fetal tissue being expelled	
Not appropriate for women with certain medical conditions such as anemia or liver disease	

Sources: Cates and Ellerston, 1998; Healthwise, 2004; Hollander, 2000; and PregnancyOptions.info (2004).

primary emotion reported by most women after having an abortion is relief, but some may also experience feelings of guilt, shame, sadness, and concern over judgment from others, including isolation and feeling as if they cannot discuss their decision with anyone (Adler et al., 1990; Arthur, 1997; Veseley, 2002). If you stop to think about it, undergoing an abortion is not something many women choose to discuss with many others in their lives. They recognize the variety of opinions people hold on the subject and that they risk being judged for becoming pregnant, for not taking proper precautions, or for choosing to abort. Some evidence suggests that antiabortion opinions are actually making women who opt for abortion feel more ostracized and isolated than ever before (Russo & Dabul, 1997). As the president of the National Coalition of Abortion Providers once remarked about women's postabortion experiences, "Feelings of isolation are almost universal. There's no Hallmark card for abortion. No one is bringing over a casserole" (quoted in Veseley, 2002).

Opponents of abortion have suggested the existence of a "postabortion stress syndrome" involving extreme negative aftereffects of abortion similar to postpartum depression and posttraumatic stress disorder (Lopez, 1999). However, social-scientific research has failed to find evidence of such a disorder (Adler et al., 1990; Major et al., 2000; Pope, Adler, & Tschann, 2001; Russo & Dabul, 1997). Numerous studies have determined that no such syndrome exists and that the best predictor of postabortion emotional adjustment is the level of the woman's adjustment in life *before* the pregnancy occurred.

Most mental health professionals today agree that when a woman is considering her options for dealing with an unwanted pregnancy, doctors, clinicians, and pregnancy counselors should attempt to provide her with nonjudgmental and empathetic support. Doctors and nurses should offer referrals to a patient for psychological or religious counseling services if they suspect she is having difficulty with the emotional effects of her decision to abort her pregnancy. She should be given as much information about *all* her pregnancy options (keeping the baby, adoption, abortion) as she personally needs and wants, to enable her to make as informed and educated a decision as possible. She should be encouraged to discuss her feelings about the pregnancy, the potential of becoming a parent or bringing a new child into the family, her ability and desire to provide for a child, and her attitudes about abortion and adoption. The medical or counseling setting should be open to discussing issues relating to the father of the baby, and if the woman wishes, he should be allowed to participate in the decision process and the termination of the pregnancy if that is what the woman ultimately decides to do. And after an abortion has occurred, attention must be placed on *nonjudgmental* postabortion support and counseling for those who may experience negative reactions following the decision to terminate pregnancy.

Reducing the Number of Abortions

Perhaps the single area of agreement between the pro-choice and pro-life factions of the abortion debate is the desire to reduce the number of abortions performed each year. The route to this goal, however, often leads to further disagreements. Pro-life advocates endeavor to limit the *availability* of abortions by making them illegal and at times engaging in tactics that frighten, intimidate, or even physically harm individuals who seek or perform abortions. Since abortions were legalized in 1973 in the famous U.S. Supreme Court decision in *Roe* v. *Wade*, numerous legal attempts have been undertaken to overturn the Court's decision and, as was the case prior to 1973, allow states to make their own laws about abortion. To date, virtually all of these attempts to override *Roe* v. *Wade* at the federal level have failed. However, in light of the conservative bent of the justices appointed to the Court by President George W. Bush in 2005, some legal scholars predict that the protection of legal abortion is at risk for being weakened or overturned. Many sexuality counselors, educators, and clinicians find this prospect distressing because, based on past experience in the United States and conditions in countries where abortion is a crime, making abortion illegal does not prevent abortion but rather drives it underground or to other countries, where the procedures are often far more dangerous and even potentially fatal for the mother. For a look at attempts in Russia to reduce the number of abortions, see "Sexuality and Culture: Russia's Legacy of Abortion."

Whether or not abortion will once again become illegal in the parts of the United States, one alternate route to reducing abortions is to decrease the number of unwanted pregnancies. To do that, efforts must be increased to educate people about making effective and safe choices about their sexual behaviors and to develop and encourage the effectiveness and consistent use of birth control (see Chapter 5, "Contraception"). Research has demonstrated a direct link in many countries between increased use of contraception and decreases in abortion rates (Marston & Cleland, 2003; Rahman, Da Vanzo, & Razzaque, 2001).

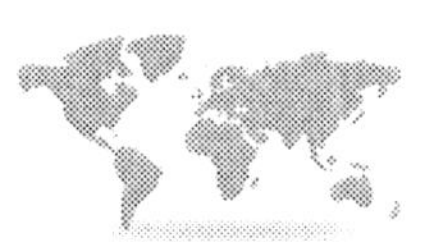

Sexuality and Culture

Russia's Legacy of Abortion

The widespread practice and acceptance of abortions throughout Russia is the leading cause of the former Soviet republic's plummeting population. During the 1990s, only three countries had higher abortion rates than Russia, and as of 1994, Russian women had undergone an average of three abortions each (La Franiere, 2003). By 2003, an estimated 1.3 abortions were performed in Russia for every live birth (Parfitt, 2003). The large number of abortions performed each year in Russia has taken a toll on the population not only through terminated pregnancies but also due to infertility caused by poor surgical care for women seeking abortions. An estimated 13 percent of Russian married couples are infertile, and of these, 75 percent of the infertility is directly attributable to the woman partner, usually due to problems arising from past abortions.

Russian views on sex and pregnancy are mixed. Although expectant single mothers receive state benefits and children born to unwed mothers are not discriminated against, sexual topics are rarely discussed either at home or in schools. Inga Grebesheva, the director of the Russian Family Planning Foundation, joked, "We've had abortions but not sex. . . . We were not supposed to talk about it. Everyone would watch sex on TV with pleasure, but to talk about it would be bad manners" (La Franiere, 2003). This lack of sexual education has played a major role in the large numbers of unwanted pregnancies and abortions in Russia.

Various events in Russian history have also influenced the current problem of abortion and unintended pregnancies there. Abortions were readily available in Russia long before modern contraceptives, and the practice was legalized during the Russian famine of 1920. Then, in 1936, as part of an effort to expand the Soviet Union's future workforce, Stalin banned abortion (Parfitt, 2003). In 1955, two years after Stalin's death, legal abortions were reinstated; however, information regarding contraceptives was intentionally withheld from the public until after the fall of the Soviet Union in the early 1990s.

Today, the Russian government is making an effort to limit legal abortions, though access to contraceptives remains limited. Government-financed family planning clinics, created in 1993, lost their funding in 1998 when, under pressure from pro-life political groups, the Russian parliament ended the program's funding. In addition, the Russian Orthodox church has routinely used its influence to impede public access to birth control (La Franiere, 2003).

In spite of these pressures, Russia is making some progress. An organization called Healthy Russia (www.healthyrussia.ru), in partnership with Western medical institutes such as Johns Hopkins University, is attempting to raise awareness concerning sexual health in Russia. Despite some successes, Healthy Russia and similar organizations are fighting an uphill battle. In the face of government and religious opposition, combined with the Russian cultural hesitance to discuss sexual matters, these groups face difficult challenges in attempting to change the Russian tradition of apathy and misinformation about abortion. But the battle is worth the effort. The physical well-being of mothers-to-be and the fertility of future couples depend on Russia's success in raising sexual awareness.

The United States is making progress in increasing the use of birth control and reducing abortions. The overall number of abortions has been decreasing in the late 1990s and 2000s (Herndon et al., 2002; "Induced abortion," 2005). New methods of contraception, including the increasing availability without a prescription of *emergency contraception* (commonly known as the "morning-after pill") will likely assist in preventing unwanted pregnancies and consequently reducing abortions. In 2000–2001 alone, emergency contraception availability decreased the number of abortions by an estimated 51,000 (Jones, Darroch, & Henshaw, 2002). These developments give us cause to be optimistic, and if current trends continue, the number of abortions will decline even more in the future.

Birth

Exactly what triggers the beginning of labor and the birth process in humans is not fully understood. We do know that under normal pregnancy conditions, changes occur in the uterus and especially in the placenta at about 40 weeks of gestation, typically just before the onset of labor, signaling the mother's brain to increase production of various chemicals and hormones including estrogen, steroids, prostaglandin, and a chemical called *corticotropin-releasing hormone* (Bainbridge, 2003). Corticotropin-releasing hormone is produced naturally in the human body and is related to our physical responses to stress. However, it is also intimately linked to the beginning of childbirth and may signal the uterus to begin contractions (Grammatopoulos & Hillhouse, 1999). The amazing aspect of all this is that the woman's body "knows" the right time to produce these physical changes in almost all births—not too early and not too late—to provide for the best chance of survival for the infant.

Labor

The various chemical changes cause an unmistakable biological signal to the baby and the mother that it is time for them to meet "face to face." The first sign of labor is usually the pain of a contraction indicating that the uterus is beginning the process of expelling the fetus. Women may also experience some blood from the vagina, called "the show," as the cervical "plug" of mucus and blood is expelled. Some women may experience a heavy flow of clear liquid (referred to as her "water breaking") as the amniotic sac containing the fetus ruptures and the fluid flows from the uterus, through the cervix, and out the vagina (Guattery, 2002). Water breaking does not necessarily imply that labor has begun, but it usually signifies that the birthing process will begin soon.

Stage One Labor

At the onset of labor, called **stage one labor**, contractions begin as the cells of the uterus, now the largest muscle in the mother's body, contract in sequence along its length, pulling and straightening the uterus and pushing the fetus down toward the cervix (see Figure 9.15a). At this point, the cervical canal is closed, but it will begin to dilate or "soften" as pressure is applied by repeated contractions of the uterus and the downward movement of the infant (Bainbridge, 2003).

As the contractions come more rapidly, the cervix begins to dilate, and the top of the baby's head will soon become visible (see Figure 9.15b). Typically, the baby's head will be facing the mother's spine, turned slightly to the left or right of the spinal column itself. This is the most common and best fetal position for moving through the birth canal, although not every infant follows the rules. A relatively small percentage

stage one labor The first stage of the birth process, involving the beginning of contractions of the uterus.

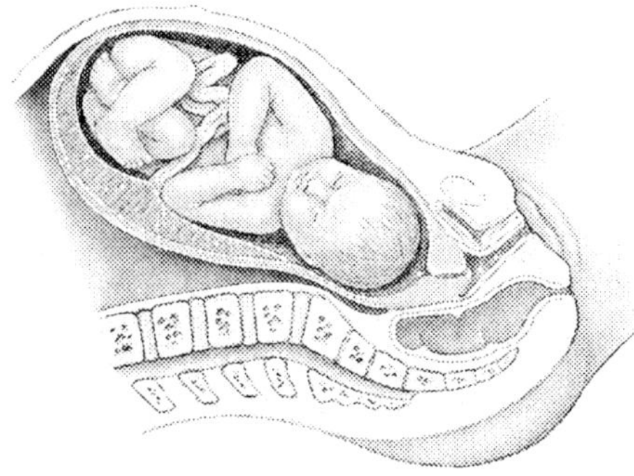

(a) Fully Developed Fetus Before Labor Begins

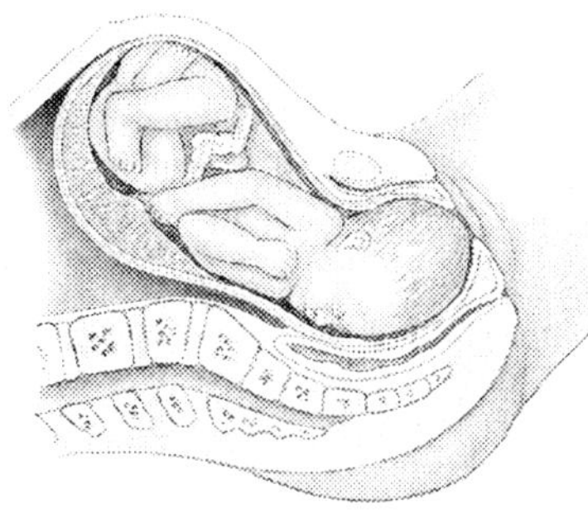

(b) Stage One Labor

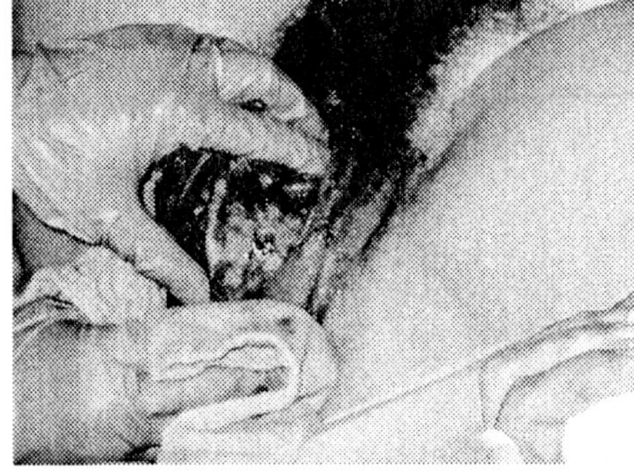

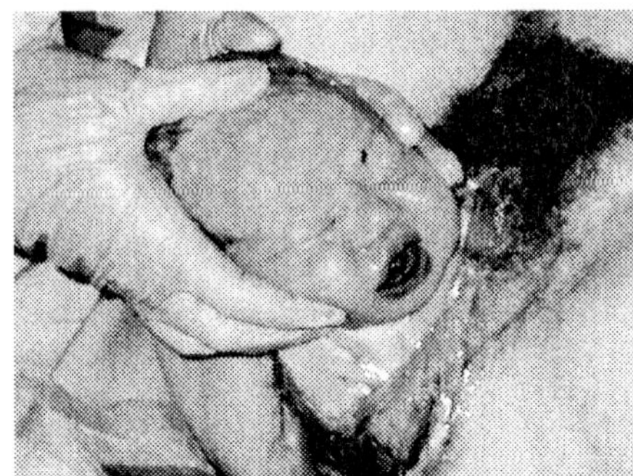

(c) Stage Two Labor

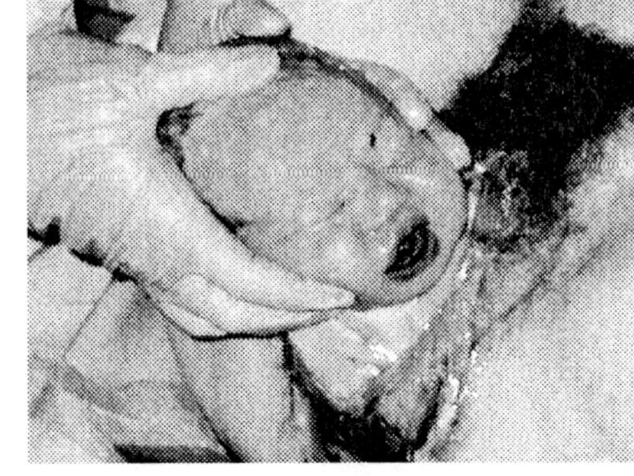

(d) Stage Three Labor

FIGURE 9.15 The Stages of Childbirth

Crowning of the baby's head (top) and delivery of the baby's head (bottom).

of infants present themselves for birth in various other positions such as bottom or leg first (called a **breech birth**; shown in Figure 9.16), face first, shoulder first, or forehead (brow) first (Wheeler, 1995).

The contractions continue, becoming increasingly frequent. This first stage of labor lasts, on average, about 12 hours for first-time mothers (although most women will tell you it *seems* considerably longer!) and closer to 8 hours for women who have previously given birth. Keep in mind, however, these are averages, and labor can in some cases proceed as quickly as a few hours or take longer than 20 hours, but these are exceptions rather than the rule (Wheeler, 1995). During the first stage of labor, the cervix will usually become "fully dilated," which is considered to be about 4 inches. At this point, the baby's head will "crown," meaning it is visible at the vaginal opening. Usually, during the entire delivery process, the infant's heart rate is electronically monitored for any signs of distress. This monitoring allows the doctor or midwife and the mother to know immediately if the infant is experiencing any major difficulties during the strenuous birth procedure; most often, it reassures everyone that all is well.

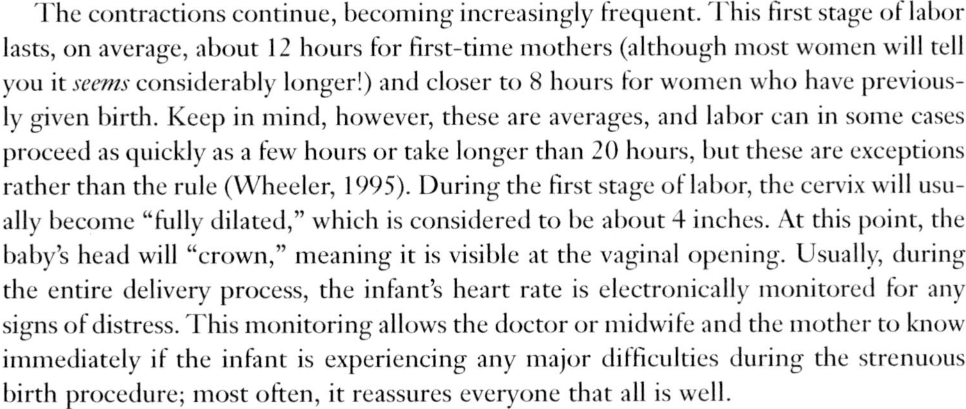

FIGURE 9.16 A Breech Birth

In a breech birth, the infant presents itself for birth in positions other than head-first, such as legs-first as shown here.

Stage Two Labor

In **stage two labor**, the contractions, in addition to occurring more often, begin to involve the muscles of the abdomen as well as the uterus itself. The mother has somewhat more control over these contractions, and many women report that this sense of control seems to reduce the amount of pain they are perceiving (Bainbridge, 2003). At this point, the woman will feel a great deal of abdominal pressure as her body is working to deliver her baby.

Typically, the woman now feels the need to become an active participant in the delivery process: to bear down and to push the baby out. With each contraction and each push, the infant rocks back and forth and inches slowly along until the head is ready to emerge from the vagina. The passage of the head is typically the most painful moment of the birth process, and once that is completed, the rest of the baby usually

breech birth Delivery of a fetus emerging with buttocks or legs first rather than head first.

stage two labor The stage of the birth process in which contractions occur closer together than in stage one, involve the muscles of the abdomen as well as the uterus, and continue until the infant has been expelled from the mother's body.

emerges with somewhat less difficulty. In the past, doctors at this stage would routinely perform an *episiotomy*, the surgical cutting of the perineum, the area between the vagina and the anus, presumed to expand the passageway for delivery. During the 1990s, however, this practice decreased dramatically, and today most medical professionals consider the routine episiotomy to offer no advantages and may even make various postpartum physical problems worse. Many researchers and health organizations have called for the routine use of episiotomies to be stopped (Hartmann et al., 2005; Wagner, 1999; A. D. Walling, 2000).

As stage two continues, the infant's head usually appears first (see Figure 9.15c), followed by one shoulder and then the other, and at that point, the baby emerges rather quickly—so fast, in fact, that the job of the doctor or midwife is often referred to as "catching" the baby. If you have the chance to see an actual birth, you will probably see exactly why this term is used. (To see an online video of a birth, visit http://www.med-help.net and click on OB/Childbirth.)

Following delivery, the umbilical cord is cut, and the newborn infant is immediately examined by the doctor, nurse, or midwife for any signs of difficulty. One widely used immediate assessment of a **neonate** (a newborn) is the **APGAR score**, developed by Dr. Virginia Apgar in 1953 and presented in Table 9.6. This test simply looks for the crucial signs of infant health with respect to skin color, heartbeat, reflexes, movement, and breathing (colleagues of Dr. Apgar assigned the acronym of her name to the test as a way of teaching it to medical and nursing students, the letters APGAR standing for appearance, pulse, grimace, activity, and respiration, respectively). As you can see in the table, the maximum score is 10 (which is fairly rare, because most newborns tend to be deficient in at least one area). However, most newborns will score between 7 and 9. You should be aware that this is a very basic test and, except for very low scores of under 4, does not predict the future health or abilities of the child. Furthermore, with today's advances in neonatal care, even babies with relatively low APGAR scores, such as between 4 and 6, typically develop well (Moster, Lie, & Markestad, 2002). One humorist has taken the APGAR one step further and developed an APGAR scoring system for fathers during delivery (H. Bennett, 1998). This is presented in Table 9.7.

neonate A newborn infant.

APGAR score A test that analyzes infant health at birth on the basis of skin color, pulse, reflexes, movement, and breathing.

Table 9.6 APGAR SCORES FOR NEWBORNS

QUALITY	SIGN	SCORE = 0	SCORE = 1	SCORE = 2	TOTAL FOR ITEM
Appearance	Color	Blue all over or pale	Acrocyanosis (blue and red patches on skin, sweating)	Pink all over	
Pulse	Heart rate	Absent	Below 100	Above 100	
Grimace	Reflex/irritability	No response	Grimace or weak cry	Good cry	
Activity	Muscle tone	Flaccid	Some flexing of extremities	Active flexing or movements of extremities	
Respiration	Respiratory effort	Absent	Weak, irregular, or gasping	Good, crying	

Score ranges: 7–10 Infant displays healthy, normal newborn responses.
4–6 Infant will need close watching and repeated APGAR evaluations.
0–3 Infant is in serious distress and its survival is in danger.

The APGAR score should be calculated at one minute and five minutes after delivery, finding the total score (0–10) each time by adding up the points in the table. Scores should be calculated every five minutes thereafter as long as the total score is less than 7.

Table 9.7 "APGAR SCORES" FOR NEW DADS

QUALITY	SIGN	SCORE = 0	SCORE = 1	SCORE = 2	TOTAL FOR ITEM
Appearance	Color	Ghostlike	Acrocyanosis: *body*: normal, *face*: pale or green	Normal all over	
Pulse	Heart rate	Greater than 200	Below 100	About 80	
Grimace	Reflex irritability (when asked to cut cord)	Faints	Hesitates; needs help	Feels confident	
Activity	Muscle tone	Bouncing off walls	Jumpy, extremities tightly flexed	Extremities normally flexed	
Respiration	Respiratory effort	Deep and very rapid	Panting	Regular	

- A score of 10 indicates that the dad is in excellent condition and will, in all likelihood, thank you profusely and donate large sums of money to your favorite charity.
- A score of 7 to 9 shows that the dad is still in pretty good shape and that at least a lawsuit is not very likely.
- A score of 4 to 6 indicates that the dad needs some medical attention. In many cases, this score results from his partner strangling him during a contraction. In other situations, a little oxygen should help tremendously. Another technique is a quick slap on the cheek accompanied by the statement, "Snap out of it, man, you're about to become a father!" Be careful about letting a dad with a score less than 7 cut the cord because he may snip off one of the nurses' (or his own) fingers instead.
- A score of 1 to 3 indicates that things are pretty dicey. Valium, smelling salts, and intravenous Coca-Cola have all been used successfully in this situation. In many cases, however, the best treatment is to prop up the dad in a recliner and turn on videos of situation comedies from the 1950s. After all, back then all dads (such as *I Love Lucy's* Ricky Ricardo) had to do was sit in the waiting room until their little bundle arrived, all clean and snug, in the nurse's loving arms.

APGAR scores for dads will help clinicians manage the one who is often the most neglected member of the family unit during delivery. Dads will appreciate the attention, and if the delivery room staff does a good job, the family might even name their pets after them.

Source: "'APGAR' Scores for New Dads" by H. Bennett in *British Medical Journal*, Vol. 317, p. 1712, (1998). Copyright © 1998. Reprinted by permission from the BMJ Publishing Group.

Stage Three Labor

In **stage three labor**, within a few minutes following the completed birth of the infant, the placenta is expelled from the uterus with the umbilical cord attached (see Figure 9.15d). The doctor or midwife will inspect the cord and both sides of the placenta to be sure that they are intact and that the placental tissue appears normal and show no signs that might indicate problems for the mother or the baby. A placental examination typically takes about a minute, and if any serious abnormalities are discovered, it is typically sent on for further pathological examination (Afriat & Coustan, 1995; Yetter, 1998). Abnormal placentas are rare.

Choices and Decisions in Childbirth

In Western cultures, giving birth was, in past decades, a passive activity, with expectant mothers heavily sedated (as described early in this chapter) and fathers, pockets stuffed with cigars, anxiously pacing in the hospital waiting room or even at work, waiting for a call from the hospital. In stark contrast, today the process of labor and delivery has become an active, shared event for most couples, especially in industrialized countries. Today, women and couples are not only deeply involved in their child's birth, but they are taking over a great deal of the control and decision making relating to labor and delivery (De Witt & Hamel, 1993; Hock, 2003).

Pregnant women and couples now often expect and demand detailed information, education, comfort, and various amenities to enhance the experience of birth itself. Parents, rather than health professionals, may be the ones to make decisions about medical procedures, such as when to shift course from a vaginal birth to a cesarean section, what type and how much pain medication the mother desires, whether an episiotomy should be performed, and whether their boy baby should be circumcised. In

stage three labor The final stage of the birth process, when the placenta is expelled from the uterus with the umbilical cord attached.

addition to the presence and participation of fathers in the delivery room, some parents are inviting even more people to attend their baby's birth, including family members such as grandparents, siblings, aunts, and uncles of the new infant and close friends. Let's take a brief look at some of the issues surrounding these various decisions.

Doctor or Midwife?

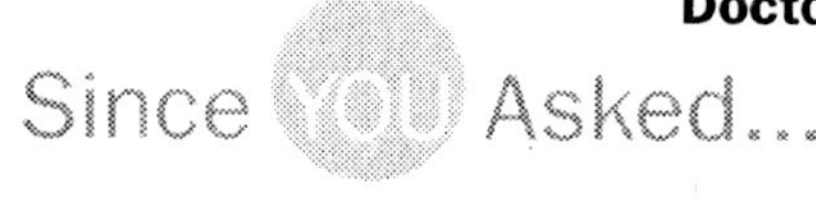

8. My sister wants to have a midwife deliver her baby. Is this dangerous compared to having a doctor handle the birth?

Women and couples may choose among several types of trained specialists to assist them in the actual process of delivery. Typically, the choices are a physician, usually an **OB/GYN** (obstetrician-gynecologist) or family practitioner; a **midwife**, usually a woman who has been trained in most aspects of pregnancy, labor, and delivery but is not a physician or registered nurse; or a **nurse-midwife** who is a registered nurse who also has completed an accredited midwifery program and has been certified by the state to become a certified nurse midwife, or CNM.

Both physicians and midwives may legally attend births in hospitals in most states, but in general, it is midwives who deliver babies in birthing centers and home births, and the popularity of midwife-assisted births appears to be on the rise ("More Episiotomies," 2004). For some deliveries, both a midwife and a physician may be present simultaneously. Research has found that births managed by physicians and by midwives do not differ in terms of delivery problems and complications, but patients sometimes report greater satisfaction with the care they receive from midwives after delivery (Turnbull et al., 1996). Of course these comparisons assume a normal, relatively uncomplicated delivery. Physicians are usually needed when complications arise that require medical intervention. One large study found that 32 percent of women in midwife-managed care were transferred to the care of a physician (Turnbull et al., 1996). On the other hand, women who give birth with midwives are significantly less likely to have an episiotomy, birth by cesarean section, or artificially induced labor ("Midwife-Assisted Deliveries," 1997).

Birthing Locations

In North America, delivery venues include hospitals, birthing centers, and home births. Most major hospitals have maternity services, and many women feel more comfortable knowing that a full range of medical care is immediately available should any problems arise during delivery. A hospital setting is especially recommended for women who have a history of medical problems during childbirth or who have medical issues with their current pregnancy (such as a predelivery decision that a cesarean section will be necessary, multiple births, diabetes, or a breech delivery). However, many hospital maternity departments today are not the sterile-looking, metal-and-plastic, impersonal places you might imagine. The "birthing business" has become very lucrative and competitive with the rise of birthing centers, so hospitals have been attempting to keep pace by offering private rooms decorated in ways that appear to be more from the pages of home decorating magazines than "hospital sterile," where the mother can stay for labor, delivery, and recovery without being shuttled from room to room. This has come to be called "one-stop birthing" (De Witt & Hamel,1993; Hock, 2003; Rogoznica, 1997).

In response to the demand for more personalized, parent-controlled childbirth, freestanding **birthing centers** are growing in number and popularity. Birthing centers are hospital-like facilities with basic medical care equipment that feature a homelike setting and have as their primary focus a natural family-centered approach to the birth process. These centers tend to promote midwife-tended births, typically have on-call physicians readily available, encourage less use of pain medications during labor and delivery (epidural and certain other medical analgesics are ordinarily not

OB/GYN Short for obstetrician-gynecologist, a physician specializing in women's health care and childbirth.

midwife A person (usually a woman) who has been trained in most aspects of pregnancy, labor, and delivery but who is not a physician or registered nurse.

nurse-midwife A registered nurse who has completed an accredited midwifery program and has been certified by the state to deliver babies.

birthing center A hospital-like facility with basic medical care equipment, focusing on a natural, family-centered approach to the birth process in a homelike setting.

available). Birthing centers offer more choices of food and drink (no alcohol, of course), more activities are permitted and even encouraged during labor (walking, stretching, etc.), and various comfort measures such as massage, relaxation exercises, and even warm tub soaks are available (Ural, 2001). Research has indicated that one in three pregnant women would choose a birthing center over a hospital and more than one in five would prefer a nurse or midwife for the delivery over a physician (Seymour, 2000).

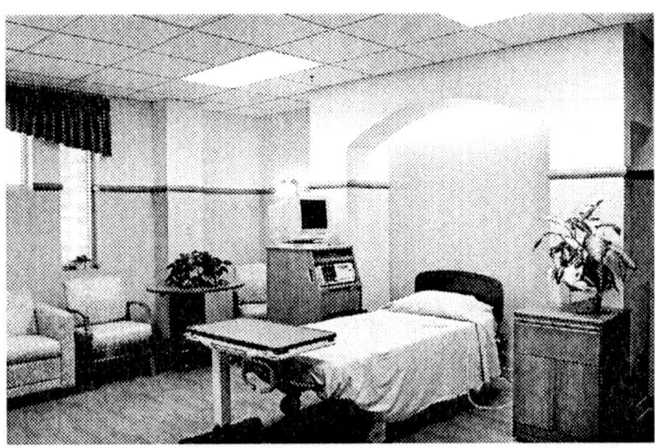

Many hospitals try to create a more comfortable, "homelike" birthing environment.

Another option that some prefer is **home birth**. This is not usually a "do it yourself" birthing process but rather involves the use of a home birth service that provides necessary equipment and personnel in the parents' home (Severns, 2000). A home birth resembles a delivery in a birthing center in that the materials that may be necessary for most normal births are present, including fetal monitors, oxygen, medications to slow bleeding, and sutures to repair tears or an episiotomy (if one is performed). A well-planned home birth requires backup plans, including prearranged transportation to a hospital and an on-call physician in case serious complications arise that may require medical attention beyond that available to the midwife in the home. The most important advantage of home birth is that it places the woman or couple in familiar surroundings where they feel more comfortable and in control of the birthing process (Harper, 2001).

Pain Medication during Labor and Delivery

In the recent past, women were placed under general anesthesia to ease the pain and trauma of childbirth. This, of course, also removed the mother from the psychological and emotional joy of seeing her baby come into the world and subjected the fetus, along with the mother, to potentially dangerous sedating effects of the drugs.

In the early 1950s, the French obstetrician Ferdinand Lamaze, on a trip to Russia, discovered a drug-free method of childbirth that used psychological techniques to allow women to limit the pain of childbirth and deliver babies naturally. When he brought the techniques back to Europe and the United States, they began to catch on. Here was a way for women to give birth not only fully conscious but also, if they chose, with no drugs at all, using special breathing exercises, visualization, massage, focused attention, and relaxation training, along with the help of a "coach" (husband or partner, friend, relative) to ease pain and increase the mother's comfort during labor and delivery.

Today, variations on the so-called Lamaze method are used by millions of women worldwide. Most women desire to be conscious, alert, and aware during the birth of their children. They want to be an active participant in giving birth, and they want to protect their baby from the negative effects of medications. Using techniques related to Lamaze's work, many women are able today to choose to make the journey through labor and birth with less or no pain medication.

However, many other women will tell you that "talk is cheap" and that the *idea* of childbirth without medication is much more attractive than actually enduring it. Fortunately, Lamaze never truly took a stand against pain medication; he simply felt that women should understand the available options and make an informed decision. One of the many decisions a woman or couple must make concerns the availability and type of pain medication during labor and delivery.

It is not at all unusual for a woman to plan on a medication-free, or "natural" childbirth but at some point in the emotionally intense, physically demanding, and painful birthing process desire a change in that plan. Many childbirth experts suggest that the expectant mother be given the *option* to receive pain medication during birth even if she fully intends to attempt an "all natural" birth.

home birth Delivery of an infant in a private home setting, usually with necessary equipment and personnel provided by a professional service.

Once the decision has been made to use pain medication or have it available during the birth process, the next consideration is the type of medication preferred. The most common pain medications in use today are *sedatives*, such as antianxiety medications; *local anesthesia*, numbing agents used in specific areas of the birth canal area; *regional anesthesia*, the numbing of the entire birth canal and pelvic area; and the *epidural*, currently the most popular method, in which pain-relieving medication is delivered "as needed" through a small tube inserted near the base of the woman's spine. These methods usually provide enough pain relief to allow the mother to deliver her baby with tolerable levels of pain and anxiety, leaving her free to participate in the birthing experience and keeping her awake, alert, and active enough to help push the baby out when the time comes to do so (Santos & Nicholson, 2002).

Birth by Cesarean Section

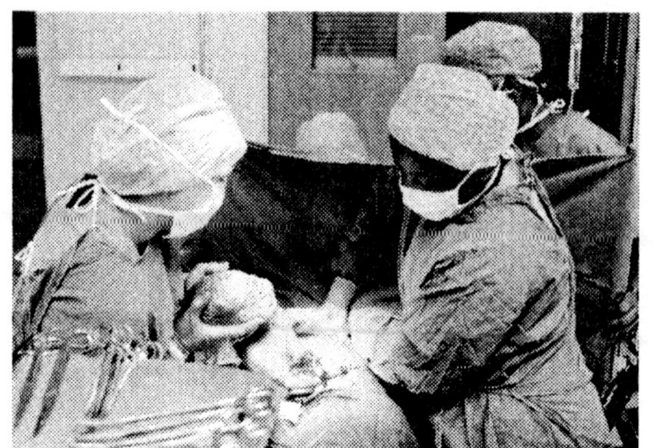

FIGURE 9.17 C-Section Birth

A Cesarean section is performed when medical complications prevent a vaginal delivery or, in some cases, if preferred by the mother.

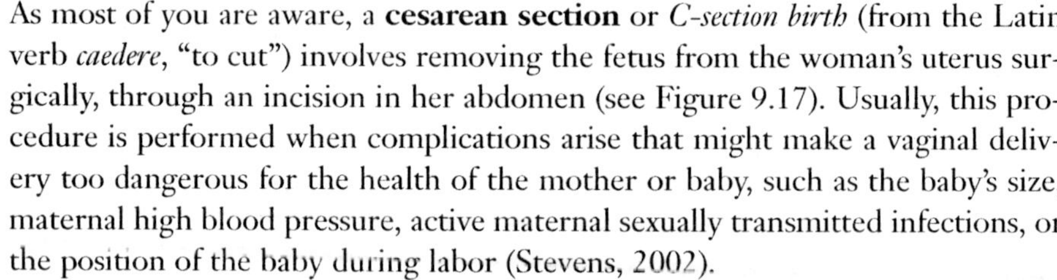

As most of you are aware, a **cesarean section** or *C-section birth* (from the Latin verb *caedere*, "to cut") involves removing the fetus from the woman's uterus surgically, through an incision in her abdomen (see Figure 9.17). Usually, this procedure is performed when complications arise that might make a vaginal delivery too dangerous for the health of the mother or baby, such as the baby's size, maternal high blood pressure, active maternal sexually transmitted infections, or the position of the baby during labor (Stevens, 2002).

However, in the United States and many other industrialized countries, the number of C-section births has been steadily rising over the past ten years or so, but the number of natural childbirth complications has not. In 2003, the U.S. cesarean birth rate reached its highest point in history, accounting for 27.6 percent of all births. Nearly a quarter of those C-sections were not medically necessary but were elected by the pregnant woman (Song et al., 2004). Why so many C-sections? Three possible reasons are currently being discussed in the birthing literature: (1) More mothers are choosing to have C-sections, (2) doctors are more willing to recommend them due to fears of malpractice litigation if any problems arise from a potentially complicated natural birth, and (3) the average age at which women give birth has risen significantly, increasing the possibility for complications that may lead to cesarean births.

Pregnant women are choosing to have C-section births (called "elective C-sections") for various reasons, including the desire to avoid labor and childbirth pain, the convenience of giving birth on a schedule set by the mother rather than by the baby, or simply as a matter of personal preference (Bouchez, 2001). In some countries, elective C-sections are even more common. In Brazil, for example, where C-sections account for 70 to 90 percent of all births, a commonly heard joke is that the only way a woman will have a vaginal delivery is if her doctor gets stuck in traffic (Finger, 2003; Sloan, 2005; Song et al., 2004). The medical community in the United States, however, is debating giving women this choice because many doctors consider an elective C-section unnecessary surgery, and avoiding unnecessary surgery is a basic tenet of the medical code promise to "do no harm." Other physicians disagree and believe it is clearly a woman's choice and may even encourage women to exercise their right to choose (Bouchez, 2001). Overall, the risks of a C-section delivery are greater than those of a vaginal delivery because a C-section is major abdominal surgery, requiring stronger anesthesia and carrying a higher risk of blood loss, infection, and damage to the reproductive tract. Moreover, C-section births require a longer recovery time. Nevertheless, the trend of pregnant women electing C-section deliveries is growing and may become one of the many routine choices of childbirth in the future.

cesarean section Removal of a fetus from the mother's uterus surgically, through an incision in her abdomen; also called a *C-section birth*.

The Challenges of Childbirth Choices

So many choices and decisions face prospective parents today! How do people cope with all that must be learned for a safe and personally satisfying birth process? A great deal of information is available from doctors, nurses, midwives, hospitals, and birthing centers, not to mention the hundreds of excellent Web sites on the Internet.

No two pregnancies are exactly alike, and perhaps the most important resource for women and couples about their very personal experience of childbirth is the comfort and trust they are able to establish with their doctor or midwife. Often that is the person who is in the best position to consult in the complex process of bringing a new life into the world. If a woman or couple does not feel that connection with their birth facilitator, they should not hesitate to obtain a referral to another who they feel better meets their needs.

Postpartum Issues

The delivery of a baby is, of course, only the first step in a lifetime of the challenges of parenting. Being an effective parent is a discussion that is well beyond the scope of this chapter and this book. Nevertheless, we should touch on a few issues that many parents face **postpartum**, that is, following the birth of a child. These include the very real and all-too-common problem of postpartum depression, the resumption of sexual activities following birth, and issues relating to the return of ovulation, fertility, and menstruation.

Postpartum Depression

After giving birth, some new mothers experience what are commonly referred to as the "baby blues," a normal, relatively mild depressed mood, usually stemming from the exhaustion from labor, hormonal shifts, the fatigue of nights with little and poor sleep, and the stress of a major lifestyle upheaval with addition of a new family member. While women often worry about these feelings of sadness, crying spells, and extra anxiety at a time when they feel they should be happy, the baby blues are short-lived and usually pass within a week or two at the most.

However, about 10 to 15 percent of new moms suffer from a much more serious problem called **postpartum depression (PPD)**. Postpartum depression is a clearly defined psychological disorder that begins within four weeks after childbirth and shares many of the symptoms of other forms of depression, such as deep sadness, emotional apathy, withdrawal from family and friends, loss of interest in favorite activities, fatigue, changes in eating habits, and feelings of failure or inadequacy. However, PPD also typically involves a troubling lack of interest in the new baby, overly intense worry about the baby's welfare, fears that she might harm the infant in some way, and often extreme anxiety or panic attacks (Suri, 2004). These symptoms may cause the relationship between the mother and infant to suffer, and both the baby's and the mother's health may be affected (Stevens & Glass, 2002).

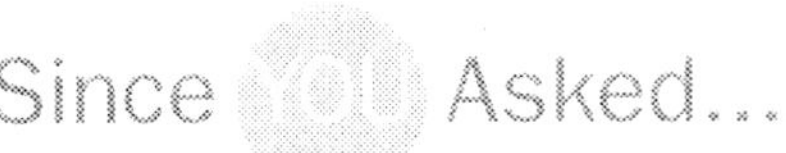

9. Why do some women get so depressed after giving birth? That seems so opposite of how a new mother should be feeling, if she really wanted the baby.

Some doctors may fail to recognize or inquire about PPD in their patients, probably because they are focused on the physical well-being of the mother and child or because they are not trained adequately in recognizing the symptoms of PPD (Heneghan et al., 2000). The "Self-Discovery: A Postpartum Depression Checklist" offers a useful guide for evaluating if you, or someone you know, might be suffering from PPD (D. Moore, 2000).

Lack of recognition and diagnosis can, in some of the most serious cases, lead to horrifying consequences, exemplified by the tragic case of Andrea Yates, who on June 20, 2001, drowned all five of her children, aged 6 months to 7 years, in the

postpartum Literally, "following birth"; typically refers to the months or first year following the birth of a child.

postpartum depression (PPD) A psychological depressive disorder that begins within four weeks after childbirth.

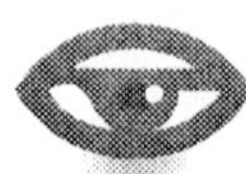

Self-Discovery

A Postpartum Depression Checklist

The following is a list of statements that relate to postpartum depression. Keep in mind that this disorder typically lasts for at least ten days after childbirth and may continue for up to a year. If you suspect that you or someone you know may be suffering from postpartum depression, take this completed form to the doctor for further evaluation and treatment. *The more statements checked, the more likely a diagnosis of postpartum depression.*

___ I don't enjoy holding and cuddling my baby.

___ I have had depression or bipolar disorder before.

___ I have frequent crying spells for little or no reason.

___ I have difficulty sleeping, even when the baby is not keeping me awake.

___ I feel extremely anxious, even when caring for my baby.

___ I have thoughts of injuring myself or the baby.

___ I have thoughts of injuring others.

___ I sometimes feel as if I just don't want to live anymore.

___ I dread or avoid nursing, feeding, or changing my baby.

___ I feel as if I'm a poor mother, even though others say I'm doing fine.

___ I have tremendous feelings of guilt (about anything).

___ I feel worthless.

___ I'm having difficulty eating (or I'm seriously overeating).

___ I have headaches that don't resolve with over-the-counter painkillers.

___ I have difficulty concentrating or remembering even the simplest things.

___ I have a history of PMS.

___ I have a family history of depression or bipolar disorder.

___ I hate or resent the baby's father.

___ I feel that if that baby doesn't stop crying, I'm going to explode!

___ I don't have a supportive relationship with the baby's father.

___ I don't have family or friends to support me emotionally.

___ I don't have support to help out with baby care or other daily tasks.

___ I had a traumatic pregnancy or delivery; it was one of the worst experiences of my life.

___ I just can't seem to get out of bed.

___ I've experienced PPD in the past.

Source: Based on D. Moore, 2002, http://www.drdonnica.com/display.asp?article=154.

bathtub of the family's Houston home (V. Elliot, 2001; Roche, 2002). Her legal defense was temporary insanity, related, in many experts' opinion, to a serious and rare form of PPD called **postpartum psychosis**, which, in addition to many of the symptoms of PPD, causes delusions, hallucinations, and extreme mental disorganization (Doherty, 2001).

postpartum psychosis A severe postpartum psychological disorder that may include delusions, hallucinations, and extreme mental disorganization.

Fortunately, effective treatments exist for PPD. These remedies are similar to established treatments for other forms of depressive illness and include psychotherapy and antidepressant medication. Usually, medications will not be prescribed for nursing mothers because they can be secreted in the breast milk and potentially harm the baby. This has been the primary reason that so many women with PPD have gone untreated or have been forced to stop nursing sooner than they wish so that they could start (or resume) medication. Studies have shown, however, that although the newer antidepressant drugs (the SSRIs, such as Prozac and Zoloft) do enter the mother's breast milk, very little, if any, enters the system of the infant, and no adverse effects on infants have been found so far (Epperson et al., 2003;

Mechcatie, 2002b). Although the potential *long-term* effects on infants whose nursing mothers took antidepressant medications is not yet known, many researchers today feel the risks of *not* treating PPD may outweigh the risk of the infant's trace exposure to a medication (L. Cohen, 2000).

Sexual Activities after Childbirth

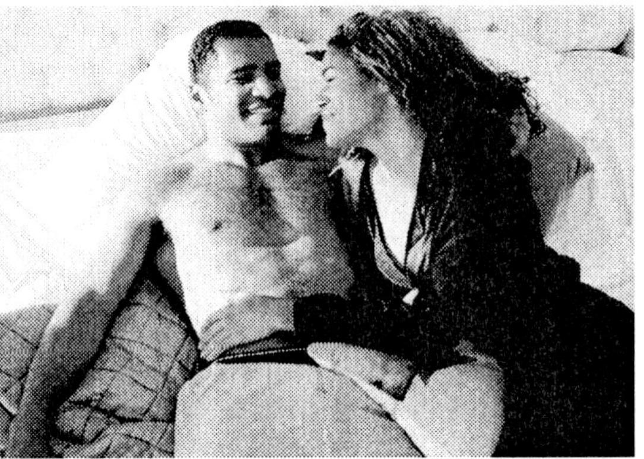
Many nonintercourse sexual activities offer ways for couples to express intimacy following childbirth.

As mentioned earlier, for most couples, sexual activity is usually considered safe during pregnancy, nearly up to the onset of labor, if the couple desires and feels comfortable with it. But what about sexual intimacy after childbirth? Most women who have recently given birth will probably not be eager to engage in some sexual activities because they are, at the very least, exhausted and sore. The exact length of time before a woman feels comfortable for sexual intimacy depends on many factors, including the length and difficulty of labor, whether she had an episiotomy, and whether the birth was vaginal or via C-section. For heterosexual couples, most doctors and midwives recommend waiting at least six weeks after birth to have intercourse in order to allow adequate time for the woman to heal and for the cervix to close fully so that bacteria that may enter the vagina during sexual activity cannot travel up into the uterus (L. Johnson, 2002). On average, couples typically end up waiting a little longer than that—about seven weeks—before resuming lovemaking involving sexual intercourse, and they many wait even longer if there were complications during delivery that make healing slower (Byrd et al., 1998; Signorello et al., 2001).

Needless to say, this can be a very trying time for some couples, especially if intercourse was suspended for a time prior to the birth as well. Sometimes a new mother's partner may feel excluded from all the attention the mother is lavishing on the baby. At the same time, however, couples need to wait an appropriate period of time to resume intercourse, and they clearly do not want to rush into something that might hurt or harm the woman. So what is a couple to do?

As mentioned throughout this book, if new parents understand and accept the full range of sexual expression, many behaviors can allow them to feel close, intimate, and sexually satisfied without physical discomfort. What kinds of behaviors? With the exception of intercourse itself, most or all of those discussed in Chapter 6, "Sexual Behaviors"—including kissing, touching, masturbation (individual, shared, and for each other), and oral sex—are the most common sexual behaviors couples use to feel close and sexually intimate during the postpartum period (Delvin & Webber, 2005). To avoid injury or infection, until the end of the postpartum recovery period, the couple should avoid inserting anything into the vagina, including a penis, fingers, "sex toys," or the tongue. None of these should come in contact with any stitches or other areas that are still healing (McKain, 2002). Other than those cautions, most sexual behaviors are safe and usually very enjoyable for couples during the postpartum waiting period or, for that matter, anytime (Gardos, 1999). Some couples even report that their sex lives become more varied and experimental during this time, and provie lasting positive effects.

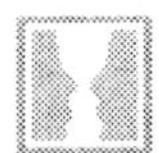
Sex is more than intercourse

Return of the Fertility Cycle

When a woman is ready to resume having intercourse after childbirth, she should not assume that just because she has recently had a baby or because she may be breast-feeding, she is not fertile. The world is full of biological siblings who are only 10 or 11 months apart in age! One common fertility myth is that a woman cannot become pregnant while she is breast-feeding (lactating).

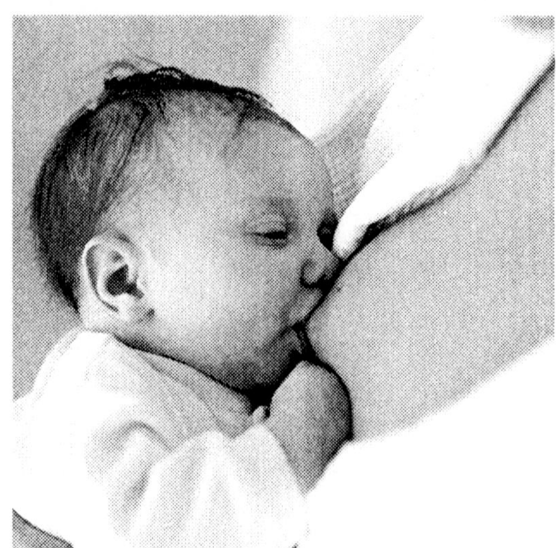

Although breast-feeding may reduce a woman's chances of becoming pregnant, ovulation and pregnancy are still possible in some cases, and lactation should not be relied upon for contraception.

Although the chances of pregnancy during lactation may be reduced, it is far from a reliable method of contraception (Kennedy & Trussell, 1998; R. Williams, 1995).

After childbirth, the woman's normal menstrual cycle usually returns in about four to six weeks. In mothers who are breast-feeding, this period of suspended menstruation, known as *lactational amenorrhea*, may be longer. However, ovulation may occur *prior* to the resumption of menstruation, and the possibility of a viable ovum being released by an ovary increases over the first six months of breast-feeding.

The best advice for most heterosexual couples is to *resume some form of birth control* rather than relying on lactation when they start having intercourse following childbirth, just to be on the safe side (assuming that they do not wish to become pregnant again soon after the birth). One or more barrier and spermicidal methods of birth control, used correctly, provide the safest contraception for new parents. In general, the use of hormonal contraceptives should be avoided by women who are nursing, at least for the first six months after birth, because small amounts of the hormones may be passed along to the infant in breast milk (Kennedy & Trussell, 1998).

Impaired Fertility

As this chapter begins to draw to a close, we arrive at the discussion at the opposite end of nearly everything we have been discussing so far: the *lack* of conception, pregnancy, and birth. As mentioned at the very beginning of this chapter, most of you who are sexually active have probably not thought very much about trying to get pregnant; you've been more concerned with avoiding or preventing pregnancy. You are undoubtedly aware of the emotional turmoil of unwanted pregnancy. You might be surprised, therefore, to learn just how many couples struggle with the emotional and psychological pain of *not* becoming pregnant when they desperately want to.

Scope of the Infertility Problem

Since YOU Asked...

10. What is sterility, and what causes it in both males and females?

Infertility, sometimes called "sterility," is typically defined as the lack of conception by a heterosexual couple over 12 consecutive months, despite trying to become pregnant, that is, having regular, unprotected intercourse (Hart, 2003; G. Stewart, 1998). In the United States, the number of couples who meet this definition of infertility it is estimated to be between 9 and 15 percent, which works out to approximately 5 to 9 million couples (Smotrich, 2002). These statistics do not imply that all of these couples will *never* become pregnant with continued trying; on the contrary, the majority will eventually conceive without any infertility intervention (Guzick, 2000).

Remember, even when both partners are fertile and making love regularly, the odds of a pregnancy occurring in any particular month are only about 20 to 30 percent (although it would be a mistake to rely on these odds for contraception!). Figure 9.18 shows the cumulative percentage rates for a normal pregnancy occurring over 13 consecutive fertility cycles, assuming a 20 percent-per-cycle rate. As you can see, pregnancy isn't a near certainty for fertile couples until after about a year of trying. Nevertheless, when a couple desire and expect to get pregnant and stop using birth control, they may begin to feel very frustrated if pregnancy does not occur over the next few months. If a couple have lower than normal fertility, the odds of pregnancy for each cycle will be lower, and their overall pregnancy rate will rise more slowly over time. In other words, it will take them longer than average to become pregnant. Typically, most fertility experts suggest that a couple try to conceive for at least a year before they consider seeking medical fertility intervention (Daya, 1998; Hart, 2003).

infertility A failure to conceive for 12 consecutive months despite persistent attempts.

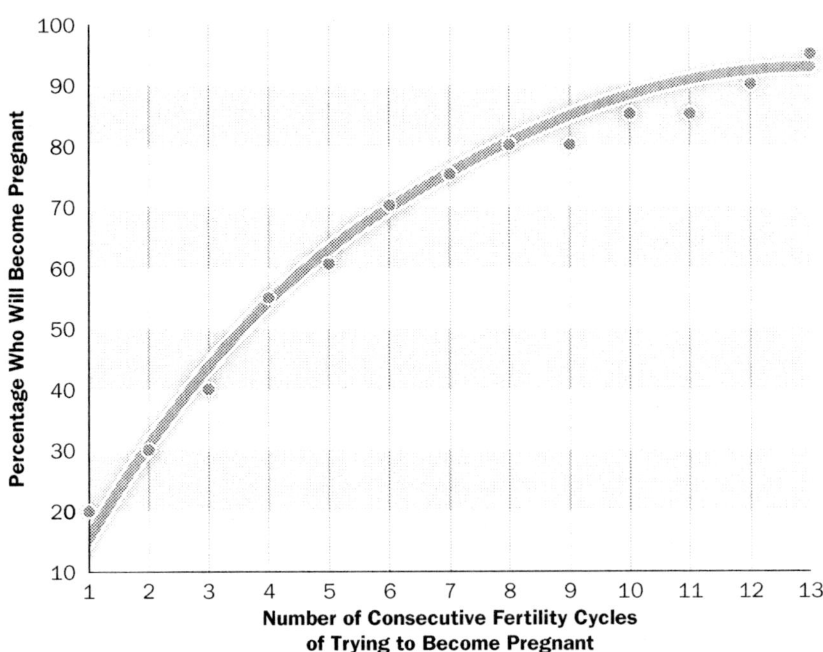

FIGURE 9.18
Probability of Pregnancy for a Couple with Normal Fertility

Causes of Impaired Fertility

One of the first questions couples ask themselves and their doctor when they seek help for difficulty conceiving is some version of "Whose fault is it?" Usually, this is not to assign blame; they are simply asking whether the problem lies with the man or the woman. If we consider all cases of impaired fertility, about 40 percent of the time a male factor is primarily responsible and in 40 percent of the cases it is a female factor. In about 5 percent of cases, the cause is shared by both partners, and in about 15 percent of the cases, the cause is simply unknown, referred to as *unexplained infertility* (Guzick, 2000; Hart, 2003). The most common causes of impaired fertility will be discussed next.

Ovum and Sperm Problems

If you think about the basics of conception as discussed earlier in this chapter, you will probably be able to figure out the most common causes on your own. For a pregnancy to occur naturally, sperm cells must encounter and be able to penetrate the ovum in the fallopian tube. If the woman is not ovulating or if her fallopian tubes are blocked in some way, conception cannot occur. Typically, the lack or irregularity of ovulation is mirrored by a similar lack or irregularity of a woman's menstrual period. Because the menstrual cycle is controlled by various hormones (discussed earlier in this chapter), any condition that interferes with normal hormonal balance, such as stress, extreme dieting, overexercising, certain medications, or the abuse of recreational drugs, may inhibit ovulation. Damaged or blocked fallopian tubes are most commonly caused by one of two conditions. Untreated sexually transmitted infections, such as chlamydia or gonorrhea, may lead to pelvic inflammatory disease, which may in turn damage and block the fallopian tubes (see the discussion of these issues in Chapter 8, "Sexually Transmitted Infections"). The other most common cause is one or more earlier tubal pregnancies that have damaged or destroyed the fallopian tubes (Daya, 1998; G. Stewart, 1998).

On the male side, the problem of infertility is related to sperm cells. If too few sperm cells are ejaculated, if the sperm cells cannot swim well enough to move up into the fallopian tube, or if they lack the enzymes required to penetrate the ovum, fertility will be impaired. Many factors may contribute to poor sperm quality, including illnesses such as mumps in adulthood, sexually transmitted infections (most commonly, gonorrhea and chlamydia), testicular infections or abnormalities, the abuse of tobacco or drugs (alcohol, cocaine, marijuana), and exposure to environmental toxins (Daya, 1998; G. Stewart, 1998).

Finally, sometimes infertility is not related to conception but rather to pregnancy. If an ovum is successfully fertilized and the zygote travels through the fallopian tube normally but for some reason fails to implant in the wall of the uterus, no pregnancy will be established. The zygote will be expelled, and the woman will begin her next period without even being aware that conception occurred during her previous cycle.

Age

Increasing age is associated with decreasing fertility, especially in women. Table 9.8 illustrates this relationship. Even though older women take longer to conceive, this does not necessarily imply that they cannot become pregnant. Approximately 45 percent of women over 40 who wish to become pregnant eventually do so, although they comprise only about 2 percent of births in the United States (Klotter, 2002; G. Stewart, 1998). The reasons for the drop in fertility prior to menopause are not clear, but most researchers agree that it is probably related to a decline in the viability of the aging eggs, which have been present in the woman's body since birth (Klotter, 2002).

A man's age, on the other hand, does not appear to affect fertility significantly. Overall, most men's sperm retain their ability to fertilize an ovum throughout the male life span (O. Smith, 1997; G. Stewart, 1998). However, emerging evidence indicates that sperm's quantity and quality (especially *motility*, or "swimming ability") may decrease as a man grows older (Brunk, 2000). In spite of these age-related changes in the sperm cells, however, a man's overall fertility does not appear to be negatively affected (Paulson, Milligan, & Sokol, 2001). For most men, the frequency of intercourse does decrease with age, which affects a couple's overall chances of pregnancy. This brings us to the next issue relating to infertility.

Frequency of Intercourse

Obviously, if a couple wants to become pregnant, they need to have intercourse often enough for sperm to be present in the fallopian tube around the time of ovulation. Therefore, you will not be surprised to learn that the percentage of couples who conceive increases right along with frequency of coitus. In the past, a common belief was that for optimum fertility, a man should abstain from ejaculation and "save up" his semen for a few days to increase the number of sperm cells in his ejaculate. However,

Table 9.8 AVERAGE TIME TO CONCEIVE, BY MOTHER'S AGE

MOTHER'S AGE IN YEARS	AVERAGE NUMBER OF MONTHS TO CONCEIVE ASSUMING AVERAGE RATES OF UNPROTECTED INTERCOURSE
20–25	4–5
26–30	5–7
31–36	7–10
36–40	10–12

Sources: Klotter (2002); G. Stewart (1998).

this does not appear to be the case. Research indicates that intercourse once every day or two is probably best for ensuring conception. Over a six-month period, only about 17 percent who have intercourse less than once a week conceive, whereas 46 percent who have intercourse twice a week conceive; and the percentage who conceive jumps to 83 percent when intercourse frequency reaches four times per week (Daya, 1998; G. Stewart, 1998). These are overall frequencies of intercourse on a regular basis. However, because a woman is fertile only for about one day each month and sperm may survive in the woman's reproductive tract for up to 5 days, *when* a couple has intercourse, in addition to how often, influences fertility rates as well.

Timing of Intercourse

The timing of intercourse in relation to ovulation is key to conception. It follows, then, that one reason a couple might be having difficulty conceiving is that they may not be engaging in intercourse near the time when the woman is ovulating. This problem may stem from a lack of understanding of the fertility cycle on the part of the couple. If a couple believes that the best time for conception is immediately after, immediately before, or during the woman's period, (and many people do have such misunderstandings), they may be focusing their lovemaking energy on precisely the times of the month when pregnancy is *least* likely to result. Remember, each woman is unique relative to her fertility cycle, but *on average*, intercourse near the middle of her cycle, typically about 14 days before the beginning of her period, will enhance the odds of conception, especially if she has fairly regular periods.

Fertility Testing

Many couples are not terribly eager to seek medical attention for fertility problems. Some people feel that these issues are intensely personal and find them difficult to discuss with anyone, even a doctor. Moreover, they are likely to feel some trepidation about the nature of any tests that might be prescribed and fearful of perhaps discovering that they may be permanently infertile (which is rarely the case). However, the problem of impaired fertility is common enough that couples having difficulty conceiving should not feel alone and should know that many dedicated professionals are available to help them.

Typically, a family doctor or a physician specializing in fertility issues will take a detailed medical history from each partner and discuss in detail what the two of them have done so far in their efforts to conceive a child. At this point, the couple is often reassured, given accurate and helpful information about their chances of becoming pregnant without any intervention, informed about the frequency and timing of intercourse, and advised to continue "doing what comes naturally" a while longer. In other cases, depending on the length of infertility, the age of the couple, and the individual couple's needs and desires, some testing may be initiated to try to determine a cause of their fertility problem.

The main test for the male is a *semen analysis*, in which a sample of the man's semen (usually gathered through masturbation into a sterile cup) is analyzed microscopically to check for adequate numbers, movement, and formation of the man's sperm cells (a do-it-yourself home semen analysis kit now exists). For the woman, tests may include a *hysterosalpingogram*, also (thankfully) referred to as the HSG, an X-ray that allows the doctor to view the interior of the uterus and fallopian tubes to check for malformations or blockages. For this test, a special dye is infused into the uterus under slight pressure so that it flows through the fallopian tubes, allowing any tubal problems to be seen on an X-ray monitor. The HSG is somewhat invasive and can cause some temporary cramping for the woman during the test itself.

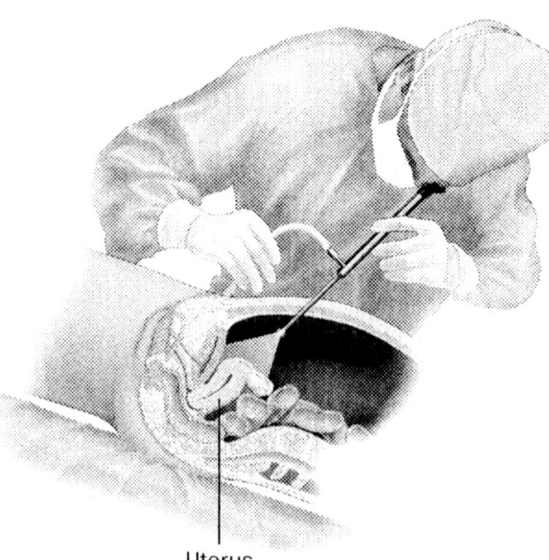

FIGURE 9.19 Laparoscopy

A laparoscopy allows a physician to check visually a woman's ovaries, fallopian tubes, and surrounding structures for any problems that may contribute to infertility.

Sometimes it is necessary for doctors to have a direct, internal look at the ovaries, fallopian tubes, and uterus. This is accomplished with a **laparoscopy**, in which a tube with a tiny camera and light is inserted through a very small incision in the abdomen (see Figure 9.19). Laparoscopies are usually performed under general or spinal anesthesia. By moving this camera inside the abdomen, the doctor is able to visually examine the woman's reproductive anatomy to check for any abnormalities of the ovaries or uterus, cysts, endometriosis, or damage to the fallopian tubes.

Solutions to Impaired Fertility

Individuals and couples who want to have children but who have difficulty becoming pregnant for any of the reasons discussed in the previous section often face a difficult emotional road (Read, 1999; Spector, 2004). They make love with the goal and the hope of pregnancy, but each time the woman's period begins, they must deal with a new wave of disappointment and start all over again. Couples in this situation often report that they are living their lives in two-week fragments: two weeks or so until ovulation when they "must" engage in frequent intercourse and then about two weeks of waiting and hoping that the next scheduled menstrual period does not arrive. For some couples on this path, lovemaking becomes a "duty" that must be performed with a dictated frequency and at predetermined days of the month to optimize the odds of conception. They feel that the spontaneity, joy, and fun of their love life has given way to a tightly scheduled obligation.

Fortunately, numerous paths to parenthood are available today to infertile couples. These include various treatments to enhance natural fertility, assisted reproductive techniques that allow pregnancies to occur using laboratory fertilization techniques, and adoption.

laparoscopy A surgical procedure in which a tube with a tiny camera and light is inserted through a small incision in the abdomen.

assisted reproductive technology (ART) Various treatments to help infertile women or couples to become pregnant and have a child.

Infertility Treatments

Various treatments have been developed that enhance the chances of conception via the process of sexual intercourse. Several fertility drugs such as *clomiphene citrate* (brand names, Clomid and Serophene) have been designed to stimulate ovulation in women or assist in sperm production and quality in men (Bozdech, 1998; Murdock, 2004). Surgical procedures may be effective in some cases to unblock fallopian tubes, repair testicular or related disorders, or remove cysts or scar tissue from the uterus, ovaries, or fallopian tubes.

Another group of treatments for infertility are collectively referred to as **assisted reproductive technology (ART)**. These technologies represent a "brave new world" of reproduction and are constantly being researched, modified, and improved.

At least six methods of ART are in current use. The cost of these methods can range from several thousand dollars to over $100,000, depending on the technique used and the number of fertility cycles during which the method is attempted. The average cost in 2005 was around $30,000. Except in a few states that mandate it, most health insurance will not cover ART. The six methods are briefly explained in the following paragraphs (Scott and White Hospital, 2002; Centers for Disease Control and Prevention [CDC], 2004a).

FIGURE 9.20 Intrauterine Insemination

Intrauterine insemination, or IUI, introduces sperm cells directly into the uterus, thereby placing them closer to the fallopian tubes and enhancing the odds of conception. This is one of the simplest and most common forms of assisted reproductive technology.

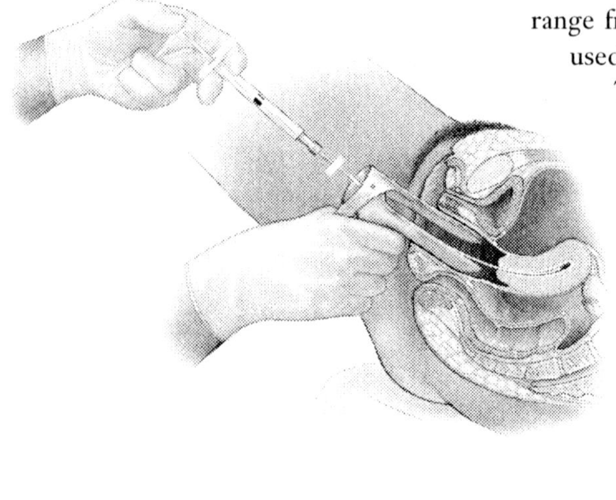

- *Intrauterine Insemination (IUI).* Often referred to as "artificial insemination," IUI is a rather simple process of inserting a small tube through the woman's cervix and injecting sperm cells directly into the uterus (see Figure 9.20). Usually the sperm for this procedure is from the woman's male partner; however, the cells may be from a sperm donor if her partner does not produce viable sperm, if she is not in a relationship but wants to conceive, or if she is in a same-sex relationship in which children are desired.

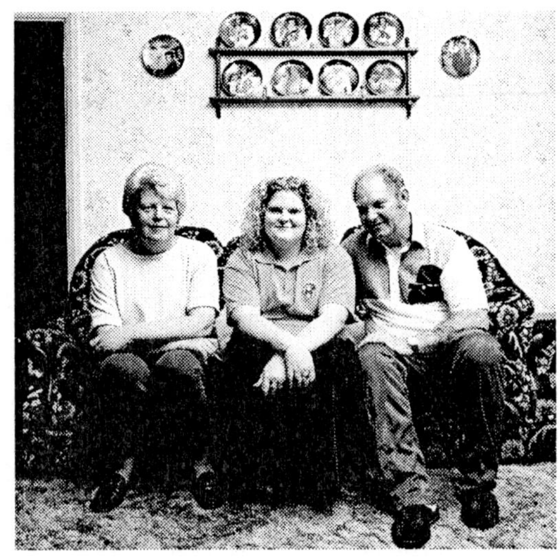

FIGURE 9.21 The World's First "Test Tube Baby"

The first in vitro fertilization baby, Louis Brown, born in 1978, is shown here with her parents in Lancashire, England.

- *In Vitro Fertilization (IVF).* This technique is probably the best known, the one said to produce "test tube babies." Its first successful use in 1978 led to a normal pregnancy and birth (see Figure 9.21). It does not involve growing a baby in a test tube, of course, but rather a process in which ova (eggs) are extracted from the woman's ovaries during a laparoscopy, fertilized with sperm in a shallow dish in the lab (*in vitro* means "in glass"), and then placed into her uterus through her cervix approximately three days later. Typically, three to five zygotes are transferred to help ensure at least one pregnancy, and thus the chances of multiple births are increased by this procedure. IVF is typically used when a woman's fallopian tubes are blocked or missing. Here, either the eggs or sperm cells or both may be from individuals outside the relationship (egg donors or sperm donors). Donor eggs or sperm are sometimes used for this and other ART procedures when the woman is unable to produce viable eggs, if the man cannot provide functional sperm, or when a gay or lesbian couple desire to have children (the issue of gay and lesbian couples having children is discussed in greater detail in Chapter 11, "Sexual Orientation").
- *Gamete Intrafallopian Transfer (GIFT).* This procedure is nearly the same as IVF except that fertilization occurs naturally in the fallopian tube. As in IVF, eggs are retrieved from the ovaries and mixed with the father's sperm in the lab. The sperm and eggs are then transferred to the fallopian tubes for conception using laparoscopic surgery. This method can be used only for women who have at least one healthy fallopian tube.
- *Zygote Intrafallopian Transfer (ZIFT).* ZIFT combines IVF and GIFT. The process for harvesting and fertilizing the ova is exactly the same as in IVF, but instead of transferring the zygotes to the uterus, they are placed into the fallopian tube using the laparoscope.
- *Intracytoplasmic Sperm Injection (ICSI).* This ART method was developed to assist a couple when the man's sperm production is very low, the cells have poor shape or motility, or some other problem exists with his sperm or semen that makes the other ART methods ineffective. In ICSI, a single sperm cell from the man is injected using a microscopic needle, directly into each harvested egg from the woman (see Figure 9.22). The resulting zygote is then transferred after a few days into the mother's uterus. All this method requires is a minimum of one viable sperm cell, which nearly all men with functional testicles can provide, even if they are unable to ejaculate.

FIGURE 9.22 Intracytoplasmic Sperm Injection

Intracytoplasmic sperm injection involves injecting a single sperm cell into an ovum.

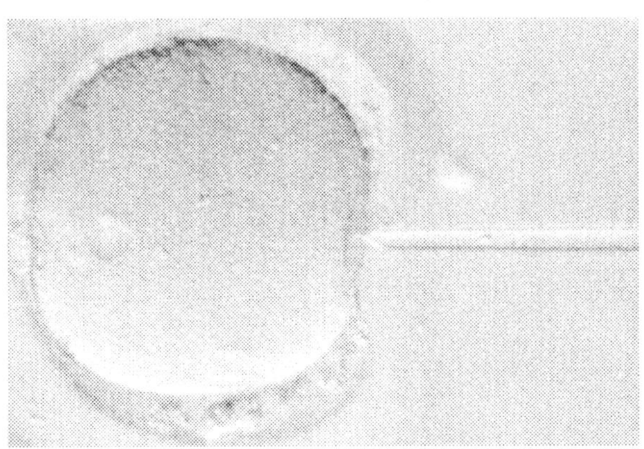

- *Embryo Cryopreservation.* The technology now exists to preserve embryos for later use through freezing (cryopreservation) and then transferring them into the uterus when pregnancy is desired. This reduces the costs to a couple for multiple ART attempts or for later attempts at having children. Also, couples who cannot conceive by any means, who need to avoid conception due to the risks of passing on genetic illnesses or other problems, who risk losing fertility due to chemotherapy or other medical regimens, or gay and lesbian couples who desire children may opt to use an embryo created by others. Embryos that have been cryopreserved for over ten years have been successfully implanted, carried to term, and born as normal, healthy infants.

FIGURE 9.23 Results of Assisted Reproductive Technology (ART) per Cycle per Couple Using Fresh Nondonor Eggs or Embryos.

Source: CDC (2004c), fig. 6.

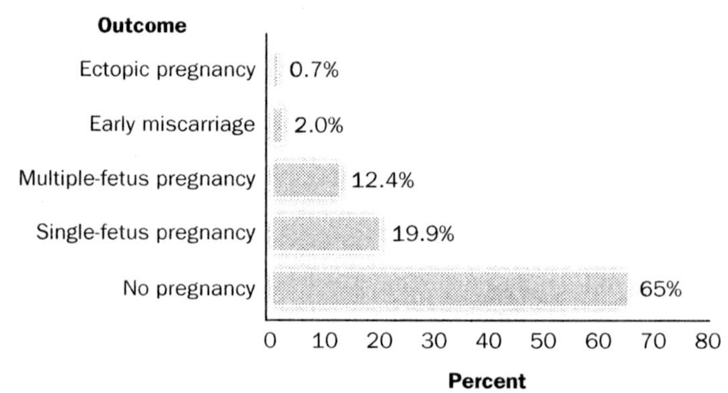

Rates of Success for Assisted Reproductive Technology

Successful pregnancies from various ART methods have been steadily climbing over the past quarter century. As you can see in Figure 9.23, the combined pregnancy rate for all ART methods, including single and multiple births, is just over 30 percent, and the live birth rate is approximately 25 percent (CDC, 2004c). This is the overall percentage *per cycle* for all couples. The percentage of pregnancies increases with more attempts to about 50 percent after three cycles. Success rates drop significantly as the age of the woman increases, from a 37 percent average success rate in women under 35 years of age to only a 4 percent average success rate for women over 42 (CDC, 2004c).

Adoption

One very common and popular route to parenthood is adoption. Many potential parents—those who are able to conceive and have conceived children, those dealing with fertility difficulties, singles, and gay and lesbian couples—choose to start or expand their families through adoption. In the United States and many other countries, one of the first decisions a couple must make once they consider adopting a child is whether they prefer to adopt a child from their home country or from a foreign country. It is important to consider the numerous pros and cons for either decision so that prospective adoptive parents make the choice that's right for them. Many excellent Web sites exist that can help advise and guide couples (and sometimes singles as well) through the complex adoption process.

The author with his daughter, whom he and his wife adopted from China in 1996.

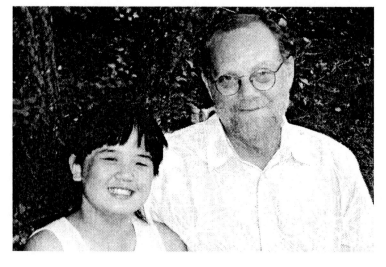

Like fertility treatments, adoption can be expensive. There are attorney fees, agency fees, potential medical fees if the birth mother has not yet given birth, social worker home-study fees, document fees, fees charged by orphanages and agencies in other countries, and travel expenses in the case of foreign adoptions. In general, total costs for an adoption from start to finish are between $10,000 and $20,000, with most domestic adoptions at the lower end of the range and foreign adoptions at the higher end. To encourage adoption, Congress has passed tax laws that provide financial help to people who adopt children. In 2005, these benefits amounted to approximately $10,000 in tax credits for most couples.

Although adoption may seem expensive, if you look back at our discussion of the costs of fertility treatments, which come with no guarantee of success, you will see why many couples struggling with conception begin to look at adoption in a new light. This is not to say adoption is for all infertile couples. To many, the deep need to have a baby who carries their own genes is so strong that adoption does not seem an acceptable option. For many other couples, however, it is the ideal solution, benefiting both the parents and providing a loving home for the child. In fact, some couples who choose to adopt are fertile and are capable of becoming pregnant and having biological children as well.

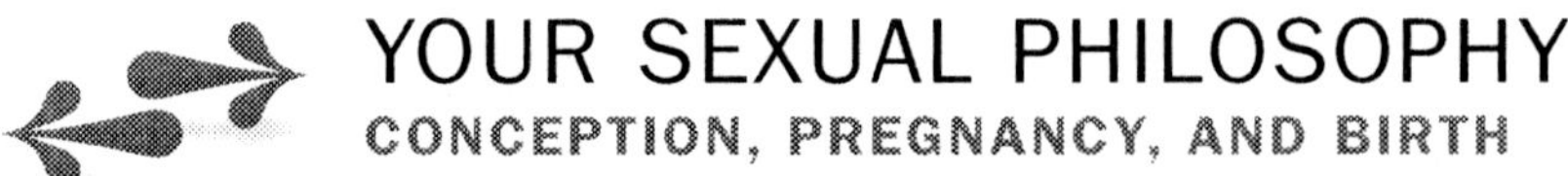

YOUR SEXUAL PHILOSOPHY

CONCEPTION, PREGNANCY, AND BIRTH

Conception, pregnancy, and childbirth should hold an important place in your sexual philosophy. If you still doubt this after reading this chapter, just ask people who have been pregnant, given birth, chosen to have an abortion, or dealt with impaired fertility. They will tell you what a big part of their life as sexual beings these experiences formed. And most of them will tell you they wish they could have been better prepared for them. Anyone who is trying to develop a rational, knowledgeable, educated map of their future sexual life—one that is harmonious with one's desires, goals, and personal values—must prepare answers in advance to address some important questions raised by this chapter:

- Do you want children, and if so, when?
- How can you best ensure that you will be able to parent healthy children?
- What would you do about an unwanted pregnancy?
- Where would you prefer your child to be born—hospital? birthing center? home?
- Would you probably prefer a physician or midwife to deliver your baby?
- How do you feel about an elective C-section birth?
- How will you deal with the possibility of postpartum depression?
- What actions do you think you would take if you or your partner were found to be infertile?

You may not be at a stage in your personal life that requires immediate answers to all these questions. But that's true of most of life's choices relating to sexuality. What's important is to give these questions some careful consideration now, to think about them *before* you are under the real-life pressure of decision making. The information in this chapter relates to major life events and decisions that are much more difficult to handle when you are actually faced with them and your rational thinking skills may be clouded by your emotions. Even if your answers to the questions change as you live and learn and share your thoughts with a partner, you will be equipped with more effective tools to address all these issues, to make choices that work for you, and to plan ahead—provided that you make them part of your ongoing sexual philosophy.

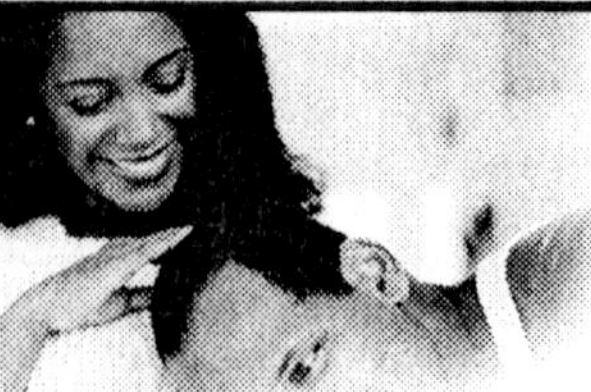

Summary

HISTORICAL PERSPECTIVES The Pain of Giving Birth

- A century ago, pain control for birth was usually achieved using general anesthesia. Today's pain control techniques allow a woman to be awake, participate in, and assist in the birthing process.

Deciding Whether or Not to Have a Child

- Many factors must be considered in the decision to have a child. For some couples, having children is a top priority; others make a conscious choice to be child-free.
- Parents may now select to have a boy or a girl using sex preselection technology. But the use of such technology is controversial due to the ethics of people's reasons for making such choices.

Conception

- In puberty, the female's ovaries begin to produce mature eggs, or ova. Once ovulation is established, most women will release one ovum per month for about 40 years. The ovum will enter the fallopian tube, where it is available for fertilization for only 12 to 24 hours. If not fertilized, the ovum is shed with the uterine lining during menstruation.
- Sperm cells generated in a man's testicles are stored in the epididymis until mature and ready to be ejaculated. The average ejaculate contains about 400 million sperm cells, but only one is necessary for conception.
- Hormonal changes in the woman's body signal whether or not conception has occurred. The fertilized ovum, or zygote, enters the uterus and attempts to implant in the rich lining that has built up on the walls of the uterus. If implantation is successful, pregnancy begins, and the zygote becomes an embryo.

Pregnancy

- Pregnancy is typically divided into three trimesters. During the first trimester (first three months of pregnancy), growth of the embryo continues until, at 8 weeks, the embryo becomes a fetus. At 12 weeks, the fetus is about 3 inches long.
- During the second trimester, the fetus begins more complex movements and by the sixth month is approximately a foot long and weighs about 2 pounds. The fetus, if born prematurely at this point, has a chance of survival with modern intensive medical care.
- During the third trimester, the fetus grows quickly, develops, and prepares for birth.

Potential Problems in Pregnancy

- Potential problems in pregnancy and birth include ectopic pregnancy, spontaneous abortion, preterm birth, and fetal abnormalities. These problems are the exception, not the rule, but any of them may cause serious health difficulties and may threaten the life of the fetus or the mother.
- Teratogens are substances that may harm a developing fetus. Teratogens include radiation, alcohol and other drugs, and some antibiotics.

Abortion

- Abortion is one of the most socially, religiously, and politically contentious issues in the world today. The two polarized sides of the abortion controversy are commonly referred to as "pro-life" and "pro-choice." Most people fall into one camp or the other, but a few see some middle ground.
- The goal of reducing the number of abortions performed each year is shared by those on both sides of the controversy. However, the methods toward reaching that goal vary greatly. As birth control becomes more widely accepted and used correctly, the number of abortions usually declines. The new morning-after pill may also significantly reduce abortion numbers by preventing unwanted pregnancies.

Birth

- The process of labor and birth is divided into three stages. In stage one, contractions begin, the cervix dilates, and the top of the baby's head becomes visible. During stage two, the muscles of the uterus and abdomen work to push the fetus out through the cervix and vagina. In stage three, the placenta, or afterbirth, is expelled from the uterus.
- Parents have many choices they must make about pregnancy and birth. These involve whether to use a physician or midwife, where to have the birth, what pain medication if any they want to use or have available, and whether to have a cesarean section or a vaginal delivery.

Postpartum Issues

- Serious postpartum (after-childbirth) depression occurs in a small percentage of women. This depression should be treated, as it can have major and even life-threatening consequences on the mother and infant.
- During breast-feeding, many women do not ovulate and are not fertile. Nevertheless, breast-feeding is not a reliable method of contraception, and a couple should not assume that birth control is unnecessary if the mother is lactating.

Impaired Fertility

- More than 10 percent of couples who wish to become pregnant find that they cannot. Infertility is due to many factors and may be either a female or a male problem or a combination of both. In 15 percent of cases, the cause of infertility is unknown.

- Many solutions to infertility are available to couples. These include simply continuing to try to conceive over a longer time period, or using one or more assisted reproductive technology methods (such as in vitro fertilization).

Adoption

- Another solution to impaired fertility is to adopt a child, either domestically or abroad. With so many children in need of loving homes, this solution is very gratifying to many prospective parents.

YOUR SEXUAL PHILOSOPHY: Conception, Pregnancy, and Birth

- A complete and accurate understanding of conception, pregnancy, and birth is crucial to everyone's sexual philosophy of life whether they have or plan to have children or not. Reproduction is, after all, one of our most basic functions as sexual beings.

Have You Considered?

1. Looking back at "Self-Discovery: Are You Ready to Be a Parent?" near the beginning of this chapter, what do you feel are the *five most important* questions people should ask themselves to determine if they are ready to have children? Explain why you picked those five.
2. What would you say are three reasons people should have as clear an understanding as possible of the events that lead up to the fertilization of an ovum by a sperm? Explain your answer.
3. Do you see any way to defuse the emotionally charged and sometimes violent debate over abortion? If so, explain your ideas. If not, explain why you feel there may be no resolution to the debate.
4. Imagine that you are expecting a child for the first time. What choices do you think you would make regarding where you would have the baby, whom you would want to deliver your baby, what pain medication you would prefer, if any, and your feelings about a C-section versus a vaginal birth. Explain your answers.
5. Explain briefly how you think you would react if you found out that you were infertile. What do you think you would do about having children? Why?
6. Discuss your attitudes and opinions about gay and lesbian couples having children through assisted fertility techniques or through adoption.

Companion Website Resources

For further chapter resources go to **www.prenhall.com/hock.** This robust text website includes polling questions for you to vote on, regular news updates, quizzes, sample tests, suggested reading lists, and more.

SCENARIOS USA Also on the website are links to videos. *Scenarios USA's* films portray real-life narratives that explore the non-biological aspects of relationships and sexual health. The films will help you consider how the themes of the text affect your own life and the lives of those around you.

10

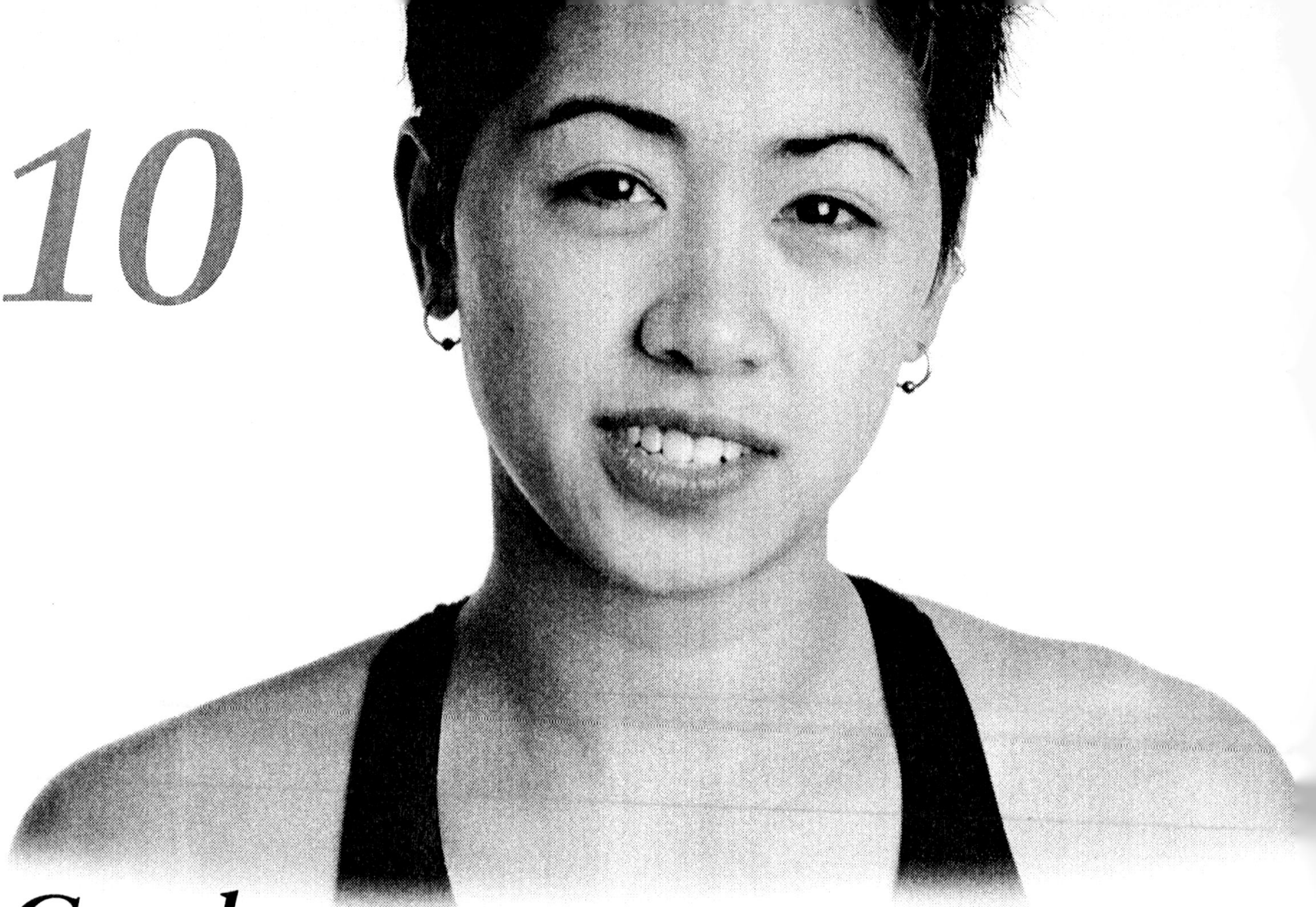

Gender

Expectations, Roles, and Behaviors

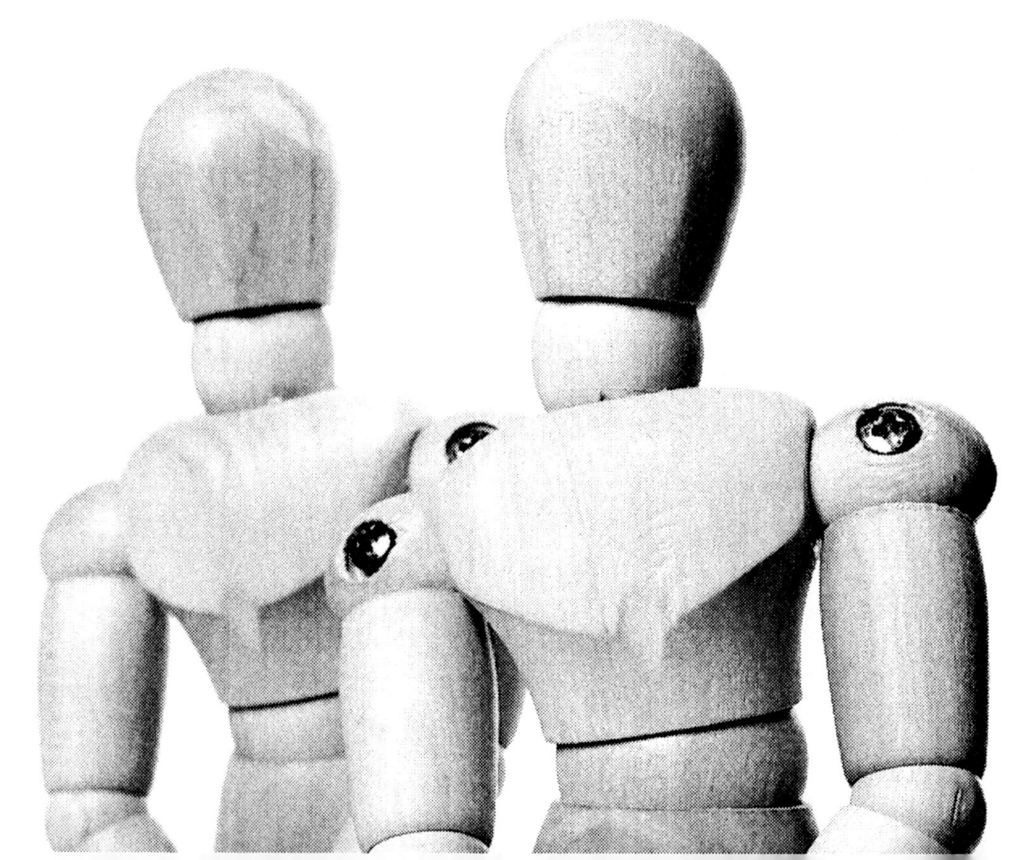

Since YOU Asked...

1. I saw pictures of hermaphrodites in a magazine. Do they really exist? How does this happen? (see page 377)

2. Are male and female sex roles and behaviors determined by genetics, or are they learned from society? (see page 378)

3. I have a friend who has a 7-year-old son who always wants to play with girls and not with other boys. Is this something she should be worried about? (see page 380)

4. I saw a commercial for a talk show with "male lesbians." Is that for real? (see page 387)

5. Why is it that men are always supposed to be the aggressors, the ones to take the lead in relationships? (see page 388)

6. Everyone always says that men are more aggressive than women, but I'm a woman, and I think I'm usually more aggressive than most men. Is everyone wrong, or am I just weird? (see page 391)

7. Why is it that men seem to want sex more than women? (see page 393)

8. Why do guys feel that they must "play the field," even after they've made a commitment to someone? (see page 393)

9. Why are women who have sex a lot seen in negative ways, while men who do the same are seen in a positive light? (see page 393)

10. I've tried talking to my boyfriend about how I feel and what I want, but he never seems to understand, even though he says he does. How can I make him understand how I really feel? (see page 395)

11. Can someone be both male and female, or masculine and feminine, at the same time? I feel as if I don't really fit into either the masculine or feminine categories of behavior. (see page 399)

gender identity The sex individuals perceive themselves to be.

gender The masculinity-femininity dimension of our basic nature as humans.

Are you male or female? Are you a man or a woman? Are you masculine or feminine? These are three seemingly similar questions, yet the range of possible answers to them may surprise you. Most people find the answer to the first question fairly clear: It is a biological answer based on a person's chromosomes, hormones, and sexual anatomical structures. Most people also have little trouble answering the second question: Virtually all people are quite sure about their **gender identity**, that is, which sex they perceive themselves to be, and they've known the answer since they were about 4 years old. Odds are good that none of you had to stop and think about whether you perceive yourself to be a man or a woman. However, the third question might not be so easy to answer. Different people possess varying amounts of "maleness" and "femaleness," or masculinity and femininity. If you think about people you know, you can think of some you would place on the extremely feminine side of the scale (these are more likely to be women), others who fit on the extremely masculine side (these are more likely to be men), and some who seem to fall somewhere in between the two (these are no more likely to be men or women). These categories are not intended to be judgmental; they simply define one important variation among people. **Gender** refers to this masculinity-femininity dimension of our basic nature as humans, and it forms the basis of our discussions in this chapter.

Gender and your gender identity are more about who you are as a person than simply about what sex you are. Few human characteristics define us more than our gender. Think about it for a moment. Imagine how you would feel if you were to wake up tomorrow morning with no idea whether you were a man or a woman, male or female. How do you think you would feel? Confused? At the least. Anxious and insecure? No doubt. You might even think to yourself, "I don't know who I am!" This is how important gender is to your identity as an individual; it is a fundamental part of who you are.

Gender is equally important in helping us understand others. Think about how most of us tend to interact differently with individuals, depending on whether we perceive them to be male or female. Now think of individuals you may know or have met who do not fit into the culture's traditional gender molds. For example, many celebrities—Annie Lennox, Grace Jones, Prince, RuPaul, to name a few—could be called "gender-benders" in that in their dress, actions, and attitudes, they challenge our social and cultural preconceptions of what it means to be male or female, man or woman, masculine or feminine.

You can see that gender is a complex component of our study of human sexuality. In this chapter, we will discuss how a person's sex and gender differ, how your *sexual identity* as a man or a woman develops in childhood, the important distinction between gender and sexual orientation, gender stereotypes, scientific evidence of real gender differences, how gender has been shown to influence communication in intimate relationships, and the concept of androgyny (the idea that people may possess both masculine and feminine traits).

Historically, the world received one of its first lessons about the complexities of gender identity from a shy, slightly built World War II army veteran named George Jorgensen, who, at the age of 26, became Christine Jorgensen.

Focus on Your Feelings

The title of this chapter provides a clue to how emotions might become involved with the concept of gender. The world, as most people know it, is divided into two, and only two, genders into which everyone is expected to fit: male and female. Yet in reality, not all people can be categorized neatly into one of those two categories. When a person defies gender expectations, he or she tends to make others uncomfortable. Try a simple experiment. The next time you meet someone or encounter a person you know, try to relate to that person as if he or she were a member of the opposite sex. Most likely, you will not be able to do it. You will find it impossible to switch a person's gender in your mind! This illustrates just how basic the notion of gender is to our view of the social world around us. When someone fails to adhere to our usual ideas about gender roles and behaviors, we are at a loss to know how to respond. And whenever our expectations about people are violated, we react emotionally: We might feel confused, uncomfortable, or even annoyed.

This chapter helps you recognize that gender is not a simple matter of dividing all people into two neat groups, male and female. Many shades, gradations, and combinations of gender exist in humans. And they are all *normal*. Suddenly, through the process of learning about the complexities of gender, we are able to see a whole new world of human sexual diversity. The concepts of male or female, man or woman, and masculine or feminine take on new dimensions of meaning and understanding. As if looking through a wide-angle lens, we are able to realize and, ideally, be more comfortable with the idea that people cannot always be neatly and conveniently stereotyped as male or female; rather, each individual must be presumed to occupy a unique place on the gender continuum.

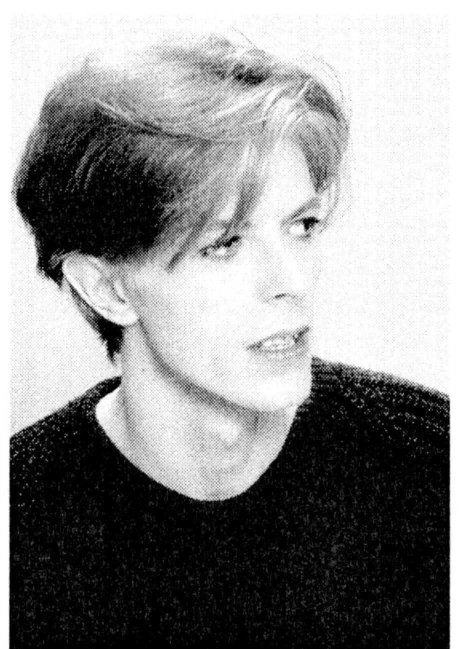

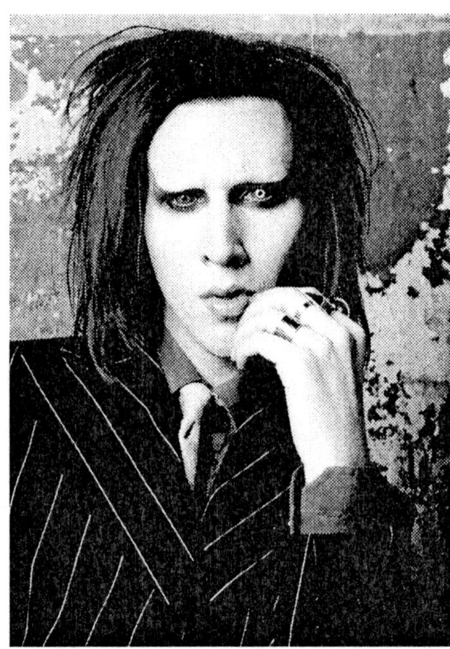

Some pop culture celebrities, such as David Bowie and Marilyn Manson, could be considered "gender-benders" in that their dress, actions, and attitudes challenge our social and cultural preconceptions of what it means to be male or female.

Historical Perspectives

The Story of Christine Jorgensen

Here is the opening paragraph of an obituary that appeared in *Newsday* on Friday, May 5, 1989:

> It was meant to be a private affair, a quiet series of operations that would change the 26-year-old Bronx photographer into a woman and, in the process, exorcize the personal demons that had haunted him since childhood. But even before she left the Copenhagen hospital in February, 1953—transformed from George Jorgensen, Jr., the 98-pound ex-GI, into Christine Jorgensen, "the convertible blonde"—word had leaked out. Overnight, it became the most shocking, celebrated surgery of the century. And even if the furor eventually waned, the curiosity lingered, following Jorgensen to her death Wednesday at San Clemente General Hospital after a 2-year battle with bladder and lung cancer. She was 62. (Ingrassia, 1989)

George Jorgensen was born a biological male. Throughout his early adult life, he never really had any doubt about his biological sex, but he never thought of himself as a man. Psychologically, he was a woman. The demons mentioned in the obituary referred to the emotional pain he felt in being forced into a gender role that was contrary to his personal gender identity. Imagine for a moment if, to avoid being socially ostracized and humiliated, you were required to begin to live your life as a member of the other sex, hiding your true gender from everyone. How do you think that would feel? You would likely feel that every minute of every day you are living a lie. This is how George Jorgensen felt until he undertook, literally, to change his sex.

Prior to his travels to Denmark seeking surgery that would make the transformation from George to Christine, Jorgensen was taking the female hormone estradiol, which caused his breasts to enlarge, his skin to soften, his beard to stop growing, and his appearance to become softer and more feminine. Although his was not the first surgical sex change operation, very little was known about such surgery, and no surgeon in the United States was willing to perform one at the time, in the early 1950s. Moreover, the surgery then was significantly more primitive than today's gender reassignment surgical techniques (to be discussed later in this chapter). Basically, the only

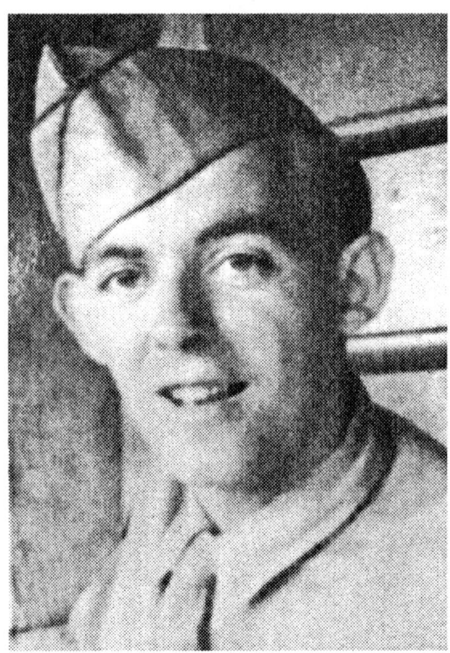

George Jorgensen before sex reassignment surgery.

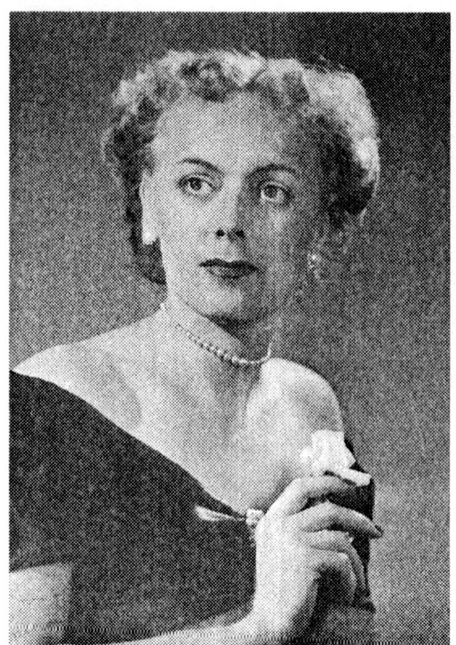

Christine Jorgensen after sex reassignment surgery.

procedures Jorgensen received was a bilateral orchiectomy (removal of both testicles), removal of the scrotum, and penectomy (removal of the penis). No reconstructive surgery was done on Jorgensen at the time to create female genitals. Several years later, Christine returned for more surgery to construct a vagina, but that surgery was only moderately successful (Bullough, 2001).

Jorgensen's sex change operation was the first to receive worldwide media attention, and she did not shy away from the publicity. The *New York Daily News* broke the story with the headline: "Ex-GI Becomes Blond Bombshell." Christine wanted publicity, chose to capitalize on her experience, and became one of the best-known names of the twentieth century. She was a performer; she had a singing and dancing road show that included monologues about herself and at times earned as much as $5,000 per week performing throughout the United States. She also became a spokesperson for transgender, gay, and lesbian causes. Most researchers credit her with pioneering the way for the development of more effective treatments and procedures for thousands of transgender people uncomfortable with their biological sex (we will return to this topic later in this chapter).

Most of us take our gender identity for granted. However, Christine Jorgensen's story points out just how powerful a force gender is in our lives. She demonstrated (as many others have) that our gender is such a fundamental part of who we are as humans that we will go to extremes to express it.

The Distinctions between Sex and Gender Identity

In popular usage, the term *gender* is often interchangeable with *sex*. However, in the world of sexuality research and education, the terms reflect separate aspects of human existence. Whereas *sex* is biologically determined, *gender* is something we learn or construct for ourselves based on our social and cultural experiences in childhood and throughout life: our gender identity. Those experiences are shaped by our biological sex and perhaps other biological or genetic factors, but biology does not solely determine gender. Sex and gender identity are two *separate* expressions of who we are as sexual beings. In fact, as demonstrated by Christine Jorgensen's story, some people's gender identity is the opposite of their biological sex: a biological male may perceive his gender as female, or a biological female may perceive her gender as male. These individuals are referred to as *transsexual* or *transgendered* (more on this later).

It is important to understand that gender is more a personality characteristic than a biological trait. To say that someone's gender is male or female is similar to saying that a person is shy or optimistic. Psychologists point out that personality may have some genetic, biological basis, but it is also strongly influenced by experience. So it is with gender as well. Also, many personality characteristics tend to be extremely stable, just like gender identity. It is precisely because gender affects our lives so strongly that many people resist the idea that gender and sex are separate. For most people, their biological sex is the same as their gender identity, and to see themselves, or anyone else, in any other way is unimaginable.

The Development of Biological Sex

As we discuss in Chapter 9, "Conception, Pregnancy, and Birth," a person's biological sex is determined at the moment of conception, based on the combination of *chromosomes* that result from fertilization. Normally, the egg, or *ovum*, from the woman's ovary contains an X sex chromosome, and the sperm cell that fertilizes the ovum carries either an

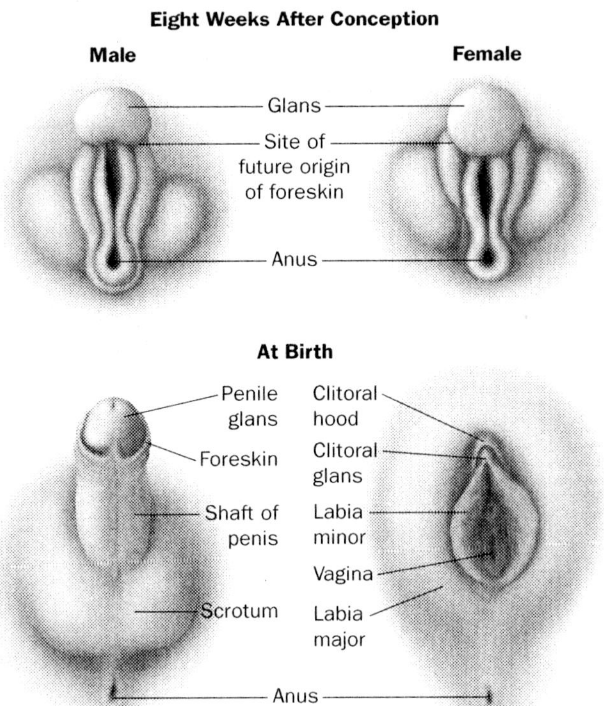

FIGURE 10.1
The genitals of normal male and female fetuses develop from the same anatomical tissues and are indistinguishable early in pregnancy, as shown at eight weeks. At about twelve weeks of pregnancy, the fetus's genitals begin to differentiate, and by birth they are fully developed as male or female.

X or a Y sex chromosome. Two X chromosomes combine to produce a female, while an XY combination produces a male. In the presence of the Y sex chromosome, male hormones, called *androgens*, are secreted, causing the fetus to develop testicles, a penis, and male internal sexual anatomy. With two X chromosomes, androgens are not produced, and the fetus develops a vulva, ovaries, a uterus, and other internal female sexual anatomy. The genitals of male and female human fetuses are indistinguishable until about the twelfth week of pregnancy. At that point, they have developed to the point that the biological sex of the fetus is distinguishable (see Figure 10.1).

The chromosomal development of sex is nature at work creating an approximate balance between the sexes to help ensure survival of the human species. The development of male or female genitals sets the stage, in most humans, for the development of gender identity in childhood; but as noted earlier, biology is not the sole determinant of a child's gender, as you will see later in our discussion of socialization influences on gender identity development. Furthermore, not all fetuses contain only XX or XY chromosomes, and not all fetuses develop clearly male or female genitals.

Variations in Biological Sex

This may seem like an odd chapter heading to you. You may be thinking, a person is either male or female, so how are *variations* in biological sex possible? The fact is that biological sex is not as simple as it may at first appear. Not all fetuses have only XX or XY sex chromosomes. Two of the most common chromosomal variations in humans are Klinefelter syndrome and Turner syndrome. In addition, some fetuses do not develop clear male or female genitals and are born with what are commonly referred to as "ambiguous genitalia." This does not imply that they have both male and female genitals but that upon examination, the genitals are not readily identifiable as male or female and may have some features of both. These genital variations are probably due

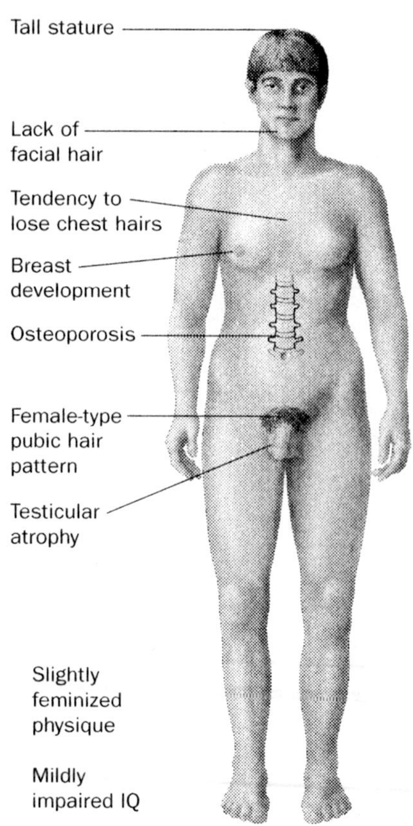

FIGURE 10.2
Characteristics of Klinefelter Syndrome

to hormonal imbalances in the uterus during fetal development. The most common of these conditions is called androgen (male hormones) insensitivity syndrome.

Klinefelter Syndrome

Approximately one out of every 500 to 1,000 male babies is born with an additional X sex chromosome. These males, instead of the typical XY pairing have an XXY chromosome configuration and are referred to in the medical community as *XXY males*. This unusual genetic makeup may result in a condition called **Klinefelter syndrome**, named after the physician who discovered it in 1942. Not all XXY males will develop the characteristics of Klinefelter syndrome, and some may never even know they have the extra X chromosome. However, when the syndrome is activated, common physical signs and symptoms include a rounded body type, lack of facial hair, breast enlargement in puberty, smaller than normal testicles, osteoporosis, and a tendency to be taller and heavier than average, as shown in Figure 10.2 (Bock, 1993).

Most, but not all, XXY males do not produce enough sperm in adulthood to be fertile. They also appear to have a somewhat higher risk of autoimmune diseases such as diabetes and lupus. XXY males who develop breast tissue have a risk of breast cancer equal to that of women, which is 20 to 50 times greater than the risk to normal XY men (Amory et al., 2000).

An early developmental concern for XXY males is that they often display delayed development of language and may have learning difficulties, especially in reading and writing. These children are not mentally retarded and eventually learn to speak and converse normally. Furthermore, their learning difficulties are treatable with proper guidance and attention.

Virtually all the symptoms of Klinefelter syndrome are treatable, and males with the disorder are usually able to live normal, relatively healthy lives. Learning problems can be overcome, assisted fertility techniques and adoption can provide children, hormone therapy can enhance masculine development in puberty and throughout life, and the typical slight breast enlargement often reverses itself naturally. More pronounced breast development may be corrected surgically (Amory et al., 2000; Bock, 1993).

Turner Syndrome

In female infants, instead of an extra chromosome, **Turner syndrome**, also named for the physician who discovered it in 1938, is caused by a lack of or damage to one of the pair of X chromosomes. This condition is far less common than Klinefelter syndrome, affecting only one in 2,000 to 2,500 female births. Nearly all cases of Turner syndrome (99 percent) result in miscarriage in the first or second trimester of pregnancy (Ranke & Saenger, 2001).

For the few fetuses who survive, the symptoms and effects of Turner syndrome tend to be more physically and psychologically serious than in Klinefelter syndrome. The most common conditions associated with Turner syndrome (see Figure 10.3) are short stature (average height of 4 feet 7 inches in adulthood), slow or no sexual development at puberty, puffy hands and feet, kidney malformations, hearing problems, extra folds of skin at the sides of the neck, heart abnormalities, lack of ovarian function (hormone and ovum production), and soft upturned fingernails (National Institute of Child Health and Human Development, 2003; Ranke & Saenger, 2001).

Due to hormonal abnormalities, virtually all Turner syndrome individuals are infertile. As they age, women with the syndrome are at a significantly increased risk of bone thinning (osteoporosis). Underdevelopment of the kidneys or the lack of one kidney is also quite common. Most worrisome are the 20 percent of Turner syndrome individuals who have heart valve and vessel malformations. These conditions may be life-threatening and require careful monitoring and treatment throughout life. As for Klinefelter syndrome, Turner syndrome patients also have twice the incidence of dia-

Klinefelter syndrome A male genetic condition characterized by a rounded body type, lack of facial hair, breast enlargement in puberty, and smaller than normal testicles.

Turner syndrome A female genetic condition characterized by short stature, slow or no sexual development at puberty, heart abnormalities, and lack of ovarian function.

betes than the general population. Cognitively, Turner syndrome individuals are of normal intelligence but may have learning difficulties, especially associated with math and spatial relationships. Although the dangers of Turner syndrome may be serious, with awareness and proper treatment, most of the effects can be controlled and mitigated successfully.

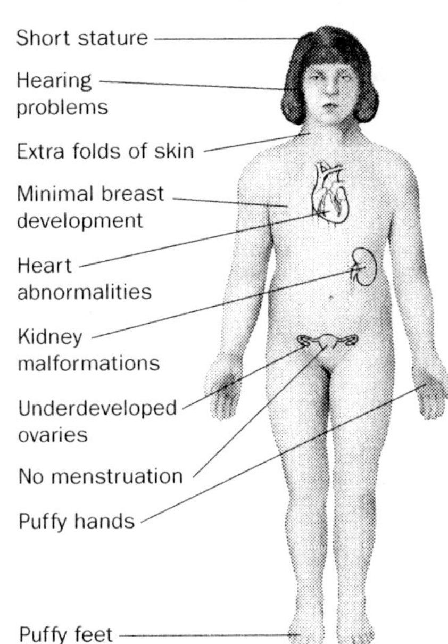

FIGURE 10.3
Characteristics of Turner Syndrome

Androgen Insensitivity Syndrome

In very rare cases (1 in 20,000), a hormonal disorder called **complete androgen insensitivity syndrome (CAIS)** results in babies who are born genetically male—that is, they possess an XY chromosome pair—but possess completely normal-appearing female external genitals (Hines, Ahmed, & Hughes, 2003). This makes biological sense in that all fetuses' genitals are identical in early pregnancy. It is not until the male fetal testicles begin to release testosterone into the bloodstream that the genital tissue begins to "masculinize," developing into a penis and a scrotum ready to receive the testicles when they descend, normally a few weeks prior to birth. However, if the XY fetus is insensitive to the androgens and does not respond biologically to them, genital masculinization will not occur, and the fetus will develop female external genitals—clitoris, labia, and vagina—but typically will not have fallopian tubes or a uterus. The baby is born externally appearing to be a girl but with internal testicles that sometimes go undetected until puberty but produce normal male levels of testosterone. These babies are ordinarily raised as girls; as they grow and develop, the testosterone insensitivity continues, and the testosterone is converted to estrogen, which continues feminization, female gender identity formation, and normal breast development in puberty. However, pubic hair will usually be absent, and menstruation will not occur (B. Wilson, 2003). It is commonly at this point when the condition is diagnosed, the internal testicles are removed, and female hormone therapy is prescribed.

A variation on CAIS is **partial androgen insensitivity syndrome (PAIS)**, which is a condition similar to CAIS, but the fetus has a lower than normal response to androgens in the uterus. PAIS, then, rather than producing a baby with female genitals, is more likely to cause genitals that are ambiguous—not clearly male or female. This is one cause of what have become known as intersex babies for whom gender identification is not as clear. We will discuss this circumstance next.

complete androgen insensitivity syndrome (CAIS) A hormonal condition that results in babies who are genetically male but possess completely normal-appearing *female* external genitals and internal testicles.

partial androgen insensitivity syndrome (PAIS) A hormonal condition in which the fetus has a reduced reaction to androgens in the uterus, producing a baby with genitals that are not clearly male or female.

intersex Born with sexual anatomy that is neither completely male nor completely female but rather a combination with features of both.

Intersexuality

Not only can we identify various "degrees" of masculinity and femininity, but even biological sex is not always neatly divided into male and female. Most sexuality and biomedical researchers today agree that a small percentage of people (just how small is a topic of debate, but somewhere between 0.02 and 1.7 percent) are born with sexual anatomy that is neither completely male nor completely female but rather a combination with features of both. People with these characteristics are referred to as **intersex** individuals (Fausto-Sterling, 1993; Sax, 2002).

Most of you are probably aware of the stereotype of the *hermaphrodite*, usually portrayed as having a functional penis, a vagina, and usually female breasts. These individuals are often part of the mythology of pornographic literature, but some males do choose to alter their breasts with hormones or implants and leave their penises intact. It is also possible for an adult man to have both a penis and femalelike breasts through naturally occurring hormone imbalances, such as may occur in Klinefelter syndrome. However, these are not examples of intersex.

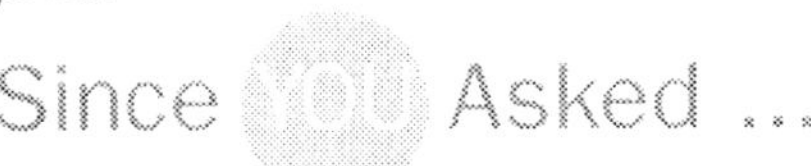

1. I saw pictures of hermaphrodites in a magazine. Do they really exist? How does this happen?

Intersex babies are born with one of three conditions (Sax, 2002): (1) They are genetically male (XY chromosomes) but have external genitals that are completely female (vagina and clitoris), (2) they are genetically female (XX

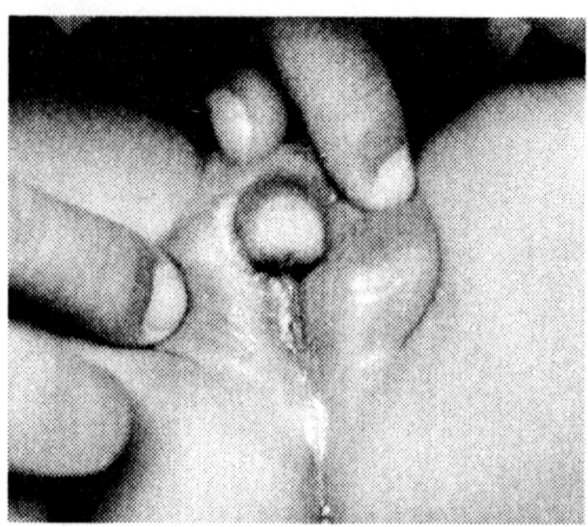

Intersex individuals may be born with genitals that are not clearly male or female.

chromosomes) but have external genitals that are completely male (penis and testicles), or (3) they are genetically female but have external genitals that are ambiguous, somewhere in between male and female. Often in the first two conditions, if no genetic testing has been done, doctors and parents may be unaware of the condition until the child reaches puberty and begins to develop the secondary sexual characteristics of the opposite sex from how the child was raised. In the third case, however, when the baby's genitals are ambiguous, the usual response by parents and doctors has been to alter the child's external sexual anatomy surgically to resemble either a "normal" male or female. The selection of genital sex in these cases has typically been based on a combination of genetic sex and the child's anatomy, so the minimal amount of surgical reconstruction is required. The child is then raised as the sex that matches the surgically reconstructed genitals.

In recent years, the practice of routine surgical alteration of intersex babies has become increasingly controversial. Critics of the procedure, including many adult intersexuals, claim that altering intersex babies against their will and without their consent is ethically and morally wrong and is done simply because society is unable to accept the notion that a person might not be either male or female but somewhere in between. These critics propose that babies should be left intact, as nature intended them, until they reach adulthood and can decide their sex for themselves (which may be male, female, or a combination). For more discussion, see "Sexuality, Ethics, and the Law: Intersexual Politics."

As is evident, the development of biological sex is far more complex than most people realize. This, of course, plays a role in the development of gender identity, a separate but interrelated process we turn to now.

Since YOU Asked ...

2. Are male and female sex roles and behaviors determined by genetics, or are they learned from society?

The Development of Gender Identity

Your genetic, biological sex was determined at conception, but your gender and gender identity—your maleness or femaleness, masculinity or femininity—developed during the months and years after conception. To study the various influences on gender development, we turn to one of the oldest debates in psychology, nature versus nurture. Today, widespread agreement exists among behavioral and biological scientists that most human traits and characteristics are influenced by an *interaction* between *nature*, meaning biological factors, and *nurture*, referring to environmental, experiential forces. This appears to be the case for gender development as well.

Biology and Gender Development

As mentioned earlier in this chapter, the presence or absence of specific male and female hormones produced during pregnancy, depending on the chromosomal sex of the fetus (XX or XY), triggers the development of either male or female genitals and internal sex organs (for more details on this process see Chapter 9, "Conception, Pregnancy, and Birth"). Some evidence suggests that hormones may also play a role in the development of a person's sexual orientation (see Chapter 11, "Sexual Orientation"). But do sex hormones also influence the characteristics in humans that are usually associated with gender? The answer appears to be that they do, but hormonal effects are difficult to study systematically in humans.

Obviously, we cannot ethically subject human fetuses, children, or adults to various amounts and types of sex hormones simply to study what effects they might have on the person's gender profile. Consequently, researchers must rely primarily on observations of people with hormonal disorders, studies of very young children whose behavior has not yet had much opportunity to be shaped by environmental forces, or animal research. Studies employing these methods provide a convincing, if not airtight, case for the influence of hormones on gender behavior.

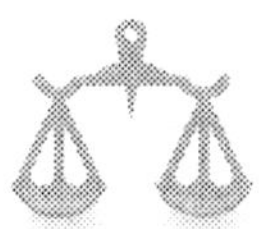

Sexuality, Ethics, and the Law

Intersexual Politics

An article published in 1998 in the *GLQ: A Journal of Gay and Lesbian Studies* had a very interesting title: "Hermaphrodites with Attitude: Mapping the Emergence of Intersex Political Activism" (Chase, 1998). You're probably thinking, "What could this title possibly mean?" The article discussed the fairly new debate over the rights of intersex people. First of all, to most people, the whole notion of hermaphrodites—individuals born with both male and female genitals—is quite strange. The idea that hermaphrodites might have an "attitude" and that a journal article might be discussing the fact that hermaphrodites, or more correctly, *intersexuals*, are becoming politically active will likely strike most of you as bizarre indeed.

As we discuss in this chapter, intersex is usually not, in reality, having both male and female genitals; rather, it refers to people who are born with genitals that are somewhat ambiguous, not clearly either male or female. Although this characteristic is more common than most people realize, the existence of true intersex is not widely known. Why? A major reason is that medical specialists have traditionally intervened in such cases soon after birth and surgically altered these infants to have the external appearance of one sex or the other. Such surgery is usually performed due to the inability of society to accept the concept of a person who does not fall into one of two categories of biological sex: male or female. We do not even have a vocabulary to accommodate an in-between, ambiguous sexual concept. Which restroom would such a person use? Which locker room? Whom might this person marry? What sexual orientation would he or she have? How would he or she dress? Would this person try out for the high bar or the uneven parallel bars? Ice hockey or figure skating? Such cultural and social worries, however unfounded, go on and on. Basically, what society is saying is that we have no place for this person. So intersex infants are surgically "fixed" without any regard, activists assert, for issues of consent or for what the person may want later in life. This, they say, amounts to a blatant violation of their rights. The intersex community is beginning to organize and speak with one voice about what intersexuals regard as great injustices that have been and are being committed against them.

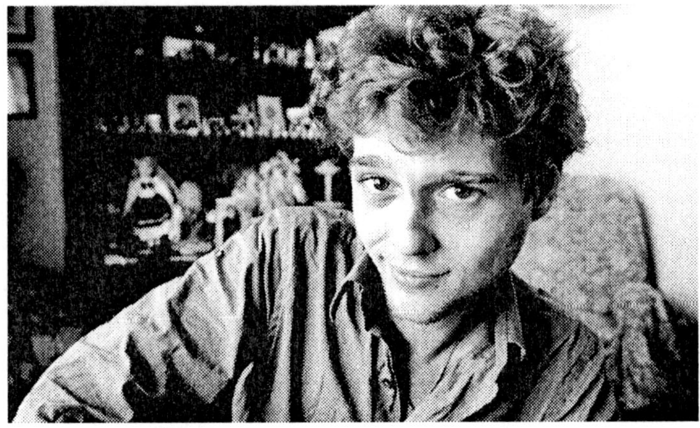

The story of David Reimer in the book As Nature Made Him *brought the issue of the treatment of intersex babies into popular culture.*

The issue of altering the sex of babies received international attention in the early 2000s with the publication of the book *As Nature Made Him*, about a boy named Bruce who, because of a botched circumcision that destroyed his penis, was surgically altered and raised as a girl, Brenda, without "his" knowledge (Colapinto, 2000). However, Brenda never felt or behaved like a girl and experienced many emotional, psychological, and behavioral problems. As a teenager, Brenda was given hormone injections to promote breast development and other typical female characteristics. However, she continued to feel confused, depressed, and eventually became suicidal. Finally, she was told of the accident and surgery in infancy. She immediately recognized the source of her turmoil, chose surgery to change sex once again, and became David Reimer. Although David was not born an intersex baby per se, his story illustrates clearly that gender is far more than anatomy and physiology. David was never able to overcome the tumult that had accumulated over his lifetime. He committed suicide on May 4, 2004, at the age of 38.

In addition to the hormone disorders discussed in the preceding section, a condition known as *congenital adrenal hyperplasia*, or CAH, causes the adrenal glands of affected individuals to produce large amounts of male hormones beginning before birth and continuing throughout their lives. Boys may have some health issues due to CAH but typically develop relatively normally. In girls, however, CAH usually produces ambiguous external genitalia, and the imbalance of male hormones must be controlled with hormone treatments.

Researchers studying the *gender* effects of CAH on children have found that boys with the condition appear to develop the usual patterns of sex-typed behaviors as their peers.

CAH girls, however, have been found to engage in many sex-atypical behaviors. These girls tend to prefer toys that are typically associated with boys (trucks, fire trucks, toy guns, etc.), seek out boys as playmates rather than girls, engage in more rough-and-tumble play activities than non-CAH girls, and reject traditional female childhood pretend roles of wife and mother. Findings such as these have been reported fairly consistently in studies over several decades (Berenbaum & Snyder, 1995; Ehrhardt & Baker, 1974). These studies lend further support to the idea that hormones play a significant role in the development of gender-typed behavior. Other evidence of this comes from systematic observations of early childhood development of normal children.

Since YOU Asked ...

3. I have a friend who has a 7-year-old son who always wants to play with girls and not with other boys. Is this something she should be worried about?

A well-established pattern of behavior in most children is a preference for friends and playmates of their own sex (Maccoby, 1988; Maccoby & Jacklin, 1987). This preference is seen as early as age 3 or 4 and extends throughout childhood until puberty, when sexual interest in the other sex awakens (if the child is heterosexual). But does this observation imply that the preference for same-sex playmates is biologically based? Not necessarily. You could easily argue that by age 3 or 4, children have already been exposed to many potentially powerful environmental behavioral influences from parents, siblings, peers, and the media, which could have molded their playmate tendencies completely separate from hormonal effects. However, several other factors lend strength to the hormonal argument for this gender-based behavior.

First, the degree of the preference for same-sex friends is very strong. Anyone who has ever observed young children over time has seen that girls and boys seem automatically to form totally separate groups in play settings and rarely allow a child of the opposite sex to participate in the group's activities. You can see one obvious example of this gender segregation at children's birthday parties: The guests are typically all girls or all boys, and the mere suggestion that the child invite even one guest of the opposite sex is soundly rejected. Moreover, by age 4, children are spending three times as many hours with same-sex peers than with other-sex peers, and by age 6, they are spending as much as 11 hours with same-sex friends for every hour spent with opposite-sex peers (Maccoby & Jacklin, 1987).

Second, the propensity for same-sex playmates is seen in nearly every culture around the world. Since we know that culture exerts extremely powerful influences on human behavior, whenever we encounter a behavior that appears to be universal, existing in all or nearly all cultures, we can assume that it may be of biological origin rather than learned through interactions with the social environment.

Third, the preference for same-sex playmates is seen in many nonhuman animals. Whenever a well-defined human behavior is found in other animals, it suggests that the behavior in humans may have a biological basis that has been passed along to us through our evolutionary heritage. This suggestion becomes stronger when the animals are closer genetically to humans, such as various nonhuman primates, such as monkeys and chimpanzees. Research has indicated that young nonhuman primates seek out the companionship of their same-sex peers and avoid playing and interacting with those of the opposite sex until they reach mating age (Beatty, 1992).

This and other related research is suggestive of how strong a role sexual biology plays in the development of gender. Clearly, however, it is not the whole story. From the moment you are born, and sometimes even before you are born, the society and culture around you influence how you develop as male or female through expectations, modeling, and societal norms for sex-role behaviors.

Socialization and Gender Identity

Society influences and molds the behavior of its members through the process known as socialization. This process affects our development in many areas of our lives, but perhaps in none more significantly than our gender identity and gender behavior.

From the moment of birth, society perceives us as different and places different expectations on us based, to a large extent, on our sex. These expectations create what are referred to as **gender roles**, the distinctive behaviors society expects and encourages us to engage in, depending on our sex. These perceptions and expectations often begin even before birth, when parents discover the sex of the fetus relatively early during pregnancy through genetic testing (such as amniocentesis) or ultrasonic imaging. They may then paint their baby's room the "right" color, purchase gender-appropriate clothes and toys, and begin to talk and fantasize about the unique joys and challenges of raising either a boy or a girl (Pomerleau et al., 1990).

gender roles The distinctive behaviors society expects and encourages its members to engage in, according to their sex.

Gender differences are so socially ingrained in most of us that we have trouble violating our expectations even if we are made acutely aware of them. For example, imagine you have been invited to visit some friends, a couple, whom you haven't seen in several years. You've kept in touch, so you know they have a child who has recently turned 3 years old. You want to bring a present for the child, so you make a trip to the toy store at your local mall. Take a moment to make a mental list of the gifts you might consider if the child is a girl and the list if the child is a boy. If you are like most people, your mental lists are not the same. While some items may appear on both lists, many will appear on only one list, depending on the sex of the child; for example, a toy truck or a football for a boy versus a baby doll or a jump rope for a girl. Almost no one would place a baby doll on the boy's list or a toy truck on the girl's list. Gender differences are so deeply embedded in our perceptions of the world that they are often assumed automatically, even without conscious thought.

One of the reasons gender is so solidly rooted in our perceptions of the social world around us is that rightly or wrongly, gender is one of the most conspicuous human differences we use to judge others. Knowing others' gender allows us to predict, or *think* we can predict, a great deal about their behavior, which in turn makes us more comfortable in social settings. Thus differences in gender are constantly reinforced through powerful influences in society. Probably the most important of these influences are parents, peers, teachers, and the media. We will consider briefly each of these societal influences on gender.

Parents

Parents' assumptions about the gender of their children are reflected in how the parents treat and interact with their sons and daughters and how their children behave in response. Studies have shown that parents describe their infants in different ways, depending on the sex of the baby. Parents tend to describe their newborn girls as soft, fine-featured, petite, delicate, and beautiful and their boys as strong, big, and determined. They also describe infant girls as little, beautiful, pretty, cute, and resembling their mothers but describe their infant sons primarily as *big* (Rubin, Provenzano, & Luria, 1974; Sweeney & Bradbard, 1988). Keep in mind that these variations in perceptions of infants occur independently of any real, objective differences among the babies in any relevant measures such as weight, length, or activity level.

The number and strength of gender-based attributions made by parents appear to be decreasing somewhat as people have become more educated about gender issues and as fathers play a larger role in the birthing and parenting process (Karraker, Vogel, & Lake, 1995). Nevertheless, parental expectations of their infants based on the baby's gender persist. It is not difficult to find examples of these attitudes throughout the culture surrounding infants. Even the cards sent out to announce births are typically gender-specific. One such story tells of a new mother who was very concerned that people be able to tell at first glance that her baby was a girl. However, the baby had no hair yet, and even though the mother dressed her in feminine baby clothes, some people would mistake her for a boy. To avoid this problem, the mother took to taping a pink bow to the child's bald head. This, it turned out, was the ideal gender "marker"; no one mistook the child's sex again.

Many parents take steps to ensure that their babies are not mistaken for the "wrong" gender, as evidenced by this baby with a pink bow taped to her head.

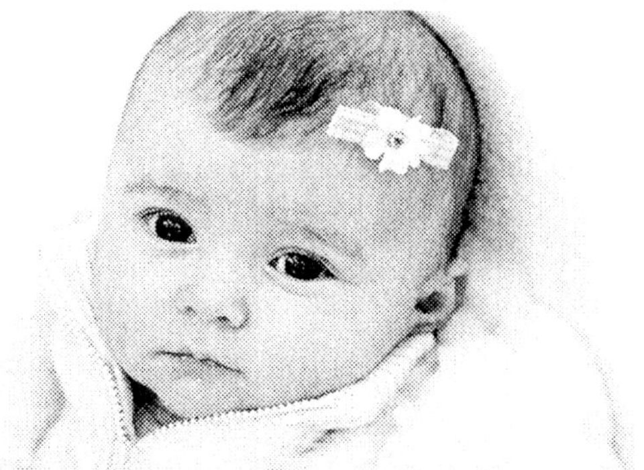

In part, children are directed into gender-appropriate activities and attitudes throughout childhood by the choices parents make for toys, room décor, and clothing the child wears. Perhaps even more important, children are rewarded by the subtle or not-so-subtle reactions of parents and others to the children's behaviors. Parents and other important individuals in a child's life reward behaviors that conform to gender expectations and either withhold rewards for or punish behaviors that appear to violate those expectations. For example, if a child asks for a birthday gift that is gender-appropriate, he or she is far more likely to receive the desired item than if the request was for a gender-inappropriate item (Robinson & Morris, 1986). Also, mothers tend to interact with greater emotional warmth and responsiveness with girls but encourage greater independence in boys. Fathers typically spend more time and engage in more physical activity with their sons than with their daughters (Karraker et al., 1995). Most parents are uncomfortable if their child engages in activities and behaviors that are gender-inappropriate. For example, if a young boy enjoys playing with baby dolls, the parents may direct the child away from the dolls and into play that is seen as more gender-appropriate (Wood, Desmarais, & Guglia, 2002).

This parental influence on children's gender development continues throughout childhood. Among school-age children, many parents maintain a distorted perception of their children's academic skills based on gender. For example, one study demonstrated that parents rated their daughters as more competent in English but rated their sons as better in math and sports. In reality, the sons and daughters in the study performed equally well in all of these areas (Eccles, Jacobs, & Harold, 1990). The authors of that study, as well as others, have suggested that these parental perceptions are communicated to the children in ways that influence the children's self-perceptions and consequently their choices of activities throughout childhood and perhaps beyond. As children grow up, these childhood gender-based experiences cause males and females to pursue different educational and professional paths, further reinforcing cultural gender stereotypes (these stereotypes will be discussed in detail later in this chapter).

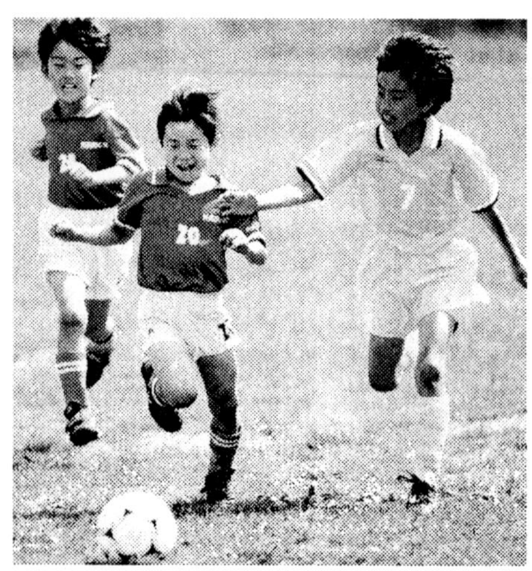

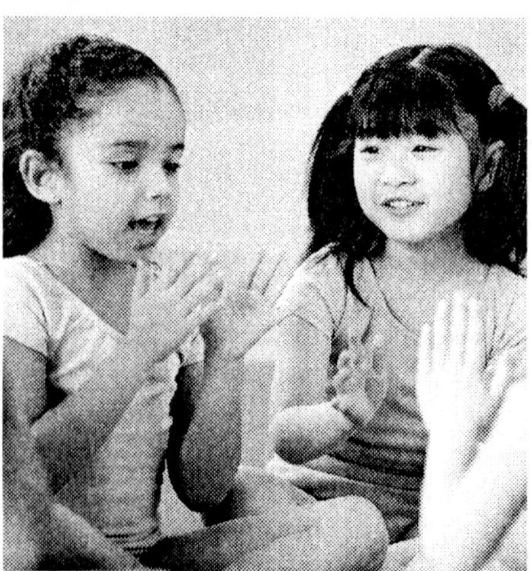

Boys and girls, without any encouragement from adults, display a strong preference for same-sex playmates beginning in early childhood.

Peers

Gender messages do not come from parents exclusively. Children typically spend a great deal of time with other children. These interactions may place equally strong or perhaps even stronger expectations on attitudes and behavior than those of parents. As noted earlier, children segregate themselves into same-sex groups in early childhood. Once this occurs, very little social interaction occurs between the groups of boys and girls. You can imagine how strong the peer pressure becomes on each child within his or her gender group to behave in ways that are appropriate for the sex of the group. Boys and girls who do not follow these behavioral norms are often ostracized by their same-sex group and may also find it difficult to gain acceptance from opposite-sex peers as well (Sandberg et al., 1993; Zucker et al., 1995).

Within these same-sex groups, very different types of behaviors are rewarded through praise, imitation, and various verbal and nonverbal indications of approval. For instance, the tactics of persuasion for boys and for girls become significantly different as children interact with their same-sex peer groups. Boys learn from their peers "controlling tactics"; that is, they use commands, threats, and physical strength to gain compliance from other children. Girls, by contrast, develop "obliging strategies" involving quieter and more refined methods for obtaining what they want, such as polite requests and other forms of subtle verbal persuasion (Leaper, 1991, 1994; Strough, Swensen, & Cheng, 2001).

Another difference typically observed in male and female peer groups relates to the quality of their same-sex friendships. Boys tend to have larger groups of friends, but the quality of their relationships is typically more distant and less emotionally involved. Girls typically have fewer friends, but their friendships are warmer, and they place a higher value on trust and emotional closeness (Leaper, 1991, 1994). These qualitative differences in peer relationships appear to become deeply entrenched and can be seen in adult friendships as well. Moreover, they may relate to gender differences in adult romantic and sexual desires and attitudes, which we will discuss shortly.

Teachers

Social scientists have long recognized that children's teachers sometimes reinforce and strengthen the gender-based attitudes that exist in the culture at large. Even today, classroom participation from elementary school to college classes appears to be influenced by student gender (Crombie et al., 2003; Jobe, 2002). Because gender is such a powerful influence on society's fundamental view of who people are, teachers often reflect those views in their teaching styles and classroom management strategies without being aware that they are doing so. In general, teachers tend to give boys more time and attention in the classroom. Often this is because boys display higher levels of activity, which, if not controlled, is disruptive to the classroom environment. Teachers may attempt to deal with boys' difficult behavior by involving them more in class activities and discussions and allowing them to break the rules more often and more blatantly than girls before administering discipline (Garrahy, 2001; Huang et al., 1998).

Teachers also tend to interact differently with boys and girls during the teaching process itself. When students have difficulties in problem solving, teachers tend to guide girls quickly toward the answer or simply give them the answer, whereas they encourage boys to keep working until they can reach a solution on their own. This has the effect of undermining girls' confidence in their academic abilities (Huang et al., 1998). Furthermore, teachers often come into the classroom with the same gender-based learning biases held by parents and other nonteachers. For example, in math and science, teachers tend to overestimate boys' abilities, maintain higher expectations for boys, and have more positive attitudes about male students overall (Jobe, 2002; Li, 1999). If you ask teachers, most will say with great confidence that they are "gender-blind" when it comes to treating their students equally. However, when their teaching practices are examined carefully, subtle yet important biases are often found throughout the culture of their classrooms (Garrahy, 2001).

The Media

In most cultures throughout the world, children are bombarded by media images and messages from movies, storybooks, music, advertising, and especially television. You have probably heard the following TV-watching statistics before, but they deserve repeating. In the United States, preschool children watch TV an average of 30 hours per week, and many spend more time watching TV than any other activity except sleeping. This amount of viewing exposes children to approximately 400 advertisements per week. At age 16, children have watched more hours of television than they have spent attending school (Aulette, 1994; Witt, 2000). Consequently, when we discuss the many influences on the development of gender roles and identity, television must feature prominently. In her review of the research on the influence of television on gender development, Witt (2000, p. 322) summarizes the process as follows:

> Children's ideas about how the world works come from their experiences and from the attitudes and behaviors they see around them. The young child who believes that only women are nurses and only men are doctors may have developed this understanding because the first doctor he or she saw was a man, who was assisted by a female nurse. This "man as doctor, woman as nurse" idea may have been reinforced further by parents, books, conversations with friends, and television. If the child frequently meets such gender biases . . ., this knowledge will be incorporated into their future [sex-role] perceptions. . . .
>
> Children who witness female characters on television programs who are passive, indecisive, and subordinate to men, and who see this reinforced by their environment, will likely believe that this is the appropriate way for females to behave. Female children are less likely to develop autonomy, initiative, and industriousness if they rarely see those

> traits modeled [by females]. Similarly, because male characters on television programs are more likely to be shown in leadership roles and exhibiting assertive, decisive behavior, children learn this is the appropriate way for males to behave.

Indeed, gender messages are sent out to all viewers of TV programs. Although the television networks and cable outlets have become more aware of gender bias in recent decades, bias persists. If you watch TV with this in mind, you will see this bias often on virtually all channels. Although exceptions exist, here is a list of the central findings of research on the content of most television programming as it relates to gender (Johnson & Young, 2002; Witt, 2000):

- Men are usually more dominant than women in male-female interactions.
- Men are often portrayed as rational, ambitious, smart, competitive, powerful, stable, violent, and tolerant; women are portrayed as sensitive, romantic, attractive, happy, warm, sociable, peaceful, fair, submissive, and timid.
- Television programming emphasizes male characters' strength, performance, and skill; for women, it focuses on attractiveness and desirability.
- Marriage and family are not as important to men as to women in television programs. One study of TV programming found that for nearly half the men, it wasn't possible to tell if they were married, a fact that was true for only 11 percent of the women.
- Television ads for boy-oriented products focus on action, competition, and destruction, and control; television ads for girl-oriented products focus on limited activity, feelings, and nurturing.
- Approximately 65 percent of the characters in television programs are male (even most of the Muppets have male names and voices).
- Men are twice as likely as women to come up with solutions to problems.
- Women are depicted as sex objects more frequently than men.
- Men are shown to be clumsy and inept in dealing with infants and children.
- Saturday morning children's programs typically feature males in dominant roles with females in supporting or peripheral roles.

Do these gender messages on TV actually affect the gender-role development in children? Evidence suggests that the answer is yes. For one thing, studies have indicated that children who grow up without television tend to be less stereotyped in their attitudes about gender. In addition, children who watch programs that violate traditional gender roles—such as those that show women in traditional male roles such as lawyers or police officers or men who are portrayed in more traditional female roles, such as stay-at-home dads or schoolteachers—tend to be less traditional in their gender roles in the culture (Witt, 2000).

Although the strength of various influences on gender development is clear, this does not automatically imply that all boys and girls will develop a gender identity that corresponds to their biological sex or conforms to society's expectations. A small percentage of people perceive that their biological sex and their gender identity are in conflict. These individuals are referred to as transgendered.

Transgenderism

The story of Christine Jorgensen at the start of this chapter illustrates how some people experience extreme discomfort with their biological sex and feel that their physical self is at odds with their gender identity. A **transgender** individual may be a biological male who perceives herself as partially or fully female and believes her male sexual body is a mistake of nature (referred to as "male-to-female," or MTF). A transgender biological female ("female-to-male, or FTM) sees himself as mistakenly born with a female body. In clinical practice, these attitudes and feelings both in children and

transgendered Individuals whose gender identity is in conflict with their biological sex.

adults are often referred to as **gender identity disorder**, a strong and persistent cross-gender identification—the desire or insistence that one is of the other sex, combined with persistent discomfort about one's biological sex or a sense of inappropriateness in the gender role of that sex (American Psychiatric Association, 2000). Some individuals who are confused, anxious, or depressed about their gender identity may indeed require the help of a therapist to understand and resolve their gender-related discomfort. For the most part, however, transgender individuals are no more confused about their gender identity than anyone else; the difference is that unlike most people, their gender identity does not conform to their biological sex.

The number of transgender people is difficult to estimate accurately because so many keep their true gender identity hidden due to fear of discrimination, ridicule, or violence that is often targeted at the transgender community. Official medical estimates place the prevalence of transgenderism at about 1 in 30,000 for MTF and 1 in 100,000 for FTM. However, many gender activists claim that these figures vastly underestimate the true prevalence and are based on statistics of the number of sex reassignment surgeries performed rather than the overall number of people who are living transgender lives. Estimates from the transgender community are that the prevalence may be at least 10 times higher (Conway, 2003b). Moreover, awareness of transgender issues has become far more mainstream in Western cultures as exemplified by feature films such as *Flawless*, *Boys Don't Cry*, and *Hedwig and the Angry Inch*, in addition to the introduction of transgender characters on popular TV programs such as *Friends* and *Six Feet Under*.

Some transgender individuals choose to suppress their true gender identity and conform to society's expected gender-appropriate behavior as best they can. However, the emotional toll of "living a lie" often proves too difficult for many transgender individuals, and they eventually decide to transition to their true gender identity (Conway, 2003a). The term **transsexual** is commonly used to describe transgender people who, in varying degrees, transition from their biological sex to the sex that conforms to their gender identity. Transsexuals may choose to remain at various stages in this sexual transition process. Many engage in cross-dressing to the extent that dressing as the opposite sex allows them to express their gender identity and achieve some gender comfort. For some, wearing a few items of opposite-sex attire from time to time might satisfy their gender comfort needs; others may choose to dress fully as a member of the opposite sex most or all of the time and seek to be perceived by society as a member of that sex. This form of cross-dressing is not considered a *fetish*, as it is when a man wears women clothes for sexual gratification (fetishes are discussed in Chapter 14, "Paraphilias"). For the transgender individual, cross-dressing is about gender comfort, not sexual thrills.

Other transsexuals may choose to alter their physical sex in part biologically through hormone treatments. Opposite-sex hormones, administered via injection or skin patch, produce significant changes in the bodies of both men and women. When male-to-female transsexuals receive the female hormones estrogen and progesterone, their bodies begin to change and become more feminine. Their breasts enlarge, fat is deposited on the hips, and the growth of facial hair decreases or stops altogether. When female-to-male individuals receive the male hormone testosterone, their bodies masculinize; the voice deepens, body hair growth increases in the usual male pattern, their overall musculature enlarges, and the clitoris usually grows larger. In male-to-female individuals, hormone treatments do not produce a change in voice pitch, but most will work to change voice patterns and inflections to sound more female. Recently, a medical procedure called *phonosurgery* has been developed to raise voice pitch in male-to-female transsexuals.

The most extreme strategy transsexuals turn to for relief from their gender conflicts is **sex reassignment surgery**, commonly known as a "sex-change operation." The thought of undergoing extensive surgery on one's genitals and other sexual

gender identity disorder A strong cross-gender identification characterized by the desire to be the other sex, combined with persistent discomfort about one's biological sex or culturally prescribed gender role.

transsexual A transgender person who makes an effort to transition from his or her biological sex to his or her self-identified gender through dress, hormone therapy, or surgery.

sex reassignment surgery Surgical procedures used to transform an individual from one sex to the other, commonly known as a "sex-change operation."

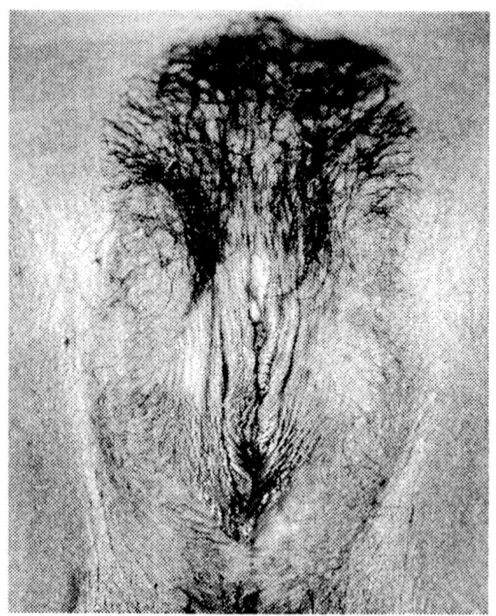

Male-to-Female Sex Reassignment

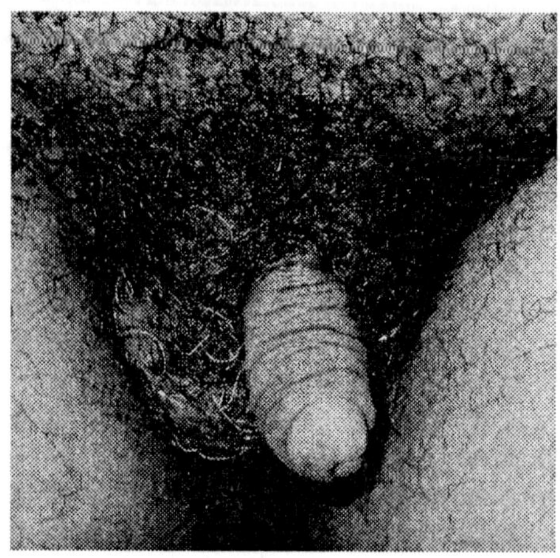

Female-to-Male Sex Reassignment

FIGURE 10.4
Outcomes of Sex Reassignment Surgery

The genitals after gender reassignment surgery are usually quite natural in both appearance and function.

anatomical structures in the name of gender identity is difficult for most people to imagine. However, the emotional pain many transsexuals feel in being "trapped" in the wrong-sex body often outweighs any hesitation they may feel, and the surgery becomes a deeply desired goal in their lives.

Over many decades, surgical procedures have been developed to allow transgender individuals to alter their sexual anatomy to resemble that of the opposite sex. The surgery is lengthy and expensive (from $18,000 to $50,000 in the United States, depending on the procedures selected) and is for all intents and purposes irreversible (Savage & Neff, 1999). Hospitals in foreign countries such as Thailand are offering sex reassignment surgeries for a fraction of the cost ($7,000 to $10,000) while providing the most modern hospital facilities and surgeons trained in major medical schools in the West (Talbot 2001; Vyas, 2004).

Transgender individuals and medical professionals alike must be sure that surgery is the best course of action before performing the surgery itself. Extensive psychological counseling, hormone therapy, and a presurgical transition period (usually defined as living full time as the opposite sex for at least a year) are typically required prior to undertaking sexual reassignment surgery. Modern medical techniques, combined with continuous hormone therapy, are now capable of altering physical sex with remarkably accurate visual results while usually preserving sexual response and orgasmic functioning. Chances are, you could meet, get to know, date, have sex with, and even marry a postoperative transsexual and be unaware of the person's transgender status unless he or she were to inform you of it. As you can see in Figure 10.4, the genitals of postoperative transsexuals are anatomically very realistic.

Male-to-female sexual reassignment surgery may involve some or all of the following procedures:

- *Penectomy* (removal of the penis)
- *Uroplasty* (rerouting of the urethra)
- *Orchiectomy* (removal of the testicles)
- *Vaginoplasty* (the use of penile skin to construct labia and a vagina)
- *Breast implants* (if the patient feels that enlargement through hormone therapy has been inadequate)
- *Chondrolaryngoplasty* (optional procedure to reduce the size of the Adam's apple)
- *Phonosurgery* (optional procedure to raise voice pitch)

Female-to-male sexual reassignment surgery may include some or all of these procedures:

- *Mastectomy* (removal of the breasts and, optionally, reduction in nipple size)
- *Hysterectomy* (removal of the uterus, fallopian tubes, and ovaries)
- *Metadioplasty* (creation of a small erectile phallus from the clitoris)
- *Phalloplasty* (formation of a penis from tissue taken from other areas of the body and transplanted using microsurgical techniques in the genital area; requires a penile implant for erection)
- *Uroplasty* (rerouting of the urethra)
- *Scrotoplasty* (reshaping and stretching of the labia to resemble a scrotum and the insertion of silicone prosthetic testicles)

Obviously, sex reassignment surgery is *not* minor surgery. A complete sex change usually requires numerous operations occurring in stages over a period of months or years. However, research has shown that most transsexuals who undergo this surgery are satisfied with the outcome and are better adjusted in life (Lawrence, 2003; Lief & Hubschman, 1993). Part of the reason for the success of sex reassignment surgery is our advanced state of medical art in transforming one sex into the other.

Gender and Sexual Orientation

sexual orientation The gender to whom a person is primarily romantically, emotionally, and sexually attracted.

Just as a person's gender identity does not necessarily match up with his or her sexual anatomy, gender may not always be predictive of his or her **sexual orientation**, that is, which gender a person is primarily attracted to, romantically, emotionally, and sexually (see Chapter 11, "Sexual Orientation," for a detailed discussion of sexual orientation issues). A person whose gender identity is male may be heterosexual, homosexual, or bisexual, just as a person whose gender identity is female may also be heterosexual, homosexual, or bisexual. Of course, the vast majority of people who self-identify as male are attracted to those who self-identify as female, and vice versa, but this is not universally the case. Gender and sexual orientation tend to function as separate expressions of human sexuality. What does this separation of gender identity and sexual orientation mean in terms of the complexities of human sexual identity? It means that a person may live life as any one of many potential combinations of biological sex, gender, and sexual orientation. To take the example of the vast majority of cases, a biological male might have a gender identity of male and be heterosexual—sexually and romantically attracted to women. Likewise, a biological female might have a gender identity of female and be heterosexual—sexually and romantically attracted to men. In a small percentage of people however, a biological male may have a gender identity of female (in other words, is transgendered) and also be attracted to women. This person may be considered a lesbian (yes, a "male" lesbian—although this designation is a topic of some debate among some scientific and lesbian groups). Conversely, transgender biological female who gender identifies as male and is attracted to women may be considered heterosexual. Confusing? Maybe, but these complex combinations, although they are exceptions, point out that most people's assumptions about human sexual identity are overly simplistic. Table 10.1 lists various combinations of the characteristics of sex, gender, and sexual orientation that may be found among the rich diversity of human sexual beings.

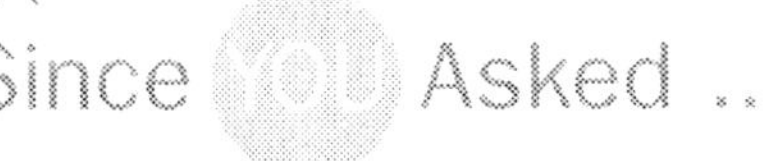

4. I saw a commercial for a talk show with "male lesbians." Is that for real?

Table 10.1 THE COMPLEXITIES OF HUMAN SEXUAL IDENTITY

Although the majority of people will identify with the characteristics in rows 1 and 2, the table illustrates that the characteristics of biological sex, gender identity, and sexual orientation are separate human characteristics and may exist in people in numerous combinations.

	BIOLOGICAL SEX	GENDER IDENTITY	PRIMARY SEXUAL OR ROMANTIC ATTRACTION	SEXUAL ORIENTATION
1	Male	Male	Female	Heterosexual
2	Female	Female	Male	Heterosexual
3	Male	Female*	Female	Lesbian†
4	Male	Female*	Male	Heterosexual
5	Male	Male	Male	Gay
6	Male	Male	Male and Female	Bisexual
7	Male	Female*	Male and Female	Bisexual
8	Female	Male*	Male	Gay
9	Female	Male*	Female	Heterosexual
10	Female	Female	Female	Lesbian
11	Female	Female	Male and Female	Bisexual
12	Female	Male*	Male and Female	Bisexual

* Transgender individuals.

† This designation is debated in some gay and lesbian communities.

Since YOU Asked …

5. Why is it that men are always supposed to be the aggressors, the ones to take the lead in relationships?

Gender Roles and Stereotypes

Our discussion of the factors that influence the development of gender roles and identity leads us directly into an examination of what these forces may produce: **gender stereotypes**. A stereotype is the assumption (usually wrong) that all people who belong to a certain group share certain characteristics, regardless of the uniqueness of each individual group member. Therefore, a gender stereotype is an assumption about a person based solely on his or her gender, without regard for his or her individuality as a person.

We grow up learning from others in society that certain behaviors and attitudes are "male" and certain others are "female." As these differences become psychologically attached to one gender or the other, we begin to incorporate them into our fundamental belief systems about men and women. The differences transform from "how a person behaves" to "who a person is." Once this happens, we then come to *expect* men and women to behave differently, and we interact with them based on those expectations. When our expectations of individuals is based on their membership in a particular group, whether the group is a certain gender, race, religion, sexual orientation, profession, or any other characteristic, this is referred to as a stereotype.

That stereotypes exist is not open to debate; they do. To get an idea of the number of gender stereotypes and how widely they are believed, take a look at the list in "Self-Discovery: Gender Stereotypes." These stereotypes are common in Western cultures, and you can see signs of them nearly everywhere you look. They form the basis for best-selling books (the hugely popular "Venus and Mars" series was based largely on gender stereotypes) and hundreds of jokes (e.g., men refusing to ask directions jokes, blonde female jokes). Stereotypes, in and of themselves, are not necessarily harmful. Rather, it is how they affect our attitudes and behavior that determines the consequences of stereotypes. Some stereotypes may be quite innocuous, such as your belief that your home team players are more talented than members of other teams in a certain sport or that all cars made by a specific manufacturer are safe and dependable. When social scientists study stereotypes, they are primarily concerned with how stereotypes develop and to what extent they are based on true rather than imagined differences.

How Do Gender Stereotypes Develop?

Earlier we discussed how society places many expectations on its members for different behavioral roles based on sex. These expectations are communicated to all of us very early in life. By the time children are 3 years old, they already have a sense of themselves and others as male or female. By age 4 or 5, most have acquired the concept of *gender stability*; that is, they believe that when they grow up, they will be either a man or a woman, a daddy or a mommy, and most dream of traditional gender-based occupations (such as fireman for boys and ballerina for girls). By this age, they have also developed very strong preferences for gender-appropriate, sex-typed behavior (most boys resist playing house, and most girls reject playing ninja warrior). Within another year or two, children understand *gender constancy*, that a person's gender stays the same even if that person violates expected, traditional sex-role behaviors (such as a man dressing up in women's clothes for a skit or a woman who is a plumber).

Gender stereotypes develop parallel with gender identity. By the time children are 5 years old, they have a remarkably clear sense of the difference between masculine and feminine sex roles in the culture, and they use people's gender as the main criterion to predict the behaviors of others. Even today, when society has developed an increased awareness of sexual inequalities, most preschoolers are confident that girls cannot be, say, firefighters and boys cannot be schoolteachers. If you watch young children pretending to go somewhere in a car, the boy nearly always drives. Interestingly, these stereotypes persist even when the child's personal experience pro-

gender stereotype An assumption about a person based solely on gender, without regard for his or her individuality as a person.

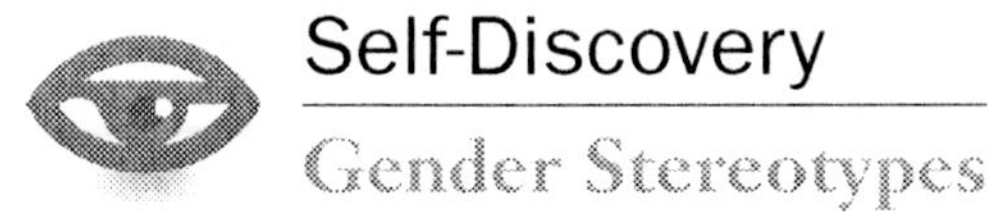

Self-Discovery

Gender Stereotypes

Below is a list of words often used to describe common human characteristics. The check marks indicate whether the trait is typically seen as a masculine or feminine characteristic in most Western cultures and whether the trait is usually perceived as desirable or undesirable. As you study the list, an interesting pattern emerges. Finally, the last two columns provide an opportunity for you to examine your own attitudes and see if you agree or disagree with society's view of these gender stereotypes.

Characteristic	Male	Female	Desirable	Undesirable	Do You Agree?	Do You Disagree?
Independent	✓		✓			
Assertive	✓		✓			
Strong	✓		✓			
Decisive	✓		✓			
Self-confident	✓		✓			
Submissive		✓		✓		
Passive		✓		✓		
Emotional		✓		✓		
Talkative		✓		✓		
Fearful		✓		✓		

As you can see, the pattern that emerges demonstrates how stereotypes usually seen as feminine are also typically judged as undesirable. This suggests how stereotypes can lead to prejudice and discrimination based on gender. If you found yourself disagreeing with many of these, that is because you are not typical. You are more highly educated than the average person, and research has shown that as education level increases, belief in gender stereotypes declines.

vides examples of exceptions to the gender expectations, such as when the child's father is a teacher or mother does all the driving or when the child's books take a nonstereotypical approach to gender roles (Diekman & Murnen, 2004; Witt, 1997).

In the United States, you can easily see these gender beliefs in children by observing the costumes they choose for Halloween. Although the costume might hide the child's true identity, 90 percent of children's Halloween costumes are conspicuously gender-appropriate, and only 10 percent are gender-neutral (Nelson, 2000). Girls dress up as beauty queens, princesses, brides, animals (butterfly, cat), and food items (lollipop, ice cream cone). Boys are more likely to wear costumes representing police officers, warriors, villains, monsters, or symbols of death (Dracula, executioner, grim reaper). The gender identities and stereotypes in young children are so strongly formed that a child might well forgo all the candy Halloween promises than set out trick-or-treating in a clearly opposite-gender costume.

As children move into the school years, gender stereotypes are further strengthened by systematic expectations about which subjects and activities are feminine and which are masculine. From kindergarten through elementary school and even beyond, children perceive math, sports, and various mechanical skills as masculine, while art, reading, and music are seen as feminine (Eccles et al., 1990). This is not to say that boys refuse to produce art or play music or that girls reject math and sports. However, if you ask most children whether these are "girl activities" or "boy activities," they are quite clear about the differences.

As children enter middle and high school, their gender stereotypes have already begun to mirror those held by adults. They see certain courses, extracurricular activities,

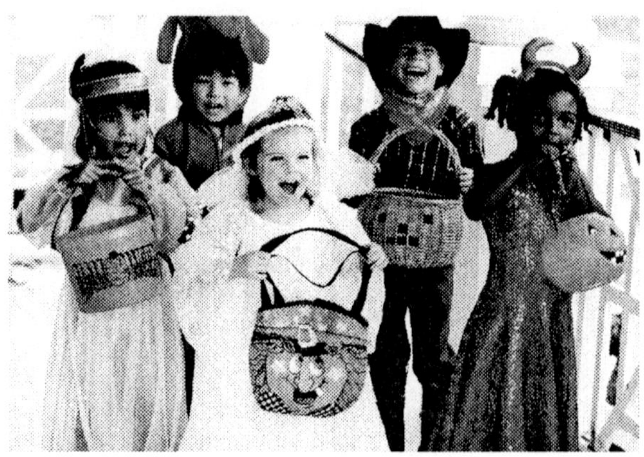

Awareness of gender expectations, roles, and stereotypes is obvious in the Halloween costumes chosen by young boys and girls.

recreational choices, and jobs as appropriate for one sex or the other. This stereotyped thinking then guides their social, educational, and professional choices throughout the teen years and into adulthood.

Gender-based stereotyped beliefs are so ingrained by adolescence that they tend to be an integral part of teens' view of the world. That said, however, older children also tend to be more flexible in the gender-violating behaviors they will accept. They become increasingly willing, as most adults are, to judge people on criteria in addition to their gender. They become aware that gender roles are social norms and that "breaking the rules" is sometimes acceptable (or even cool). However, this does not imply that as adults we become "gender-blind." Various gender-role expectations and the resulting stereotypes remain strong throughout life. For example, many adults are still surprised—and some are uncomfortable or even disapproving—upon encountering, say, a female airline captain or a male nurse. This explains why many professions continue to be dominated by one sex or the other, as can be seen in Table 10.2.

The "Truth" about Gender Stereotypes

Accepting the reality of gender stereotypes brings us to another important question: Are they true? It is one thing for individuals or cultures to believe that certain characteristics and behaviors are appropriate for one gender or the other, but to what extent are gender stereotypes based on real differences between the sexes? Look again at "Self Discovery: Gender Stereotypes" on page 389. You may disagree with some or even most of the items listed as gender stereotypes. For example, your personal opinion may

Table 10.2 OCCUPATIONS BY GENDER

Gender stereotypes continue to influence people's choices of occupations.

OCCUPATION	PERCENTAGE WHO ARE MEN	PERCENTAGE WHO ARE WOMEN
Airline pilot	95.8	4.2
Truck driver	95.1	4.9
Aerospace engineer	91.9	8.1
Dentist	80.6	19.4
Architect	79.9	20.1
Lawyer	70.8	29.2
Physician	69.4	30.6
College and university teacher	57.3	42.7
Psychologist	34.1	65.9
Occupational therapist	29.8	70.2
Waiter, waitress	29.3	70.7
Librarian	18.3	81.7
Legal assistant	17.8	82.2
Elementary school teacher	17.0	83.0
Registered nurse	7.1	92.9
Preschool and kindergarten teacher	2.3	97.7
Dental hygienist	1.9	98.1
Secretary	1.4	98.6

Source: Bureau of Labor Statistics (2002).

be that women are just as capable of being independent as men or that men are just as sensitive as women. You may even believe that some of the stereotypes should be reversed—that women are actually stronger than men in many ways or that men can be more talkative than women. The reason for these discrepancies is that two levels of gender stereotypes exist: cultural and personal. **Cultural gender stereotypes** are the beliefs about gender roles held by a majority of people in a given cultural setting and communicated through parenting, schooling, mass media, literature, and advertising, as discussed earlier. In addition, people hold **personal gender stereotypes**, beliefs about gender that are unique to each individual and may or may not agree with cultural stereotypes. Personal gender stereotypes are shaped by individual life experiences such as those that caused you to disagree with some of the stereotypes in the Self-Discovery.

cultural gender stereotypes Beliefs about gender roles held by a majority of people in a given cultural setting.

personal gender stereotypes Beliefs about gender that are unique to each individual and may or may not agree with cultural stereotypes.

Who is right? The culture? You? Both? Neither? Social scientists have been working for many decades to tease apart scientific fact from cultural and personal beliefs about gender. Most people believe that every stereotype must contain a grain of truth or it would never have come into existence. Overall, research has shown this to be true for some gender stereotypes, but the differences between the sexes are usually smaller than most people expect. To illustrate, let's look at what the research tells us about two of the most common gender stereotypes, aggression and intuition. Then we will look a bit more closely at one stereotype that is very relevant to many of our discussions in this book: gender differences in sexual drive.

Aggression

One of the strongest and most widely accepted stereotypes is that male humans are more aggressive than female humans. A great deal of evidence seems to support that this stereotype represents a real gender difference (Eagly & Steffen, 1986; Knight, Fabes, & Higgins, 1996; Knight et al., 2002). Men engage in significantly more aggressive behaviors in nearly all cultures worldwide. Among very young children, boys typically display higher levels of physical and verbal aggression than girls during play activities. As children enter school, this gender difference in aggression continues. As shown in Figure 10.5 based on data from one large, diverse urban school district, boys demonstrate significantly higher levels of aggressive behaviors than girls throughout the school years of first through seventh grade. In addition, Figure 10.6 demonstrates a clear difference in the types of aggression engaged in by boys and girls by the time they reach seventh grade.

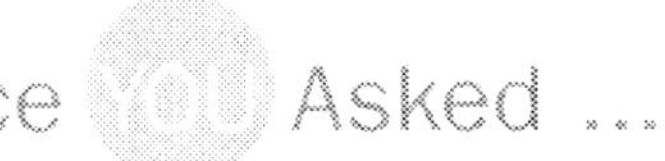

6. Everyone always says that men are more aggressive than women, but I'm a woman, and I think I'm usually more aggressive than most men. Is everyone wrong, or am I just weird?

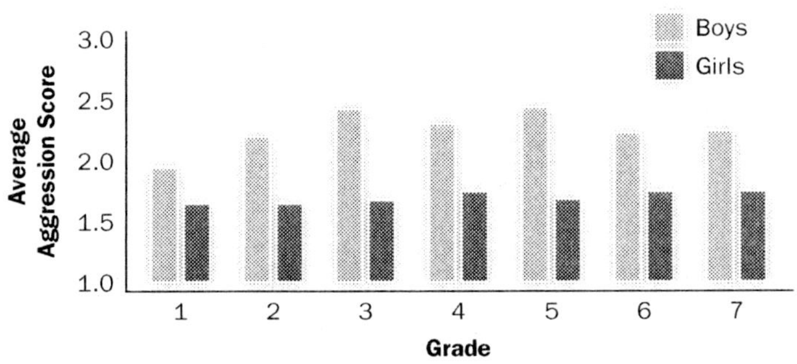

FIGURE 10.5 Boys' and Girls' Aggressive Behavior in Grades 1 through 7 Boys tend to display consistently higher overall levels of aggression throughout childhood.

Source: Adapted from "Gender and Aggression." Graph, "Boys' and Girls' Aggressive Behavior, Grades 1-7." The Institute for Teaching and Research on Women, 2002.

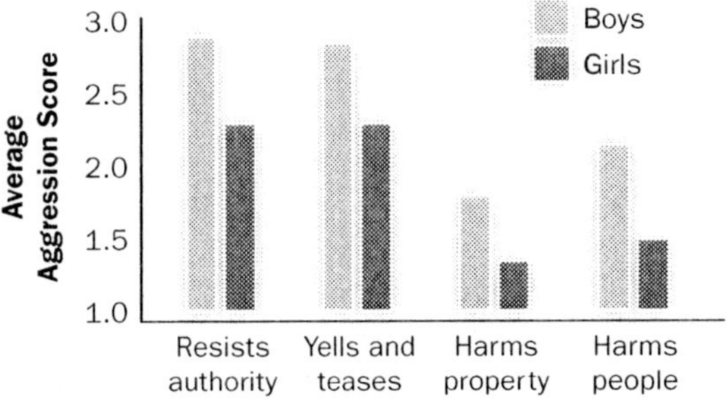

FIGURE 10.6 Aggression by Gender among Seventh Graders Boys have been shown to display greater levels of aggression across various behaviors.

Source: Adapted from "Gender and Aggression." Graph, "Types of Aggression by Gender, 7th Grade." The Institute for Teaching and Research on Women, 2002.

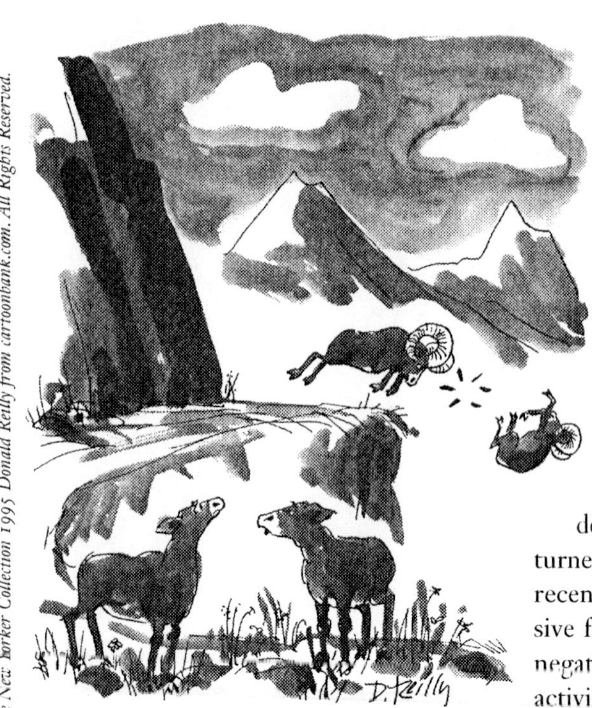

"It's a guy thing."

Men appear to be more physically aggressive well into adulthood. One demonstration of this difference lies in comparing violent crime statistics. The fact is that men commit the vast majority of violent crimes worldwide. In the United States, men commit 80 percent of all violent crimes, including 88 percent of murders, 93 percent of robberies, 83 percent of aggravated assaults, and 93 percent of sexual assaults (Bureau of Justice Statistics, 2001). We must be cautious, however, and avoid jumping to conclusions (or stereotypes!) in how we interpret the research on aggression and gender. Although most researchers agree that men are, overall, more aggressive than women, a closer examination of some of the findings reveals that men may not *always* be more aggressive. In fact, when the definition of aggression is expanded and the context in which the aggression occurs is considered, gender differences diminish and even reverse themselves.

Most studies of aggression focus on verbal and physical aggression. If the definition of aggression is broadened a bit, the typical gender differences may be turned upside-down. One type of aggression that researchers have focused on more recently is a type of relational aggression called **social alienation**. This is a more passive form of aggression that includes behaviors such as malicious gossip, spreading negative rumors, and *shunning* (the exclusion of someone from social groups and activities). When studies of children of all ages include these forms of aggression, girls have been found to engage in significantly more relational aggression than boys, and this finding appears to hold true across cultures (Crick, Casas, & Mosher, 1997; Crick & Grotpeter, 1995; French, Jansen, & Pidada, 2002). Furthermore, this same gender difference in social alienation forms of aggression has been found in adult populations such as college students (Werner & Crick, 1999). Figure 10.7 graphically illustrates this profound difference in aggression styles by gender. Men typically respond with greater aggression in situations involving frustration, negative feedback concerning their intelligence, physical attack, and no provocation at all. Women demonstrate greater aggressive responses to insults such as insensitive or condescending actions, impolite treatment by others, and rude comments (Bettencourt & Miller, 1996). Also, in contexts where provocation is present and aggression is seen as justified, the difference between men and women in aggression is minimal.

social alienation A passive form of aggression that includes behaviors such as malicious gossip, spreading negative rumors, and shunning.

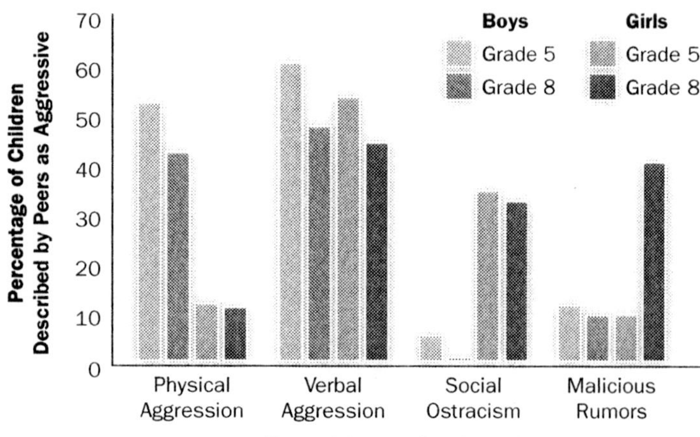

FIGURE 10.7 Gender Differences in Aggression in Fifth- and Eighth-Grade Children

Boys are far more aggressive than girls in overt forms of physical and verbal aggression; but for relational aggression behaviors of social ostracism and the spreading of malicious rumors, gender differences are reversed.

Source: Adapted from French, D., Jansen, E., & Pidada, S. (2002). United States and Indonesian children's and adolescents' reports of relational aggression by disliked peers.

You can see how the gender stereotype of aggression may represent very real differences between the sexes but may also lead us to assume that more or greater differences exist than actually do. Even for the most widely believed and accepted stereotype of aggression, if you factor in broader definitions and context, the differences are far more complex than the stereotype would have us believe.

Intuition

You have no doubt heard comments about "women's intuition." That simple phrase refers to another commonly held stereotype, that women are better than men at "reading people" nonverbally, based on facial expressions, body language, tone of voice, and situational cues. Do you think this stereotype is based on a real gender difference in people's ability to sense others' thoughts, feelings, and desires and to decode nonverbal signals? Research has indicated that the answer is yes. This is not to say that men are never able to intuit the feelings of others, but women, on the whole, do indeed appear to be better at it.

Researchers have conducted many studies in which women and men are asked to interpret the emotions in films or videos of people in various emotional states and situations without any verbal cues. In audio studies, men and women listen to people's voices in recordings that have been filtered so that the words are removed and only the tone of voice remains. In the vast majority of these studies, women perform better than men (Hall, 1984, 1998).

One important aspect in the overall skill of intuition is the ability to read facial expressions, referred to as *facial expression processing*. Over the past several decades, findings of studies looking at gender and facial expression processing have been mixed, with some research finding females performing better than males but other research showing no gender difference. However, a study from 2000 used a research technique called *meta-analysis* to attempt to resolve these contradictions in the literature. A meta-analysis gathers together the data from many previous studies, combines them, and reanalyzes them to see if any systematic differences emerge. "Evaluating Sexual Research: The Meta-Analysis" discusses this type of research in greater detail. When meta-analytic techniques were applied to gender effects on intuition, researchers found a clear female advantage in the ability to read nonverbal communication and facial expressions (Hall, 1978; McClure, 2000). Interestingly, we can see this advantage in facial expression processing from infancy all the way through adolescence. That very young girls show greater skill in decoding nonverbal communication lends support to the notion that this gender difference may have a biological basis. We will discuss the possible origins of gender differences later in this chapter.

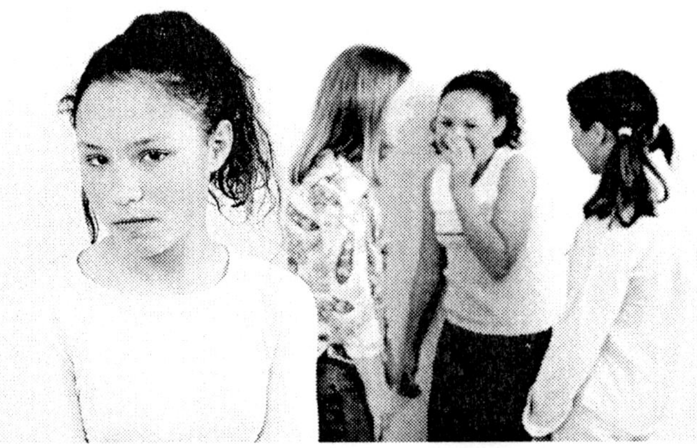

Females are far more aggressive than males when the aggression involves social alienation.

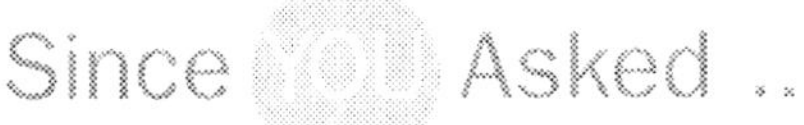

7. Why is it that men seem to want sex more than women?
8. Why do guys feel that they must "play the field," even after they've made a commitment to someone?
9. Why are women who have sex a lot seen in negative ways, while men who do the same are seen in a positive light?

Sexual Attitudes and Desire

Differences between males and females in various aspects of sexuality are included in discussions throughout this book. Clearly, many stereotypes exist about the sexual differences between men and women. Some of the differences people

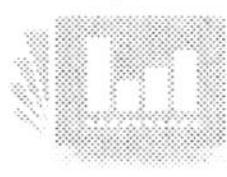

Evaluating Sexual Research

The Meta-Analysis

In the field of human sexuality as well as other areas of research, a technique called *meta-analysis* has often been used to organize research and resolve disputes in the scientific literature. With the aid of computers, meta-analysis takes the results of many individual studies that may appear inconsistent and integrates them into a larger statistical analysis so that the evidence forms a more meaningful whole. This research strategy was first proposed in 1976 by Dr. Gene Glass of Arizona State University.

For example, to determine the validity of the stereotypes discussed in this chapter, such as gender effects on aggression or intuition, a multitude of individual studies have been conducted, yielding many conflicting findings. Subsequent meta-analyses combining hundreds of studies on male and female aggression, however, have consistently found that male humans are more physically and verbally aggressive than female humans. As for intuition, one meta-analysis of 75 gender and intuition studies found that in 68 percent of the studies, women were better at decoding nonverbal messages; in only 13 percent were men better; and 19 percent found no gender difference. If you were to read a random sampling of those 75 studies, you could end up quite confused or even draw incorrect conclusions about what the overall research has actually shown.

With over 40,000 scientific journals and the number of new scientific articles appearing at the unbelievable rate of nearly 3,000 per day, you can see that the job of making sense out of the literature can be overwhelming. Through meta-analysis, many studies can be combined into one, and a larger, more organized picture of the research as a whole may be revealed.

believe are based in fact. Specifically, research has tended to support the following gender differences in sexual attitudes and desire. Most of these probably won't surprise you; they may already be part of your gender expectations and personal stereotypes (Laumann et al., 1994; Peplau, 2003):

- Women focus more on the relationship aspects of sexual activities; men have a more physical or recreational orientation toward sexuality.
- Men are more tolerant than women of casual sexual encounters.
- A greater number of men than women masturbate, and men masturbate more frequently.
- Men are more likely than women to be accepting of premarital sex and tend to feel less guilty having it.
- Men are less disapproving than women of extramarital sexual behaviors.
- Men think about sex more often than women on a daily basis.
- Men are more likely than women to engage in intercourse without an emotional attachment.
- Men are more likely than women to assume that others are interested in sex.
- When describing sexual experiences, women are more likely to romanticize them, while men are more likely to sexualize them.
- Women tend to see the goals of sex as building intimacy and expressing affection; men cite sexual variety and physical gratification as the goals of sexual activity.
- Men have stronger sexual drive and desire than women.

As with other gender stereotypes, however, we must consider these sexual differences with caution. For example, consider the last difference on the list. One of the most enduring stereotypes about human sexuality is that male sexual interest and desire is stronger than female sexual interest and desire. Virtually all the research on this difference tends to support this stereotype. However, if such a universal difference does exist, how large a difference is it? And how can we account for the many heterosexual couples who report a higher sex drive for the woman than the man? The answer to these questions lies in how the differences in male and female sexual desire are statistically determined.

When researchers find gender differences—for example, that men's sexual interests and desires are greater than women's—they are basing their conclusion on *averages*. An average reveals nothing about how much the two groups may overlap. Although the *average* level of sexual desire among men is higher than that of women, the variation in sexual desire in both men and women is quite large and overlaps considerably. Men and women are not polarized or opposite in their sex drive. In other words, some women's sex drives are higher than some men's, and some men's sex drives are lower than some women's (Baldwin & Baldwin, 1997). Figure 10.8 graphically illustrates this point. You can see that the curve for male sexual desire is skewed toward the higher range of sexual interest (the blue area) and the female curve is skewed toward the lower range (the red area). However, the largest area under the two curves is the overlapping area (shown in purple), representing higher sex drive for women and lower for men. Two people in an intimate relationship might come from the red and blue ranges respectively, but it is more likely they will both fall somewhere in the purple range of sexual desire.

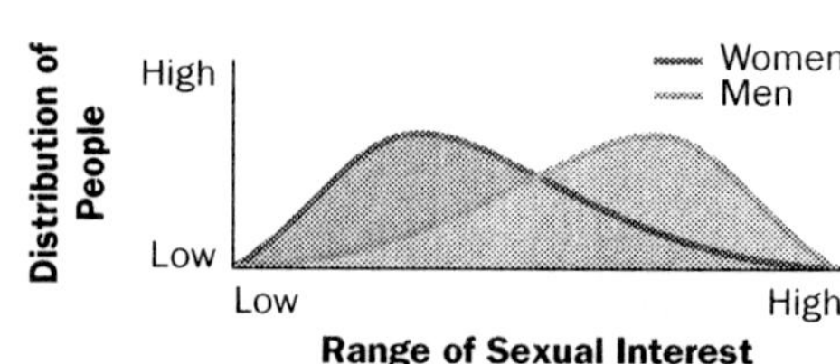

FIGURE 10.8 Male and Female Levels of Sexual Desire
Although levels of sexual desire are somewhat higher for men than for women overall, a great deal of overlap exists between the sexes.

Source: Adapted from Baldwin and Baldwin (1997), p. 182.

This overlapping-curve model of gender differences in sexual interest can be applied to all true gender differences in behavior. For example, although males are more physically aggressive than females overall, some women are more physically aggressive than some men, and some men display less aggression than some women. The male and female "curves of aggression" overlap, as do the gender curves for intuition and other sexual differences. The degree of difference between males and females determines the extent of the overlap. That is, the physical aggression curves probably overlap less than the sexual desire curves, meaning that we see a greater gender difference for physical aggression than for sexual desire. It is safe to say that most, if not all, gender differences have at least some overlap. Moreover, some research has reviewed numerous studies on gender and found that for most human characteristics gender differences are relatively small (Hyde, 2005). Such findings argue for more of a "gender similarity" model than a view expounding major gender differences overall.

Gender and Intimate Communication

One area relating to sexuality in which gender plays a crucial role is communication. As you may know from your personal experience, masculine and feminine patterns of communication differ in significant ways, and these differences can have far-reaching effects on intimate relationships.

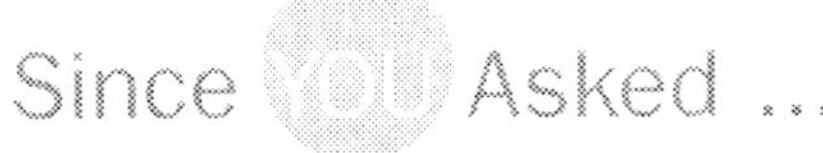

10. I've tried talking to my boyfriend about how I feel and what I want, but he never seems to understand, even though he says he does. How can I make him understand how I really feel?

One of the most common stumbling blocks in heterosexual love relationships relates to fundamental gender differences in communication styles. An awareness of these differences can go a long way in helping a couple reach deeper and more effective levels of communication. The problem is not that men and women are purposely trying to communicate poorly with each other. On the contrary, both want the same thing: to be understood, to understand, and to arrive at mutually satisfying communication outcomes. However, a great deal of research has pointed to the unavoidable conclusion that men and women, especially in intimate relationships, are just not talking the same language.

You may be able to recognize the essence of this problem from one very common example that often occurs when male-female partners are attempting to discuss personal problems. Women tend to express personal problems to those they are close to because they want support and understanding for whatever it is they are going through. However, when men confide personal difficulties, they are typically looking for solutions. When a woman expresses her issue to her male partner, typically, his first reaction is to try to "fix it"—give advice, problem-solve—when what she wants is support and understanding and may not want him to "fix it" at all. Conversely, when a man confides his problem to his female partner, she is likely to empathize—ask questions, offer support, understanding, and sympathy—which he may not want at all; he is looking for suggestions for how to "fix it." Both partners feel they are offering the partner the help they are seeking when in reality they are offering what they themselves would want in the same situation. Often this communication breakdown leads to frustration, distancing, and anger at the other's insensitivity, even when both are well intended and trying to be sensitive to each other's needs. Deborah Tannen, one of the leading researchers in the field of gender and communication, offers the following example of this particular problem in her famous book, *You Just Don't Understand: Men and Women in Conversation* (1991, pp. 49–50):

> Eve had a lump removed from her breast. Shortly after the operation, talking to her sister, she said that she found it upsetting to have been cut into, and that looking at the stitches was distressing because they left a seam that had changed the contour of her breast. Her sister said, "I know. When I had my operation, I felt the same way." Eve made the same observation to her friend Karen who said, "I know. It's like your body has been violated." But when she told her husband, Mark, how she felt, he said, "You can have plastic surgery to cover up the scar and restore the shape of your breast."
>
> Eve had been comforted by her sister and her friend, but she was not comforted by Mark's comment. Quite the contrary, it upset her more. Not only didn't she hear what she wanted, that he understood her feelings, but, far worse, she felt he was asking her to undergo more surgery just when she was telling him how much this operation had upset her. "I'm not having any more surgery!" she protested. "I'm sorry you don't like the way it looks." Mark was hurt and puzzled. "I don't care how it looks," he protested. "It doesn't bother me at all." She asked, "Then why are you telling me to have plastic surgery?" He answered, "Because you were saying *you* were upset about the way it looked."
>
> Eve felt like a heel: Mark had been wonderfully supportive and concerned throughout her surgery. How could she snap at him because of what he said . . .? She had perceived his words as [messages] that cut to the core of their relationship. . . . He thought he was

> reassuring her that she needn't feel bad about her scar because there was something she could *do* about it. She heard his suggestion that she do something about the scar as evidence that *he* was bothered by it. . . .
>
> Eve wanted the gift of understanding, but Mark gave her the gift of advice. He was taking the role of problem solver, whereas she simply wanted confirmation of her feelings.

Is this sort of dialogue familiar to you? It sounds suspiciously close to the old gender stereotype that men are socialized to be rational problem solvers while women are expected to be focused on feelings and connecting emotionally with others. Yet this communication pattern is pervasive. When most people, both men and women, first learn about it, a look of dawning recognition spreads across their faces. Barriers to communication such as this do not imply that men and women are consciously trying to avoid mutual understanding, but rather they usually have different basic, and deeply ingrained, goals in their interactions based on their gender. Even after learning about this advice-support communication disparity, men and women continue to have great difficulty learning and remembering to incorporate the knowledge into their relationships.

Again, this is only one example of the many gender differences in communication styles that interfere with mutual understanding. Table 10.3 lists some other gender differences in communication goals and strategies.

Origins of Gender Revisited

Earlier in this chapter, we discussed the influences of biology and environment (socialization) on gender development. How do these forces affect the development of the gender differences that form the basis of gender stereotypes? To answer that question, we must return to the nature-nurture debate.

Table 10.3 GENDER AND COMMUNICATION GOALS*

MEN'S GOALS	WOMEN'S GOALS
Give help; solve problems	Offer emotional support; empathize
Establish status	Seek harmony
Demonstrate authority	Strive for cooperation
Provide or receive information	Establish interaction
Avoid disagreement	Avoid being "cut-off"
Gather information, formulate rules	Draw from others' personal experience
Avoid asking questions	Ask questions, explore, show interest
Provide information	Provide encouragement
Avoid private conversations	Seek private conversations
Avoid talking about feelings	Seek talking about feelings
Seek debate	Seek agreement
Seek respect	Seek acceptance
Challenge others' expertise	Accept others' expertise
Keep active and busy	Maintain companionship and interaction
Avoid personal discussions with friends	Discuss personal issues with friends
Obtain big picture	Obtain details
Display knowledge and expertise	Conceal knowledge and expertise
Seek opportunities to speak in public	Avoid public speaking
Find personal independence	Find sense of shared community

*These are general findings and exceptions exist for both men and women.

Source: Adapted from Tannen (1991).

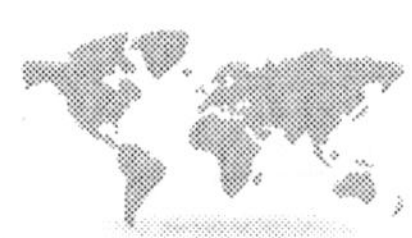

Sexuality and Culture

The Hijras: The Third Sex of India and Pakistan

The Hijras, primarily found in India and Pakistan, are a religious sect of biological males who dress and assume the role of women. Although they do not consider themselves male or female—but rather "neither man nor woman," a "third sex"—they are generally referred to with feminine pronouns and treated by the culture as women. Their religious practices focus on the worship of the mother goddess Bahuchara Mata (Slijper, 1997). Those who consider themselves true Hijras undergo the ritualistic surgical removal of the penis and testicles. This emasculation ritual is illegal and potentially life-threatening, causing it to be performed in great secrecy by a designated member of the sect, called a *dai ma*, who is not medically trained. During their six-hundred year existence in these countries, the Hijras have been discriminated against, ridiculed, and marginalized as a low class subculture.

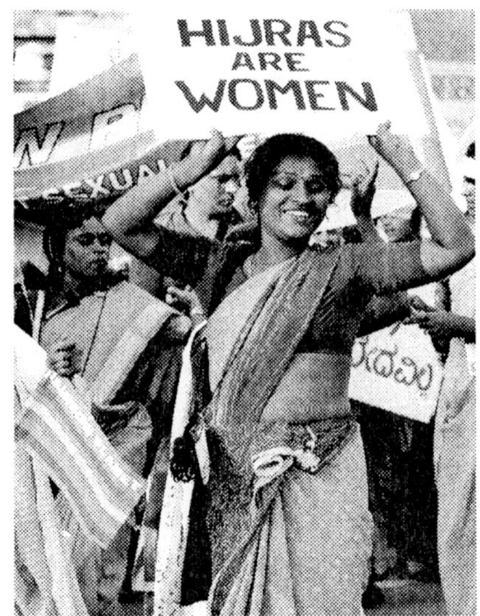

Hijras define themselves as neither male nor female, neither man nor woman, but rather as asexual or a "third sex."

However, Hijras are believed to have the power to bestow fertility on others, so they often are hired to perform songs, dances, and blessings at weddings and the births of male infants. Many are not able to earn enough money this way and also engage in prostitution (Slijper, 1997).

Recently, Hijras have begun to organize and demand greater personal and civil rights. Hijras are running for and winning local, state, and national elections and are poised to become increasingly politically powerful. Moreover, they are not denying their cultural practices to do so. Instead, they are using their non-sexual identities for political advantage, as demonstrated by a Hijra campaign slogan: "You don't need genitals for politics; you need brains and integrity" (Reddy, 2003).

Nature

The nature argument contends that gender differences are rooted in our biology and are passed down to us through our genetic heritage. Embedded in this position is the idea that these differences exist in humans as part of nature's grand design that has enabled humans to survive and evolve as a species. From this perspective, the reason that men are more aggressive, women are more intuitive, or men are more interested in sex is that these characteristics are survival strategies or *adaptive mechanisms*: Greater aggression in men stems from the evolutionary role of males to be protectors of females and infants, to fight for food and status, and to defend territory. Women, then, are more intuitive because females, over the course of evolution, were placed in the role of caring for infants whose needs must be recognized without the benefit of language in order to survive and thrive. The male's greater sexual drive relates to "reproductive strategies" and the biological need for the male to impregnate multiple partners to ensure continuation of his genes and the species in general. On the other hand, the female's best strategy for reproducing is to select the best, strongest, healthiest male and keep him around for protection and support. Although these mechanisms are probably no longer needed for our survival as a species, supporters of the genetic position contend that they continue to function and cause gender differences such as those we have discussed here. Interestingly, however, a few cultures worldwide draw the universality of these contentions into question (see "Sexuality and Culture: The Hijras").

Nurture

The nurture side of debate downplays genetic influences and focuses on sociocultural factors as responsible for producing gender differences. This argument maintains that strong social and cultural factors, such as we discussed earlier, begin to

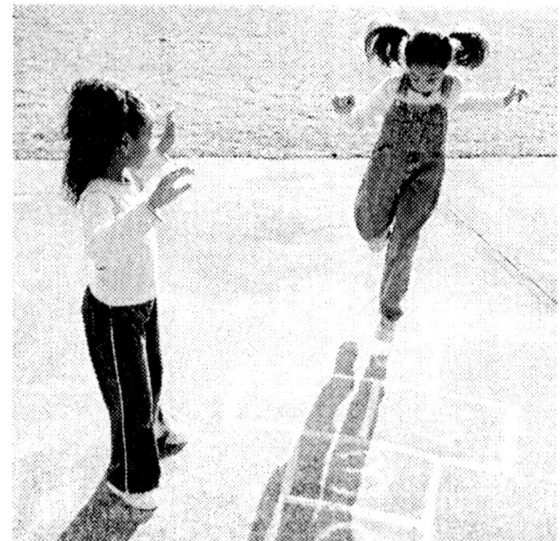

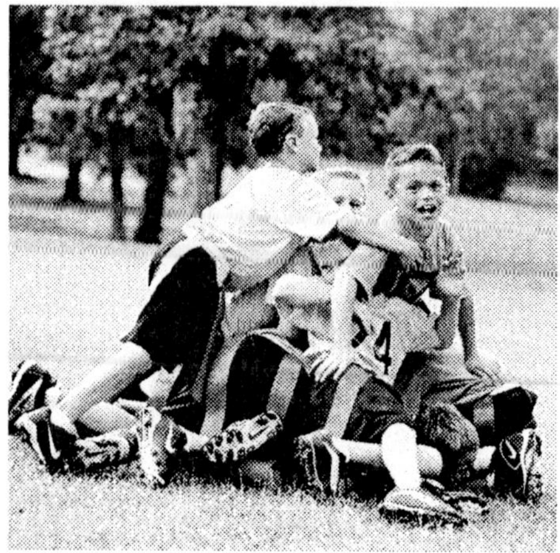

Many researchers contend that gender differences are learned through sociocultural expectations.

mold male and female behavior nearly from the moment of birth and continue to exert pressure on the behavior of men and women throughout their lives. From this point of view, males are more aggressive than females because society *expects* and *allows* boys and men to display greater aggression but expects girls to behave in less (overtly) aggressive ways and does not allow them to display as much aggression. The female's greater intuitive skills may be explained by society's expectation that girls and women should be focused on the emotional side of social interactions and therefore learn to be skilled at reading nonverbal expressions of various emotional states. The nurture position might explain differences in sexual interest as stemming from the different messages boys and girls receive from the culture about sex. In most cultures, boys are "given permission" to be sexual, while girls receive the message that behaving in certain sexual ways is inappropriate and unacceptable. It follows, then, that boys and girls will grow up with different levels of sexual interest, desire, and behaviors, such as masturbation.

The central question becomes, which side of the nature-nurture debate is right about gender? As you think about these two approaches, you may find yourself leaning more toward one or the other; most people do. However, you are probably also thinking that the truth may lie somewhere in between, that both genes and environment may be functioning together in some way. This is probably the case, and yet the debate over the relative influence of nature and nurture remains quite divided. In one study of gender differences in sexual interest, the authors explain the level of the controversy as follows:

> This debate often becomes so polarized that no compromises seem possible. Many people see women and men as opposite sexes and tend to explain the oppositeness in terms of biological differences in the form and function of the two sexes. Other people believe that the two sexes are basically similar, except for minor differences resulting from cultural factors. . . . When biological and cultural extremes are pitted against each other, discussions about female-male differences often turn into debates over "nature vs. nurture," and the advocates from each side attempt to explain all—or at least all the important—male-female differences in terms of *either* biological or cultural variables. Although behavioral scientists have been advised for decades to avoid the either-or arguments that pit nature against nurture and focus instead on developing models that unify nature and nurture, this goal is often not attained in analyzing sex and gender differences. (Baldwin & Baldwin, 1997, pp. 183–184).

Perhaps one way of turning down the volume of this controversy over gender differences is to return to the idea that genders overlap rather than directly oppose each other. In fact, research has shown quite clearly that some people do appear to exhibit both masculine and feminine traits. These individuals are often referred to as **androgynous**.

Androgyny

androgynous Exhibiting both masculine and feminine traits.

two-dimensional model of gender An approach to defining gender suggesting that gender is not an either-or proposition but that people may manifest elements of both genders simultaneously.

Early theories of gender assumed a mutually exclusive view: that people have a gender role identity that is either primarily masculine or primarily feminine and that masculinity and femininity are at opposite ends of a one-dimensional gender scale. If you were to complete a test measuring your gender identity based on this view, your score would place you somewhere along a single scale, either more toward the masculine or toward the feminine end of the scale.

During the 1970s, psychologists proposed a groundbreaking **two-dimensional model of gender**. This approach allowed for the possibility that gender is not an either-or proposition but that people may manifest elements of both genders (Bem, 1974, 1994; Constantinople, 1973). This two-dimensional view of gender measures people on two *separate* scales, one for masculinity and one for femininity. Instead of being either masculine or feminine, a person can rate high on *both* masculinity and femininity. This may not sound very surprising to you now, but at the time it was revolutionary. One of the leading figures in gender research, Sandra Bem, described people who perceive themselves as having both strong masculine and feminine traits as *androgynous* (from *andro*, meaning "male" or "masculine," and *gyn*, meaning "female" or "feminine"). Here is how she framed the issue in her now-famous 1974 article:

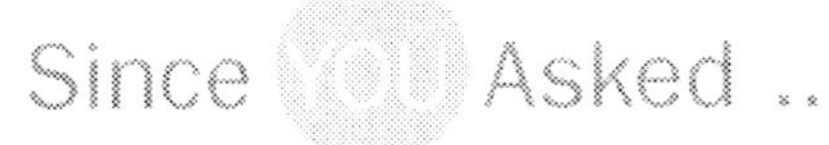

11. Can someone be both male and female, or masculine and feminine, at the same time? I feel as if I don't really fit into either the masculine or feminine categories of behavior.

> Both in psychology and in society at large, masculinity and femininity have long been conceptualized as bipolar ends of a single continuum; accordingly, a person has had to be either masculine or feminine, but not both. This sex-role dichotomy has served to obscure two very plausible hypotheses: first that many individuals might be "androgynous"; that is, they might be both masculine and feminine, both assertive and yielding, both instrumental and expressive, depending on the situational appropriateness of these various behaviors; and conversely, that strongly typed individuals might be seriously limited in the range of behaviors available to them as they move from situation to situation. (p. 155)

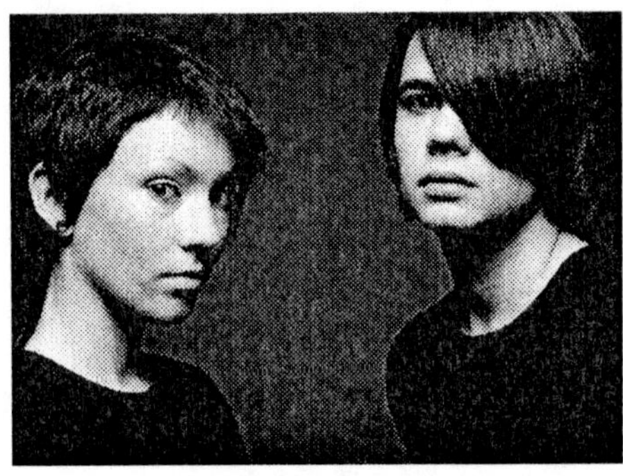

The concept of androgyny suggests that some people possess a balance of traditional masculine and feminine qualities.

Measuring Androgyny

Interestingly, Bem was not simply theorizing a new way of looking at gender but also suggesting that some *advantages* might exist for people who are less strongly sex-typed and more able to behave in either masculine or feminine ways, depending on the situation. In her article, Bem developed a new instrument for measuring gender that incorporated her two-dimensional approach. The Bem Sex-Role Inventory contains a list of 60 characteristics that are masculine (e.g., acts as leader, ambitious, assertive, dominant, independent, self-reliant, willing to take risks), feminine (e.g., affectionate, childlike, sympathetic, understanding, yielding, shy), or gender-neutral (e.g., adaptable, conscientious, friendly, reliable, truthful, adaptable) on which people can rate themselves on a 7-point scale (Bem, 1974). By examining the differences among the feminine, masculine, and gender-neutral scores, a person can determine his or her degree of masculine, feminine, or androgynous gender identity.

Research on Androgyny

A great deal of research was generated by the new conceptualization of gender as two-dimensional, allowing for the existence of androgyny in addition to the traditional divisions of masculine and feminine. Prior to the 1970s, the prevailing belief was that people would be most well-adjusted in life if their "gender matched their sex"; that is, boys and men should display masculine attitudes and behaviors, and girls and women should display feminine attitudes and behaviors. However, the recognition of androgyny shifted this focus.

Studies began to show that people who are more androgynous appear to be happier and better adjusted than those who are strongly sex-typed. For example, research has shown that androgynous children and adults tend to have higher levels of self-esteem and are more adaptable in diverse settings (Taylor & Hall, 1982). Other research has suggested that androgynous individuals have greater success in heterosexual intimate relationships, probably due to their greater ability to understand and accept each other's differences and needs better than couples in which the man is highly masculine and the woman is highly feminine (Coleman & Ganong, 1985). More recent research has revealed that people with the most positive traits of androgyny tend to be psychologically healthier and happier overall (Woodhill & Samuels, 2003).

Today, the basic theory of androgyny as developed by Bem and others has undergone various changes and refinements over the years. Numerous researchers have suggested that the psychological advantages experienced by people who score high in androgyny may be due more to the presence of masculine traits rather than a balance between male and female characteristics (Whitley, 1983). If you think about it, this makes sense. Looking back at the Self-Discovery about gender stereotypes, you will notice that many traits associated with femininity are regarded by most Western societies as undesirable. Based on this, we can assume that people who possess more masculine than feminine characteristics will probably, in most circumstances, receive more favorable treatment by others, which in turn creates greater levels of self-confidence and self-esteem in the individual.

Of course, not all masculine qualities are positive or feminine qualities negative. Positive and negative traits exist for both genders. The suggestion of positive and negative gender traits has led researchers to propose a further refinement of the androgyny concept to include *four* dimensions: *desirable femininity, undesirable femininity, desirable masculinity*, and *undesirable masculinity* (Ricciardelli & Williams, 1995). Qualities such as firm, confident, and strong are seen as desirable masculine traits, while bossy, noisy, and sarcastic are undesirable masculine traits. On the feminine side, patient, sensitive, and responsible are desirable traits, and nervous, timid, and weak are undesirable traits. Depending on how someone's set of personality traits line up, a person could be seen as positive masculine, negative masculine, positive feminine, negative feminine, positive androgynous, or negative androgynous. Table 10.4 illustrates these differences and how they could combine to produce positive and negative androgyny.

When gender characteristics are more carefully defined to consider both positive and negative traits, the advantages for *positive androgynous* individuals become even more pronounced (Woodhill & Samuels, 2003). People who combine the best of male and female gender qualities are more likely to be more well-rounded, happier, more popular, better liked, more flexible and adaptable, and more content with themselves than those who are able to draw on only one set of gender traits or who combine negative aspects of both genders. Just imagine someone (male or female) who is patient, sensitive, responsible, firm, confident, and strong (positive androgyny) compared to a person who is nervous, timid, weak, bossy, noisy, and sarcastic (negative androgyny), and you'll easily get the idea behind this theory.

Table 10.4 SETS OF GENDER TRAITS CREATING POSITIVE AND NEGATIVE ANDROGYNY: SOME EXAMPLES

POSITIVE FEMININE TRAITS	POSITIVE MALE TRAITS	NEGATIVE FEMININE TRAITS	NEGATIVE MALE TRAITS
Patient	Firm	Nervous	Bossy
Appreciative	Confident	Timid	Showing off
Loves children	Competitive	Self-critical	Noisy
Responsible	Strong	Nervous	Aggressive
Loyal	Outspoken	Bashful	Sarcastic
These two columns combine to create: *Positive androgyny*		**These two columns combine to create:** *Negative androgyny*	

Note: Some individuals may have various combinations of positive and negative masculine or feminine traits, giving them various degrees of positive or negative androgyny.

Source: Adapted from Ricciardelli and Williams (1995), pp. 644–645.

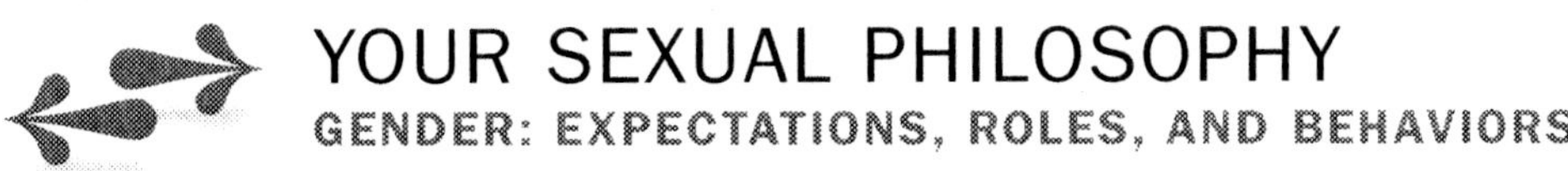

YOUR SEXUAL PHILOSOPHY
GENDER: EXPECTATIONS, ROLES, AND BEHAVIORS

If you are like most people, you have probably not given very much thought to your gender or, for that matter, anyone else's. Most likely, you have simply made assumptions about gender all your life: People are male or female, masculine or feminine, man or woman. But the concept of gender is not nearly as simple as it seems, and the influence of gender on our understanding of human sexuality is powerful and far-reaching. Gender plays a role in virtually every part of life, and an awareness of the complexities of masculinity and femininity are crucial to each individual's journey through life as a sexual being.

Consequently, gender also has a very important place in everyone's sexual philosophy. Although you may not have given a great deal of thought to your or other people's gender in the past, you probably will now, after reading this chapter. One of the reasons an awareness of gender issues is important relates to the range of behaviors you perceive as available to you as an individual. As we discussed in the chapter, people who are most sex-typed, meaning those who display behaviors that are at the extremes of masculine or feminine characteristics, may be less flexible in their behavior in a given situation. In other words, very masculine or very feminine individuals may have fewer options available to them for dealing with the world around them.

For example, people who are mainly feminine might have difficulty being assertive or taking a leadership role, but they might be an ideal choice for caring for a child or an elderly person. On the other hand, highly masculine people might feel utterly lost if asked to care for a young child or help a friend with emotional difficulties but might be ready, willing, and able to assume the role of leader when necessary. Both of these skills are culturally desirable, and that is why it is important to understand that male and female, masculine and feminine, are not opposite ends of a single scale but rather two separate scales on which each person may be either high or low. The possibility exists for someone to embody both masculine and feminine sides of personality—to be androgynous. The flexibility of androgyny may allow for a fuller, more varied set of options for dealing effectively with many of life's complex situations.

Can people learn to be androgynous if they are not already? Or is it something people are born with or develop throughout life? The answer is yes to both questions. Many people seem to grow up feeling easy and comfortable displaying behaviors and characteristics commonly associated with both masculinity and femininity. Others enter adulthood with a very rigid, one-sided masculine or feminine self-concept. However, many of those who seem unable to accept androgynous behaviors and attitudes in themselves can learn to do so if they wish. And the learning begins with becoming educated about cultural expectations for gender-appropriate behavior and recognizing that violating those expectations, under the right conditions, can be seen as a strength and is often very rewarding. When the "macho man" discovers his capacity for tenderness, caring, and affection or when the ultrafeminine woman realizes her ability to be strong, independent, and assertive, both have grown and have become more effective people in life and in love.

Incorporating awareness and acceptance of gender diversity in yourself and others is a basic and compelling component of everyone's sexual philosophy. After all, the whole point of pursuing a clear, personal sexual philosophy is to know who you are, what you want and don't want for yourself in your life, and planning ahead to be the most effective and satisfied person possible. Breaking free of some of society's limiting gender expectations is one of the many challenges along that path.

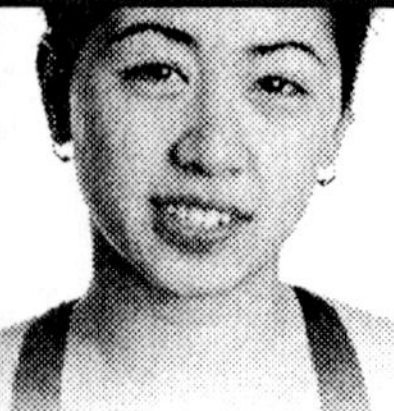

Summary

HISTORICAL PERSPECTIVES The Story of Christine Jorgensen

- George Jorgensen in 1953 became Christine Jorgensen as a result of the first widely publicized sex reassignment surgery. Through her willingness to go public with her transsexualism and sex reassignment process, Christine Jorgensen is today considered by many a pioneer in the social awareness of transgender issues.

The Distinctions between Sex and Gender Identity

- Gender and sex are two separate human dimensions. Biological sex is related to hormonal levels and genes. In a small percentage of births, the biological sex of the infant is not always obvious. Some infants are born with ambiguous genitalia, referred to as intersex. Abnormal levels of hormones may also produce sex- and gender-based disorders such as Klinefelter syndrome in males and Turner syndrome in females.
- Gender and gender identity tend to be a more socially constructed characteristic relating to a person's degree of perceived masculinity or femininity.

The Development of Gender Identity

- Development of gender identity is believed by many experts to be primarily influenced by biological and environmental factors. These influences include genes and hormonal levels in the uterus during fetal development.
- Others hold that socialization primarily determines gender through society's overt and hidden influence on gender-appropriate behaviors, which are heavily influenced by parents, peers, teachers, television, and other media.
- Some individuals, referred to as transgendered, feel that their biological sex does not accurately represent their gender identity, and some, often called transsexual individuals, take steps—including dress, hormone therapy, and surgery—to align their appearance with their gender identity. Current medical procedures for altering a person's physical sex are quite effective and produce realistic and functional sexual structures.

Gender and Sexual Orientation

- Gender identity is not always predictive of a person's sexual orientation. A person who perceives his gender as male may identify as heterosexual, gay, or bisexual, just as a person whose gender identity is female may self-identify as heterosexual, lesbian, or bisexual. Most people who self-identify as male are attracted to those who self-identify as female and vice versa, but this is not universally the case. Gender and sexual orientation may function as separate expressions of sexual identity.

Gender Roles and Stereotypes

- Gender stereotypes exert a powerful influence on a culture's perceptions of men and women. Stereotyped expectations of masculine and feminine behaviors begin in early childhood. Many gender stereotypes contain a grain of truth, but differences are smaller and more overlapping than typically believed.
- The stereotype that males are more aggressive than females is generally true for physical and verbal aggression. However, females are found to be more aggressive than males when the definition of aggression is broadened to include relational aggression such as social rejection and malicious gossip. Overall, girls and women are found to be better than boys and men at intuition, the reading nonverbal communication signals. Males are found to have higher overall levels of sexual desire and interest, but the ranges of male and female sexual desire overlap significantly.
- Communication patterns and goals are different for men and women, often interfering with effective communication between the genders.

Origins of Gender Revisited

- Origins of sexual orientation tend to revolve around the larger nature-nurture controversy.
- The nature argument contends that gender differences are rooted in our biology and are passed down to us through our genetic heritage. Embedded in this position is the idea that these differences exist in humans as part of nature's grand design that has enabled humans to survive and evolve as a species.
- The nurture side of the debate downplays genetic influences and focuses on social and cultural factors as primarily responsible for producing gender differences. This position maintains that strong environmental factors begin to mold male and female behavior from the moment of birth and throughout life.
- Strong proponents of the nature and nurture sides of human development continue to polarize the debate over the exact origins of gender differences.

Androgyny

- In the 1970s, the concept of gender was redefined to include androgyny, the notion that both masculine and feminine characteristics may exist in the same person at the same time. Research suggests that androgynous individuals are generally happier and better adjusted. However, an androgynous person may possess masculine and feminine traits that are either socially positive or negative that combine to determine his or her overall gender personality.

YOUR SEXUAL PHILOSOPHY: Gender: Expectations, Roles, and Behaviors

- Gender is a major component of human sexual identity. Gender roles and behavioral expectations play a role in virtually every part of life. Awareness and understanding of the complexities of masculinity and femininity are crucial to each individual's journey through life as a sexual being.

Have You Considered?

1. Think for a few minutes about a typical week in your life. List eight or ten activities that you would be likely to engage in during that week. Now imagine that your gender identity is suddenly reversed and you are a member of the opposite sex. Go back over your list to see how many of your usual activities might change and in what ways. What does this exercise tell you about gender?
2. Imagine you are filling out a job application on which you are asked to check whether you are "male," "female," or *"other."* Discuss how you think you might react to seeing such a question. Do you think your reaction would be similar to others'? Why or why not?
3. Think of one gender-related behavior or activity that is likely to vary greatly from culture to culture. Now think of one that you would expect to be fairly consistent across cultures. Why do you think the first behavior varies while the other remains constant? What might this tell you about the two behaviors?
4. Picture groups of kindergarten boys and girls playing on the playground at recess. List at least three clear differences you are likely to see in the groups' activities, interactions, and behaviors. Based on what you've read in this chapter, what might explain these differences?
5. On a Saturday morning, set aside an hour or so to watch children's programming on TV. Choose any program or channel you wish. While you watch, pay close attention to any gender differences and stereotypes you see in the writing and production of the shows, and make note of them. Discuss your findings from this brief observations study. What gender differences and stereotypes did you observe? If you observed none, why do you think the shows you watched were different from most?
6. Imagine you are looking for a new romantic relationship and you meet someone with whom you really hit it off. You enjoy the same activities, you share similar attitudes and beliefs, and you find each other physically and sexually attractive. As the relationship progresses and begins to grow more intimate, your new partner confides in you that he or she is transgendered and has undergone sex reassignment surgery. How do you think you might react to this news? What do you think might happen from that point on in the relationship?
7. Research finds that overall, men display greater levels of sexual drive, desire, and interest than women. Why might this difference exist from both the nature and the nurture perspectives?
8. Think of three people you know who are very masculine, very feminine, or androgynous (no names, please!). For each person, list three aspects of their personality or behavior patterns that reflect their gender identity. Which of the three individuals do you feel is the best adjusted? Explain your answer.

Companion Website Resources

For further chapter resources go to **www.prenhall.com/hock**. This robust text website includes polling questions for you to vote on, regular news updates, quizzes, sample tests, suggested reading lists, and more.

SCENARIOS USA Also on the website are links to videos. *Scenarios USA's* films portray real-life narratives that explore the non-biological aspects of relationships and sexual health. The films will help you consider how the themes of the text affect your own life and the lives of those around you.

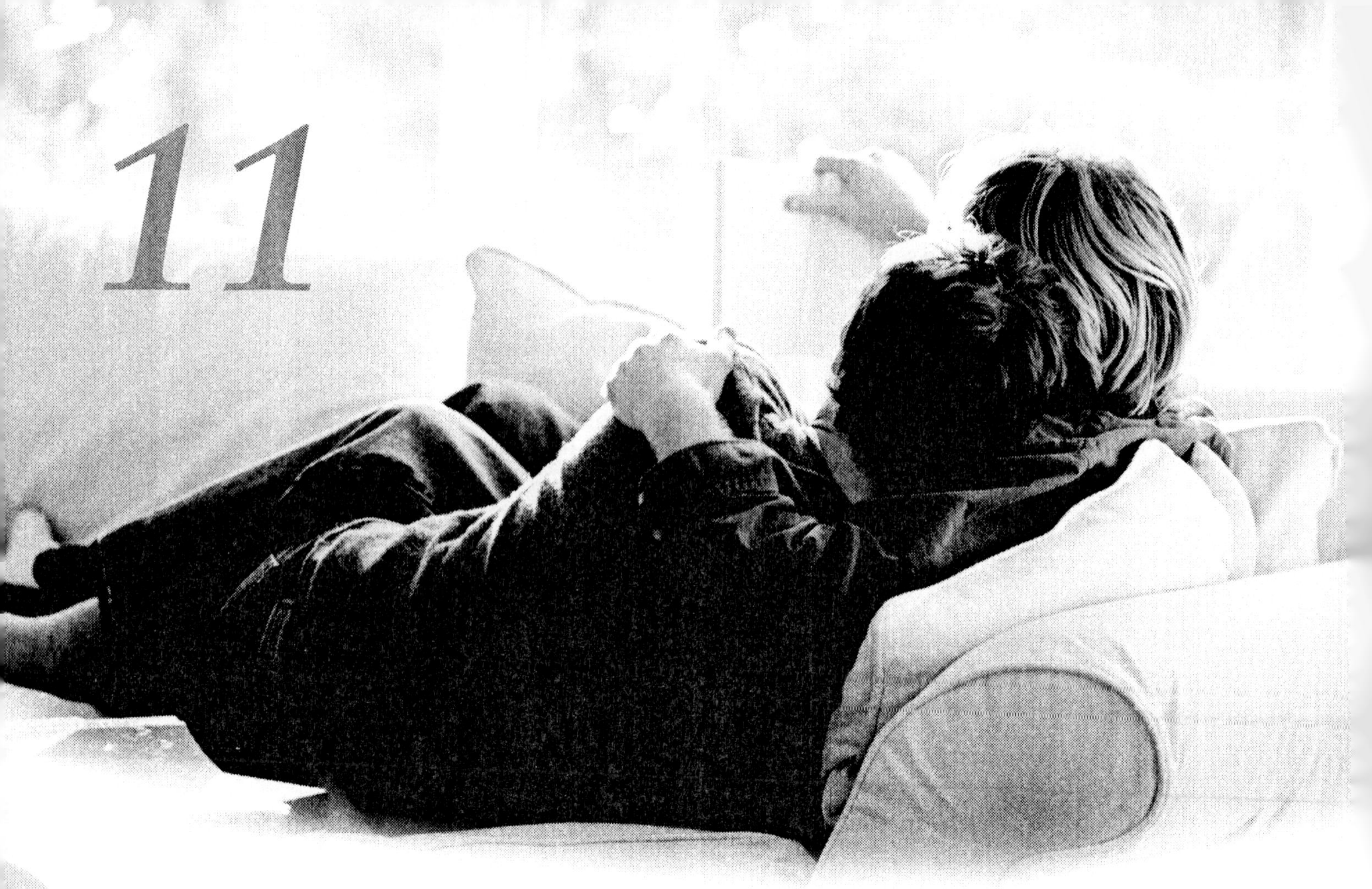

11

Sexual Orientation

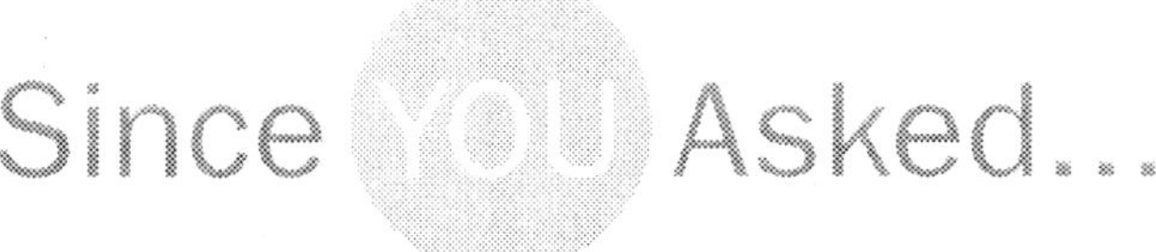

Since YOU Asked...

1. I have gay friends who often refer to something called "Stonewall," but I don't know what they are talking about and I don't want to ask and seem stupid or offend them. (see page 407)

2. Are gay and lesbian people ever attracted to members of the opposite sex? (see page 408)

3. Is bisexuality only a stage in getting to know oneself as a gay individual, or is it a sexual orientation in itself? (see page 409)

4. It seems to me that male sexual anatomy is designed to "fit" with female sexual anatomy and vice versa. So what's the deal with homosexuality? (see page 411)

5. How do people know or decide to be homosexual or heterosexual or bisexual? (see page 412)

6. I have no problem with homosexuals. I say live and let live. But I don't see why they are so concerned with getting married. I mean, if they can have their relationship, why do they have to get married? (see page 413)

7. Do gay and lesbian couples really love each other in the same way as straight couples? (see page 414)

8. How do gay and lesbian relationships differ from heterosexual ones, if they do? (see page 415)

9. Why are some people gay? Is it something they're born with or just bad experiences with their parents or the opposite sex? (see page 415)

10. How old are most people when they come to terms with or understand that they are homosexual? Do they usually tell people right away? Are they usually comfortable with the realization? (see page 424)

11. Do homosexual people feel comfortable holding hands and showing other public displays of affection with their partner? How often are they ridiculed or threatened? (see page 426)

The following is an excerpt from a second-year college student's paper written for a human sexuality class and reprinted here with his permission.

I have known I was gay for as long as I can remember. I hear stories of people saying that they didn't know until high school or college, but I really find that hard to believe. A person's sexuality is a very important part of his or her life, and I always think to myself, "How can you not know?" It has always been with me and I have always been aware of it.

Early in my life, I lived a lie. I behaved in ways that everyone would like and accept, and nobody, not even my parents, would suspect I was gay. I have to tell you I was miserable. Can you imagine going through life having to hide your true self? It was absolute torture. I was so upset because we only have one chance at life and I was given a major "handicap." I kept asking, "Did I do something to deserve this?". " And I would have given anything to be like everyone else. I just knew that for the rest of my life, I would be forced to live this lie.

Never in my wildest dreams did I imagine that I would be able to talk freely and openly about my sexuality. My friends would have rejected me instantly if I had told them I was gay. When I entered college, everything changed. In college, I made new and wonderful friends who taught me it is all right to be who I am and I shouldn't worry about what other people think about me. But the real event that changed everything occurred over the summer. My best friend introduced me to a guy who was also gay. We hit it off right away, and one thing led to another and we started dating. This posed a lot of problems. I felt guilty about hiding it from my parents and everyone else, but I was afraid someone would find out. Soon, as my boyfriend and I became closer and closer, I realized that my happiness was more important than what other people thought. I was proud of who I was, and I didn't want to change.

I finally decided to tell my brother and my mom. Afraid of what might happen and hoping they would not reject me, it took a while for me to spit it out; but after I did, their response could not have been better. They were very accepting of the fact that I am gay and were sorry that I did not feel comfortable enough to tell them sooner. My boyfriend and I are still together, and we are doing great!

I must say, my life has been a roller coaster of emotional highs and lows. I would not change a thing, however, because I love the person I am today. I have realized that it doesn't matter what other people think about me as long as I am happy. I believe I am a stronger person because of what I have had to go through. Now, at twenty years old, I feel like my life is just beginning, and I know that it is going to be filled with happiness.

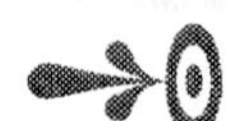

Focus on Your Feelings

Like many of the topics throughout this book, issues of sexual orientation often provoke various intense emotions. For many, feelings tend to run high in response to gay and lesbian individuals themselves, but for others, the strongest emotions are triggered by the prejudice and discrimination that still exist in our society today. These feelings may include confusion, sadness, fear, anger, outrage, hostility, and even violent intentions. As a culture, we are working through negative stereotypes, prejudices, and discriminatory behaviors targeted at nonheterosexual individuals. But events all around us make it clear that we still have a long way to go.

Reading about and studying sexual orientation in this book and in class is an opportunity for each of you to reveal (to yourself) and examine (within yourself) your feelings about this important topic. Some questions you might want to think about are these: Do you feel comfortable with your emotional reactions? Do your reactions truly reflect the attitudes you want to hold toward people of all sexual orientations? If you are unsure of or unhappy with your feelings as you read this chapter, can you identify where your attitudes came from and how they developed in you? How will you go about altering the feelings you do not like? And finally, after you have read the chapter, have your feelings about these topics changed? If so, how did they change? What do you think triggered those changes?

Remember, emotions are based on knowledge and experience, and it is a fact that many people simply have very little experience with people of various sexual orientations. Taking time to study and understand these topics, especially those that evoke the strongest negative emotions, can help us grow, change, and learn to respond to the world in productive and constructive ways. This is, as much as anything, what all education is all about.

Sexual orientation refers to the sex of the individuals to whom a person is romantically, emotionally, and sexually attracted. **Heterosexual** or **straight** refers to individuals who are primarily attracted to members of the opposite sex. **Homosexual** or **gay** and **lesbian** apply to those whose primary attraction is to members of their own sex—*gay* is often used for both men and women, while *lesbian* refers to homosexual women. **Bisexual** refers to people who are attracted to members of both sexes. The excerpt just presented recounts one student's journey as he discovered and accepted his sexual orientation.

Most of our attention in this chapter will be on the sexual orientations of nonheterosexuals. Why? Because most people in most cultures are **heterocentric**. That is, they take heterosexuality for granted and often have difficulty understanding and accepting nonheterosexual orientations. To understand nonheterosexual orientations better, we will examine what it means to be gay, lesbian, or bisexual in a heterocentric culture and explore the sociopolitical storm over the concept of gay marriage. We will analyze various theories about the origins of a person's sexual orientation. We will consider the challenges a person may face when acknowledging that he or she is not heterosexual, a process called *coming out*, including such topics as the stigma of HIV. We will conclude with a look at the disturbing nature of prejudice, discrimination, and violence against nonheterosexuals in our society and the emergence and growth of the gay rights movement.

Nonheterosexual orientations have been identified in writings and other art forms throughout the world for millennia. But in the next section, we will look back only a few decades to an event considered to be a turning point in the history of gay life in the United States.

sexual orientation Term describing the sex of those to whom a person is primarily romantically, emotionally, and sexually attracted.

heterosexual A person who is attracted romantically and sexually primarily to persons of the opposite sex.

straight Heterosexual.

homosexual A person who is attracted romantically and sexually primarily to persons of one's own sex.

gay Homosexual; often applied to both men and women.

lesbian A female with a homosexual orientation.

bisexual A person who is attracted romantically and sexually to members of both sexes.

heterocentric The assumption of a universal heterosexual orientation.

Historical Perspectives

The Stonewall Riot

In 1969, homosexuality was against the law in the United States and most other countries. The prohibitions went so far as to include a ban on serving alcohol to homosexuals. At that time, the Stonewall Inn in New York City was one of the few night spots where gay people could meet each other, flirt, hang out together, order drinks, dance, and just be uninhibited or romantic. Once a month or so, the police would raid the bar, rough up and ridicule the patrons, make numerous arrests, and cart large numbers of patrons away to jail in police vans.

June 27, 1969, was just another evening at the Stonewall Inn. No one knows why, but when the police once again raided Stonewall in the early morning hours of June 28, the patrons fought back. They were fed up with being harassed, beaten, and arrested for simply being who they were. They began yelling at the police to get out and leave them alone. As the police punched, dragged, and otherwise forced the patrons out into the street toward the paddy wagons, the yelling turned into fistfighting, and then beer bottles and garbage cans were hurled at the police. Crowds began to gather outside the bar, and more people, seeing the patrons being victimized, joined the fight against the police. Astonished that "these kind of people" would actually fight back, the police drew their guns and called in SWAT teams in full riot gear. Remarkably, by the time the dust cleared, no one had been killed or seriously injured, but the course of gay history had been changed forever. As word of the Stonewall riot spread, gays and lesbians across the country were emboldened to resist and even fight the prejudice and discrimination they had endured for so long. Four months after the riot, both *Time* and *Newsweek* ran cover stories on homosexuality in America, gay "be-ins" began to be held in New York's Central Park, and the gay rights movement had been born (Cusac, 1999).

Today, the Stonewall Inn still stands, although now as a men's clothing store. Most historians trace the true beginning of the now powerful gay rights movement to the

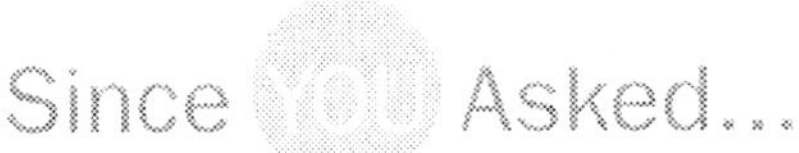

1. I have gay friends who often refer to something called "Stonewall," but I don't know what they are talking about and I don't want to ask and seem stupid or offend them.

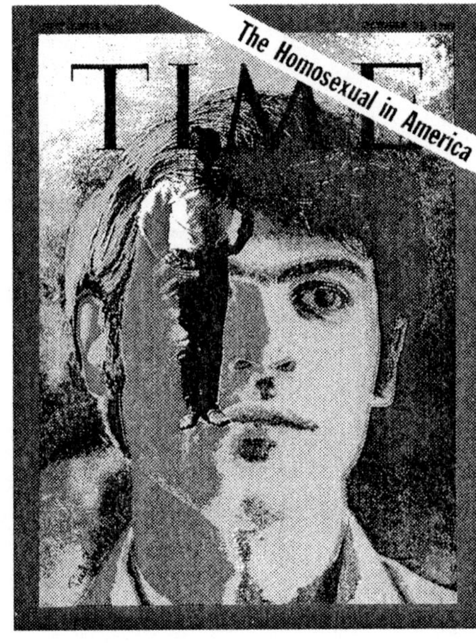

Four months after the Stonewall riot, Time *magazine published its first issue focusing on the rights of homosexuals.*

Stonewall riot of 1969. Each year, parades and other celebrations are held around the end of June in nearly every large city in the United States commemorating the Stonewall Inn riot and the antidiscrimination campaign it started. Clearly, prejudice and discrimination based on nonheterosexual orientation still exist, but now the *discriminators* are the ones more likely to be breaking the law. We will return to today's ongoing issues about gay rights later in this chapter.

Straight, Gay, Lesbian, Bisexual: A Closer Look

Regardless of your personal sexual orientation, you probably feel you have a pretty good idea of what it means if someone is referred to as "straight," "gay," "lesbian," or "bisexual." In fact, you are probably quite sure that your own sexual orientation falls into one, and *only* one, of three categories: *heterosexual, homosexual, or bisexual.* However, these labels are not as clearly differentiated as you may think. A person's sexual orientation, just like his or her sexuality in general, is complex and multifaceted and not always neat, clear-cut, or well defined.

The American Psychological Association (2004) defines sexual orientation in this way:

> Sexual orientation is an enduring emotional, romantic, sexual or affectional attraction to another person. It is easily distinguished from other components of sexuality including biological sex, gender identity (the psychological sense of being male or female) and the social gender role (adherence to cultural norms for feminine and masculine behavior). Sexual orientation exists along a continuum that ranges from exclusive homosexuality to exclusive heterosexuality and includes various forms of bisexuality. Bisexual persons can experience sexual, emotional and affectional attraction to both their own sex and the opposite sex. Persons with a homosexual orientation are sometimes referred to as gay (both men and women) or as lesbian (women only). Sexual orientation is different from sexual behavior because it refers to feelings and self-concept. Persons may or may not express their sexual orientation in their behaviors.

Sexual Orientation as Defined by Alfred Kinsey

One of the earliest attempts at defining sexual orientation was undertaken by Alfred Kinsey in his reports on sexual behavior that were published in the middle of the twentieth century. As noted in Chapter 1, Kinsey conducted large surveys of Americans in which participants were asked about virtually every aspect of their sexual practices. His reports on these interviews, *Sexual Behavior in the Human Male* (Kinsey, Pomeroy, & Martin, 1948) and *Sexual Behavior in the Human Female* (Kinsey et al., 1953), were intended for medical and other professionals, but as you might guess, they became runaway national best-sellers. People were eager to read about the sexual behaviors of others and compare themselves to the statistical findings revealed in the Kinsey Reports. Kinsey's studies were conducted at a time in American history when homosexuality was concealed and rarely discussed, much less written about. Yet here were the Kinsey researchers asking respondents the extent to which they had ever engaged in same-sex behaviors.

Since YOU Asked...

2. Are gay and lesbian people ever attracted to members of the opposite sex?

Based on responses from participants in the surveys, Kinsey asserted that very few people could be classified as totally heterosexual or totally homosexual. He maintained that most people fell somewhere in between or, as the modern definition puts it, "along a continuum." Kinsey found that most people who identified themselves as heterosexual had at least some same-sex experiences (including fantasies, dreams, thoughts, emotions, and

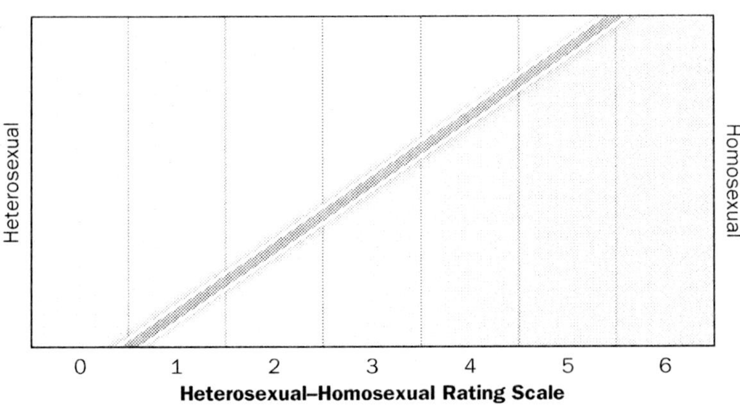

0 Exclusively heterosexual
1 Predominantly heterosexual, only incidentally homosexual
2 Predominantly heterosexual, but more than incidentally homosexual
3 Equally heterosexual and homosexual
4 Predominantly homosexual, but more than incidentally heterosexual
5 Predominantly homosexual, only incidentally heterosexual
6 Exclusively homosexual

FIGURE 11.1 Kinsey's Sexual Orientation Rating Scale

According to Kinsey's sexual orientation scale, most people cannot be classified as exclusively heterosexual or homosexual; rather, they fall somewhere in between, along a continuum.

Source: Kinsey, Pomeroy, and Martin (1948), p. 638.

behaviors) and, conversely, that many of those who perceived themselves as homosexual had some experiences involving the opposite sex. Therefore, Kinsey developed a sexual orientation rating scale that places each person on a scale of 0 to 6 where 0 indicates "exclusively heterosexual" and 6 reflects "exclusively homosexual" (see Figure 11.1). According to Kinsey, most people would fall somewhere above 0, but below 6 (rather than exactly on 0 or 6).

Using this scale as a guideline, some people, based on their sexual feelings and experiences (rather than their overall self-identification) might be categorized as primarily homosexual (5 or 6 on the scale) or primarily heterosexual (0 or 1). Someone who falls in the middle categories (2, 3, or 4) might be categorized as bisexual. To allow you to develop a clearer idea of this type of analysis, "Self-Discovery: A Sexual Orientation Worksheet" is an opportunity for you to see where on Kinsey's scale you might fall.

Bisexuality

It may seem as if *gay*, *lesbian*, and *bisexual* all fit neatly into a single category of "nonheterosexual orientations." However, in some ways, bisexuality is a unique sexual orientation, different from being gay, lesbian, or heterosexual. Kinsey's efforts to place sexual orientation on a continuum notwithstanding, most people continue to see people as either straight or gay. It appears, however, that bisexuality is a clearly defined sexual orientation in which a person may be emotionally, psychologically, and physically attracted to members of either sex.

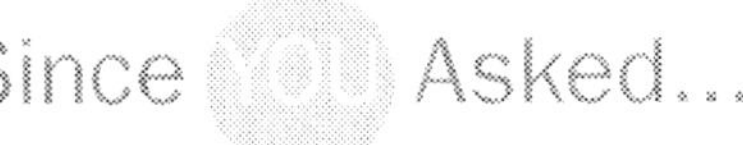

3. Is bisexuality only a stage in getting to know oneself as a gay individual, or is it a sexual orientation in itself?

Historically, many people and even some researchers believed that individuals who self-identified as bisexual were in reality tying to hide the fact that they were actually gay or lesbian or were simply on their way to coming out as gay or lesbian. Consequently, they have been given little attention in the scientific research and have been brushed aside by both straight and gay groups (Morgenstern, 2004). Many people assume that when bisexual individuals are in a relationship with someone of the other sex, they must be

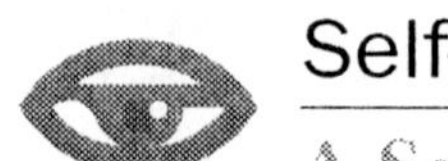

Self-Discovery

A Sexual Orientation Worksheet

This worksheet is designed to help you explore your own sexual orientation and to gain some insight into the idea that sexual orientation is rarely "all or nothing" in one direction or the other. Many of you may want to use a blank sheet of paper to complete this exercise. It is for your own self-discovery and needn't be shared with anyone. There are no right or wrong answers, and the scoring categories are rough approximations. You'll be able to understand the complexities of sexual orientation simply by looking at the distribution of your answers.

Use the following scales to respond to the categories in the table as indicated. In accordance with the scoring key following the scale, lower overall scores indicate a heterosexual emphasis, higher scores relate to homosexual leanings, and scores in the middle may imply a bisexual orientation.

Scale 1	Scale 2
Other sex only = 1	Heterosexual only = 1
Other sex mostly = 2	Heterosexual mostly = 2
Other sex somewhat more = 3	Heterosexual somewhat more = 3
Both sexes equally = 4	Heterosexual or homosexual = 4
Same sex somewhat more = 5	Gay/Lesbian somewhat more = 5
Same sex mostly = 6	Gay/Lesbian mostly = 6
Same sex only = 7	Gay/Lesbian only = 7

Self-Analysis Category	Scale to use	Past (ever)	Present (currently)	Ideally (if you could choose freely)	
1. Attraction to others (sexual, physical)	1				
2. Sexual behavior (kissing, touching, sexual interactions)	1				
3. Sexual fantasies (dreams, during masturbation, daydreams)	1				
4. Emotional preference (infatuation, love, romance)	1				
5. Social preference (friendships, confidants, hanging out)	1				
6. Self-identification (how you see yourself)	2				
7. Lifestyle (how you live your life as a sexual person)	2				
	Totals	______ +	______ +	______	= ______

Scoring

Possible scores range from a low of 21 to a high of 147 and may be interpreted as follows:

21–38 = Exclusively heterosexual
39–56 = Predominantly heterosexual, only incidentally homosexual
57–74 = Predominantly heterosexual, but more than incidentally homosexual
75–92 = Equally heterosexual and homosexual
93–110 = Predominantly homosexual, but more than incidentally heterosexual
111–128 = Predominantly homosexual, only incidentally heterosexual
129–147 = Exclusively homosexual

Source: Adapted from "Sexual Orientation Scale" from p. 38 in "Sexual Orientation: A Multi-Variable Dynamic Process" by F. Klein, B. Sepekoff, and T. Wolf in Two Lives: Bisexuality in Men and Women ed. by F. Klein and T. Wolf. Copyright © 1985. Reprinted by permission of The Haworth Press.

straight, but when they are involved with someone of their own sex, they are gay or lesbian. Self-proclaimed bisexual individuals are subject to prejudice and discrimination by the heterosexual majority (Eliason, 1997), but they encounter it in the gay world, too, with derisive phrases such as "Pick a lane" or "Choose a team." As one bisexual individual put it:

> We feel even more hurt when gays reject us than when straights do, since we feel that gay people know better. Many bisexuals have fought on the front lines of the gay rights movement, yet it seems like we have only token representation in the community; the word "bisexual" has been added to the masthead, but we don't feel truly included or accepted. (Morgenstern, 2004, p. 47)

Bisexual people are not more highly sexed or promiscuous than any other group of people (or in less delicate language, they are not out to "sleep with just anyone"). Their sexual orientation is not about being indiscriminate about their sexual or relationship partners (Evans & Wall, 1993). Some bisexuals might define themselves as more attracted to women than to men or vice versa, while others feel an equal romantic and sexual attraction to both sexes. Regardless, most bisexual individuals will tell you that they feel open to relationships with a potential partner regardless of his or her biological sex, rather than some compulsion to have loving relationships with both sexes simultaneously.

Nonheterosexual Orientations: Issues and Attitudes

To paraphrase (greatly) a former presidential campaign slogan: "It's not just about the sex, stupid!" Think about it: Is your sexual orientation determined by whom you have sex with and how you have it? Of course not. Imagine that from this moment on, you decide to be celibate, not having sex of any kind, for the rest of your life. I know, for many of you that's not easy to contemplate, but try. Would that decision change your sexual orientation? No. If someone were to engage in zero sexual behavior, would the person cease to have a sexual orientation? No. The answers to these questions are obvious, but one of the most common mistakes many heterosexuals make about nonheterosexuals is assuming that what defines people as gay or lesbian is simply their sexual *behavior*. However, straight people are not straight only because they engage in sexual behaviors with members of the opposite sex. In the same way, gay and lesbian people are not gay and lesbian only because they engage in sexual behaviors with members of their own sex.

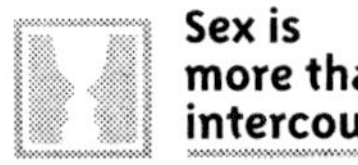
Sex is more than intercourse

Sexual orientation is about who you are; the sex of the people you want to date, fall in love with, have a romantic relationship with, spend the rest of your life with; and all things being equal (which, of course, they are not in most places in the world), the sex of the person you would choose to marry.

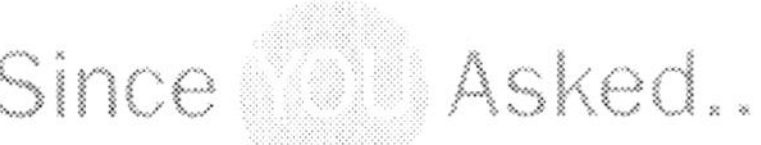

4. It seems to me that male sexual anatomy is designed to "fit" with female sexual anatomy and vice versa. So what's the deal with homosexuality?

Individuals of all sexual orientations experience similar attractions, emotions, and attitudes with respect to love, romance, and relationships. The following quote from Malcolm Boyd, a gay man and chaplain of the AIDS Commission of the Episcopal Diocese of Los Angeles, will help demonstrate the point. The feelings he expresses are universal and not limited to any particular sexual orientation, which is, after all, the point.

> My lover and life partner, Mark, and I had watched the end of the 10 o'clock news, turned off the lamp, and snuggled into our warm, nurturing good-night hug. Shortly Mark fell asleep. I didn't drift off right away. Instead I found my thoughts drifting to Mark and me. What did it mean that we were a gay couple, living in a gay home, after 12 years? What had kept us going in the face of so much societal negativity and rejection? I knew I loved him. I also liked him. It wasn't simply a body connection. There was an awesome soul connection. I thought of some of the things that give it a context.
>
> A sense of humor is certainly right up there. I like to see Mark's face break into a grin or hear his sudden laughter. We both see humor in all sorts of situations that would otherwise remain humorless, from standing in the supermarket checkout line to the aftermath of a domestic crisis, from problems in our families of origin to a newly discovered leak in the roof.
>
> Tenderness is central to our bonding. This means vulnerability. So is listening (as well as speaking) and letting silences be opportunities for soul communication; maintaining solid friendships; volunteering our time to work in our community; being patient; striving for inner relaxation—which means we try to leave the day's agendas at the front door when we walk into our home; physically demonstrating affection; and empathizing. (Boyd, 1997, p. 11)

Is Sexual Orientation a Choice?

We will soon be discussing various theories about sexual orientation, which may shed additional light on the question of whether sexual orientation is a conscious choice people make. The important point here is to realize that heterosexual individuals are rarely, if ever, asked if their sexual orientation was a choice. This question appears to be reserved for gay or lesbian people, and it is nearly always asked by heterosexuals. If you define yourself as heterosexual, as most of you do, try answering these questions: *When did you decide to become a heterosexual? Why did you choose your straight sexual orientation? At what age did you first realize you were heterosexual?* If you are like most heterosexual people, not only are the questions difficult to answer, but they seem nonsensical. Your answers were probably along the lines of *I never really decided; I didn't choose to be straight; it's just who I am!* and *I don't recall any particular age; I just always sort of knew.*

Since YOU Asked...

5. How do people know or decide to be homosexual or heterosexual or bisexual?

It is probably because nonheterosexual orientations are in the minority that such a fascination exists about when, where, why, and how those sexual orientations came to be. If you are straight, Table 11.1 will help you understand how difficult it is for gay and lesbian individuals to answer the kinds of questions often posed to them.

Gay Marriage

The issue of same-sex marriage has become front-page news in recent years. Many gay and lesbian couples who are deeply committed to each other have a strong desire to confirm that commitment personally, publicly, and legally through marriage. Beyond that personal and emotional desire, however, is the very real problem faced by nonheterosexual couples' inability to obtain the same legal rights and privileges that heterosexual cou-

Table 11.1 A HETEROSEXUAL QUESTIONNAIRE

Turnabout is fair play! Here is a list of questions that are frequently asked of gay and lesbian individuals, but the orientation in each question has been altered to *heterosexual*. It won't take long for you to realize how odd these questions must seem, unless you are gay, lesbian, or bisexual; then you already know.

1. When did you first decide you were a heterosexual?
2. What do you think caused you to be heterosexual?
3. Is it possible your heterosexuality is just a phase you may grow out of?
4. If you've never slept with a person of the same sex, how do you know you wouldn't prefer that?
5. Why do you insist on being so obvious with public displays of affection? Can't you just be what you are and keep it quiet?
6. Whom have you informed about your heterosexual tendencies? How did they react?
7. Do heterosexuals hate or distrust others of their own sex? Is that what makes them heterosexual?
8. Why are heterosexuals so promiscuous?
9. There seem to be many unhappy heterosexuals. Techniques have been developed to help you change your sexual orientation if you want to. Have you considered trying conversion therapy?
10. Why do heterosexuals place so much emphasis on sex?
11. How can you enjoy a fully satisfying sexual experience with a person of the opposite sex when the physical, biological, and psychological differences between you are so great? How can a man possibly understand what pleases a woman sexually or vice versa?
12. Why are heterosexuals always trying to seduce others into their sexual orientation?

ples take for granted. These include such rights as inheritance if a partner dies, participation in medical decisions, insurance coverage from a partner's employment, child custody rights, family leave benefits, domestic violence protection, and community property rights in the case of divorce, to name a few.

As this book goes to press, only one state, Massachusetts, had legalized marriage for same-sex couples (the law applies to legal residents of that state only). Conversely, more than 37 states have passed "defense of marriage" acts that specifically limit marriage to opposite-sex couples and forbid same-sex marriages. In 1996, the federal Defense of Marriage Act defined marriage as the union of a man and a woman and allowed states not to recognize gay marriages performed in other states where it has become legal.

However, these laws only apply to *marriage*. Many people who support limiting marriage to heterosexual couples also support gay and lesbian couples' right to equal or similar protections, rights, and privileges that are granted couples through marriage. In the United States, gains continue to be made toward legalizing **domestic partnerships** or **civil unions** between members of the same sex that confer all or most of the legal benefits of marriage but are not legally or religiously identical to heterosexual marriage.

As of 2006, several states—Vermont, Connecticut, California, Maine, Hawaii, and New Jersey, and the District of Columbia—have passed civil union or domestic partnership laws that allow for same-sex unions. Oregon is close to passing a similar law, and many other states are moving in this direction. Although these states maintain that marriage is an exclusively heterosexual institution, the new laws extend at least some of the rights of marriage to same-sex couples. To be eligible, same-sex couples must obtain a license and have their union officially certified. If a civil union fails, the couple must file for divorce or dissolution just as is required for married couples.

In the first 18 months after the Vermont civil union law was enacted in 2000, nearly 3,500 civil unions had been granted, 2,291 to lesbian couples and 1,180 to gay male couples. In the first eight months following Massachusetts' legalization of gay marriage, more than 6,000 same-sex couples were wed.

Overall, the legal status of gay marriage in the United States is in turmoil. The future of same-sex marriage and the legality of those marriages already performed in the United States will most likely be decided, eventually, by the U.S. Supreme Court. Until then, across the United States, many same-sex couples are exchanging or hoping to exchange wedding vows while state and local governments are either allowing or revoking these rights as litigation on both sides of the issue abounds.

Legalization of same-sex marriage has moved swiftly in several other countries. As of 2005, gay and lesbian couples in Canada, Germany, Belgium, the Netherlands, and Spain could marry and obtain all the rights bestowed on heterosexual married couples.

Sexual Orientation and Having Children

One of the many judgmental and often prejudiced statements gay and lesbian couples may hear goes something like this: "You can't have children, so what's the point of your relationship?" Of course, one of many weaknesses in this particular antigay sentiment is that it fails to consider all the heterosexual couples who either cannot conceive due to infertility issues or choose to be child-free. One generally does not hear those same people saying "What's the point of your relationship?" to them.

The reality is that many gay and lesbian couples do have children and typically make excellent parents; furthermore, the children of

Since YOU Asked...

6. I have no problem with homosexuals. I say live and let live. But I don't see why they are so concerned with getting married. I mean, if they can have their relationship, why do they have to get married?

domestic partnership A legal contract between two members of the same sex that imparts all or most of the legal benefits of marriage but is not socially or religiously equated with heterosexual marriage.

civil union Another term used for domestic partnership.

In the near future, marriage in many parts of the United States may no longer be limited to the union of a man and a woman.

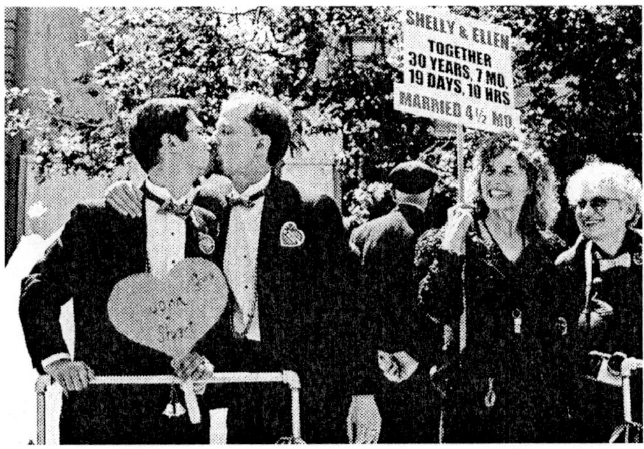
SHELLY & ELLEN
TOGETHER
30 YEARS, 7 MO.
19 DAYS, 10 HRS
MARRIED 4½ MO.

nonheterosexual parents grow up as well adjusted as those raised by heterosexual couples and are no more or less likely than any other child to have any particular sexual orientation (American Civil Liberties Union, 1999; Clarke, 2001; Fitzgerald, 1999). You may be wondering how gay and lesbian couples have children. Sometimes, individuals who come out or accept their sexual orientation as gay or lesbian later in life may have been in a heterosexual marriage and may have one or more children from that marriage. They do not cease to be parents when they come to grips with their true sexual orientation. Beyond this, however, many gay and lesbian couples feel a deep desire to have and raise children of their own. Such couples cannot conceive children on their own, of course, but the various assisted reproduction technologies (ART) discussed in Chapter 9, "Conception, Pregnancy, and Birth," are now making it possible for them to conceive children, with assistance from others, just as would be the case for some straight couples.

This is not really as new an idea as you may think. In the past, one member of a gay or lesbian couple might have a friend help them achieve pregnancy through intercourse. However, because of the personal and interpersonal significance of asking and agreeing to such a suggestion, many gay and lesbian couples today prefer to rely on artificial insemination techniques to realize their desire for children. This may involve "do-it-yourself" artificial techniques involving collecting sperm from a donor and transferring it to the vagina of the designated mother-to-be using a needleless syringe or placing the man's semen into a diaphragm or cervical cap and inserting it into the vagina. However, many gay and lesbian couples are uncomfortable with such casual methods, do not have ready and willing friends or acquaintances, or feel that defining (or denying) the third party's parental rights is ethically too complicated. In these cases, they often turn to the various ART techniques carried out in a medical setting using donated sperm or eggs. In most states, adoption for nonheterosexual couples is also an option.

Because the laws affecting nonheterosexual relationships vary greatly from state to state, gay and lesbian couples who decide to have children through any means should be sure to obtain the services of an attorney to ensure that both parents' rights are protected as well as the rights of the child. When gay and lesbian couples choose to conceive or adopt, many resources are available in most states and large cities to help them avoid legal problems that might arise in the future (Crawford et al., 1999; Sultan, 1995).

Interpersonal Qualities of Nonheterosexual Relationships

Many myths and misconceptions exist about the ways in which gay and lesbian relationships differ from heterosexual ones in the quality of the interpersonal interactions. For example, many people hold the following beliefs—all of them FALSE:

- Most gays and lesbians are unable to form close, enduring romantic relationships and prefer to be promiscuous.
- Gay and lesbian relationships are more likely than heterosexual relationships to be unhappy and dysfunctional.
- In same-sex relationships, one partner chooses or is assigned the role of "husband" and the other takes on the role of "wife."
- Most gay and lesbian couples are isolated from society and do not have meaningful social support networks.

All of these notions have been shown to be no more true of gay and lesbian couples than of straight couples. In 2001, the results of a 12-year study of gay and lesbian couples provided the best evidence to date of the similarities and differences between gay and straight romantic relationships (Gottman et al., 2003). This study, along with others (Gottman & Levenson, 2001; Kurdek, 2001), found that overall relationship satisfaction and quality are about the same regardless of the makeup of the couple. The main differences relate to the couples' emotional

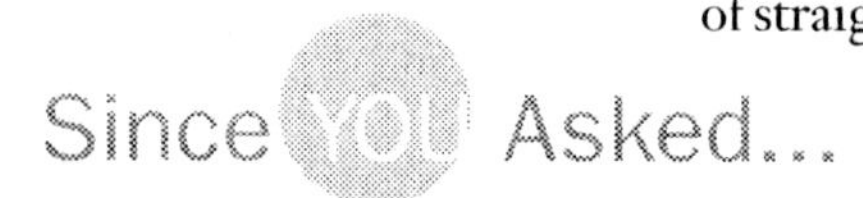

7. Do gay and lesbian couples really love each other in the same way as straight couples?

interactions, especially their handling of conflict, and difficulties related to the amount of social support received (or withdrawn) from family members.

For example, gay and lesbian couples tend to be generally more upbeat about their relationships than their heterosexual counterparts. They use more humor and withdraw affection less when conflicts arise, and they continue to view their relationships in more positive terms following discord (Gottman & Levinson, 2001). Gay and lesbian couples tend to be less hostile and controlling toward one another overall; they establish an equal balance of relationship power more readily. Another difference is that gay and lesbian couples appear to be able to calm down after conflict, soothe each other, and move past a problem more quickly compared to straight couples. Table 11.2 summarizes some of the differences between gay and straight romantic relationships.

Since YOU Asked...

8. How do gay and lesbian relationships differ from heterosexual ones, if they do?

Theories of Sexual Orientation

One of the hottest debates in the field of human sexuality has been about the causes of sexual orientation. This debate, in all its complexities, leads us back to the old familiar nature-versus-nurture controversy. Overall, this debate has not been particularly focused on the causes of heterosexuality or on sexual orientation in general but rather on determining the causes of homosexuality. As you will see, none of the theories proposed thus far is convincing

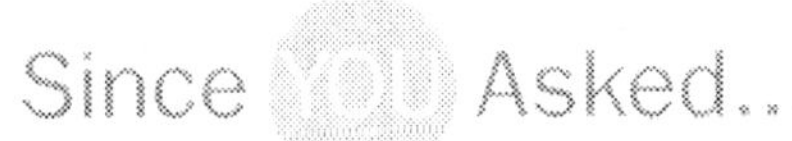

9. Why are some people gay? Is it something they're born with or just bad experiences with their parents or the opposite sex?

Table 11.2 DIFFERENCES IN EMOTIONAL QUALITIES BETWEEN GAY AND LESBIAN VERSUS HETEROSEXUAL COUPLES

QUALITY	DESCRIPTION
Gay and lesbian couples are more upbeat in the face of conflict.	Compared to heterosexual couples, gay and lesbian couples inject more affection and humor into their disagreements and conflicts, and same-sex partners are more positive in how they receive messages about conflict. Gay and lesbian couples are also more likely to remain positive about the relationship after a disagreement.
Gay and lesbian couples use fewer controlling or hostile emotional tactics.	Gay and lesbian partners display less belligerence, domineering, and fear with each other than straight couples. They use fewer controlling tactics and recognize the importance of fairness and of a balance of power than heterosexual couples.
In a fight, gay and lesbian couples take things less personally.	In heterosexual couples, a partner may be more easily hurt by a negative comment and less likely to feel uplifted with a positive comment. The opposite seems to be the case in gay and lesbian couples. Gay and lesbian partners' positive comments have more impact on feeling good, and their negative comments are less likely to produce personal hurt feelings.
Gay and lesbian couples tend to show lower levels of physiological arousal during conflict.	Again, this is generally the opposite for heterosexual couples, for whom the physiological arousal (including elevated heart rate, sweaty palms, and jitteriness) produced by conflict signifies ongoing aggravation. The ongoing aroused state makes it difficult for the partners to calm down and move past the conflict. Gay and lesbian couples' lower level of psychological arousal allows them to soothe one another during or soon after the conflict.

Source: Adapted from Gottman and Levinson (2001).

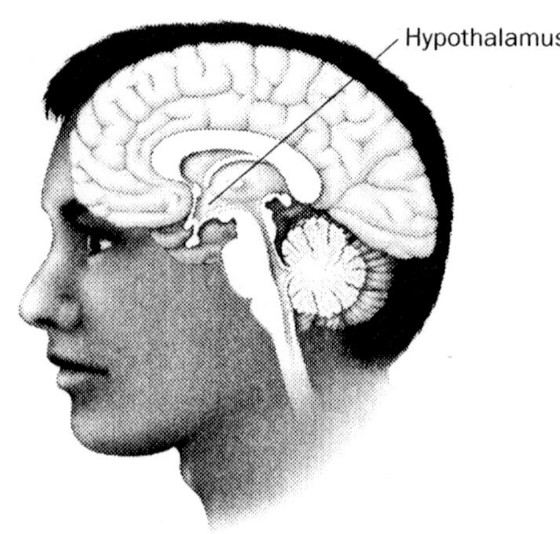

FIGURE 11.2 Sexual Orientation and the Brain

In the early 1990s, Simon LeVay found that the third interstitial nucleus in the hypothalamus of the brain appeared to be smaller in gay men than in straight men.

from a scientific perspective, so we will review the recent directions of relevant research. Finally, we will close this section with a brief look at the possible motivations behind this rather intense "search for a cause."

Biological Influences on Sexual Orientation

Arguments that sexual orientation results from biological factors usually fall into one of three categories: brain structure and function, hormones, and genes. All have been implicated in the roots of sexual orientation, yet none has managed to lay claim to a central role.

Brain Structure and Function

In 1991, Simon LeVay, a neurobiologist at the Salk Institute in La Jolla, California, made international headlines when he published in the journal *Science* that he had found a measurable, consistent difference in the brains of a small group of heterosexual and homosexual men (see Figure 11.2). It was a minute difference in the *third interstitial nucleus*, a very small part of the brain structure called the *hypothalamus*, which is known to play a central role in emotions and sexual urges (LeVay, 1991; Pfaff, Frolich, & Morgan, 2002). The third interstitial nucleus is normally larger in men than in women. What LeVay found, in essence, was that this structure was larger in his sample of straight men than in gay men. The size of this section of the hypothalamus in his gay male sample was about the same as is typically found in women. Although this was not the first finding that the brains of men and women are different, it was the first to find a potential gay-straight variation.

LeVay's research did not prove that sexual orientation is *caused* by a brain difference, but it did suggest a biological difference that is, in his view, related in some way to a person's sexual orientation (Barinaga, 1991). However, LeVay's study was considered flawed by groups with widely varying positions on the origins of sexual orientation. Those who view nonheterosexual orientations in negative terms pointed to this brain structure as a biological defect. Some went so far as to envision the discovery as a way potential parents might screen for homosexuality during pregnancy and abort "gay fetuses." Conversely, the findings were seen by many gay individuals, gay activists, and their supporters as proof that sexual orientation, whether gay or straight, is a natural biological variation in humans and not a lifestyle choice, in the same way that one is male or female, nearsighted or farsighted, tall or short. Indeed, some gay rights supporters saw that if LeVay's findings could be interpreted as proof that sexual orientation is a biological, inborn characteristic, laws forbidding discrimination based on such differences might become easier to legislate by modeling legislation after similar statutes relating to race and gender.

Before LeVay's research could be put to such social and political uses, other scientists questioned his findings on methodological grounds (Byne, 1994; Nimmons, 1994). The most convincing of these criticisms related to the subjects of LeVay's research and to his assumptions about the sexual orientations of the men whose brains were studied (Fausto-Sterling & Balaban, 1993). The size of the brain structure under study was so minuscule (less than the head of a pin) that it could not be seen with any available brain X-ray or scanning technology. The only way to study it was through autopsies after the men had died. Consequently, LeVay's sample of subjects was small: only 19 gay men and 16 heterosexual men.

Furthermore, the gay men in his sample had died of AIDS. You are, no doubt, already guessing the nature of the criticism. One of the many devastating effects of AIDS on the human body is often destruction of brain tissue. Consequently, LeVay could not be sure if the smaller size of the interstitial nucleus was due to the subjects' sexual orientation or their illness. LeVay contested the validity of this criticism, and later he examined the brain of one gay man who did not have AIDS but had died of lung cancer. He found the same small-sized structure as was typical for all of the subjects in his studies (Nimmons, 1994). Nevertheless, this criticism of his findings in general has not been silenced by this single non-AIDS case (Byne, 1994).

The other most common criticism of LeVay's research relates to the discussion earlier in this chapter about sexual orientation as a continuum rather than discrete categories of gay and straight. In his brain research, LeVay seemed to be dividing his subjects along a strict gay-straight dichotomy (Fausto-Sterling & Balaban, 1993). But sexual orientation cannot be so clearly divided into "camps." The reasoning behind this criticism goes, if people cannot be divided into purely heterosexual or homosexual groupings, then what do variations in brain structure really mean? Would bisexual individuals, for example, have interstitial nuclei that are of a size in between gay and straight brains? These questions have never been fully answered, and LeVay's findings on the gay male brain continue to be met with skepticism in the scientific community. It must be said, however, that LeVay's research opened the scientific door on the possibility that sexual orientation might be rooted in biological rather than environmental causes.

Since LeVay's findings, other researchers have suggested various additional biological differences relating to sexual orientation. For example, several studies have demonstrated that right- and left-handedness may be linked to sexual orientation (Bode, 2000; Lalumiere, Blanchard, & Zucker, 2000). Findings have shown that lesbians are 91 percent more likely to be left-handed than heterosexual women, and gay men are 34 percent more likely than straight men to be left-handed, although the *overall* percentages of left-handed people regardless of sexual orientation is only about 10 percent (Blanchard et al., 2006). Researchers have also found a connection between sexual orientation and how the brain processes sound (Jensen, 1998). Apparently, all people's ears make faint noises in response to clicking sounds, called "click-evoked otoacoustic emissions." However, lesbians' ears make significantly softer sounds than the ears of heterosexual women. In addition, research has demonstrated that visual-spatial abilities may also be related to measures of sexual orientation in men (K. M. Cohen, 2002). These findings may not sound particularly interesting or important, and perhaps they are not earth-shaking scientifically, but they represent additional pieces of the puzzle that sexual orientation may have a biological basis.

Hormones

Hormonal changes or imbalances in adulthood may change sexual behavior, sexual desire, or even male and female sexual anatomy (see Chapter 10, "Gender," for more detail on this topic), but they do not appear to alter sexual orientation. Hormonal explanations for gay, lesbian, and bisexual orientations focus on the exposure of the *fetus in the uterus* to male or female hormones, in combinations or levels that vary from those of heterosexuals.

Separating hormonal influences from other biological factors is extremely difficult. Any physiological differences found in different sexual orientations, such as the brain differences discussed in the previous section, may be preprogrammed by genes (to be discussed next); influenced by behavior, environment, or illness; or caused by hormones during fetal development (Heino et al., 1995). In fact, the researchers who found the spatial ability and auditory differences in gay versus straight orientations acknowledged the possibility of prenatal hormone exposure as a potential cause (K. M. Cohen, 2000; Jensen, 1998; Lalumiere et al., 2000).

One example of the hormonal hypothesis for the development of nonheterosexual orientations involves the fingers. You are probably not aware of this, but the length of the ring finger is more similar in length to the index finger in women than in men. In other words, the difference in length between the index finger and ring finger is greater in men than in women. This difference is measurable at age 2 and is stable into adulthood. You can now amaze your friends by bringing up this bit of trivia at your next party. Seriously, beyond this male-female difference, a similar difference exists between lesbian and straight women. That is, the index-to-ring-finger ratio in lesbian women is more similar to that of men. Research has also revealed that the ratio is even smaller (meaning the difference in finger lengths is greater) in lesbians who self-identify as "butch" (more masculine) than in those who self-identify as "femme" (more feminine) (Brown et al., 2002). Add to this the fact that the index-to-ring-finger ratio is a marker for fetal exposure to male hormones, and you have evidence for a potential hormonal cause of sexual orientation—not conclusive proof but an interesting, suggestive correlation.

One study was concerned not with fingers but with penis size. Researchers at the Kinsey Institute for Research in Sex, Gender, and Reproduction obtained data about length and circumference of the penises of more than 900 gay men and more than 4,000 straight men (Bogaert & Hershberger, 1999). On average, penis size was found to be slightly larger for gay men than for straight men (about 0.33 inch longer and 0.15 inch greater circumference). The authors of the study speculate that "these findings provide additional evidence that variations in prenatal hormonal levels affect sexual orientation" (p. 213). This study has not been widely reported, probably due to concerns about how the media would spin such findings (can't you just imagine?).

Another study investigated women whose mothers were given the drug *diethylstilbestrol* (DES) while pregnant (Meyer-Bahlburg, Ehrhardt, & Gruen, 1995). DES is a form of synthetic estrogen that was thought to prevent miscarriage and premature labor and was widely prescribed to pregnant women between 1938 and 1971 (Cornforth, 2002). Not only did the drug not work as advertised, but it caused an increased risk for cancer and infertility in the daughters of women who took the drug. The exposed daughters have been followed and studied extensively for years. One consistent finding has been that women exposed to DES in the womb are significantly more likely as adults to be bisexual or homosexual than nonexposed controls. This lends additional correlational evidence that atypical hormonal exposure in the womb may indeed play a role in the development of nonheterosexual orientations.

Finally, researchers have discovered a new possible biological basis of sexual orientation that has become known as the "big brother effect" (Motluk, 2003). A statistically significant association has been found that as the number of older brothers a man has increases, so do his chances of being gay (regardless of the brothers' sexual orientation). Each additional older brother increases the odds of a gay sexual orientation by one-third (Cantor et al., 2002). No such relationship has been found for lesbians regardless of how many older sisters or brothers they may have. What might be the reason for the "big brother effect"? After all, the male fetus in the womb hasn't the slightest idea how many brothers he has. But the child's mother's body does. Various scientific studies across cultures have confirmed this finding (Zucker, Blanchard, & Siegelman, 2003). Although the *correlation* between birth order and sexual orientation is real, the reasons for it are more difficult to ascertain. The theory most often suggested by researchers relates to immune systems in some women (Motluk, 2003). A few fetal cells can sometimes pass from the womb into the mother's bloodstream during pregnancy or the birthing process. Researchers speculate that these cells interact with the mother's immune system and begin to develop antibodies against male fetal cells. The more male babies the mother has had, the stronger the immune response against them. Her body, then, at least in some cases, may react by changing something (probably the hormonal balance) in the uterine environment for later-born males that in turn leads to a tendency toward a gay sexual orientation. A comprehensive explanation for the "big brother effect" theory remains to be elaborated.

Genetics

The genetic theory proposes that a person's sexual orientation is *preprogrammed* at conception when the genes from the mother's egg and the father's sperm merge to create the blueprint for a new person. Historically, researchers had difficulty separating genetic from environmental influences on human characteristics because most people grow up in the same environment as their genetic donors, that is, their parents. Therefore, any behavior or personality similarities between children and parents might be either inherited or learned. However, over the past 30 years or so, research methods have become increasingly sophisticated, allowing researchers to tease apart the forces of environment and genes, and consequently researchers have been placing an increased focus on genes as a potential source of human behaviors and personality traits, including sexual orientation.

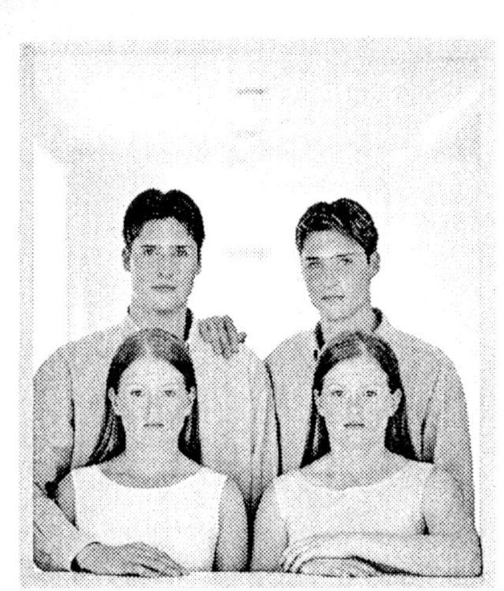

Research with identical twins has suggested clear genetic influence on sexual orientation.

The most promising genetic studies involve pairs of identical twins, some of whom were adopted at birth, or very soon after, into different families and therefore different environments. If two individuals with the same genetic makeup (that is, identical or *monozygotic* twins) share certain personality characteristics far more often than fraternal (*dizygotic*) twins or nontwin brothers and sisters, this argues that genetic influences most probably account for those shared characteristics.

This avenue of research has been applied to sexual orientation, and the results have been quite consistent. Numerous studies have shown that when one member of a pair of identical twins is gay or lesbian, the chances are far higher that the other twin will share that same sexual orientation than would be expected among fraternal twins or nontwin siblings (Bailey & Benishay, 1993; Bailey & Pillard, 1991; Blum, 1997; Hershberger, 1997; Kendler et al., 2000; Pillard, 1998). In other words, as the degree of genetic relatedness increases, the similarity of siblings' sexual orientation also increases, regardless of their environment. Figure 11.3 summarizes representative findings from two studies.

Today, widespread scientific support exists for the notion that genes play an important role in sexual orientation. But has science uncovered a true "gay gene"? Not yet. Although researchers have demonstrated convincingly that sexual orientation is influenced by a person's genetic makeup, finding the actual gene or complex of genes responsible for that influence is far more difficult. Some researchers maintain that a gene on the X chromosome may be linked to sexual orientation, indicating that sexual orientation is passed along through maternal genes (Hamer et al., 1993) but this theory has yet to be widely accepted (Sardar, 1999; Wickelgren, 1999). Furthermore, as you can see in Figure 11.3, at the most only about 50 percent of sexual orientation can be explained by genetic influences, so genes are not the whole story and environmental influences certainly cannot be ignored. Moreover, many scientists question whether the need to prove that a "gay gene" exists at all (we will return to this issue toward the end of this section).

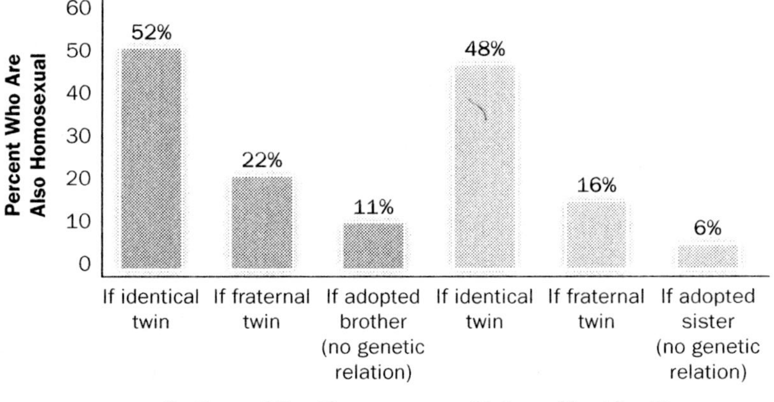

FIGURE 11.3 Twin Studies and Sexual Orientation

As genetic relatedness increases, the similarity of same-sex siblings' sexual orientation also increases.

Source: Bailey and Benishay (1993); Bailey and Pillard (1991).

Experiential and Environmental Influences on Sexual Orientation

Researchers appear to be closer to identifying meaningful potential biological causes of sexual orientation than to uncovering consistent evidence of specific environmental or experiential influences. In fact, most of the environmental "causes" for nonheterosexual orientations that were popularly believed during the second half of the twentieth century have been resoundingly rejected by more advanced research techniques. How many of these scientifically rejected beliefs about family and environmental origins of homosexuality have you heard?

- Homosexual men are more likely to have had domineering or overly protective mothers and weak, distant fathers (and hence no masculine role model).
- Homosexual women were more likely to have had cold, unloving, rejecting mothers and absent fathers.
- Homosexuals grew up hating or fearing members of the opposite sex, which caused them to turn to members of their own sex for love and intimacy.
- Most homosexuals were molested during childhood by a same-sex adult, which turned them toward homosexuality as they became adults themselves.
- Homosexuals are more likely to have engaged in sex play as children with peers of their own sex.
- Homosexuals are more likely to have a gay mother or father.

All of these assumptions have been shown in numerous studies to be FALSE. The methodology used to study psychosocial origins of sexual orientation have been fairly straightforward: Ask a large random sample of homosexual and heterosexual people about their experiences with all of these issues and compare the answers of the two groups. When researchers have done this, they nearly always find no significant differences among the groups for any of the influences on the list (Bell & Weinberg, 1978; Bell, Weinberg, & Hammersmith, 1981; Golombok & Tasker, 1996). In other words, nonheterosexual individuals are just as likely or unlikely as straight people to have experienced any of the listed circumstances during their lifetime.

The question we must ask is, have any purely experiential explanations for sexual orientation been supported by scientific evidence? The answer is no. The research that attempts to refute the biological evidence for sexual orientation does not claim any *exclusively* environmental model in its place. Rather, most of the criticism takes the position that the biological findings are not yet sufficient to conclude that biology is solely responsible for sexual orientation and that any complete explanation of such a complex human quality will likely include both nature and nurture (Byne, 1994, 1997; Herron & Herron, 1996; Veniegas & Conley, 2000).

A Biological-Environmental Interactive Approach

Most people have difficulty imagining that whether a person is straight, gay, lesbian, or bisexual could be a result of either biological or environmental factors exclusively. Yet few have meshed these two sides of the discussion into an integrated, interactionist theory to explain the development of sexual orientation. One attempt to do so has received a great deal of attention over the past several years. Daryl Bem (1996, 2000a), a psychologist at Cornell University, has proposed what he has termed the **exotic becomes erotic (EBE) theory** of sexual orientation.

exotic becomes erotic (EBE) theory Psychologist Daryl Bem's explanation for the interaction of biology and environment in determining a person's sexual orientation.

Bem suggests that people are not born with a genetic predisposition for a certain sexual orientation per se but for varying childhood temperaments such as aggression, activity level, or shyness. Indeed, these *temperamental variables* have received a great deal of scientific support outside of the sexual orientation arena (Caspi & Silva, 1995;

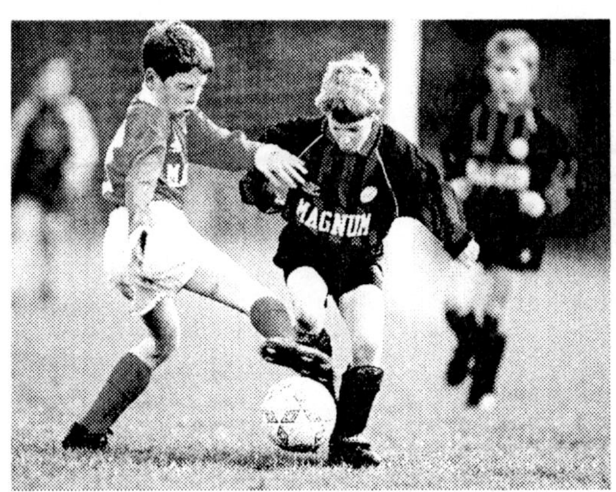
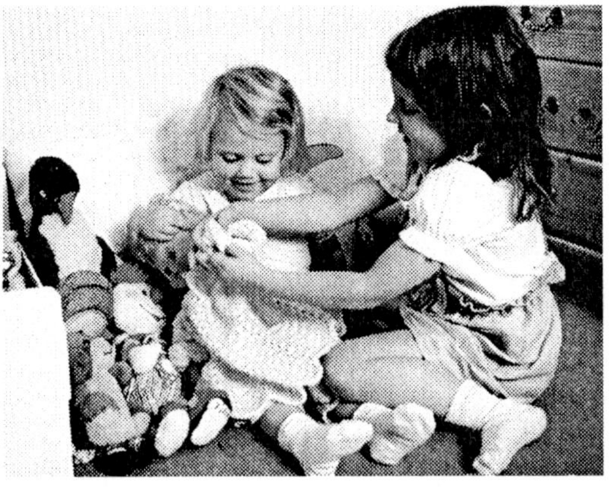

Children may naturally be drawn to same-sex playmates and gender-conforming activities.

Kagan, 1992). According to Bem, these temperamental variations prime the child to prefer some early childhood activities over others. Usually, Bem points out, preferences in play behaviors track with the child's sex: Boys prefer male-typical activities such as rough-and-tumble play or competitive sports, whereas girls gravitate toward female-typical, quiet, cooperative play such as jacks or hopscotch. This is referred to as **gender-conforming behavior**.

Moreover, Bem contends, children will seek out other children who share the same play preferences, that is, children who like to play jacks or hopscotch will seek out girls to play with while children who prefer rough, competitive sports will prefer to play with boys. Sometimes, however, a child will engage in **gender-nonconforming behavior**, meaning that the child prefers play activities that are typical of opposite-sex children and will seek out those children as friends and playmates.

Bem's theory proposes that nonconforming children will then feel increasingly different from their "outgroup" of peers. In other words, children who primarily have playmates of their own sex (the vast majority of children) will feel different from opposite-sex children, while children whose playmates are of the other sex (a small minority) will feel different from same-sex peers. Each will see the "other group" as strange and "exotic." These feelings of difference create increased levels of emotional (not sexual) arousal toward children of the outgroup sex that might be expressed in statements such as "I hate girls" or "Boys are *so* weird!" This arousal may occur below conscious awareness, or sometimes it might be very obvious. "A particularly clear example," Bem suggests, "is the 'sissy' boy who is taunted by male peers for his gender-nonconformity and, as a result, is likely to experience the strong physiological arousal of fear and anger in their presence" (2000b, p. 533).

You may be thinking that this theory is heading in the wrong direction, that it will lead to repulsion of the outgroup sex rather than attraction to it. However, Bem maintains that later, in puberty, as sexual feelings begin to surface, this perceived difference and "exoticness" in the gender outgroup and the accompanying emotional arousal transform into erotic feelings toward that group. Hence the theory's name, *exotic becomes erotic*. Figure 11.4 illustrates Bem's theory step by step.

Bem maintains that his theory serves to link the biological (whether genetic or hormonal) and environmental influences that lead to a person's sexual orientation in adulthood. He also argues that even though a child's environment plays a major role in the formation of sexual orientation, this does not imply that sexual orientation is a choice or that it is "changeable" in adulthood any more than if it were found to be exclusively biological (D. J. Bem, 1997). Consistent childhood experiences may be just as deeply ingrained in a person as genetic heritage.

As you may imagine, the EBE theory has not been without controversy. It has been criticized on the grounds that it does not accurately represent the experiences of girls

gender-conforming behavior Behavior that is consistent with traditional cultural expectations for a child's sex.

gender-nonconforming behavior Behavior that is inconsistent with traditional cultural expectations for a child's sex and considered more appropriate for children of the other sex.

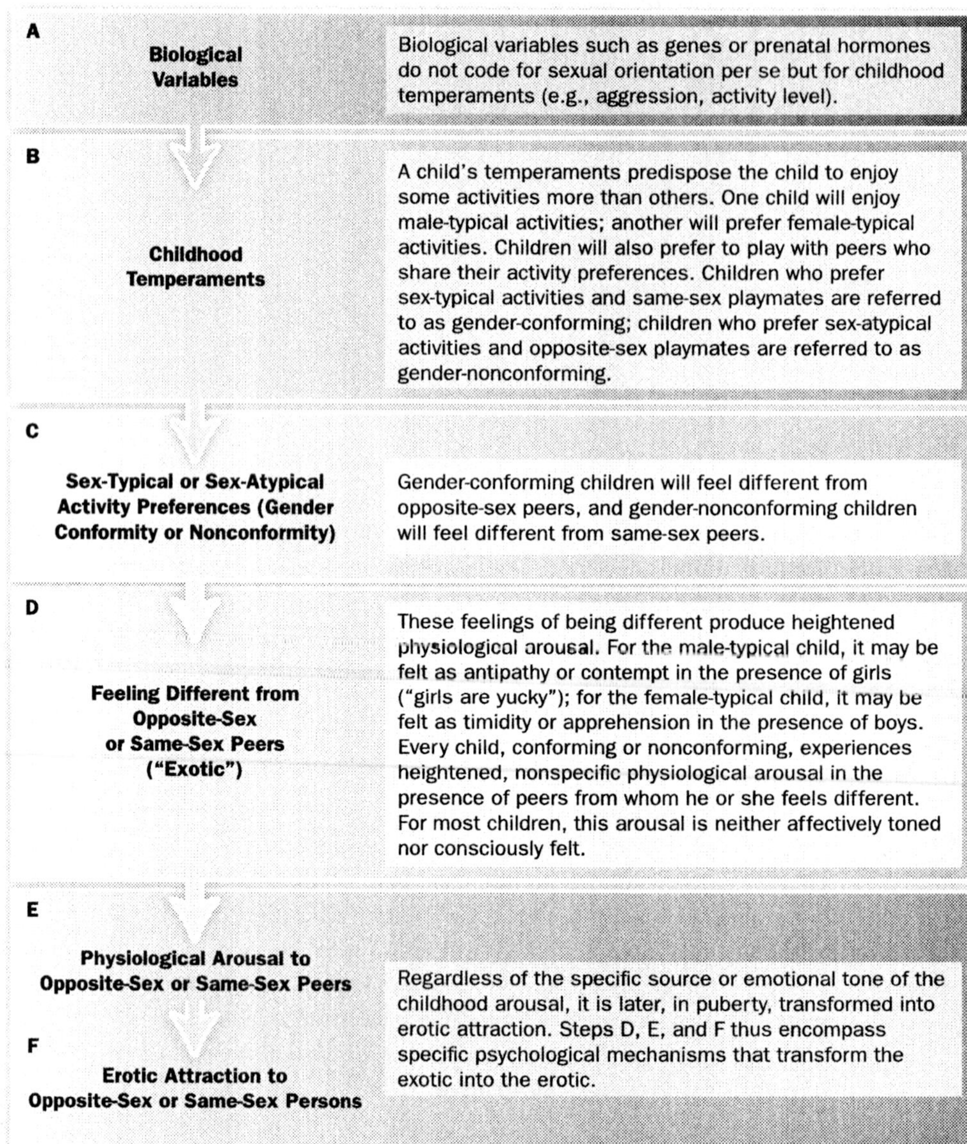

A
Biological Variables
Biological variables such as genes or prenatal hormones do not code for sexual orientation per se but for childhood temperaments (e.g., aggression, activity level).
B
Childhood Temperaments
A child's temperaments predispose the child to enjoy some activities more than others. One child will enjoy male-typical activities; another will prefer female-typical activities. Children will also prefer to play with peers who share their activity preferences. Children who prefer sex-typical activities and same-sex playmates are referred to as gender-conforming; children who prefer sex-atypical activities and opposite-sex playmates are referred to as gender-nonconforming.
C
Sex-Typical or Sex-Atypical Activity Preferences (Gender Conformity or Nonconformity)
Gender-conforming children will feel different from opposite-sex peers, and gender-nonconforming children will feel different from same-sex peers.
D
Feeling Different from Opposite-Sex or Same-Sex Peers ("Exotic")
These feelings of being different produce heightened physiological arousal. For the male-typical child, it may be felt as antipathy or contempt in the presence of girls ("girls are yucky"); for the female-typical child, it may be felt as timidity or apprehension in the presence of boys. Every child, conforming or nonconforming, experiences heightened, nonspecific physiological arousal in the presence of peers from whom he or she feels different. For most children, this arousal is neither affectively toned nor consciously felt.
E
Physiological Arousal to Opposite-Sex or Same-Sex Peers
F
Erotic Attraction to Opposite-Sex or Same-Sex Persons
Regardless of the specific source or emotional tone of the childhood arousal, it is later, in puberty, transformed into erotic attraction. Steps D, E, and F thus encompass specific psychological mechanisms that transform the exotic into the erotic.

FIGURE 11.4 Bem's Exotic Becomes Erotic Theory of Sexual Orientation

Bem's theory considers the interaction of biological and environmental factors in the development of sexual orientation.

Source: Adapted from D. J. Bem (2000b).

and women (as evidenced by his examples of playing jacks and hopscotch as female gender-conforming behavior), that it is not supported by the very scientific evidence Bem himself cites, and that it is too limited in its application of psychoanalytic theory because it omits the influence of early boyhood trauma (Nicolosi & Byrd, 2002; Peplau et al., 1998). Nevertheless, Bem continues to research and build support for his theory (J. D. Bem, 1998, 2000a), and the discussion goes on. The validity of the EBE theory may never be completely settled, but as one of the few theories attempting to integrate biological and experiential influences on sexual orientation, it is providing material for a worthwhile debate among social scientists on this complex issue.

Do the Origins of Sexual Orientation Matter?

In the midst of the research and controversy over the question of the origins of sexual orientation, many experts are questioning the importance of finding the answer. Some researchers have suggested that the underpinnings of the search for the cause of sexual orientation lie in widespread prejudiced attitudes and hostile actions targeted at gays and lesbians in Western cultures. It has been suggested that these negative attitudes and acts are based on four basic, unenlightened, and erroneous assumptions about homosexuality (Marmor, 1998): It is immoral and sinful, it is unnatural, it is a chosen behavior and therefore can be "unchosen," and it is potentially "contagious."

Some analysts assert that the basis for all of these assumptions can be challenged by demonstrating that sexual orientation is determined, by and large, naturally, biologically, and genetically, just like sex, hair color, and race. If you think about it, clear proof that sexual orientation is inborn could pose a dilemma for people who base their antigay attitudes on religious teachings, in that they also claim that humans are made in God's image. However, others contend that those who espouse such prejudice will find a way to distort the research, no matter what causes are finally established, to strengthen their position ("The Causes of Homosexuality," 2001). In fact, most gay and lesbian individuals themselves appear to downplay the importance of finding the cause of homosexuality.

Finally, one of the leading researchers who has questioned the conclusions drawn from the current accumulation of biological evidence offers the following caution:

> Perhaps . . . we should also be asking ourselves why we as a society are so emotionally invested in this research. Will it—or should it—make any difference in the way we perceive ourselves and others or how we live our lives and allow others to live theirs? Perhaps the answers to the most salient questions in this debate lie not within the biology of human brains, but rather in the cultures those brains have created. (Byne, 1997, p. 79)

In other words, as we learn more about how the human brain works, we see that as much as our brains may be able to come up with ways of changing the world around us, our environment is also able to make very real changes in the structure and functioning of our brains. Therefore, as Byne and others are saying, the important question may be not if a biology-environment interaction exists but how can science explore and define such an interaction.

Coming Out

Regardless of how sexual orientation develops, nonheterosexual individuals face a life event that straight people never even imagine: *coming out*—short for "coming out of the closet," and which reflects the fact that in a society that is largely rejecting at best and dangerously hostile at worst, nonheterosexuals typically spend a portion of their lives hiding their true sexual orientation from everyone, sometimes including themselves. They keep their sexual identities "in the closet." Most people with nonheterosexual orientations eventually find that living such a lie and hiding their true sexuality is too stressful and emotionally unbearable (as was expressed in the student's essay that began this chapter), so they make the often painful and difficult decision to come out. If you are gay or lesbian, you already know how it feels to be in the closet and the complex emotions usually linked to the coming-out process. If you are heterosexual and have close friends or relatives who have come out, you may have some sense of the intensity of their experiences.

Heterosexuals never feel any need to hide their sexuality, of course, because society as a whole assumes that everyone is straight. They are able simply to be who they are, at least as it relates to their sexual orientation, and are not in any sort of closet to begin with. Furthermore, heterosexuals often ask why gay and lesbian individuals need to come out at all, especially if it is so difficult and risks exposing them to the negative fallout of society's antigay attitudes. However, if you talk to nonheterosexuals who have come out, virtually all of them will tell you that the pain and frustration of "living a lie" about their true sexual identity was far more difficult, more painful, and more stressful than dealing with whatever adverse consequences may have accompanied their decision to come out. And when gay people choose to live a life that is honest and open about their sexual orientation, they are happier, physically healthier, psychologically better adjusted to life in general, and better able to develop close and mutually satisfying friendships and romantic relationships with others (Jordan & Deluty, 1998; Scasta, 1998).

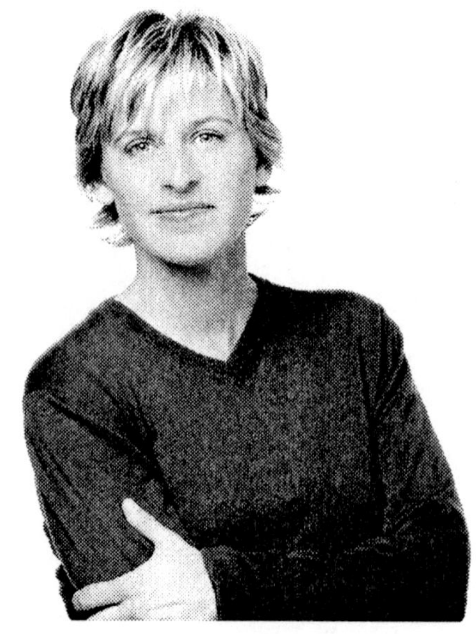

Originally, the network sitcom Ellen *was not a show about a lesbian bookstore owner. It was a show about a straight woman who owned a bookstore and was looking for a relationship with a man. When the show's star, comedian and actress Ellen DeGeneres, came out in real life, she made the decision that her character must do the same. When the* Ellen *"coming-out episode" aired on prime-time TV (to a great deal of press and controversy), the impact on the attitudes and emotions of people of all sexual orientations was significant. It helped inspire tens of thousands of people to accept themselves for who they are, come out of the closet, and stop hiding their true sexuality (Ryan & Boxer, 1998).*

When Do People Come Out?

Coming out is not typically a single moment, a single decision, or a single act in someone's life. Usually coming out as gay, lesbian, or bisexual person is a process that takes place gradually, over time, in a step-by-step fashion (to be discussed in the next section). Most people begin to realize, or at least suspect, that they may have a nonheterosexual orientation in adolescence, around the time when puberty arrives and everyone begins to have erotic feelings toward others. This is not to say that sexual orientation begins in adolescence—that debate is ongoing, as we noted earlier in this chapter—or that most people will come out to themselves or others during adolescence. However, most self-aware gay and lesbian individuals are quite clear that they always knew they were "different" from the other kids in some fundamental ways for as long as they can remember.

In the "coming-out" episode of *Ellen*, one of Ellen's friends, a gay man named Peter, was helping Ellen gather the courage to tell her straight friends that she had finally realized she was gay. Peter tells her, "Ellen, it's *never* easy. I remember when I decided to tell my parents, I sat them down and said, 'Mom, Dad, I'm gay, and if you can't accept that it's too bad because it's who I am.' And the next year, when I entered kindergarten, they were behind me 100 percent!" This line produced a great deal of laughter from the audience, even though it is probably a bit of an exaggeration. Young children are not aware of such complex sexuality issues at all, much less able to analyze and recognize their sexual orientation. However, once a person begins to acknowledge his or her gay or lesbian orientation, that feeling of difference felt throughout childhood begins to make a great deal more sense.

Still, no exact timeline exists for beginning the process of coming out. It might begin as early as the onset of puberty or as late as old age (Altman, 2000). Indeed, many people have lived heterosexual lives, dated members of the opposite sex, fallen in love with them, married them and had families, only to realize later in life what it was that had been bothering them all those years, what had been making them feel unhappy, unfulfilled, and somehow "off track." They had been forcing their lives into a mold expected by society but one that was not true to themselves. They are among the many who will tell you of the intense relief and inner peace they felt when, finally, they came out.

The Coming-Out Process

Many theories have been proposed to explain the process nonheterosexuals go through as they come out of the closet to themselves and to others. All of the theories share certain common characteristics in that they assume a gradual, developmental process that involves various stages. Two of the more widely accepted models of the coming-out process—one proposed by Vivienne Cass and another by Richard Troiden—reflect some of the current thinking on this issue (Floyd & Stein, 2002). Both models share certain characteristics but also incorporate some uniquely different factors to explain the stages many people go through as they navigate through their

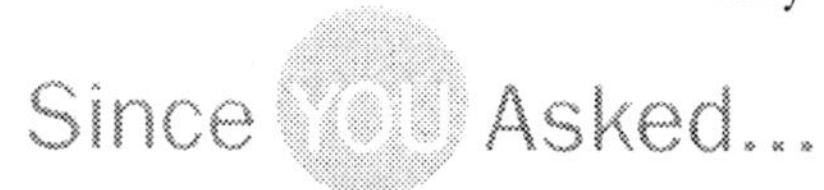

10. How old are most people when they come to terms with or understand that they are homosexual? Do they usually tell people right away? Are they usually comfortable with the realization?

coming out experiences. As you will see, they both focus on the formation of personal sexual identity. Moreover, both end with acceptance and integration of one's sexual orientation into overall self-identity and life satisfaction, as well as being open to others about his or her sexual orientation.

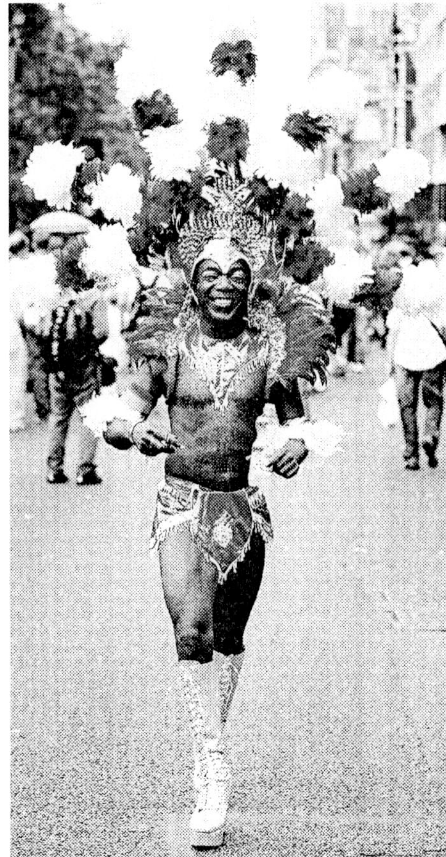

During the coming-out process, many gay and lesbian individuals will feel the need to identify strongly with their sexual orientation and rebel against societal attitudes.

Cass's Model of Homosexual Identity Formation

Cass's model (1984) demonstrates how nonheterosexual individuals move from a state of denial, confusion, or discomfort through increasing degrees of realization about their sexual orientation and to increasing acceptance of themselves as nonheterosexual individuals, greater comfort with themselves, and clearer commitment to their true sexual orientation.

Stage 1: Identity Confusion. In this stage, individuals begin to wonder if they may be homosexual. They may consider the possibility or reject it. If they choose to consider the possibility, they will move to the second stage.

Stage 2: Identity Comparison. Individuals begin looking at others and comparing themselves to homosexuals and nonhomosexuals in the surrounding environment. At this point, individuals may make contact with another homosexual person.

Stage 3: Identity Tolerance. Individuals are becoming increasingly committed to the homosexual identity and may seek out more and more homosexual contacts. The self-image is still one of merely "tolerating" the homosexuality rather than embracing it.

Stage 4: Identity Acceptance. At this point, a more positive view of homosexuality begins to develop. Individuals may feel they fit into the homosexual society. However, they will generally attempt to pass for heterosexual, and self-disclosure will be limited.

Stage 5: Identity Pride. Individuals in this stage characteristically feel a great deal of pride about their homosexuality. They will identify strongly with other homosexuals and feel anger at the way society treats homosexuals as a whole. They are often very conspicuous in their sexuality.

Stage 6: Identity Synthesis. Finally, the influence of positive gay and lesbian role models helps individuals become aware that homosexuality is not a negative trait. At this point, they may feel "settled in" to their identity, neither ashamed of it nor needing to flaunt it.

Troiden's Formation of Homosexual Identities

In Troiden's model (1989), similar assumptions to Cass's are expressed about the stages of development, but his theory begins at younger ages, is more age-specific, and is summarized in four rather than six stages.

Stage 1: Sensitization. This stage occurs before puberty and involves often being marginalized and made to feel different from peers. Teasing and negative labeling, whether experienced directly or witnessed, contribute to the internalization of a negative self-concept.

Stage 2: Identify Confusion. This stage usually occurs during late adolescence (ages 16 to 18) as individuals begin to recognize feelings and behaviors that they or others may see as homosexual. They may feel unable to find a clear category for themselves in the sexual world. Individuals may employ certain strategies to reduce the stress of feeling like an outsider, including denial, avoiding homosexual situations, pretending to be heterosexual, or in some cases, accepting their homosexuality.

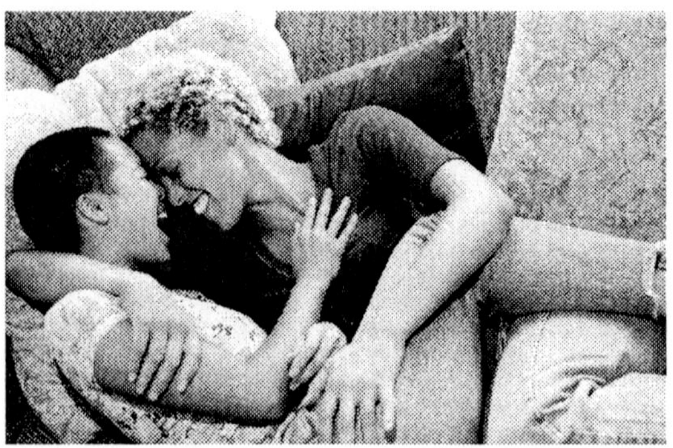

In the final stage of coming out, gay and lesbian individuals typically feel a high level of happiness, self-acceptance, and satisfaction with life.

Stage 3: Identity Assumption. This stage occurs in the early 20s; typically somewhat later for women than for men. Individuals begin to increase their contact with other homosexuals. A major task in this stage is learning to cope with the prejudice and discrimination associated with nonheterosexual orientation in the culture. Strategies employed here include agreeing with the negative stereotyping (but not denying being gay or lesbian), becoming exaggeratedly gay or lesbian ("flaming" or "butch"), "passing" or hiding one's true orientation from most others, and becoming immersed in the gay or lesbian subculture and rejecting heterosexual activities and associations.

Stage 4: Commitment. This final stage involves accepting that sexual orientation is a major part of self-identity and not simply a preferred set of sexual behaviors. Sexual orientation becomes part of the choices and commitments the person makes in life and in love. Self-identification as gay, lesbian, or bisexual becomes routine. Typically this produces a greater level of happiness and satisfaction with life in general. This stage typically occurs before the age of 25.

The Dangers and Pitfalls of Coming Out

Research mentioned earlier has shown that nonheterosexuals who come out live happier, better-adjusted lives. However, this does not imply that coming out is easy. On the contrary, many gay and lesbian individuals approach each step in the coming-out process with apprehension and even fear. It is no secret that being gay in a heterocentric society (in which heterosexuality is the "norm") carries with it the potential for very real emotional, psychological, and physical harm. Just some of the potentially negative consequences faced by individuals grappling with coming out include harassment and ridicule from peers, fellow students, or coworkers; rejection by friends, parents, and other family members, and even one's church; eviction from and denial of housing; loss of current job, denial of access to military service, and other forms of prejudice and discrimination; and intimidation or physical violence that may result in destruction of property, serious injury, or even death (Davison, 2001, 2005; Murdoch & Price, 2001; Scasta, 1998).

Although few gay or lesbian individuals will experience all of these, it's safe to say that most will encounter some of them as they move through the coming-out process. The reality or merely the expectation of these negative outcomes of choosing to live an openly gay life often takes a serious emotional toll. For example, teens who are struggling with the realization that they may be gay and the prospect of coming out to themselves and others have a significantly higher rate of psychological and adjustment problems, including depression, drug abuse, eating disorders, and homelessness (Came, 1993; Gilman et al., 2001; Russell & Keel, 2002). The psychological effect of greatest concern is a significantly increased risk of suicide among gay and lesbian teens as they realize their true sexuality and face the prospect of how their sexuality will "play" in a largely intolerant world.

Homosexuality and Suicide

Numerous studies have pointed to the unfortunate fact that gay and lesbian teens attempt and complete suicide in significantly greater proportions than straight teens (Came, 1993; Halpert, 2002; Paul et al., 2002). If you think about it, this is probably not so difficult to understand. Regardless of your own sexual orientation, imagine for a moment that you are subjected to ridicule, rejection, verbal abuse, and the threat of physical violence on a daily basis simply because of something about yourself over which you have no control, such as your height or the size of your feet. You can see how life under those circumstances might at times seem out of control and not worth living. This is often how young gay and lesbian individuals feel.

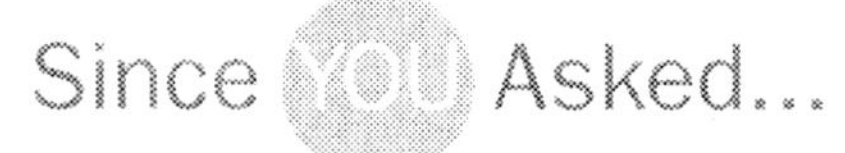

11. Do homosexual people feel comfortable holding hands and showing other public displays of affection with their partner? How often are they ridiculed or threatened?

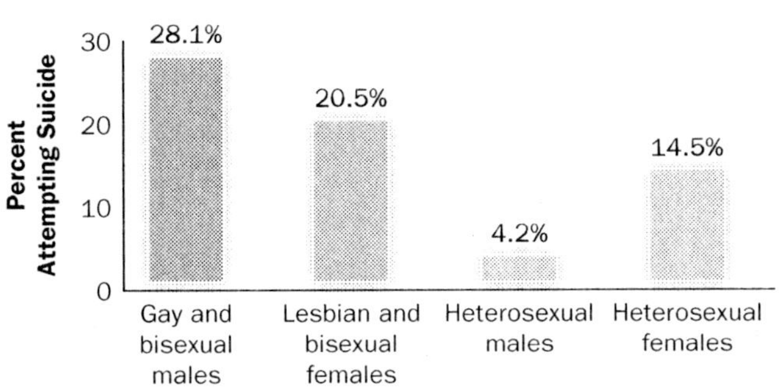

FIGURE 11.5 Attempted Suicide Rates among Gay, Lesbian, and Straight High School Students

Source: Data from Remafedi (1998)

The path to developing a personal identity and a comfortable sense of self during adolescence is difficult enough for straight teens. But gay and lesbian adolescents must also face a society that is often hostile and rejecting of the central teen issue they are facing: their sexuality. Just at a time in our lives when we all want to be seen as individuals and begin to express ourselves as young adults, gay and lesbian youth represent an "invisible minority" in a culture that makes the assumption of heterosexuality. Most feel they must hide, at least temporarily, their true nature or face ostracism, isolation, loneliness, abuse, stigma, and oppression (Halpert, 2002; Nichols, 1999). These perceptions may understandably lead to feelings of anxiety, hopelessness, and depression often accompanied by self-destructive behaviors such as alcohol and other drug abuse. Add to this the very real experiences of victimization and rejection by friends, family, and even teachers, and you have a strong recipe for suicidal thoughts, behaviors, and attempts (Garofalo et al., 1999; Russell & Joyner, 2001).

When rates of attempted suicide among gay and straight teens are compared, the differences are striking. One study in the late 1990s found that 28 percent of gay or bisexual male teens had attempted suicide, compared to 4 percent of straight male teens (Remafedi, French, & Story, 1998). Other research has found suicide rates for gay teens ranging from 20 to 42 percent, a rate 3 to 14 times higher than for straight adolescents (Bobrow, 2002; Garofalo et al., 1999; Paul et al., 2002). Figure 11.5 summarizes some of these alarming findings.

Teens who endure the stresses and strains of working through their nonheterosexual orientation during adolescence often find that the process of coming out and being themselves becomes easier upon entering college. Nearly all colleges and universities today are working to educate all students about nonheterosexual issues and to provide supportive and safe environments for gay, lesbian, and bisexual students. However, this is not to imply that it's easy to be gay in college. Coming out and being openly gay on campus remain difficult challenges for many.

Coming Out on Campus

In general, gay and lesbian students' experience of college life is different in some important and fundamental ways from their heterosexual counterparts. In spite of efforts on the part of most colleges and universities to reduce homophobic and antigay attitudes within their educational community, research demonstrates that nonheterosexual students continue to experience hostile campus environments (Howard & Stevens, 2000; Waldo, 1998). You can get an idea of the genuine attempts by colleges and universities to accommodate their nonheterosexual students by examining the pages on their Web sites devoted to gay, lesbian, and bisexual issues (most address these issues).

However, these efforts by colleges and universities to provide support and encourage tolerance among students for all sexual orientations, while commendable and probably sometimes helpful, may not be adequate to solve the innumerable problems that nonheterosexual college students face. One large university study of nearly 2,000 students (Waldo, 1998) found that gay, lesbian, and bisexual students tend to rate their overall campus climate in more negative terms than heterosexual students do. This study concluded that the hostility they encounter causes them to feel less able to fit in, and this in turn lowers their satisfaction with academic life overall.

Specifically, nonheterosexual students felt less accepted and respected by heterosexual students and by the campus environment in general. Lesbians reported experiencing these feelings more strongly than gay men. Also, lesbian, gay, and bisexual students rated themselves as less confident than their heterosexual peers and perceived that they were treated less fairly in various academic settings. Moreover, nonheterosexual students reported more negative relationships with their instructors and advisers. Although this study was carried out at only one university, similar experiences have been reported by students on many campuses (Eisenberg & Wechsler, 2003).

The inhospitable campus atmosphere for gay students was further revealed by this study in the observation that heterosexual students were generally *not* in favor of official college efforts to institute policies that are more supportive of nonheterosexual students and were opposed to programs designed to promote greater interpersonal contact between gay and straight students (Eisenberg & Wechsler, 2003). Furthermore, specific subgroups of students appeared to exacerbate the antigay biases more than others. Students who identified themselves as Christian or politically conservative expressed less concern for the negative college experiences of lesbian, gay, and bisexual students and were found to hold stronger antigay attitudes. Members of fraternities and sororities, while acknowledging the hostile campus climate for nonheterosexual students, had greater negative attitudes about interpersonal contact with gay and lesbian students than students who were not part of the Greek system.

Finally, the antigay bias on campus appears to extend beyond attitudes directed toward gay, lesbian, and bisexual students to the teachers themselves. Another study found that when students are aware that their instructor is gay, they perceive the teacher as less believable and feel that they will learn significantly less than students in a class taught by a straight professor (Russ, Simonds, & Hunt, 2002).

Sexual Orientation and HIV

One of the most challenging hurdles facing nonheterosexuals, especially gay men, is the stigma of HIV and AIDS. It is true that when AIDS first appeared in the United States in the early 1980s, the illnesses and deaths associated with this terrible virus were occurring primarily in the gay male communities in large U.S. cities, especially New York and San Francisco. In fact, when researchers at the Centers for Disease Control (CDC) in Atlanta and the National Institutes of Health (NIH) first began working to identify and isolate the cause of the growing epidemic, the illness was named *gay-related immune deficiency* (GRID). That designation lasted only about a year before heterosexual men and women began to become infected, and the official name of the disease was quickly changed to *acquired immune deficiency syndrome* (AIDS). Today, while the majority of existing cases are still among males, everyone knows that HIV and AIDS are clearly not limited to any one sexual orientation. The number of new U.S. cases of AIDS grew among women during the 1990s while the number was declining among men (CDC, 2001b). Moreover, the vast majority (80 percent) of HIV infections worldwide are due to heterosexual, not homosexual, contact (National Institute of Allergy and Infectious Diseases, 2002).

Although HIV is not a "gay disease," gay people, regardless of whether they are HIV-positive or not, are discriminated against based on irrational and misinformed beliefs about the illness. This form of discrimination has become known as **AIDS stigma**. The belief that gay individuals are to blame for the AIDS epidemic and are an ongoing threat to spread the disease increases the overall level of prejudice and discrimination that already exists in society. "In Touch with Your Sexual Health: AIDS Stigma" summarizes some of the effects of AIDS stigma.

AIDS stigma Prejudice and discrimination against nonheterosexual individuals based on the erroneous belief that gay individuals are solely to blame for the AIDS epidemic and are the primary threat to the continuing spread of the disease.

What can be done to ease the many difficult barriers typically faced by gay, lesbian, and bisexual individuals struggling with coming out? Perhaps the place to begin to answer that question is to educate as many people as possible about the prejudice, discrimination, and intolerance targeted at nonheterosexuals that continues to permeate society and then find ways of reducing or eliminating it. This is the focus of the next section.

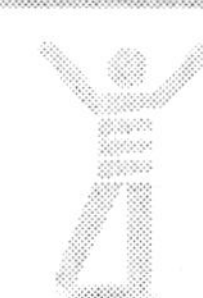

In Touch with Your Sexual Health

AIDS Stigma

AIDS stigma refers to a specific set of prejudicial and discriminatory beliefs and practices directed against people who are perceived to have AIDS or HIV and especially against individuals who are associated with groups who are believed to be more likely to have or spread HIV, such as the gay male community. Below are the main prejudicial beliefs and discriminatory effects of AIDS stigma, based on a survey of 7,500 adults in the United States.

Prejudicial Beliefs of AIDS Stigma

- People who are infected with HIV "get what they deserve" (18.7 percent).
- All gay male behavior transmits HIV, even between two *infected* men with or without the use of condoms (19 percent).
- All gay male behavior transmits HIV, even between two *uninfected* men without the use of condoms (47 percent).
- HIV can be transmitted by a sterilized drinking glass used by someone with AIDS (27.1 percent).
- HIV/AIDS can be transmitted by a sweater that had been worn by an infected person after it has been dry-cleaned and repackaged like new (27.5 percent).
- HIV can be transmitted by being coughed or sneezed on (41.1 percent).
- People with HIV/AIDS are personally responsible for their own illness (55.1 percent).

Discriminatory Effects of AIDS Stigma

- Increased discrimination toward nonheterosexual individuals regardless of HIV status
- Fear, delay, and avoidance of HIV testing
- Avoidance and ostracizing of people with HIV
- Hiding infection from potential sexual partners
- Less support for AIDS prevention programs
- Support for sodomy laws (discussed later in this chapter)
- Interpreting nonheterosexual orientations as pathological (sick)
- Reduced seeking of health care by gays and lesbians due to fear of disclosure and rejection
- Isolation and lack of support for infected individuals regardless of sexual orientation
- Calls for public disclosure of individuals with HIV
- Call for quarantining HIV-positive people

Sources: Carr and Grambling (2004); CDC (2000c); Herek and Capitanio (1999); Herek, Widaman, and Capitanio (2005); and Lopes (2001).

Prejudice, Discrimination, and the Gay Rights Movement

As you learned at the beginning of this chapter, the gay rights movement, which officially began with the Stonewall riot of 1969, discussed at the beginning of this chapter, already has multiple decades of history behind it. However, the gay rights movement is far more than a single event. It is a complex web of efforts by gay, lesbian, bisexual, and straight people using various social and political strategies to eliminate all forms of prejudice and discrimination based on sexual orientation. The fight for gay rights is being waged on several fronts, including working for formal antidiscrimination laws, fighting to overturn laws forbidding specific sexual acts that are aimed at nonheterosexuals, preventing violent attacks on gay and lesbian individuals, attempting to interact with and educate people about nonheterosexual orientations, and working to establish equal rights for nonheterosexuals with regard to marriage (as discussed earlier).

Laws against Discrimination Based on Sexual Orientation

The campaign to establish antidiscrimination laws regarding sexual orientation is just beginning. Fewer than 10 percent of the world's countries have passed national legislation forbidding discrimination based on sexual orientation. Of those that have, the United States is conspicuously absent. Many political, social, and religious factors may account for the lack of federal U.S. laws designed to protect people from discrimination based on sexual orientation, but one that stands out is the debate over whether granting specific antidiscriminatory rights to nonheterosexual groups bestows on them "special rights."

Opponents of such laws claim that current laws against discrimination are adequate to protect all minority groups including gays and lesbians. Proponents claim that people are routinely discriminated against in numerous ways, in various settings, solely because of their nonheterosexual orientation and therefore should be specifically protected by law. Legally naming nonheterosexuals as a "protected class" of people in the same vein as members of a particular sex, religion, and race is a hot political potato, and emotions on the subject run high. The official policy statement of the American Civil Liberties Union (2002) says, in part:

> The struggle of lesbian, gay, bisexual and transgender (LGBT) people for full equality is one of this generation's most important and galvanizing civil rights movements. Despite the many advances that have been made, however, LGBT people continue to face discrimination in many areas of life. No federal law prevents a person from being fired or refused a job on the basis of sexual orientation. The nation's largest employer—the U.S. military—openly discriminates against gays and lesbians. Mothers and fathers still lose child custody simply because they are gay or lesbian. And gay people are still denied the right to marry. . . .
>
> Discrimination based on sexual orientation still permeates many areas of American life. Businesses openly fire LGBT employees, and every year, lesbians and gay men are denied jobs and access to housing, hotels and other public accommodations. Many more are forced to hide their lives, deny their families and lie about their loved ones just to get by.

While it is difficult to locate a specific policy statement on the other side of the debate, one opposing argument claims that the Fourteenth Amendment to the U.S. Constitution forbids *all* discrimination against *any* group, including, by default, people of any sexual orientation. Therefore, the argument maintains, additional protections are unnecessary (Sowell, 1994). However, many lawmakers in both the federal and state governments do not consider nonheterosexuals one of the groups that is protected by this constitutional amendment. Therefore, supporters of gay rights point to many cases of discrimination that go unaddressed and believe that more specific language is necessary in state constitutions to guarantee nonheterosexuals the same rights afforded other protected groups. Where within this polarized debate does the "truth" lie? Of course, truth tends to be relative to one's convictions, but some statistics might help clarify the issue.

You are probably aware that discrimination in employment, housing, education, credit practices, and so on, is illegal according to various federal and state statutes. But this begs the question: Discrimination is illegal against *whom*? In general, state and federal antidiscrimination laws specify certain characteristics of groups that are protected under these laws, such as race, religion, sex (male or female), country of origin, age, or disability. These are referred to as **protected classes**. Some states have passed laws adding sexual orientation to their list of protected classes that receive some protections under the states' antidiscrimination laws. However, even in those states with legal protections based on sexual orientation, many have extended that protection to very specific settings, such as state employment or education, but not across the board, as is the case for other protected classes. Figure 11.6 identifies the states that have enacted laws prohibiting employment discrimination based on sexual orientation. In addition, Table 11.3 gives you an overall picture of which states have enacted sexual orientation protection laws (31 in all) and the areas of protection they provide.

protected classes Specific groups of people protected under federal and state antidiscrimination laws, identified by race, religion, sex, age, or other characteristics.

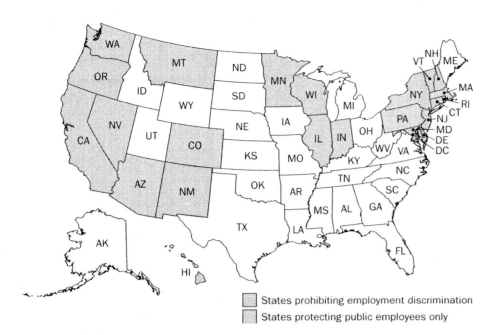

FIGURE 11.6 States with Laws Prohibiting Employment Discrimination on the Basis of Sexual Orientation

Source: Lambda Legal Defense and Education Fund (2005).

What does this mean for nonheterosexuals in states that do not provide any legal protections against discrimination based on sexual orientation? It means that they can be denied housing, be evicted from rental housing, be denied a job, be fired from a job, be denied an equal education, be denied credit, and so on, based solely on the fact that they are gay or lesbian, without any legal recourse. You may be thinking to yourself, "Yeah, but these things never really happen, do they?" Yes, they happen frequently, but significantly more frequently in those states that do not have antigay discrimination laws (Heubner, Rebchook, & Kegeles, 2004).

sodomy laws Laws prohibiting specific sexual activities between adults, even in private and with their consent.

Laws Prohibiting Gay and Lesbian Sexual Behaviors

In the past, all U.S. states enacted **sodomy laws**, which prohibited people from engaging in certain sexual acts that were deemed strange, deviant, or immoral. These laws referred to nonreproductive, noncommercial, consensual sexual acts between adults in private and included oral and anal sex at a minimum and in some cases virtually any sexual behavior other than sexual intercourse between a married man and woman in the "missionary position." During most of the twentieth century, these laws were rarely enforced, and when they were, they were usually applied only against gay and lesbian individuals. But times change, and between 1962 and 2001, 36 states either repealed their sodomy laws or decriminalized all sexual behaviors engaged in by consenting adults in private.

In 2003, a U.S. Supreme Court decision in effect negated all sodomy laws in the remaining 14 states. The case, known as *Lawrence v. Texas*, stemmed from a 1998 event in which the Houston police were called out on a domestic disturbance complaint (which later turned out to be a false report) by a neighbor of the defendants. When the police arrived, they did not find a disturbance, but did discover two men, Geddes Lawrence and Tyron Garner engaged in, according to the police report, "deviate sexual conduct, namely, anal sex," and arrested them for violating Texas's sodomy laws (Gibbs, 2003). The case was eventually heard by the Supreme Court which in a 6 to 3 verdict, struck down all of Texas's remaining sodomy laws (which had applied only to nonheterosexual couples), basing their decision on the defendants' constitutionally guaranteed right to privacy. In the majority ruling, Justice Anthony Kennedy stated: "The petitioners are entitled to respect for their private lives. The state cannot demean their existence or control their destiny by making their private sexual conduct

Geddes Lawrence and Tyron Garner were the defendants in the case of Lawrence v. Texas *that overturned the last of the sodomy laws in the United States.*

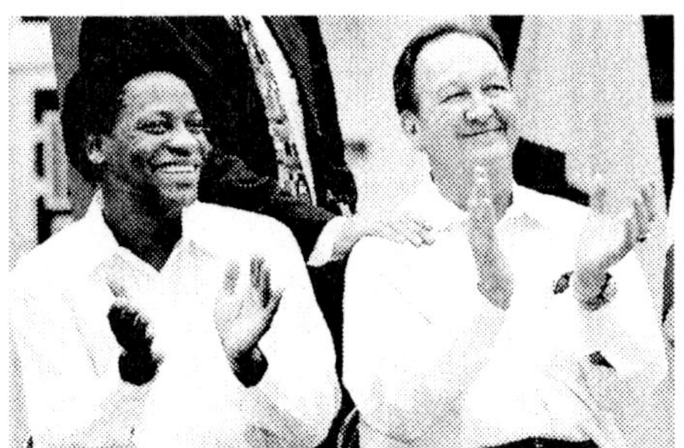

Table 11.3 STATE LAWS PROHIBITING DISCRIMINATION BASED ON SEXUAL ORIENTATION

	DISCRIMINATION PROHIBITION						
State	Public Employment	Public Accommodation	Private Employment	Education	Housing	Credit	Union Practices
Alaska	√[a]			√[b]			
Arizona	√[a]						
California[c]	√		√	√	√		√
Colorado	√						
Connecticut[c]	√	√	√	√	√	√	√
Delaware	√[a]						
Florida				√[b]			
Hawaii	√		√		√		√
Illinois[c]	√	√	√		√	√	√
Indiana[c]	√[d]						
Iowa	√[a,e]						
Kentucky[c]	√[a]						
Lousiana	√[a]						
Maine[c]	√	√	√	√	√	√	√
Maryland	√	√	√		√		
Massachusetts	√	√	√	√	√	√	√
Michigan	√[a]	√[f]					
Minnesota[c]	√	√	√	√	√	√	√
Montana	√[b]						
Nevada	√		√				√
New Hampshire	√	√	√		√		√
New Jersey	√	√	√	√	√	√	√
New Mexico[c]	√	√	√		√	√	√
New York	√	√	√	√	√	√	√
Oregon	√[g]		√[g]				
Pennsylvania[c]	√[a]			√[b]			
Rhode Island[c]	√	√	√	√	√	√	√
Utah				√[b]			
Vermont	√	√	√	√	√	√	√
Washington	√[a]						
Wisconsin	√	√	√	√	√	√	√

[a] Executive order only (not a law).

[b] Administrative code or rules (not a law).

[c] Includes gender identity.

[d] State employment policy only (not a law).

[e] Executive order affirms commitment to equal employment opportunity and affirmative action and creates a state workforce diversity program and a task force for equal opportunity in employment.

[f] Applies to health care facilities only.

[g] Oregon Court of Appeals ruling, December 9, 1998.

Source: Myers (2005).

a crime" (Gibbs, 2003; Jurand, 2004). This precedent-setting ruling is widely seen as rendering unconstitutional all sodomy laws still in effect anywhere in the United States, and for everyone, regardless of their sexual orientation. Since the ruling, however, several reports have surfaced indicating that some states, including Kansas, Virginia, and North Carolina continue to enforce their discriminatory sodomy laws against nonheterosexual behavior (Allen, 2003; Han, 2005). The decision in *Lawrence v. Texas*, although highly influential, may not mark a final end to sodomy laws in the United States. Future interpretations of the case and potential legal maneuverings have the potential to dilute the Court's ruling and reverse its antidiscriminatory influence (Adler, 2005).

As with antidiscrimination laws, discussed earlier, the legal status of sexual behaviors among same-sex couples varies considerably around the world. At one end of the spectrum are countries in which sexual activities among adults are simply legal regardless of the sexes of the participants. At the other extreme are countries in which homosexual activities are crimes punishable by death. Most countries fall somewhere inbetween these two ends of the legal scale. A sampling of these laws appears in "Sexuality and Culture: Laws Applying to Same Sex Behaviors in Selected Countries."

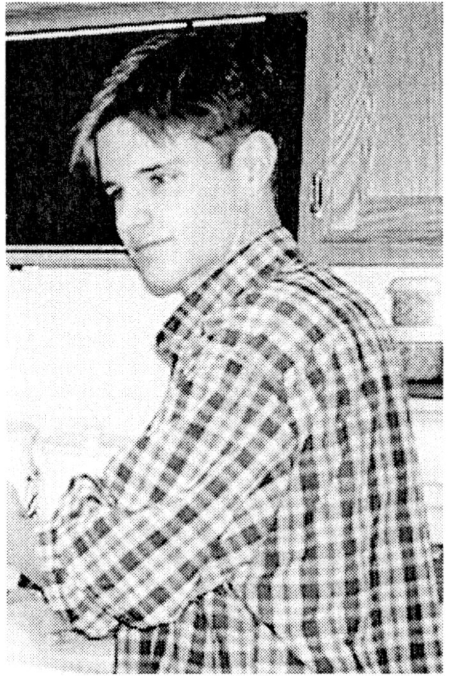

The brutal abduction, beating, and killing of Wyoming college student Matthew Shepard in 1998 brought the issue of violence directed at those with nonheterosexual orientations to a higher level of public awareness in the United States and around the world.

Hate Crimes and Sexual Orientation

Homophobia refers to an extreme fear, discomfort, or hatred of gay and lesbian people. In its most extreme forms, homophobia may lead to verbal abuse and even physical violence toward nonheterosexual individuals. In October 1998, Matthew Shepard, a gay college student at the University of Wyoming, was kidnaped by two men he had met in a bar, driven to a deserted field, brutally beaten, tied to a fence in freezing temperatures, and left to die (Bull, 1999; Hock, 2003). Four months later, Billy Jack Gaither, a 39-year-old gay man who worked at a clothing company in Alabama, was brutally beaten to death. His throat was cut and his body beaten with an ax handle before he was thrown on top of a pile of automobile tires and set on fire (Bull, 1999; *Frontline*, 2002). These horrible, ruthless murders focused renewed national attention on violence against gays and lesbians. However, as you can see in Figure 11.7, extreme

homophobia Extreme fear, discomfort, or hatred of nonheterosexual individuals.

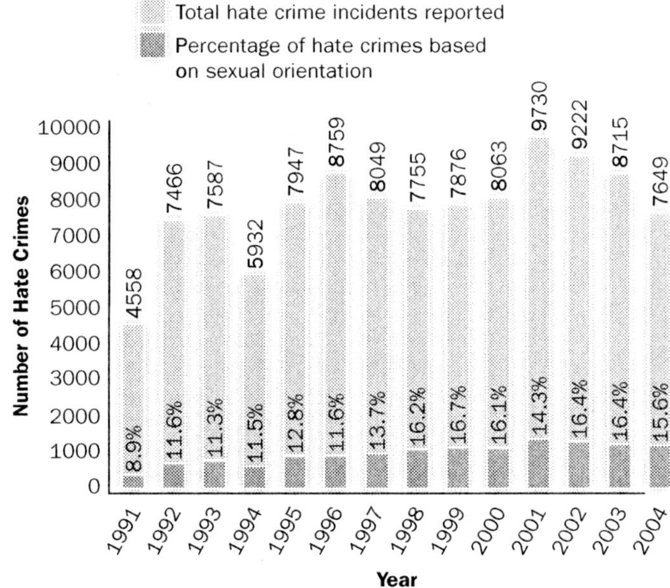

FIGURE 11.7 Hate Crimes against Gay, Lesbian, and Bisexual Individuals, 1991–2004

Source: Federal Bureau of Investigation (2004b, 2005).

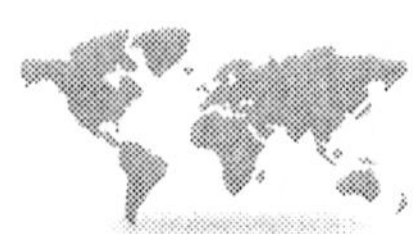

Sexuality and Culture

Laws Applying to Same-Sex Behaviors in Selected Countries

Country	Lesbian	Gay Male	Maximum Penalty
Africa			
Algeria	✖	✖	3 years, fine
Egypt	✖	✖	Various
Ethiopia	✖	✖	3 years
Kenya	✓	✖	14 years
Mauretania	✖	✖	Death
Morocco	✖	✖	3 years, fine
Nigeria	✓	✖	Death
South Africa	✓	✓	
Sudan	✖	✖	Death
Americas			
Argentina	✓	✓	
Aruba	✓	✓	
Bahamas	✓	✓	
Barbados	✖	✖	Unknown
Bermuda	✓	✓	
Brazil	✓	✓	
Canada	✓	✓	
Costa Rica	✓	✓	
Cuba	✓	✖	1 year
Guatemala	✓	✓	
Jamaica	✓	✖	10 years, hard labor
Mexico	✓	✓	
Nicaragua	✖	✖	3 years
Panama	✓	✓	
Puerto Rico	✓	✓	
United States (most states)	✓	✓	
Asia-Pacific			
Afghanistan	✖	✖	Death
Australia	✓	✓	
Bangladesh	✖	✖	Life in prison
China	✓	✓	
Fiji	✓	✖	14 years
India	✖	✖	Life in prison
Japan	✓	✓	
Nepal	✖	✖	Life in prison
New Zealand	✓	✓	
Pakistan	✖	✖	Death
Philippines	✓	✓	
Singapore	✖	✖	Life in prison
South Korea	✓	✓	
Taiwan	✓	✓	
Vietnam	✓	✓	
Europe			
Belgium	✓	✓	
Czech Republic	✓	✓	
Denmark	✓	✓	
France	✓	✓	
Germany	✓	✓	
Greece	✓	✓	
Hungary	✓	✓	
Ireland	✓	✓	
Italy	✓	✓	
Netherlands	✓	✓	
Norway	✓	✓	
Poland	✓	✓	
Portugal	✓	✓	
Romania	✓	✓	
Russia	✓	✓	
Spain	✓	✓	
Sweden	✓	✓	
Switzerland	✓	✓	
Turkey	✓	✓	
United Kingdom	✓	✓	
Vatican City	✓	✓	
Middle East			
Iran	✖	✖	Death
Iraq	✓	✓	Legal but taboo
Israel	✓	✓	
Jordan	✓	✓	
Kuwait	✖	✖	7 years
Lebanon	✖	✖	1 year
Palestinian territories	✖	✖	10 years
Saudi Arabia	✖	✖	Death

Key: ✓ = legal; ✖ = illegal

Source: Adapted from Sodomy Laws (2005a).

Table 11.4 FBI HATE CRIME STATISTICS FOR 2004

CATEGORY	INCIDENTS	PERCENTAGE OF ALL HATE CRIMES
Race	4,042	52.8%
Religion	1,374	17.9%
Sexual orientation	**1,197**	**15.6%**
Ethnicity/National origin	972	12.7%
Disability (physical or mental)	57	0.75%
Multiple bias incidents	7	0.09%
Total	7,649	100.0

Source: Federal Bureau of Investigation (2006), Table 1.

and violent forms of prejudice and discrimination targeted at people of nonheterosexual orientations, often referred to as **gay bashing**, did not by any means begin or end with those high-profile stories. Antigay beatings and killings happen far more often than most people know or would want to admit (Bull, 1999).

During the 1990s and early 2000s, violent crimes in the United States, especially homicides, that targeted specific groups of individuals began to receive special legal consideration. They came to be called **hate crimes**. These violent crimes are motivated by strong feelings of fear and hate toward members of a certain protected class of people. Typically, the perpetrators of these crimes are weak individuals who feel threatened by the mere existence of the group at which their violence is targeted. **Hate crimes laws** have allowed for more stringent penalties for violent crimes that can be shown to have been motivated by bias or prejudice toward a protected class of people, such as a racial or religious minority.

More than half of all hate crimes in 2004 were motivated by racial bias, and another 17.9 percent are motivated by religious bias. Crimes against gay and lesbian individuals are the third most common category of hate crimes, comprising over 15 percent of such crimes in 2004, up from just under 9 percent in 1991 (FBI, 2006). Table 11.4 provides a breakdown of the various categories of hate crimes in 2004.

The Psychology of Violent Crime against Nonheterosexual Groups

Murders and beatings of gays, lesbians, and bisexuals tend to be among the most gruesomely violent of all violent crimes. Typically, the victims are tortured, brutally beaten, or stabbed numerous times. The degree of hate evidenced by these crimes is difficult for most people to comprehend. But anyone who is openly gay or lesbian will tell you that nonheterosexual individuals are routinely aware and vigilant of the possibility that they could be physically attacked at any moment. What is behind such extreme reactions to homosexuality that some people resort to physical beatings and even murder to express their fear and hatred?

Most psychologists will agree that it is one thing to object to homosexuality on moral, philosophical, or religious grounds but that these over-the-top reactions of violence and murder are vastly out of proportion to any real threat the victim poses. These overreactions suggest that deeper psychological mechanisms may be at work in people who commit violent acts against nonheterosexuals. One of the motivations for irrational antigay attitudes and behaviors that has been proposed is a

gay bashing Criminal acts or violence, motivated by homophobia, committed against nonheterosexual individuals.

hate crimes Violent crimes motivated by prejudice and discrimination, targeting specific groups of individuals.

hate crime laws Laws prescribing more stringent penalties for crimes motivated by bias or prejudice.

psychological defense mechanism called a **reaction formation**, in which a person engages in extreme and exaggerated behaviors in the *opposite* direction of the person's unacceptable internal urges. How does this translate into violence toward gays and lesbians? The theory says that when some individuals with strong antihomosexual attitudes are forced to confront, consciously or unconsciously, their *own* homosexual urges, the fear that those urges generate drives them to beat or kill a homosexual person to "prove that they could not possibly be gay." In other words, gay bashers may themselves be in deep denial that they themselves are closeted homosexuals and will resort to extreme behaviors (form extreme reactions) to try to alleviate the anxiety their urges are creating in them.

psychological defense mechanism Originally suggested by Freud, a psychological distortion of reality serving to defend against personally unacceptable thoughts or urges.

reaction formation A type of defense mechanism in which a person engages in exaggerated behaviors in the *opposite* direction of internal urges felt to be unacceptable or intolerable.

penile plethysmograph An electronic device that records blood flow into the penis to detect sexual arousal.

Does any scientific evidence exist for this theory? The answer is yes. In the mid-1990s, an article titled "Is Homophobia Associated with Homosexual Arousal?" appeared in the *Journal of Abnormal Psychology* (Adams, Wright, & Lohr, 1996). The article created quite a stir in human sexuality and psychology circles and continues to be heatedly discussed today because it reported on a study that seems to support the reaction formation explanation of homophobia.

The method the researchers used was relatively simple. They first gave heterosexual male subjects a written scale to determine their level of negative attitudes toward homosexuality, a "homophobia scale." They then asked each subject to watch sexually explicit videos of heterosexual and homosexual activities and measured degree of sexual arousal using a penile strain gauge, called a **penile plethysmograph**, (see Chapter 1) that records blood flow into the penis to detect sexual arousal.

The researchers found that only the men who scored highest on the measure of homophobia became sexually aroused in response to the gay male video. Furthermore, those same homophobic men rated their level of sexual arousal to the gay male videos significantly lower than the nonhomophobic participants did. This implies that men with stronger antigay attitudes may indeed be experiencing homosexual feelings in themselves but denying them. It follows, then, that gay bashers, who clearly hold the strongest antigay feelings, may be resisting the strongest gay tendencies of all within themselves.

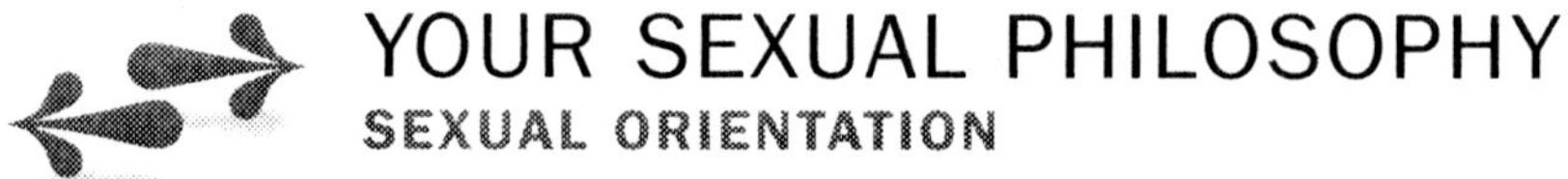

YOUR SEXUAL PHILOSOPHY

SEXUAL ORIENTATION

We live in a heterocentric society in which most straight people place the assumption and expectation of heterosexuality onto most, if not all, others. If you are gay, lesbian, or bisexual, you already know this, perhaps all too well. But if your self-defined sexual orientation is heterosexual, you have probably not had to deal personally with many of the topics discussed here. However, nearly every straight person has friends, acquaintances, or family members who are gay, lesbian, or bisexual, whether they know it or not. A clear and accurate understanding of the issues they face is crucial to your personal journey through our sexually diverse world.

Issues relating to sexual orientation play important roles in everyone's basic sexual philosophy. An awareness of these issues contributes to the development of understanding and tolerance of sexual diversity. The material presented in this chapter relates to the development of your ability to feel comfortable yourself and with those who may have sexual orientations different from yours.

If you are heterosexual, some of you may believe some of the misconceptions and stereotypes about gay, lesbian, and bisexual individuals examined in this chapter. If so, now that you have more accurate information about sexual orientation, your challenge is to begin to discard those erroneous beliefs and start becoming a person who is more tolerant of the richness of human sexual diversity. Tolerance of all kinds of human differences is usually a matter of education and learning to see others as individuals rather than solely as members of a stereotyped group. People with sexual orientations other than your own do not pose any serious threat to you, your sexual orientation, your health, or your life as a sexual being. As you acknowledge and accept these facts, which some of you have already, you will be able to plan ahead to interact with others, all others, from a position of tolerance, equality, and empathy, based on who they are as fellow humans and not as people with a certain sexual orientation.

If you are not heterosexual, your challenges are different but equally important. You have to be emotionally prepared for the unfortunate fact that others may view you through a lens of prejudice and discrimination and treat you accordingly. It is hoped, of course, that most of the people you care about in your life will not take these views, but for most of you, it is bound to happen, if it hasn't already, and you must be ready for it. How will you react to the homophobia that exists in others? Here is your chance to think about it now, analyze your position, develop strategies, plan ahead, and clarify your sexual philosophy about your sexual orientation and others' reactions. That will help you avoid being taken by surprise by prejudiced attitudes or discriminatory or violent acts. This is not to imply that you should not work to fight injustice and bigotry and to be comfortable and proud of who you are. Everyone should do that. You will also have the opportunity to educate others about sexual orientation, and education is the very best weapon against the ignorance on which bigotry is based.

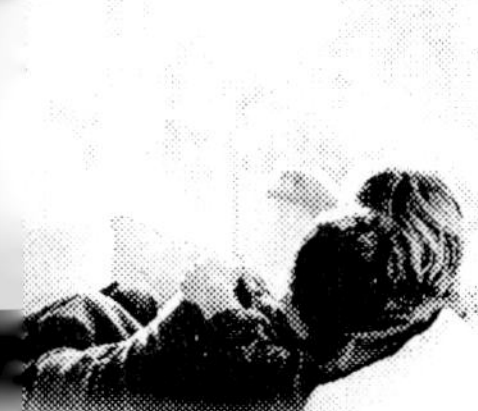

Summary

HISTORICAL PERSPECTIVES The Stonewall Riot

- The 1969 Stonewall riots sparked the beginning of the gay rights movement. Patrons of the Stonewall Inn, one of the country's few gay bars at that time, rose up and fought violently against police harassment. This event is marked by many as the beginning of the gay rights movement in the United States.

Straight, Gay, Lesbian, Bisexual: A Closer Look

- Sexual orientation is not categorical; straight and gay exist on a continuum. Most people have thoughts, feelings, fantasies, or experiences involving both sexes.
- Alfred Kinsey developed a rating scale for measuring degrees of sexual orientation rather than placing it into distinct categories.

Nonheterosexual Orientations: Issues and Attitudes

- Sexual orientation is about more than simply sexual behavior. Sexual orientation relates to which sex you are primarily attracted to, want to date, are likely to fall in love with, want to establish long-term relationships with, and perhaps marry.
- Marriage is legally defined in most states as a union between one man and one woman. In recent years, however, some states were beginning to liberalize laws against gay unions, and gay marriage has become legal in at least one state.
- The quality of gay and lesbian relationships is similar to those of heterosexuals, but research shows that nonheterosexual couples tend to experience less hostility and are generally more upbeat than straight couples overall.

Theories of Sexual Orientation

- The scientific consensus is that sexual orientation not a choice. Most anecdotal and scientific research indicates that sexual orientation is a basic and probably inborn characteristic.
- Researchers have found differences between heterosexual and homosexual brain structure and functioning. These biological findings combined with twin studies have provided evidence that sexual orientation may be genetic in origin. Research also indicates that differences in the balance of hormones in the uterine environment during pregnancy may relate to a person's sexual orientation.
- Research has not found that gay men are more likely than straight men to have domineering mothers or absent fathers. The family backgrounds of gay individuals, and of heterosexuals differ very little, if at all.
- The exotic becomes erotic theory attempts to integrate nature and nurture approaches to sexual orientation. It suggests that inborn tendencies, combined with early nonsexual play experiences with peers, may determine sexual orientation in puberty and adulthood.
- Some people argue that the origins of sexual orientation are unimportant and that nonjudgmental acceptance of nonheterosexual individuals is more important than finding an exact cause.

Coming Out

- Heterosexuals never have to "come out" because they are never "in the closet." Most cultures assume heterosexuality as the "default orientation."
- Coming out is a gradual, step-by-step process, often occurring over years.
- Coming out is a risky and difficult yet emotionally satisfying process for most nonheterosexual individuals, who find "living a lie" more difficult than facing the possible prejudice, discrimination, and stigma of coming out.
- Suicide rates among gay youth are many times higher than among their heterosexual peers. Societal and peer pressures cause increased rates of serious depression among gay and lesbian teens.
- Gay, lesbian, and bisexual students experience college life more negatively than straight students. Bigoted peer attitudes and antigay campus climates may have a chilling effect on nonheterosexual students' college life.

Sexual Orientation and HIV

- AIDS stigma negatively affects gays and heterosexuals. This is one type of prejudice and discrimination based on gay and lesbian sexual orientation that often poses problems for those who have come out.

Prejudice, Discrimination, and the Gay Rights Movement

- The United States has failed to pass a law protecting citizens from discrimination based on sexual orientation. No federal law identifies sexual orientation as a characteristic of a protected class of individuals in cases of discrimination.
- Twenty-four states omit sexual orientation from antidiscrimination laws. Conversely, approximately half of all states have specifically added sexual orientation as a protected class in at least some of their discrimination laws.
- Sodomy laws are still on the books in some states. However, the 2003 U.S. Supreme Court ruling in *Lawrence vs Texas* has drawn the constitutionality of all these laws into question.
- Violence against nonheterosexuals is the second most common hate crime in the United States. Only violence based on race is more common.
- Gay bashing may be a defense mechanism against the bashers' own homosexual desires. Research indicates that men who deeply fear their own gay tendencies may be the most likely to commit violent acts against gay men to "prove" that they are straight.

YOUR SEXUAL PHILOSOPHY: Sexual Orientation

- Developing an understanding of and sensitivity to the complex issues relating to sexual orientation is one of the keys to developing tolerance for sexual differences and appreciating human sexual diversity.

Have You Considered?

1. Imagine for a moment that you are the parent of a son or daughter (your choice) who informs you that he or she is gay. How do you think you would react? What would be the three most important things you would want to tell your child after hearing this news?
2. Now turn the question on yourself. Imagine that you wake up tomorrow morning and your sexual orientation has changed (from straight to gay, from gay to straight, from either to bisexual, etc.). Discuss how you might feel about such a change and how such a transformation would alter your life and your view of the world around you.
3. What do you think are the three best strategies for reducing prejudice and discrimination targeted at nonheterosexual individuals? Explain your ideas.
4. Do you think it is important for researchers to get to the bottom of what causes homosexuality? Discuss at least three reasons for your answer.
5. Suppose you were placed in charge of gay, lesbian, and bisexual student services at your college or university. Discuss what actions you would take and what strategies you would propose for improving the climate on your campus for nonheterosexual students.
6. Do you think marriage should be legalized for nonheterosexual couples? Discuss at least three reasons for your answer.
7. What do you think are some strategies for reducing violence targeted at gays and lesbians? Explain why your idea might be effective.

Companion Website Resources

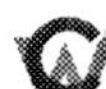

For further chapter resources go to **www.prenhall.com/hock.** This robust text website includes polling questions for you to vote on, regular news updates, quizzes, sample tests, suggested reading lists, and more.

SCENARIOS USA Also on the website are links to videos. *Scenarios USA*'s films portray real-life narratives that explore the non-biological aspects of relationships and sexual health. The films will help you consider how the themes of the text affect your own life and the lives of those around you.

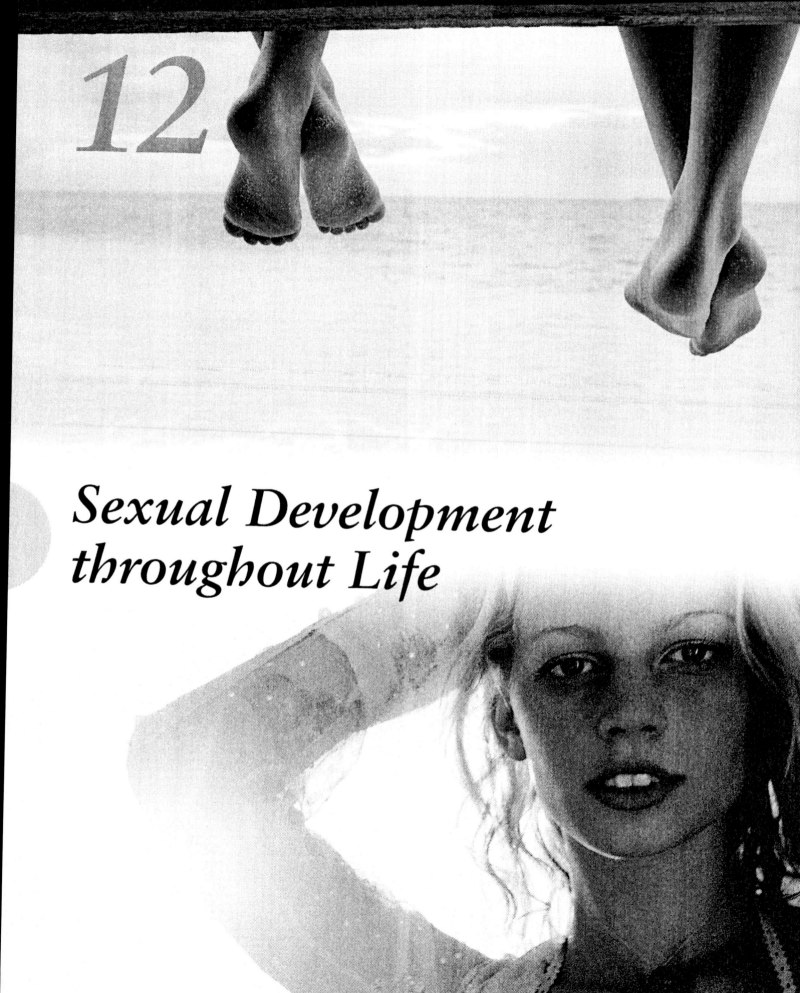

12

Sexual Development throughout Life

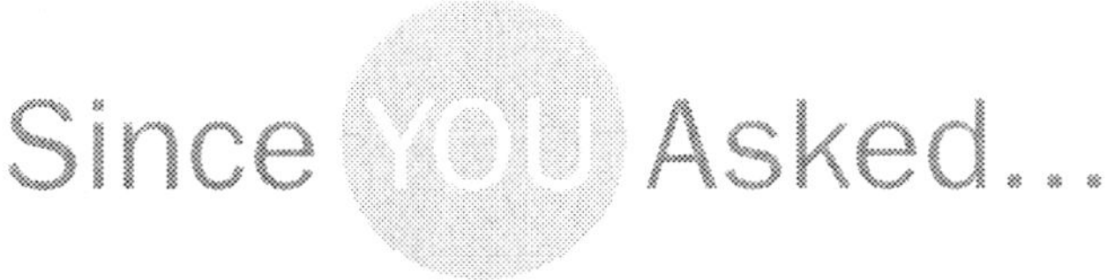

1. Is it unhealthy to masturbate at an early age? (see page 444)

2. I recently caught my 4-year-old daughter playing "doctor" with the neighbor boy (both naked). Is this a sign of a problem, or should I not be concerned? (see page 446)

3. If a child between the ages of 5 and 7 acts out sexual acts, specifically lying down on top of another child and imitating movements of intercourse, does this indicate a problem, or is it part of normal childhood curiosity? (see page 448)

4. What prevents parents from talking to their kids about sex? My parents never had "the talk" with me, and I had to find out from friends, or even worse, boyfriends. Now, two abortions later, I'm finally taking this class. (see page 449)

5. I started puberty very late (around age 15). All my friends were already getting their periods and breasts and everything. It was very embarrassing. Why do some people start puberty so late? (see page 452)

6. In high school, a lot of my friends were having oral sex but not intercourse. Is it true that oral sex doesn't spread diseases? (see page 458)

7. Women reach their sexual peak at 35, right? And men at 18? Why did nature create such a discrepancy? (see page 463)

8. My roommate went to a party and drank too much. She had sex with two guys (that she remembers), but she says she didn't really want to. Was this rape? (see page 465)

9. I've heard that when people get married, their sex life goes right down the tubes. Is this true? (see page 469)

10. At what age do most elderly people stop being interested in sex? (see page 471)

If you ask most people what they think of when you say "sexual development," they will probably respond with something relating to puberty, the time in our lives when we mature sexually and develop secondary sexual characteristics such as breasts, pubic hair, and penis and testicular growth. However, this is only a part of the larger picture of sexual development. We are developing sexually throughout our life span. As has been noted often in this book, we are by nature sexual beings.

Sex, at its most fundamental level, is required for the human species to survive and not become extinct. Beyond the biological inevitability of certain sexual acts, we develop in many ways as sexual beings surrounded by powerful social and cultural influences. These environmental forces combine with our genetic predispositions to mold our sexual identities, attitudes, and preferences. All of these factors combine to make us what are probably the most sexually complex creatures on earth.

As you read this chapter you will notice that we touch on many of the topics from other chapters in this book. Virtually all the topics of human sexuality intersect with our lives at one or many points as we develop as sexual beings. This is easy to see if you simply turn to the table of contents and think for a moment about how each chapter topic has played a role in your sexual development or the sexual life of people you have known or learned about: sexual anatomy, sexual responding, love and intimacy, birth control, sexual activities, sexual problems, STIs, pregnancy, gender expectations, sexual orientation, sexual aggression and violence, atypical sexual behaviors, prostitution, and pornography. All of these topics influence, or are influenced by, human sexual development.

When social scientists study human development, whether focusing on sexuality or on other aspects of life, their goal is to examine the changes that unfold in all of us, under normal circumstances, in a somewhat predictable way. In other words, they are not usually trying to focus on one particular individual and his or her specific development, but rather they are looking for universals, changes and milestones that happen to most of us at approximately the same age or stage in life. For example, most children acquire the concept of gender (that is, they know whether they are girls or boys and become aware of gender-role expectations) between the ages of 3 and 5; children enter puberty with all of its accompanying physical, emotional, and social changes between 10 and 15; most people form a loving, lifelong relationship (or try to) in their early 20s; and we all experience sexual changes as we age. These common and expected developmental events occur in fairly predictable patterns for all humans and form the basis of the

Focus on Your Feelings

Children experience strong feelings relating to normal sexual exploration, either through masturbation or sex play with other children. They know it feels good, and they want to experiment, but societal expectations often cause them to feel guilt and shame. Then, as children enter puberty, hormones surge and create new feelings of sexual attraction and desire. Most of you can probably remember the intensity of those early teen years, filled with highly charged emotions that are a normal part of adolescent sexual development but that sometimes may have felt too powerful and perhaps made you feel out of control.

As you entered college, you were probably faced with new feelings that went along with sexually focused university student cultures. Moreover, you were more often regarded as an adult, expected to make your own decisions about life and about sex. College students must learn how to deal as an adult with the feelings that are generated by sexual relationships. This is an integral and valuable part of the educational process for college students (although it's not in the catalog!), and it can be more challenging than any academic major.

The feelings associated with sexuality in adulthood can seem, at times, overwhelming. In early adulthood, most people will take one of the most important steps of their life: choosing a mate; the mix of emotions that comes with making such a commitment are all normal reactions to facing such a major life change. Then, moving through adulthood, most of us will face one or more of such emotionally charged issues as sexual problems, marital discord, infidelity, divorce, or the death of a spouse. Working through the emotions we feel during these experiences is part of human growth, learning, and developing.

Sexual responses and abilities change as we grow older, and we will likely experience feelings of sadness and loss, as if somehow our bodies are failing us, in more ways than one. An awareness that certain changes are a normal part of aging can help us cope rationally with them and take whatever steps are necessary to resolve problems that arise. The process of aging, sexually speaking, does not need to lead us into despair; knowing what to expect allows each of us to keep a positive outlook, adapt to the natural changes, and continue to live a sexually fulfilling life.

topics in this chapter. Of course, many variations to the usual motifs can occur, but they tend to be exceptions.

We will proceed chronologically in our discussion of human sexual development, and that means we must begin *before* birth, with sexual development and sexuality in the womb. By the time this chapter is done, we will have traveled from the womb all the way to sexuality in old age, with a number of stops in between. First, we will take a brief look at some of the theories suggested by the person who first put the "sex" in development: Sigmund Freud.

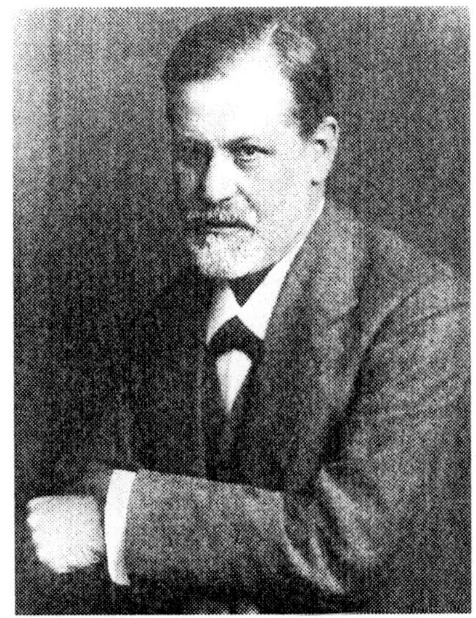

Sigmund Freud believed that all human development is sexually motivated.

Historical Perspectives

Freud's Psychosexual Stages of Development: Oedipus and Electra?

In the late 1800s, Sigmund Freud was revolutionizing how the world thought about human nature. Freud saw the development of our personality—*who we are*—as occurring in a series of **psychosexual stages** during the first 12 years or so of life, each focusing on a different sexual body part. He called the stages: the oral stage (birth to 18 months), the anal stage (18 months to 3 years), the phallic stage (3 to 6 years), the latency stage (6 years to puberty), and the genital stage (adolescence).

One major developmental milestone in children's lives is the realization of which sex they are. This is a process called **gender identification**, which typically occurs between the ages of 3 and 5 and is discussed in detail in Chapter 10, "Gender." Freud also saw this as an important event in the developmental process. He believed that for a young boy to self-identify as male and learn to behave according to cultural expectations for men is a very difficult task. After all, the boy has been under the nurturing care of his mother since birth, so what possible motivation could he have, Freud asked, to leave her side and identify with his father? (If this sounds sexist to you, remember that Freud was living in late-1800s Victorian Europe, where such roles were very strictly delineated.) Freud contended the boy's motivation must be very compelling, as evidenced in his theory of the **Oedipus complex**, named for the hero of the Greek tragedy *Oedipus Rex*, in which Oedipus unknowingly kills his father and marries his mother.

psychosexual stages Freud's theory that the development of human personality occurs in a series of stages during childhood.

gender identification A developmental stage in children between the ages of 3 and 5 during which they begin to understand which sex they are.

Oedipus complex A Freudian notion explaining how a young boy comes to identify with his father.

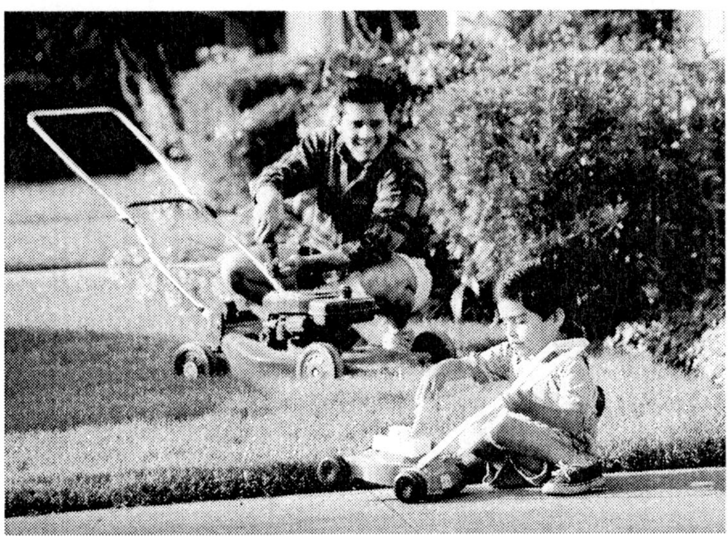

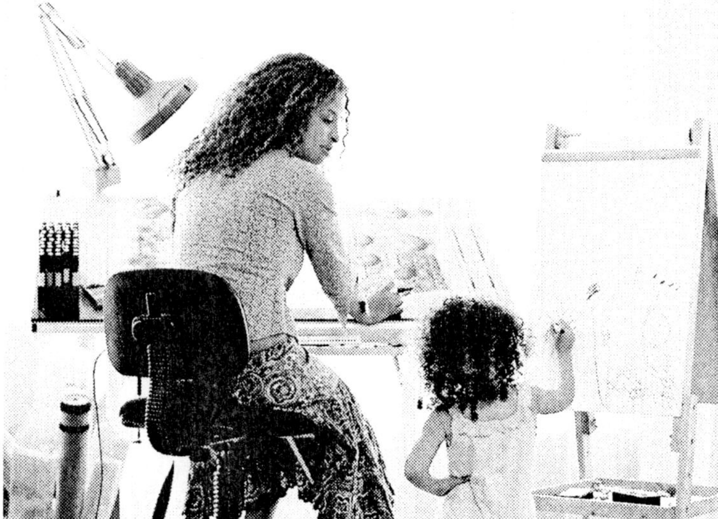

Gender identification is the process through which children discover their gender and begin to behave in socially prescribed, gender-appropriate ways.

In Freud's theory, all boys at about 3 or 4 years old develop unconscious sexual desires for their mothers. They yearn, literally though unconsciously, to have sexual intercourse with her. However, every boy soon realizes (through unconscious processes at work) that he cannot have his mother in this way because someone else already does, namely, his father. He begins to see himself as competing with his father for the mother's affection, even though he knows he has no chance of winning because his father is so much bigger and more powerful. At the same time, the boy becomes terrified that the father might find out about the boy's feelings for the mother and punish him by cutting off the boy's penis (what Freud referred to as "castration anxiety"). The only way he can figure out to avoid this terrible fate is to identify with the father—to become "just like Dad." By identifying with the father, by imitating and emulating him, the boy comes to understand his gender identity as male, develops appropriate male social behaviors, and suppresses his desires for his mother until he can be as big and strong as his father, be able to do away with his father, and then possess his mother. Of course, by the time he becomes "as big as his father," those urges are fully repressed and he seeks out a wife of his own (who, according to some interpretations of Freud, is as close a likeness to his mother as possible).

You may be asking yourself, "What about girls?" Freud later developed a theory of female gender identification through what became termed the **Electra complex** (in the Greek tragedy *Electra*, the title character convinces her brother to kill her mother so that she can possess her father). In Freud's theory, girls at about 3 years old become aware that her father has a penis, something she and her mother are lacking. This feels unjust to her and makes her feel castrated (Freud called this "penis envy"). Her reaction, according to Freud, is to reject the mother and identify with the father until she realizes that she cannot possess his penis because it already "belongs" to her mother. So she returns to identify with her mother so that when she grows up, she will be able to find a penis of her own. And in some interpretations of Freud's notion of penis envy, when she finds the right penis, she marries it.

You can see why most modern-day psychologists reject the Oedipus and Electra explanations for gender identification. They are overly complex and not subject to scientific study to be proved or disproved. Moreover, simpler and testable theories exist that seek to explain gender identification in less fanciful ways. And Freud never studied children but developed his ideas through recollections of his adult patients in analysis, who were probably not typical of all human beings.

Freud's theories are fascinating to read and think about, but they do not carry a great deal of scientific weight. As we begin our discussion of *current* thinking about sexual development, we will see how modern psychological and sexuality research sheds more direct and believable light on this complex topic.

Sexuality in Infancy and Childhood

Since YOU Asked ...

1. Is it unhealthy to masturbate at an early age?

Many parents and other adults become concerned when infants, toddlers, or young children engage in sexual behaviors such as masturbation or explorations of each other's sexual bodies, as in "playing doctor." Child development specialists, however, are quick to reassure them that such behaviors are usually normal signs of childhood curiosity and healthy enjoyment of activities that feel good. Moreover, there is no evidence that early childhood sexual experimentation is predictive of any particular sexual attitudes or behaviors later in life. In fact, sexual behaviors in children have been shown to *decrease* as age increases. In other words, 12-year-olds tend to engage in significantly *fewer* sexual behaviors than 2- or 3-year-olds (Friedrich et al., 1991).

Electra complex A Freudian notion explaining how a young girl comes to identify with her mother.

Part of the problem for parents may be the overall lack of adequate research into and discussion of childhood sexuality. A common perception in most Western societies is that humans are not "supposed" to be sexual until they enter puberty. This is simply not true. Although the interpersonal, emotional, and psychological components of sexuality begin to play a larger role during adolescence, many of the physical responses were always there. Studies examining childhood sexual experiences have found similar and very common sexual behaviors among most children between the ages of 2 and 12 (De Latimer & Friedrich, 2002; Friedrich et al., 1991). However, lack of awareness of these norms among the general population means that parents sometimes perceive their children's behaviors as abnormal. Consequently, they may avoid talking to other parents or professionals about them out of embarrassment or denial. However, if they did discuss them, they would find great comfort in the fact that most parents have experienced and dealt with similar issues and situations relating to childhood sexuality.

Childhood Masturbation

As noted earlier, the human body is designed to be sexual; it is normal for stimulation of sexual body parts to feel good. This is part of the evolution process to ensure our survival as a species. It should not be surprising that children begin to touch their genitals as soon as their motor development allows them to do so and to respond to those touches in sexual ways. Both male and female infants are capable of sexual arousal in response to stimulation soon after birth. Male infants have erections and female infants vaginally lubricate within the first 24 hours after birth (De Latimer & Friedrich, 2002). Five-month-old male infants have been found to have between 5 and 40 erections per day.

The first signs of rhythmic movements that we associate with masturbation usually appear in children between the ages of 2 and 3 (Martinson, 1994). By age 3 or 4, children understand that genital self-stimulation is pleasurable and by this age are capable of experiencing orgasm through masturbation (Leung & Robson, 1993). Based on adult memories of childhood sexual experiences, approximately 43 percent of men and 34 percent of women report exploring their genitals between the ages of 6 and 10, and 6 percent of men and 7 percent of women recall masturbating to orgasm during this age range (Larsson & Svedin, 2002). Research relying on mothers' observations has shown that among children between 2 and 10 years old, 30 percent of boys and 21 percent of girls engage in hand-to-genital masturbation (Friedrich et al., 1998).

Perhaps the most important point frequently made in the research about childhood sexuality is that virtually all child development specialists, psychologists, physicians, and other professionals consider masturbation a natural, harmless, and extremely common childhood behavior. Furthermore, childhood masturbation itself has not been linked to any sexual problems in later life. On the contrary, some evidence suggests that children who are punished or made to feel shameful for their natural sexual feelings may be more uncomfortable and less able to enjoy their sexuality as adults (Leung & Robson, 1993).

In most Western societies, parents and other caregivers have become increasingly accepting of children's masturbation behaviors, but many still express surprise, shock, anger, and concern when they see it in their own children. Typically, a concerned parent will mention the behavior to the child's pediatrician or the family doctor and will be reassured that the behavior is normal and harmless. However, children need to learn that cultural expectations dictate that such behavior is personal, private, and should not be done in public. "Self-Discovery: Masturbation in Young Children" offers advice to parents or caregivers of young children who are masturbating.

Note that childhood masturbation *can*, in some cases, become a problem. The behavior may become overly compulsive and interfere with the child's other normal childhood activities, or the child may be unwilling to limit the behavior to private settings. In these cases, parents should seek treatment and counseling, but these are unusual exceptions to normal masturbation behaviors in children.

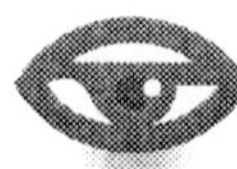

Self-Discovery

Masturbation in Young Children

Occasional masturbation is a normal behavior of many infants and preschoolers. Up to one-third of children in this age group discover masturbation while exploring their bodies, just as they explore all their parts of their bodies eventually. They find it feels good to touch their genitals and sometimes continue to do so. Genital or urinary infections do not cause masturbation; they cause pain or itching, inciting the child to scratch the area, but this is different from masturbation.

By age 5 or 6, most children have learned that genital touching is not to be done in public places, and they masturbate only in private. Masturbation becomes increasingly common in puberty in response to the surges in hormones and sexual drive that occur at that time.

How should a parent deal with masturbation in their young children? Here are some suggestions:

1. Once your child has discovered and enjoys masturbation, it is not realistic to eliminate it entirely. A reasonable goal is to control where it occurs. Perhaps limit it to the bathroom or bedroom. Tell your child that it is something that should be done only in private. Don't ignore it completely; if you do, your child may think it's acceptable anytime and anyplace, which may result in criticism by adults and chiding by other children.
2. Ignore masturbation at naptime and bedtime. Keep in mind that this is often a self-comforting activity.
3. When masturbation occurs outside of the child's bedroom, try distracting the child with a different activity. If this fails, remind the child that you know it feels good, but it is not allowed in front of other people.
4. Discuss your views on the behavior with others who may care for the child so that everyone is on the same page. Consistency among caregivers is key to success for all child behavior management.
5. Call the child's physician if you suspect that the masturbatory behavior may have been learned from someone else, if your child tries to masturbate others, or if your child continues to masturbate in front of others.

Masturbation does not cause physical injury to the body, promiscuity, or sexual deviance later in life. Masturbation in children is normal. Masturbation is not a problem or considered excessive unless it is deliberately done in public places after the age of 5 or 6. Masturbation generally leads to negative emotional consequences only if adults overreact to it and make it seem dirty or forbidden.

Source: Adapted from Steele (2005).

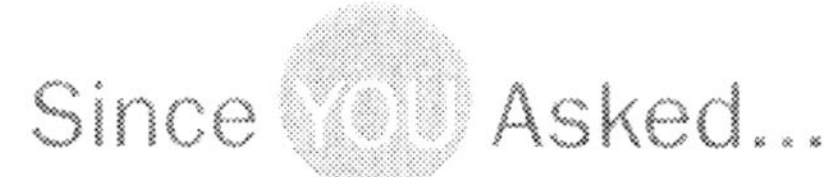

2. I recently caught my 4-year-old daughter playing "doctor" with the neighbor boy (both naked). Is this a sign of a problem, or should I not be concerned?

Childhood Sex Play

Although it is very common, masturbation is only one of many sexual behaviors normally seen in children. Not only are children curious about their own bodies, but beginning at about 3 years of age, they begin to become very interested in other people's bodies, especially those of the opposite sex, an interest that is evident until about age 7. This curiosity probably stems from children's developing cognitive awareness of their own gender and the realization that boys and girls are of different genders. They learn quickly that the most obvious difference between boys and girls are their genitals. Their natural curiosity leads them to want to see other children naked and engage in sexual games such as playing "doctor." Children also typically display a keen interest in adults' sexual bodies and will often make efforts to see their parents and other adults naked.

As with masturbation, when parents, teachers, or other caregivers discover that children are engaging in mutual sex play, they often become upset, worried, or angry. Their concerns typically revolve around the effect such play will have on the children's emotional, psychological, and sexual development later in life. However, no evidence exists that early peer-to-peer sex play of any type has negative consequences for later sexual adjustment (Okami, Olmstead, & Abramson, 1997).

What should parents and caregivers do if they discover that their child is engaging in sex play with other children? Most childhood development experts recommend approaching the situation gently, avoiding any extreme emotional responses. For example, one leading researcher on effective parenting suggests the following steps for parents in dealing with uncomfortable sexual events involving their children (Pantly, 1999, pp. 239–240):

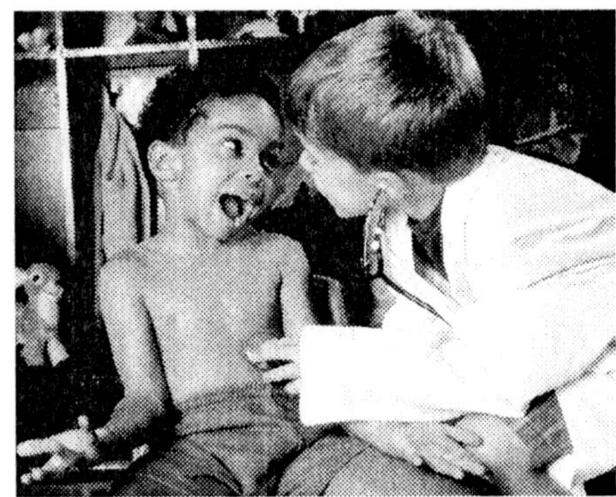

A curiosity about other children's sexual bodies is a normal part of early childhood development.

1. **Think about it.** If you found the kids eating candy before dinner or playing with a baseball in the house, you'd handle the situation easily. If, however, they were eating candy or playing ball *with their clothes off*, you'd suddenly feel confused and concerned. That's because you're viewing the situation from an adult point of view. Usually, childhood nudity and mutual curiosity are normal and natural. You just need to teach kids what's appropriate and what's not.
2. **Stay calm.** If you actually walk into a room and catch children playing with their clothes off, it's best to remain calm. Make a statement such as "It is not appropriate to play with your clothes off." Help them get dressed and find a different fun activity. Later, at a quiet time, have a brief conversation with your child about what is and is not appropriate. Teach that private areas (bathing suit areas) must always be kept covered. If you discover the same two children playing naked more than once, don't let them play together unsupervised. (Don't make a major announcement, just monitor their time together.)
3. **Pay attention.** Take the situation as a cue that your child is ready for more sex education. Spend a brief amount of time answering any of your child's questions. Let your child's interest and questions lead the discussion, and don't overwhelm your child with too much information. Give straightforward answers in accurate but simple terms. Address the issue of appropriate versus inappropriate touching so that your child will learn how to be respectful of his or her own privacy and that of others.
4. **Read about it.** Purchase a book about sexuality and development. Read it yourself first, because there's lots of stuff you may have forgotten and some things you may not even know! Share it with your child at an appropriate time. Let your child know that you're available to answer any questions.
5. **Take note.** Excessive interest in sexual topics or repeated occurrences of sexual play may be a warning sign of other problems. There may also be cause for concern if one of the children is several years older than the other. Discuss your concerns with a pediatrician, school counselor, or family therapist.

Although some exceptions exist (which we will discuss next), the vast majority of the sexual activities of children are an integral part of normal, healthy early development and should not be cause for concern. Moreover, many of these sexual behaviors decline or change on their own as children discover society's expectations of activities that are public versus private. Table 12.1 indicates the frequency with which children of varying ages engage in common sexual behaviors within view of their parents.

Now that we have discussed how most childhood sexual behaviors are part of normal and healthy child development, it is important to touch on behaviors that may not be normal or may signal unhealthy situations in a child's life. Again, these are exceptions, but an awareness of them on the part of all adults, whether parents or not, is important for protecting and helping children who may be experiencing difficulties.

When Childhood Sexual Behavior Is *Not* "Normal"

As parents and other caregivers become more relaxed and comfortable with healthy childhood sexuality, they must also be alert to certain forms of sexual acting out that may be a red flag that a problem exists relating to sexual abuse (see Chapter 13, "Sexual Aggression and Violence," for more on this issue). But how are caregivers to know the difference? Unfortunately, the answer to that question is not as clear as we might wish. The best way parents and other adults in children's lives can care for and protect them

Table 12.1 FREQUENCY OF CHILDREN'S OBSERVABLE (PUBLIC) SEXUAL BEHAVIORS

The percentages in the table represent a sample of observations made by over 800 mothers of children between 2 and 12 years of age using a survey device called the Child Sexual Behavior Inventory. All of the children were screened to ensure the absence of any sexual abuse. Keep in mind that these are parental observations, so private behaviors are not reflected in the data. You can see that children learn as they grow which behaviors are socially acceptable and which should be private.

	BOYS EXHIBITING BEHAVIOR (%)			GIRLS EXHIBITING BEHAVIOR (%)		
BEHAVIOR	2–5 YEARS	6–9 YEARS	10–12 YEARS	2–5 YEARS	6–9 YEARS	10–12 YEARS
Touches own breasts	42.4	14.3	1.2	43.7	15.9	1.1
Touches genitals at home	60.2	39.8	8.7	43.8	20.7	11.6
Touches genitals in public	26.5	13.8	1.2	15.1	6.5	2.2
Attempts to see others undressed	26.8	20.2	6.3	26.9	20.5	5.3
Masturbates with hand	16.7	12.8	3.7	15.8	5.3	7.4
Shows genitals to adults	15.4	6.4	2.5	13.8	5.4	2.2
Shows genitals to children	9.3	4.8	0.0	6.4	2.4	1.1
Exhibits great interest in opposite sex	17.5	13.8	24.1	15.2	13.9	28.7
Touches other children's genitals	4.6	8.0	1.2	8.8	1.2	1.1
Masturbates with toy or object	3.5	2.7	1.2	6.0	2.9	4.3
Attempts to look at pictures of nude people	5.4	10.1	11.4	3.9	10.2	3.2
Touches adults' breasts or genitals	7.8	1.6	0.0	4.2	1.2	0.0
Tries to have intercourse	0.4	0.0	0.0	1.1	0.0	0.0

Source: Adapted from table #3 & #4 from "Normative Sexual Behavior in Children: A Contemporary Sample" by W. N. Friedrich, et al., in *Pediatrics*, April 1998, Vol. 101, No. 9.

is to become as educated as possible about sexual development and as skilled as they can in communicating with children. These two abilities combine to allow us to observe children intelligently and analytically for signs of problems and to talk and listen to them when they attempt to communicate with us in their own childlike ways.

Usually, normal childhood sexual behaviors and problematic sexual behaviors can be distinguished by the pervasiveness and intensity of the activities and by linking them to other troubling aspects of the child's behavior. For example, an excessive preoccupation with genital self-stimulation or the touching of other children, doing so in public, or refusing to stop or alter the behavior when told to do so may indicate that a child is feeling emotionally deprived or is imitating behaviors others may have inflicted on him or her. "Normalcy" boils down to a matter of degree and the context of the behavior. Also, certain sexual behaviors that signal a child knows "too much" about sexual acts should receive extra attention and concern. These include acts of oral sex, imitations of adult sexual acts, engaging in sexual contact with animals, sexual behaviors aimed at adults that cause discomfort for the adult involved, and sexual actions that produce fear, anxiety, or shame on the part of the child (T. C. Johnson, 2001).

Since YOU Asked...

3. If a child between the ages of 5 and 7 acts out sexual acts, specifically lying down on top of another child and imitating movements of intercourse, does this indicate a problem, or is it part of normal childhood curiosity?

Another way to distinguish between healthy sexuality in children and sexual acting out that may be a sign of a problem is to consider the sexual behavior in the larger context of other problems the child may be manifesting. For example, when a young child appears to be engaging in troubling sexual behaviors, caregivers should think about how the child seems to be adjusting in other areas of his or her life. Consider whether the child is showing an unusual interest (or avoidance) of all things of a sexual nature; experiencing uncharacteristic sleep problems; withdrawing from friends or family; resisting to going to school; portraying sexual molestation themes in drawings, games, or fantasies; engaging in excessive masturbation or unusual levels of aggression; displaying overly adultlike sexual behaviors or vocabulary; or expressing suicidal thoughts, ideas, statements, or behaviors (Putnam, 2003; Sexual Abuse, 2002).

Sexual behaviors themselves form only one component of many factors that may combine to indicate a problem. The point here is that parents and caregivers need to make an effort to know the child and to view his or her sexual behaviors in the larger context of overall adjustment to better gauge if they might be a sign of a problem. However, the bottom line is that if an emotional problem or sexual abuse is suspected, professional help should be sought to either uncover and resolve the problem or to ensure that the child is safe and healthy.

How Children Learn about Sex

Virtually everyone, including most older children, agrees that parents should be the main source of sexual information for their children. However, this attitude assumes that parents are both willing and able to provide adequate, accurate, and timely information so that children will have the tools they need, when they need them, to deal with a complex sexual world. In some cases, parents take on this role responsibly and conscientiously. However, a great deal of evidence suggests that overall, parents are relinquishing the duty to various other sources, including schools, the media, and peers.

Parents' avoidance of responsibility for sex education may be contributing to an overall increase in young people's beliefs in sexual myths, poor sexual decision making, and reduced sexual knowledge among children and teens. Only half of all teenagers report having had a meaningful talk about sex with their parents during the preceding year, and whereas most parents (72 percent) claim to have had a "good talk" with their teens about sex, only 45 percent of those teens felt that such a talk had occurred (M. Edwards, 2003). It appears parents may *think* they are providing the information their children need, but the children disagree.

In a study done in the early 2000s, researchers asked boys and girls between the ages of 14 and 18 where they received their information about sex (Somers & Gleason, 2001). The participants were asked where they had received information about various sexual topics ranging from sexual anatomy (the reproductive system) to masturbation to sexually transmitted diseases. Their information sources were school, peers, media, parents, and professionals (doctors, nurses, counselors, etc.), in that order. For virtually every topic, school was the most common source of their current knowledge (see Table 12.2).

This is not to say that parents do not recognize the importance of talking to their children about sex. One national survey found the vast majority of parents (82 to 96 percent) agreed that it is very important for parents to talk with their children about such issues as reproduction, becoming sexually active, pregnancy and STI prevention, and saying no to sex. And the same percentage say they feel comfortable talking to their kids about sex. However, the survey found that only about half of the parents had actually had such discussions with their children by age 10, and only 60 to 70 percent had done so by age 12 (Lake Snell Perry & Associates, 2002). Why the gap between what parents feel they *should* do and what they actually do? Part of the reason may lie in the fact that many parents feel unsure that they possess adequate and correct knowledge to provide their children with the information they need. This is especially true for parents of younger children. Therefore, as noted in Chapter 1 of this text, if parents (and prospective parents, such as most of you) first work to educate themselves as thoroughly as possible about all aspects of

Since YOU Asked ...

4. What prevents parents from talking to their kids about sex? My parents never had "the talk" with me, and I had to find out from friends, or even worse, boyfriends. Now, two abortions later, I'm finally taking this class.

Table 12.2 TEENS' SOURCES OF SEX INFORMATION

This table lists the percentage of 157 teenage boys and girls who reported receiving information from various sources on each of the sexual topics listed.

SEXUAL TOPIC	SOURCES OF INFORMATION FOR TEENAGE BOYS AND GIRLS				
	SCHOOL (%)	PEERS (%)	MEDIA (%)	PARENTS (%)	PROFESSIONALS (I.E., DOCTORS, NURSES, ETC.) (%)
Reproductive system	89	26	33	43	2
Father's part in conception	78	25	25	34	1
Menstruation	82	32	22	43	1
Nocturnal emissions	71	30	17	14	2
Masturbation	48	37	22	10	<1
Dating	57	48	26	44	<1
"Petting"	39	49	15	11	0
Sexual intercourse	82	46	35	34	<1
Birth control	66	30	29	29	1
Birth control use	27	15	8	16	1
Pregnancy risks	82	26	35	36	3
STIs	89	22	40	30	3
Love and/or marriage	48	29	33	43	2
Morality of premarital sex	42	27	19	32	3

Source: Adapted from table, "Children's Sources of Sex Information" from "Does Source of Sex Information Predict Adolescents' Sexual Knowledge, Attitudes, & Behaviors?" by C. L. Somers and J. H. Gleason, *Education*, 121, (2001), pp. 674–681. Copyright © 2001. Reprinted by permission of Project Innovation, Mobile, AL and C. L. Somers.

sexuality, they will be prepared to discuss sex with their children at all stages of development. "In Touch with Your [Children's] Sexual Health: Guidelines for Talking to Children about Sex" offers guidelines for parents and caregivers for communicating effectively with children about sex.

Sexuality in Adolescence

As childhood draws to a close, an entirely new world (or perhaps it is better described as a "new planet") appears in sexual development: the world of adolescence. This begins as the many physical and hormonal changes of puberty combine with the psychological, emotional, social, and cultural changes and expectations that accompany the magical, stormy, and sometimes turbulent transition from child to adult. **Adolescence**, usually defined as the period of life between 12 and 19 years old, is an identity-seeking time of life. It is a time of psychological, emotional, and sexual changes as teens awaken sexually and experience the beginnings of romantic ideals and fantasies of love. If anything is more difficult than the changes of adolescence itself, it is the culture's response to them. Studies have shown that Western cultures, and especially U.S. society, appear bewildered about how to nurture and support teens as they attempt to maneuver through those difficult years. Nevertheless, on their way through adolescence, teenagers must try to avoid many common sexual pitfalls, such as accidental pregnancy and sexually transmitted infections, to name just two of the most common and most serious.

adolescence The period of life between the ages of approximately 12 and 19 years, often a tumultuous, self-identity-seeking stage of life.

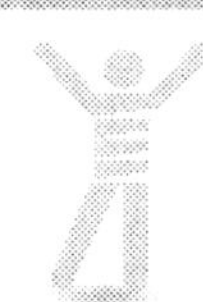

In Touch with Your [Children's] Sexual Health

Guidelines for Talking to Children about Sex

The Sexuality Information and Education Council of the United States (SIECUS) offers the following guidelines to help parents and caregivers communicate with their children effectively about sexuality.

1. *You are the primary sexuality educator of your children.* They want to talk with you about sexuality and to hear your values.
2. *Find "teachable moments."* Make use of TV shows even if you believe they send the wrong message. Say, "I think that program sent the wrong message. Let me tell you what I believe."
3. *Remember that it is okay to feel uncomfortable.* It is often hard to talk about sexual matters. Relax and tell your children you are going to talk to them because you love them and want to help them.
4. *Don't wait until your children ask questions.* Many never ask. You need to decide what is important for them to know and then tell them before a crisis occurs.
5. *Be "ask-able."* Reward a question with "I'm glad you came to me." It will teach your children to come to you when they have other questions.
6. *Become aware of the "question behind the question."* The unspoken question, "Am I normal?" is often hiding behind questions about sexual development, sexual thoughts, and sexual feelings. Reassure your children as often as possible.
7. *Listen, listen, listen.* Ask them why they want to know and what they already know. That may help you prepare your answer.
8. *Remember that facts are not enough.* Share your feelings, values, and beliefs. Tell your children why you feel the way you do.
9. *Talk about the joys of sexuality.* Tell your children that loving relationships are the best part of life and that intimacy is a wonderful part of adult life.
10. *Remember that you are telling your children that you care about their happiness and well-being.* You are also sharing your values. This is one of the real joys of parenthood.
11. *Know what is taught about sexuality in your schools, faith communities, and youth groups.* Other groups can help. It is often helpful when professionals lead talks.

Source: M. Edwards (2000), p. 3.

Adolescents probably receive more confusing messages about sex than any other age group. Some of the confusion no doubt stems from two opposing approaches to a long-standing debate about what to "teach" teens about sex. On the one side are people who suggest that adolescents should be encouraged to practice abstinence (usually meaning they should not have sexual intercourse) and therefore should have little need for education about sexual behavior, contraception, or STIs. The effectiveness of this approach is not supported by research (Hubler, 2004; Sparks, 2005). On the other side of the debate are those who see better education about sexual behavior as the solution—who believe that the more teens know about all aspects of sex, the more informed and intelligent their choices will be. Research appears to support this approach (Schaalma et al., 2004). This sexual education controversy finds its way into all areas of adolescents' lives, from what they hear from their parents to what sexual education programs, if any, receive funding in their schools to what they see and hear in the media. In the meantime, biological and social pressures exert powerful influences as many teenagers are left to figure it all out for themselves.

Summarizing the complexities of adolescent sexuality in one brief section is a challenge. We will touch on some of the more important issues of this developmental stage as we review the physical changes of puberty, the surge of sexual interest in teens' lives, the many sexual firsts that occur during this time, the use (or nonuse) of contraception, unwanted pregnancy, and teens' risks for STIs.

Since YOU Asked...

5. I started puberty very late (around age 15). All my friends were already getting their periods and breasts and everything. It was very embarrassing. Why do some people start puberty so late?

Physical Changes of Puberty

You are already personally familiar with the physical changes that occur during puberty; you have experienced or are experiencing them. Outward signs of puberty normally unfold between the ages of 11 and 16 for boys and 8 and 16 for girls. However, the exact age when puberty normally begins varies greatly and can be anytime within these ranges. Rarely, puberty may begin earlier (*precocious puberty*) or later (*delayed puberty*), but these are exceptions and may indicate a medical condition requiring treatment. The onset of puberty is stimulated when the **pituitary gland** in the brain releases a hormone called **gonadotropin**, which in turn signals the testicles to release testosterone and the ovaries to release estrogen. Although these are the primary hormones influencing sexual development in boys and girls, small amounts of female hormones are present in boys and small amounts of male hormones are secreted in girls. The secretion of testosterone and estrogen causes the internal and external physical changes associated with puberty (Cool Nurse, 2004; Figgs et al., 2001).

Internal biological changes in both sexes begin slightly before any of the familiar external, more obvious signs of puberty appear. In boys, as the testicles mature, they begin to manufacture and release testosterone. The testicles enlarge during puberty, and internal structures, such as the prostate gland and seminal vesicles, mature. The combination of these changes prepares the boy's body to manufacture sperm cells, produce semen, and ejaculate. In other words, during puberty, boys become fertile and able to create a pregnancy through unprotected intercourse. However, it is common for a boy's early ejaculations, whether through masturbation or wet dreams (which typically begin at this time), to contain few sperm cells. However, this is no guarantee that he is not fertile during this time.

Internally, a girl's ovaries mature during puberty, and increases in estrogen secretion cause the building up of the uterine lining, leading to **menarche**, her first menstrual period. The age of menarche varies considerably among girls and may occur normally any time between 8 and 16 years of age; the average age is about 13 years (Chumlea et al., 2003). Within a year after a girl's first period, hormonal changes also cause the ovaries to begin to release mature eggs, or ova. At first, the release of an ovum and the accompanying menstrual period may be very irregular both in frequency and amount of fluid. For example, a girl may have her first period and then no period for two or three months, then another period and skip a month, and so on for the first year or so. Soon, however, barring illness or unhealthful levels of dieting or exercise, her periods will begin to follow a regular monthly cycle. Prior to her first period and in between periods, a clear or whitish discharge may be noticeable from the vagina. This is normal. Usually, a girl is considered to be fertile and able to become pregnant with the occurrence of her first menstrual period. You can find a more thorough discussion of menstruation in Chapter 2.

Boys and girls who begin puberty very early or very late sometimes experience social or emotional difficulties due to the obvious body differences that exist, temporarily, between them and their peers. However, barring any physiological abnormalities, nearly all boys and girls will complete the physical changes of puberty by their seventeenth birthday. External physical changes, referred to as the development of **secondary sexual characteristics**, vary in timing and in sequence among boys and girls. Many teens who are entering, are in the midst of, or have recently completed this transition wonder what is considered "normal" development during puberty. To help answer this question, "In Touch with Your Sexual Health: The Physical Changes of Puberty" outlines the physical process of the observable bodily changes associated with puberty.

pituitary gland A gland in the brain that at the onset of puberty releases hormones necessary for the physical changes of puberty.

gonadotropin A hormone released by the pituitary gland that signals the testes to release testosterone and the ovaries to release estrogen.

menarche The onset of menstruation; a girl's first period.

secondary sexual characteristics Physical changes not biologically related to reproduction that occur during puberty.

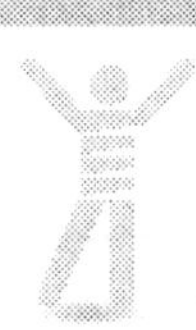

In Touch with Your Sexual Health

The Physical Changes of Puberty

PUBERTY IN GIRLS

Average Age*	Physical Features	Description of Changes
8–10	Growth, breasts, pubic hair	Height spurt begins. Breasts are *prepubertal*; no glandular tissue. Usually no pubic hair.
11–12	Breasts	The *areola* (pigmented area around the nipple) enlarges and becomes darker. It raises to become a mound with a small amount of breast tissue underneath. This is called a *bud*. Girls vary a great deal in the size, shape, and coloring of breast buds.
11–13	Pubic hair, growth	Maximum growth rate is reached. Body fat continues to increase normally.
11–13	Growth	*Peak height velocity* (maximum growth rate) is reached. Body fat continues to increase normally.
12–14	Breasts	Breast tissue grows to varying degrees past the edge of the areola.
12–14	Pubic hair	Hair is close to adult pubic hair in curliness and coarseness. Area of pubis covered is smaller than in adults, and there are no hairs on the middle surfaces of the thighs. Menarche occurs in 50 percent of girls.
13–14	Breasts	Continued development of breast tissue; areola and nipple protrude to varying degrees.
13–14	Growth	End of growth spurt. Normal body fat reaches adult proportions. After menstruation begins, girls gain at most 3 to 4 more inches in height, usually less.
14–15	Pubic hair, body fat	Adult levels. It is normal for some long pigmented hairs to grow on the inner thighs. Natural body fat stabilizes.
15–16	Breasts	Usually a girl's breasts have reached their adult size by age 16.

PUBERTY IN BOYS

Average Age*	Physical Features	Description of Changes
11–14	Growth of body hair and pubic hair	Hair begins to grow on various parts of the body. (Hair can continue to spread to other parts of the body until about age 20.) Sparse growth of slightly pigmented pubic hair at base of penis around age 12.4 years. Adult-type hair spreads to the inside of thighs but not up the abdomen yet (15.3 years). Hair begins to grow on the face, underarm area, pubic area, abdomen, chest, arms, legs, and buttocks. The amount and distribution of hair can vary considerably and may be genetic.
11–15	Voice changes	As a result of increased testosterone, vocal cords become longer and thicker, and the voice deepens. While these changes are occurring, it is not unusual for the voice to change pitch abruptly or "crack" at times. Voice change begins around 13.5 years, completed in about a year.
12–16	External genital development	Growth of penis and scrotum often starts about age 13 and continues until adult size is reached two to three years later. Thinning and reddening of scrotum begins around age 12 years.
11–20	Oil glands	Oil glands in the skin become more active. This can cause acne. Many people will have problems with acne into adulthood.
10–17	Growth, muscularity	The growth spurt in boys usually occurs about two years later than in girls. About age 12.5 years, the boy's body takes on a more muscular and angular shape when testosterone causes muscle mass to increase. The greatest effect can usually be seen in the upper chest and shoulder muscles. Testosterone also causes bones to lengthen, giving young men a heavier bone structure and longer arms and legs.
12–18	Penile erections	Males have spontaneous erections throughout their lives (even as infants). During puberty, boys tend to get erections more frequently. Erection can occur with or without any physical or sexual stimulation. Though sometimes embarrassing, it is a normal, spontaneous event.

* Average ages can vary widely; one or two years earlier or later than most of these listed ages is usually considered within the normal range.

Source: Adapted from Coleman and Coleman (2002); *Puberty*, (2004).

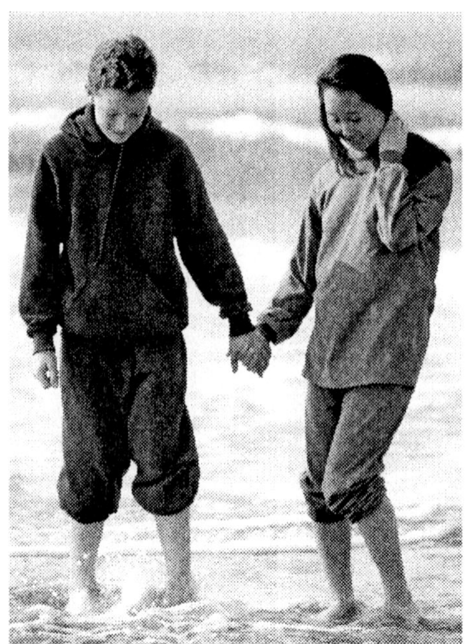

Romantic partners become the most important relationships in adolescents' lives.

Romantic Relationships in Adolescence

The biological changes of puberty lead to a flood of new emotions and attitudes. Typically, the most noticeable and powerful of these is the newly discovered interest in romantic relationships and sex. Most boys and girls begin to show an intense emotional and sexual interest in others as they enter and proceed through puberty and adolescence. This change is often quite surprising because it appears on the heels of a period of development in which not only is sexual interest at a lifetime low, but such matters are typically met with opinions such as "eew!" and "gross!" As puberty and adolescence occur, however, nature and nurture team up to facilitate adolescents' romantic and sexual feelings. The nature side relates to the hormonal and other biological changes just discussed. In addition to producing the physical developments of puberty, hormones also appear to affect cognitive factors that create sexual feelings and sexual attractions to others.

However, biology is only part of the story. The social and cultural effects on adolescents—the nurture side—must not be underestimated. Adolescence is perceived by most societies throughout the world, and by adolescents themselves, as one of the most important stages of life: the passage from childhood to adulthood. Adolescence is a time of individuation, when young people are moving out of the orbit around their parents and becoming individuals in their own right, with their own personal beliefs, values, goals, and responsibilities. It is during the teen years when a sense of self develops, when people attempt to discover their identities and roles in life, when they begin to answer the question "Who am I?"

Adolescence is also the stage in life when most people become sexually active. Part of the larger questions of overall personal identity is the more specific question of "Who am I as a sexual person in relationships with others?" Most of the research on adolescent sexuality has focused on heterosexual intercourse and its accompanying consequences of accidental teen pregnancy and sexually transmitted infections. We will discuss these important issues shortly. However, teenagers are not, as many people believe, preoccupied by sex exclusively. Researchers are only now discovering what adolescents have known all along: teen *romantic* relationships are not trivial instances of "puppy love" but constitute a very important and meaningful part of their lives.

The potentially negative consequences of teen sexual activity do not exist independent of the interpersonal relationships in which the sexual behavior occurs. Dating and romantic relationships may be the most important interpersonal connections in the social lives of heterosexual adolescents, but until recently, this side of teenagers' sexual development has been virtually ignored (Furman, 2002). Over half of all adolescents report having been involved in a romantic relationship during the previous 18 months, and by age 16, teens are socializing more frequently with romantic partners than with parents, siblings, or nonromantic friends (Furman, 2002). By the end of high school, boys spend an average of five hours a week with girls, and girls spend ten hours a week with boys (Richards et al., 1998). These romantic relationships appear to be based on more emotional involvement than mere sexual interest and are often characterized by caring, friendship, and companionship.

Understanding the romantic aspect of heterosexual teenage relationships is vitally important because it is within these relationships that most adolescent sexual activity occurs. In fact, the most accurate predictor of first sexual intercourse is involvement in a romantic relationship during the previous 18 months (Furman, 2002). A national survey conducted in the mid-1990s found that for 35 percent of males and 86 percent of females, the primary reason for having intercourse for the first time was feelings of affection for their partner (Michael et al., 1994). When we talk about teen sexual behavior, we must also acknowledge the context of the romantic relationship in which the sexual activity is most likely to begin.

Relationships and sexual behavior among gay, lesbian, and bisexual teens have received even less attention. However, one of the leading researchers in the field of adolescent romantic relationships suggests that nonheterosexual teens may follow a somewhat different path during early adolescence:

> Most have same-sex sexual experiences, but relatively few have same-sex romantic relationships because of both the limited opportunities to do so and the social disapproval such relationships may generate from families or heterosexual peers. Many sexual minority youths date other-sex peers; such experiences can help them clarify their sexual orientation or disguise it from others. (Furman, 2002, p. 178)

However, as nonheterosexual adolescents continue through their teens and into their early 20s, they usually become more comfortable with their sexual orientation and more ready to establish meaningful same-sex relationships.

That teens tend to form romantic relationships may come as a positive and hopeful sign that sexual behavior is more than a result of purely hormone-driven physical desires. Romantic experiences appear to facilitate adolescents' personal identity development and their understanding of intimacy. However, these same relationships also form the backdrop for early sexual activities, unwanted pregnancy, and the spread of STIs. We will discuss each of these next. Another unfortunate and sad consequence of some adolescent dating relationships is abuse and violence. Abusive and violent relationships in adolescence mirror those of adults (as we discuss in Chapter 13, "Sexual Aggression and Violence"), but can sometimes be even more devastating because teens are new to intimacy and often very emotionally fragile. "In Touch with Your Sexual Health: Teen Dating and Violence" explores this important problem in detail.

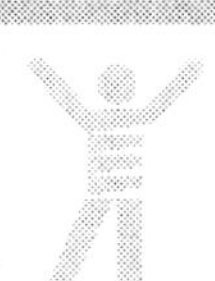

In Touch with Your Sexual Health

Teen Dating and Violence

The following information about teen dating violence is based on a true story.

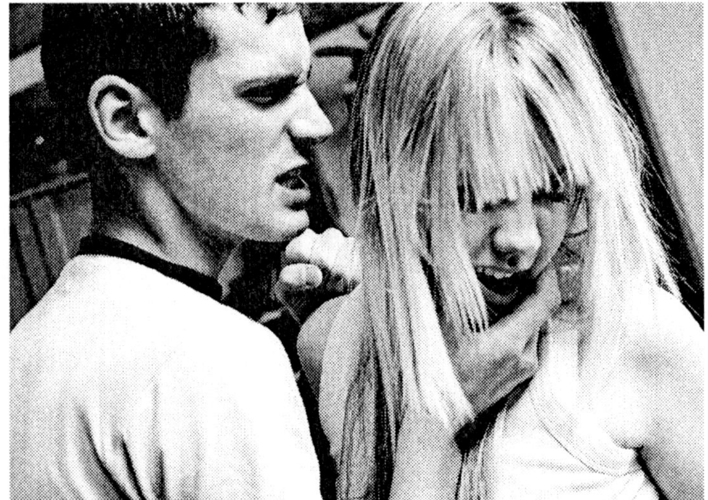

> Brenda is 15 and has never had a boyfriend before. She recently started dating Frank. She thinks he is so cute. Her friends all tell her how lucky she is because she has a boyfriend. At first, Brenda thought it was sweet that Frank began calling her all the time. He always wants to know whom she is with, where she is, and when she'll be home. He has told her that she was meant to be with him and him only, forever.
>
> Recently, Frank has started belittling her in front of his friends, insulting her, and telling her she is fat. He doesn't want her to spend time with certain of her friends—he thinks they are a bad influence. He threatens to break up with her if she won't do what he says and warns that no one else will ever want her. Brenda wants to make Frank happy. In fact, she'll do anything to keep her boyfriend. She thinks this is what being in a relationship is all about.

Unfortunately, many teens have faced or are dealing with situations similar to this. Relationship violence often starts as emotional or verbal abuse but can quickly escalate into physical or sexual violence. The following can help you better recognize if you or someone you know may be involved in a violent relationship.

Continued . . .

Relationship abuse and violence are not about having a disagreement or getting angry over something. What *is* relationship violence?

- A *pattern* of behavior used by someone to maintain control over his or her partner.
- Verbal, physical, emotional, or even sexual abuse.
- One partner being afraid of and intimidated by the other.

How often does it happen?

- Relationship violence is the number one cause of injury to women between the ages of 15 and 44.
- Seventy percent of severe injuries and deaths occur when the victim is trying to leave or has already left the abusive relationship.
- Thirty-eight percent of date rape victims are young women between the ages of 14 and 17.
- Seventy percent of pregnant teenagers are abused by their partners.

Who is involved?

- Relationship violence occurs between two people who are currently or formerly involved in a dating relationship.
- The abuse can begin at a very young age, as young as 11 or 12 years old.
- Friends of the couple are usually aware of the abuse but are unsure how to stop it.

Where can it happen?

- Relationship violence can occur at school—in the hall, in the classroom, in the parking lot, on the bus, at after-school activities, at a student's workplace, at a school dance, or at a student's home.
- In teenage dating relationships, the abuse is often public with peers witnessing the abuse; however, the abuse can also occur in private.

What are signs of an abusive teen dating relationship?

- Is one partner afraid of the other or scared to break up?
- Does one partner call the other names, make the other feel stupid, or tell the other that he or she cannot do anything right?
- Is one partner excessively jealous?
- Does one partner tell the other where he or she can and cannot go or whom he or she can and cannot be with or talk to?
- Does one partner tell the other that no one else would ever go out with him or her?
- Is one partner being cut off from friends and family by the other partner?
- Does one partner feel that saying no to sexual activities will result in trouble or danger?
- Does one partner feel pushed or forced into sexual activity?
- Does one partner say that the other *caused* the abuse?
- Does one partner shove, grab, hit, pinch, hold down, or kick the other?
- Is one partner *really* nice sometimes and *really* mean at other times (almost like two different people or personalities)?
- Does one partner make frequent promises to change or say that he or she will never hurt the other again? Does one partner say that the other is "making too big a deal" out of the abuse?

Answering yes to ***any*** *of the above questions probably indicates an abusive relationship.*

What can you do to help someone you think may be in an abusive relationship?

- Remember, anyone can be a victim.
- If you or someone you know might be affected by relationship violence, look for resources that can provide help. School counselors, parents, teachers, women's shelters, and clergy are all potential sources of assistance.
- Tell someone you trust and who you feel can intervene, such as a local domestic violence agency. Try to get help as soon as possible before the violence increases.
- By reaching out, you may literally save your or someone else's life.

Source: Adapted from Washington State Medical Association (2003), "Teen Dating Violence" (2004)

The Beginnings of Sexual Activity

The vast majority of teens become sexually active prior to graduating from high school. The average age of first intercourse in the United States, for both boys and girls, is approximately 16 years old. About 35 percent will experience their first heterosexual intercourse in grade 9, and slightly over 60 percent will have had intercourse by grade 12. The overall percentages of high school students who have engaged in intercourse tend to run somewhat higher for African Americans than for Caucasians and Hispanics. Table 12.3 summarizes some recent statistics on adolescent intercourse (Grunbaum et al., 2002). It should be noted that these statistics are based on what teens report about their sexual activities, so the possibility of under- or overreporting must be taken into account when evaluating these findings.

Table 12.3 PERCENTAGE OF HIGH SCHOOL STUDENTS REPORTING THAT THEY HAVE HAD SEXUAL INTERCOURSE

GRADE	FEMALE	MALE	TOTAL
9	29.1	40.5	34.4
10	39.3	42.2	40.8
11	49.7	54.0	51.9
12	60.1	61.0	60.5
Total	42.9	48.5	45.6

Source: Grunbaum et al. (2002), p. 60.

As mentioned earlier, the research literature about adolescent sexual behavior has been preoccupied with heterosexual intercourse. That this has been the focus is understandable in that coitus is the behavior primarily responsible for accidental pregnancy and the transmission of many sexual infections. Moreover, most people, and this is especially true for teens, equate the word *sex* with intercourse. However, as has been pointed out frequently throughout this book, intercourse is only one form of sexual behavior. A significantly larger proportion of adolescents engage in various sexual activities other than intercourse either in addition to or instead of penis-vagina sex. For example, a study of one Los Angeles County high school found that just over 50 percent of males and 45 percent of females had engaged in sexual intercourse, but many other sexual behaviors were also reported: 64 percent of males and 55 percent of females had experienced mutual masturbation, 45 percent of males and 30 percent of females had engaged in fellatio with ejaculation; 41 percent of males and 38 percent of females had experienced cunnilingus (more on oral sex in a moment), and 18 percent of males and 6 percent of females had engaged in anal intercourse (Schuster et al., 1998). Furthermore, the study reported that of males between the ages of 15 and 19 who reported experience with vaginal intercourse, 78 percent also reported having been masturbated by a female partner, the same percentage had received oral sex from a female partner, and 61 percent had performed cunnilingus.

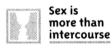

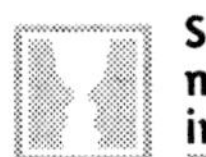
Sex is more than intercourse

Perhaps even more meaningful was a finding that among males who had never had intercourse, 22 percent had been masturbated by a female partner, 15 percent had received fellatio, and 12 percent had performed cunnilingus (Gates & Sonenstein, 2000). We will discuss the significance of this in the next section on teen oral sex. These findings are summarized in Table 12.4.

Teen Oral Sex

During the late 1990s and early 2000s, researchers began reporting a new and alarming trend in the sexual behavior of adolescents: a significant increase in oral sex (Halpern-Felsher et al., 2005). In addition to the statistics mentioned in the preceding section, another study found that over 50 percent of both boys and girls engaged in oral sex at least once prior to their first sexual intercourse and over 25 percent participated in oral sex on numerous occasions before ever having intercourse (Schwartz, 1999). A study done by *Seventeen* magazine, marketed to teenage girls, found that 55 percent of readers said they had engaged in oral sex (M. O'Brien, 2003). To many, these statistics alone are worrisome, but here's the alarming part: 40 percent of those same teens claim that oral sex "doesn't count" as sex. So if you say to adolescents, "Are you having sex?" they may answer no honestly,

Table 12.4 PERCENTAGE OF HETEROSEXUAL MALES AGED 15–19 WHO REPORTED HAVING EVER ENGAGED IN SEXUAL ACTIVITIES OTHER THAN INTERCOURSE

AGE	WERE MASTURBATED BY A FEMALE	RECEIVED ORAL SEX FROM A FEMALE	GAVE ORAL SEX TO A FEMALE	HAD ANAL INTERCOURSE WITH A FEMALE
AMONG THOSE WHO HAD ALSO ENGAGED IN INTERCOURSE				
15–16	70.4	67.3	48.2	19.4
17–19	80.8	81.5	65.9	18.1
Total	77.8	77.4	60.8	18.5
AMONG THOSE WHO HAD NEVER HAD INTERCOURSE				
15–16	19.0	12.1	9.6	0.4
17–19	25.6	20.1	14.8	1.7
Total	21.7	15.4	11.7	0.9

Source: Gates & Sonenstein (2000), Table 1.

even though oral sex may be a regular occurrence in their lives. (This may remind some of you of a past president of the United States who also did not equate oral sex with sex.) Furthermore, when parents and schools attempt to teach abstinence to teens as part of sex education, many teens take the message to heart and substitute oral sex for intercourse, thinking this constitutes abstinence as it has been explained to them.

Since YOU Asked . . .

6. In high school, a lot of my friends were having oral sex but not intercourse. Is it true that oral sex doesn't spread diseases?

This oral sex trend appears to be a direct response to an increased awareness among teens of the risks of STIs, especially HIV and AIDS, and unwanted teen pregnancy. Girls as young as 12 and 13 are performing oral sex on their boyfriends as a "substitute" for sexual intercourse, and they are not using condoms. Many girls feel pressured to be sexually active in order to be accepted and not rejected by boys. However, they feel too young and not yet ready for intercourse. They see oral sex as a way of remaining a virgin while satisfying the demands of boyfriends. More important, however, is that some teens equate oral sex with safe sex ("Oral Sex," 2001; Remez, 2000). Of course, oral sex itself carries no risk of pregnancy, but many teens believe they are safe from STI infection if they refrain from vaginal or anal intercourse and limit their insertive sexual activities to oral sex. As we discuss in detail in Chapter 8, "Sexually Transmitted Infections," this belief is seriously misguided. While HIV appears to have a low rate of transmission through oral-genital contact, other STIs transmit routinely through oral-genital contact, including gonorrhea, syphilis, chancroid, herpes, hepatitis B, and human papilloma virus (HPV, genital warts). Genital warts have been diagnosed in the mouth and throat, and many cases of oral herpes are actually the genital form of the virus.

Nearly half of all teens believe that oral sex doesn't count as real sex.

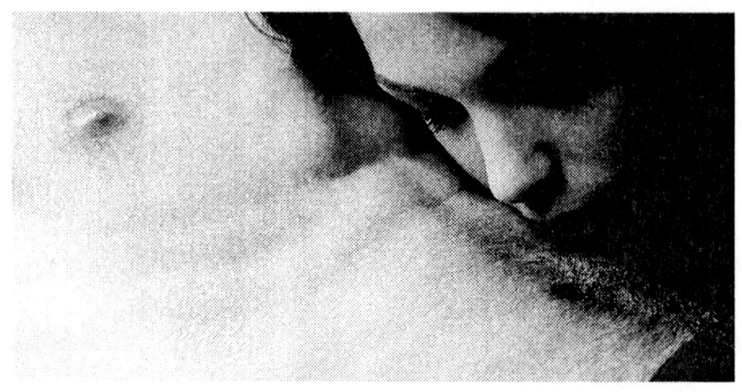

Public health officials are calling for renewed efforts to educate teens about the dangers of nonintercourse sexual activities, especially oral sex. These efforts appear necessary in the face of the widespread casual attitudes among adolescents about oral sex. For example, interviews with junior high and high school students in California produced the following comments (Goldston & Wong, 2003):

"It's a way to take the relationship to a different level without going all the way. It's a step in between" (boy).

"I could have done it. I'll probably do it before I go to high school. I know girls who will do it" (boy).

"In seventh grade we didn't even talk about oral sex, but I think things have evolved. . . . Kids are introduced to things at a younger age" (girl).

"I had oral sex when I was 15 with a male friend. It was wanting to fit in, so you make the choice" (girl).

"It's not like having sex. It's not as big a commitment" (boy).

"It's not like being all committed. It's just basically friends with benefits" (girl).

Oral sex is often a precursor to sexual intercourse, which carries with it the additional dangers of pregnancy and STIs. As one teenage girl said, "If you're having oral sex with someone, you will have sex with them. In two months or a few days, but you will" (Goldston & Wong, 2003).

Birth Control and Pregnancy in Adolescence

A long-standing problem in the United States and in many other parts of the world is teenage pregnancy. The rate of births among adolescents increased steadily through the 1980s, but the trend then reversed during the 1990s and early 2000s. Between 1991 and 2000, the overall teen birthrate in the United States decreased by 22 percent (Ventura, Matthews, & Hamilton, 2001). Figure 12.1 shows the trends in teen birthrates since 1980. The drop has been attributed to a combination of the development of more effective hormonal contraceptive methods, an increased use of condoms due to fears of STI transmission, and an increase in the number of teens postponing sexual intercourse or engaging in other sexual behaviors. The decline does *not* appear to be due to higher rates of abortion because abortion rates for teens also fell during the same years (Moore & Sugland, 1999).

The statistics suggest a positive social trend but do not in any way imply that the problem of unwanted pregnancy among teens is abating. On the contrary, even at current levels, hundreds of thousands of teenage girls become pregnant each year. And the majority of teen pregnancies and births do not lead to happy, healthy outcomes.

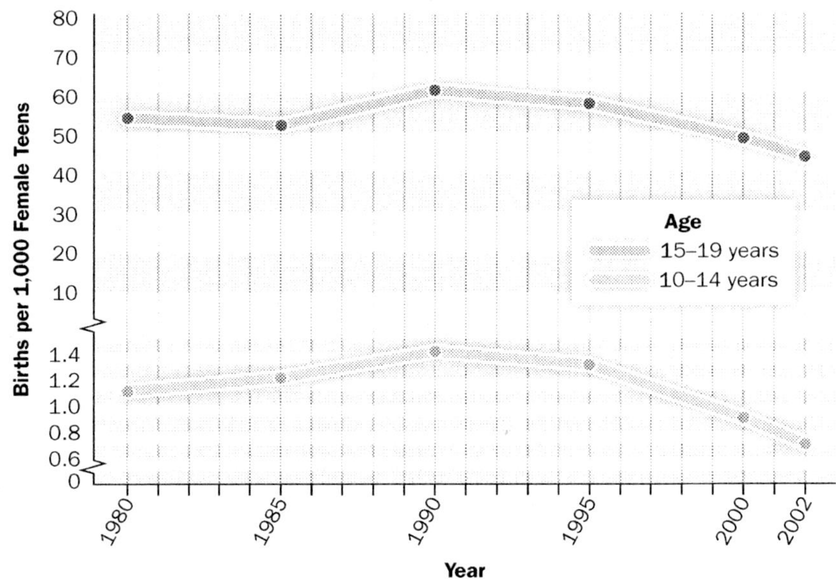

FIGURE 12.1 Teen Birthrates in the United States, 1980–2002

Since the 1990s, birthrates among teens have been on the decline, due in part to the greater use of condoms among teens.

Source: Martin et al. (2003), tab. 4.

Instead, they often end in abortion or lead to major life difficulties. For example, 30 percent of girls who become pregnant never finish high school; 81 percent of teens who give birth are unmarried; 56 percent of teen mothers must rely on public assistance; 60 percent of teens who give birth are living in poverty at the time; and 50 percent of teen pregnancies result in abortion (SIECUS, 2002).

The drop in teen pregnancies and births is partly attributable to a greater acceptance and use of condoms among teens. This increase in condom use is due to a combination of factors including, the greater availability of condoms to teens, the reduced stigma previously associated with buying and using them, and the desire to reduce the risk of contracting incurable STIs, such as HIV, herpes, HPV, and hepatitis B. Statistics show that the percentage of female high school students who used a condom during their most recent intercourse increased from 38 percent in 1991 to 51 percent in 2001. For males, the increase was from 55 percent in 1991 to 65 percent in 2001 ("Trends in Sexual Risk Behaviors," 2002).

Beyond condom use, various new developments in contraceptive technology have helped reduce the rate of adolescent pregnancy. For example, in addition to the hormonal birth control pill, which carries the risk of missed doses and inconsistent use, adolescents may now choose injectable forms of hormonal contraceptives that have a continuous effectiveness of 30 or 90 days. Hormonal implants, such as Norplant and Norplant-2, provide highly effective protection from pregnancy for three to five years. In addition, teens are taking increased advantage of **emergency contraception pills**, also known as the "morning-after pill." This method of preventing pregnancy, while not a substitute for before-intercourse birth control, is more than 80 percent effective in preventing a pregnancy if taken correctly within 72 hours of intercourse (Sadovsky, 2000a). All of these methods of birth control are discussed in detail in Chapter 5, "Contraception: Planning and Preventing Pregnancy."

The key to maintaining the strides made over the past decade in reducing unwanted pregnancy among adolescents is to ensure that teens receive the education necessary to employ birth control methods successfully. Although many people believe that teaching teens about sexuality and contraception leads young people toward sexual experimentation, the opposite has been shown to be the case. In reality, **comprehensive sex education** for adolescents leads to better decision making, delay of first sexual activity, more effective contraception use, and decreases in unhealthy and risky sexual behavior (Kirby, 2001). Moreover, **abstinence-only sex education** approaches have failed to show these positive effects and in some cases may increase teens' tendencies toward unhealthy sexual activities (Collins, Alagiri, & Summers, 2002).

emergency contraception pills Hormonal contraceptives that help prevent pregnancy after an unprotected act of intercourse; also known as the *morning-after pill*.

comprehensive sex education Sexual education programs for adolescents that provide information about abstinence and about preventing STIs and unwanted pregnancy.

abstinence-only sex education Sexual education based on the assumption that adolescents will not engage in sexual activities until after marriage; may have the paradoxical effect of increasing teens' tendencies toward engaging in unhealthy sexual activities.

Adolescents and STIs

The intersection of sexual activities and low condom use among adolescents leads directly to the problem of sexually transmitted infections among adolescents. Although condom use among teens has increased, the fact remains that almost half of adolescent males and more than a third of females did not use a condom during their most recent sexual intercourse ("Trends in Sexual Risk Behaviors," 2002). Furthermore, research indicates that about a third of all teens use no birth control at all the first time they have intercourse, and only 55 percent use condoms consistently. And as discussed earlier in this chapter, many teens are engaging in oral sex in the false belief that it is a low-risk behavior for contracting STIs. All of these factors contribute to the high rate of STIs in the adolescent community.

One study of adolescent girls seeking care at a health clinic tested participants for various STIs at the beginning of the study and again after six months (Bunnell,

Dahlberg, & Rolfs, 1999). Overall, the girls in the study typically were engaging in low- to moderate-risk sexual behaviors. At the initial screening, 40 percent of the girls tested positive for an STI. At the six-month follow-up, 23 percent had acquired an STI or an additional infection. Overall, 53 percent of the girls in the study tested positive for more than one STI. Chlamydia was the most common infection (38 percent), followed by herpes simplex type 2, gonorrhea, and trichomoniasis (these are explained and discussed in Chapter 8, "Sexually Transmitted Infections"). The participants were not tested for HIV. Interestingly, the vast majority of the girls (88 percent) were at the clinic for other health issues and were unaware that they had an STI.

Other research has demonstrated that STI infection is disturbingly high in adolescents. Each year, about 3 million teens (25 percent) become infected with an STI. Adolescents have the highest rates of all age groups of gonorrhea, chlamydia, and syphilis. Teenage rates of HPV (genital warts), which has been shown to cause cervical cancer, are rising quickly. HIV is the seventh leading cause of death among people aged 15–24 (Aggarwal & Rein, 2003). Clearly, sexually transmitted infections among adolescents is a serious public health problem. Researchers and educators are working to find solutions, but progress is slow due to the power exerted by the hormones of puberty and the pressures of the teen sexual culture.

Numerous strategies for increasing STI awareness among teens have been suggested (Campaign for Our Children, 2003). Some efforts include establishing sex and STI education programs in schools and communities for young people while at the same time creating opportunities for educating parents about STIs and how to talk with their children about them. Other efforts focus on reducing the spread of STIs among teens and young adults by establishing private, confidential avenues for STI testing and treatment where teens can feel safe and comfortable; educating health care providers about creating a trusting environment with their teen patients; stressing efforts to make condoms readily available to teens; educating children about strategies for safe sexual expression either through solo masturbation or safe activities with a partner; ensuring that teens understand the STI dangers of oral sex and recognize that it is not a safe substitute for intercourse; and helping teens understand that consensual sexual activity in the context of a loving, monogamous relationship is the most satisfying *and* safest sex of all. Any or all of these strategies can be started by parent groups, schools, or youth organizations. Of course, many of the proposals are controversial, and not all parents would support them. However, as mentioned earlier, the research is quite clear that comprehensive sex education increases effective and safe choices among teens.

Sexuality in College

As puberty and adolescence are drawing to a close, most teens will be thrust into the next sexual stage of their life: college. Many of the same issues of pregnancy, STIs, and choices about sexual behavior teens faced in junior high and high school continue into college, but the challenges become greater because college is typically a highly sexual environment. Young people who were considered children in the eyes of the culture a year earlier are suddenly, upon entering college, considered adults. They are increasingly independent of their parents' influence and must often make sexual decisions on their own. And in college, a pervasive influence is added to the sexual mix: alcohol. Although many high school students have experimented with alcohol and other drugs, on most college and university campuses, alcohol is an integral part of the social culture, and it is associated with sexual activities in a variety of very important ways.

Sexual Activity on College Campuses

From our discussion of adolescent sexuality, you already know that most college students are sexually active, in one way or another, before they enter college. During college, sexual activity becomes more pervasive, more frequent, and more expected. Eighty percent of college students, both male and female, between the ages of 18 and 24 have engaged in heterosexual intercourse. Among college students over 24 years of age, the percentage who have had intercourse increases to 98 percent (CDC, 1997).

As discussed in relation to adolescents, college sexual activity is clearly not limited to intercourse. Most college students have also engaged in solo masturbation, sexual touching, oral sex, mutual masturbation, and a variety of other sexual activities (Hsu et al., 1994). Table 12.5 gives an indication of the sexual practices of college students. You will note that contrary to most people's beliefs, approximately the same percentage of college men and women have experienced nearly all of the sexual behaviors on the list (these behaviors are discussed in greater detail in Chapter 6, "Sexual Behaviors: Experiencing Sexual Pleasure"). Part of the reason people are surprised to see such a similarity between college males' and females' sexual activities is due to the commonly believed myth of differing "sexual peaks" for men and women. This myth suggests that males reach their sexual peak at around 18, whereas females reach their peak closer to 30. This popular belief, however, is not supported by scientific research; its source is probably the early findings of Kinsey's surveys (discussed in Chapter 1) that measured sexual peak as the age of highest frequency of orgasm from all forms of stimulation including masturbation (Schmitt et al., 2002). When it comes to sexual desire, lust, and pleasure with a partner, you can see that this definition of "sexual peak" is very misleading. A look at Table 12.5 shows that sexual activities are not very different for college-age men and women. So the claim that college-age men are at their peak but

Table 12.5 SEXUAL BEHAVIORS OF STUDENTS AT A LARGE WEST COAST UNIVERSITY

EVER EXPERIENCED	PERCENTAGE OF MALES	PERCENTAGE OF FEMALES
Sexual intercourse	91	91
Masturbating	83	71
Naked caressing and embracing	96	92
Stroking/petting partner's genitals	96	93
Genitals caressed by partner	94	92
Mutual petting of genitals to orgasm	89	82
Having your genitals orally stimulated	94	89
Oral stimulation of partner's genitals	89	89
Mutual oral stimulation of genitals	78	83
Caressing partner's anal area*	61	37
Having anal area caressed	61	50
Anal intercourse	22	27

*This is the sole activity for which the difference between males and females was found to be statistically significant.

Source: Data from Hsu et al. (1994), Table 1.

college-age women are still ten years from theirs doesn't hold up. The truth is that sexual activity is much more a function of people's readiness for sexual activities, their comfort level with their own bodies, and their feelings of attraction and desire for a partner. When these psychological and social elements are factored into the notion of a "sexual peak," the differences between men and women largely disappear. Figure 12.2 illustrates how the sexual peaks of men and women, when measured in terms of self-reports of sexual desire, tend to rise and fall more or less together throughout life. The slight separation in the desire curves during people's 20s may be related to biological, reproductive factors or possibly due to society's greater acceptance of male sexuality and the fact that many women are busy with childrearing, with precious little time or energy for sexual desire.

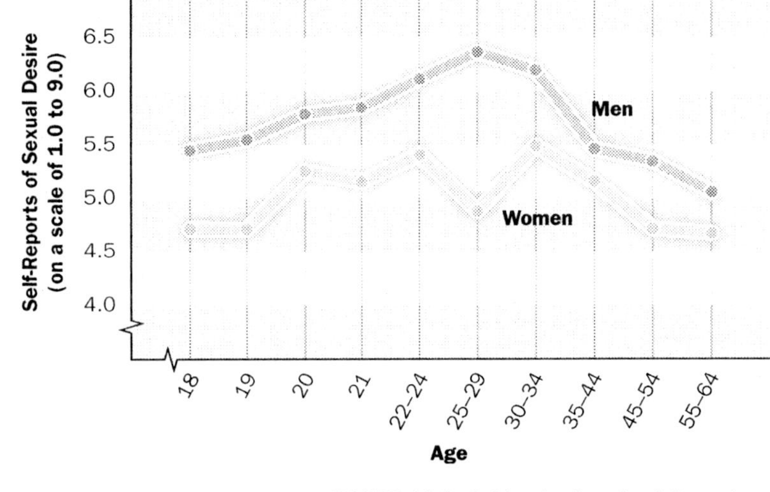

FIGURE 12.2 Subjective Levels of Sexual Desire in Men and Women

The differences between the sexual peaks of men and women tend to largely disappear when psychological and social factors are considered.

Source: Adapted from Schmitt et al. (2002, p. 6).

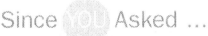

With so many college students engaging is such a wide variety of sexual practices, you might suspect that sexually transmitted infections would be a major problem on campuses. Unfortunately, your suspicions are correct.

Sexually Transmitted Infections among College Students

Most high school students who go on to college have finally heard the message about birth control. A large majority of college students (86 percent) use some form of effective birth control, most commonly oral contraceptives (the pill) (CDC, 1997; Murray & Miller, 2000). Although the pill and other hormonal contraceptives provide excellent protection against pregnancy, they offer no protection from sexually transmitted infections (STIs). Although not perfect, the consistent use of male or female condoms provides the most reliable method for sexually active college students to reduce their risk of STIs. However, research indicates that most college students are not using condoms when they engage in intercourse. In a major national surveys, less than half of college students (43 percent) reported consistent use of condoms during heterosexual intercourse, and nearly a quarter (24 percent) said they never used condoms (Eisenberg, 2001).

Since YOU Asked . . .

7. Women reach their sexual peak at 35, right? And men at 18? Why did nature create such a discrepancy?

Add to these statistics the fact that 25 percent of college students have had six or more sexual partners, and you can easily see why they have one of the highest rates for STIs of all groups in the United States (Abbey, Saenz, & Buck, 2005). Although HIV and AIDS are not rampant on university campuses, they do exist, and the risk of transmission is very real. The most common STIs among college students, however, are chlamydia, herpes, and HPV (genital warts). Two of the most important reasons these STIs spread so easily among college populations are that the infections are often asymptomatic, so awareness of even having the infection is low (see Chapter 8, "Sexually Transmitted Infections"), and many students resist being tested for them, even though the tests themselves are not particularly painful or difficult. This is unfortunate because the majority of those who are tested for STIs test negative, and the relief they feel makes their initial hesitation about being tested seem exaggerated. On the other hand, those who do test positive are able to obtain treatment to cure or reduce the symptoms and dangers of the infection sooner, thereby maximizing the success of the treatment. On the surface, it is difficult for anyone to defend a decision not to be tested, especially if the person is sexually active. Nevertheless, the number of students who seek STI testing is far lower, statistically, than the number who are at risk and *should* seek testing. Why does this discrepancy exist? Most people may feel some embarrassment at the notion of asking to be tested, but many other health issues cause some embarrassment, yet treatment for those is not so persistently avoided.

A study examining the reasons behind college students' attitudes about STI testing found that a number of factors are influencing their decisions. On the positive side are factors such as the relief gained from a negative test, the knowledge that treatments are available if a test is positive, and the desire to avoid infecting partners. However, a multitude of negative factors often override these positives for many students. These include fear of a positive test, the social stigma associated with having an STI or being tested for one, denial, underestimation of vulnerability, and characteristics of the clinic and the provider (Barth et al., 2002). "In Touch with Your Sexual Health: STIs: Why Students Decide to Be Tested . . . or Not" lists the various factors that influenced one group of college students' decisions about STI testing. When this list was shown to other students in human sexuality classes, their response was nearly unanimous that the reasons for avoiding testing were too weak to justify such a decision. What do you think?

Taking effective steps to avoid contracting STIs in the first place is significantly more effective than worrying about whether or not you may be infected. Most colleges and universities provide students with various resources on campus and on their Web

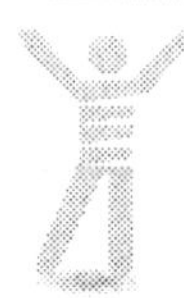

In Touch with Your Sexual Health

STIs: Why Students Decide to be Tested . . . or Not

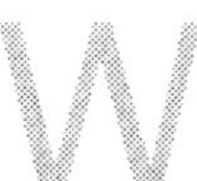

When asked during interviews about the factors that influenced their decisions whether or not to seek STI testing, college students cited the following factors.

Negative Perceptions or Personal Characteristics	Beneficial Personal Perceptions	Personal Vulnerability	Social Factors	Health System Factors
What others would think (88%)	Low severity of STIs vs. HIV (66%)	Characteristics of sexual partner(s) (93%)	Lack of knowledge about STIs (76%)	Gender of health provider (41%)
Embarrassment (61%)	Better to know for sure (44%)	Existing symptoms (88%)	Stigma of STI (56%)	Health provider's knowledge (27%)
Fear of positive test result (56%)	Relief if test negative (42%)	Type of sexual encounter (80%)	Privacy about sex and STIs (49%)	Comfort with physician (20%)
Negative emotions (29%)	Health benefits (39%)	Past sexual history (73%)	Low media coverage of STI dangers (15%)	Reputation of test site (78%)
Fear of procedures (24%)	Concern for partner (10%)	Nonsexual exposure (10%)		Cost (60%)
Negative effect on future life (12%)				Confidentiality (60%)
Denial (29%)				Convenience (68%)
Would rather not know (22%)				Availability of testing services (37%)
				Not sure where to be tested (20%)

Source: Adapted from Barth et al., 2002, p. 156.

sites to help inform and educate them about STIs and the behaviors that transmit them. Make a point to examine your own college's efforts to provide this information to students, and if you feel it is insufficient, consider taking action to improve it.

The Alcohol-Sex Link in College Students

Another important reason for the high rate of STIs among college students is that sex and drugs, mainly alcohol, are intimately linked on college and university campuses. Alcohol is routinely a part of college social interactions, and sex is clearly one form of social interaction. If a couple are drinking small to moderate amounts of alcohol in the course of an evening and as that evening progresses, they mutually agree that they want to make love, that is their choice as consenting adults. The problem comes when larger amounts of alcohol (or some other drug) twists the scenario so that they make irresponsible sexual choices, such as unsafe, unprotected sexual activities. Alcohol may also render one member of the couple unable to consent freely (or legally) to sexual advances. Without that consent, if sexual penetration occurs, it is rape (incapacitating and raping women using alcohol and other drugs is discussed in detail in Chapter 13, "Sexual Aggression and Violence").

Since YOU Asked ...

8. My roommate went to a party and drank too much. She had sex with two guys (that she remembers), but she says she didn't really want to. Was this rape?

Alcohol use has been shown to contribute significantly to college students' decisions to engage in sexual intercourse and to participate in various indiscriminate sexual behaviors such as casual sex and sex with multiple partners (Cooper, 2002). Also, studies have found that the likelihood of safer sexual behaviors such as condom use or other contraceptive practices is reduced under the influence of alcohol (Cooper & Orcutt, 2000; MacDonald, Zanna, & Fong, 1996). When intoxicated, some students tend to become single-minded, focusing on the pleasure and excitement of the sexual behaviors of the moment, and lose sight of long-term risks involved in those activities.

Sexuality in Adulthood

As people enter their 20s, whether attending college or not, they begin the next stage of development, adulthood. Adult sexuality is characterized by less sexual experimentation and typically focuses on lasting relationships, having children, and establishing a satisfying sexual life.

Adult Intimate Relationships

Adults perceive their romantic relationships in very different ways compared to those of adolescence. You are probably thinking they look back fondly on the simplicity and carefree days of adolescence, but just the opposite is true. Adults typically see their relationships as characterized by stability, mutual support, and mutual trust. Moreover, they find them more enjoyable and burdened with fewer problems than during adolescence (Shulman & Kipnis, 2001). Of course, adults have many more choices about their intimate relationships than do adolescents. Adults may freely choose to stay single, get married, live together, and start a family (or not), in almost any order and combination. One major decision many couples will make during early adulthood is whether to get married or to live together without being formally and legally married. A romantically involved couple who live together without marriage is called **cohabitation.**

Cohabitation

A clear trend in Western societies is an increase in the number of couples choosing to cohabit. The majority of couples who are getting married as you read this have lived together prior to their decision to marry (Bumpass & Lu, 2000). In 2000, 5.5 million couples were living together, compared to 3.2 million in 1990 and about 400,000 in 1960 (U.S. Census

cohabitation Living together as if married without legally marrying.

Bureau, 2003). The reasons researchers suggest for this striking increase probably won't surprise you. One is the desire on the part of young people to wait longer before getting married in order to pursue personal or professional goals (see the next section on marriage patterns). Among those who wish to wait for marriage, living together becomes an increasingly attractive option as their relationship with a significant other grows. Another frequently cited reason for the trend toward more cohabitation relates to the examples of married life young people see around them in society today. As one prominent researcher in the field notes, "High levels of marital disruption can increase the likelihood that people will cohabit as they learn either through observation or experience that marriage may not be permanent" (Smock, 2000, p. 5). In other words, when you see couples divorcing all around you, or when you have experienced a divorce yourself, cohabiting might begin to look more attractive than marriage. Research has shown that children whose parents were divorced are indeed more likely to cohabit prior to marriage (Axinn & Thornton, 1993).

Of the 5.5 million cohabiting couples in the United States, 600,000 are gay or lesbian couples (U.S. Census Bureau, 2003; "What Happened," 2003) for whom legal marriage is not an option, although this is beginning to change (see Chapter 11, "Sexual Orientation," for a discussion of gay marriage and its alternatives).

Race and ethnicity appears to influence who decides to live together instead of marrying. Native Americans and African Americans are significantly more likely to cohabit than White non-Hispanic and Asian Americans (U.S. Census Bureau, 2003). Figure 12.3 shows the percentages of cohabiting couples according to racial background.

Only a small percentage of couples who choose to cohabit will do so for the long term. Nearly all cohabiting relationships (95 percent) will end within five years. Now, before you run and tell all your cohabiting friends that their relationships are doomed, this statistic is not nearly as pessimistic as it sounds. Within those first five years, only 40 percent of these relationships will break up; 55 percent of the couples stop cohabiting because they get married (Smock, 2000). Interestingly, about 75 percent of cohabiting individuals say they *plan* to marry their partner.

Most people asked say they consider cohabitation an acceptable alternative to marriage, at least for the short term. As of 1999, only 25 percent of people surveyed in the United States defined the traditional family as a married couple with children. Also, in 2002, over 25 percent of all employers provided benefits to their workers' domestic partners, married or not (U.S. Census Bureau, 2003).

FIGURE 12.3 Cohabiting Couples by Race

Source: U.S. Census Bureau (2003).

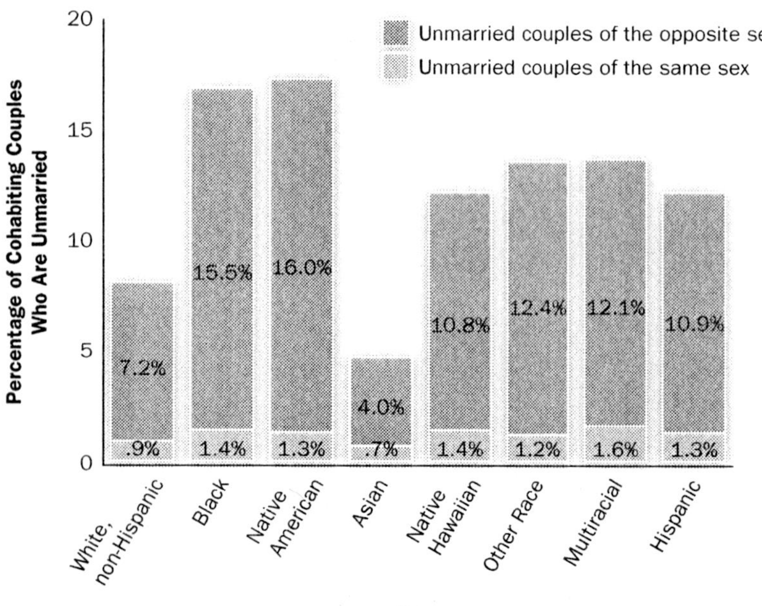

Although a great deal of support exists for cohabitation for the adults who choose it, most people feel that marriage is the preferred situation for child rearing. That said, an increasing number of children are born into, living with, or being raised by cohabiting couples. Over 40 percent of all births in the United States that are to "single mothers" are in reality to women who are part of a cohabiting couple. About 40 percent of all American children will live in a cohabiting household at some point in their lives (U.S. Census Bureau, 2003).

People who have reservations about this trend toward greater numbers of children growing up in cohabiting households may have a valid point. Research has suggested that children raised by cohabiting couples may experience increased behavioral and developmental difficulties compared to those raised in the context of marriage (Dunifon & Kowaleski-Jones, 2002). Keep in mind that these children in cohabiting households may be living with both biological parents or one bioparent and one stepparent. However, studies have shown that for children living with cohabiting parents—whether biological or nonbiological—is associated with greater behavior problems and reduced engagement in school, compared to those living with married biological parents. In addition, children who live with cohabiting parents tend to experience more academic difficulty and more serious behavior problems compared to those living with a married or a single parent (Dunifon & Kowaleski-Jones, 2002).

These findings, however, must be interpreted with care. That children of cohabiting couples have been found to have certain difficulties does not imply that *all* such children will experience those problems. Clearly, there are many happy, healthy, academically successful children raised by cohabiting parents. Also, because all the findings are correlational, we cannot assume that it is the cohabitation that *causes* the children's problems. For example, parents who choose to cohabit rather than marry may be less willing and able to form emotional attachments to other people such as an intimate partner or a child. Therefore, it may be attachment issues that lead to *both* cohabitation and less effective parenting, rather than the cohabitation causing the children's problems. "Evaluating Sexual Research: Self-Selecting Couples: Not Exactly Apples and Oranges, but . . ." further explores this problem of inferring cause and effect from correlational data.

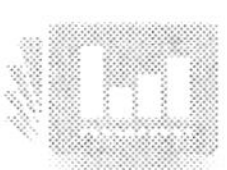

Evaluating Sexual Research

Self-Selecting Couples: Not Exactly Apples and Oranges, but . . .

One of the difficulties in doing research about different types of couples is that we cannot, as researchers, arbitrarily assign people to be members of certain couple groups in order to study the outcome. For example, if we want to study the effect of cohabiting couples on child rearing or on the success of their future marriages, we obviously can't take, say, 100 people and assign 50 of them to cohabit and the other 50 to get married. All we can do is study couples who independently *chose* to live together and compare them to couples who independently *chose* to marry, and neither group may represent the population in general. In other words, the researchers can't decide which study group to place the subjects in; they select it themselves before they volunteer for the study. Therefore, they are what are called "self-selected" participants. Since we have no choice about it, this is OK with us as researchers; we can, if they agree, ask them lots of questions about their relationships, interview them about their sex lives, have them fill out surveys about anything we think is interesting, study how their kids are doing in school, find out how happy or unhappy they are, learn how long their relationships last, and so on. And we can compare our married couple group's findings to our live-together group's findings.

However, we must contend with a basic flaw built into this research method, and there is really no way around it. *The people who comprise our two groups are not the same.* They are not different simply because they are married or cohabiting; they are very likely different in lots of other ways, too. Ask yourself the following question: In what ways might people who choose to cohabit be different from those who choose to marry, other than the mere fact that they are either married or cohabiting? You can probably come up with several possible differences fairly quickly: they avoid commitment, they have more (or less) money, they had parents who divorced, they don't love their partner as much, they are younger, they are more focused on a career than on a relationship, they don't want to have kids, they are less mature, and so on. These differences may or may not be true, but some or all of them might be. So comparing cohabiting and married couples is really trying to compare two different groups of people, and anything you find may be due to the fact that they are cohabiting or married *or* due to the individual differences in people who cohabit and people who marry. In other words, when studying a self-selected group of people, they may not represent the larger, overall population. This is called the *self-selection bias*.

The self-selection problem means that if we are not careful, we might be comparing apples and oranges and coming up with conclusions that *sound* right but may not be valid at all, such as the problems experienced by children of cohabiting parents or the higher divorce rate in couples who previously cohabited. Some of these problems can be overcome by controlling for as many extraneous variables as possible in our groups. For example, we can limit our comparisons to couples of the same average age or same average annual income or whose parents did or did not divorce. These controls help, but we can never really eliminate all the built-in differences when subjects of our study are self-selected.

Another question researchers have examined relates to whether cohabitation increases a couple's chances for a lifelong successful marriage. The conventional wisdom contends that living together is a way for couples to get to know each other in a "real-life," marriagelike setting and discover how compatible they are (or are not) prior to becoming legally married. This "trial run" should, many believe, pave the way for a better, happier marriage with less chance for discord and divorce. Does the scientific research support this common view? In a word, the answer is no. Most research finds that people who cohabit have marriages that are less happy, less harmonious, and more likely to end in divorce. How can we explain this striking discrepancy between common sense and scientific "fact"?

The most likely reason for these findings is not related to cohabitation at all, but like the effects of cohabiting on children discussed previously, it is due to the characteristics of the individuals who choose to cohabit prior to marrying (Smock, 2000; Woods & Emery, 2002). It is not much of a stretch to see that people who choose to cohabit may have different views about marriage from those who marry prior to living together. The fact that when cohabiters do marry, they are less happy and more divorce-prone is not due to the fact that they previously cohabited but that they were not prime marriage candidates to begin with. They may, on average, be less supportive of the institution of marriage or have poorer relationship skills (Axinn & Barber, 1997; Smock, 2000; Woods & Emery, 2002). However, some evidence supports the notion that negative attitudes toward marriage may develop during the time a couple cohabits prior to marriage (Axinn & Thornton, 1993; Hall & Zhao, 1995). This would indicate that the cohabitation experience itself may negatively influence marriage outcomes.

Marriage

An old joke tells of the young man who is trying to decide whether to ask his girlfriend to marry him. He is conflicted about this big step in his life and decides to make a list of all the pros and cons of marriage. On the con side of the list are "less freedom," "never date again," "less time out with the guys," and many other items. On the pro side is a single item, "regular sex." Of course, marriage is about far more than sex, but sexuality in marriage is the primary focus of our discussion here of married couples.

Although cohabitation has risen dramatically and is therefore a topic of recent research interest and focus, marriage remains the most likely lifestyle choice of adults. About 90 percent of all adults in the United States will marry at some point in their lives, but the current trend is for couples to wait longer than ever before. In 1980, the median age for marriage was 24.7 for men and 22.0 for women. In 2000, those ages had risen to 26.8 and 25.1, respectively (U.S. Census Bureau, 2003). This trend reflects several possible causes, including a greater interest by women in establishing a career before committing to marriage, a greater social acceptance for staying single longer, the poor success rate of marriage based on rising divorce statistics, and greater social and economic support for cohabitation, as noted earlier.

Ninety percent of all adults will marry at some point in their lives.

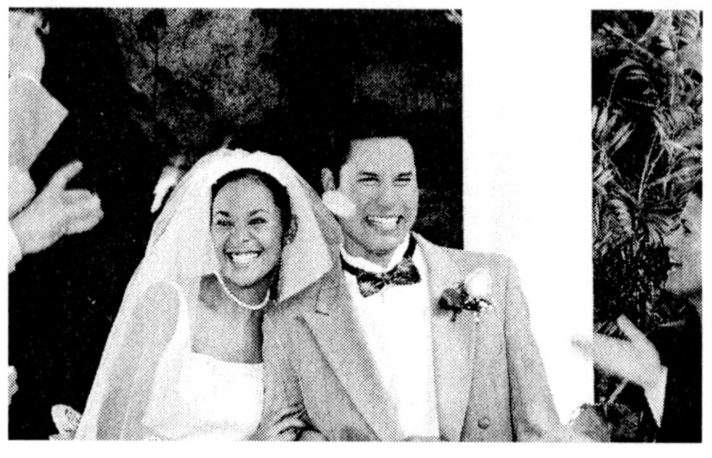

Married couples have always been the primary focus of research about sexuality. Most of the studies about sexual behavior and attitudes you will read deal primarily with married people. The reason for this is simply that married couples are the single largest group of people who are dealing with the largest number of sexual behaviors and issues.

Sexual Behavior in Marriage

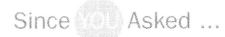

9. I've heard that when people get married, their sex life goes right down the tubes. Is this true?

Approximately 80 percent of married couples have sexual intercourse on average between 3 and 12 times per month, 7 percent report a frequency of 4 times a week or more, and 13 percent report intercourse a few times a year (Laumann et al., 1994). Does that sound like a little or a lot to you? In comparison, about 76 percent of cohabiting couples with similar demographics have intercourse 3 to 12 times per month, 15 percent or so report 4 times a week or more, and 8 percent a few times per year. So the difference in intercourse frequency for cohabiting and married couples is minimal. The larger numbers on the high end and fewer on the low end probably reflect that cohabiting relationships tend to be newer, and newer relationships tend to be more sexually charged in general.

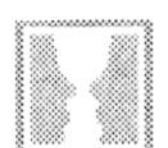

Sex is more than intercourse

We must keep in mind, however, that sex, even in marriage, is not limited to intercourse. Many couples engage in a wide range of sexual activities either along with intercourse or, at times, instead of it (Laumann et al., 1994). Research has shown that over 70 percent of both married men and women have engaged in oral sex and 25 percent of men and 16 percent of women report that oral sex was part of their most recent lovemaking with their spouse. Married couples also engage in anal intercourse more than most people realize. Approximately 27 percent of married men and 21 percent of married women have experienced anal intercourse, and 10 percent of men and 7 percent of women report anal sex during the previous year. Many individuals continue to masturbate after marriage, and masturbation tends to enhance, not detract from, sexual activities between married partners. At least 60 percent of husbands and 40 percent of wives masturbate (Laumann et al., 1994).

The next important question concerns whether these couples who are satisfied and happy with the sexual aspects of their marriages are also happily married. Not surprisingly, the answer is yes. Married couples who report greater sexual satisfaction with their partner also report higher levels of happiness with the marriage. The problem arises in attempting to determine which is causing which. Obviously, couples who get along well, enjoy each other's company, are more harmonious, and experience less discord are likely to feel more sexual attraction within the marriage. On the other hand, a satisfying sexual life may contribute to the couple's ability to get along, feel greater harmony, and find each other more sexually attractive. One study of 5,000 married adults from 49 U.S. states examined various factors that might play a role in married couples' sexual satisfaction. The factors studied were couples' overall satisfaction with the marriage, their satisfaction with the nonsexual aspects of the marriage (i.e., shared goals, mutual respect, and shared recreational preferences), their frequency of orgasm during sex, their frequency of sexual activity, their degree of sexual experimentation, and their religious beliefs (Young et al., 1998). The factor that accounted for the greatest amount of couples' sexual satisfaction was their rating of their overall satisfaction with the marriage in general, followed by their ratings of the nonsexual aspects of their relationship. Other factors also played significant yet less powerful roles with the exception of couples' religious beliefs, which were not related to sexual satisfaction. Figure 12.4 summarizes the study's findings for all the factors measured.

FIGURE 12.4 Factors Predicting Sexual Satisfaction in Marriage

Source: Data from Young et al., (1998), Table 3.

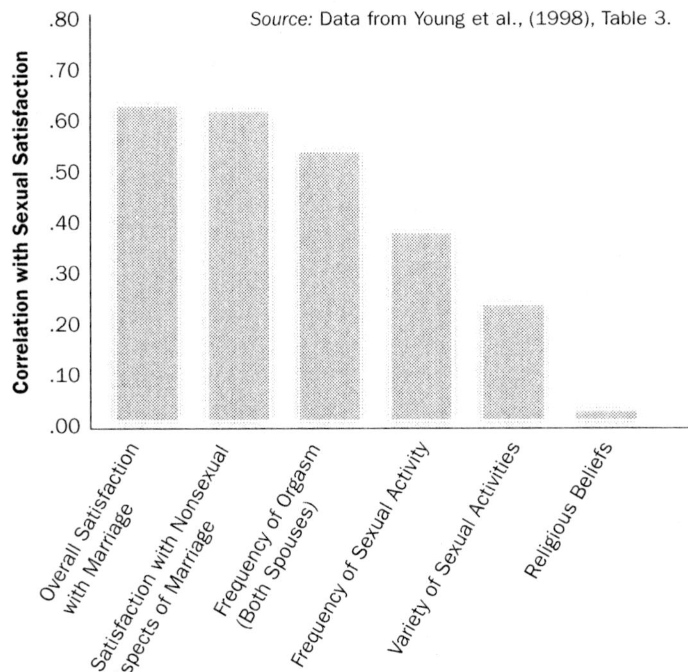

If sexual satisfaction and marital happiness are closely linked, is the opposite true? That is, are sexually inactive marriages *less* happy? Again, the answer appears to be yes, overall. Marriages in which no sexual activity had occurred over the previous month (16 percent of those surveyed) were associated with less marital

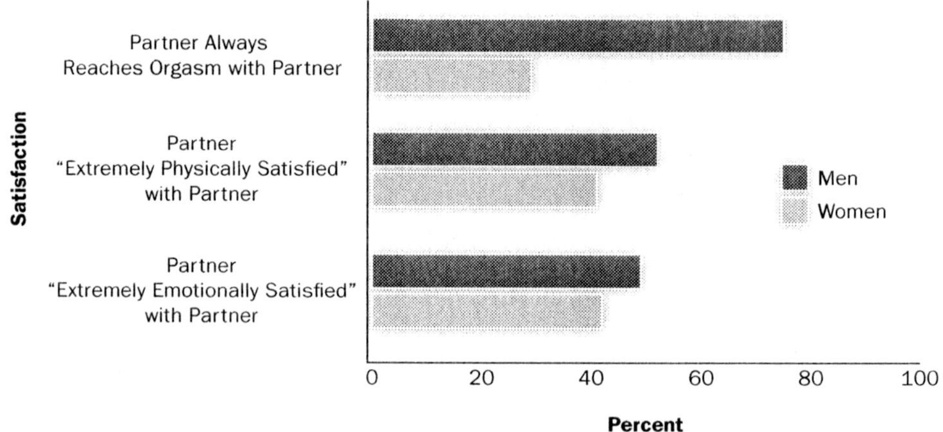

FIGURE 12.5 Sexual Relationship Satisfaction among Married Couples

Source: Data from Laumann et al. (1994), pp. 115–117.

satisfaction, greater likelihood of separation, and a lack of shared activities (Donnelly, 1993). Indeed, a lack of sex in a marriage may be a more powerful influence on the relationship's demise than satisfying sex is on a marriage's success.

How many married couples feel that their sexual relationship is both physically and emotionally satisfying? One large survey of married couples conducted in the mid-1990s found that about 75 percent of men and 29 percent of women reported having an orgasm every time they make love with their spouse. When men were asked how physically and emotionally satisfied they were in their marriage, about 52 percent said they were extremely physically satisfied and 49 percent said they were extremely emotionally satisfied. For women, the numbers were 41 and 42 percent, respectively (Laumann et al., 1994). See Figure 12.5 for a summary of these findings.

Sexual Problems in Adulthood

As people move from adolescence into adulthood and settle into more stable and meaningful intimate relationships, most expect to enjoy satisfying, relatively carefree sexual lives. This expectation stems from a common, yet mistaken, belief that sexual behavior and responses are naturally occurring events and that everything should "work" just as nature intended. Unfortunately, the majority of couples run into sexual problems of one sort or another at some point in their relationship. These sexual difficulties are typically the result of changing conditions in the couple's life, such as children, busy work schedules, stress, and fatigue. The most common sexual problems are a loss of sexual desire in one or both partners, problems achieving or maintaining an erection, lack of sexual arousal, lack of orgasm, delayed orgasm, rapid ejaculation, and painful sex. All of these problems are far more common than most people think. We discuss sexual problems and solutions in detail in Chapter 7.

The important point to make here is that couples need to know that their sexual problems are common, usually reversible, and do not signal the end of a satisfying sexual life. Approximately 43 percent of women and 31 percent of men report experiencing at least one sexual problem during the previous 12 months (Laumann, Paik, & Rosen, 1999). Figure 12.6 summarizes the frequency of occurrence of the most common sexual problems. Couples should understand that these and other sexual problems often resolve on their own when conditions in the couple's life become more accommodating to sexual intimacy. Moreover, those that do not resolve are nearly always successfully treated with counseling, medications, or a combination of the two (various treatments are also discussed in Chapter 7).

Finally, couples should realize that certain changes in sexual responding occur as a part of the aging process. When we examine data on sexual problems by age groups,

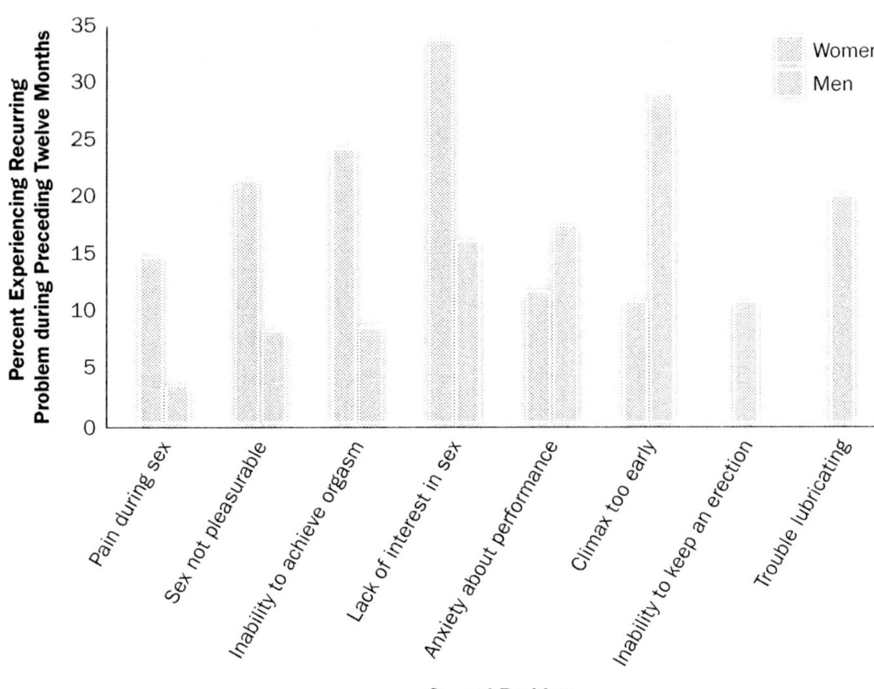

FIGURE 12.6 Common Sexual Problems in Intimate Relationships

Source: Data from Laumann et al. (1994), p. 369.

some clear trends emerge. For example, the percentage of men in their 20s and 30s who have difficulty maintaining erections is under 10 percent, whereas this problem is reported by about 20 percent of men in their 50s. For women, difficulty becoming physically aroused as indicated by vaginal lubrication is reported by approximately 18 percent of women in their 20s and 30s; this increases to about 24 percent for women in their 50s (Laumann et al., 1994).

For these and other reasons, the frequency of lovemaking tends to decline with age, but not by as much as many (especially younger) people think. Our ability to enjoy life as sexual beings continues into late adulthood and throughout the aging process. This chapter is called "Sexual Development *throughout Life*" because our capacity for sexual responding, enjoyment, and pleasure is truly lifelong.

Sexuality and Aging

When you try to imagine your parents making love together, do you think, "Yuck!"? How about your grandparents? "Double yuck!" Well, you might as well get used to it. Many older people continue to be sexual and enjoy sexual activities well into their 50s, 60s, 70s, 80s, and 90s. In fact, some senior citizens may be having more sex than some busy, two-career parents in their 20s! Very often, older couples find that being alone with their spouse after the kids have left the nest and no longer needing to be concerned about birth control allows them to rekindle a sexual life together that may have diminished over the years.

Women and men have the capacity for sexual desire and sexual activity throughout their lives. They are physically able to express their sexuality well beyond their reproductive years. Women and men who maintain a sexually active life throughout later life years seem to be more sexually responsive in old age than those who have not. The key to maintaining sexual function in later years is to continue a pattern of regular sexual activity. This is one instance in which the "use it or lose it" rule applies.

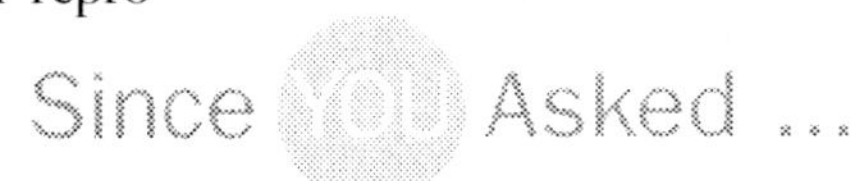

10. At what age do most elderly people stop being interested in sex?

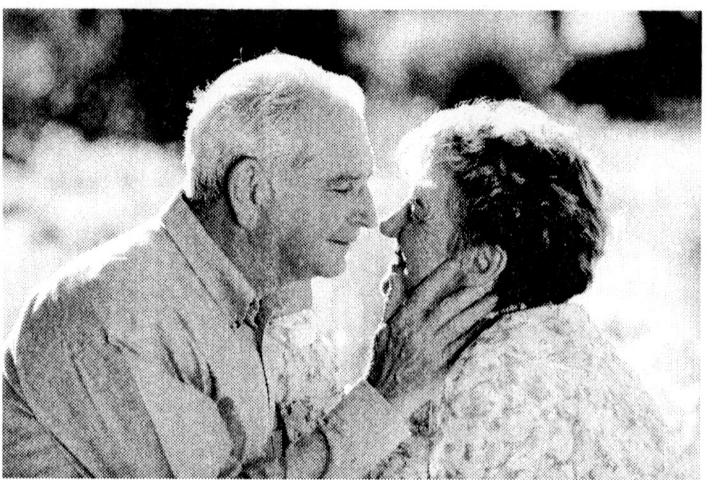

Intimacy and sexual interactions are important to us throughout our lives.

However, one of the most widely believed human sexuality myths is that when people get old, they stop desiring and having sex. This is simply not true. Humans are sexual beings from birth to death, and most elderly individuals continue to have sexual feelings, desires, and in many cases, active sexual lives. In fact, there are few, if any, physical reasons that anyone should ever have to stop being sexual. The most common reason that older individuals stop having sex is that they buy into cultural expectations that it is inappropriate for the aged to "behave that way."

Apart from depriving older adults of the enjoyment and intimacy sexual interactions bring, these myths and expectations can also prevent older adults from receiving adequate health care. For example, health care providers often neglect to deal with issues related to sexually transmitted infections when they are treating older clients because they automatically, and often mistakenly, assume that older clients are not engaging in risky sexual behaviors. Similarly, doctors often do not consider the possible effects on sexual activities and response of chronic medical conditions and medications when dealing with older clients. Consequently, they may not anticipate that some of these older patients may become frustrated with the sexual side effects of prescribed medications and may discontinue treatment without notifying their doctor (Engender Health, 2003). This, of course, can have serious and even fatal consequences.

Normal Age-Related Changes in Sexual Responding

Although sexual activity can continue well into one's 90s and beyond, the aging process does have some predictable effects on sexual responding. In general, the response cycle slows down. The stages of response take longer to achieve, the intensity of sensation may be reduced, and the genitals may become somewhat less sensitive. Sexual excitement and orgasm are somewhat subdued but no less pleasurable. Indeed, for many people, the later years can offer a rich sex life without the worry of pregnancy and the inconvenience of contraception. However, it is important to remember that the risk of acquiring HIV and other STIs does not disappear with age.

In older women, menopause results in drops in estrogen and progesterone, causing physiological changes that affect sexual function. These hormone-related changes include thinning of the vaginal lining, reduced elasticity of the vagina, and decreased lubrication, sometimes resulting in discomfort or pain during intercourse. Urinary incontinence may also occur (because of reduced estrogen), as well as loss of libido (because of reduced testosterone). All of these changes are reversible and treatable if they are interfering with enjoyment of sexual activities. In men, the time to achieve erection increases, and the period of time between orgasms lengthens. Most men as they age require more direct stimulation of the penis for erection, whereas at younger ages, mere visual or fantasy images were sufficient. Normal physiological changes for men and women associated with aging may be divided into the stages of sexual arousal shown in Table 12.6.

Aging and Dating

Western cultures have always seen romance, passion, and sex as reserved for the young. However, the reality is that the group we commonly refer to as "senior citizens" are often as interested and active in dating as people decades younger. Cultural attitudes about aging, romance, and sex are just plain wrong. Single adults over 60 report that dating is an important and meaningful part of their lives. Moreover, as

Table 12.6 AGING AND NORMAL CHANGES IN SEXUAL RESPONSE

Age-related changes that may interfere with a satisfying and pleasurable sexual life are normal and can be treated effectively. For many people, their later years can offer a rich sex life without the worry of pregnancy and the inconvenience of contraception. However, it is important to remember that the risk of contracting STIs does not disappear with age.

STAGES OF SEXUAL AROUSAL	FOR OLDER MEN	FOR OLDER WOMEN
Desire	– A decrease in sexual desire may be experienced by either partner, which may be due to changes in hormone levels or cultural expectations about sex and aging. – Certain chronic illnesses or other physical conditions may require adjustments in the sexual behaviors and desires shared by older couples.	– A decrease in sexual desire may be experienced by either partner, which may be due to changes in hormone levels or cultural expectations about sex and aging. – Certain chronic illnesses or other physical conditions may require adjustments in the sexual behaviors and desires shared by older couples.
Excitement	– Erections are slower to develop with increasing age. A younger man may be able to experience erection in a matter of seconds, while some older men may need several minutes of direct stimulation to become erect. – Erections may be less firm.	– There is less blood engorgement of the genitals than in younger women. – Vaginal lubrication may take longer to occur and the amount of lubrication may be reduced. Use of artificial lubricant may increase ease of intercourse. – Nipple erection is slower. – Elasticity of the vagina may decrease with age.
Plateau	– Older men may have less overall muscle tension, than younger men. – Complete erection may not be achieved until near end of the plateau phase. – The testes do not elevate as far up toward the body. – The older man is able to stay in the plateau phase longer. This may enhance his and his partner's sexual pleasure—one of the positive changes that occurs with aging.	– Enlargement of the inner vagina (tenting) is slightly less than in younger women. – The uterus elevates slightly less.
Orgasm	– Older men may experience a somewhat lowered level of intensity during orgasm. – Orgasm sometimes produces fewer contractions. – The seminal fluid may be thinner in consistency and somewhat reduced in volume.	– Women may experience fewer muscle contractions during orgasm. – The uterine contractions that take place with orgasm may become uncomfortable. – Sexual flush may be less pronounced.
Resolution	– This phase progresses faster in older men. – The testes lower away from the body more rapidly. – Nipple erection lasts longer than in younger men. – The refractory period tends to lengthen.	– This phase occurs more rapidly. Older women have less vasocongestion than younger women, so less time is needed for the body to return to the unaroused state. – Some older women may experience vaginal discomfort or pain if lubrication is insufficient

Sources: Meston (1997) and Sex Info (2003).

people live longer and healthier lives, an increasing proportion of the population is over 60. In 2000, 16.3 percent of the U.S. population was over 60, an increase of nearly 10 percent from 1990 (Administration on Aging, 2001). And an increasing number of older Americans are single due to divorce or the death of a spouse. The traditional notion that older people cease to be interested in love, intimacy, and passion is fading quickly, and rightly so. A great deal of evidence exists demonstrating that remaining romantically and sexually active into old age provides a wide range of emotional and physical health benefits.

You might think that when the elderly date, the feelings and behaviors associated with meeting someone new, going out, and becoming involved would be significantly different from dating among people in their teens and 20s. However, the emotions older people experience surrounding dating are remarkably similar. As the authors of one study of dating among those over 65 wrote:

> One of our major findings was the similarity between how older and younger daters feel when they fall in love—what we've come to call the "sweaty palm syndrome." This includes all the physiological and psychological somersaults, such as a heightened sense of reality, perspiring hands, a feeling of awkwardness, inability to concentrate, anxiety when away from the loved one, and heart palpitations. A 65-year-old man told us, "Love is when you look across the room at someone and your heart goes pitty-pat." A widow, aged 72, said, "You know you're in love when the one you love is away and you feel empty." Or as a

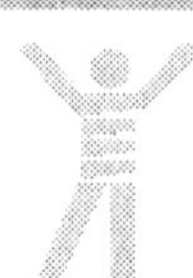

In Touch with Your Sexual Health

Sex and Nursing Homes

Over 1.5 million elderly U.S. citizens reside in nursing homes. Talk to any nursing home staff member, and you will hear stories about the sexual exploits of their clients. This is a controversial topic, due in part to society's expectation that "old people aren't supposed to be sexual." Families of residents are often shocked to discover that their aging relative has been spending several nights each week in another resident's room and bed. However, with few exceptions, these senior citizens are consenting adults with the right to express themselves sexually if they choose.

Nursing homes are required by law to provide for the privacy needs of their cognitively competent residents, just as any other consenting adult would expect in U.S. culture. In a nursing home care setting, this may include

> knowing which behaviors are and aren't staff business; dealing with a variety of moral and religious beliefs; providing privacy; protecting observers from potentially offensive behaviors; coping with families' opposition; and handling residents' needs for information and materials on all aspects of sexuality, diseases, and erectile dysfunction. (Bonifazi, 2000, pp. 22–23)

Although nursing home staff and physicians have become increasingly accepting of the reality of sexuality in elder patients and residents, families still often have problems accepting it. In the words of one researcher in the field:

> Sixties-generation baby boomers aren't clamoring for change: many are aghast at senior sexuality and worried about its impact on finances and family loyalties. Instead, residents in their seventies, eighties, and older are requesting everything from pornography to double beds. (Bonifazi, 2000, p. 22)

For an example of just how important love, intimacy, and sexuality are to some elderly nursing home residents, consider the following example from one nursing home:

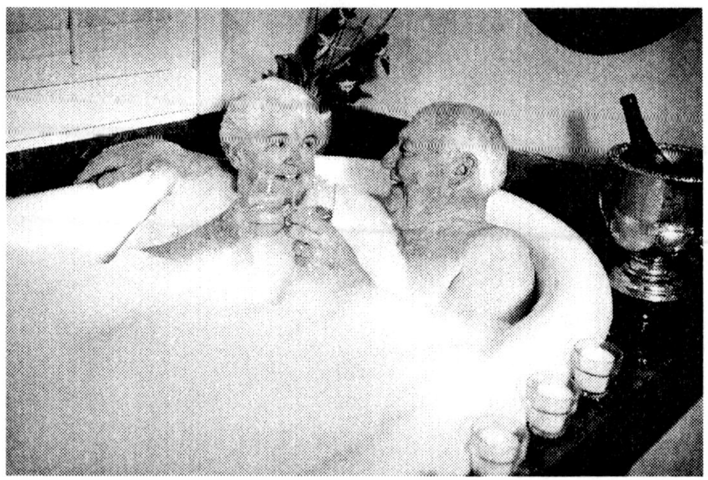

> June, 75, met fellow resident Charles "Chico" Byars, 65, last year while helping the former Golden Gloves boxer at bingo.
>
> "Thank God, he woke me up to love and desire, things I thought I put away forever," says June. "We're very proud of ourselves. We accept each other wholeheartedly."
>
> "With our souls," Chico concurs. "We're very much in love." Staff members and other residents followed their courtship with fascination and curiosity.
>
> "Our relationship turns some of them on," says June. "They assumed we were intimate."
>
> They were, but it was challenging for June, completely paralyzed on one side since a stroke, and Chico, an amputee.
>
> "We spent 10 months kissing, fondling, and making love as best we could in our wheelchairs," says June. "But there wasn't enough room in my bed. Chico fell out twice."
>
> After their facility wedding this past winter, the couple considered tying two beds together. In January they got a double bed, which brings them even closer, says Chico.
>
> "There are no legal code issues, because our rooms accommodate the bed and wheelchairs, and there aren't side rails because we're restraint-free," says the home director, sounding as delighted as the couple. "I wouldn't be surprised to see more of it. Everyone likes to be close and say goodnight." (Bonifazi, 2000, p. 26)

68-year-old divorcee said, "When you fall in love at my age there's initially a kind of 'oh, gee!' feeling . . . and it's just a little scary." (Kris & O'Connor-Roden, 1986, p. 66)

Dating for older individuals is not merely platonic companionship. Sex, including intercourse, plays an important role for many. One 71-year old widower told researchers, "You can talk about candlelight dinners and sitting in front of the fireplace, but I still think the most romantic thing I've ever done is to go to bed with her" (Kris & O'Connor-Roden, 1986, p. 66). For many in their 60s, 70s, and 80s, a dating partner is their only source of physical affection and touching. Just as is true throughout life, sexual intimacy is a way for people to continue to feel loved, attractive, and needed as they enter old age. As one 77-year-old woman said, "Sex isn't as important when you're older, but in a way you need it more" (p. 67).

The main roadblock older daters face is society's discomfort with romance and sexuality among the elderly. Many senior citizens who have a dating partner are not interested in marrying again. They are happy with the mix of independence and romance that they have established. However, being sexual outside of marriage often goes against the values they believed throughout their lives and evokes embarrassment or guilt. In an ironic role reversal, some elderly daters hide their dating intimacy from their grown children. But that does not mean that love and intimacy are any less important to them. For many older people, dating is a happy and central part their lives. In the words of one 65-year old man, "I'm very happy with life right now. I'd be lost without my dating partner. I really would." Or as a 64-year-old woman summed it up, "I suppose that hope does spring eternal in the human breast as far as love is concerned. People are always looking for the ultimate, perfect relationship. No matter how old they are, they are looking for this thing called love" (Kris & O'Connor-Roden, 1986, p. 69).

Unfortunately, not all elderly people live independent lives that allow them to meet others and form dating relationships. Many, who reach a point in life where they need extra care, move to assisted living facilities or nursing homes. It may surprise you to learn that the human need, desire, and perhaps instinct for an intimate connection with another is not extinguished in these circumstances either. Sexual relations among nursing home residents is a reality that requires sensitive understanding from management and nursing staff. "In Touch with Your Sexual Health: Sex and Nursing Homes" elaborates on this important issue.

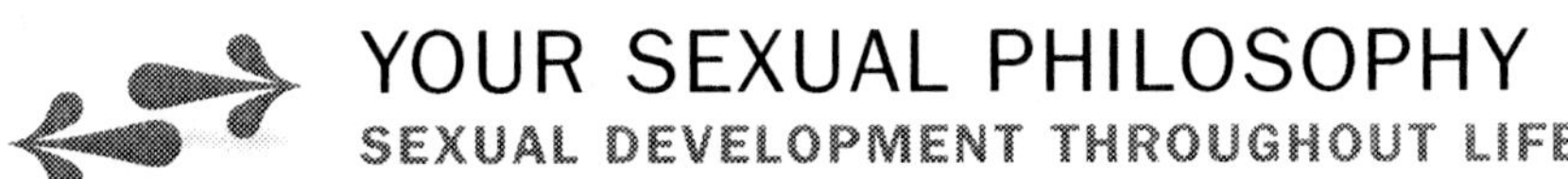

YOUR SEXUAL PHILOSOPHY

SEXUAL DEVELOPMENT THROUGHOUT LIFE

We have come full circle. We have taken a look at our sexual development from before birth to the last stages of life. As mentioned at the beginning of this chapter, we are intended by nature to be sexual, to respond sexually, and to desire intimacy with others. For better or for worse, these human capacities are present in all of us throughout our entire life span.

This chapter relates directly to the importance of developing a sexual philosophy as early in life as possible. Everyone experiences the various phases of sexual development discussed in this chapter, and each sexual passage presents new and different challenges for healthy sexual adjustment. Even children will benefit from some guidance in developing their own version of a sexual philosophy that includes an understanding of appropriate and inappropriate sexual behavior in public, respect for their own and others' bodies, the difference between good and bad touches by an adult, and knowing how to communicate to trusted adults any uncomfortable sexual encounters they may experience.

Adolescence is perhaps the stage in most people's lives when focusing on their sexual philosophy becomes most important. There is probably no other time in life during which sexual issues exert more power over us. You know this is true from the way people talk about "raging hormones" causing teens to lose all control over their sexual desires and actions. However, adolescents' hormones do not, in reality, have the power to cause any specific sexual behaviors. They merely awaken natural sexual feelings and motivations. What a person does with those feelings still requires conscious choices. Teens who have developed at least the beginnings of a personal sexual philosophy are much better equipped to make safe and healthy choices when faced with sexual situations, because they have had the opportunity to think about them before they are in the heat, and the peer pressure, of the moment.

The value of a well-developed sexual philosophy does not end with adolescence. Major life decisions will be made during adulthood involving relationships, living together, marriage, having children, sexual satisfaction, and sexual problems. This does not imply that you should have all the answers to these life events before you are faced with them. No one can predict the future, and everyone's sexual philosophy evolves and changes through learning and experience. However, just think how much easier and more effectively you will be able to approach sexual issues in adulthood if you have taken some time to think about them; to consider your own personal needs, wishes, and desires; and to become educated about them.

Finally, continuing to expand and develop your sexual philosophy is important as a lifelong process. Sexuality does not end with old age, but it does change in various ways. Preparing for those changes and knowing what is a normal part of aging will give you the best chance of staying sexually active throughout your later years, which will in turn make the aging process a healthier and happier experience.

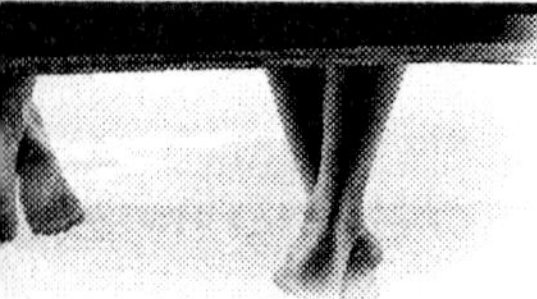

Summary

HISTORICAL PERSPECTIVES Freud's Psychosexual Stages of Development: Oedipus and Electra?

- Freud contended that all human development is sexually based. Although many of his ideas have not held up well to modern scientific research methods, Freud's five psychosexual stages of human development were widely accepted in the early 1900s.

Sexuality in Infancy and Childhood

- Childhood masturbation and sexual exploration are normal activities in childhood. When parents or other caretakers find children masturbating or "playing doctor," they usually need not be concerned. However, extreme sexual acting out in childhood may indicate emotional problems or sexual abuse issues.
- Most children do not receive adequate information about sex from their parents. Studies show that many children rely on school, peers, and the media for sex education.

Sexuality in Adolescence

- Puberty may begin at any time between about 8 and 15 years of age.
- Many teens report that an intimate partner is the most important relationship in their lives.
- Most teens will experience their first intercourse by grade 12, but teen sex is not limited to intercourse. Oral sex among teenagers is becoming increasingly common, based on their false belief that oral sex is safe sex.
- Although the teen pregnancy rate is declining, the rates of sexually transmitted infections remain high among adolescents.

Sexuality in College

- Nearly all college students are sexually active. The rates of most sexual experiences among college students are similar for males and females.

- College students appear to be protecting themselves fairly well from unwanted pregnancy but not taking adequate precautions against STIs. Less that half of college students use condoms, and the majority of college students resist being tested for STIs.
- Sexual assault, acquaintance rape, and date rape on college campuses are often associated with the use of alcohol or other drugs.

Sexuality in Adulthood

- Adults report that intimate relationships become more enjoyable as they grow older and they feel less conflicted about them than during adolescence.
- Research has shown a striking increase in the number of couples choosing to cohabit before or instead of marrying.
- Cohabitation is associated with less happy subsequent marriages and higher divorce rates. Over 90 percent of all adults in the U.S. will marry, although they are waiting longer to marry. The median age for marriage in the United States is now around 27 for men and 25 for women.
- Sex in marriage is not limited to intercourse among heterosexual couples; oral and anal sex are also common. A couple's sexual satisfaction and the happiness of their relationship are closely linked.

Sexuality and Aging

- Although sexual responses change as we age, few physical reasons exist for the elderly to forgo satisfying sexual interactions. Sexual intimacy among the elderly is an important part of their happiness.

YOUR SEXUAL PHILOSOPHY: Sexual Development throughout Life

- Sexuality is a lifelong part of human nature, which changes as we age.
- Understanding and preparing for sexual changes—knowing what to expect and what is normal—allows us to stay sexually healthy throughout life, which in turn makes our lives healthier and happier.

Have You Considered?

1. Imagine you are babysitting for two 5-year-old children. You notice they have become "too quiet" in the other room, and you go in to find the kids naked and "playing doctor." Describe how you think you would react to this, and what actions you would take, if any?
2. Discuss when childhood masturbation is not a cause for concern and when it might indicate a problem.
3. Imagine that you are the parent of a precocious 13-year-old girl, and you are having a serious parent-daughter talk with her about sexual issues. She tells you that she has never had intercourse, but upon further discussion, she admits that she is having oral sex with boys. What do you think your response to this would be, and what information would you want to give her?
4. What do you think are the three most important sex education issues for young teens to understand as fully as possible? Explain your answer.
5. If you were a sexuality educator hired by a large urban school district to develop programs to reduce unwanted pregnancy and the spread of STIs among teens, discuss at least three strategies you would propose to accomplish these goals.
6. Discuss what you feel are the main advantages and disadvantages of a couple's choosing to live together without getting married.
7. As the statistics quoted in this chapter indicate, fewer than half of married couples say they are extremely physically and emotionally satisfied with their partners. Discuss at least three possible suggestions you might make to help more married couples move up into the ranks of the extremely satisfied.
8. Discuss the various barriers elderly people face in maintaining sexually intimate and active lives. How would you suggest some of these barriers might be removed?

Companion Website Resources

For further chapter resources go to **www.prenhall.com/hock.** This robust text website includes polling questions for you to vote on, regular news updates, quizzes, sample tests, suggested reading lists, and more.

SCENARIOS USA Also on the website are links to videos. *Scenarios USA's* films portray real-life narratives that explore the non-biological aspects of relationships and sexual health. The films will help you consider how the themes of the text affect your own life and the lives of those around you.

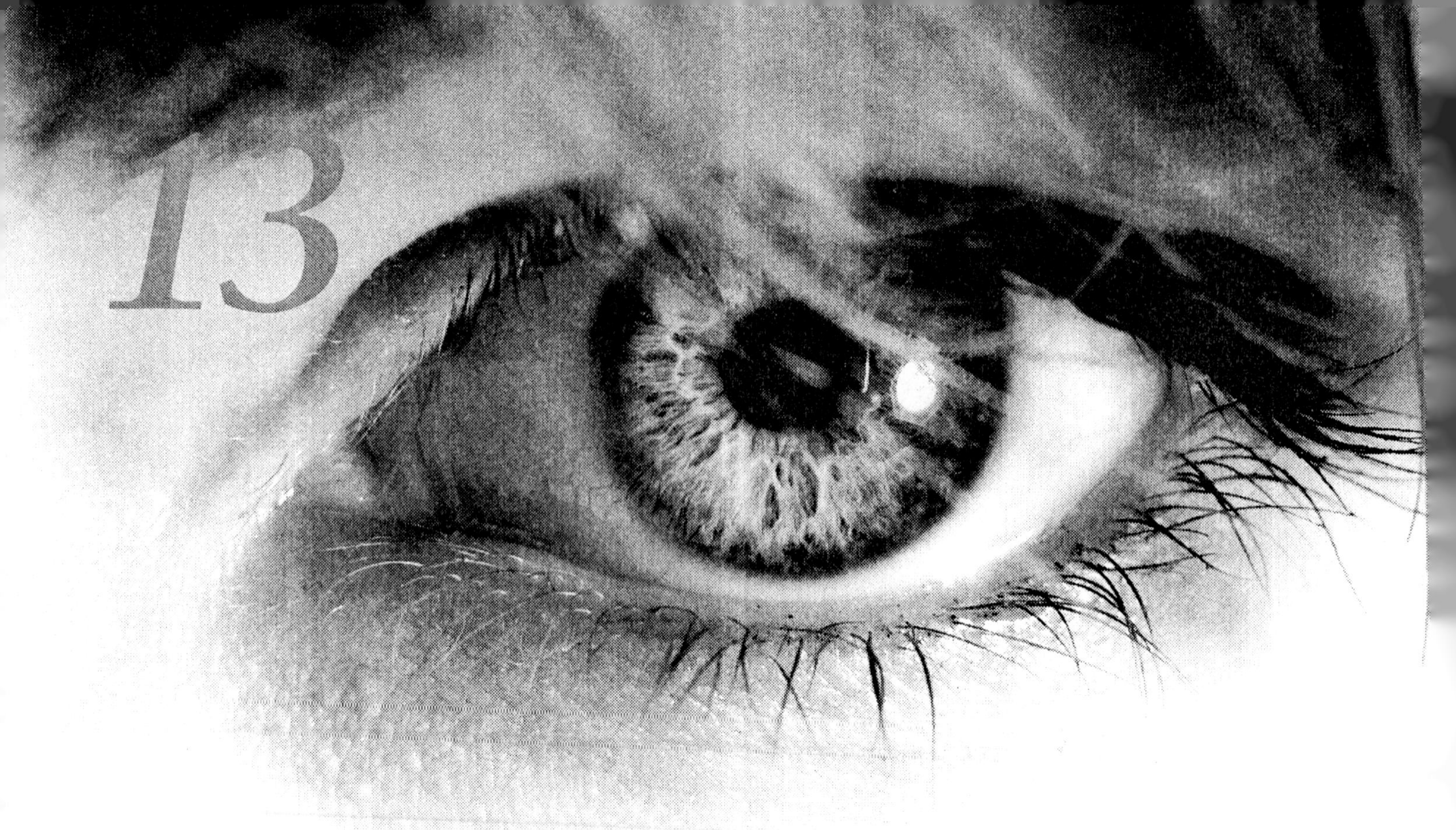

13

Sexual Aggression and Violence

Rape, Child Sexual Abuse, and Harassment

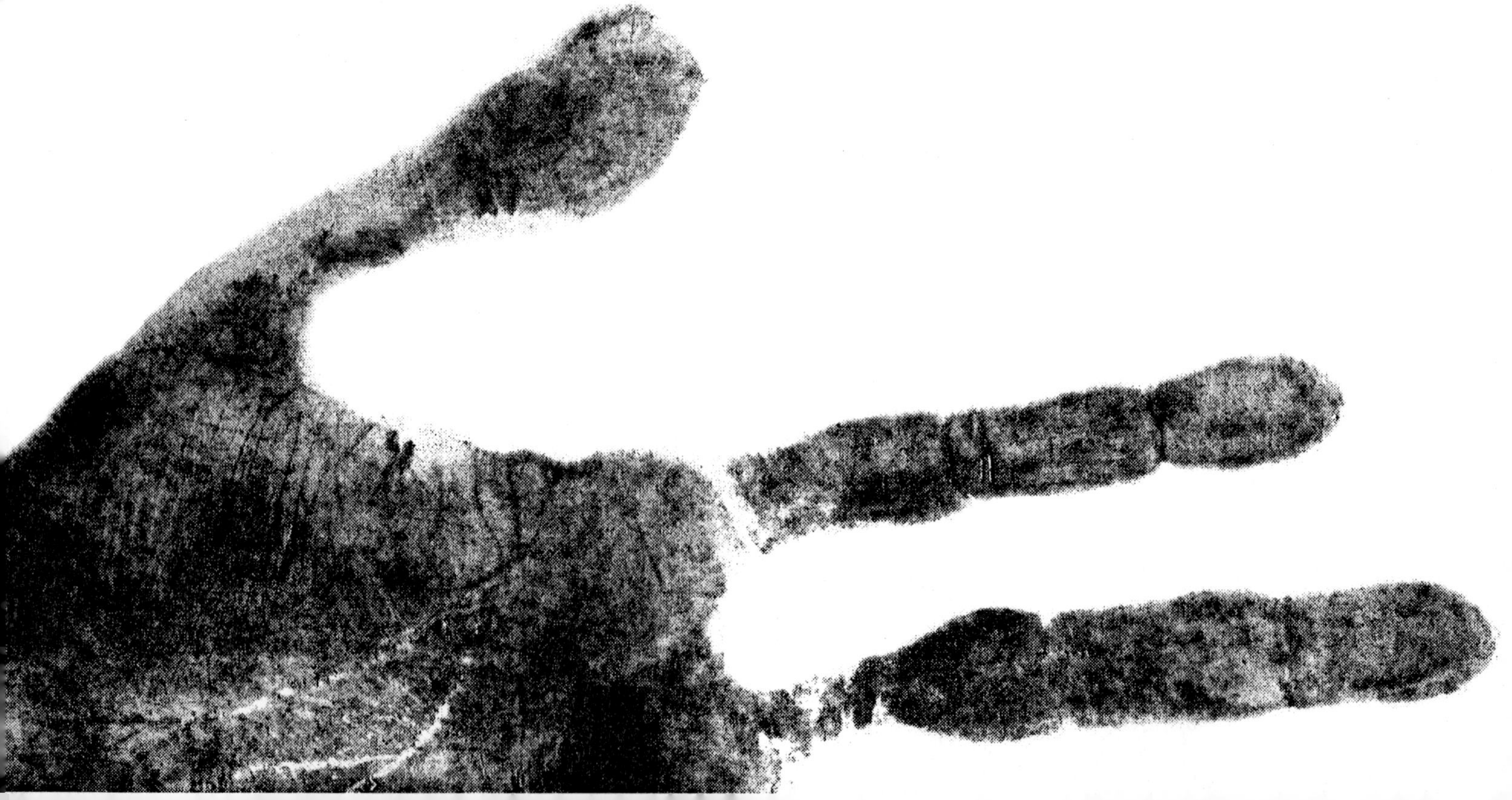

Since YOU Asked...

1. My friend's husband wants to have children, but she is not ready. She told me he is forcing her to have sex and not using protection. I told her this is rape, but she doesn't think so because they are married. Is that true? (see page 481)

2. Why do guys feel that a woman's body is theirs, but the guy's body is never the woman's? (see page 481)

3. I read a story about a man being raped by a woman. Is this possible? What about his erection? (see page 484)

4. If women don't want to be sexually attacked, why do they dress like they do? (see page 485)

5. I've heard that some women really want to be raped because that way they can have sex without taking any responsibility for it. (see page 486)

6. Someone told me that all men, if they got the chance and knew they would never be caught, would commit rape. Is that true? (see page 487)

7. My roommate went to a party last weekend and got totally wasted (drunk). Two of the guys at the party told her that two other guys had sex with her while she was passed out, but she has no memory of this. Could this really have happened? Why would guys want to have sex with someone who is passed out? (see page 488)

8. Is there any way to tell if someone has slipped a roofie into your drink (I mean, before you drink it)? (see page 490)

9. My sister was raped over three years ago, but she's still very upset and angry about it. What can she do to get over it? Will she ever get over it? (see page 495)

10. Can being sexually abused as a child prevent a person from having good relationships in adulthood? Do the effects of the abuse really last so long? (see page 504)

11. I heard that a professor was fired for sexual harassment. Is that true? What did he do? (see page 510)

Marci had liked him. When she met Kirk two weeks ago after a party at a fraternity house, he was attentive, caring, and eager to know all about her. He was willing to talk about himself and his feelings. They had gone out twice during the next week, and on their second date, they had spent almost an hour kissing in his car in front of her campus apartment. Just kissing, that's all; she was pleased that he didn't seem particularly aggressive or interested just in sex like so many of the other guys she had dated. The next weekend, she invited Kirk over to her room for pizza and a movie. After dinner, they began kissing on the bed, and his hands began to wander. Marci stopped him and told him that she wasn't ready to be sexual with him. He said he was sorry, but as the kissing continued, he began to force his hands under her clothing. The more she protested, the more forceful he became. She told him no and pleaded with him to stop, but he was bigger and stronger, and with all his weight on top of her, she just felt powerless. She tried to fight but couldn't. For some reason, she didn't call out for help. He got her panties off and his pants down and pushed himself into her. When he was done, he told her how great it was and actually wanted to kiss her. When she told him to get out, he acted hurt, as if nothing wrong had happened.

* * *

It is a beautiful campus, framed by rolling hills and pine-covered mountains. The main entrance into the library, theater, student union, and classroom buildings is a red brick path through blue spruce and pine. On either side of the walk are benches and tables where students gather to eat, study, or just hang out, especially on warm days. Over the past couple of years, this walkway has become, at times, an obstacle course of sexual harassment. On hot days, groups of male students congregate on the benches to leer, gesture, and make inappropriate sexual remarks to female students as they walk by on their way to and from the campus. A few of the women have complained to trusted faculty and staff about this sexually harassing behavior. Two women students even cited this harassment as a reason for transferring to other colleges, explaining that their discomfort was so great that they did not want to come to the campus at all. Several women have been followed to their cars by one or more of the gawking men and asked out on dates. When the women refused, they were subjected to scorn and ridicule on subsequent trips along the walkway. The men involved have been warned by the administration, fraternity sponsors, and coaches, but the behavior continued. Last week, the local police came onto campus and arrested 12 of the male students and charged them with sexual harassment. They have all been suspended from the college and are awaiting trial.

* * *

These stories, adapted from actual events on college campuses, portray the dark side of human sexuality. It is difficult to comprehend that the human capacity for physical intimacy can, in some people, become so corrupted as to produce their opposites: sexual assault, child sexual abuse, and sexual harassment. The reality is that these acts happen all too often. They are acts of violence and control and usually have little to do with the intimacy of sexual expression. Yet the fear and trauma of these acts often create painful obstacles to a survivor's ability to experience the joy of healthy sexual intimacy with a partner. That is why this chapter is crucial to this book. We will examine each act—rape, child sexual abuse, and sexual harassment—in turn, but first we will review briefly a period in our recent history relating to sexual aggression that might just surprise you.

Focus on Your Feelings

Undoubtedly, most of the feelings you will experience while reading this chapter will not be particularly pleasant ones. High on the list will probably be anger, fear, sadness, and outrage. Considering the terrible acts discussed in this chapter, all of these emotional reactions are normal and understandable. Such strong emotions may serve a positive function in that they can help you identify with the seriousness of the problems of rape, child sexual abuse, and sexual harassment, even if you have not been victimized by any of them yourself. Furthermore, these strong negative emotions often incite people to take action aimed at reducing or eliminating their source, and everyone would agree that the world would be a better place without sexual aggression. From this perspective, what you do with your feelings can be recast in a reasonably positive light.

Strong emotional reactions alone are insufficient to bring about needed social change. For that, we must channel our emotional energy into rational, organized actions. Movements such as "take back the night" marches against rape, "men against rape" organizations, Megan's law (requiring notifying communities of residential convicted sexual offenders), and the passage of antiharassment laws with real teeth are examples of how people's feelings about these terrible acts have been redirected into concrete social action for change. If some of you who read this chapter, upon feeling these emotions, choose to become involved in similar movements, society will continue to change for the better.

Historical Perspectives

Marital Rape

Can a man rape his wife? If you are like most people, you are probably nodding an emphatic yes. So you'll probably be surprised to learn that until quite recently, states' rape laws did not prohibit forcible sexual acts between a husband and wife. Many state statutes, in fact, provided specific exceptions that protected husbands from arrest and prosecution for raping their wives (Wellesley Centers for Women, 1998).

Where does this rape "double standard" come from? It probably stems from English common law, in which a wife was seen as the property of her husband. Such "ownership" included the husband's sexual rights over his wife; that is, as his legal wife, she was obligated to submit to sex on his terms, whenever he desired it. Within this framework, if she refused and he forced her, the blame for the assault lay with *her*. Moreover, if a woman were raped, it was considered a property crime that victimized the woman's husband! This notion of "wife as property" is implied if not actually stated in rape laws in the United States. It probably sounds like ancient history to you, but such laws began to change only in the late 1970s.

The current legal environment in all 50 states regarding marital rape (also referred to as "wife rape") varies. All states now provide for criminal penalties for rape within marriage, but only a minority view marital rape as indistinguishable from other forms of rape. As of 2005, thirty states continued to make exceptions for husbands who rape their wives if it is found that they did not use extreme physical force (see Figure 13.1). In other words, the rape of a woman by her husband is still seen by most states as somehow "less serious" compared to rape by an acquaintance or a stranger.

Nothing could be further from the truth. Rapes occurring in the context of an ongoing intimate relationship (including marriage or cohabitation) are

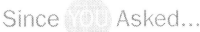

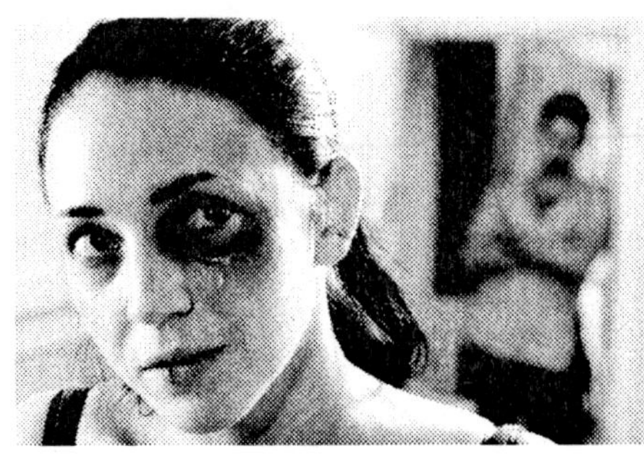

Sexual violence is the "dark side" of human sexuality.

1. My friend's husband wants to have children, but she is not ready. She told me he is forcing her to have sex and not using protection. I told her this is rape, but she doesn't think so because they are married. Is that true?

2. Why do guys feel that a woman's body is theirs, but the guy's body is never the woman's?

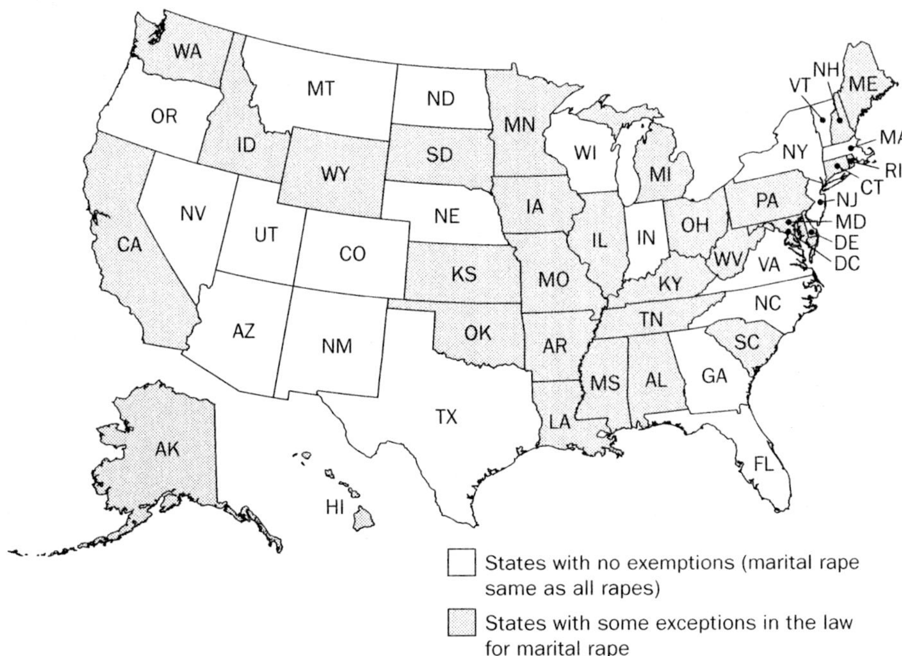

FIGURE 13.1 Marital Rape Laws in the United States

Notes: In all states, federal statutes may apply in certain circumstances. All exemptions in military courts were repealed in 2005.

Source: National Clearinghouse on Marital and Date Rape (2005).

equally or even more traumatic; they are less likely to be reported, however, because the victims themselves often do not understand that they have been raped, or they are unaware that it is against the law. Women often blame themselves for the attacks and erroneously assume that what they are experiencing is rare. It is not. Estimates of marital rape range from 8 to 14 percent of married women, and this number is probably low due to underreporting of the crime (Finkelhor & Yllo, 1985; D. E. H. Russell, 1990). Moreover, the psychological pain, physical injury, and loss of self-worth that accompany all forms of rape are at least as intense in marital rapes. Injuries associated with wife rape include broken bones, black eyes, knife wounds, miscarriages, infertility, depression, and various sexual dysfunctions (Bergen, 1999). Often sexual assault and rape occur as part of a larger pattern of violence in the relationship. Many abusers use coercive sexual tactics along with other forms of physical and verbal abuse to maintain a position of power and control over their partners (Dugan & Hock, 2006).

While it may seem a stark contrast with the strides that have been made in the area of women's rights, today, as you are reading this, many groups continue to work to convince state legislatures and governments around the world that marital rape should carry the same crime status and sentencing consequences as any other form of rape.

Rape

Until the 1980s, most people thought of rape as a crime committed by a strange and deranged man lying in wait for his female victim, attacking her, overpowering her or threatening her with a knife or gun, and forcing intercourse and other sexual acts on her. Of course, such rapes do occur, but they are much less common than rapes in which the victim has some sort of relationship with the rapist. In fact, among the many myths and misconceptions about rape, one of the most widely believed is that most rapes are committed by strangers; this is not so—most rapes are committed by someone the victim knows. Moreover, the crime of rape is more common than most people believe. For the decade ending in 2003, the average number of rapes was over 230 per day in the United States alone (see Table 13.1). As is also evident in the table, the number of rapes has changed very little over the years.

Table 13.1 FBI RAPE STATISTICS UNITED STATES 1994–2003

YEAR	TOTAL POPULATION	NUMBER OF RAPES
1994	260,327,021	102,216
1995	262,803,276	97,470
1996	265,228,572	96,252
1997	267,783,607	96,153
1998	270,248,003	93,144
1999	272,690,813	89,411
2000	281,421,906	90,178
2001	285,317,559	90,863
2002	287,973,924	95,235
2003	290,809,777	93,433

Source: Based on FBI Uniform Crime Reports, 2004a.

Defining Rape

In the United States, legal definition and prosecution of the crime of rape is left to each individual state. Therefore, the exact wording of the behaviors that constitute rape varies. In general, however, the act of **rape** usually refers to nonconsensual sexual penetration of the body using physical force or the threat of bodily harm (Cowan, 2000). Historically, this definition of rape referred to unwanted penetration of a woman's vagina by a man's penis, but most states now include in their legal definitions of rape, forced penetration by objects other than a penis and penetration of the anus and mouth in addition to the vagina (Tjaden & Thoennes, 1998). This change in the definition of rape has come about due to the recognition that forced sex may involve various acts and that the victims of rape are sometimes men (to be discussed shortly). Most states also have specific laws against other forms of unwanted sexual contact that usually fall under one or more categories of *sexual assault*. Perhaps more important than technical, legal definitions, however, are the behaviors that fall into most people's working understanding of rape.

rape Nonconsensual sexual penetration of the body using physical force or the threat of bodily harm.

stranger rape Rape by an assailant who is not known to the victim.

acquaintance rape Rape by an assailant the victim knows or is related to but is not dating.

date rape A rape that occurs in the context of a planned or spontaneous date.

partner rape A rape that occurs in the context of an ongoing romantic and sexual relationship.

Types of Rape

Rape can be divided into several types—**stranger rape**, a rape in which the assailant is a stranger to the victim; **acquaintance rape**, a rape by an assailant the victim knows or is related to but is not dating; **date rape**, a rape that occurs in the context of a planned or spontaneous date; and **partner rape**, a rape that occurs in the context of an ongoing romantic and sexual relationship (see Table 13.2). No matter what type, rape is one of the most devastating traumas anyone can experience. Some women have stated that they would rather be murdered than raped. Rape is, literally, a brutal invasion of a person's most intimate territory: her or his body. Psychologists, sexuality educators, and counselors are in general agreement that the act of rape usually has little to do with sex but arises out of a misplaced, warped desire to overpower, aggress against, humiliate, control, and victimize another person. In other words, most rapists are not sexually deprived; they are violent criminals.

The vast majority of rapes are committed by men against women. There are, of course, rapes of men by men and even rare cases of women raping men. But it is women who must carry with them, often on a daily basis, the burden of the possibility of being raped. In a rape-awareness workshop in 2000, university men and women were asked separately to list the steps they take on a daily basis to minimize the chance of their being sexually assaulted or raped (Ottens, 2001). "In Touch with Your Sexual Health: Daily Precautions Taken to Prevent Being Sexually Assaulted or Raped" shows how the two sexes' lists looked at the end of the exercise. This eye-opening exercise demonstrates that women must maintain nearly constant vigilance against the threat of rape, while men, it seems, rarely give it a thought. When the men who participated in this exercise were asked if they were aware of the steps women routinely take to avoid sexual assault, most said they were not (O'Brien, 2001).

Table 13.2 STATISTICS FOR TYPES OF RAPE

TYPE OF RAPE	ESTIMATED PERCENTAGE OF ALL RAPES*
Stranger rape	10–30
Acquaintance rape	15–25
Date rape	20–50
Partner rape	10–20

*Estimates vary due to research methodology and how rape is defined for a particular study.

Sources: Counseling Center for Human Development (2001), Laumann et al., (1994), National Crime Victims Center (2001).

Can a Man Be Raped?

The answer to that question is an unequivocal *yes*. Male rape is becoming an increasingly recognized crime, and over the past two decades, most states have revised their rape laws to be gender-neutral; in other words, rape may be perpetrated against either sex by either sex.

Statistics on male rape are thought to be very unreliable because men may feel a greater sense of shame and stigma than women do, and so even more men than women may choose not to report being raped. Keeping that in mind, recent statistics show that

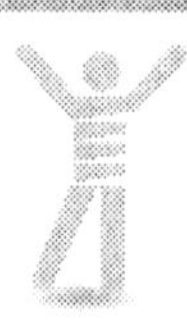

In Touch with Your Sexual Health

Daily Precautions Taken to Prevent Being Sexually Assaulted or Raped

Here are the results of a workshop during which men and women, separately, were asked to generate a list of the precautions they take nearly every day to protect themselves from being sexually assaulted.

Men	Women
	Lock all doors
	Check backseat of car
	Avoid eye contact
	Check under car
	Be aware of potential danger in surroundings
	Dress conservatively
	Park in well-lit areas
	Carry pepper spray
	Monitor drinks while out or at party
	Not wear high heels when walking alone
	Carry keys as weapon
	Alternate jogging routes
	Cross to other side when male is approaching
	Lock car doors when driving
	Leave lights on
	Notify friends of plans when going out

Source: Adapted from "Daily Precautions Taken to Prevent Being Sexually Assaulted or Raped" from "THE MVP Program: Focus on Student-Athletes" by J. O'Brien in *Sexual Violence on Campus* ed. by A. Ottens & K. Hotelling. Copyright © 2001. Reprinted by permission of Springer Publishing Company.

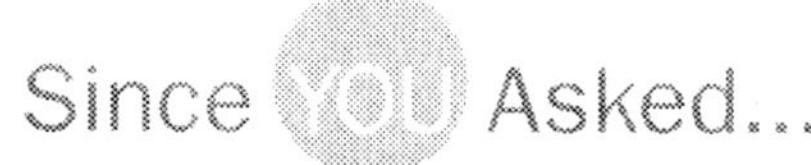

3. I read a story about a man being raped by a woman. Is this possible? What about his erection?

approximately 3 percent of men report being the victim of rape or attempted rape at some point during their lifetime, compared to approximately 20 percent of women (Laumann et al., 1994; Tjaden & Thoennes, 1998). Although the percentage is probably artificially low, it represents nearly 3 million men. At least one study found significantly higher percentages of rape among college men, with 16 percent reporting one or more episodes of forced sex in their lifetime, compared with 22 percent of women in the same college sample (Struckman-Johnson, 1988).

The majority of male rapes are committed by other men and usually involve anal or oral penetration (or both). These perpetrators and victims may be gay or heterosexual, and the attacks may happen in various settings including prisons, in the victim's or assailant's home, in a car, or out of doors. As with female rapes, most male victims are acquainted with their attackers (King & Woolett, 1997).

The effects of rape on the male victim tend to parallel those of female victims (to be discussed later in this chapter). Men who are raped by other men are at higher risk for greater physical injury and often fear for their lives during the attack. They frequently feel guilt, shame, and confusion about their sexual orientation, sometimes lasting for years after the attack, and yet are less likely to report the crime or to seek help than female victims are (King & Woolett, 1997).

Rape of men by women is the exception, not the rule, but it does happen (King & Woolett, 1997; Laumann et al., 1994; Struckman-Johnson, 1988). You may be thinking, "No way! No man would be able to have an erection if he was being violently or otherwise coerced, right?" Well, not exactly. Men have been coerced into nonconsensual sex by women through psychological pressure (such as blackmail), physical force (holding down, tying up, etc.), threats with weapons, and intoxication (Krahe, Waizenhofer, & Moller, 2003; Struckman-Johnson, 1988). The point is that it's possible, under some circumstances, for a woman to rape a man, and all rape needs to be recognized and taken seriously and the perpetrators held accountable. However, it would be a mistake to allow ourselves to become preoccupied with the relatively minuscule number of women who rape men (however curious this may appear to you) lest our attention and resources be diverted from the larger problem of men raping women.

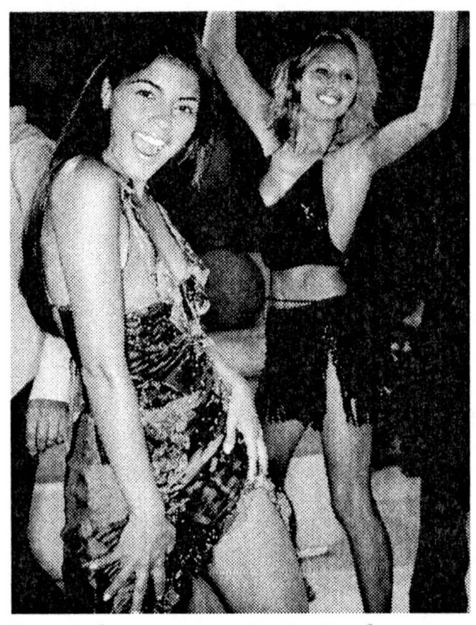
Sexy clothes are not an invitation for rape.

Rape Myths

You have seen that nearly all areas of human sexuality have their share of myths and misunderstandings. You may have discovered some of your own along the way. Unfortunately, rape is no different. In fact, rape myths may be among the worst because in many ways they place the blame on the victim and absolve the perpetrator. This has the effect of supporting a cultural acceptance of rape that leads to a staggering number of victims of this violent crime. Let's go through some of the more common and dangerous rape myths and set the record straight.

Myth: *Women encourage rape by their dress and actions.* "If she didn't want sex, why did she dress so hot?" "She kept touching my arm and resting her hand on my shoulder. We started kissing and she was totally into it. The signals were clear that she wanted it." "When she agreed to come over to my apartment for more drinks, I just assumed she wanted to have sex." These statements are typical of the thinking of many men who rape. The mistaken assumption they make is that certain clothing and behaviors on the part of a woman actually lead to her being forced into intercourse. The perpetrator feels justified in forcing sex because he's thinking "she's asking for it" by her choice of clothing or other actions.

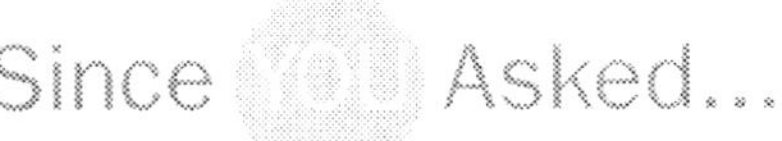

4. If women don't want to be sexually attacked, why do they dress like they do?

Truth: Can you think of any reason someone would *want* to be raped? Of course not. That's like asking if someone would like to be mugged for wearing a Rolex watch, beaten up for wearing a street gang's color in the wrong neighborhood, or robbed because you don't have bars on your windows. A woman may dress and behave in certain ways because she is interested in appearing sexually attractive or wants to have consensual sex with someone. But no one wants to be raped. All people (in the United States, at least) have the right to dress and behave as they choose without giving others permission to commit a crime against them. Conversely, women will often avoid certain modes of dress or potentially vulnerable situations, but this is not because they are concerned about "causing" a rape. Rather, they know that some men believe in the "victim as cause" myth and are taking steps to protect themselves. The only person who can cause a rape is, by definition, the rapist (Powell, 1996; Warshaw, 1994).

Myth: *Men who rape simply lose control over their sexual urges.* This misconception relates closely to the preceding one. If men are seen as compelled to rape by the strength of their sexual drive, then it seemingly becomes the woman's responsibility to avoid any behavior that might provoke him. Once provoked, this myth contends, he becomes so crazed by sexual desire that he is unable to control himself (Powell, 1996; Cowan, 2000).

Truth: There are two main problems with this way of thinking. First, as mentioned earlier, rape is not primarily a sexual act. It is the rapist's attempt to exert power and control over a victim through force, coercion, and violence. Most rapists are not sex-deprived, and many have an ongoing relationship with a consensual sexual partner. Furthermore, when people commit other crimes involving violence, we do not attempt to excuse their acts because, as men, they are unable to control their violent urges. Second, if men really were helpless puppets of their sexual urges, rape would be more universal than it is. While rape is all too common, men with healthy sexual drives do not rape.

Myth: *Men who rape are mentally ill.* This falsehood takes us back to the stereotype of the rapist as a deranged stranger hiding in the bushes or coming through a bedroom window in the middle of the night. Although repeat rapists may have psychopathic tendencies, which is a form of psychological disorder, they are not generally out of touch with the reality of the crime they are committing (Helfgott, 1997).

Truth: Only a very small percentage of rapes are by strangers, mentally ill or not. The vast majority of rapes, 80 to 90 percent in fact, are committed by someone the victim knows, is dating, or is involved with in a romantic relationship. Believing that all rapists are mentally ill leads to a dangerous perception that potential rapists can be identified by their deviant behavior. This may lull potential victims into a false sense of safety with acquaintances, dates, or partners who are clearly not mentally ill but with whom the threat of rape is, statistically, the greatest.

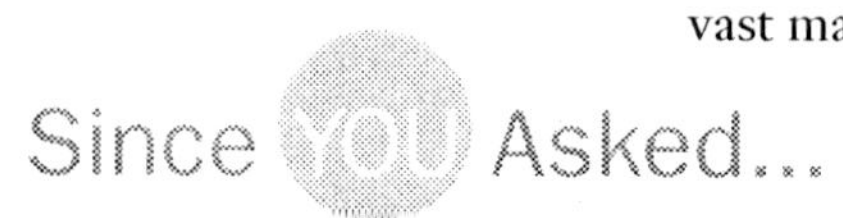

5. I've heard that some women really want to be raped because that way they can have sex without taking any responsibility for it.

Myth: *Women secretly want to be raped.* This belief stems from fictional novels, movies, and magazine stories as well as from the fact that some women's sexual fantasies involve rape motifs. The reasoning is that if women fantasize about being raped, they must, "deep down," really want to be forced to have sex.

Truth: Although it is true that some women have reported fantasies involving rape and that such fantasies are sometimes exploited in various media, this in no way implies that women want to be raped in real life (see Chapter 6, "Sexual Behaviors," for a more detailed discussion of this issue). First of all, many people entertain fantasies, sexual or otherwise, that they would never want to happen in reality (Leitenberg & Henning, 1995; Reinisch, 1990). Furthermore, in a fantasy of forced sex, the fantasizer knows that it is not real and that she is not at any real risk of bodily harm. In fantasy, the fantasizer is in control, whereas in a real rape, all control is taken away by the rapist. Most women who fantasize about being raped actually maintain control in the fantasy by luring or seducing the pretend "attacker" and playing the role of victim, knowing she is ultimately in control of the entire episode (Strassberg & Lockerd, 1998).

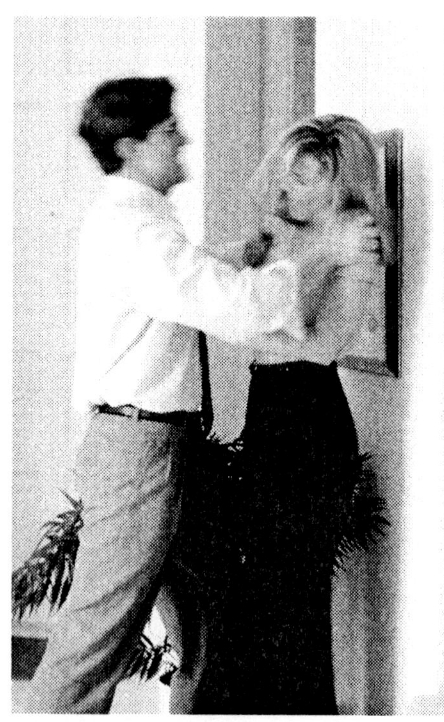

Threats of physical harm or death may intimidate a sexual assault victim to submit rather than fight back.

Myth: *Any woman can resist if she really wants to.* This ties in directly with the misguided belief that women who are raped in reality want to give in and that clearly saying no, repeatedly demanding that the attacker stop, and physically struggling and fighting against the attacker are only token resistance. This false belief assumes that a woman who truly wants to avoid being raped can do so by fighting, running, or repositioning her body.

Truth: This myth is full of flaws. First, men, on the whole, are physically stronger and heavier than women and are capable of pinning a woman down, forcibly removing her clothes, and penetrating her. Beyond this, however, rapists use threats of violence, actual violence such as hitting and punching, and weapons to create a situation in which fighting back is obviously futile and to intimidate their victims into submission. In addition, a common tactic of some rapists is to prey on women who are unable to resist due to extreme alcohol or other drug intoxication.

Myth: *Women falsely accuse men of rape.* The thinking here is that a woman may regret or feel guilty about having intercourse with a man, be angry with him, or be seeking revenge against him for some past offense, so she accuses him of raping her when no rape has taken place.

Truth: False reporting of rape is no more common than the false reporting of any violent crime; it is very rare. When it does happen, the woman nearly always recants before it is prosecuted. The exact opposite of this myth appears to be true. Many survivors of rape choose not to report the crime to authorities due to shame, guilt, fear of retaliation, or confusion over whether what happened to them was truly rape.

Myth: *Most rapes are committed by strangers.*

Truth: This is simply not true. To underscore the extent to which this myth fails to represent real life, take a look at Figure 13.2, which identifies the relationships of women to the men who forced them to engage in sexual acts of any kind against their will. Only 4 percent of the men were strangers; the rest were known to the victim—as acquaintances, dates, or intimate partners. Rapes committed by strangers are terrible and traumatic, but they are the exception, not the rule. The extent to which people perceive rape as primarily committed by strangers can reduce women's awareness of the much larger problem of rapes committed by men they already know.

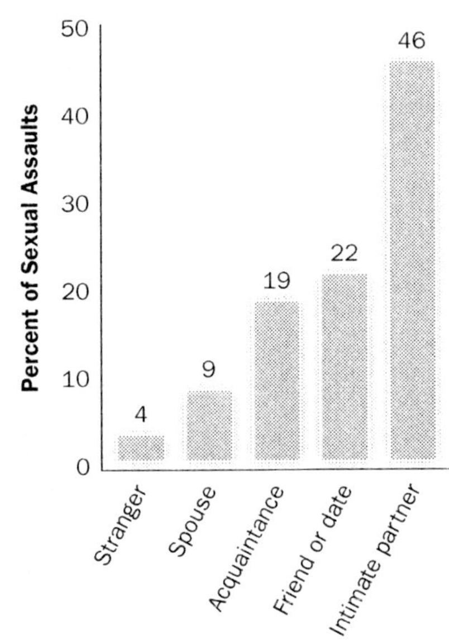

FIGURE 13.2 Relationships between Victims of Sexual Assault and Their Attackers

Source: Data from Laumann et al. (1994), p. 338.

Myth: *All men are capable of rape.* Again the subtext of this myth is that it is in men's nature to force sex and therefore it is up to the woman to protect herself from it.

Truth: The majority of men have not and would never engage in any sexually assaultive behaviors, including rape (Maxwell, Robinson, & Post, 2003). The number of victims of sexual assault is significantly higher than the number of perpetrators. Nevertheless, about a third of college men engage in behaviors that comprise sexual assault. This is a disturbingly high statistic, and we explore it in more depth next.

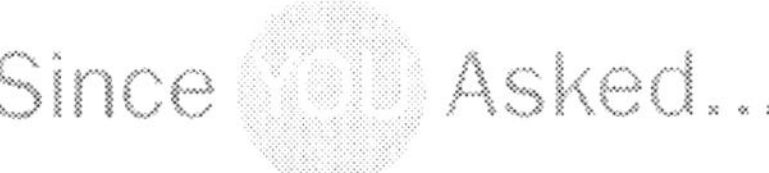

6. Someone told me that all men, if they got the chance and knew they would never be caught, would commit rape. Is that true?

Rape on Campus

Two facts about rape are clear: it is predominantly committed by a rapist who is acquainted, to some degree, with the victim, and the victims of rape are primarily young. While women of any age can be and are raped, nearly 62 percent of female victims are between the ages of 12 and 24; nearly 30 percent are aged 18 through 24 (see Figure 13.3). These two facts are due in large part to the unfortunate reality that rape is a widespread and serious problem on college campuses. During their college years, more than half of all college women are the victims of some form of sexual assault or sexual coercion, and between 20 and 25 percent are raped (Fisher, Cullen, & Turner 2000; Ottens, 2001). Moreover, stranger rape is even more uncommon on campus than in the general population; only 3 percent of college rapes are committed by strangers. It follows, then, that nearly all rapes on college and university campuses occur between people who know each other (Binder, 2001). Why? What is turning college life into an environment of rape? Research has focused on several factors that contribute to the problem of rape on college campuses.

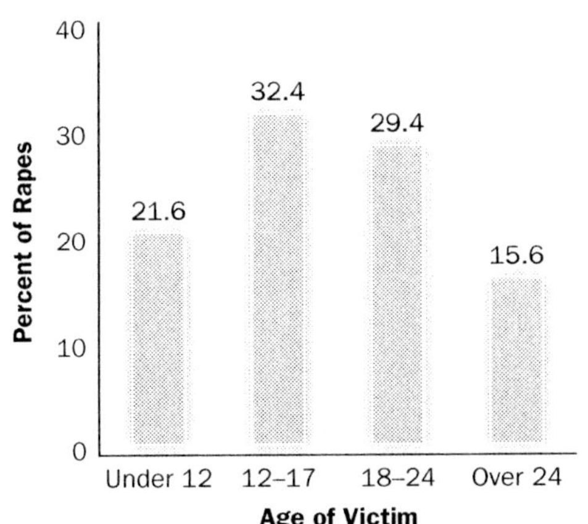

FIGURE 13.3 Female Victims of Rape, by Age

Source: Data from Tjaden & Thoennes (2000), p. 36.

The Alcohol-Rape Connection

Alcohol should never be seen as *causing* rape. Clearly, many men and women drink alcohol as a routine part of their social interactions and are never involved in sexual assaults. Conversely, rapes happen when neither the perpetrator nor the victim has had any alcohol at all. However, alcohol appears to play a frequent and

Since YOU Asked...

7. My roommate went to a party last weekend and got totally wasted (drunk). Two of the guys at the party told her that two other guys had sex with her while she was passed out, but she has no memory of this. Could this really have happened? Why would guys want to have sex with someone who is passed out?

important role in some rapes, especially acquaintance and date rapes, and in college rapes in particular (as do other drugs, which will be discussed shortly). Studies have shown that alcohol use by the victim or perpetrator is involved in up to 75 percent of all rapes (Abbey et al., 2001). A great deal of research suggests that alcohol facilitates rape on college and university campuses through a combination of the following factors (Abbey, 2002; Abbey, McAuslan, & Ross, 1998; Abbey et al., 2001; Carr & Van Deusen, 2004; Marchell, & Cummings, 2001; Mohler-Kuo et al., 2004; Ottens, 2001):

- Drinking alcohol goes hand in hand with college life. The percentage of college students who drink in excess is significantly higher than in the general population.
- Most alcohol use occurs in social settings, primarily parties at off-campus apartments or fraternity houses, where men and women go with the express purpose of meeting others, having fun, and getting drunk.
- Alcohol, as a drug, inhibits brain centers that are responsible for judgment, problem solving, impulse control, and recognizing the future consequences of behavior. When drinking, men are more likely to interpret a woman's friendliness as sexual interest and become less able to choose nonaggressive routes to sexual satisfaction.
- Alcohol is known to increase the tendency toward all forms of interpersonal aggression, especially in men, who are more aggressive in general.
- Alcohol increases a potential victim's vulnerability, mentally and physically. It interferes with a woman's ability to read a date's intentions and may cause her to assume he understands that she is not interested in sex when, also due to alcohol, he understands just the opposite. Furthermore, alcohol interferes with physical coordination and may limit a woman's ability to effectively resist a sexual attack. College judicial files are full of cases of rape in which the victim was too drunk to walk, had passed out, or was throwing up during the rape.
- Men use alcohol to exploit the vulnerability of potential victims. A common shared goal of men at fraternity parties is to get women drunk in order to loosen up their sexual inhibitions. Some male predators prey on women by keeping tabs on those who are drinking the most and becoming the most intoxicated and targeting them for sexual assault.
- Men believe that alcohol enhances their sexual prowess. Physiologically, of course, this is not true, but the *perception* of greater sexual abilities through alcohol use increases the likelihood of rape.
- Women who have been drinking at the time they were raped are often seen as less credible when reporting the assault. This is because many people mistakenly believe that if a woman was drinking, she shares the responsibility for being raped. In addition, alcohol in larger quantities often produces memory blackouts regardless of whether there was a loss of consciousness. A spotty memory of the events surrounding and during the rape makes investigation and prosecution of the perpetrator difficult. Knowing this, the victim is less likely to report the rape to authorities.
- Men who rape often use alcohol as an excuse to justify their behavior. According to one study, "A sexually predatory male who has stereotypic beliefs about gender roles and rape is inclined to view women as sexual objects . . . and misperceive friendliness as a sexual come-on because that is what he is hoping to find. He then feels comfortable forcing sex, especially if he feels led on or can attribute his actions to the effects of alcohol" (Abbey et al., 1998, p. 186).

Alcohol use and abuse contributes significantly to sexual aggression on college campuses.

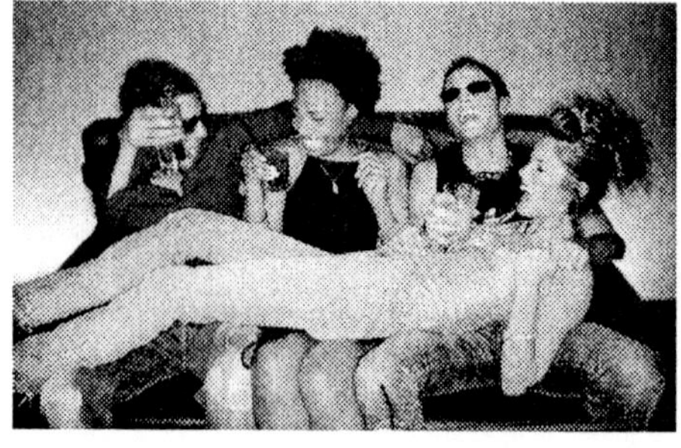

- A perception held by many sexually aggressive men is that women who drink moderate to heavy amounts of alcohol are fair game for sexual coercion in that by drinking they bring it on themselves.

Date Rape Drugs

Alcohol is not the only drug that plays a role in rape on college campuses, although it is the most common one. One of the most disturbing trends in sexual assault over the past decade has been the increased use of so-called **date rape drugs**, also sometimes referred to as "club drugs." These are powerful sedatives that render a potential victim unconscious or unable to move. They are referred to as date rape drugs because a sexual predator will sometimes slip a dose into a date's drink, making her defenseless against a sexual assault. When combined with alcohol, these drugs can be deadly.

Rohypnol pills, commonly known as "roofies," contain the tranquilizer flunitrazepam, which suppresses the wakefulness and pain receptors in the brain. In Europe, Rohypnol is prescribed as a sleeping pill or surgical preanesthetic; in the United States, it is illegal but is the most common date rape drug in current use (Abramovitz, 2001). In pill form, Rohypnol is white or off-white; when dissolved in liquid, it is impossible to detect by odor, taste, or color. It may also be obtained in a clear liquid form. In an effort to make the use of these drugs more discernible, the manufacturer now makes Rohypnol tablets that contain a blue dye and dissolve more slowly.

Gamma hydroxybutyrate (GHB), sometimes called "liquid ecstasy," is another drug that can be used to incapacitate a potential rape victim. This drug was legal in the United States, primarily as a body-building food supplement (Marsa, 2002), until the early 1990s, when the FDA banned its sale after studies revealed that it could be deadly. GHB comes in the form of an odorless, colorless liquid that tastes salty or a white powder or capsule. The strength of the drug varies according to who is manufacturing it and how it is formulated, but overall, the effects of GHB begin within ten minutes to one hour after ingestion. Low doses may have various effects including sleepiness, increased sex drive, memory loss, hallucinations, headache, and loss of muscle reflexes. Larger amounts may lead to nausea, vomiting, difficulty breathing, seizures, unconsciousness, coma, and even death (especially when combined with alcohol).

Ketamine, or ketamine hydrochloride, sometimes called Special K on the streets, is yet another drug used for rape. It was developed in the 1970s as a surgical anesthetic for humans and animals; it is now illegal to use in the United States except under a doctor's supervision. Taken orally, ketamine begins working in 10 to 20 minutes and can last up to 48 hours. Ketamine causes increases in heart rate, blood pressure, and oxygen consumption (Long, Nelson, & Hoffman, 2002). It has increased in popularity as a club drug because it may also cause hallucinations, memory loss, dreaminess, numbness, paralysis, and out-of body experiences. Recreational users of the drug call these out-of-body feelings "entering a K-hole."

In addition to sedating properties, these drugs produce an amnesia effect, so victims of a rape that occurred while under the drug's influence typically have no memory of the event. These are, obviously, dangerous drugs. They are physically and psychologically addictive and can lead to death, especially when used in combination with alcohol or other recreational drugs. When people ingest one of these drugs, they rarely know the exact dose they are receiving or what other dangerous chemicals may have been added, such as methamphetamines, LSD, or even drain cleaners. Moreover, some of these club drugs may cause long-term brain impairment, difficulties in balance and movement, and alterations in the senses (Abramovitz, 2001; Yambo et al., 2002).

date rape drugs Powerful sedatives that render a rapist's potential victim unconscious or otherwise unable to resist; also known as *club drugs*.

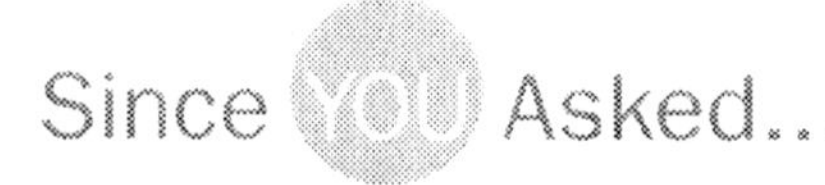

8. Is there any way to tell if someone has slipped a roofie into your drink (I mean, before you drink it)?

Federal and state laws have been enacted that provide severe penalties for the crime of drug-facilitated rape, and the drugs themselves are illegal substances in the United States. However, because the drugs are metabolized quickly by the body and are difficult to detect in the bloodstream the following day, combined with the fact that the victims have very vague memories or no memory at all of the attack, prosecution of drug rapists has been difficult. Interestingly, laws are being enacted on the state and federal levels to define alcohol as a rape drug; this could significantly increase prosecutions and penalties. "Sexuality, Ethics, and the Law: The Knockout Punch of Date Rape Drugs" offers a closer look at these drugs and how women can reduce their risk of victimization.

Underreporting of Rape

Rape is one of the most underreported crimes, and this is especially true on college campuses. Estimates of rapes that are not reported by victims range from 60 to 90 percent, and on some college and university campuses, the number may even be higher. One study of 140 women at Skidmore College in New York found that of the women who had experienced rape at the college, not a single one reported it to the authorities (Finkelson & Oswalt, 1995). Nonreporting is most common for acquaintance and date rapes. This is because many victims assume, wrongly, that maybe the assault "wasn't really rape," or that somehow she led him on or gave him "mixed signals" or "it was her fault" because she had been drinking. The judicial system that is in place on college campuses may also deter people from reporting sexual assaults. Victims may fear becoming involved in a long, public judicial or legal court proceeding; they may fear being harassed or threatened on campus by their assailant; or they may wish to avoid being judged negatively by friends, peers, or future potential dating partners. In short, victims choose not to report rape out of a perhaps justifiable fear of being victimized again. Perhaps more important from a psychological perspective, as many as one-third of rape victims never discuss the experience with anyone (Counseling Center for Human Development, 2001).

Whatever the reason, underreporting of rape is a serious problem for reducing rape on campus, for several reasons. First, without accurate statistics about the prevalence of rape on campus, school officials will be less likely to give the problem the attention and resources it clearly needs. Second, underreporting may lull potential victims into a false sense of security and cause them to fail to take the precautions to protect themselves from sexual assault that they would take if they were aware of the true numbers. Finally, and perhaps most important, men who rape rarely do so only once. For most, sexual violence represents a pattern of behavior over time and across situations. Obviously, as noted earlier, not all men rape. But when a rape goes unreported, the rapist goes unpunished for his behavior and is not only free to rape again but may even feel encouraged to do so, believing he has done nothing wrong.

The Sexual Coercion Culture of Some Fraternities

Not all fraternities and certainly not all fraternity members support rape. In fact, many fraternities have begun to take steps to reduce the incidence of rape both within the fraternity and throughout the larger college community. However, historically, fraternities and frat houses have been notorious for creating environments where rapes have been tolerated or even encouraged (Humphrey & Kahn, 2000). Although this sexually aggressive culture in fraternities is beginning to change, it continues to be the case at some colleges and universities.

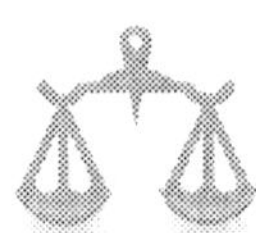

Sexuality, Ethics, and the Law

Date Rape Drugs

Jenna was having a great time at the off-campus party. Trevor, a cool and good-looking guy, was paying a lot of attention to her. She thought he might offer to drive her home.

"How about another beer?" Trevor asked.

"Sure," replied Jenna, a college sophomore new to the party circuit.

"Be right back with it," Trevor said

As she sipped the drink Trevor gave her, Jenna chatted happily and was surprised when she started feeling dizzy and drunk. This was only her second beer, and she usually didn't feel this way at all.

"Are you OK?" Trevor asked. "You look a bit shaky."

Jenna held her head in her hands. "No. . . . I don't feel well. I think I'd better go home."

"Why don't I give you a ride?" Trevor suggested.

"OK, thanks," Jenna said.

By the time they reached Jenna's house, she could barely stand up. Trevor carried her inside and put her on her bed. Then she passed out and woke up eight hours later feeling nauseated and shaky.

Jenna was surprised to find her clothes on the floor. She also ached all over, as if someone had hit her repeatedly. She tried desperately to remember what had happened, but her last memory was of Trevor driving her home from the party.

"Oh no, he must have raped me!" she whispered. "But how can I prove it? I don't remember anything."

Jenna had indeed been raped. Trevor had slipped a tablet of the drug Rohypnol into her drink at the party. The tablet had dissolved quickly, leaving no taste, odor, or color. Knowing what the drug would do to Jenna, Trevor had offered to drive her home with the intent of raping her.

Unfortunately, Jenna's experience has been happening more frequently to other women since Rohypnol and the other so-called date rape drugs (GHB and ketamine) were introduced into the United States in the early 1990s. Not only are these drugs themselves extremely dangerous, but the people who use them knowingly or unknowingly are subject to rape and other forms of abuse because of the powerful sedative effects. It's also difficult to prosecute those who commit rape after forcing their victims to ingest the drugs because these substances tend to erase the victim's memory of what happened. The drugs also move quickly through the body and often cannot be detected in blood or urine tests by the time the person gets to a hospital. . . .

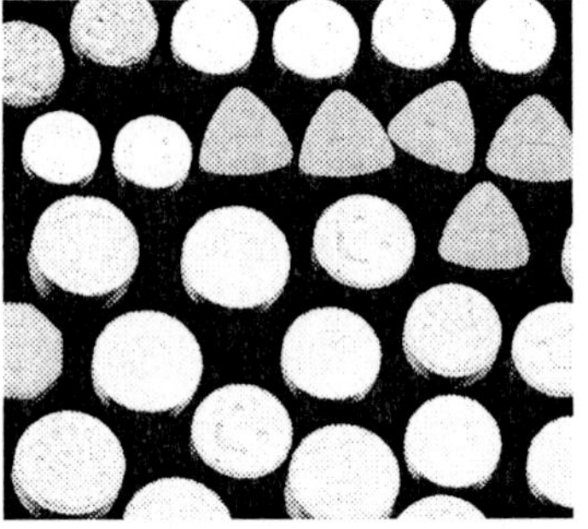

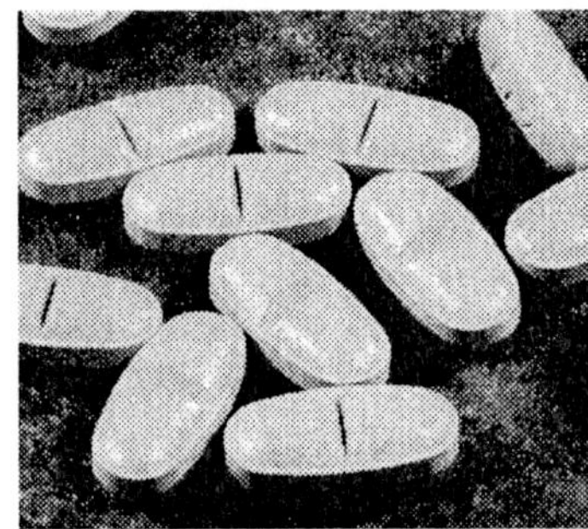

Date rape drugs come in many shapes and sizes, as well as in liquid form.

In 1996 the federal government passed a law called the Drug-Induced Rape Prevention and Punishment Act of 1996. This law makes it a felony to give an unsuspecting person a date rape drug with the intent of committing violence, including rape, against him or her. The law also imposes penalties of large fines and up to 20 years in prison for importing or distributing more than one gram of these drugs. However, even with this law in effect, the use of date rape drugs is growing. . . . These drugs are out there, and it's up to you to make sure you aren't a victim.

- Avoid parties where you know everyone will be drinking alcohol. It's more likely you would encounter date rape drugs on such occasions.
- Always keep your eye on your drink at any party or on a date. Don't put the drink down and leave it unattended, even to go to the restroom or to greet a friend on the other side of the room.
- Don't accept a drink of any sort from someone else, particularly if you don't know the person well.
- Never drink anything from an open container unless you opened it yourself.
- Don't drink anything from a punch bowl or other communal container like a keg.
- Go to parties with close friends and watch out for each other. If you leave the party, tell a friend where you're going and with whom.
- If you think someone drugged you, call 911 and get someone to take you to the hospital to be tested for drugs—and for rape treatment, [evidence collecting,] and counseling.

Source: Excerpted from Abramovitz (2001), pp. 18–21.

Researchers have suggested that some fraternities may encourage a "culture of rape" by rewarding coercive sexual behavior directly or indirectly through membership, acceptance, camaraderie, and a sense of belonging (Brown Sumner, & Nocera, 2002; Foubert & McEwan, 1998). Furthermore, the use of alcohol as a date rape "tool" may often be observed in the fraternity party setting. You can imagine how a fraternity party, where young adults are gathered for the purpose of meeting others, in an unsupervised location full of bedrooms and beds and where alcohol is flowing freely might combine to create an environment for rape (Ottens, 2001).

Various programs for reducing rape within the Greek system have been suggested and evaluated. Binder (2001) has pointed out that any rape prevention approach, to be effective, must be comprehensive and must address risk reduction strategies as well as alcohol and substance abuse issues and provide sexual assault awareness training. In addition, schools must develop clear policies, procedures, and consequences for sexual assault, and these must be distributed repeatedly and actively (that is, not merely stated in the student handbook) to everyone in the college community.

Binder also recommends greater monitoring of social events that may provide rape opportunities. This does not necessarily imply the presence of chaperones, something that most college students would avidly resist, but rather suggests that student leaders be responsible for specific controls such as selecting locales for social events so that overnight stays are not necessary, avoiding "common container" events ("keggers"), prohibiting alcohol at events on campus property, and challenging inappropriate party themes that may promote sexual aggression, such as wet T-shirt contests, drinking competitions, or games that involve removing articles of clothing as penalties.

Finally, Binder proposes that colleges and universities *anticipate* problem situations for sexual violence. Addressing the problem of rape on campus in proactive ways such as requiring workshops on sexual aggression for high-risk groups, including first-year women and new fraternity members, may help head off potential problems before they have a chance to occur.

A recent program designed to reduce the incidence of sexual assault focuses on all-male, high-risk groups such as fraternity members and college athletes. Mentors in Violence Prevention (MVP) concentrates on raising awareness of sexual violence, altering beliefs about women and sex, providing opportunities for open dialogue about sexual violence issues, motivating participants to become leaders in reducing sexual assaults, and inspiring immediate, on-the-scene bystander intervention in potential rapes and sexual assaults (O'Brien, 2001). The following exercise occurs early in the Mentors in Violence Prevention program. It is a visualization in which the team, fraternity members, or other all-male group is given the following instructions:

> "Take a few deep breaths. . . . Close your eyes and imagine the woman closest to you—your daughter, sister, mother, or girlfriend. . . . She may be at a party, in a room, or walking down the street when she is approached and sexually assaulted by a man. . . . Now imagine that there is a third person at the scene, a bystander who sees what's happening to the woman you love and is in a perfect position to help, but chooses to do nothing. . . . The bystander either watches or walks away." (O'Brien, 2001, p. 147)

The group is then asked: How did it feel to imagine the woman you care about being assaulted by that man? Ask yourself the same question. The response most commonly given by participants in this workshop are "helpless," "vengeful," "furious," and "confused." When asked to describe the bystander, typical characterizations are "gutless," "just as guilty as the attacker," "a punk," "a coward," and "scared." Later, members of the group are asked to place themselves in various scenarios in which they become the bystander to a sexual assault. You can see how their view of such a situation is often changed by the first visualization.

Another program targeting high-risk groups has been developed at the University of Maine; called Male Athletes Against Violence (MAAV), it is becoming a model for similar programs across the country. The mission statement for MAAV reads, in part:

> Change will come when we challenge the social norms and institutions that actively or implicitly condone and promote violence. MAAV is an effort to involve men so that we can begin to understand that [sexual] violence is very much a "man's issue" (MAAV, 2006).

Can We Predict Who Will Rape?

In taking precautions to protect themselves from sexual assault, many women want to know if warning signs exist that might alert them if an acquaintance or date might be a potential rapist. The answer appears to be a resounding maybe. Men who rape share some characteristics, attitudes, and behavior patterns, but little evidence exists that the tactic of "profiling" is an effective rape prevention strategy. Nevertheless, as part of an overall awareness of the risk of rape that exists for women, a general working knowledge of some of the possible "warning signs" of a "rapist personality" might raise a red flag of caution. These are admittedly generalizations, but a woman should be extra careful if a man she's seeing seems to be a very impulsive or aggressive person overall—for example, if he displays a need to dominate and control events around him; is emotionally abusive, discounts her opinions, insults or belittles her; is excessively and irrationally jealous; exhibits any physical violence toward her or others even if it's minor pushing, grabbing, or "pretend" fighting; believes in very traditional male and female roles; has a very short anger fuse; intimidates her by crowding her, blocking her way, or touching her in intimate ways without her consent; is fascinated with various weapons; abuses alcohol or other drugs; or bullies others or is cruel to animals or children (Harney & Muehlenhard, 1991; Prentky & Knight, 1991; Warshaw, 1994; Women's Services and Gender Research Center, 2005).

It is important to note here that a great many men have some of these characteristics but would never dream of sexually assaulting anyone. However, rapists seldom possess only a few of these traits; they will usually exhibit many of them. A working knowledge of this list will help women avoid risky situations with potentially dangerous men.

What to Do If You Are Raped

Ideally, neither you nor anyone you know or care about will ever have to face the trauma of rape. However, the reality is that nearly a quarter of all college students, primarily women, will be raped at some point by the end of their college years. Rape is a traumatic and terrifying event at the very least. Victims frequently have difficulty thinking clearly and are unsure what steps to take in the immediate aftermath of being victimized by rape. The truth is, what survivors *should* do is often quite different from what they probably *feel like* doing. The first reaction of many rape survivors is often denial and withdrawal. They want to be alone, shower or bathe, wash away any traces of the terrible event. The emotional jumble of confusion, pain, humiliation, embarrassment, anger, and powerlessness that typically accompanies rape often causes victims to wish they could just disappear and avoid seeing or talking to anyone. Although all of these reactions are understandable and normal, rape survivors should try to follow certain specific postrape guidelines (see "In Touch with Your Sexual Health: Guidelines for Rape Survivors"). Why? Because these guidelines can help survivors deal with and heal from the trauma of rape, and they may assist authorities in catching and prosecuting rapists and perhaps preventing them from victimizing others.

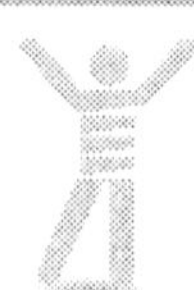

In Touch with Your Sexual Health

Guidelines for Rape Survivors

Many of the steps suggested here for survivors in the immediate aftermath of rape are difficult and often feel exactly the opposite of what the victim is emotionally inclined to do. However, following these guidelines can often help the survivor cope with the trauma and assist in the arrest and prosecution of the rapist, thereby preventing him from victimizing others. (Rape, Abuse, and Incest National Network, 2005).

1. **Call the police**. Reporting the assault as soon as you are safe allows the authorities to take an immediate description and collect evidence. Most police departments today are trained in proper and sensitive handling of survivors of rape and will not pressure you into any actions against the rapist that you are hesitant to take.
2. **Don't wash or douche**. Bathing, showering, douching (cleansing of the inside of the vagina with water or other solutions), washing hands, brushing teeth or hair, or changing bed linens or clothes may destroy evidence that will be important in charging, prosecuting, and punishing your attacker. Even if you feel you do not want to press charges or pursue the matter further, preserve evidence anyway, just in case you change your mind in the future (as many victims do).
3. **Seek medical attention immediately**. Here are four very important reasons why you should seek medical care as soon after the attack as possible:
   - You should be evaluated for physical or emotional injuries that may need professional attention.
   - Quick medical care allows for careful collection of various specimens and physical evidence that is crucial to any charges against and prosecution of your attacker.
   - While adding insult to injury, tests for some STDs can be done soon after the event, and many may be prevented with quick treatment.
   - Emergency contraceptive pills are now available if you were not using birth control and wish to reduce the risk of an unwanted pregnancy resulting from the attack.
4. **Seek counseling**. Remember rape is *never* the victim's fault. Call a local rape hotline in your area (they are listed in the phone book), and discuss your feelings with friends, family, religious advisers, or college counselors. If you feel uncomfortable talking to people near you, call the National Sexual Assault Hotline at (800) 656-HOPE (4673), or visit the Rape, Abuse, and Incest National Network Web site at http://www.rainn.org. Do not try to cope with this alone.

Again, if you are a victim of rape, you will probably be tempted to ignore all of these steps. Your hesitancy is normal and understandable. But if you follow these guidelines, you'll be much more likely to enhance your healing, speed your recovery, and help prevent a rapist from preying on other victims.

The Aftermath of Rape

Rape can profoundly affect its victims. Survivors of rape may experience shock over what happened to them, fear of their attacker or of a future such event, anxiety and depression due to the denial of personal control over their body that suffered, anger at the perpetrator or themselves that this could have happened, and even embarrassment, guilt, and shame stemming from the victim's (false) perception that the rape was somehow her fault (Funderburk, 2001; Lyons, 1997; Nordenberg, 2000; Wellesley Centers for Women, 1998). All of these feelings are normal reactions to a traumatic event. Any survivor of rape who is consumed by these feelings for a prolonged period should seek professional help. Sexual assault is a trauma that is often very hard to learn to live with. Survivors should ask for and accept help from people who care about them.

During the 1970s, the emotional, psychological, and physical reactions were at one time combined into a model that describes and explains the aftermath of rape, called the **rape trauma syndrome**. Survivors of rape and sexual assault were often diagnosed with this syndrome, which was considered a psychological disorder. Although rape trauma syndrome was controversial in that it appeared to pathologize the victim and is no longer an official clinical diagnosis, it offers a helpful framework for understanding some of the normal psychological and physiological responses of a victim of rape.

rape trauma syndrome A two-stage set of symptoms that follow the trauma of being raped, consisting of physical, emotional, and behavioral stress reactions.

The symptoms accompanying the trauma of rape may be divided into an immediate acute phase, typically lasting several weeks, and a longer reorganization and recovery phase, which may continue for many months or years. Rape trauma typically includes physical, emotional, and behavioral stress reactions that result from facing the life-threatening, violent, and traumatic event of rape (Burgess & Holmstrom, 1974; Washburn, 2003). In the acute phase, survivors experience intense and overt emotions of fear, anxiety, and anger. They typically also feel deeper, less obvious feelings of shock and numbness, which may in some cases hide survivors' true emotions. This phase also includes physical responses to the traumatic event, such as sleep disturbances, appetite and digestion problems, and various other pains and symptoms relating to the attack. As the acute phase progresses, survivors begin to experience more complex emotions that may alternate unpredictably between the fear and anger mentioned earlier and humiliation, degradation, shame, and guilt.

As more time passes, survivors enter the second, longer-term reorganization phase of recovery. This phase often includes changes in lifestyle—moving away, changing one's phone number, hiding out—anything that helps victims feel safer. They may get a dog, install alarms on their residence, find friends or family members to stay with, and even obtain weapons such as pepper spray, knives, or guns for personal protection.

In the reorganization phase, survivors also typically experience frightening nightmares reenacting the rape itself or portraying other situations in which the victims feel helpless and at the mercy of others. Fortunately, in most cases, as survivors heal emotionally and physically, the nightmares decrease, and as they become psychologically stronger, the images become less frightening. Survivors should know that it is OK to talk about the feeling and nightmares with friends and family or a counselor. Talking them through often reduces their power and renders them less scary.

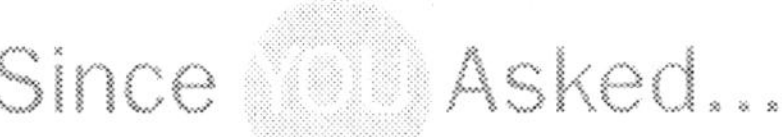

9. My sister was raped over three years ago, but she's still very upset and angry about it. What can she do to get over it? Will she ever get over it?

Finally, in the reorganization phase, survivors may develop phobias, irrationally strong fears of situations such as being in crowds, being alone, or beginning new potentially intimate relationships. The important point for survivors of rape to remember is that if the anxiety begins to control their life—for example, an irrational fear of dating or extreme social withdrawal—they need to seek professional help.

Preventing Rape

No one deserves to be raped, and as stressed before, it is *never* the victim's fault. However, every person is a potential victim, regardless of behavior, lifestyle, or personal characteristics. Some danger signs to watch for that may offer clues to potential rapists were listed earlier in this chapter. Beyond that awareness, everyone should incorporate as many strategies as possible to reduce the chances of being sexually assaulted. In "Self-Discovery: Staying Safe from Rape" are actions you can take to minimize your risk in various situations. The goal here is not to frighten or to suggest that you are somehow to blame but simply to enhance your safety.

Clearly, the issues of sexual assault and rape are seen far differently for most men and women. The precautions each sex takes and the attitudes and emotions of each sex surrounding these issues are as different as night and day. In fact, on this point, and perhaps various others relating to human sexuality, men and women have what could be described as separate cultures. Women have taken various actions to raise awareness of rape and to reduce its incidence (self-defense training, "take back the night" marches, alcohol and other drug dangers, etc.). The necessity of taking so many safety precautions against sexual assault may seem exasperating and terribly unjust. The frequency of these crimes, however, turns the cliché "better safe than sorry" into an unfortunate truism.

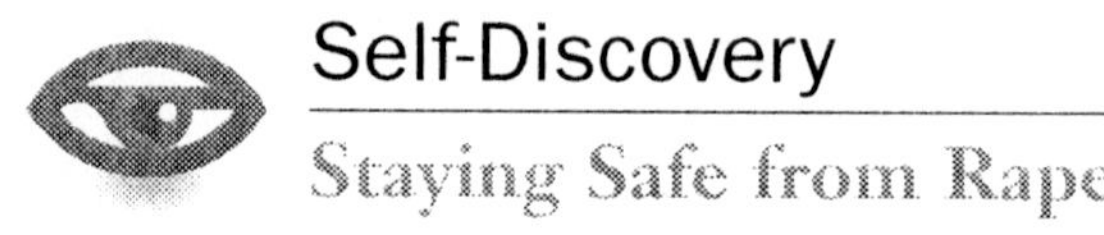

Self-Discovery

Staying Safe from Rape

Below are a number of precautions you can take to help protect yourself from becoming a victim of a sexual assault.

Safety While Dating	Safety at Home	Safety While Walking	Safety While Driving
Go to parties and other social events with friends, and agree to keep an eye on each other. Never leave your friend alone at a party, especially if she has been drinking, even if she tells you to do so.	List only your last name and initials in the phone directory and on your mailbox.	*Be aware and alert.* Always look around to see if you are being followed. If someone suspicious is behind or ahead of you, cross the street. Walk toward other people or lights. Don't be afraid to run.	When possible, travel on well-lighted streets.
Never leave a gathering with a man you do not know well. If you do leave with someone, be sure to tell a friend you are leaving and with whom.	Be sure to lock your doors when you are at home, even during the day.	Make eye contact with strangers. Don't look away or down.	Keep windows closed and doors locked at all times.
Make sure someone knows where you are, and check in with that person at a prearranged time.	Never open the door to your home automatically after a knock; require the caller to identify himself or herself. Use a deadbolt and door viewer for identification.	Walk near the curb, and avoid passing close to shrubbery, dark doorways, and other places of possible concealment.	Lock your doors immediately upon entering your car. This is a common moment of attack.
Avoid isolated areas. Be cautious of areas such as empty houses, abandoned buildings, "parking spots," and so on.	Leave a light on at night. Set a timer so a light will be on if you will be returning home after dark.	Avoid shortcuts through isolated areas.	Keep your car in gear while stopped at traffic lights and stop signs.
Trust your intuition. If someone scares you or creeps you out in any way, steer clear.	If a stranger asks to use your phone, do not let the person enter your home. Offer to make the call on his or her behalf.	Have your keys ready in your hand so that your house or car can be opened immediately. Lock the door *immediately* upon entering.	If you believe you are being followed, pull over to the curb where people are present and let the car pass. Wait a few minutes before proceeding. If the other car stays behind you, drive to the nearest police station, campus security office, fire station, or drive-through fast-food restaurant.
If you have concerns, consider double-dating the first few times you go out with someone you do not know well.	Do not leave your name or any unnecessary details about yourself or whereabouts on your answering machine. Consider using a prerecorded message in a male's voice and use "we" instead of "I."	When arriving home by taxi or in someone else's car, ask the driver to wait until you are safely inside.	If you are followed into your driveway at night, stay in your car with the doors locked until you can identify the occupants of the other car. If you are unsure, call the police.

Safety While Dating	Safety at Home	Safety While Walking	Safety While Driving
Be aware of your decreased ability to judge and react under the influence of alcohol or drugs; stay sober.	If a door or window is found forced open while you were away, do not enter. Silently leave and use a neighbor's phone or a cell phone to call the police. Wait until they arrive before entering.	Get to know the areas where you are likely to be walking. Know which stores and restaurants are open late in the evening. Watch for homes with lights on. If an attempt is made to attack you, run to these places.	Check under your car and in the backseat before entering. When parking, select a place that will be well lighted if you return after dark. After dark, always try to walk to your car with others. If no one is available, call campus security for an escort. Check for loiterers before leaving or entering your car. If you feel you are in danger, run away for help or sound your horn to get the attention of others.
Find out as much as possible about your date, particularly if it is a blind date or someone you do not know well.	Never hide a key on top of a door frame, in a flowerpot, under a door mat, or in any other obvious location.	Do not give directions or talk to strangers, even if they are well dressed or seem harmless.	
Never be afraid or hesitant to communicate *no* firmly and forcefully. When you say *no*, mean it, and don't change your mind. Set sexual limits, and communicate them clearly to your date.	Secure all doors and windows against forced entry as best you can. Keep emergency phone numbers posted for easy access. Call 911 if you fear someone is trying to break in.	If someone in a car pulls alongside and orders you to get in the car, don't go, even if the assailant has a weapon. Yell, scream, and run away in a zigzag pattern toward a barrier such as a tree or another car.	Never leave your keys in the ignition. Even if you park for only a short time, take them with you and be sure your car is locked.
Find out where you are going and what time you will be home, and then tell someone.	Ask local law enforcement to make regular drive-bys of your home for increased security. If you are in a sexually abusive (or any form of abusive) relationship, begin the process of leaving your abuser. (see Chapter 4, "Love, Intimacy, and Sexual Communication").	Get and carry a cell phone. If cost of a cell phone is a problem, low-cost phones for emergency-only use are available.	

Sources: Houston Area Women's Center (2005); Powell (1996).

It is important to add that it is not only women who should take precautions to reduce sexual violence. Men can play an important role as well. In fact, strong, caring men are often in the best position to help reduce the occurrence of rape. Men who rape are typically insecure and believe in the myth that sexual aggression is a way to express their masculinity to themselves and to their peers. Furthermore, as discussed earlier, some all-male settings, such as fraternities and men's athletic teams, tend to promote a culture of rape acceptance. If more men understand how they can help in toppling the systems and attitudes that support rape, some of the motivation for committing rapes will likely disappear. Here are some suggested guidelines that men might use to reduce or prevent sexual assaults and rape (Powell, 1996, p.150).

1. Get to know your date as a person (what a concept!). There is always time for sex; it doesn't have to be tonight. Besides, sex is better and safer when two people know each other first.

2. Avoiding making comments that treat women like sex objects; don't brag about sexual activities, and do not accept other men doing so. Call them on it. Ignore them. Or say, "I really do not want to hear that crap!"
3. Do not try to get women drunk for sexual manipulation, and don't allow others to do so either. Watch out for women's welfare at parties or other occasions where alcohol is present.
4. If your date is drunk, do not have sex with her. She is legally unable to consent to sex (or any other agreement) while intoxicated, and intercourse under those conditions may be considered rape, no matter what she says or does.
5. Remember that *no* means *no*, and if you're not sure, ask her what she does and does not want to do.
6. Never assume that she wants the same amount of sexual intimacy as you do. To you, kissing and touching may communicate a desire to move on to intercourse, but it may not mean that at all to her. Ask, "Are you comfortable with how things are going?" "How far do you want this to go?" It may sound corny, but most women love feeling honored and respected. In other words, don't assume that silence means "yes." Ask.
7. Communicate what you want. Are you unwilling to go out with her if there is no possibility of sexual intercourse? If not, you need to let her know that. If you are willing to wait for sex in the relationship, she needs to know that too.
8. If she doesn't want to have intercourse, that doesn't mean she doesn't want you. She is making choices about her sexual behavior, which may be very different from her romantic feelings about you.
9. You can stop! Things with your date may be hot and heavy; your desire for sex may be at a fever pitch. But if there is any doubt about her full consent, just stop. It might be frustrating, but it won't kill you. Consider this: imagine that your mother were to burst in on you when your desire was at its peak. You could stop, right?
10. Understand and be sensitive to the size and strength advantage you probably have over most women. Some women may feel intimidated and frightened by your physical presence without your even being aware of it. She might *feel* forced, even if you had no intention of forcing.
11. Spread this information to other men. Not only is rape violent and wrong, but it also carries major criminal penalties. Determining and proving the identity of a rapist today is as simple as a DNA test. Most rapists today and in the future will be caught, tried, and convicted. The days of "getting away with it" are over.
12. Support organizations of men that adopt antirape policies, and work to promote antirape policies in groups of men to which you belong.
13. If you know or suspect that a rape is being committed or may be committed, do everything in your power to intervene and stop it.

Child Sexual Abuse

Looking back at Figure 13.3, you will notice the stunning statistic that over 50 percent of female rape victims are under the age of 17 (Tjaden & Thoennes, 1998). Tragically, rape is only one of many types of sexually coercive behavior perpetrated by adults against children, both boys and girls. The sexual acts committed on children by adults include inappropriate kissing, fondling of the child's genitals, forcing the child to fondle the genitals of the adult, oral sex on the child, forcing the child to perform oral sex on the adult, vaginal penetration with the child, and anal sex with the child.

child sexual abuse (CSA) The sexual victimization of a child by an adult or a significantly older child.

pedophilia Uncontrollable sexual compulsions involving children.

Child sexual abuse (CSA) typically falls into three main categories, all of which involve the sexual victimization of children. **Pedophilia** is a psychological disorder in which a person experiences uncontrollable sexual compulsions involving children (see also Chapter 14, "Paraphilias"). **Child molestation** refers to sexual acts with a child by an adult or a much older child, regardless of a clear diagnosis of pedophilia. Both of these involve the sexual abuse of a child by a nonrelative. The third type of child sexual abuse, **incest**, involves a perpetrator who is a relative, such as a parent, aunt, uncle, grandparent, brother, or sister.

Sexual abusers of children typically do not use violence or physical force to achieve their goals; rather they rely on their position of greater power and threats of punishment if the child refuses or threatens to expose the adult's acts. Like rape, child sexual abuse is commonly less an act of sex than an expression of power and control over someone of weaker status physically, emotionally, and socially. And also as is true of rape, the vast majority of abusers are male, and they are almost always members of the victim's family or nonrelatives whom the child knows well (Gorey & Leslie, 1997; Knudsen, 1991; Laumann et al., 1994). Table 13.3 details the breakdown of the adult abusers' relationship to their child victims. You can see that only 7 percent of the women and 4 percent of the men reported that their childhood sexual abuser was a stranger, similar to the percentage of stranger rapes discussed earlier in this chapter.

As you might imagine, child victims of sexual coercion typically experience terrible fear, trauma, guilt, and the sad loss of innocence that accompanies such a betrayal by adults that they know, trust, and love. Let's take a closer look at this horrendous crime.

Who Are the Abusers?

Do sexual abusers of children share any predictive characteristics other than the high likelihood that they know or are related to their victims? The answer is yes, but no characteristic appears to be consistent enough to predict for sure who will prey sexually on children. You can probably remember news reports in which someone known as a "pillar of the community," a "wonderful parent," someone "trusted with children" or in some other respected position was discovered to be a child molester. When these stories appear, they invariably shake our trust in our ability to identify adults who might victimize our children. With that caution, here is what we do know about perpetrators of child sexual assault (Murray, 2000; R. Rodriguez, 1999; Seto, Lalumiere, & Kuban, 1999). Most are shy and relatively immature males who probably have been sexually abused themselves as children.

child molestation Any sexual act performed with a child by an adult or a much older child.

incest Molestation of a child by a blood relative such as a parent, aunt, uncle, grandparent, brother, or sister.

Table 13.3 ABUSERS' RELATIONSHIP TO THEIR VICTIMS

ABUSERS' RELATIONSHIP TO CHILD VICTIM	PERCENTAGE OF FEMALE VICTIMS	PERCENTAGE OF MALE VICTIMS
Family friend	29	40
Older brother	9	4
Father	7	1
Other relative	29	13
Stepfather	7	1
Older friend	1	4
Mother's boyfriend	2	1
Teacher	3	4
Stranger	7	4
Other	19	17

Note: Differences in frequencies between female and male victims were not statistically significant.

Source: Data from "Abusers' Relationships to Their Victims" from *The Social Organization of Sexuality* by E. Laumann, J. Gagnon, R. Michael, and S. Michaels. Copyright © 1994. Reprinted by permission of The University of Chicago Press.

They usually report that they are sexually aroused by children of both sexes and fear sexual relationships with adults. Most suffer from a number of psychological problems, especially anxiety disorders and depression. Typically, they know their victims and are usually family members or friends of the victim's family. Child sexual abusers live in relative isolation or with a parent and may abuse alcohol or other drugs. They are often unemployed or work in menial, low-paying jobs. It is not unusual for them to also engage in other atypical sexual behaviors, such as exhibitionism or sadomasochism. Ironically, some are devoutly religious and moralistic. Finally, the vast majority have engaged in a pattern of child sexual abuse with more than one victim and often many.

If you use this general description to construct an overall profile of a typical child molester, you may be slightly better prepared to suspect if someone in your child's circle is likely to victimize your child. But because predicting child sexual abuse is far from an exact science, suspecting innocent adults of such behavior is unjustifiable and harmful. The best advice is to be alert and attentive to the warning signs and never allow children to be alone with any adult you are suspicious of or do not know reasonably well. Awareness of the profile is probably worthwhile for parents, child care workers, and other adults who are responsible for the safety of children.

How Common Is Child Sexual Abuse?

Recently, in a sexuality class, during a discussion about childhood sexual abuse, a female student stated that she felt very lucky she had not suffered incest or molestation in her lifetime. Several other women in the class agreed that they felt fortunate as well to have escaped the trauma of sexual abuse. At that moment, the discussion abruptly ceased while the implications of what these women had said dawned on most of the class (a real discussion stopper!). Think about it: they felt lucky *not* to have been the victim of a crime that no child should ever have to face. Their feeling of being lucky grew out of the fact that they all knew at least one other woman who had been molested as a child (one student knew four). This was a nonscientific yet powerful demonstration of just how common child sexual abuse is.

Statistics for child molestation do exist, but as is true for adult rape, researchers agree that the numbers from any study are likely to distort the truth about child sexual abuse due to underreporting and variations in definitions. With that in mind, here are some estimates for the prevalence of child sexual abuse. Historically, surveys of adults conducted in North America have produced estimates for the prevalence of childhood sexual abuse ranging from 2 percent to 62 percent (Gorey & Leslie, 2001). Two studies from the late 1990s attempted to reanalyze data from numerous previous studies (a technique, you may recall, known as *meta-analysis*) also disagreed on the numbers. One study found 30 to 40 percent rates among women and 13 to 16 percent rates among men (Bolen & Scannapieco, 1999), while the other estimated 13 to 17 percent for women and 5 to 8 percent for men (Gorey & Leslie, 1997). A large survey from the mid-1990s found that 12 percent of the men and 17 percent of the women reported that they had experienced sexual contact with one or more adults when they were children (Laumann et al., 1994). A 2001 report from the Office of the Surgeon General (2001) estimates that 104,000 children become new victims of sexual abuse each year.

Because the numbers are so variable, perhaps the issue would be best served if researchers focused less on exactly how many children are victimized and concentrated more energy and resources on prevention and intervention. Regardless of the percentage that is closest to the truth, we know that a staggering number of victims were sexually abused as children in the United States alone. And of course, child sexual abuse is not limited by any means to this country. "Sexuality and Culture: Prevalence of Child Sexual Abuse in Selected Countries" summarizes statistics for this crime in various parts of the world.

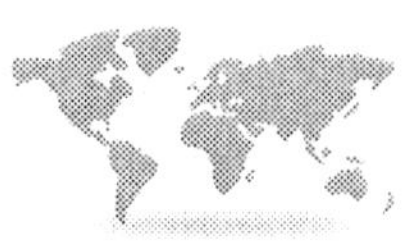

Sexuality and Culture

Prevalence of Child Sexual Abuse in Selected Countries

Country	Year of Study	Size and Description of Sample	Method	Any Child Sexual Abuse*	Contact-Only Sexual Abuse
Canada	1984	2,000; representative population aged 18+	Hand-delivered questionnaires	42% of women 25% of men	10% of girls under 14
Canada	1997	9,953; general population survey of Ontario residents aged 15+	Health survey: self-administered questionnaire as part of interview	12.8% of women 4.3% of men	11.1% of women 3.9% of men
Finland	1994	7,349; random sample of 15- and 16-year-olds in schools	Self-administered questionnaire in school nurse's room or classroom	8% of girls 3% of boys	—
Ireland	2003	3,118; random selection of adults	Telephone interviews	30.4% of women 23.6% of men	20.4% of women 16.2% of men
New Zealand	1996	1,019; community sample of 18-year-olds	Face-to-face interviews	17.3% of women 3.4% of men	13.0% of women 3.0% of men
Switzerland	1996	1,116; representative sample of Geneva adolescent school population, aged 13 to 17	Self-administered questionnaire	33.8% of girls 10.9% of boys	20.4% of girls 3.3% of boys
United Kingdom	2000	2,869; random probability sample of young adults aged 18 to 24	Computer-assisted personal and self-interviewing	21% of women 11% of men	16% of women 7% of men
United States	1987	3,132; two-stage probability sample of adults in Los Angeles	Mental health survey; face-to-face interviews	—	6.8% of women 3.8% of men
United States	1994	2,000; nationally representative community sample of 10- to 16-year-olds	Telephone interviews	15.3% of girls 5.9% of boys	6.9% of girls 1.0% of boys

*Includes noncontact instances of child sexual abuse, such as exposure (exhibitionism) and covert observation of children (voyeurism).

Source: Adapted from Creighton (2004).

Rather than overall numbers, more precise breakdowns of the abuse itself might be more useful and instructive. Table 13.4 details the specific behaviors comprising the sexual contact from a national survey published in 1994 (Laumann et al., 1994). From that same survey, we also have some information about the ages in childhood at which the sexual abuse occurred. These are contained in Table 13.5.

Table 13.4 CONTACT BEHAVIORS REPORTED BY SURVIVORS OF CHILD SEXUAL ABUSE

		PERCENTAGE REPORTING				
Sex of Survivor	Sex of Perpetrator	Kissing	Genital Touching	Oral Sexual Activities	Vaginal Intercourse	Anal Intercourse
Male	Male	10	82	30	—	18
Female	Male	31	90	10	14	1
Male	Female	64	82	10	42	0
Female	Female	25	92	0	—	—

Source: Data from "Percentage of Specific Contact Behaviors Among Survivors of Child Sexual Abuse" from *The Social Organization of Sexuality* by E. Laumann, J. Gagnon, R. Michael, and S. Michaels. Copyright © 1994. Reprinted by permission of The University of Chicago Press.

Table 13.5 AGE AT WHICH SEXUAL ABUSE OCCURRED

		VICTIM'S AGE		
Sex of Victim	Sex of Abuser	Percentage 6 Years and Under	Percentage 7 to 10 Years	Percentage 11 to 13 Years
Female	Male	33	40	27
Male	Male	30	46	24
Male	Female	31	26	43

Note: There were too few reports of abuse of females by females for meaningful statistical analysis.

Source: Data from Table, "Age at Which Sexual Abuse Occurred" from *The Social Organization of Sexuality* by E. Laumann, J. Gagnon, R. Michael, and S. Michaels. Copyright © 1994. Reprinted by permission of The University of Chicago Press.

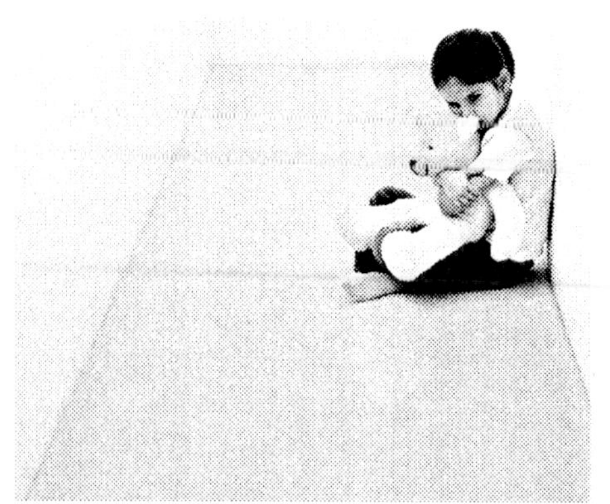

The trauma of child sexual abuse typically continues far into the child's future life.

Effects of Child Sexual Abuse on the Victims

The list of short- and long-term negative consequences of childhood sexual abuse is depressingly lengthy. Nearly all research on the effects of CSA supports the fact that reverberations of the trauma last far beyond the abusive events—often for the victim's entire life. Specific reactions may be divided into several categories, including emotional distress, psychological disorders, relationship problems, and physical or medical complaints. While no survivor of CSA is likely to exhibit all of the effects discussed here, most will experience at least one; many will suffer from a combination of symptoms.

Emotional Distress

Most of the emotional disturbances manifested by CSA survivors stem from the perception, however false, that the abuse was somehow the victim's fault. Many victimized children are haunted into adulthood with the notion that they somehow allowed the abuse to happen; that they didn't report the abuser and that due to their silence, no one rescued them; or that perhaps in some way they had enjoyed it. Many survivors see themselves as bad, immoral, or sexually perverted—"damaged goods," not worthy of being loved or treated well by an intimate partner. In many cases, this may lead them into abusive relationships in adulthood.

The emotional distress experienced by survivors is usually increased by the fact that they keep the abuse a closely guarded secret. One study found that the average time span between the end of the abuse and the survivor's disclosure of it was 14 years (Roesler, 2000). Failure to disclose the abuse does not imply, of course, that it was in any way the child's fault. On the contrary, the child's motivation to keep the secret may be an integral part of the abuser's tactics. Abusers will convince children that telling anyone will cause great trouble, and the child (or the child and the abuser, if the abuser is a beloved family member) will be punished. Or the abuser will threaten the child with physical harm or harm to other family members or the family pets if the child tells anyone. Beyond this, however, children learn from experience that when there are two conflicting reports about anything, sexual or not, the adult is usually the one who is believed. When children do disclose the abuse, often events begin to unfold that in the child's eyes are even worse than the abuse, such as a father arrested and jailed, fights between parents, or the complete collapse of the family unit. These dynamics put tremendous pressure on children who report sexual abuse to retract their accusations, and research has indicated that as many as 80 percent of such children will withdraw all or part of their initial report (Roesler, 2000).

The burden of feeling at fault combined with minimal support over many years almost always leads to emotional problems for the victim, which include the following (Ray, 2001; Roberts, 1996; Roesler, 2000):

Anger—toward self, the abuser, or some other party who should have stopped the abuse but did not.

Poor self-esteem—due to the feeling that something must be wrong or bad in their character to have allowed the abuse to occur and to continue.

Self-blame—because the abuser was a beloved family member who "could do no wrong," and to blame the perpetrator would destroy the victim's ideal image of the abuser.

Shame—stemming from self-blame.

Guilt—over engaging in forbidden, immoral, sinful acts, the failure to tell anyone, or the perception of causing the abuse.

Self-hatred—as the feelings of self-blame, shame, and guilt erode self-esteem and self-image over time.

Isolation and loneliness—stemming from the belief that the victim is unworthy of love, closeness, and intimacy with another person.

Psychological Disorders

In addition to emotional suffering, the trauma of childhood sexual abuse leaves long-lasting psychological scars years and decades after the abuse has ended. Childhood sexual abuse, like rape, robs victims of their personal power and sense of control over their lives and their bodies. When we feel powerless and unable to control our own destinies, we invariably suffer from a wide range of psychological disorders, most notably, depression. In fact, depression may be defined as an individual's perception that personal control is gone; that no matter what actions one takes, one is powerless to control or change the outcomes in one's life (Dugan & Hock, 2006). Adding to the depression stemming from powerlessness is the sadness victims often experience over the loss of innocence and the loss of trust once held for the adult responsible for the violation. Virtually all of the following identified psychological effects of CSA are related to or follow directly from this depression (Bridgeland, Duane, & Stewart, 2001; Dugan & Hock, 2006; Kendall-Tackett, 2000; Lang, 1997; Laumann et al., 1994; Ray, 2001; Roberts, 1996; Roesler, 2000):

Self-destructive behavior—such as dangerous risk taking, self-mutilation (cutting, burning, etc.), unsafe promiscuous sexual behavior, eating disorders, or reckless or intoxicated driving.

Abuse of alcohol and other drugs—often as an attempt at self-medication to deaden depression, pain, or unpleasant emotional reactions.

Anxiety, panic, and phobic disorders—stemming from the abuse itself, from the fear that others may discover the past abuse that the victim feels compelled to keep hidden, from the fear and mistrust felt in all current relationships, or from the loneliness and isolation from which victims often suffer.

Denial—pretending, distorting reality, glossing over the truth, or refusal to accept or acknowledge having experienced CSA.

Dissociation—using various psychological escape mechanisms that alter or block out awareness and memory; symptoms may include "out of body" experiences; fantasies or daydreams that seem real; loss of awareness of blocks of time, from minutes to days; or in some cases of especially violent and sadistic abuse, the development of multiple personalities.

Posttraumatic stress disorder—a syndrome characterized by reliving the abuse ("flashbacks"); avoiding situations, thoughts, and feelings related to the abuse; "emotional numbing"; sleep disturbances; a heightened startle response; "hypervigilance"; and difficulty concentrating.

Learning disabilities—more common among CSA survivors than among the general population.

Suicidal behavior—including thinking about or planning suicide, attempting suicide, and succeeding at suicide, all more common among CSA survivors than among the population in general.

Since YOU Asked...

10. Can being sexually abused as a child prevent a person from having good relationships in adulthood? Do the effects of the abuse really last so long?

Adult Intimate Relationship Problems

It should come as no surprise that survivors of CSA often experience difficulty with close relationships in adulthood. In fact, of the four categories discussed here, relationship problems are the most commonly encountered aftereffects of CSA (physical and medical complaints run a very close second, however). Interpersonal problems experienced by former victims include unsafe sexual behaviors, sexual disorders, and sexual violence. Numerous specific relationship issues are more common among CSA survivors than among the general population (Dugan & Hock, 2006; Hollander, 2001b; Lang, 1997; Laumann et al., 1994; Meston, Heiman, & Trapnell, 1999; Ray, 2001; Roberts, 1996; Roesler, 2000):

Revictimization—a significantly greater chance of becoming a victim of sexual violence such as rape and partner abuse as adults.

Emotional distance—from intimate partners and often friends and family.

Less trust—in others in general, and in intimate partners in particular.

Feelings of danger in intimate relationships—an inability to feel safe and secure in an intimate relationship for fear of betrayal or harm.

Lack of enjoyment in sex—which for many survivors, reactivates the emotional trauma of the abuse, resulting in low or absent sexual desire; moreover, the body may react in ways that inhibit sexual responding altogether.

Anxiety over sexual performance—due to memories of abuse.

Specific sexual problems—such as those discussed in Chapter 7, "Sexual Problems and Solutions," including erectile disorder, inability to achieve orgasm, inhibited sexual arousal, vaginismus, and dyspareunia.

Forcing sex on a partner—as perpetrators of sexual assaults, rapes, and child sexual abuse.

Increased promiscuity—due at least in part to such factors as low self-esteem, lack of trust in intimate relationships, emotional distance, and the lack of feelings of a secure attachment.

Medical Consequences

Of course, if the abusive behaviors are particularly aggressive and violent, physical injury of the genitals, anus, rectum, mouth, and throat, as well as trauma to other parts of the body, may result, sometimes requiring medical treatment immediately or at some point later in life. Just as victims will work to keep the abuse a secret, they will suffer physical injuries in silence for fear of being "found out."

Beyond these acute medical injuries, however, recent research has demonstrated a variety of additional long-term medical consequences of CSA. All of the following medical ailments are found more frequently in survivors of CSA than in people in general. This does not necessarily imply that the abuse caused these problems directly; some of them may be secondary to the emotional and psychological issues associated with the abuse. Nevertheless, most of the long-term aftereffects among CSA survivors are medical (Berkowitz, 1998; Hollander, 2001b; Kendall-Tackett, 2000; Laumann et al., 1994; Ray, 2001; Roberts, 1996). The following are among the most common.

Alcoholism—possibly stemming from depression, anxiety, or low self-esteem.

Obesity—perhaps secondary to low self-worth, self-blame, avoidance of romantic or sexual entanglements, or self-destructive behavior.

Tobacco use—likely due to such issues as low self-worth, self-blame, avoidance of romantic or sexual entanglements, stress, or self-destructive behavior.

STIs—probably related to the combination of the greater number of sexual partners and the self-destructive practice of unsafe sexual behaviors.

Gastrointestinal problems—such as irritable bowel syndrome and others commonly precipitated by chronic anxiety.

Gynecological disorders—possibly related to the combination of greater number of sexual partners and the avoidance by survivors of gynecological exams due to reactivation of past sexual abuse experiences.

Chronic pain—such as headache, stomach pain, and pelvic pain, for which CSA survivors are treated by physicians and hospitalized in exceptionally high numbers.

Insomnia—often linked to stress, anxiety, and depression.

Eating disorders—perhaps arising from issues of powerlessness and lack of control, poor self-esteem and body image, self-destructive behavior, or depression.

Asthma—which may be triggered by psychological factors.

One further and very important health-related consequence of child sexual abuse is *avoidance of routine medical care*, especially gynecological exams or other exams such as breast exams, mammograms, dental exams, prostate exam, and colonoscopy, and tests that require any type of confinement, restriction, or other situations of powerlessness, such as MRIs and CT scans. These exams may remind survivors of specific abusive experiences. Paradoxically, survivors of CSA also tend to overuse other medical services. This relates to a phenomenon known as *somatization*, expressing traumatic psychological issues through physical complaints that produce real symptoms. These health differences between survivors and nonsurvivors are not subtle. One study of women members of an HMO found that among those who reported a history of sexual abuse, 83 percent suffered from depression, 35 percent were obese, 64 percent reported frequent gastrointestinal problems, 45 percent suffered from chronic headaches, and 13 percent had been diagnosed with asthma (Felitti, 1991). Some women suffered from more than one of these ailments. All of these rates were approximately twice the prevalence in nonabused women. In addition to the problems experienced by the survivors, many health medical practitioners, including physicians, nurses, and some counselors, are themselves uncomfortable when dealing with survivors of childhood sexual abuse (Roberts, 1996).

Reducing Child Sexual Abuse

The consensus regarding sexual abusers of children is that the behaviors tend toward compulsivity. That is, perpetrators find it very difficult to stop victimizing children, even if they sincerely want to. Typically, when a child molester is arrested and convicted, the "treatment" is jail or prison time. Very few penal systems offer therapy to offenders, and after their release, repeat offending is extremely common. One study found that within a period of 10 years following release from prison, 30 percent of child molesters are rearrested and, after 20 years, approximately 50 percent have become repeat offenders (Prentky et al., 1997). Furthermore, some child molesters have victimized hundreds of children. These offenders are referred to as *career sexual predators*.

Success in the treatment of child molesters has been notoriously poor. How can society prevent child molesters from victimizing more children? In the United States, three approaches are usually taken, either individually or in combination: (1) alter the abuser's behavior, (2) prevent abusers from gaining access to potential victims, and (3) help children understand how to recognize, avoid, resist, and report attempted molestation by an adult.

Surgical and Chemical Castration

Because child molesters tend to exhibit defensiveness and denial about their crimes and because they are often ordered against their will into treatment by the courts, therapy and counseling have shown poor treatment success overall. Consequently, voters and their elected representatives have begun to get tough. In 1996, California passed a law *requiring* surgical or chemical castration for repeat child molesters. The law took effect in January 1997, and since that time, several more states have passed similar statutes.

These laws provide that any child molester convicted two or more times must voluntarily agree to surgical or chemical castration as a condition of parole (Brienza, 1997). **Chemical castration** refers to regular injections of female hormones that effectively block the production of testosterone (usually the hormone is Depo-Provera, which is also used for contraception for women). In most states, if the inmate chooses, he may serve out his entire sentence rather than submit to the castration requirement. Several studies have demonstrated that the hormone injections are helpful, especially in conjunction with counseling, in reducing the risk that child sexual abusers and rapists will offend again. This is probably due to the fact that blocking testosterone significantly reduces male drives toward sex and aggression, which in turn helps them to control their violent urges toward children (Bradford & Greenberg, 1997). A newer drug, *triptorelin*, which produces the same testosterone-blocking effect but fewer negative side effects, is now available (Rosler & Witztum, 1998). As you might imagine, this treatment of child molesters is extremely controversial, and many legal rights groups, lawyers, and ethicists have denounced any form of castration as cruel and unusual punishment for any criminal no matter how horrific society views the crime. On the other side of the debate, victims and victims' families argue that these criminals must be stopped, and the welfare of their potential victims far outweighs any concern for the molesters' rights.

Isolating Child Molesters from Contact with Children

Child molesters are prevented from contact with children in two ways: imprisonment and notification laws. Repeat child molesters are often sentenced to lengthy prison terms. This, of course, removes them from society at large so that they are unable to victimize more children. However, in general, no attempt is made during incarceration to rehabilitate molesters, largely because of the widespread belief that such attempts are usually ineffectual. Some molesters themselves have admitted that if and when they are released, they will almost surely molest again.

The crime of child sexual abuse, if it does not involve extreme physical violence, is usually punishable with prison terms of five years or less. A disturbing question, therefore, is what should society do when these criminals have served their time and are released? Currently, in the United States, one answer is *Megan's law*. This law was named after Megan Kanka, a 7-year-old girl who in the early 1990s was raped and

chemical castration Blocking the production of testosterone in repeat sex offenders through the regular injection of female hormones.

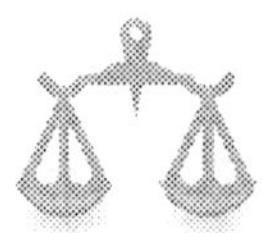

Sexuality, Ethics, and the Law

Megan's Law

Are convicted child molesters living in your community? All 50 states now have child molester notification laws, commonly referred to as "Megan's laws." All states post the names and addresses of convicted sex offenders on the Internet. If you want to know who and where convicted child molesters are in your community, the best place to begin is with your state's attorney general's office's Web site, or call your local police or sheriff's office for instructions. Here, for example, is a portion of such a Web site from California.

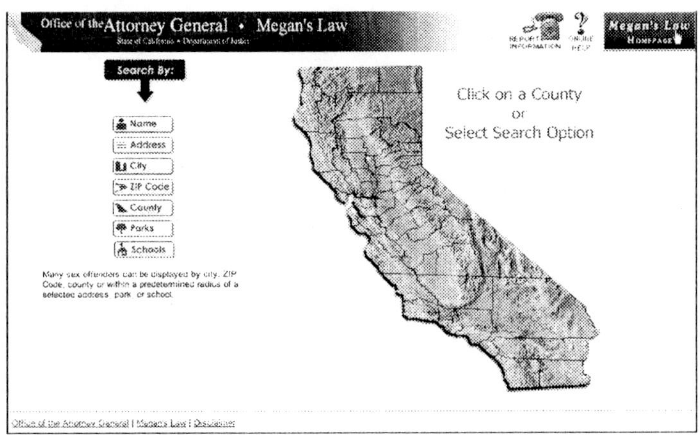

killed by a convicted child molester on parole who had moved into her neighborhood without anyone's knowledge. Since then, most states have enacted laws that require local communities to be notified when sex offenders are living in their residential area. The idea of this is not necessarily to punish the perpetrator but to allow residents to be aware and alert to the offenders' presence and protect their children accordingly. For more on this notification law, see "Sexuality, Ethics, and the Law: Megan's Law."

Teaching Children to Protect Themselves

Finally, many believe that child molestation may be effectively prevented in many cases through increased and improved education of children and their parents. Studies have suggested that when children participate in school- or home-based child sexual abuse prevention programs, they are less likely to be victimized (Putnam, 2003). Among college women, 8 percent of those who had participated in such a program had experienced sexual abuse, compared to 14 percent who were not involved in prevention education (Gibson & Leitenberg, 2000). Prevention programs typically include "good touch, bad touch" awareness, helping children understand that they have the right to say no if anyone attempts to touch them inappropriately and impressing on children the importance of telling a trusted adult if anyone touches them, asks them to do something, or behaves in a way that makes them uncomfortable and insisting that they should tell even if the offending adult is a relative or warns the child not to tell anyone. Children also need to know that it is OK to take action to get away or to find help if a situation feels dangerous or uncomfortable: yell, scream, run away, seek help from a trusted adult. This information should be on an appropriate age level for the child, but parents should start them at a very young age, probably 3 or 4 years old. Then information should be updated and expanded on a yearly basis as the child and the potential dangers grow. Of course, many parents find discussion such as these difficult and fear scaring their child away from healthy relationships and touching. Many resources exist in books and on the Internet to assist parents and educators in this awareness education process.

Two of the best Web sites on CSA are from the Canadian Ministry of Health at http://canada.justice.gc.ca/en/dept/pub/ssh/, which includes an excellent downloadable book for children about child sexual abuse, *The Secret of the Silver Horse*, and the Child Abuse Prevention Center of Dutchess County in New York at http://www.child-abuse-prevention.org.

Sexual Harassment

The third and final category of victimization in this chapter is sexual harassment (relationship abuse and domestic violence are discussed in Chapter 4, "Love, Intimacy, and Sexual Communication"). Sexual harassment has become a common problem in work and educational environments throughout North America and elsewhere in the world. Some people might argue that compared to other forms of sexual aggression, sexual harassment is less serious and less damaging to victims. Although this may be true in some cases, many individuals who have been the victim of sexual harassment in school or on the job would emphatically disagree. The trauma and life disruption caused by sexual harassment may affect an individual in ways comparable to those discussed in relation to rape and child sexual abuse.

Defining Sexual Harassment

The crime of **sexual harassment** is defined by the U.S. government's Equal Employment Opportunity Commission (EEOC) as follows:

> Unwelcome advances, requests for sexual favors, and other verbal and physical conduct of a sexual nature constitute sexual harassment when (1) submission to such conduct is made explicitly or implicitly a term or condition of an individual's employment; (2) submission to or rejection of such conduct by individual is used as a basis for employment decisions affecting such individuals; or (3) such conduct has the purpose or effect of substantially interfering with an individual's work performance or creating an intimidating, hostile, or offensive work environment. (Stoddard et al., 2000, p. 1498)

If you stop for a moment to analyze this legal definition, you will notice that although it covers many behaviors and actions, we can boil it down to two categories of sexual harassment. The first is the requiring of sexual favors in exchange for some beneficial event (a job promotion, a raise, a good job evaluation, etc.). This form of sexual harassment is commonly referred to using the expression **quid pro quo**, a Latin phrase meaning "this for that," or something required in exchange for a benefit or reward. The second category is the creation of a **hostile environment** due to unwanted, overt or covert sexually related activities. These definitions apply equally to educational environments where academic decisions (admissions, grades, letters of recommendation, etc.) may be on a quid pro quo basis between an instructor and a student or where an offensive or hostile educational environment has been created through words or actions. Notice that the definition is not gender-specific and applies to a person of either sex harassing a person of either sex.

The difficulty here, as with most definitions, lies in interpreting the components of the definitions for a specific situation. For example, when do friendly or seemingly *consensual* interactions cross the line into sexual harassment territory? In an attempt to clarify this sticky problem, various refinements of the definition have been offered (Stoddard et al., 2000). Conduct of a sexual nature is more likely to be considered harassing if

- It is unwelcome, unsolicited, and offensive to the victim(s)
- It is repeated or becomes a pattern of behavior, particularly after a warning from the receiver that it was unwelcome or offensive
- The behavior involves any supervisor-subordinate relationship where the harasser is in a position of power over some aspect of the receiver's educational or professional career
- The conduct is extremely and flagrantly verbally hostile, physically abusive, disruptive, continuous, pervasive, or provoking
- Preferential treatment of some individuals in the workplace or classroom, based on their sexual actions, has a negative impact on others in the same environment

sexual harassment A pattern of unwelcome sexual advances, requests for sexual favors, or other verbal and physical conduct that is coercive or create a hostile work or educational environment.

quid pro quo Something given in exchange for a benefit or reward; with reference to sexual harassment, a situation in which a person in a position of power over another requires sexual favors in exchange of some beneficial outcome for the victim.

hostile environment A distressing work or educational environment resulting from overt or covert sexually related activities or intrusions.

- a "reasonable person" (in the legal definition) would likely be affected negatively by similar conduct in a similar situation. (Stoddard et al., 2000, p. 1498)

If you consider these various guidelines, you can see that sexual harassment is rarely a charge made for the occasional inappropriate sexual joke, an innocent flirtation, or a single friendly touch. Most sexual harassment charges are in response to very clear-cut and usually blatant offenses. By way of example, here are two case summaries of sexual harassment, the first demonstrating a quid pro quo situation and the second the creation of a hostile classroom environment.

Henry, a gay man, was hired at a bookstore in the town where he attended the state university, majoring in history. He knew and loved books and quickly became popular with the shop's customers for the advice and assistance he could offer them. Hester Grant, the store's owner and manager, seemed pleased with him and his work until she discovered his sexual orientation. Henry had never tried to hide that he was gay, but he had never seen any need to mention it to his boss. One day, Henry introduced Hester to his partner when he stopped by the store to go to lunch with Henry. From that day on, Hester's attitude toward Henry underwent a clear change. She became less flexible about his working hours, stopped seeking his advice about books to stock that would be in the high-demand area, and began spending less time in the store when Henry was there. Paradoxically, she also became flirtatious toward him. She would brush her hand across his back when she walked past and make remarks such as "Heeeey, Henry . . . " in a tauntingly inviting tone of voice or compliment him on his "sexy" clothes. Henry would try to make light of these events with comments such as "Watch it, Hester!" or "Hester, give me a break, would you?" and even, "Careful, Hester. That's sexual harassment, you know." But her teasing escalated. She began to suggest that the only reason he liked men was that he had never been with a really talented woman—like her. "Come on, Henry. Come to my apartment tonight; I'll show you just what you're missing." Henry finally quit his job, sued Hester for sexual harassment, and was awarded $700,000 in compensatory and punitive damages.

Professor Richard Flemming (not his real name) taught contemporary literature part time at a small private college in New England. One of his in-class activities was to have students read specific passages of novels and plays for class discussion and interpretation. He would call on individual members of the class and ask them to begin reading on a certain page and continue until he stopped them. He would then lecture or lead a discussion of the passage. Usually, his selection of students to read appeared to be random, except when a particular passage contained sexually explicit material. In these cases, he would invariably call on one of several attractive women students in the class. As the woman was reading the sexual passage aloud, he would smile and wink and raise his eyebrows at the men in the class, especially the athletes, who would smile, chuckle, and exchange glances with one another in response. As this pattern became established over several weeks, some of the women became so uncomfortable with the hostile environment in the classroom that they either stopped attending or dropped the course. Near the end of the semester, two of the female students who had stayed in the class reported Flemming's behavior to the sexual harassment mediators on campus. A review board was convened so that the identity of the students would be concealed because they feared reprisals from the instructor. The instructor was ordered to stop the behavior in question and undergo eight weeks of sexual harassment training before being allowed to teach another class at the college. He left the college at the end of that semester and never returned to his part-time position.

Little doubt or gray area may be found in these accounts of sexual harassment. Typically, most sexual harassment cases demonstrate this level of clarity.

Sexual Harassment Settings

As awareness of sexual harassment as a form of victimization has grown over the past 20 years, the variety of settings in which sexual harassment is commonly found has increased as well. Harassment used to be seen as primarily occurring between two people of unequal social power, such as supervisor-subordinate or professor-student (or president-intern). However, today it is generally accepted that sexual harassment may also occur between peers of equal or nearly equal power, regardless of the setting. Although the fact of one person sexually harassing another may occur virtually anywhere, several specific venues should be discussed. These are: K–12 schools, colleges and universities, and the workplace.

Sexual Harassment in Schools

Recently, awareness has been growing that adults are not the only ones to harass or to suffer from sexual harassment. Today, sexual harassment situations have been identified and supported by state and federal court findings in elementary, middle, and high schools. Sometimes the harassment takes the form of teachers or administrators discriminating against certain students because of their sex, but more often sexual harassment in the K–12 arena is about kids sexually harassing other kids. Believe it or not, approximately 80 percent of adolescent boys and girls report experiencing sexual harassment from their peers, and most of it occurs right under the noses of their teachers (D. Smith, 2001). Recent research suggests that some of what we have traditionally referred to as "bullying" appears to fit quite well into the definition of sexual harassment (Dickenson, 1999; Woods, 2001).

Sexual harassment in our schools appeared on the national radar screen in 1999 when the U.S. Supreme Court ruled that a school district that fails to prevent or is "deliberately indifferent" to student-on-student sexual harassment may be held financially responsible for the emotional and psychological damage caused by the harassing events (Taylor, 1999). The original suit was brought by the mother of LaShondra Davis against a school board in Georgia for the suffering her daughter endured over a five-month period during the fifth grade, caused by a fifth-grade boy. The boy allegedly touched the girl's breasts, rubbed against her suggestively, and repeatedly told her he wanted to have sex with her (although those were not the exact words he used). The lawsuit stated that LaShondra and her mother reported each incident to school officials, but the boy was never disciplined. Other common forms of peer harassment in schools include sexual graffiti about specific individuals, verbal taunting, rumor spreading, sexual teasing, intimidation, unwanted touching, sexual assault, and rape.

The Supreme Court decision placed all K–12 school districts in the United States on notice that they must take affirmative steps to protect their students, regardless of age, from possible peer sexual harassment. Peer sexual harassment is relatively uncommon in the elementary grades but appears to increase dramatically through the middle and high school years (Fuertes, 1998; Timmerman, 2004). Many schools have responded by enacting antiharassment and antibullying measures for preventing, identifying, intervening, and punishing harassing conduct (American Association of University Women; 2002; Meraviglia et al., 2003). However, many researchers contend that schools, especially at the secondary level, need to do more to stop the continuing high levels of peer sexual harassment (Stone & Couch, 2004).

Sexual Harassment at Colleges and Universities

Sexual harassment in higher education may take either form, quid pro quo or the creation of a hostile environment. And it may be perpetrated by individuals in positions of power, usually faculty members, on those with less power, the students; perhaps much more commonly, it takes the form of peer harassment, student on student. The problem is of epidemic proportions. Research has estimated that 30 percent of college students are sexually harassed each year,

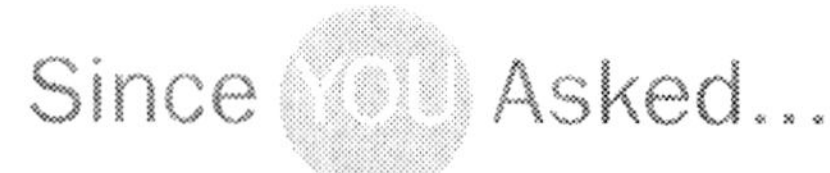

11. I heard that a professor was fired for sexual harassment. Is that true? What did he do?

and the number who have experienced at least one instance of sexual harassment while in college may be as high as 60 to 70 percent (Hippensteele & Pearson, 1999).

Reports of sexual relations between faculty (usually male) and students (usually female) are innumerable. Sometimes these liaisons grow out of an honest, free attraction between two people who just happen to be an instructor and a student. Unfortunately however, some college professors prey on their vulnerable students.

Today most colleges and universities have specific policies that limit or outright forbid faculty from engaging in such relationships, and college professors are beginning to get the message. However, some researchers, instructors, and college students themselves believe that it is not the university's business; they argue that if two consenting adults wish to become involved voluntarily in a relationship of any sort, it is their choice and indeed their right to do so (Paglia, 1998). However, the arguments against such relationships focus on the question of whether such relationships are truly voluntary; does the student really feel free to consent or refuse? If the student is currently in the faculty member's class, may be in the future, or may need to rely on the faculty member at some point for advice, academic counseling, letters of recommendation, and so on, the possibility always exists that the student will feel pressured, either subtly or explicitly, to submit to an instructor's advances. This is a clear example of sexual harassment based on different degrees of social power. If someone has the power to control your future, how free are you to say no to that person's request of you? Therefore, rather than try to judge who is being harassed and who is choosing freely, colleges and universities tend to avoid that labyrinth and simply make policies against such relationships.

Far more common is peer sexual harassment on college campuses. Both college men and women may be victims of peer sexual harassment, but the majority of cases reported involve a male harasser and a female victim. Typical behaviors associated with student-to-student harassment include such things as continually asking for dates even when the answer has been a clear no; an unwelcome pattern of waiting outside of classrooms, dining halls, and residence halls to "walk her home" or simply "say hi"; or even repeatedly stopping by her room, classroom, or apartment without consent. In addition, the harasser may make unwelcome sexual remarks about the woman's appearance or body and may suggestively rub against her and even touch her breasts or buttocks. Other harassing behaviors may include unwanted kissing; intimidating her by leering, making suggestive gestures, or blocking her freedom of movement; telephoning at all hours of the day or night; spreading unflattering sexual rumors about her ("bad-mouthing"); stalking her; sending numerous unwanted e-mails or voicemails; verbally abusing her following rejection; and rape or attempted rape.

Most colleges and universities have instituted policies that specifically prohibit sexual harassment between students, and a student perpetrator may be suspended, expelled, or arrested. The problem here is that most sexual harassment on campuses is hidden and insidious, so proving it is often difficult. However, if potential victims understand what constitutes sexually harassing behaviors, they will be in a much better position to prevent or stop such behaviors. Moreover, potential harassers need to be better informed about exactly what comments and behaviors are likely to be considered sexual harassment. Often men will make comments such as "I just can't say or do anything around here without someone accusing me of sexual harassment!" But this is usually far from the truth. Such statements simply underscore the lack of understanding many men still have about sexual harassment. "Self-Discovery: Defining Sexually Harassing Behaviors" offers guidelines for judging whether your behavior toward another person might be harassment.

Sexual Harassment at Work and in the Military

The workplace was where sexual harassment awareness originally began. Typically it took the form of a superior (boss, supervisor, ranking officer) using his or her position of power to intimidate and coerce subordinates into providing sexual favors as a condition of or in

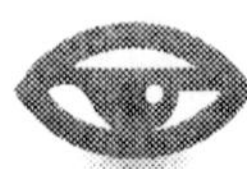

Self-Discovery

Defining Sexually Harassing Behaviors

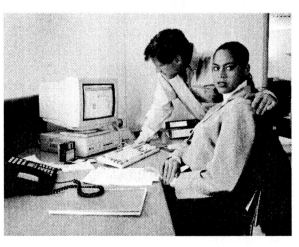

Sometimes a person may unintentionally engage in a sexually harassing behavior. Ask yourself the following questions to help you determine if your comments or actions toward another person might be interpreted as unwanted, inappropriate, or sexual harassing.

1. Would I want my comments and/or behaviors to appear in the newspaper or on TV so that my family and friends would know about them?
2. Is this something I would say or do if my mother, father, girlfriend, boyfriend, sister, brother, wife, or husband were present?
3. Would I be comfortable if someone else said or did this to my mother, father, girlfriend, boyfriend, sister, brother, wife, or husband?
4. Is this something I would say or do in front of the other person's boyfriend, girlfriend, wife, or husband?
5. Is there a commonly accepted difference in social status or power between me and the other person? Am I the person's boss, teacher, professor, counselor, priest?
6. Am I physically bigger or stronger than the other person?

If you are unsure about a certain action or comment, applying these questions *before* doing or saying it will probably help you make the right choice. If you answered yes to any of these questions, it should raise a red flag of warning. Remember, avoiding harassing behavior is about respect for others' feelings and comfort level, and when you substitute people you care deeply about for the target person, the appropriateness of your actions quickly becomes clearer.

Source: Excerpted and adapted from *Sexual Harassment and Teens: A Program for Positive Change by Susan Strauss*. Copyright © 1992. Published by Free Spirit Publishing. Reprinted by permission of Susan Strauss, http://www.straussconsult.com.

return for raises, promotions, better working conditions or schedules, or keeping a desirable position. While this quid pro quo form of power-based workplace sexual harassment continues to be a problem, the circumstances that may be defined as creating a hostile, intimidating, or offensive work environment have received greater attention recently. Anyone, at any level in an organization, may engage in behaviors that create a hostile environment, including military officers, executives, managers, supervisors, and peers.

Over the past decade, legal decisions involving sexual harassment have significantly broadened the scope of what constitutes sexual harassment and under what circumstances an organization may be held legally and financially responsible for it. For example, the U.S. Supreme Court has ruled that a business may be responsible for proven claims of sexual harassment regardless of whether it had any knowledge of the behavior in question. Also, if a manager threatens a subordinate who refuses sexual advances, the company is liable even if the threats are never carried out and the subordinate experiences no losses in income or job benefits. Furthermore, contrary to what most people believe, sexual harassment doesn't have to be about sex per se. Any actions that generate a work environment that is hostile, intimidating, or offensive to one gender may be defined as harassment (McGarvey, 1998).

As you might imagine, the laws prohibiting sexual harassment on the job and the penalties accompanying them have begun to sink into the national consciousness. The courts' advice to business, the military, and schools is this: "Have a clearly stated policy against sexual harassment, widely publicize it, and rigorously implement it, following up on all complaints. . . . In taking these steps, you're sending an unmistakable message: . . . Sexual harassment will not be tolerated" (McGarvey, 1998, pp. 86–87). Most U.S. businesses, corporations, and the armed forces now enact strict antiharassment policies and engage in extensive education programs for executives, managers, and workers in general to prevent harassment or, if it happens, to intervene and stop it as soon as possible (T. S. Nelson, 2003).

Effects of Sexual Harassment on the Victim

Many of the effects of sexual harassment on the victim are similar to those of rape and child sexual abuse discussed earlier in this chapter. However, sexual harassment clearly differs from other forms of sexual victimization in many ways, and consequently, the overall effects are unique. Victims of sexual harassment, regardless of the setting in which it occurs, experience a wide range of negative emotional and psychological repercussions, including a greater likelihood of depressive and anxiety disorders, higher rates of alcohol and drug abuse, insomnia, poor self-esteem, anger, poorer work or academic performance, greater absenteeism at work or in the classroom, and an increased probability of resigning from a job or dropping out of school (Hippensteele & Pearson, 1999; D. Smith, 2001; van Roosmalen & McDaniel, 1998).

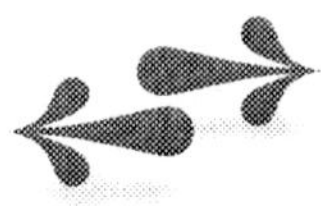

YOUR SEXUAL PHILOSOPHY

SEXUAL AGGRESSION AND VIOLENCE: RAPE, CHILD SEXUAL ABUSE, AND HARASSMENT

This chapter has been about a dark side of human sexuality, and now you know just how dark it can be. However, there is a brighter side to all this; it's called *prevention*. It's probably quite clear to you how the material in this chapter can be incorporated into your sexual philosophy. All you need to do is ask yourself a few basic questions: What steps will you take to help ensure that you or anyone you care about will never (or never again) be the victim of sexual aggression? How can you be totally sure that you will never (or never again) sexually victimize anyone else? How can you help yourself or others who are victims of sexual aggression or have been in the past? What will you do, personally, to contribute to reducing rape, child sexual abuse, and sexual harassment in our culture and around the world?

Working now to develop a clear sexual philosophy about the disturbing topics in this chapter will help you predict when a sexually dangerous situation exists or could develop. You will be able to make the best possible choices in situations where sexual aggression might unfold, and you will be more likely to take effective steps to prevent or intervene in it, whether you or someone else is the potential target. Those who are aware and vigilant about sexual aggression are significantly less likely to become victims or to victimize others.

You will also be more attuned to the possibility that child sexual abuse may be occurring within a family or other setting where children might be vulnerable. You'll be better able to notice suspicious signs of abuse and take action to protect children who are or might be sexually abused.

Finally, you will be able to spot sexual harassment wherever it might occur: in the classroom, on the campus, in the workplace, or in schools. Incorporating this knowledge into your sexual philosophy will not only reduce the chances that you will be sexually harassed but also help you determine what to do about it if you are. Furthermore, you will be far less likely to sexually harass others, you will be in a position to help those who are being harassed, and you will be able to contribute to the creation of policies in your school or workplace that reduce and eliminate sexual harassment.

Although all chapters in this book contain information that is crucial to your sexual philosophy, it's just possible the material in this chapter about *preventing* violence and abuse may be the most critical.

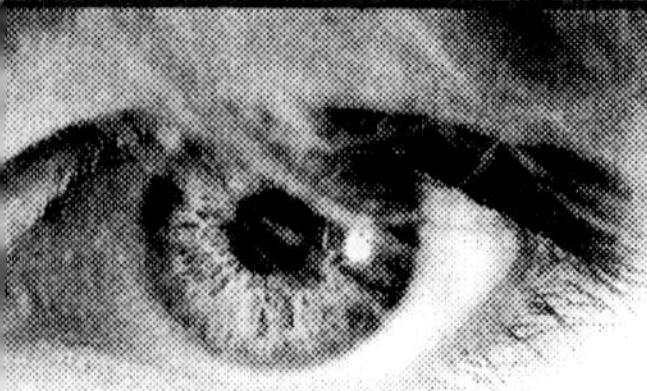

Summary

HISTORICAL PERSPECTIVES Marital Rape

- Forced sex in marriage was not considered rape in the past. Not until 1993 did the last of the 50 states include husband-wife rape in laws against rape. Prior to 1973, husbands who forced sexual acts on their wives were exempt from rape laws, as wives were considered their husband's "property."

Rape

- Rape may be defined as forced penetration of the vagina, mouth, or anus by a penis or any other object, although definitions may vary by state. Other nonconsensual sexual acts are often referred to as sexual assault.
- Most rapists are known to their assailants. By far the most common types of rapes (approximately 70 percent) occur between a perpetrator and victim who know each other through dating, friendship, or an intimate relationship. Only about 3 percent of rapes on college campuses are committed by strangers.
- Rapists and victims may be of either sex, but most rapes are committed by men against women. Rapes of men by men and, although rare, rapes of men by women do occur. Studies have found that approximately 22 percent of women and 2 percent of men have been victims of a forced sexual act.
- Rape myths typically blame the victim and remove responsibility for the crime from the perpetrator. Two common examples are "If she didn't want it, how come she dressed like that?" and "Women secretly want to be raped."
- The vast majority of rapes on college campuses occur in an atmosphere of heavy use of alcohol by the victim and usually also by the perpetrator.
- A diabolical trend on the dating scene is rapists who slip so-called date rape drugs into women's drinks, rendering them unconscious and unable to resist or even remember the sexual assault that follows.
- Some women who are victims of rape, in an attempt to put the trauma behind them, resist reporting the crime and having tests to collect evidence to arrest and convict their attackers.
- Unfortunately, the underreporting of rape is widespread and leaves rapists free to prey on more victims.
- A disproportionately large number of acquaintance rapes occur at fraternity house parties.
- Studies reveal that some college fraternities turn a blind eye to their "culture of rape," in essence encouraging rape through subtle or overt social rewards to their members for sexual assaults.
- Many emotional and psychological difficulties stem from the rape trauma syndrome. Effects on the victim may include shock, depression, shame, anger, guilt, embarrassment, posttraumatic stress disorder, and difficulties in forming and maintaining future intimate relationships.
- In a positive trend, more men are joining rape prevention efforts. Men may have a great deal of power to discourage behaviors among their peers and discourage environments that contribute to the incidence of rape.

Child Sexual Abuse

- The vast majority of child molesters are relatives of the child or people the child knows.
- The effects of child sexual abuse tend to be long-lasting and include emotional distress, psychological disorders, future relationship problems, and numerous medical conditions.
- All 50 states now have laws requiring repeat sexual offenders to undergo surgical or chemical castration as a condition of receiving parole.

Sexual Harassment

- Requiring sexual favors by a person in a position of power in exchange for a positive event or outcome for the subordinate is known as quid pro quo sexual harassment. When a person is made to feel uncomfortable in a work, military, or school setting due to a pattern of unwanted sexual behaviors, advances, or language, this form of sexual harassment is referred to as the creation of a hostile environment. Both types are illegal, and perpetrators are subject to criminal prosecution and civil remedies.
- The characteristics of bullying and sexual harassment have been shown to be similar, and both have been found in primary schools as well as in higher grade levels.
- Student-on-student sexual harassment is common on college campuses. When one student persists in unwanted advances toward another student, this often creates a hostile environment for the victim and is considered illegal under sexual harassment laws.
- The effects of sexual harassment are often similar to those of rape.

YOUR SEXUAL PHILOSOPHY: Sexual Aggression and Violence: Rape, Child Sexual Abuse, and Harassment

- Rape, child sexual abuse, and sexual harassment represent the dark side of human sexuality.
- Incorporating an understanding of factors related to sexual aggression and violence into your sexual philosophy may at first seem unnecessary. But such knowledge is power—in this case, the power to help stop the violence.

Have You Considered?

1. Imagine you are at a party and you notice a woman you do not know drinking beer after beer and a man whom she has met at the party encouraging her to drink more. He is watching her, touching her, and cheering her on. A little later, you see them off in corner where he rubbing against her and trying to kiss her. She is laughing but attempting, without much success, to push him away. Discuss how you think you would react to this situation. What are at least two courses of actions you might take?
2. If you were asked to give a workshop to first-year college *men* about dating violence and date rape, what three topics would you want to cover in the most detail? Why did you pick those three?
3. If you were asked to give a workshop to first-year college *women* about dating violence and date rape, what three topics would you want to cover in the most detail? Why did you pick those three?
4. Discuss at least three reasons why it is important for male or female victims of rape to go immediately to the hospital emergency room, preserve evidence, and press charges against their attackers.
5. How do you think society should deal with repeat sexual child molesters? Explain your answer.
6. Discuss what actions you might take if you suspected that someone in your neighborhood could be a pedophile.
7. Create a realistic scenario of student-on-student sexual harassment in a college setting in which the harasser is female and the victim is male. Include in your scenario how the problem might be resolved.

Companion Website Resources

For further chapter resources go to **www.prenhall.com/hock.** This robust text website includes polling questions for you to vote on, regular news updates, quizzes, sample tests, suggested reading lists, and more.

SCENARIOS USA Also on the website are links to videos. *Scenarios USA*'s films portray real-life narratives that explore the non-biological aspects of relationships and sexual health. The films will help you consider how the themes of the text affect your own life and the lives of those around you.

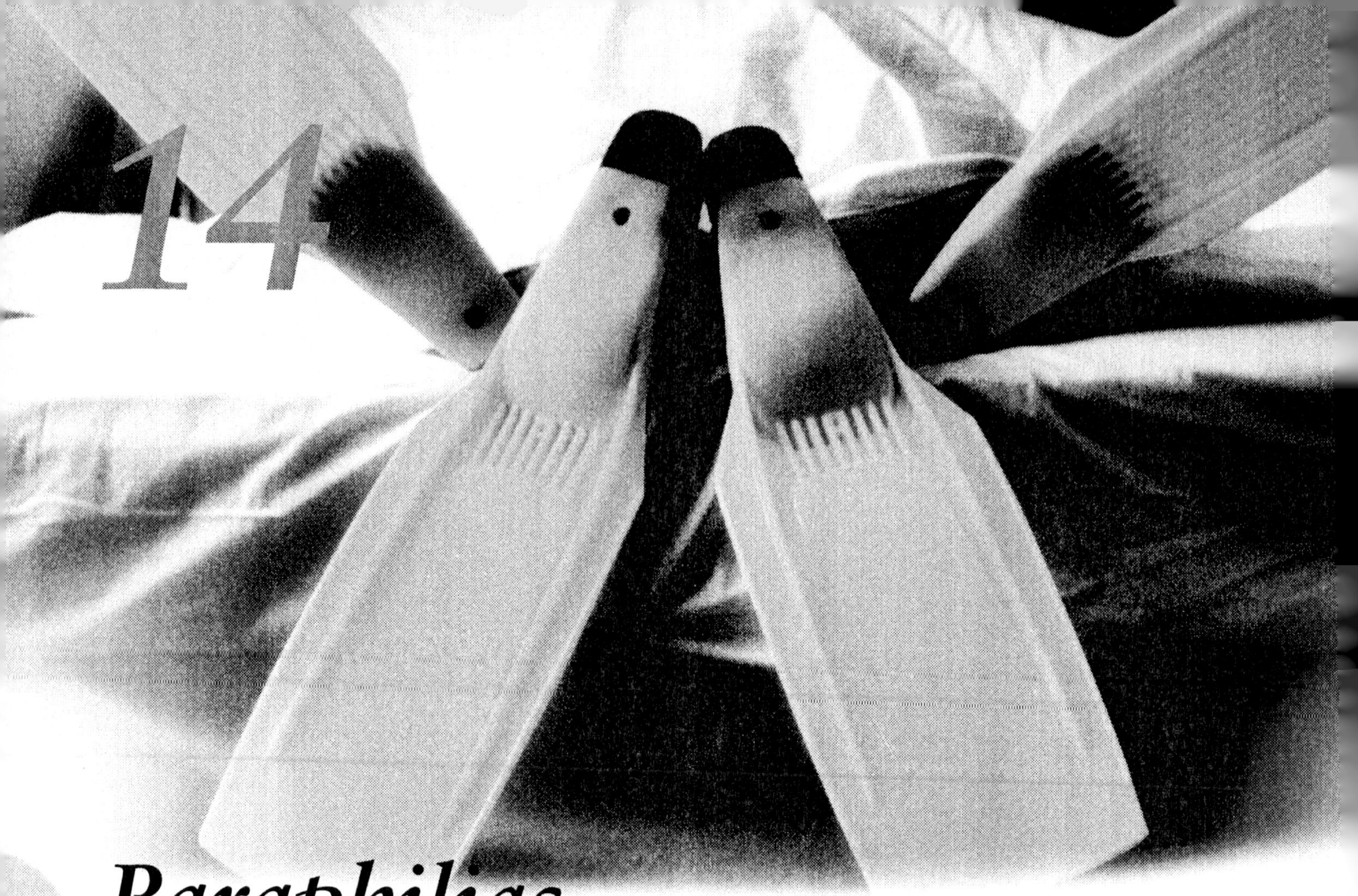

14

Paraphilias

The Extremes of Sexual Behavior

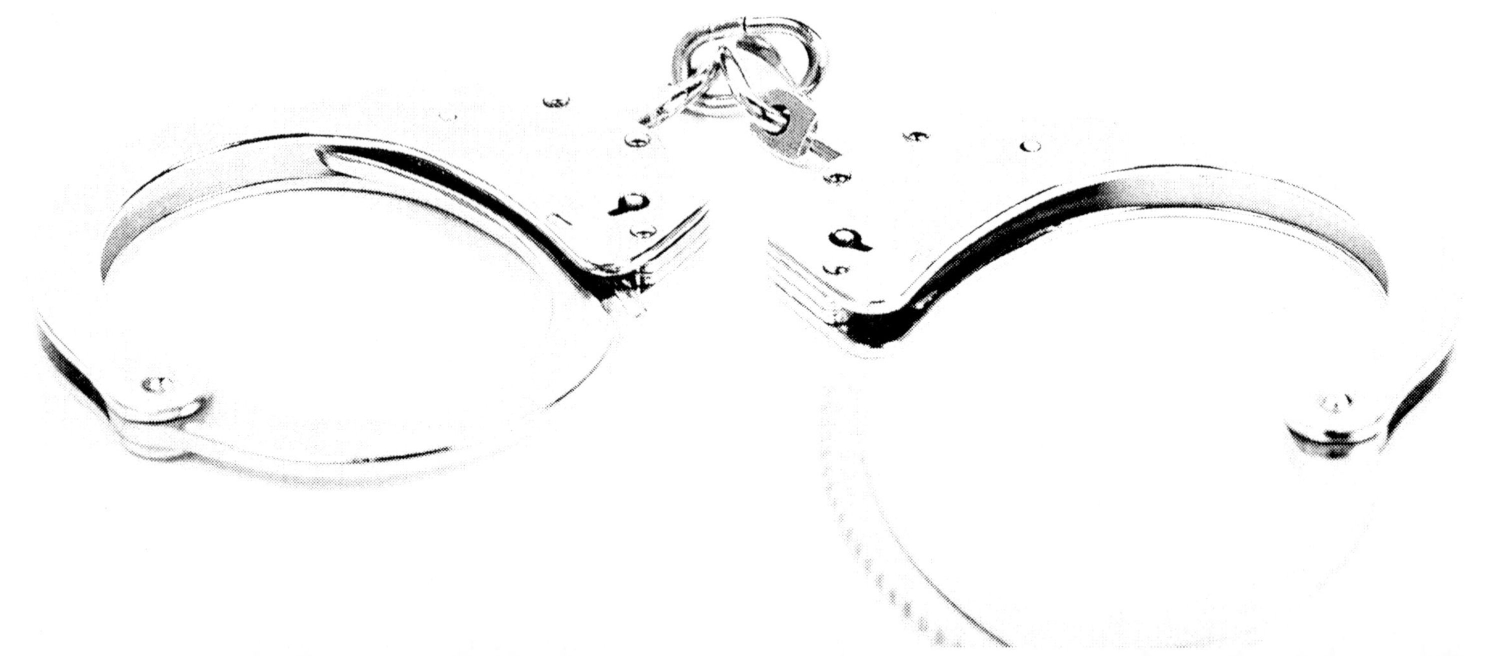

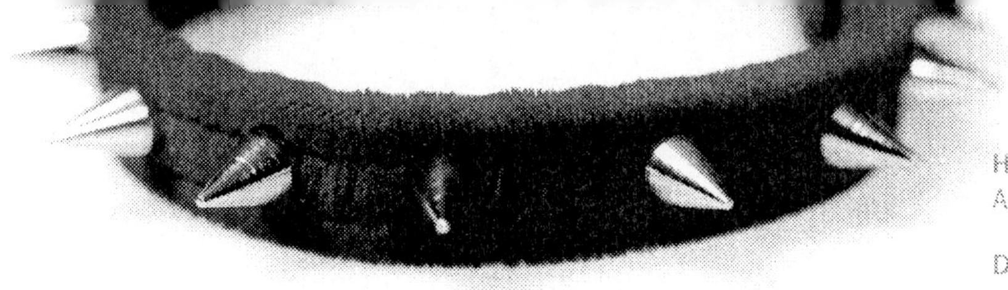

Since YOU Asked...

1. Sometimes my girlfriend and I like to do some things that are a little strange (like tying each other up and stuff). Is this really weird and perverted? (see page 519)

2. I get so angry reading about all the child abusers out there! Why don't we just lock them all up for life? (see page 521)

3. Last year, there was this guy who kept looking into girls' windows in the dorms (peeping Tom, right?). What is that all about? (see page 529)

4. I saw this movie (not porno) where a guy got off by rubbing up against women at concerts when everyone was crowding and pushing up to the stage. What is up with that? (see page 530)

5. I was sexually molested as a child. I never told anyone (until now). With all these stories about priests molesting kids, I think about it a lot and wonder why it happened. Do you think I should get some counseling to work through it? (see page 534)

6. I met a woman at a party. She told me that "on the side," meaning not her main job, I guess, she's a dominatrix. Does that mean what I think it means? (see page 537)

7. My mom has this friend who shops for shoes constantly. It's like if she's not eating or sleeping, she's shoe shopping. Is this what is meant by a shoe fetish? (see page 538)

8. I saw a movie on TV called *Rising Sun*. In the movie, a man strangles a woman during sex. It seemed that she wanted him to do it, but he did it too hard and killed her. Why would anyone want to be choked during sex? (see page 541)

9. Everyone in my neighborhood has received a notice that a convicted sex offender has been released from prison and will be moving near us. Of course, this news is scary. Can sex offenders be cured (I think he's an exhibitionist)? What are the chances he will do those acts again? (see page 544)

To understand the full range of human sexuality, we must extend our discussion out to the extremes of sexual behavior, to activities that are practiced by a small percentage of people and that most people would consider very odd and perhaps deviant or pathological. In this chapter, we explore a group of behaviors called **paraphilias**, sexual practices that may fascinate, repel, or even anger you. The prefix *para-*, from the Greek, means "faulty" or "abnormal," and *philia* means "attraction" or "love." Thus *paraphilia* literally means "abnormal love."

paraphilias Compulsive sexual activities that are practiced by a small percentage of people and that most members of a given culture would consider abnormal, deviant, or pathological.

In this chapter, we will explore in detail the criteria that define paraphilias, including their origins and the role of gender in these behaviors. We will consider each of the paraphilias individually within the context of two categories: those that are coercive and those that are noncoercive. We will follow with a discussion of treatments available. Finally, we will close with a look at how, perhaps surprisingly, even the paraphilias can be incorporated into your personal sexual philosophy. Before that, however, let's take a brief look at historical reports of some behaviors that are known today as paraphilias.

Historical Perspectives

An Early Account of Paraphilias

One of the first detailed accounts of paraphilic behaviors was in a medical text written in 1886, called *Psychopathia Sexualis*, by psychiatrist Richard von Krafft-Ebing. His 600-plus-page book consisted of 237 case studies of the kinds of sexual activities we will discuss in this chapter. *Psychopathia Sexualis* was a groundbreaking scientific study of sexual pathology that influenced many medical and psychiatric writers and researchers of his day, including Sigmund Freud. Most of the terms for various unusual sexual activities you will see in this chapter were developed by Krafft-Ebing. The book was republished in its entirety in 1998 (Rosen-Molina, 2001). Here are just two examples of the cases he describes (Krafft-Ebing & Klaf, 1998). The first involves a paraphilia called *zoophilia*:

> In a provincial town a man was caught having intercourse with a hen. He was thirty years old, and of high social position. The chickens had been dying one after another, and the man causing it had been "wanted" for a long time. To the question of the judge, as to the reason for such an act, the accused said that his genitals were so small that coitus with women was impossible. Medical examination showed that actually the genitals were extremely small. The man was mentally quite sound. There were no statements concerning any abnormalities at the time of puberty. (case 229)

Another case from *Psychopathia Sexualis* is about a type of behavior we now call a *fetish*:

> Z began to masturbate at the age of 12. From that time he could not see a woman's handkerchief without having orgasm and ejaculation. He was irresistibly compelled to possess himself of it. At that time he was a choir boy and used the handkerchiefs to masturbate within the bell tower close to the choir. But he chose only such handkerchiefs as had black and white borders or violet stripes running through them. At age 15, he had coitus. Later on he married. As a rule, he was potent only when he wound such a handkerchief around his penis. Often he

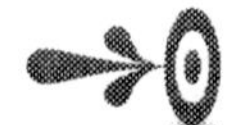

Focus on Your Feelings

Discussions about strange sexual behaviors known as paraphilias usually stir up strong emotional reactions in most of us. These feelings may include embarrassment that anyone would ever want to try such an activity, shock at how "abnormal" the behavior seems, anger at the people who engage in the activity, disgust over how disgusting the behavior sounds, and perhaps even arousal—because the idea of the activity, no matter how strange, may sound exciting to some people. Any of these and many other reactions to the material in this chapter are common and perfectly normal.

As you read this chapter, you may experience these or other strong feelings yourself. If you do, think about which paraphilias evoke your reactions and why you feel the way you do. Think about how your reactions to the various paraphilias might compare to those of your friends or others in your class. Talk to them about your feelings; compare "emotional notes." Understanding your reactions to unusual or "abnormal" sexual behaviors is extremely valuable if you ever find yourself confronting that particular behavior in your life. You can learn a lot about yourself by analyzing your reactions and thinking about whether they are appropriate and effective responses. This self-knowledge is also essential to understanding how you will incorporate learning about paraphilias into your sexual philosophy, which is discussed at the end of this chapter.

preferred coitus between the thighs of a woman where he had placed a handkerchief. Whenever he espied a handkerchief, he did not rest until he was in possession of it. He always had a number of them in his pockets and around his penis. (case 110)

From these examples, you can see that our knowledge of paraphilias is not at all new. However, exactly what behaviors qualify as paraphilias has changed markedly throughout history. Although many of Krafft-Ebing's sexual pathologies are still seen as paraphilias, others that Krafft-Ebing strongly condemned, including masturbation, oral sex, anal sex, and nonheterosexual activities, are seen today by nearly all sexuality educators, psychologists, and medical professionals as normal variations in sexual behaviors (Szasz, 2000).

Defining Paraphilias

Paraphilias are far more complex than "strange sexual acts" or than the word's more literary definition of "abnormal love." However, in general, it is usually fairly easy, using a few simple criteria, to analyze a particular behavior to see if it is likely to be a paraphilia. Beyond this, society applies standards to unusual sexual behaviors to determine how pathological, or deviant, they are. In addition, mental health professionals have their own set of formal criteria for diagnosing paraphilias.

Basic Criteria for a Paraphilia

A sexual activity may be considered a paraphilia if it meets *all three* of the following criteria:

1. The behavior is engaged in for the purpose of sexual arousal or gratification.
2. The behavior tends to be compulsive.
3. A clear majority of people in a given cultural setting would consider the behavior to be strange, deviant, or abnormal.

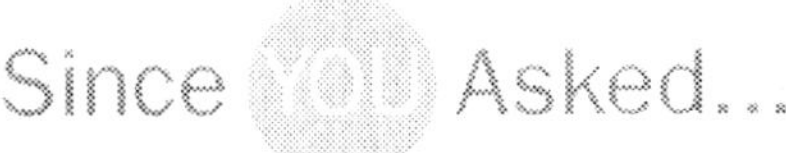

1. Sometimes my girlfriend and I like to do some things that are a little strange (like tying each other up and stuff). Is this really weird and perverted?

The first criterion is obvious: at least one of the primary reasons a person is engaging in the behavior is because it is a sexual turn-on. If a man sometimes slips into women's clothes but doing so is unconnected to sexual arousal or gratification, his cross-dressing is unlikely to be defined as a paraphilia (transvestism). Or if a person enjoys, say, walking around the house naked without bothering to close the curtains, this would not be a paraphilia (exhibitionism) unless the person is doing it with the goal of sexual excitement.

The second criterion of paraphilias is that they tend to be **compulsive behavior**. Any behavior, sexual or not, may for some people become compulsive. In essence, a compulsive behavior is one that controls the person instead of the other way around. Usually, it is a behavior that the person would like to stop doing but feels powerless to control. The destructive effects of compulsions may be seen in many behaviors, including compulsive drinking, compulsive gambling, and compulsive drug use.

The compulsive component of paraphilias is manifested in the inability to stop the undesirable behavior; even if the person is distressed by it and wants to stop it, he or she is unable to control it. Some people with paraphilias find themselves tormented after each occurrence of the act, vowing and promising themselves that they will never do that again. But then, as time passes, the obsessive thoughts creep back, the desire and need escalate, and they are irresistibly drawn back to the behavior once again. This compulsive aspect of paraphilias typically causes distress and dismay at being unable to resist the impulse. However, if a person

compulsive behavior Any behavior, sexual or otherwise, that a person is unable to control regardless of repeated attempts to do so.

engages in a strange sexual behavior once or twice and never has the desire to do so again or simply chooses not to, the behavior would not be characterized as a paraphilia.

The third criterion of paraphilias is what sets them apart from other sexual behaviors (even those that might meet the first two criteria). Paraphilias are sexual behaviors that would strike most people in a particular cultural setting as strange or abnormal. This judgment sounds subjective—you may be thinking, "What's strange to one person is mainstream to another" or "Who's to say what's abnormal anyway?" This is true of many human behaviors, but defining paraphilias is not as tricky as it seems. It is important to take into account the culture in which the behavior occurs, because societies are often surprisingly diverse in their social and sexual customs. That said, if you ask 100 people about virtually any of the paraphilias discussed in this chapter, the vast majority will agree that they are, indeed, strange or abnormal. Here we are not discussing a formal diagnostic meaning of abnormal but rather a cultural one (more on this in the next section). Table 14.1 lists some of the common and not-so-common paraphilias, just to give you a clearer idea of the types of behaviors we are discussing in this chapter.

With these criteria, you have the tools necessary to analyze any sexual behavior to decide if it meets the informal criteria for a paraphilia. Questions from students (usually in the anonymous "sex questions box") often ask if a particular behavior they have heard about or engaged in is a paraphilia. When the class applies the three criteria discussed here, usually (but not always) the behavior in question does not make the cut. The "Self-Discovery: Do *You* Have a Paraphilia?" applies these criteria to two paraphilias and will help you obtain a clearer idea of

Table 14.1 SOME WELL-DOCUMENTED PARAPHILIAS

NAME OF BEHAVIOR	TARGET OF SEXUAL ATTRACTION	TYPE OF ACTIVITY
Autoerotic asphyxia	Choking or strangulation during sexual activities and intercourse	Noncoercive
Coprophilia	Feces; excrement	Usually noncoercive
Exhibitionism	Displaying genitals or sexual acts to others without consent	Coercive
Fetishism	Nonliving objects or nonsexual body parts	Victimless
Formicophilia	Insects or other small crawling creatures	Victimless
Frottage or frotteurism	Rubbing genitals against another person without consent	Coercive
Gerontophilia	Elderly people	Coercive or noncoercive
Infantilism	Being treated as an infant	Noncoercive
Klismaphilia	Enemas	Victimless
Masochism	Receiving pain	Usually noncoercive
Necrophilia	Human corpses	Coercive
Pedophilia	Children	Coercive
Sadism	Inflicting pain on another	Coercive
Stigmatophilia	Piercing or scarring of genitals or nipples	Noncoercive
Telephone scatalogia	Obscene telephone calling	Coercive
Transvestism	Dressing in clothes of opposite sex	Victimless
Urophilia	Urine	Usually noncoercive
Voyeurism	Without consent, watching others undress or engage in sexual behavior	Coercive
Zoophilia	Animals	Debatable

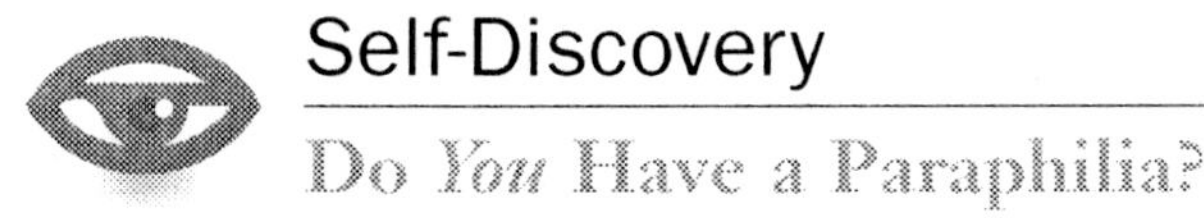

Self-Discovery

Do *You* Have a Paraphilia?

First of all, you probably *don't* have a paraphilia. Paraphilias are not all that common. However, many people worry that a sexual activity they enjoy, either in reality or in fantasy, might be "abnormal." Here is a self-test to help you get an idea if the sexual behavior you are concerned about might be diagnosable as a paraphilia. You can substitute any sexual behavior into the questions to get an idea if it might qualify as a paraphilia.

Paraphilia Self-Test

Question	Yes	No
1. Over a time period of at least six months, have you experienced strong, repeated urges, desires, or fantasies involving this sexual behavior?	____	____
2. Have you acted on your sexual urges or fantasies and actually engaged in this sexual behavior?	____	____
3. Have you been troubled, upset, guilty, or otherwise distressed about these urges or acts?	____	____
4. Have these urges or acts ever interfered with your education, occupation, or relationships with others?	____	____
5. Have these sexual urges or acts interfered with your ability to form and maintain *mutually* satisfying intimate or sexual relationships with others?	____	____
6. Do these activities involve nonconsenting victims, or have you ever been arrested or otherwise had trouble with the authorities due to these sexual behaviors?	____	____

Scoring: If you answered yes to question 1, yes to questions 2 or 3, and yes to 4, 5, or 6, you may have a paraphilia or a tendency toward developing one.

Source: Adapted from Cormier (1993).

how to judge for yourself whether a certain sexual behavior might be defined as paraphilia.

Society's Criteria for Judging Paraphilias

As a member of society, you are constantly making judgments about behavior, your own and that of others. But have you ever really thought about exactly what criteria you are applying when you make such judgments? When a culture or society looks at any human behavior, it does so through a lens of broadly shared norms and standards. The members of a given society apply those criteria in making a judgment about whether or not the behavior, in the eyes of the broader social context, is normal, moral, or acceptable (Goodman, 2001; Victor, 1998). Although not every individual member of a society necessarily agrees with the larger group's judgment, most clearly do. You probably already know about social judgments because at some point (or perhaps many points) in your life, you have engaged in a behavior (sexual or not) and felt extreme discomfort as those around you negatively judged you for whatever it was you did. Indeed, there are few categories of behavior on which members of societies place greater social judgment than sex.

Within the category of sex, the paraphilias probably receive among the most intense negative social judgments of all human behaviors. For judging "strange" sexual practices, all societies invoke numerous, often unspoken, guidelines. However, for the purposes of our discussion here, a paraphilia will be more likely to be judged negatively by a *society* when it is seen as

Since YOU Asked ...

2. I get so angry reading about all the child abusers out there! Why don't we just lock them all up for life?

meeting one or more of the following four criteria (refer as necessary to Table 14.1 for definitions of the paraphilias mentioned here):

1. *The behavior is harmful or destructive to the person engaging in it.* When a paraphilia is seen by society as harmful, either physically or emotionally, to the person doing it, that behavior will be judged in significantly more negative ways. Examples of paraphilias that fit into this category are a person who participates in extreme sexual masochism to the point of serious injury, scarring, or broken bones; a man who dresses in women's clothes in public and is ridiculed, scorned, rejected by his family, and fired from his job; or a teenager involved in autoerotic asphyxia behaviors (near strangulation during sexual activity).
2. *The behavior is illegal.* Laws are one way a society makes overt statements about acceptable and unacceptable behavior. It make sense that if the paraphilia involves behavior that is against the formal, written laws of the state, people will tend to judge it more harshly than if it is strange but not illegal. Illegal paraphilias generally involve victimization, as in the case of voyeurism, exhibitionism, pedophilia, and frottage (frotteurism).
3. *The behavior interferes with the person's ability to form and maintain loving, intimate, and sexual relationships with others.* In other words, if a person engages in paraphilic behavior *instead of* forming healthy intimate relationships with others, the sexual activity will be judged more negatively. On the other hand, if a person engages in certain *victimless* paraphilias and is able to develop and maintain a close loving relationship, he or she is typically judged less harshly by society for the strange sexual behavior.
4. *The behavior involves another person without that person's consent.* This standard may be the most important in determining how most societies will judge the "wrongness" of a paraphilia. As you will see when we discuss specific paraphilias, some are typically **consensual**, meaning entered into voluntarily by a partner, or **victimless**, meaning not harming or even involving a partner at all. An example of a typically consensual paraphilia is sexual masochism; by contrast, fetishism and transvestism are victimless paraphilias. Nonconsensual paraphilias, by definition, involve victimization and coercion of another person; examples include voyeurism, exhibitionism, frotteurism, and pedophilia. Nonconsensual paraphilic behaviors are likely to be illegal, whereas the legal status of consensual and victimless paraphilias varies from state to state and country to country.

Clinical Criteria for Paraphilias

If a person's behavior meets all three of the criteria for a paraphilia, does that imply that the person may be diagnosed with a psychological disorder? Although many or even most members of a society might feel that certain paraphilias are abnormal or "sick," formally diagnosing a psychological disorder is a more rigorous process. The *Diagnostic and Statistical Manual of Mental Disorders* of the American Psychiatric Association (2000), referred to as DSM-IV-TR, lists specific criteria for the diagnosis of certain paraphilias, including voyeurism, exhibitionism, fetishism, pedophilia, sexual masochism, sexual sadism, frottage (or frotteurism), and transvestic fetishism. These criteria are listed in Table 14.2. As you can see, they all share some similar characteristics: The person has experienced recurring, intense sexually arousing fantasies, sexual urges, or behaviors related to the paraphilia for a period of at least six months, the person has acted on those

consensual A behavior entered into voluntarily by all parties.

victimless Harming no one with the possible exception of the person performing the action.

Table 14.2 PSYCHOLOGICAL DIAGNOSTIC CRITERIA FOR PARAPHILIAS

PARAPHILIA	CRITERIA
Exhibitionism	• Over a period of at least six months, recurrent, intense sexually arousing fantasies, sexual urges, or behaviors involving the exposure of one's genitals to an unsuspecting stranger. • The person has acted on these urges, or the sexual urges or fantasies cause marked distress or interpersonal difficulty.
Fetishism	• Over a period of at least six months, recurrent, intense sexually arousing fantasies, sexual urges, or behaviors involving the use of nonliving objects (such as female undergarments). • The fantasies, sexual urges, or behaviors cause clinically significant distress or impairment in social, occupational, or other important areas of functioning. • The fetish objects are not limited to articles of female clothing used in cross-dressing (as in transvestic fetishism) or devices designed for the purpose of tactile genital stimulation (such as a vibrator).
Frotteurism	• Over a period of at least six months, recurrent, intense sexually arousing fantasies, sexual urges, or behaviors involving touching and rubbing against a nonconsenting person. • The person has acted on these urges, or the sexual urges or fantasies cause marked distress or interpersonal difficulty.
Pedophilia	• Over a period of at least six months, recurrent, intense sexually arousing fantasies, sexual urges, or behaviors involving sexual activity with a prepubescent child or children (generally age 13 years or younger). • The person has acted on these urges, or the sexual urges or fantasies cause marked distress or interpersonal difficulty. • The person is at least age 16 years and at least 5 years older than the victim. (Does not include an individual in late adolescence involved in an ongoing sexual relationship with a 12- or 13-year-old.)
Sexual Masochism	• Over a period of at least six months, recurrent, intense sexually arousing fantasies, sexual urges, or behaviors involving the act (real, not simulated) of being humiliated, beaten, bound, or otherwise made to suffer. • The fantasies, sexual urges, or behaviors cause clinically significant distress or impairment in social, occupational, or other important areas of functioning.
Sexual sadism	• Over a period of at least six months, recurrent, intense sexually arousing fantasies, sexual urges, or behaviors involving acts (real, not simulated) in which the psychological or physical suffering (including humiliation) of the victim is sexually exciting to the person. • The person has acted on these urges with a nonconsenting person, or the sexual urges or fantasies cause marked distress or interpersonal difficulty.
Transvestic fetishism	• Over a period of at least six months, in a heterosexual male, recurrent, intense sexually arousing fantasies, sexual urges, or behaviors involving cross-dressing. • The fantasies, sexual urges, or behaviors cause clinically significant distress or impairment in social, occupational, or other important areas of functioning. • If the person has persistent discomfort with gender role or identity, diagnosis becomes "Transvestic fetishism with gender dysphoria."
Voyeurism	• Over a period of at least six months, recurrent, intense sexually arousing fantasies, sexual urges, or behaviors involving the act of observing an unsuspecting person who is naked, in the process of disrobing, or engaging in sexual activity. • The person has acted on these urges, or the sexual urges or fantasies cause marked distress or interpersonal difficulty.

Source: Adapted from American Psychiatric Association (2000).

urges, and the urges have caused marked distress or interpersonal difficulties. The DSM-IV-TR allows for several of the victimizing paraphilias (exhibitionism, frotteurism, pedophilia, sexual sadism, and voyeurism) to be diagnosed as disorders if they are acted on, even if they do *not* cause distress or interpersonal difficulties for the person who engages in the behavior. The eight paraphilias in Table 14.2 are currently the only ones with *formal* psychological diagnostic criteria, but if you applied similar guidelines to any of the paraphilias mentioned in this chapter, you would be on the right track in making a determination about the behavior's level of psychological pathology.

Origins of Paraphilias

Upon first hearing or reading about paraphilias, your first question might be "How could someone acquire such an unusual sexual compulsion?" Explanations exist, but the research, or lack of it, points to one inescapable conclusion: Nobody really for sure knows what causes paraphilias. About all we can do here is consider some of the theories proposed to explain the development of paraphilias and let you draw your own conclusions.

First, it is probably safe to start with the assumption that no one is born with any particular sexual eccentricities but that unusual sexual attractions develop in one way or another during a person's life. Genetics may play a role in that some people may inherit a predisposition, a slight push from nature, toward compulsive behaviors in general, which in some may manifest in sexual acts. However, at this point in genetic research, it is doubtful that anyone is, say, a "born exhibitionist" (Bouchard, 1999).

That said, at least three theories—psychodynamic, behavioral, and biological—have been suggested to account for the development of a paraphilia (Barbaree, Marshall, & McCormick, 1998; Brannon, 2002; Friedrich & Gerber, 1994; Price et al., 2001; Wise, 1985).

Psychodynamic Theories of Paraphilias

Psychodynamic theories of human nature rest on the basic psychoanalytic ideas of Sigmund Freud, who contended that all dysfunctional or problematic behaviors in adulthood, sexual or otherwise, are caused by traumatic events that occurred in early childhood. The fundamental assumption here is that major developmental traumas or conflicts you may have encountered during your early formative years, from birth through about age 10, have been repressed into your unconscious in order to protect you from their disturbing nature. Because you repressed them into your unconscious, you are even now totally unaware that those conflicts exist. However, later, in adulthood, the theory maintains, those repressed traumas may exert powerful forces on your behavior and cause you to engage in socially unacceptable behaviors as your unconscious tries to resolve the tension they create.

In simplistic terms, for example, the psychodynamic approach might attempt to explain how a man who engages in voyeurism may have been severely punished or abused when, as a young child, he unknowingly walked into his parents' bedroom when they were naked or engaging in sexual activity. The theory claims that although the voyeur is unaware of the unconscious conflict caused by that childhood trauma, his compulsive desire to observe people undressing or engaging in sexual interactions may stem directly from it. Of course, any psychoanalyst would be quick to point out that the connections between childhood traumas and dysfunctional adult behavior are rarely so simplistic (L. J. Kaplan, 1997; Schott, 1995; Seth, 1997). Here is a summary of an article about a pantyhose fetish that appeared in a psychoanalytic professional journal called *Gender and Psychoanalysis* that will help you appreciate the flavor of the psychoanalytic approach to explaining paraphilias:

> In this paper . . . it is suggested that the wearing of pantyhose by males serves a range of functions, including, but not limited to, repairing psychic structure, an expression and defense against underlying aggression, enabling the development of symbol formation, allaying annihilation and separation anxiety, acting as a type of transitional object in terms of serving as a "second skin" component, soothing primitive anxieties related to the damaged body ego, and serving an erotic function involving desire and excitement. The function of pantyhose as a kind of "magic skin" or "second skin" suggests a relationship between perverse symptom

formation and the *development* of a "skin ego." Implications for the symbolizing function of this "magic or second skin" as a bridge to the mother figure is discussed in terms of theoretical and treatment issues. The functional use of pantyhose is viewed as a creative solution to a seemingly unresolvable interpersonal-intrapsychic dilemma. (Lothstein, 1997, p. 103)

Note that a strict psychoanalytic approach to studying and explaining human behavior has faded from favor as modern scientific psychology has grown and developed over the past century. Most modern-day psychologists find little validity in Freud's conceptualizations of human nature. Nevertheless, when sexuality researchers and educators discuss the possible causes of paraphilic compulsions, many allow that they may be rooted, at least to some extent, in certain childhood experiences (Suriano, 2002).

Behavioral Theories of Paraphilias

The behavioral approach to explaining the origins of paraphilias relies on the various components of classical and operant conditioning. If you have studied these learning theories in psychology classes, you'll recall that in *classical conditioning*, a response to a particular stimulus is learned (or conditioned) when that stimulus is paired with another event that naturally produces the response. An example of this as it relates to sexual behavior would be a person who finds a particular perfume fragrance to be an intense turn-on. This seemingly involuntary (or reflexive) physical response, from a behaviorism perspective, is not due to anything inherent in the perfume itself but rather came about through repeated pairings of the perfume with sexually arousing events, such as sexual touching, oral sex, or masturbation. And probably no one needs to tell you, these can be *very* powerful stimuli. Behaviorists contend that our personal, individual sexual histories determine our unique set of sexual likes and dislikes, preferences, and characteristic sexual inclinations. In other words, this is why no two people are sexually aroused by exactly the same patterns of situations and events. Behaviorists believe that this same process explains why some people engage in paraphilias. Somehow, somewhere during their sexual life, they learned to associate strong, highly pleasurable sexual arousal with the paraphilic behavior.

According to behaviorism, the sexual learning process is further strengthened through *operant conditioning*, in which a voluntary behavior is learned because it is followed by a rewarding consequence, referred to as *reinforcement*. This principle is, in essence, quite simple: Any behavior that occurs in a particular setting and is followed by a rewarding event (reinforcement) will be more likely to reoccur in the future in a similar setting. It's probably obvious to you how this form of conditioning plays a role in the development of paraphilias. Few events in life are more rewarding (reinforcing) than an orgasm!

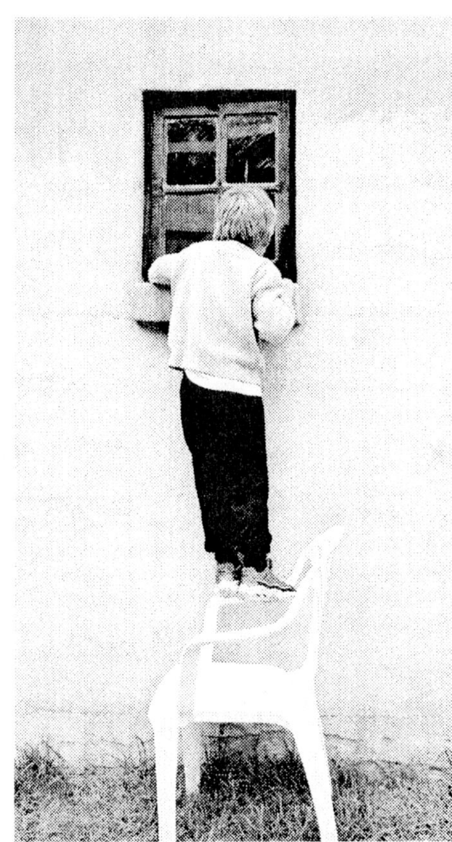

Behavior theories propose that paraphilias begin with the pairing of a particular event with sexual arousal.

Combining these two basic principles of behaviorism provides a pretty clear picture of how they might account for some people's tendency toward paraphilias. First, a person learns to associate sexual arousal with objects or unusual activities, and then those interactions are reinforced strongly with sexual pleasure and orgasm. The result? A paraphilia. For example, imagine a teenage boy sitting at his desk in his bedroom who happens to see a woman who forgot to close her blinds undressing in a window across the street. He becomes sexually aroused as he watches and masturbates to orgasm. After this first experience, he begins to watch and wait for the woman to undress again, and masturbates again. He may then begin to fantasize about spying on the woman when he masturbates at other times as well. Over the next few months or years, his desire to watch unsuspecting women undress may become increasingly strong, and he may begin to seek out opportunities to satisfy his urges. He may, for instance, prowl neighborhoods at night looking in windows for victims and, upon finding them, may masturbate on the spot as he watches, or he may use the experience for later masturbatory fantasies. He has now acquired the paraphilia we call voyeurism.

Biological Theories of Paraphilias

Biological theories of paraphilias derive from the assumption that something physiological has malfunctioned and is leading to the person's strange and compulsive behaviors. These theories focus primarily on imbalances in two biochemical systems: hormones and neurotransmitters (Kafka, 1997; Langevin, 1992; Rosler & Witztum, 2000). The hormone hypothesis suggests that compulsive sexual behavior may be related to an overproduction of male hormones, mainly testosterone (Bradford, 2001), but other hormones, such as epinephrine (adrenaline) and norepinephrine, have been implicated as well (Maes et al., 2001). The neurotransmitter serotonin, which is known to be involved in various psychological disorders, especially depression, anxiety, and obsessive-compulsive disorder (OCD), has been connected to paraphilias as well (Bradford, 2001; Kafka & Hennen, 2000).

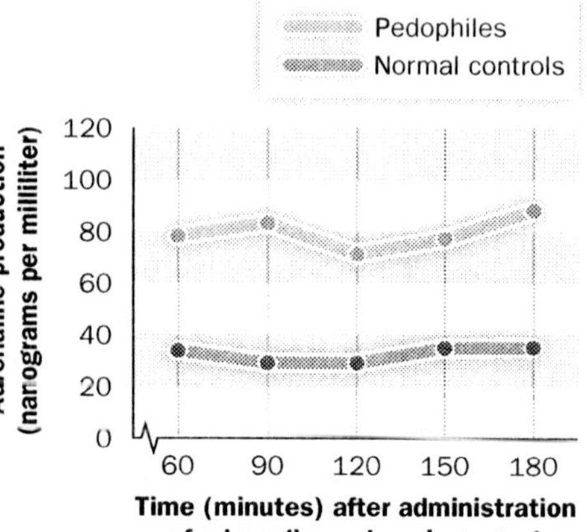

FIGURE 14.1 Adrenaline Levels in Pedophiles versus Normal Controls

Convicted pedophiles produced more adrenaline than a normal control group, which may provide evidence for a biological foundation in pedophilia.

Source: Data from Maes et al. (2001), p. 46.

Most studies on the relationship between hormones, neurotransmitters, and paraphilias have provided evidence of a link by administering medications designed to change the balance of these chemicals in men with uncontrollable paraphilic urges. By blocking the action of, say, testosterone or enhancing the effects of serotonin with medications such as Prozac, Zoloft, Luvox, Paxil, and Celexa, some individuals with paraphilias find that their compulsions are reduced to more controllable levels, and they are better able to resist acting on their urges (Abouesh & Clayton, 1999; Kafka & Hennen, 2000). This finding fits with discoveries that these same medications have also been successful in treating nonsexual obsessive-compulsive disorders (Abouesh & Clayton, 1999; Jenike, 2001). We will discuss the use of these drugs in treating paraphilias later in the chapter.

Finally, at least one study measured levels of adrenaline in men with pedophilia (sexual attraction to children) and compared them to normal men (Maes et al., 2001). The researchers found significantly higher levels of the hormone in the pedophilia group in the three hours following the administration of an adrenaline-enhancing agent (see Figure 14.1). This suggests a biological foundation in pedophilia: the sympathetic nervous system, which triggers the release of adrenaline in highly emotional situations, may be overly active in pedophiles.

Reconciling the Three Theoretical Approaches

Which theory is the correct one, you ask? Well, as with most competing opinions about anything, it depends on whom you ask. However, if you think about it, any two or even all three approaches to explaining paraphilias may be combined into a more global, cohesive explanation. For example, few psychologists would dispute that certain experiences in childhood cause us to pay more or less attention to and react in more positive or negative ways to specific sexual events, activities, and situations in our adult life. These tendencies may in turn lead us to be attracted to, enjoy, and engage in a personally unique set of sexual behaviors (psychodynamic theory). As we do so, we learn to associate those activities with sexual arousal and are rewarded for engaging in them with sexual pleasure and orgasm. Clearly, the range of sexual association is so great that for a minority, the connections formed may be seen as quite strange and bizarre in the culture (behavioral theory). Add to this set of events one or more biological or genetic factors that create in some people obsessive-compulsive tendencies (biological theory). If those obsessive-compulsive propensities become focused on certain atypical sexual inclinations, the ones that have been conditioned through association and reinforcement, what do you have? Correct! A paraphilia.

Many behavioral scientists and sex researchers would resist such a melding of views. However, little scientific research supports or even suggests a single, clear, definitive answer to the causes of paraphilias. Finding ways of combining proposed theories simply allows us to broaden, rather than restrict, our thinking on this subject.

Gender and Paraphilias

You may have noticed as you've been reading this chapter that whenever the sex of a person with a paraphilia has been mentioned, it has always been male. The reason for this is that *nearly* all those who engage in paraphilias are men. The one possible exception to this rule is sexual masochism (sexual gratification from receiving pain), which is found in women more often than other paraphilias, but is still more common in men (American Psychiatric Association, 1994). Why do we see such a gender gap for these behaviors?

Many sexuality theorists throughout history, including Krafft-Ebing (discussed in "Historical Perspectives") have applied the overly simplistic explanation that men have a stronger sexual drive than women do, and this "overdeveloped" sexual appetite leads them uncontrollably into strange compulsive sexual behaviors. However, this explanation fails to address why it is that if men have a high sex drive, only a small minority become involved in paraphilias, while most men are content with more mainstream sexual behaviors.

The relative prevalence of paraphilias among men as compared to women may be understood better from a larger cultural perspective. In most Western cultures, males are given greater "permission" to be sexual in their thinking, language, and behaviors. Most societal attitudes consider overt sexuality in men not only normal but also desirable, something to be encouraged and rewarded. You can easily see this in the language used to talk about sexuality in men and women. A highly sexually oriented man is typically referred to in positive terms such as "stud" or "hottie," while a woman who talks or behaves in similar ways is usually labeled in negative terms such as "slut" or "whore." It may be that as males are given more latitude in Western cultures to be sexual, some of them will learn to express that freedom in paraphilic ways.

This is not to imply that women never engage in paraphilias. As noted, a small but significant percentage of women practice sexual masochism. And one study found a few examples (12 in all) of women pedophiles, exhibitionists, and sexual sadists (Fedoroff, Fishell, & Fedoroff, 1999). However, by all accounts, these cases represent the exception, not the rule. In addition, some research has indicated that in cultures where sexual activity is regarded as serving primarily a reproductive function (as opposed to an attraction-based function, as in the United States), paraphilias among men and women are significantly less common (Bhugra, 2000).

Finally, it is important to understand that all research into paraphilias is extremely challenging, to say the least. Take, for example, trying to determine the relative frequency of paraphilic behavior in men versus women or among various diverse cultures. How can a researcher gather data on such a personal and socially proscribed behavior? The answer is that doing so is not impossible, but we must always think analytically about such findings, as explained in "Evaluating Sexual Research: How Biased Are the Data?"

Specific Paraphilias

Now that you have an overall picture of the important definitions, characteristics, and features of paraphilias in general, let's take a closer look at some of the more common ones. We will limit this detailed discussion, with one important exception, to the paraphilias that are defined formally in the DSM-IV-TR, which is used to help mental health professionals identify psychological disorders. Each discussion opens with a brief case study that is fairly typical of the paraphilia, followed by a description of the behavior. Again, keep in mind that some paraphilias are clearly coercive and victimizing while others are relatively victim-free and engaged in either solo or by mutual consent. We will divide our discussion of the more common paraphilias into these two categories.

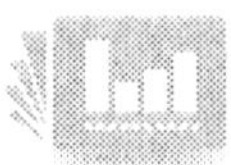

Evaluating Sexual Research

How Biased Are Sexual Data?

When researchers are trying to obtain data about sexual behavior differences between males and females or among diverse cultures, one of the few ways to do so is to ask people what they do and how often they do it (we cannot, of course, ethically peep into windows or set up hidden camcorders!). But when you ask people to tell you about their intensely personal, perhaps embarrassing, or socially questionable sexual activities, you have to assume that many, if not most, are likely to fudge their answers in ways that make them look as socially acceptable as possible. We discussed this problem, called the *social desirability bias*, in Chapter 6, as it relates to the content of people's sexual fantasies. You can imagine, if people tend to be less than truthful about their sexual fantasies, how much more likely they might be to distort the truth when asked about their paraphilias! It is important to keep in mind that self-report data always have the potential to be biased, especially when interpreting research findings showing, for example, that a certain percentage of people participate in a certain paraphilia, that few women appear to engage in paraphilic behavior compared to men, or that paraphilias are practiced more or less frequently in various cultures. This does not imply that all self-report sexual research is worthless; rather, it must always be examined with a critical eye.

However, in many countries, we have a source of data other than self-reports for paraphilias that we do not have for many other sexual behaviors: criminal justice records. Because many paraphilias victimize others and are therefore illegal, some perpetrators are caught and arrested. When we examine those arrest records, almost all the perpetrators are males. That would suggest that dramatic gender differences do indeed exist for nonconsensual paraphilias. Still, we must ask ourselves whether those crime statistics might reflect a cultural bias in the criminal justice system that focuses on male offenders and casts a blind eye toward female perpetrators of nonconsensual paraphilias. For example, consider the following: Would a man looking into a window where a woman is undressing be viewed in the same way as a woman looking into a window where a man is undressing? Or might the man be perceived in the first case as a voyeur and in the second case as an exhibitionist, and the woman as the victim in both cases? It's something to think about.

coercive paraphilias Sexual activities involving an unsuspecting, nonconsenting, or unwilling victim as the target of the atypical, compulsive behavior.

voyeurism Secretly watching others undress or engage in sexual activities without their knowledge or consent for the purpose of achieving sexual arousal.

Coercive Paraphilias

Coercive paraphilias involve an unsuspecting, nonconsenting, or unwilling victim who is the target of the compulsive behavior. Indeed, the presence of a nonconsenting victim is often a motivating factor, part of the "thrill" experienced by the person engaging in the paraphilic act. It is primarily due to the coercive nature of these behaviors that most states in the United States and most countries worldwide have enacted laws against these paraphilias.

Voyeurism

J.W. is a 22-year-old college student. For several years, he has been having persistent fantasies of secretly watching various female classmates in their dorm rooms or apartments undressing or engaging in sexual activities. He finds these fantasies especially exciting because of the fact that the women are completely unaware that he is watching them. Over the past couple of semesters, J.W. has been taking walks through campus housing areas at night looking for open blinds or cracks in curtains through which to sneak a peak. Lately, he has found several "watching posts" with views into windows and surrounded with trees and bushes that protect him from being seen. He has taken to going to these places two or three nights a week to sit, watch, and masturbate. After each foray, he feels guilty and swears never to do it again, but within a few days, is drawn back to the behavior once more.

The voyeur achieves sexual arousal through watching unsuspecting others undressing or engaging in sexual activities.

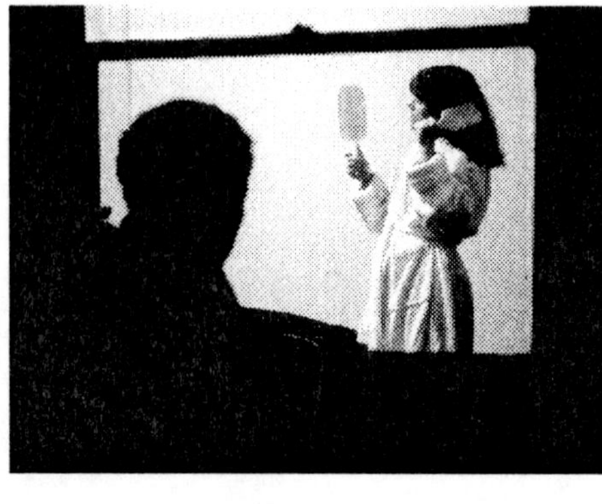

Voyeurism refers to the paraphilia of secretly watching others undress or engage in sexual activities without their knowledge or consent. You have undoubtedly heard of this rather common paraphilia; you may know someone who was watched, or perhaps you discovered that someone had been watching you. The common term for this person is a "peeping Tom." Remember, this peeping is without the victim's consent. If someone is sexually aroused watching his partner undress prior to having sex, going to clubs with sex shows, or watching sexually explicit videos, these acts would *not* qualify as voyeurism. The true voyeur's sexual experience is defined and *enhanced* by the nonconsensual nature of the act.

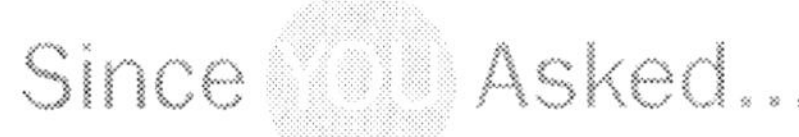

3. Last year, there was this guy who kept looking into girls' windows in the dorms (peeping Tom, right?). What is that all about?

For the victim, voyeurism can be extremely upsetting. Discovering that you have been secretly watched during your most private moments, sometimes over long periods of time, can be very frightening and may increase feelings of vulnerability in other areas of life. Some researchers contend that voyeurism is one of many forms of sexual assault and exploitation and may carry with it some of the effects of more physical forms of sexual assault such as rape (Allies Program, 2000; Wisconsin Coalition, 2000).

Although the practice of voyeurism is centuries old, recent developments in technology and the Internet have sharply refocused attention on this paraphilia. New and relatively cheap, tiny spy cameras and "Web cams" are allowing voyeuristic predators alarming new access to their victims' private worlds. Web sites exist that claim to contain images that are the product of nonconsensual voyeurism, secretly capturing people in intimate acts with these new technological tools. An increasing number of reports are appearing of apartment or hotel managers, store employees, women's dates and acquaintances, or other voyeurs setting up hidden video cameras in hotel rooms, apartment bedrooms, bathrooms, locker rooms, and dressing rooms to spy on unsuspecting victims either for the voyeur's own pleasure or for distribution for profit over the Internet (Hawaleshka, 2001). As this text goes to press, many states and provinces in the United States and Canada, as well as the U.S. Congress, are working to broaden the definition of voyeurism and enact new laws to slow the spread of this new high-tech form of a paraphilia (Dlouhy, 2003).

Exhibitionism

S.N. is a 41-year-old male. He is married with one child and has a successful accounting business. Over the past several years, he has been exposing himself while masturbating as he tries to make eye contact with unsuspecting women in relatively public places such as the beach, the park, or the mall. This behavior has become so compulsive, he can now become sexually aroused only by exposing himself or by fantasizing about his most recent episode of exhibitionism. S.N. feels totally unable to control this impulse and has been arrested twice for indecent exposure and lewd and lascivious acts. He is separated from his wife and is currently forbidden by the court to visit his daughter except under strict supervision by a court-appointed social worker.

Exhibitionism is the flip side of voyeurism in that the focus for sexual arousal and gratification is displaying one's genitals to others without their consent. A common term for someone who engages in this paraphilia is a "flasher." The stereotypical image of an exhibitionist is a "dirty old man" in a knee-length raincoat, throwing the coat open like a cape to reveal his genitals. In reality, most exhibitionists are men between the ages of 16 and 40 who experience high levels of sexual gratification from exposing their genitals to women they do not know, in various settings, and who usually masturbate at the same time (de Silva, 1999). As with voyeurism, part of the arousal of this paraphilia is the shock value of the behavior on the victim. Most exhibitionists do not engage in other predatory or violent acts such as rape and usually desire no physical contact at all with their victims.

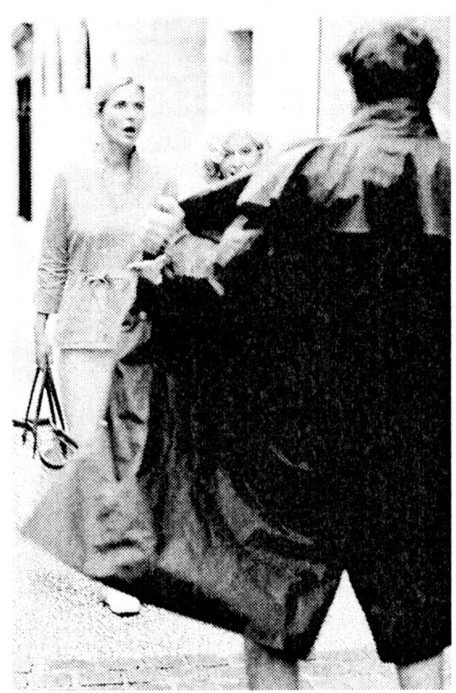

The exhibitionist is sexually aroused by exposing his genitals to unsuspecting victims.

exhibitionism Achieving sexual arousal and gratification by displaying one's genitals to others without the victims' consent.

New technology and the Internet are playing an increasing role in exhibitionism just as discussed earlier regarding voyeurism. Some people choose to place

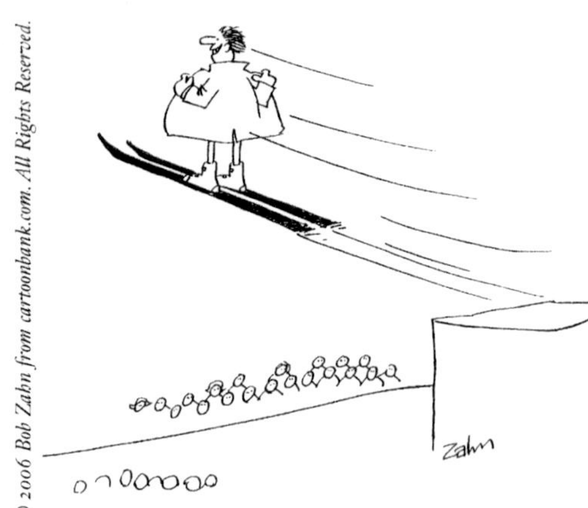

cameras in their homes and allow others to watch them on line in a sort of consensual "exhibitionism-voyeurism" way of satisfying their curiosity about how others live and love.

In most Western cultures, people take their clothes off in front of others for a wide variety of reasons, ranging from exotic dancing to acting in film or theater to undressing in provocative ways for their partners. However, as you now understand, these people are not engaging in the paraphilia of exhibitionism (or voyeurism) because the undresser and the observer are consenting to the act and, in some cases, the undresser is doing so for reasons other than his or her own sexual arousal and gratification.

Frotteurism

E.S. is obsessed with rush hour in Manhattan. The crowded subways are the highlight of his day. At peak traffic time, E.S. enters the subway, spots a woman he is attracted to, and follows her onto the train. He finds a way to get close enough in the crush of people to rub his penis against her while attempting to maintain a casual, matter-of-fact outward demeanor. It arouses him even more to know that the act is his secret; no one knows what he is doing except his trapped victim. He fantasizes that he and his victim share a special sexual bond, and he often has an orgasm through this experience. He also uses these interactions as a basis for fantasies while masturbating.

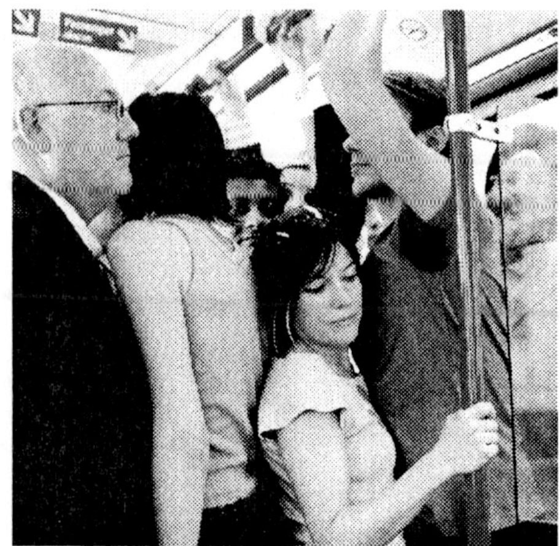

Frotteurism involves rubbing one's genitals against a nonconsenting victim.

As you can tell from the case of E.S., **frotteurism** is the compulsion to rub one's genitals against a nonconsenting person for sexual arousal and, typically, orgasm. The perpetrator usually fantasizes that he has a close, caring, loving relationship with his victim, but he will make every effort to run away and escape detection following the act. Virtually all frotteurists are men. Often when a woman learns of this paraphilia, she can remember a time or two in her life when a man had crowded her too closely in a situation tightly packed with people. It made her very uncomfortable at the time, and now that creepy feeling makes a lot more sense!

Typically, men who become involved in this paraphilia are most active between the ages of 15 and 25 and tend to decrease and stop the behavior as they age (Miller, 2000). Frotteurists often believe that due to a lack of any response, their victims are unaware or enjoying the act, but in truth, they are usually too shocked, afraid, or embarrassed to take action, or the act happens so fast that they do not have a chance to react at all. However, this, as with the other coercive paraphilias discussed here, is an illegal act and is considered a form of sexual assault (see "Sexuality, Ethics, and the Law: A Reformed Frotteurist's Confessions" for a firsthand account of frotteurism).

Since YOU Asked...

4. I saw this movie (not porno) where a guy got off by rubbing up against women at concerts when everyone was crowding and pushing up to the stage. What is up with that?

Sexual Sadism

A.R. is a 35-year-old electronics salesman. He is unable to become sexually aroused unless he is causing intense pain, suffering, and humiliation to another person. These acts are not in any way playful, and his victims' lives have at times been in danger. Last year, he was finally caught and arrested on charges of kidnaping, assault, sexual assault, and rape. His latest victim was found in A.R.'s basement, caged like an animal, with evidence of sexual and other physical abuse. A.R. has stated that for all of his adult life, he had persistent fantasies about abducting, binding, cutting, sexually assaulting, and humiliating women. He gave in to his most extreme urges and is now facing life in prison for his crimes.

Sexual sadism, the inflicting of pain and humiliation for sexual gratification, is named for the Marquis de Sade, an eighteenth-century French author and aristocrat

frotteurism Rubbing one's genitals against a nonconsenting person for sexual arousal and, typically, orgasm.

sexual sadism Inflicting pain, injury, or humiliation on another person for the sexual gratification of the person performing the action.

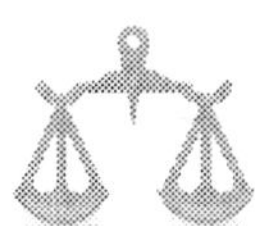

Sexuality, Ethics, and the Law

A Reformed Frotteurist's Confessions

Back when I was a teenager, my best friend and I would go out on Friday nights to rub up against college women. Our venue of choice was the Fish Market, a long, narrow place with a U-shaped bar that had high-top tables and stools running along the perimeter by the windows. Between the bar and the tables, dozens of women stood trapped in a mass of clammy bodies. Armed with fake IDs, we would begin: We circled the bar, arms raised over our heads like soldiers wading a creek. There was no room to pass through the crowd, really, so you had to squeeze in between and around the women, getting sandwiched by their breasts and butts. By pretending we had to get through to go to the bathroom or the bar, we could usually make three or four circuits before anyone started getting suspicious.

Frotteurism, as clinicians call it, is the practice of rubbing up against an unconsenting—and usually unsuspecting—person for the purpose of sexual gratification. In the *Diagnostic and Statistical Manual of Mental Disorders*, frotteurism is found in the category of sexual and gender identity disorders. Unlike other disorders in that category—exhibitionism, voyeurism, transvestic fetishism, and so on—frotteurism is a strictly male pursuit. No cases of the disorder have ever been reported in females.

Sure, I'm ashamed to admit that I wallowed in such wanton sexploitation, but back then it seemed more like schoolboy mischief than hardcore perversion. Eventually I quit rubbing up against women and moved on to more socially acceptable courtships—conversation, dating, marriage. What's so uniquely pathetic about frotteurists is the underhandedness of their transgression. Precisely because she's unaware that anything untoward is happening to her, the victim can't even begin to defend herself. Frotteurism is basically this: low-grade molestation for the chicken-hearted deviant, who dreams—while he's brushing his erection against some unaware person's backside—of a soft-focus Hallmark future with his darling victim.

What can a woman do to protect herself against the sly frotteurist slinking around the bars, subways, and shopping malls? Jane Kelly, a 32-year-old Washington, D.C., native who commutes daily on the capital's jam-packed subway, has developed elaborate techniques for defending herself. "I create a strict personal space," Kelly says. "I back into a corner and open the newspaper about 12 inches from my face. I build a wall, and nobody gets inside."

"Elevators and escalators are bad," says Martha King, a 34-year-old from Virginia. "But bars are the worst. It happens all the time: You're sitting at a bar and some guy reaches over you from behind to get his drink from the bar, and he'll rub up against you. It usually happens so quick you're not even aware of it."

Everyone seems to agree that frotteurism is rampant, but among the women I surveyed, not one has ever reported an incident to law enforcement authorities. "I've never felt physically threatened to the point that I would go to the police," King says.

What type of compulsive behavior did this old schoolboy urge morph into? A quick inventory of me finds a guy pretty normal on all sexual fronts, faithfully married, with a relaxed and wholesome approach to masturbation, no nude corpses in the closet, and no transvestic tendencies beyond the occasional craving to wear my wife's sweaters.

Most of your reformed junior-league frotteurists would make the same claim: I'm grown up now. I don't go there anymore. Then again, one of the traits commonly associated with sexual compulsion is a tendency toward denial. So play it safe, gentle reader: Keep your back to the wall.

Source: Adapted from Bowen (1999).

who spent much of his adult life imprisoned for engaging in and writing about his particularly violent form of sexual expression.

The clinical definition of sexual sadism clearly involves innocent victims and is often one of the most violent paraphilias, as you can see from the case of A.R. Sadism takes many forms, including dominating, restraining, tying up, blindfolding, beating, cutting, whipping, strangling, mutilating, and even killing another person, usually during sexual activities. Part of the attraction and excitement for the sadist is the terror experienced by the victim. Sexual sadism is seen in the pattern of behaviors of some serial rapists.

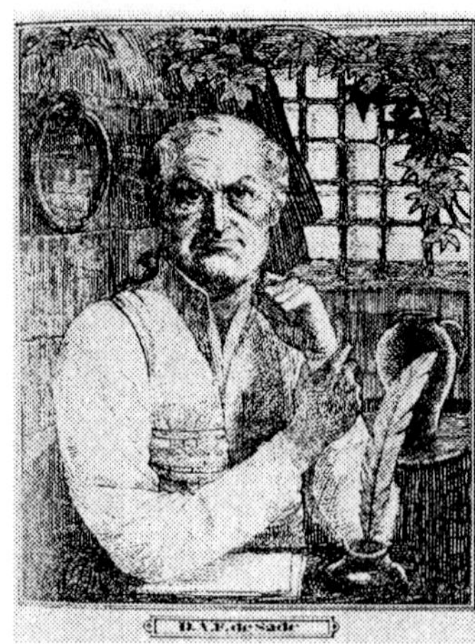

"Every man wants to be a tyrant when he fornicates." This quote has been attributed to The Marquis de Sade (1740–1814), from whose name we derive the word sadism.

Less severe forms of sexually sadistic activities also exist; usually they are combined with masochistic behavior (which is discussed with the noncoercive paraphilias), and this combination is referred to as **sadomasochism** or **BDSM** (for bondage, discipline, and sadomasochism). Some people are sexually aroused by bondage—tying up or being tied up by a partner (with consent); discipline—dominating and humiliating or being dominated or humiliated by a sexual partner (with consent); or light sadism or masochism—the giving or receiving minor pain such as spankings: However, these acts, although appearing to be paraphilic in nature, are done as sexual play, usually with strict rules and agreements to ensure that the activities never cross any undesired boundaries (as discussed in "In Touch with Your Sexual Health: Bondage and Discipline"). These activities appear to be quite popular and fairly common compared to other paraphilias (Apostolides, 1999). A thriving industry exists in the United States and around the world for S&M- or BDSM-related products such as leather costumes, dog collars, handcuffs, and so-called soft restraints. Entire catalogs and Web sites are devoted to such sexual products and paraphernalia (such as www.sirenssecrets.com/ or www.akaara.com/).

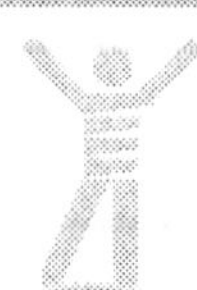

In Touch with Your Sexual Health

BDSM for "Fun"

Columbia University in New York City has a rather unusual support group that is probably not found on many college campuses. Here are just a few excerpts from its Website, http://www.columbia.edu/cu/cv.

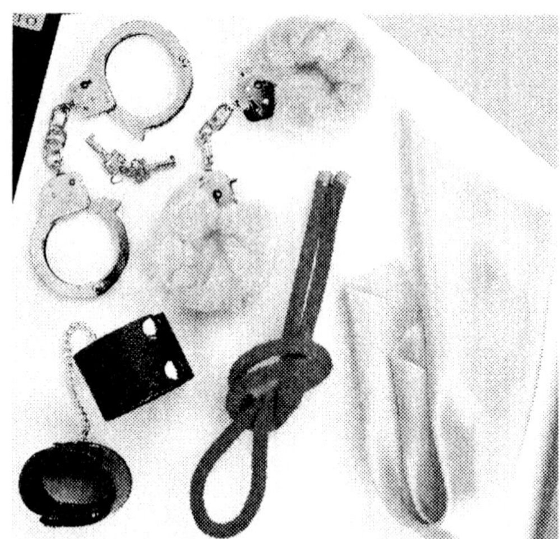

Mild, consensual sadomasochism has become a major worldwide industry.

Conversio Virium

Conversio Virium (CV) is a Columbia University student organization dedicated to discussion, education, and peer support concerning BDSM issues. CV is open to all races, ethnicities, and sexual orientations. All meetings are confidential.

Conversio Virium does not promote, support, or engage in violence of any sort. What it attempts to promote and support is safe, sane, and consensual BDSM play. The only things that CV engages in are discussion and listening. No BDSM play occurs at CV's meetings; they are for discussion, education, and peer support only.

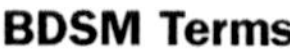

BDSM Terms

BDSM: bondage and discipline (BD), domination and submission (DS), and sadomasochistic play (SM) *between responsible and consenting adults*; just as consent separates sex from rape, consent also separates BDSM from abuse. *BDSM is not a psychological disorder*. The paraphilias of sexual sadism and sexual masochism have specific and limited criteria that differentiate them from BDSM as we define it. . . . BDSM, when done properly, may cause intense feelings but *not* physical or emotional damage. In fact, organized sports can cause far more damage than BDSM. What constitutes damage depends on what is acceptable to the recipient; however, if a person comes in with repeated or long-term or permanent effects or ones that impede daily life, keep an eye on the situation, make sure that the activities were consensual, and give the person safety information.

bondage: use of physical restraints to achieve various degrees of immobilization.

discipline: practice that produces discomfort for the purpose of sexual or emotional arousal.

domination: imposing one's will on another for the enjoyment of both partners; high level of psychological play.

Pedophilia

O.L. is 24, and his only sexual interest is in young children. He has never been sexually attracted to anyone beyond the age of puberty. O.L. is a teacher at a day care center and loves his work. The center has no knowledge of his paraphilia. He enjoys the company of children and has never been able to interact very well, sexually or otherwise, with people his own age. He has used his job as a way to be near children and to receive the only kind of love he feels safe in accepting: the love of children. More than once, this closeness has crossed the line into sexual expression. He has encouraged the children in his care to play touching games with one another while he watches, and he sometimes involves himself in the touching games as well.

O.L. suffers tremendous guilt about his actions and is terrified of being found out, fired from his job, arrested, and ostracized. Yet he has little control over his impulses. O.L. himself was sexually abused at an early age, and he has recently sought treatment to attempt to overcome his sexual compulsions toward children. He desperately desires to be able to develop a healthy expression of his sexuality with an appropriately aged partner. So far, however, the therapy has been unsuccessful.

sadomasochism Sexual activities that combine sadism and masochism.

BDSM Sexual activities that combine bondage, discipline, and sadomasochism.

submission: yielding to another's will for the enjoyment of both partners; high level of psychological play.

sadomasochism/SM: intense physical sensations enjoyed by the masochist and given by the sadist; this term is uncomfortable for many people because of its association with historical figures of disputable moral character.

scene: the period of time, either defined beforehand or during the course of the interaction, where BDSM roles and activities take place; as a verb, *scene* refers to engaging in BDSM activity. "The scene" refers to people who feel they are part of a BDSM community.

negotiation: the process of expressing interest in a BDSM scene, exchanging information about preferences and limits, and deciding whether or not to play and for what duration of time.

limit: activities, words, or scenarios that the person does not wish to experience for either physical or emotional reasons.

safeword: a code word, often a word not used in everyday or sexual contexts, that indicates that the interaction needs to stop or that an activity needs to be changed.

top: one who takes control of the activities of a scene; can refer to both physical and psychological play.

bottom: one who gives over a degree of power to another; can refer to both physical and psychological play.

Source: Adapted from http://www.columbia.edu/cu/cv. Reprinted by permission.

Facts about BDSM

- *Mutual consent* is what distinguishes BDSM from abuse and assault, just as consent distinguishes sex from rape.
- *Context* is what determines whether or not pain is experienced as pleasurable, though the context depends on the individual. An example of "good" pain may be getting scratched during sex, while an example of "bad" pain may be stubbing your toe.
- Not all BDSM play is between heterosexual couples.
- BDSM may or may not include sexual contact. People who are submissive with their partner in a BDSM scene may not be necessarily submissive in other aspects of their lives.
- BDSM can encompass both physical and psychological interactions.
- Ligature marks around wrists or ankles cause safety questions to be raised. Warn patients about erotic asphyxiation. Choking play or hanging play is very dangerous but common.
- Accidents can happen in BDSM, just as in any other physical activity, but this isn't abuse.
- Some people are proud of their bruises, marks, or cuts, just as they might be proud of a hickey on their neck. Don't assume that these are evidence of a problem or a mistake.
- Partners who know each other very well may sometimes negotiate a scene without a safeword. This is still not abuse but a matter of profound trust.

This paraphilia is probably the most reviled compulsive behavior of all. **Pedophilia** refers to the exploitation of prepubescent children for an adult's sexual purposes. Most people cannot begin to fathom what would cause someone to victimize children in this way. However, as everyone is acutely aware, it is an all too common occurrence. Because pedophilia is clearly an abusive act perpetrated against children, the specific characteristics of child sexual molesters and the effects of this crime on their victims are detailed in Chapter 13, "Sexual Aggression and Violence." Here we focus on child sexual abuse as a paraphilia called pedophilia, a diagnosable psychological disorder.

No single profile of a typical **pedophile** exists, although there are some commonalities (de Silva, 1999). Most pedophiles are men, but numerous individual cases of women engaging in an extensive pattern of child molestation have been reported. The majority of pedophiles are heterosexual (regardless of the sex of their victims), and many are married with children of their own. Pedophiles commonly experience marital difficulties, and alcohol addiction is frequently found among this group. One of the most notable characteristics shared by the majority of pedophiles is that they were themselves sexually abused as children (Lee et al., 2000; de Silva, 1999). The number pedophiles has been estimated at 4 percent of the population (Cloud, 2002). In the United States, that percentage represents well over a million people. We should note that not all diagnosable pedophiles abuse children. Some are able to suppress their urges or find ways to satisfy their compulsive tendencies through fantasy or with child pornography (which, of course, in itself, often victimizes children; this is discussed further in Chapter 15, "The Sexual Marketplace").

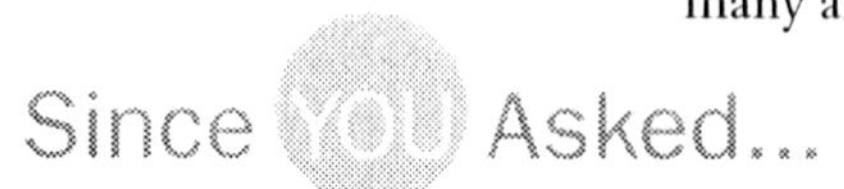

5. I was sexually molested as a child. I never told anyone (until now). With all these stories about priests molesting kids, I think about it a lot and wonder why it happened. Do you think I should get some counseling to work through it?

The victims of pedophiles also share some characteristics. Approximately 65 percent are girls between the ages of 8 and 11, and an estimated 90 percent either know or are related to their abuser (de Silva, 1999). The aftereffects victims experience vary greatly, depending on the nature and duration of the sexual abuse, the age of the child, and other psychological variables. However, research has found that those who were sexually abused as children are at greater risk for depression, suicide, alcohol addiction, anxiety disorders, rape, subsequent sexual victimization as teenagers and as adults, and divorce (Hollander, 2001c; Nelson, Heath, & Madden, 2002; Wise et al., 2001). For a more detailed discussion on the nature and effects of child sexual abuse, see Chapter 13, "Sexual Aggression and Violence."

In 2000, just under 90,000 children were estimated to have been sexually abused in the United States alone (Finkelhor & Jones, 2004). This was a significant decrease from 150,000 in 1992. Figure 14.2 shows the trend in the 1990s of substantiated cases of child sexual abuse. Some researchers contend, however, that at least some of this decline may be due to changes in the way child sexual abuse is

pedophilia The exploitation by an adult of prepubescent children for the adult's sexual gratification.

pedophile An adult, usually male, whose sexual focus is on children.

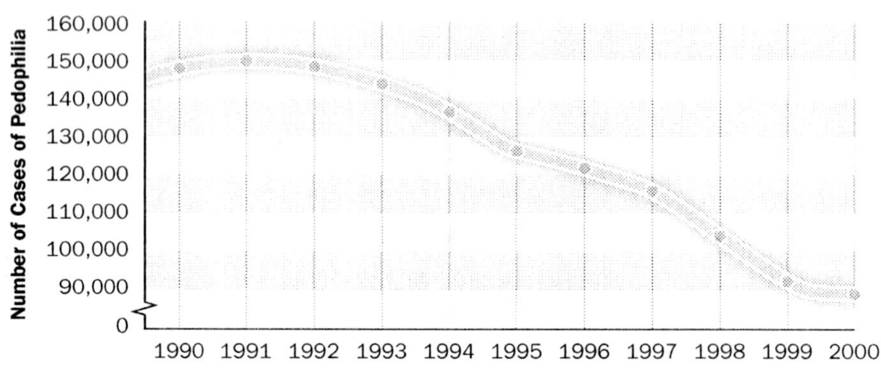

FIGURE 14.2 Substantiated Pedophilia Cases in the United States, 1990–2000

Source: Data from Finkelhor and Jones (2004).

defined or how data are reported, so the more recent statistics may underrepresent to some extent the true number of cases of pedophilia in the United States (Finkelhor & Jones, 2004).

Although the decline in cases of pedophilia strikes an optimistic note, we should remind ourselves that during those same years and into the 2000s, the dismaying flood of reports of pedophilia among Catholic priests has brought the horrors of this paraphilia to a new level of public awareness. The loss of trust in individuals long thought to be the most trustworthy has shaken many people's faith in human nature and in the church. Around the world, accusations and convictions of Catholic priests who engaged in child sexual abuse have become front-page news. Estimates place the number of Catholic priests who have been sexually involved with minors over the past 50 years at between 3,000 and 5,000. The number of boys (now men) who were abused by these priests is estimated at approximately 11,000 (Goodstein, 2004; Plante, 2004) and could be more than 20,000 victims worldwide. The Catholic church has paid out hundreds of millions of dollars, to the point of requiring several Catholic dioceses to declare bankruptcy to settle lawsuits brought by the victims of the abuse.

Probably the highest hurdles now facing the church and its leadership involve resolving the current crisis, finding ways of preventing such abuse in the future, and regaining the confidence and trust of a disillusioned religious world. Many believe that psychology must play a key role in developing solutions to this complex and painful problem. One suggestion is that psychologists must view the Catholic church and the priesthood as cultures unto themselves and adopt a multicultural perspective, just as one might do in helping any cultural subgroup overcome an internal problem that threatens its internal social structure. "Sexuality and Culture: Overcoming Child Sexual Abuse Scandals" dispels some of the common myths about the scandals and discusses specific strategies that psychology might offer for developing solutions to this Catholic "culturewide" crisis.

Noncoercive Paraphilias

If you look back at the characteristics of paraphilias discussed earlier in this chapter, you will see that the presence of a nonconsenting victim is not a necessary criterion in the definition. Many paraphilias (refer to Table 14.1) are noncoercive, by virtue of the fact that they are solitary activities or that they involve adults who have given their consent. Therefore, these paraphilias are often considered victimless, unless you support, as many people do, the notion that the person engaging in the paraphilic act is victimizing himself or herself due to the strange, degrading, or even potentially dangerous nature of the behavior. However, this use of the term *victim* is not how it is usually applied to sexual acts. The fact that these acts do not *compel* others to participate against their will is why most authorities refer to them as victimless and noncoercive.

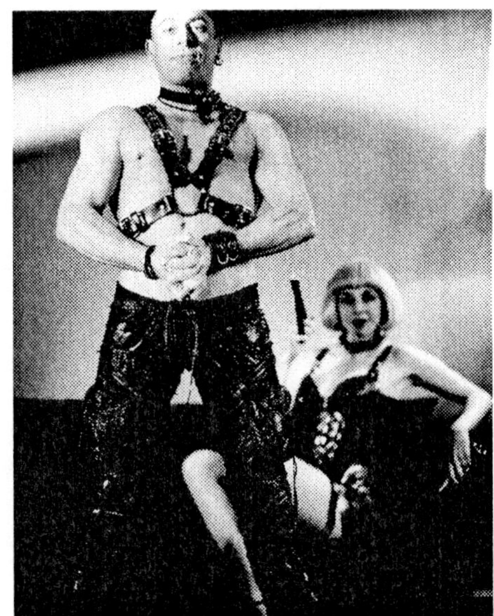

Sadomasochists are sexually aroused by games involving pain, bondage, and humiliation.

Sexual Masochism

T.W. is male, 47, a banker, stockbroker, real estate tycoon, and millionaire. At least once or twice a month, T.W. feels an overwhelming desire for a sexual partner who will make him feel worthless, powerless, and insignificant. He often pays a dominatrix, a woman who knows exactly how to engage in behaviors that humiliate, demean, and hurt him. His favorite and most sexually exciting acts are being tied up, blindfolded, spanked with a wooden paddle, and having hot wax dripped onto his penis and scrotum. T.W. reports that after a session with his "mistress," he often feels relieved and "in balance," ready to face the world as a power broker. His desire for such a masochistic session tends to increase as the stress in his life rises.

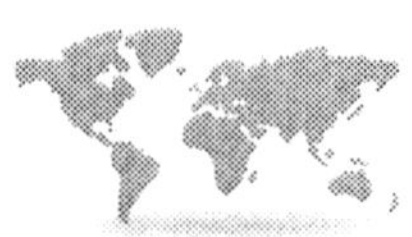

Sexuality and Culture

Overcoming the Catholic Priest Pedophilia Scandals: How Psychology Can Help

Most psychologists agree that part of the task of stopping and preventing pedophilia among Catholic priests is to understand the origins and causes of the problem. It is not enough simply to uncover, report, and expel those priests who have engaged in sexual abuse of minors because other pedophiles are very likely either presently in the priesthood or will be coming up through the training process in the future. Therefore, in addition to stopping the abuse and removing the perpetrators, we must focus on long-term prevention. Psychologists are working to dispel the many myths surrounding the scandal, shed light on the possible causes of the abuse, and offer proactive strategies for avoiding future abuse.

Two Persistent Myths

Two common beliefs about this problem are not grounded in fact and have taken the focus away from real solutions. The first is that the pedophilic behavior of priests has been due to the church's culture of celibacy (the renunciation of marriage and the vow of chastity). You can see that this argument is misguided in that although celibacy may cause a buildup of sexual tension for some people (whether in the priesthood or not), most of those individuals will not make children the focus of their desire or their sexual acting out.

The second myth is that the church scandals are related to a culture of homosexuality in the church, in that men with homosexual tendencies are drawn to the all-male culture of the priesthood, which in itself is not based in fact. Moreover, the notion that sexual orientation of priests is connected to the church's pedophilia scandals is founded in the belief that most child molesters are gay males, a belief that is simply untrue. The vast majority of adults who sexually abuse children are heterosexual, regardless of the sex of their victims. In fact, a study in the 1990s found that in 82 percent of child molestation cases, the molester was the heterosexual partner of a close relative of the child, and the chance of a child molester's being a homosexual male was between zero and 3.1 percent (Jenny, Roesler, & Poyer, 1994).

Commonalities

We do see several common characteristics in many or most of the priests who have abused children. Usually, as with most pedophiles, abusing priests were typically abused themselves as children. Psychologically, various characteristics and disorders are found among pedophile priests in significantly larger proportions than in the general population, including poor impulse control, underdeveloped social skills, substance abuse, depressive and bipolar disorders, and various personality disorders, especially narcissistic disorder (grandiose sense of self-importance, constant need for external adoration, and marked lack of empathy for others) and dependent disorder (the excessive need to be taken care

Sexual masochism refers to sexual arousal and gratification that is associated with acts or fantasies of being hurt, humiliated, or otherwise made to suffer. The masochist engages in such acts voluntarily and often seeks them out. As in the case of T.W., a wide range of behaviors are enticing and sexually arousing to masochists, including being tied up or otherwise restrained (called **bondage**); piercing with pins or needles; affixing clothespins or clamps to nipples or genitals; hanging weights from genitals; being spanked, whipped, beaten, strangled, slapped, electrically shocked, or verbally degraded; branding of the skin; and applying ice to the bare skin (Santtila et al., 2002).

As mentioned in our discussion of sexual sadism, the sadomasochism subculture typically engages in very ritualized behavior in which the partners make agreements about the acts they desire, assign specific roles to be enacted, and carry out "scripted" sequences of behaviors from very simple acts, such as making love while blindfolded or in handcuffs, to complicated and complex scenarios that may include role-playing, elaborate costumes, and a wide variety of painful or humiliating acts (Baumeister, 1995; Santtila et al., 2002).

Usually, the humiliation and pain involved do not draw blood, break bones, or leave permanent scars. Because these acts are carried out by adults with the consent of all involved, they are typically not illegal. However, such "consenting adult laws" have

sexual masochism Sexual arousal and gratification that is associated with acts or fantasies of being hurt, humiliated, or otherwise made to suffer.

bondage Being bound, tied up, or otherwise restrained during sexual activity; typically a consensual activity.

of and always looking to others for comfort and solutions to all personal problems) (Bryant, 2002).

In addition, many priests chose their profession at a relatively young age when they may not yet have achieved full psychosocial maturity or may have used the church culture as a way of retreating from or avoiding normal social and sexual development. "For these men, at the age of their ordination in their mid- to late twenties, they were intellectually and physically adults, but emotionally they remained far younger" (Donna Markham, quoted in Daw, 2002). Such emotional immaturity is often associated with pedophilia.

Finally, priests are typically not taught anything about sexuality in general during their education and training at the seminary. Seminaries make the often erroneous assumption that they have already dealt with those issues prior to their decision to become priests (Bill Mochon, in Daw, 2002). Priests who have not dealt with sexuality issues are left to their own devices to figure it all out, and some, obviously, end up making very inappropriate choices.

Possible Solutions and Prevention Strategies from Psychology

Psychology has developed various treatments for paraphilias in general in the form of psychotherapy and medication. These will be discussed in greater detail later in this chapter. Beyond this, psychologists working alongside those who are part of the culture of the church may assist in the prevention and treatment of sexual abuse among priests in a number of ways (Daw, 2002):

- Develop strategies to help priests in training and in practice develop healthy interpersonal relationships that are nonsexual. The idea behind this is that in some cases at least, psychological intimacy with others may reduce or eliminate the need for priests with pedophilic inclinations to turn to sexually abusing children.
- Provide valid psychological assessment and evaluation instruments that may be used prior to admission to seminary or ordination to screen out prospective priests who may have compulsive tendencies toward pedophilia.
- Offer effective consulting, counseling, and therapy services for priests, bishops, and parishes. This may involve one-on-one counseling with at-risk clergy, priest wellness or therapy groups, or community education with parishioners about keeping children safe or identifying warning signs of potential sexual misconduct.
- Provide training workshops for priests on maintaining appropriate boundaries with parishioners, raising awareness of warning signs of potential problems, working with challenging clients, and dealing with stress, anxiety, or conflict.
- Engage in substantive scientific research to enhance understanding, prediction, and treatment of sexual abuse within the ranks of the clergy.

Source: Adapted from Daw, 2002.

been tested from time to time, especially when the sadomasochistic acts are more extreme. For example, in England in 1990, several members of a sadomasochistic sex club were arrested for behaviors that the prosecutors claimed violated the United Kingdom's Offenses against the Person Act of 1861, which states, "Whoever shall unlawfully and maliciously wound or inflict any grievous bodily harm on any other person, either with or without any weapon or instrument, shall be liable to imprisonment."

Since YOU Asked...

6. I met a woman at a party. She told me that "on the side," meaning not her main job, I guess, she's a dominatrix. Does that mean what I think it means?

The specific acts for which the men were arrested were videotaped for distribution to other members of the club and consisted

> mainly of maltreatment of the genitals, sometimes with hot wax, sandpaper, fish hooks, and needles, plus ritualistic beatings, either with bare hands or implements including stinging nettles, spiked belts, and cat-o'-nine tails. There was branding and infliction of injuries which bled. All of the acts in question were consented to by all parties and no injury caused infection or permanent injuries. (Green, 2001, p. 543)

The men involved were convicted and sentenced to four years in prison. However, the convictions were later reversed and the case dismissed by the appeals court, which compared the consensual injurious behavior with the sport of boxing. "Each boxer

fetish A sexual preference for a nonhuman object or a body part that most members of a culture do not consider sexual.

aims to end the contest . . . by infliction of brain injury serious enough to make the opponent unconscious . . . or cutting his skin to a degree which would ordinarily be well within the scope of the Act of 1861" (Green, 2001, p. 545).

This case provides an excellent example of exactly the confusion many people feel about consensual sadomasochism. To many, it *feels* somehow wrong that people should be allowed to inflict pain and injury on each other in the name of sexual gratification. However, many others acknowledge that if these are truly consenting adults, it is probably no one's business but their own if they choose to participate.

Fetishism

B.R. is a 38-year-old naval officer. He loves women's high-heeled shoes. He is very sexually aroused by seeing women wear them, by touching them, and by collecting them. He routinely asks his sexual partners to wear them when they make love. In fact, he would just as soon have sex with the shoes as with any of his partners. Lately, he has taken to stealing his preferred type of shoes from his girlfriends in order to masturbate with them.

The first time B.R. can remember becoming sexually aroused was at a young age watching his aunt remove her high heels, before taking off the rest of her clothes in front of him. As he matured, high heels were always a significant part of B.R.'s sexual fantasies and experiences. In recent years, he has become dependent on high heels for sexual arousal and is unable to achieve orgasm with a partner unless high heels are a component of the act.

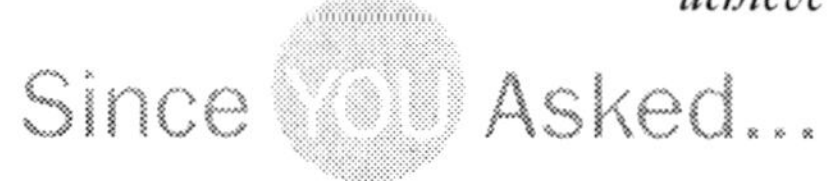

7. My mom has this friend who shops for shoes constantly. It's like if she's not eating or sleeping, she's shoe shopping. Is this what is meant by a shoe fetish?

Everyone has a unique set of sexual preferences, desires, and turn-ons. What is a sexy, exciting behavior, an arousing setting, or a provocative item of clothing or part of the body to one person might inspire boredom or even avoidance in someone else. Such differences are part of the normal diversity of human sexuality. However, when a sexual preference intensifies to the point that a person obsesses almost exclusively on a nonhuman object or sometimes on a body part that most members of a culture do not find sexy, such as feet or toes, this is called a **fetish** (de Silva, 1999; Seligman & Hardenberg, 2000).

Sometimes the line between a "normal" sexual preference and a fetish may seem blurred. However, if you apply the guidelines for defining a paraphilia discussed at the beginning of this chapter, the distinction will probably become clearer. For example, take the case of B.R. The progression of his fetish may have gone something like this: At first, he found women's high-heeled shoes to be a very attractive part of female

Shoes, lingerie, and typically nonsexual body parts are among the most common fetish objects.

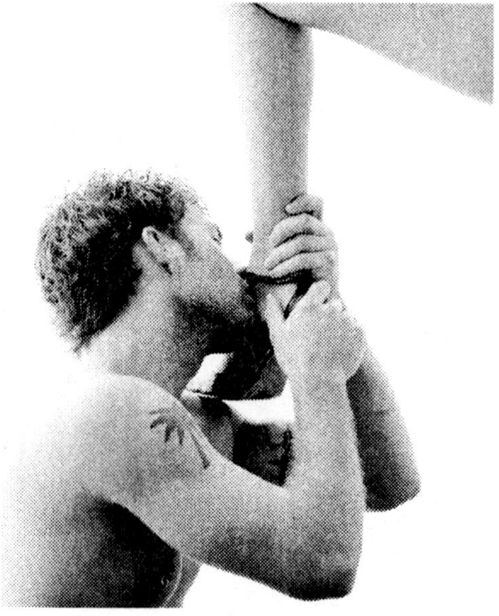

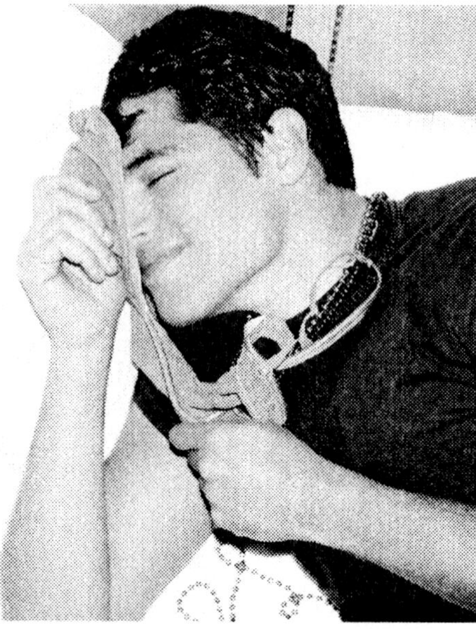

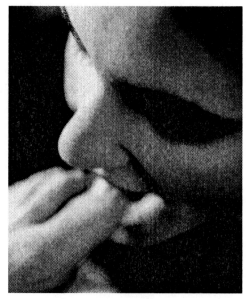

attire. He enjoyed it very much whenever a woman would wear extra-high heels on a date, and he found that he was sexually aroused more easily and more intensely when she did. Soon he began asking his sexual partners to leave their shoes on when they made love and found this very exciting. While this preference may seem a little odd to some, it is doubtful that his degree of preference for high-heels would be considered a fetish. However, over time, his fascination for high-heeled shoes increased until he reached the point that he was unable to become sexually aroused unless high-heeled shoes were worn by his partner or were at least present on the bed. At that point, the fetish object, in this case a certain type of shoes, had become a *necessity* for sex and had moved more clearly into the category of a fetish. He then advanced to the most extreme level of a fetish when his obsession for high-heeled shoes became so strong and primary that he actually began preferring sexual interaction with his partner's shoes to making love with her.

Most sexual fetishes are probably not particularly harmful, and a fetish, by definition, is noncoercive. However, in its most extreme form, a fetish may become a psychological or social problem. If B.R.'s partners are comfortable with his insistence on high-heeled shoes during sex and he is able to form close, loving relationships in spite of his fetish, his obsession with high heels would probably not be considered a psychological disorder. However, if his fetishism is causing discord in his relationships, eliciting anger and resentment from his partners, preventing him from forming healthy relationships, provoking extreme feelings of guilt and self-hate in him, or creating other difficulties, some form of therapy might be appropriate.

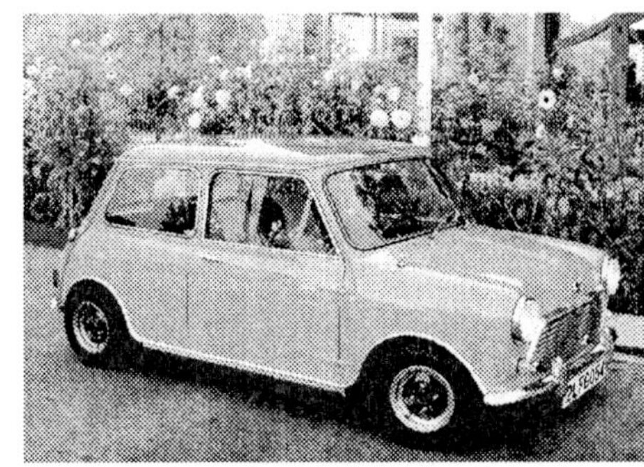

Given certain sexual developmental experiences, anything can become a fetish object, even a particular type of motor vehicle.

The development of fetishes probably stems from experiences in childhood or early adulthood in which some body part, article of clothing, or object was paired with sexual arousal and orgasm (in keeping with the behavioral theories regarding paraphilias discussed earlier in this chapter). After one or more pairings of the object and sexual responding, the object itself becomes a trigger for sexual feelings.

The most common fetish objects are shoes and boots, women's underwear and lingerie, rubber or latex objects, and feet and toes (Freund, Seto, & Kuban, 1996; Seligman & Hardenberg, 2000). If you think about it, you can see why these objects would be more likely to become associated with sexual arousal and orgasm in someone's sexual development. Theoretically, however, *anything* can become the object of a sexual fetish given the relevant sexual experiences. For example, one study reported on a very unusual fetish focusing on, believe it or not, a particular small car: the Austin Metro Mini. The man was described as very shy with very little social interaction, sexual knowledge, or sexual experience and whose main sexual outlet was masturbating in, on, or behind this particular make of car (de Silva & Pernet, 1992).

cross-dressing Dressing in clothes traditionally associated with the opposite sex.

transvestite A man who obtains sexual satisfaction by wearing female clothing.

Transvestic Fetishism

J.T. is a factory foreman, a deacon in his church, and a respected member of the community. He is quiet, seemingly well adjusted, and happily married. Once a month, J.T. tells his wife he's going fishing for the weekend. Instead, he books a hotel room in the next town and spends the weekend lounging in women's lingerie. He loves the feel of the delicate lace, the smooth, soft silk, and the sheer texture of stockings. He sips champagne, watches television, and masturbates. When he returns, he feels refreshed and happy, but his happiness is tinged with guilt and anxiety. He is constantly concerned that his wife will find out about his cross-dressing, assume he must be gay or crazy, and leave him. He doesn't like sneaking around, and he wishes he could share this side of himself with his wife, but he's terribly afraid she'll be disgusted with his behavior and file for divorce.

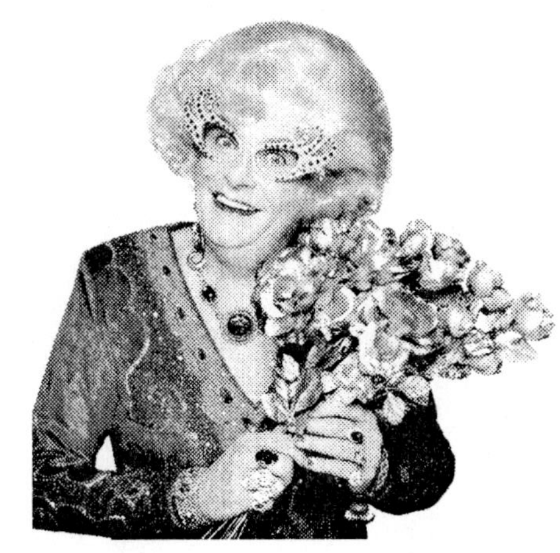

Cross-dressing for show business or to get laughs (as does the famous Dame Edna) is usually not considered transvestism.

You are probably aware that the term **cross-dressing** refers to wearing clothes traditionally associated with the opposite sex. But cross-dressing is not a paraphilia; it is not the same as *transvestism*, which is a paraphilia. Remember that paraphilias are behaviors that have a *compulsive* component and are engaged in for sexual arousal and

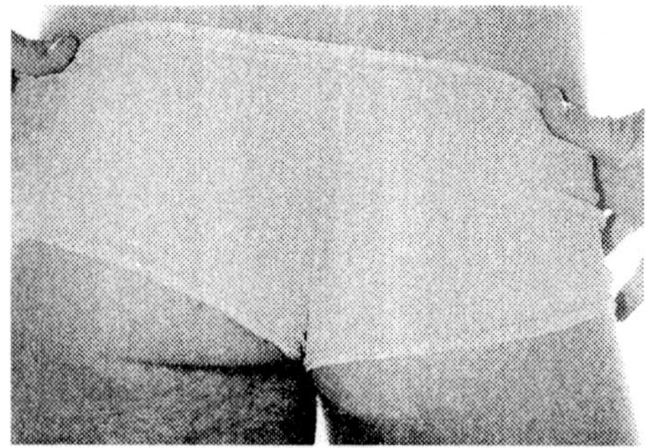

Most transvestites feel that cross-dressing allows them to express a different part of their personality.

transvestic fetishism The paraphilia engaged in by a transvestite.

transsexual A transgender person who desires and often attempts to change his or her body into the body of the opposite sex through dress, hormone therapy, and surgery.

transgender persons Individuals who self-identify as the opposite gender from their biological sex; not considered a paraphilia.

gender identity The sex (male or female) that a person identifies himself or herself to be.

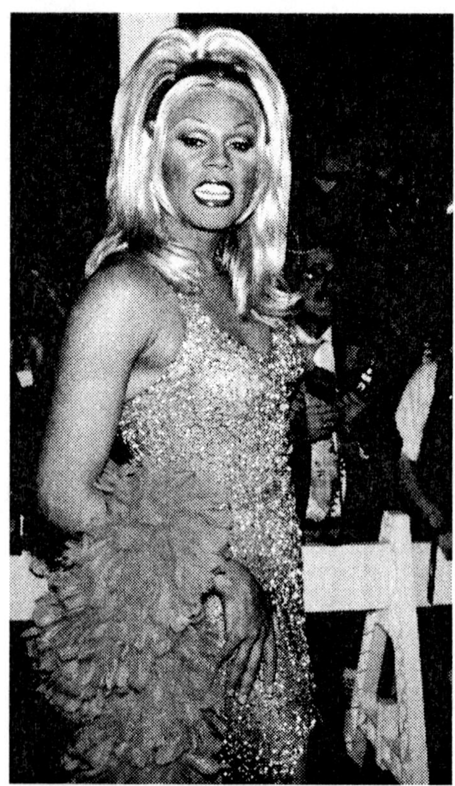

Transgender individuals are not transvestites and are not engaging in a paraphilia. They are people who self-identify as the gender other than their biological sex.

gratification. People cross-dress for many nonsexual reasons, such as a Halloween costume, a disguise, a costume for a movie, or for laughs on stage.

A **transvestite**, however, according to the DSM-IV-TR, is a man who obtains *sexual satisfaction* by wearing female clothing. Often simply referred to as *fetishism*, the psychological term for this paraphilia is **transvestic fetishism**, which makes sense when you think about the definition. The women's clothing is, in essence, the fetish object, but in this case it is the act of actually wearing it, not just touching or fondling it, that produces the sexual thrill.

One of the most pervasive myths about human sexuality is that transvestites are gay men. This is, for the most part, simply wrong. Studies indicate that most transvestites (70 to 90 percent) are heterosexual men, not gay and not bisexual (Bullough & Bullough, 1997; Docter & Prince, 1997). In fact, the DSM-IV-TR diagnostic definition for transvestism (see Table 14.1) is limited to heterosexual males. It is true that some gay men cross-dress, but this is typically for fun, for political statement, or for show, not for sexual arousal. Approximately 80 percent of transvestites either are or have been married and come from a wide variety of religions, professions, and family backgrounds. Most say that cross-dressing allows them to express different parts of their personalities and excites them sexually.

Transvestites are typically not interested in changing their behavior, but most hide their cross-dressing from wives, friends, and family and are afraid of being caught or found out. The fears transvestites cite include rejection by the people close to them and by society (47 percent); being labeled a "sissy," "queer," or "faggot" (23 percent); being seen as mentally ill (22 percent), and sinning against God (5 percent) (Bullough & Bullough, 1997).

Another common misconception is that men who dress as women for sexual purposes do so because they want to be women. Again, this is almost always false. Ninety-five percent of transvestites perceive themselves, without hesitation, as male (Docter & Prince, 1997). It should be stressed here that transvestism is not to be confused with *transsexualism* or *transgenderism*. **Transsexuals** and **transgender persons** typically self-identify with the opposite gender from their biological sex. That is, transgender men and women feel that they have been born in the wrong body; that their correct gender is the opposite of their biological sex. They identify with their perceived gender just as you identify with yours. They are not confused or in doubt, even though the bodies they were born with did not reflect their **gender identity** (International Foundation for Gender Identification, 2002). Transgenderism is *not* a paraphilia. A transgender person does not dress in the clothing of the opposite sex primarily for a sexual thrill but rather because the clothes reflect his or her gender identity. The issue of transsexualism and transgenderism is discussed in greater detail in Chapter 10, "Gender."

Autoerotic Asphyxia

R.G. is 19 years old and on his college wrestling team. He has recurrent fantasies of self-strangulation. He has lost consciousness several times during a stranglehold on the wrestling mat and has found the sensation of falling, weightlessness, and darkness to be extremely compelling. Several years ago, he began to experiment with ways of limiting oxygen to his brain during sexual fantasy and masturbation. He is very aroused by the risk he takes in courting possible death, and he loves the lightheaded feeling that he gets when he cinches his belt around his neck, attaches it to his headboard, and strangles himself almost to the point of unconsciousness while he masturbates to orgasm.

This is the one exception mentioned earlier of a paraphilia that does not have its own classification in the DSM-IV-TR. It is included here, however, because it is more common than most people think and because it can be deadly. Physically, this is the most personally dangerous of all the paraphilias. Some paraphilias may be psychologically damaging to the person performing them and to a potential victim, but most do not carry with them a high risk of death. This paraphilia, however, is often fatal. **Autoerotic asphyxia** (also sometimes referred to as *sexual hypoxia* and *hypoxyphilia*) involves depriving the brain of oxygen, usually through some form of strangulation or hanging, during masturbation (Hock, 2003b; A. P. Jenkins, 2000). This behavior is most typically engaged in by and most commonly fatal in men between the ages of 15 and 30, but autoerotic asphyxia has been found in a small number of women as well (Hucker & Blanchard, 1992; Martz, 2003). The motivation for this behavior appears to be the belief that oxygen deprivation enhances the arousal and orgasmic sensations during masturbation. However, loss of oxygen to the brain only causes lightheadedness and dizziness and is not in reality connected to enhanced sexual arousal. In other words, *do not try this at home!* It is extremely dangerous and potentially deadly. It is estimated that nearly one-third of all deaths by strangulation among teenagers are due to this activity. The total number of cases is estimated to be well over 1,000 a year in the United States, and this figure is without doubt low due to underreporting. Often such deaths are reported as simple suicides to avoid the potential embarrassment and stigma that may accompany the family's already intense grief (Gosink & Jumbelic, 2000; A. P. Jenkins, 2000).

Since You Asked...

8. I saw a movie on TV called *Rising Sun*. In the movie, a man strangles a woman during sex. But it seemed that she wanted him to do it, but he did it too hard and killed her. Why would anyone want to be choked during sex?

As with all paraphilias, people who engage in autoerotic asphyxia do so as a pattern, repeatedly, over time. The usual method is for the person to arrange some sort of hanging or other strangulation device that will cut off the supply of oxygen just up to, but not including, complete loss of consciousness. The danger, as you no doubt have guessed, is that sometimes these devices are too effective and cause unintentional unconsciousness and death.

Obviously, this is a potentially tragic sexual compulsion. Usually, no one other than the victim is aware of the behavior because it is nearly always performed in secret and in solitary, private locations. Sadly, the first sign the family has that this behavior is occurring is the discovery of the body. Consequently, intervening in the behavior of those at risk is extremely difficult.

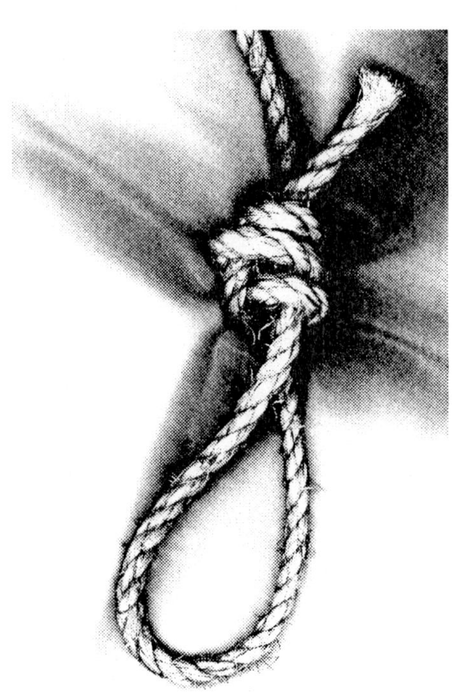

Typically, victims of autoerotic asphyxia devise some sort of apparatus that will cut off oxygen but release prior to full unconsciousness.

Warning signs that someone might be engaging in this potentially deadly behavior include a combination of the presence of pieces of short rope, padded ropes, or neckties with unusual knots; unusual marks around the neck; bloodshot eyes; marks on bedposts, headboards, or closet rods from ropes or belts; locks on bedroom doors; signs elsewhere on the body suggesting participation in bondage or other masochistic activities; and recent visits to Web sites on "scarfing" or "asphyx" (A. P. Jenkins, 2004; Tough, Butt, & Sanders, 1994). Your awareness of these warning signs will help you better recognize if someone you know may be engaging in this dangerous behavior and take appropriate steps to help the person stop through education and counseling.

Treatment of Paraphilias

Not everyone who has a paraphilia wants or even needs to alter the paraphilic behavior. However, many paraphilias create significant problems for the perpetrator, the victims, friends and family members, and society at large. For this reason, sexuality educators and mental health professionals have developed many strategies for intervening and helping clients control their dysfunctional and destructive paraphilic behaviors.

autoerotic asphyxia Depriving the brain of oxygen, usually through some form of strangulation or hanging, during masturbation (also sometimes referred to as *sexual hypoxia* and *hypoxyphilia*).

Who Seeks Treatment

People who seek treatment for a paraphilia may do so for a variety of reasons and come from a wide range of life situations. Their reason for obtaining help usually falls into one of the following four categories (de Silva, 1999):

- *Court-ordered treatment.* Individuals who have engaged in illegal acts involving paraphilias are often ordered by the court to undergo treatment as part of their sentence or probation. These individuals may or may not be motivated to make the changes the judge is demanding, so the potential success of treatment is highly variable.
- *Self-distress.* These individuals are embarrassed by behaviors they cannot seem to control; are worried that they will be caught or arrested; feel that they are unworthy, sick, or unnatural; or are afraid that they may be risking their life and career if they continue the behavior. These clients, by definition, are motivated to change, and although success rates vary (to be discussed shortly), they have a higher likelihood of successful treatment.
- *Relationship distress.* Many seek help for a paraphilia because it is creating discord or other problems in their primary relationship. The client is distressed because of the emotional pain the behavior is causing the partner and the discord it is causing in the relationship. In general, these clients come from long-term, stable relationships and are very motivated to change.
- *Distress due to sexual dysfunction.* When a paraphilia becomes well established, it often begins to interfere with sexual functioning. For example, as we discussed under fetishes earlier, some fetishists are unable to become sexually aroused or cannot achieve an orgasm without touching or interacting with the fetish object. Another example might be a transvestite who loses interest in making love with his partner because he cannot, in those situations, wear women's clothing without revealing his paraphilia. These individuals may seek treatment for the sexual dysfunction, which of necessity will involve treating the paraphilia that underlies it.

Types of Treatment

Various treatment approaches may be used in an effort to modify unwanted paraphilic behaviors. In the past, the goal of such therapy was to extinguish the behavior completely. This strict and inflexible goal, combined with the limited techniques available in the past, usually led to disturbingly poor success rates. Today, although success rates are far from perfect for most paraphilias, the effectiveness of newer therapies is improving. Obviously, for some of the most dangerous and coercive paraphilias discussed in this chapter, rapid and successful treatment is of utmost importance. The current therapeutic strategies for paraphilias includes a variety of approaches. The method employed depends on what paraphilia is being treated, the severity or danger of the behavior, and the characteristics of the client. Treatment approaches include incorporation of the behavior in acceptable ways, psychotherapy, orgasmic reconditioning, group therapy, and drug therapy (Brannon, 2002; de Silva, 1999).

Incorporation Therapy

Incorporation therapy is, in a way, a compromise, in that the frequency of the paraphilic behavior will be decreased or modified but not completely abolished. This approach is often successful when the partner of the paraphile is distressed and unwilling to accept the intensity of the paraphilic behaviors but can learn to endure a milder

incorporation therapy A treatment for paraphilias in which the paraphilic behavior is decreased or modified to acceptable levels but not completely abolished.

form of them. For example, imagine a transvestite who has a compulsion to wear women's underwear when making love with his partner, but the partner is too shocked or embarrassed to go anywhere near him when he does so. On the other hand, if he forgoes the women's lingerie, he is unable to become aroused at all. In an incorporation treatment approach, the couple might work together to reach the point where he wears only, say, a silky T-shirt or a garter on his arm, which is adequate for his arousal but mild enough not to turn her off.

Psychotherapy

Of course, standard, well-known forms of talk therapy may be used in treating paraphilias. The most successful approach appears to be **cognitive-behavioral therapy**, which combines techniques designed to modify unwanted behaviors with altering the client's thinking patterns that lead to the unwanted behaviors. The behavior component of this strategy has often included **aversion therapy**, in which behaviors and images associated with the paraphilia are paired with an unpleasant stimulus such as an electric shock or a noxious odor.

Due to ethical considerations, therapists today more often employ a technique called **covert sensitization**, in which, instead of shocks or bad odors, the client repeatedly fantasizes the unwanted behavior and then adds an extremely aversive event to the fantasy. For example, a pedophile might engage in various fantasies of sexual behavior with a child, and just before the event, a squad of police bursts in, guns drawn, and takes him to jail. This technique has been shown in some cases to be effective with certain paraphilias, including exhibitionism and sexual sadism (Brannon, 2002).

Other forms of psychotherapy that have found some success alone or in combination with other techniques include group therapy (which helps break down denial and avoidance by surrounding each client with others who engage in the same behaviors), social skills training to help the client learn to develop healthy relationships with others, and 12-step programs similar to Alcoholics Anonymous based on the assumption that paraphilias have at their core a compulsiveness similar to that of alcohol addiction (Brannon, 2002).

Orgasmic Reconditioning

Sexual arousal and orgasm are very powerful reinforcements for whatever behavior becomes associated with them. If a person who desires to modify his paraphilic behavior could be conditioned to become aroused and have orgasms in settings that bear no resemblance to the paraphilia, his maladaptive associations and behaviors might be altered. Here's how **orgasmic reconditioning** typically works. The client is told to masturbate using objects, fantasies, or images related to his paraphilia, but as orgasm approaches, he is instructed to switch completely to objects, fantasies, and images of more mainstream, socially acceptable sexual behaviors. Eventually, if successful, his sexual desires and urges will become redirected, or reconditioned, toward the new, more acceptable activities.

Drug Therapy

As noted in our discussion of biological theories of paraphilias, scientists now suspect that bio-chemical factors are involved in the development and maintenance of paraphilias. If an imbalance in brain and glandular chemicals is leading to unwanted, inappropriate sexual behavior, it makes sense that it might be treated with medications that alter, in some way, the production or effects of those chemicals.

Historically, drug treatment for paraphilias consisted of medications that would reduce the action of testosterone, based on the logic that if male hormones are

cognitive-behavioral therapy Psychotherapy combining techniques to modify unwanted sexual behaviors and the thinking patterns that lead to the behaviors.

aversion therapy Psychotherapy in which unwanted sexual behaviors and images are reduced by associating them with an unpleasant stimulus such as electric shocks or noxious odors.

covert sensitization A type of aversion therapy in which instead of actual shocks or bad odors, the client repeatedly fantasizes the unwanted behavior and then adds an extremely aversive event to the fantasy.

orgasmic reconditioning A type of therapy for paraphilias in which a person is conditioned to become aroused and have orgasms in socially acceptable settings that bear no resemblance to the paraphilia.

responsible for sex drive, less of it should decrease sex drive and paraphilic behavior along with it. Hormone-blocking drugs such as Depo-Provera and Lupron have been used with some success (de Silva, 1999; Krueger & Kaplan, 2001; Meston & Frohlich, 2002). Although such drugs do decrease paraphilic behavior in most men, they also inhibit sex drive and sexual functioning altogether, and they have the potential for other side effects (such as breast growth and erectile difficulties), which cause many men to discontinue treatment.

More recently, a newer class of medications called selective serotonin reuptake inhibitors (SSRIs) are showing promise in treating more resistant and serious cases of paraphilias. SSRIs with trade names you may recognize, such as Prozac, Zoloft, and Paxil, were originally developed and approved for the treatment of depression. However, the effective use of these drugs has been expanding to include such psychological conditions as obsessive-compulsive disorder, attention deficit disorder, and various anxiety disorders (Hollander & Rosen, 2000). It is logical to assume that paraphilic behaviors may be linked to some or all of these other disorders, and therefore, these drugs have been used in paraphilia treatment regimens. Several studies on SSRI treatments have shown positive outcomes, including reduced paraphilic fantasies, impulses, and behaviors (Abouesh & Clayton, 1999; Birken, Hill, & Berner, 2003; Meston & Frohlich, 2002).

Effectiveness of Treatment for Paraphilias

Since YOU Asked...

9. Everyone in my neighborhood has received a notice that a convicted sex offender has been released from prison and will be moving near us. Of course, this news is scary. Can sex offenders be cured (I think he's an exhibitionist)? What are the chances he will do those acts again?

Success rates of the various therapies for stopping or limiting paraphilic compulsions are difficult to determine with a high degree of accuracy. The primary source of statistics is the criminal justice system, where sex offenders who have been arrested are usually sent to jail, placed in treatment, or both. If, after serving their sentence, they reoffend and are arrested again, those treatment failures can be tracked. Beyond that, we have reports from therapists about the extent to which their clients say that the treatment has been successful.

Nevertheless, studies seem to indicate that treatment of paraphilias is significantly better than no treatment in reducing unwanted behaviors. For example, one study that followed sex offenders for many years (reported in Kokish, 2001) found the following success rates (success defined as no rearrest, self-report by the offender of no paraphilic behavior, reduced arousal to paraphilic images, and ratings by the offenders' partners): pedophiles; 95 percent; exhibitionists; 92 percent; zoophiles; 100 percent; and frotteurs; 80 percent. Another study found that overall, 11 percent of treated sex offenders reoffended, compared to 18 percent of those who received no treatment. Overall, the success rate for most paraphilias is not optimistic. High rates of reoffending are common following most treatment regimens. The most successful treatments appear to be found among individuals who are treated early in their history of paraphilic behaviors and who are the most motivated to stop the deviant behavior and involve themselves in normal adult sexual relationships (Seligman & Hardenberg, 2000).

As biomedical, psychological, and sexual research continue to refine treatment methods and strategies, the outlook for increasingly effective therapies for paraphilias is optimistic (Rosler & Witztum, 2000). However, we must keep in mind that sexual arousal and responding are compelling motivators that have the power to lead people either to heights of great pleasure to the depths of strange, antisocial, and dangerous actions. Power that strong is never easy to overcome.

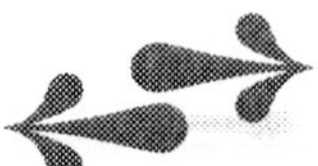

YOUR SEXUAL PHILOSOPHY

PARAPHILIAS: THE EXTREMES OF SEXUAL BEHAVIOR

As mentioned at the beginning of this chapter, our study of human sexuality would not be complete without discussing the world of strange sexual practices, and by now, you may understand them better than you ever wanted to! But paraphilias are a very real component in the landscape of human sexuality. You already know about the rich diversity of human nature; now you also have some insight into the farthest reaches of the complexity and variation of human sexuality.

How the heck, you may be thinking, can these very strange and sometimes victimizing sexual behaviors possibly find a place in my sexual philosophy? If you consider them carefully, you'll see that a knowledge of paraphilias is an important piece in the complex puzzle that allows you to know who you are, to be clear about what you want and don't want in your life as a sexual person, and to plan ahead so that you can make the choices that are right for you.

For example, you might at some point in your life find yourself in a situation involving a person who may want to engage in one of the behaviors discussed in this chapter. You will need to figure out, maybe without a lot of time for reflection, how you feel about that. Is the behavior OK with you? Are you willing to be a participant? Do you need to remove yourself from the situation quickly? Do you need to take immediate actions (such as intervening or calling the police) to protect yourself or others? These are questions that you should have some ready answers to instead of trying to figure out how you feel and what to do in the highly pressurized moment when they may arise.

Moreover, what if you find yourself attracted to sexual acts that would be considered paraphilias? How would you handle that? A clearer understanding of what these behaviors are and which ones are dangerous, victimizing, or just "different" is crucial in your decision to act on your impulses, work to reject them from your life, or seek professional help to stop or avoid them.

Finally, the material in this chapter *must* be part of your sexual philosophy so that you are as well educated and equipped as you can be to protect others, such as friends, relatives, and especially children, from sexual victimization at the hands of individuals who seem to be unable to control their coercive sexual compulsions.

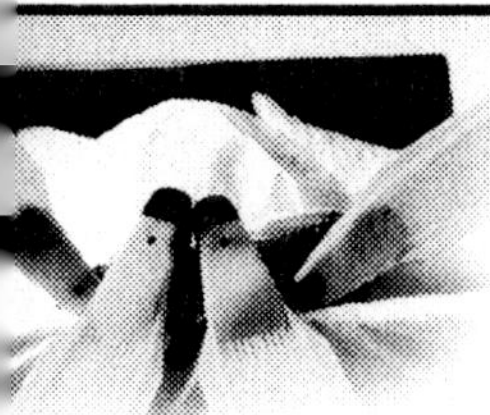

Summary

HISTORICAL PERSPECTIVES An Early Account of Paraphilias

- Among the earliest written accounts of the unusual behaviors known as paraphilias dates back to the late 1800s when Richard von Krafft-Ebing published his 600-page book *Psychopathia Sexualis,* which detailed 237 case studies of strange sexual activities, including reports of a man who had intercourse with a hen and a teenage boy who had what we would now call a handkerchief fetish.
- Some of the behaviors Krafft-Ebing condemned as pathological are today considered common and normal by most health professionals and people in general; these include masturbation, oral sex, and nonheterosexual orientations.

Defining Paraphilias

- Paraphilia, literally meaning, "abnormal love," refers to acts that most people would consider strange or abnormal that are performed for the purpose of sexual gratification and tend to be compulsive, meaning the person is helpless to stop the behavior.

- Societies tend to gauge the degree of abnormality of a paraphilia using various criteria, including the legality of the act, whether or not the act victimizes others, how harmful the act is to the person performing it and to others, and whether the person engaging in the act is able to maintain normal, intimate relationships with others.
- In professional practice, a sexual behavior may be diagnosed as a paraphilia if the person has experienced recurring, intense sexually arousing fantasies, sexual urges, or behaviors related to the paraphilia for a period of at least six months *and* the person has acted on those urges *and* the urges have caused marked distress or interpersonal difficulties.
- When a paraphilia victimizes others, it may be diagnosed regardless of whether or not the person engaging in the behavior feels distressed by it.

Origins of Paraphilias

- Though the exact cause of paraphilias is not known, various theories have been proposed to account for why some people engage in these sexual anomalies. These include psychodynamic theories that contend that paraphilias stem from early childhood conflict, behavioral theories that propose a learning theory approach to the development of paraphilic behavior, and biological hypotheses that place the source of paraphilic behavior within human biology, focusing on brain chemical or hormonal imbalances.

Gender and Paraphilias

- Nearly all paraphiles are men. The one possible exception is sexual masochism (sexual gratification from receiving pain), which is found in both men and women but is nevertheless far more common in men.
- The greater prevalence of paraphilias in men may be due to the fact that in most Western cultures, males are given greater "permission" to be sexual in their thinking, language, and behaviors and therefore have a greater opportunity to experiment with unusual sexual activities.
- Determining exact numbers of people who engage in any specific paraphilia is difficult due to the necessity of relying on self-report data, which is easily subject to bias when dealing with such socially disapproved behaviors.

Specific Paraphilias

- Paraphilias may be divided into two definitive categories: coercive and noncoercive. Coercive paraphilias involve the victimization of another person. They include voyeurism, exhibitionism, frotteurism, sexual sadism, and pedophilia and tend to be punishable by law.
- Noncoercive paraphilias are either individual (solo) activities or involve other consenting adults. These include masochism, fetishism, transvestism, and autoerotic asphyxia (self-strangulation during masturbation).

Treatment of Paraphilias

- Paraphilic behaviors are among the most difficult behavior problems to treat or cure among adults. This is probably due to the fact that the sexual arousal and orgasm that typically accompany the behaviors are among the most rewarding events a person can experience, and the behavior therefore becomes deeply ingrained.
- Types of therapy include incorporation therapy, cognitive-behavior therapy, aversion therapy, covert sensitization, orgasmic reconditioning, and medications. Success rates for treatment are generally poor, with high rates of repeat arrests of paraphilic sexual offenders.

YOUR SEXUAL PHILOSOPHY: Paraphilias: The Extremes of Sexual Behavior

- The information in this chapter must be part of your sexual philosophy so that you are as well educated and equipped as you can be to deal with atypical sexual behaviors should you be confronted with them and so that you are in the best position possible to protect others, such as friends, relatives, and especially children, from sexual victimization at the hands of individuals who are unable to control their coercive sexual compulsions.

Have You Considered?

1. Which of the four criteria listed in the section titled "Society's Criteria for Judging Paraphilias" do you feel are the most important in determining whether a certain sexual behavior is abnormal? Explain your answer.
2. Of the various theories of the origins of paraphilias, which one makes the most sense to you? Why, in your opinion, does that one seem to explain paraphilias better than the others?
3. Explain why, in your opinion, paraphilias are much more common in men than in women.
4. Which of the noncoercive paraphilias, if any, do you think should be illegal? Explain your answer.
5. How do you think the Catholic church should handle the sex scandals involving pedophile priests in the future? How can the church try to ensure that these abuses of power and position do not happen again?
6. In the chapter's discussion of masochism, you read about the arrests made in England of members of a masochism club. The appeals court, in overturning their arrests, compared sexual masochism to the sport of boxing. Does this comparison make sense to you? Why or why not?
7. Using the theories discussed in the chapter, discuss how someone might develop a fetish for watermelons.
8. Imagine that you are sexually and romantically involved with someone who has a paraphilia. Would you be willing to try incorporation therapy as a treatment strategy? If so, explain which paraphilias you think it would be suited for and why. If not, why not?

Companion Website Resources

For further chapter resources go to **www.prenhall.com/hock**. This robust text website includes polling questions for you to vote on, regular news updates, quizzes, sample tests, suggested reading lists, and more..

SCENARIOS USA Also on the website are links to videos. *Scenarios USA*'s films portray real-life narratives that explore the non-biological aspects of relationships and sexual health. The films will help you consider how the themes of the text affect your own life and the lives of those around you.

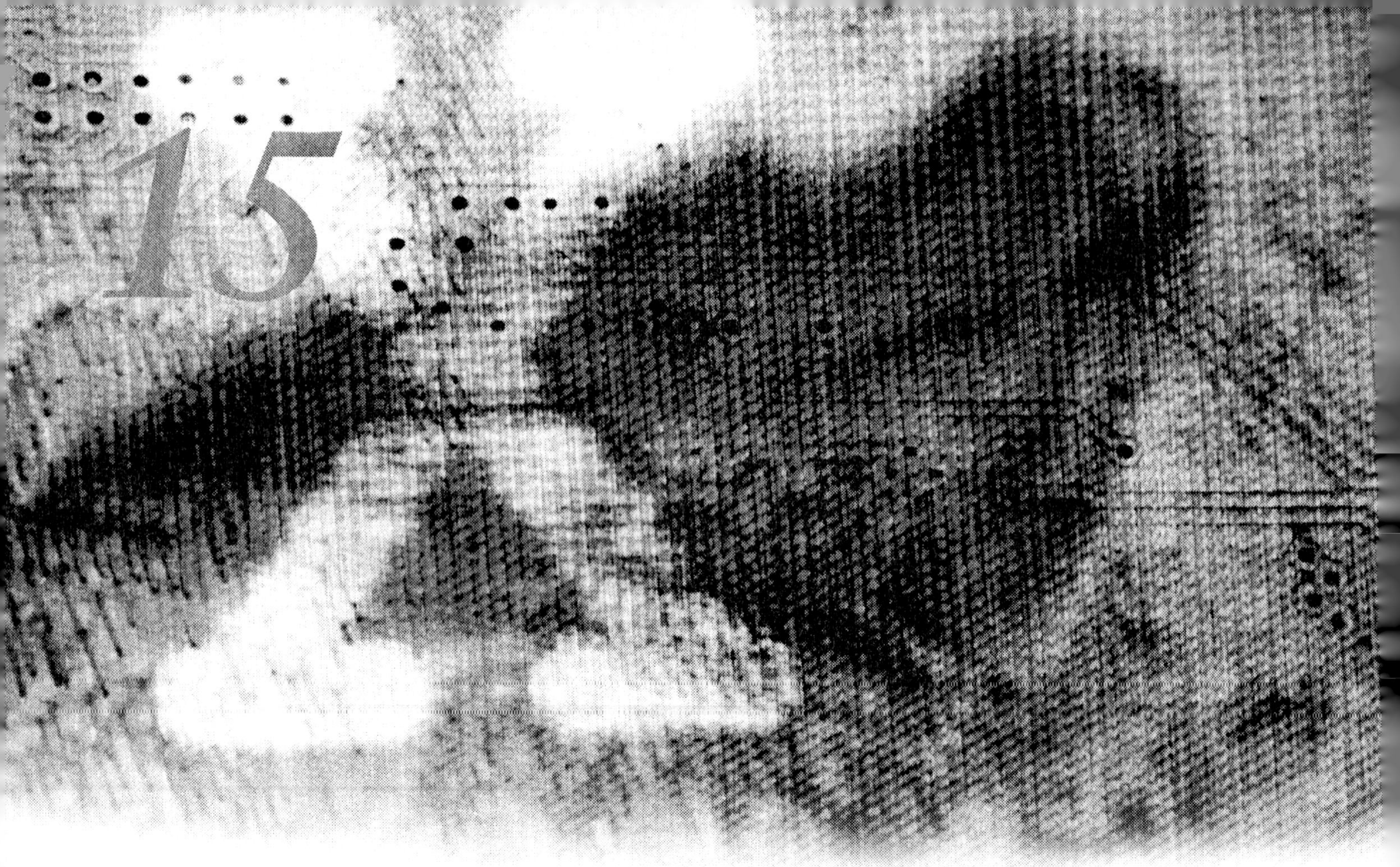

15

The Sexual Marketplace

Prostitution and Pornography

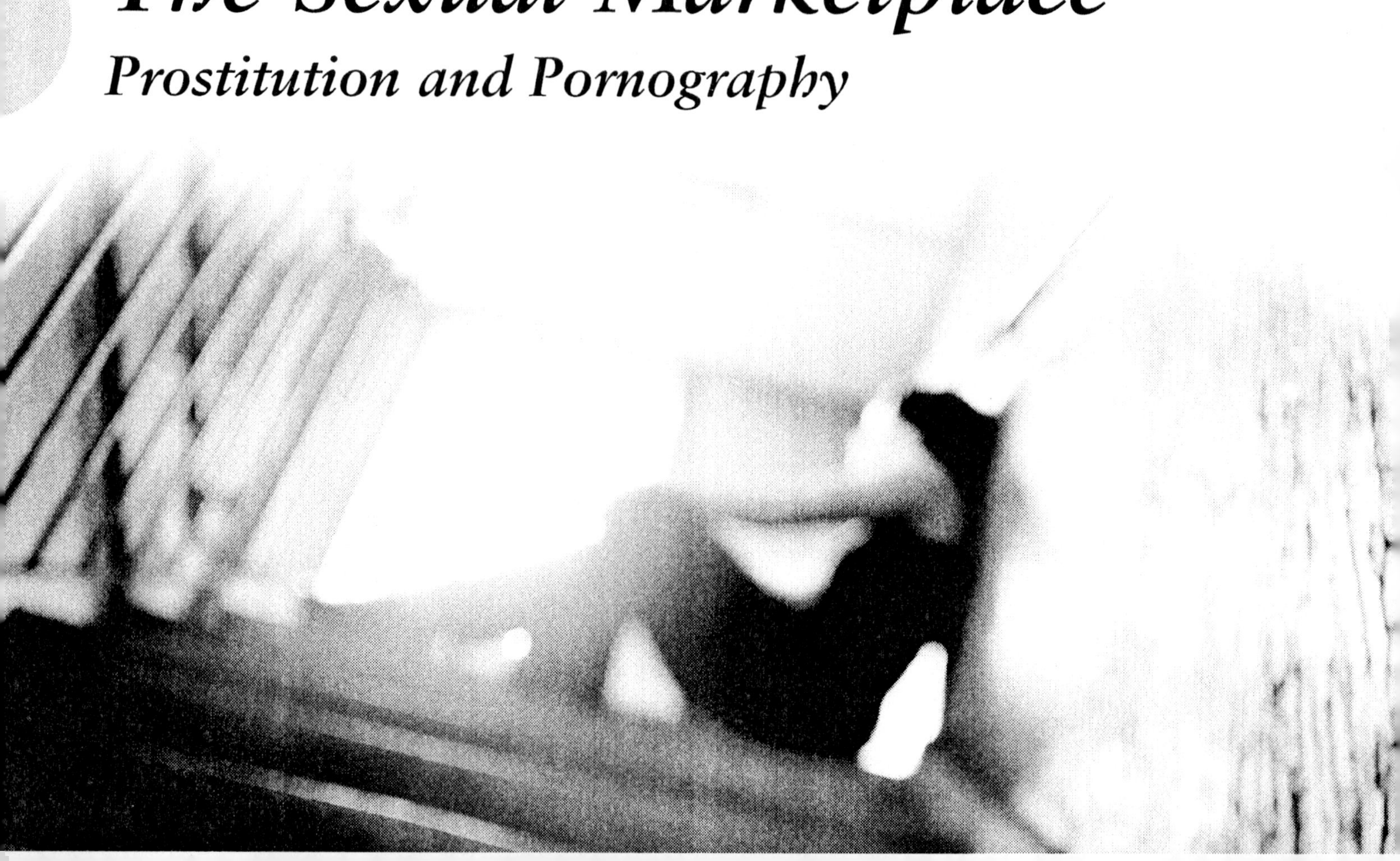

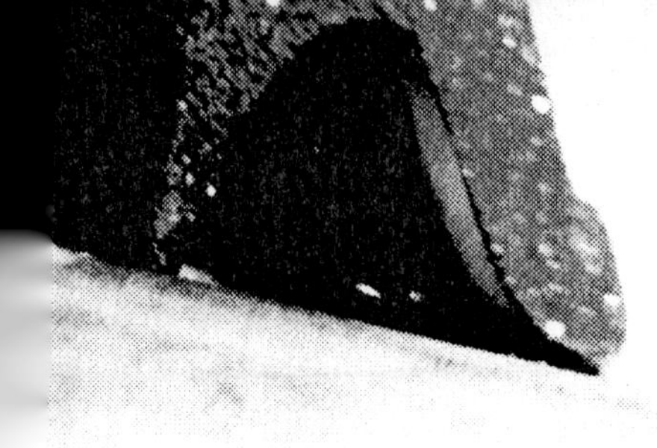
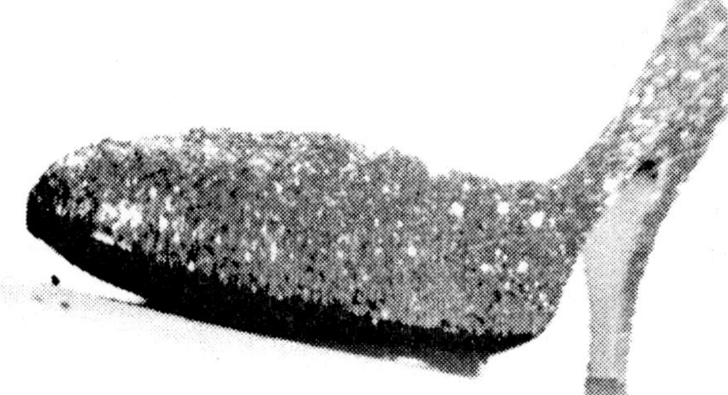

Since YOU Asked...

1. Why is prostitution called the world's oldest profession? Is it really? (see page 551)

2. My roommate is sleeping with a guy so that he will do her math homework for her. Isn't that the same as being a prostitute? (see page 552)

3. Is prostitution legal in all of Nevada or just in Las Vegas? How does it work there? (see page 553)

4. I cannot understand why any woman would ever become a prostitute. Is there something psychologically wrong with these women? (see page 557)

5. Is it true that AIDS and other diseases are spread mostly by prostitutes? (see page 562)

6. What are the main reasons men go to prostitutes? Is it usually because they can't get sex any other way? (see page 566)

7. I like to look at magazines like *Playboy* and *Hustler*, but my girlfriend says they are pornographic trash. I think pornography refers to much worse kinds of magazines and videos. Who is right? (see page 569)

8. Everybody's always saying how bad pornography is because it is violent toward women. But I've seen a lot of XXX videos that don't have any violence against women in them at all. So is that not pornography? (see page 572)

9. Can looking at pornography cause guys to want to do weird or sick things sexually? (see page 576)

10. I read that child pornography is everywhere on the Internet. I think this is just so sick. What is being done to stop it? (see page 581)

You have probably heard the claim that "sex sells." Usually, that particular cliché is applied to the use of sexual images, words, and fantasies in the advertising and promotion of products. Although "sexual marketing" may be pervasive—you can hardly turn on the TV or open a magazine without seeing it—that is not the focus of this chapter. Rather, in this chapter, we will focus on the two main markets for selling sex itself: prostitution and pornography.

Sex is big business in the United States and throughout the world. A staggering amount of money changes hands both legally and illegally in the buying and selling of sexual services and sexually explicit materials. Both prostitution and pornography are controversial topics because they weave together sexuality, law, censorship, and morality in a highly charged emotional mix. The questions raised by this mix have been asked for decades, if not centuries, and continue to be asked today. Should states enact laws that determine what people can and cannot do with their own bodies? Is prostitution a "victimless" crime? What are the factors that cause someone to become a sex trade worker? Why does someone choose to pay for sexual activities? Would decriminalizing prostitution help reduce the spread of HIV and other STIs? How do sexually explicit materials fit into the freedom-of-speech protections in the First Amendment to the U.S. Constitution? Is there a difference between *erotica* and *pornography*? Should sexually explicit films, videos, magazines, and books be censored or banned? If so, which ones? Where should societies draw the line between what is legal and illegal? Does pornography discriminate against certain groups? Does it promote rape and other sexual violence? What can be done about child pornography? Do sexually explicit materials ever serve a socially positive purpose?

These and countless other questions are the focus of some of the most heated controversies in the field of human sexuality. Chances are that these debates may never be resolved fully because history has shown us that attitudes toward pornography and prostitution are continuously reshaped by ever-changing cultural influences. For example, as you will read in this chapter, at a time in history when the debate over the legalization of prostitution was relatively quiet, the feminist movement in the 1960s and the frightening pandemic of HIV/AIDS in the 1980s and 1990s reenergized and redirected that dialogue. When at last some fairly reasonable and effective systems had been developed in the United States for dealing with the complex legalities of sexually explicit materials, along came the Internet to draw them into question once again. Therefore, we can probably assume that these issues and controversies are here to stay in one incarnation or another. That fact may be the best possible reason for all of us to continue to pursue the most complete understanding of them that we can have.

Focus on Your Feelings

Few topics in this book will generate as complex a mixture of emotions as those in this chapter. Why? Because they represent a crossroads of sex, morality, the law, and victimization. That's a powerful mix of emotion-producing themes.

Virtually no one is indifferent when it comes to prostitution. You may feel anger as you read of the uncaring people and circumstances that sometimes conspire to force a girl or woman into prostitution and keep her there. That anger may turn to distress when it becomes clear that drug addiction and coercion by pimps, and even sometimes by boyfriends and husbands, leaves some prostitutes little choice about exchanging their bodies for money or drugs, or that a vast international sex-slave-trafficking market, focusing on children, is thriving despite efforts to stamp it out. And what about your reactions to the men who choose to buy sex from prostitutes? You may feel moral outrage that those men must abuse others to satisfy their own selfish sexual urges. You may be surprised to learn that the characteristics of clients of prostitutes match quite closely the characteristics of men in general. Finally, an ongoing debate is whether prostitution should be either legalized or decriminalized. Whichever side you take, that debate is usually highly emotionally charged.

Emotional reactions to pornography tend to run as high as they do to prostitution. When you read about the difficulties in defining pornography, you may feel frustrated that people can't seem to come up with a usable working definition. Moreover, the difficulty defining pornography leads directly to the debate over what sexually explicit materials, if any, should be censored or legally banned. Opinions run the gamut from the argument that all explicit sexual images should be illegal to the belief that nothing at all should be censored. Whatever you believe, you can easily find someone to debate it with you.

Finally, this chapter covers what may be the most emotionally wrenching topic of all: child pornography. It is rampant on the Internet, yet virtually everyone not involved in that depraved market reacts to such materials with revulsion. So get ready. Of all the "Focus on Your Feelings" boxes in this text, this one is warning you most strongly of emotions you probably won't be able to escape.

With that in mind, we should perhaps start at the beginning. Prostitution has often been referred to as the world's oldest profession. That claim is probably arguable (wouldn't hunting and gathering have come first?), but it is a cliché that has become inescapably linked with prostitution. In the first half of this chapter, we will explore the current state of prostitution, also referred to as the **commercial sex trades**, analyzing what prostitution is and the profiles of prostitutes and their clients. We will also consider the risks of STIs in the sex trades and some of the ongoing legal controversies that surround prostitution. Next we will turn to the topic of pornography, its definition and what we know about its possible effects, especially in the cases of child pornography and cyberporn. As always, we will close with a consideration of how and why the topics of this chapter are important to your personal sexual philosophy.

commercial sex trades Prostitution and related sexual activities for commercial purposes.

Historical Perspectives

The Oldest Brothel?

How old is prostitution? What evidence do we have to say that prostitution is the oldest profession? A recent archaeological find might help answer these questions. In 1996, archaeologists were excavating the ruins of an ancient Roman forum in Salonika, in the ancient area of northern Greece known as Macedonia. As the digging took the scientists underneath the forum, they happened upon a remarkable discovery: a bathhouse and brothel from more than 2,000 years ago. The artifacts, rooms, and decor they found left very little doubt about the purpose of the structure:

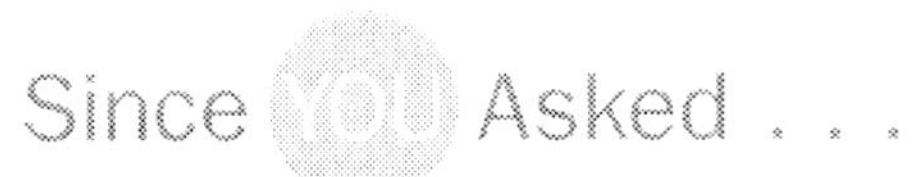

1. Why is prostitution called the world's oldest profession? Is it really?

> Experts have dug out and pieced together hundreds of rare 1st century BC clay artifacts, glass objects and erotic paraphernalia. On them are hundreds of depictions of sexual intercourse in myriad forms and combinations, including human orgies with goats. The treasure trove also includes a clay dildo, two red-and-green colored clay masks and a glass cup trimmed with a relief depicting *Fortuna*, a fertility deity and capricious dispenser of good and bad luck. Lighting up the scientists' eyes—in shock, they say—are at least 700 oil lamps decorated with explicit sexual scenes, all pieced together from millions of clay shards found on the tavern's ground floor. The designs and the abundance of lamps provide additional proof that the complex operated heavily in the after-hours. (Bird, 1999, p. 52)

Many other similar finds have demonstrated that prostitution is indeed a very old, if not the "oldest" profession. From the archaeological evidence, social scientists are able to piece together vivid scenarios that go beyond the visible, concrete discoveries to the actual behaviors that may have transpired among the people visiting these facilities devoted to sexual and sensual pleasure. Brothels such as the discovery in Salonica were not disreputable, seedy, back-street sex parlors. On the contrary, they were high-class social clubs that were visited as a normal part of a day in the life of ancient Roman men, in much the same way as, say, a health club might be frequented today. Sexual activities were only one of a variety of pleasures available to patrons:

> They would dine lavishly before stepping into one of the 25 tubs to enjoy a relaxing steam bath. . . . Given the length of the bathing procedure—with its series of immersions in pools of various temperatures, from frigid to hot—customers also may have been served food and drink while they soaked. . . . The women were respected companions. They may have worn masks and teased with sexual games of pantomime, but they also knew how to recite poetry [and] perform comedy and tragedy. They were refined and treated as intellectual equals by their customers. (Bird, 1999, p. 52)

Artifacts from ancient brothels in Greece and Italy add legitimacy to the cliché that prostitution may be the "oldest profession."

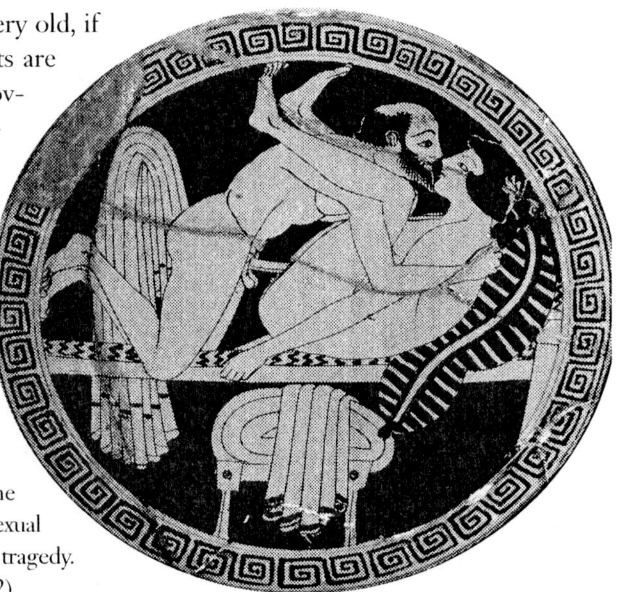

Although this quote assumes that all the prostitutes working at the brothel were female, many researchers believe that both boys and girls were available to patrons for sexual favors at that time in ancient history. The Salonica brothel site was opened for public viewing in 1999 and excavation continues into newly discovered rooms.

Prostitution

Hooker, hustler, cocotte, cruise, whore, harlot, bawd, tart, cyprian, fancy woman, working girl, streetwalker, strumpet, trollop, sporting lady, woman of the street, chuspanel, chippy, commercial sex trade worker—the list of slang and street terms for female and male prostitutes seems never-ending and unrelentingly derogatory. As we have discussed elsewhere in this book, language reflects the attitudes of a society. Clearly, most cultures throughout the world condemn the profession of prostitution as evidenced by language, laws, and punishments, which range from misdemeanors (San Francisco and New York) to flogging (Iran) to public beheadings (pre-2003 Iraq). However, when viewed from the perspective of people who work in the commercial sex trades, prostitution often takes on a different feel. In this section, we will look at prostitution from various perspectives, including how it is defined, the many and varied approaches sex trade workers take in practicing their profession, the characteristics of prostitutes, the characteristics of their customers, and the issue of STIs in the sex trades. We will also look at the laws surrounding prostitution and the debate over its legalization.

Defining Prostitution

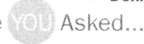

Since YOU Asked...

2. My roommate is sleeping with a guy so that he will do her math homework for her. Isn't that the same as being a prostitute?

The definition of prostitution depends on the context in which it is used. For example, various legal jurisdictions may use differing definitions, psychologists and sociologists may have specific definitions for research purposes, and even individuals rarely agree on a definition if you pin them down on specifics. Most people would say that prostitution means "sex for money." However, this straightforward interpretation is probably oversimplified and may be misleading. What exactly is meant by "sex"? Sexual intercourse? Manual stimulation? Oral sex? Kissing? Stripping? Posing for sexual photographs? All of the above?

Moreover, payment of money is not technically necessary for sexual acts to be considered prostitution. Sexual services exchanged for virtually anything—money, valued objects, personal property, drugs, shelter, or another service of some sort—probably qualify as prostitution. In fact, if you think about it, the only exchange that would likely never be defined as prostitution is sex for sex.

Sex is more than intercourse 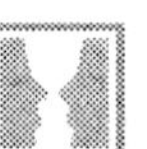

Taking all these factors into account, a general, working definition of **prostitution** for our purposes is "providing or receiving sexual acts by specific agreement between a prostitute, the client, and sometimes the prostitute's employer ('pimp') in exchange for money or some other form of remuneration." Prostitutes and their clients may be male or female and of the same or opposite sex.

This definition describes the overall practice of prostitution and says nothing about the legal definition or criminal penalties related to providing or partaking of such practices. You will also notice that the definition does not specify how much money or what the other forms of remuneration might be. It does, however, apply the definition of prostitution to both the prostitute and the client and clarifies that those involved in prostitution are not limited to any particular combination of sexes of the participants. This is an important point because historically, prostitution has been thought of and often legally defined as "acts furnished by a female to a male."

prostitution Providing or receiving sexual acts between a prostitute, a client, and sometimes the prostitute's employer ("pimp") in exchange for money or some other form of remuneration.

In most states, however, laws have been expanded to include both sexes and both the sex worker and the client. "Sexuality, Ethics, and the Law: Comparison of State Criminal

Definitions of Prostitution" compares criminal statute definitions in two rather disparate states, Utah and New Jersey. As you can see, their laws bear many more similarities than differences. One important exception to laws about prostitution is the state of Nevada, where in many counties prostitution is not a crime and is under state control. Nevada is one of the very few areas in the world where prostitution is not outlawed or prohibited in some formal way. The special case of Nevada is discussed in detail in "Sexuality and Culture: Prostitution in Nevada."

3. Is prostitution legal in all of Nevada or just in Las Vegas? How does it work there?

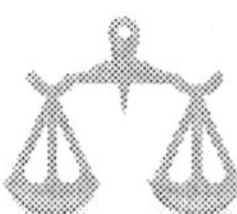

Sexuality, Ethics, and the Law

Comparison of State Criminal Definitions of Prostitution

These excerpts from the Utah and New Jersey criminal codes demonstrate how states tend to agree in their definitions and language pertaining to prostitution. You can see that both states' views of prostitution for criminal justice purposes are quite similar, even though the overall social and political climate of the two states is significantly different.

Utah

76-10-1301. Definitions. For the purposes of this part:

1. "House of prostitution" means a place where prostitution or promotion of prostitution is regularly carried on by one or more persons under the control, management, or supervision of another.
2. "Inmate" means a person who engages in prostitution in or through the agency of a house of prostitution.
3. "Public place" means any place to which the public or any substantial group of the public has access.
4. "Sexual activity" means acts of masturbation, sexual intercourse, or any sexual act involving the genitals of one person and the mouth or anus of another person, regardless of the sex of either participant (as last amended by Chapter 199, Laws of Utah 1988) 76-10-1302.

Prostitution.

1. A person is guilty of prostitution when: (a) he engages in any sexual activity with another person for a fee; (b) is an inmate of a house of prostitution; or (c) loiters in or within view of any public place for the purpose of being hired to engage in sexual activity.
2. Prostitution is a class B misdemeanor. However, any person who is convicted a second time, and on all subsequent convictions, under this section or under a local ordinance adopted in compliance with Section 76-10-1307 is guilty of a class A misdemeanor, except as provided in Section 76-10-1309 (as last amended by Chapter 179, Laws of Utah 1993) 76-10-1303.

Patronizing a prostitute.

1. A person is guilty of patronizing a prostitute when: (a) he pays or offers or agrees to pay another person a fee for the purpose of engaging in an act of sexual activity; or (b) he enters or remains in a house of prostitution for the purpose of engaging in sexual activity.
2. Patronizing a prostitute is a class B misdemeanor, except as provided in Section 76-10-1309 (as last amended by Chapter 179, Laws of Utah 1993)

New Jersey

2C:34-1. Prostitution and Related Offenses.

a. As used in this section:

1. "Prostitution" is sexual activity with another person in exchange for something of economic value, or the offer or acceptance of an offer to engage in sexual activity in exchange for something of economic value.
2. "Sexual activity" includes, but is not limited to, sexual intercourse, including genital-genital, oral-genital, anal-genital, and oral-anal contact, whether between persons of the same or opposite sex; masturbation; touching of the genitals, buttocks, or female breasts; sadistic or masochistic abuse and other deviate sexual relations.
3. "House of prostitution" is any place where prostitution or promotion of prostitution is regularly carried on by one person under the control, management or supervision of another.
4. "Promoting prostitution" is: (a) Owning, controlling, managing, supervising or otherwise keeping, alone or in association with another, a house of prostitution or a prostitution business; (b) Procuring an inmate for a house of prostitution or place in a house of prostitution for one who would be an inmate; (c) Encouraging, inducing, or otherwise purposely causing another to become or remain a prostitute; (d) Soliciting a person to patronize a prostitute; (e) Procuring a prostitute for a patron.

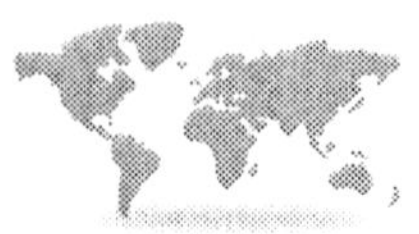

Sexuality and Culture

Prostitution in Nevada

Nearly everyone knows that prostitution is illegal in the United States and most other countries. It is true that laws forbidding prostitution exist in all 50 states. However, in most parts of one state, Nevada, prostitution is practiced legally, in state-licensed brothels. Other forms of prostitution—including streetwalking, escort services, and massage parlors—are illegal in all other states. As of 2005, all prostitutes in Nevada brothels were women, and all customers were men. Although nothing in Nevada state law prohibits male prostitutes, brothels designed for men to service women clients, or gay and lesbian brothels, none of these has yet been established (Brents & Hausbeck, 2001). The only exception to this rule is that some brothels allow a male-female couple to hire a prostitute together for a "threesome" or allow a man to hire two prostitutes simultaneously.

By 2001, Nevada had licensed 36 brothels. Interestingly, none of them are where one might expect to find them—Las Vegas and Reno; in fact, these famous gambling spots are located in parts of Nevada where prostitution is *not* legal. Because each city is allowed to determine whether to make brothels legal, some have opted to restrict them. Although prostitutes may look for business in the state's two major gambling towns, official, state-sanctioned brothels are not found there.

Nevada brothels are regulated by the state in terms of location. They may not be in highly populated areas, on a main traffic thoroughfare, or anywhere near a school or church. These regulations imply that Nevada brothels are hidden from Nevada society in general, but in reality, they are often quite obvious and even brazenly conspicuous.

One of the most common concerns raised about legalized prostitution is the potential for spreading STIs—HIV, HPV, hepatitis, gonorrhea, and so on. In Nevada brothels, all prostitutes are required to use condoms for all insertive sexual activities, including vaginal, oral, and anal sex. Furthermore, in 1985, Nevada instituted very strict laws governing the health testing for women working in brothels, mandating frequent testing for HIV and other STIs in order to receive a state health permit for brothel work. Any positive STI result prohibits her from sex work until treated and cured. If any Nevada sex worker tests positive for HIV, she is no longer legally allowed to work legally as a brothel prostitute (Brents & Hausbeck, 2001).

Of course, none of this means that everyone in Nevada, or certainly anywhere else, approves of the existence of legal prostitution in Nevada. Every few years, some Nevada lawmakers introduce new bills designed to outlaw all forms of prostitution in the state. However, legal prostitution is deeply ingrained in the social, cultural, and economic foundations of Nevada; it is unlikely it will ever be outlawed. In fact, as discussed in this chapter, the debate over decriminalizing or legalizing prostitution in other states is a much more hotly debated issue than any attempt to ban brothels in Nevada.

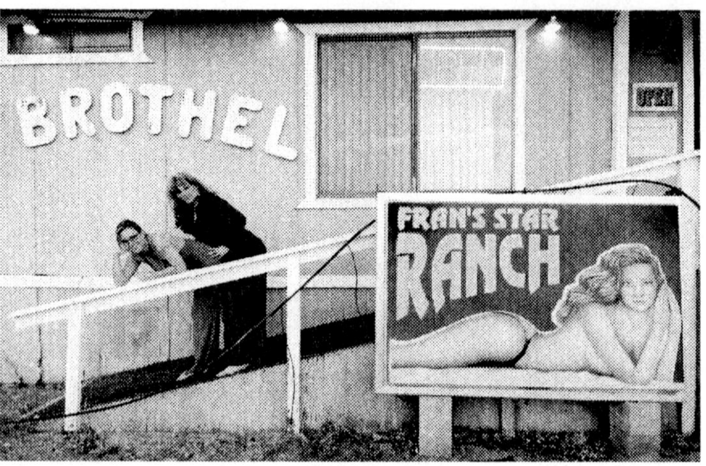

In Nevada, not only is prostitution legal, but it has become a big business. Although brothels in Nevada are required by law to be inconspicuous, often the opposite is true.

Types of Prostitutes

Individuals who work in the sex trades are often divided into various categories depending on where they work, how they procure their clients, and what activities they engage in. Without being overly specific, three main categories cover most of those who are engaged in the profession of prostitution: streetwalkers, call girls, and brothel workers. These typically apply to female prostitutes; we will discuss male prostitution later in this chapter.

Streetwalkers

As the name implies, **streetwalkers** sell their services on the street, typically to customers driving up in cars. The women in this category typically make the least money overall and per customer, and for most, a large percentage of their earnings go to their pimp. The streetwalkers' income usually averages under $20,000 per year ("Sex Trade Workers," 2001). In addition, streetwalkers are in the greatest danger of arrest, violence, and contracting STIs. Streetwalkers tend to be less educated and are very commonly involved with illegal drug abuse (Dalla, 2002; Erickson et al., 2000). The sexual behaviors provided by streetwalkers are typically less varied and of shorter duration than those provided by other prostitutes. The most common behaviors are manual masturbation, oral sex, or quick vaginal intercourse.

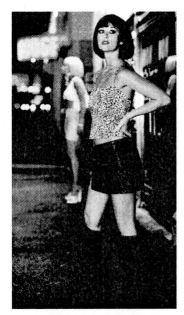

Streetwalkers are at the greatest risk for violence, drug addiction, and STIs.

Call Girls

The **call girl**, as the name implies, is usually contacted by a client when her services are desired. Typically, call girls maintain a list of clients whom they see on a regular basis, ranging from once or twice a week to once a year or less. Some call girls work for a "madam" who introduces them to clients and schedules dates for a percentage of the fee. Call girls will typically see far fewer clients than streetwalkers, often no more than one or two per day, but will charge more per client. High-priced call girls can earn from several hundred dollars for a date of an hour or two to several thousand or more for an entire night with one client. Many call girls earn hundreds of thousands of dollars per year. For example, here is a (disguised but accurate) sample of information provided from one California call girl's Web site:

> My charges are based on hourly rates. We can spend as little as one hour together or all day or all night. These prices are firm, so please do not try to negotiate with me. Pricing information is available for longer periods of time or for travel, so please give me a call or e-mail me.
>
> *Rates:* $300 first hour + $200 every hour thereafter; $400 dinner + 1 hr; $550 dinner + 2 hrs; $1,500 overnight
>
> *Prepaid Rates:* Prepaid rates can save you money by purchasing your dates with me in advance. When you purchase my hours, you can divide them up however you like. For example, if you purchase 12 hours, you could have two 2-hour appointments and eight 1-hour appointments. These prepaid hours are good for up to one year after purchase. 3 hrs—$750 (up to 3 one-hour shows); 6 hrs—$1,350 (up to 6 one-hour shows); 9 hrs—$1,800 (up to 9 one-hour shows); 12 hrs—$2,200 (up to 12 one-hour shows); 18 hrs—$3,150 (up to 18 one-hour shows)
>
> *Monthly Rates:* Monthly rates and discounts are available for regular clients. Please call me for more information.

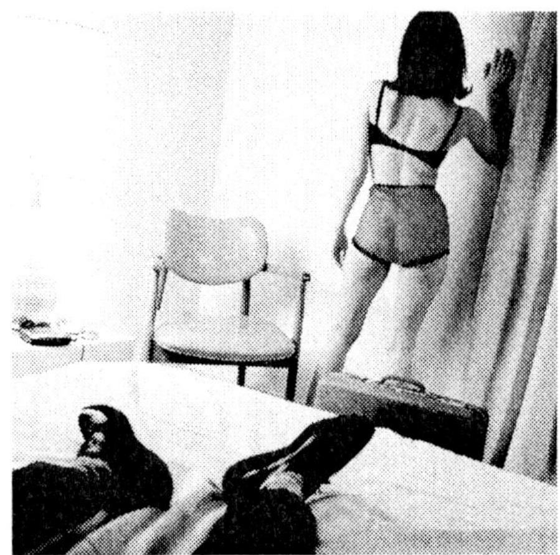

Call girls maintain a list of regular clients and are often very highly paid for their services.

Once a call girl has a consistent list of regular clients, she typically no longer needs to "hustle" to find customers. Call girls are much less likely to be drug abusers and are at significantly less risk of violence, especially once they get to know their regular customers. Some call girls are listed in the phone book or place ads in magazines, under the heading "Escort Services."

Brothel Workers

Brothel workers or **house prostitutes** are women who work in "houses" that receive paying customers. These houses of prostitution are referred to by many names and euphemisms, including brothels, bordellos, and massage parlors. In Nevada, where brothels are legal and state-controlled, prostitutes typically work under the safest conditions of all sex trade workers. These brothels are closely monitored for any signs of danger to the workers, and clients are screened before the outside gate to the entrance is opened.

streetwalker A prostitute who sells her services on the street, typically to customers who are driving by, soliciting sexual acts.

call girl A prostitute who is contacted in private by clients when her services are desired and who generally charges more and provides a wider range of services than streetwalkers, such as serving as an escort or offering overnight stays.

brothel worker A prostitute who works in a house of prostitution—such as a brothel, bordello, or massage parlor—and receives paying customers.

house prostitute A brothel worker.

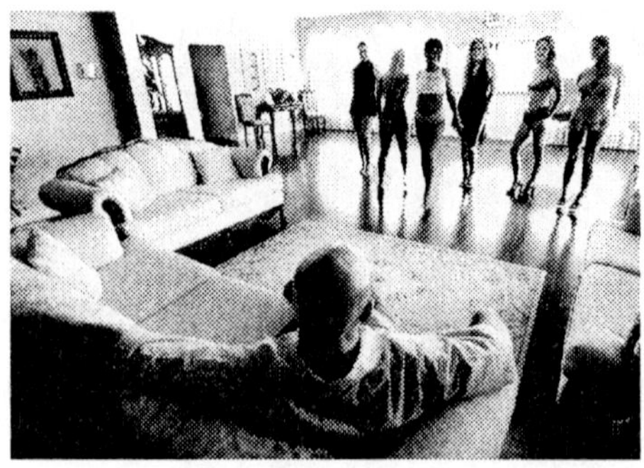

Brothel workers or house prostitutes work in an environment where they are usually protected from violence and STIs.

House prostitutes, who share fees with the house manager or madam, typically earn more money than streetwalkers but considerably less, on average, than call girls. Due to the requirements of the state, in the case of Nevada, or of the brothel itself, house prostitutes are far more likely than streetwalkers to receive regular medical exams and use condoms consistently. Therefore, they are less likely to contract STIs, even though they may see as many as or more clients than the typical streetwalker.

Male Prostitutes

Some people argue that a prostitute is a prostitute regardless of gender. In a very strict interpretation of prostitution, this may be true; however, many of the characteristic, specifics, and activities involved in male prostitution are unique and require some separate discussion. First of all, unlike female prostitutes, male prostitutes sell their services primarily to other males. Male prostitutes who service women are rare and are usually referred to as **gigolos** or **male escorts**. These men tend to function in a similar fashion to call girls as discussed earlier, but with more emphasis on the escort role and less on sexual acts.

The vast majority of male prostitutes employ professional business tactics that are very similar to female streetwalkers. These men are most commonly referred to as **hustlers**. Most will hang out on street corners or in bars waiting for customers to approach them. The sexual interactions typically take place in a car, a public restroom, an outdoor location hidden from public view, a motel room, or less often, in the prostitute's or client's residence. The most common behaviors are oral sex, manual masturbation, and anal intercourse. The actual number of male prostitutes is difficult to gauge, but they account for more than a third of all the arrests made for prostitution in the United States (FBI, 2002).

Although male prostitutes are selling sex to other males, only 18 percent self-identify as gay. The rest self-identify as either heterosexual (46 percent) or bisexual (36 percent). However, their sexual relations with women tended to occur outside of their professional activities (Altman & Aggleman, 1999; Miller, Klotz, & Eckholdt, 1998).

Male hustling appears to be linked more strongly than female prostitution to various drug abuse and health issues. Studies have found high rates of HIV infection (28 percent), syphilis (37 percent), herpes (67 percent); and hepatitis B (38 percent) among active male sex workers (Elifson, Boles, & Sweat, 1993; Jones et al., 1998). Moreover, in related findings, rates for drug abuse are very high among this group of men, with between 40 and 53 percent reporting a history of injection drugs use, 76 percent cocaine abuse, and 61 percent crack abuse (Boles & Elifson, 1994; Reitmeijer et al., 1998).

Now that you have an idea of the various types of sex trade workers, the next question that should be addressed is why? Why do people become prostitutes? To answer that question, we also must consider the extent to which men and women *choose* prostitution versus being forced into the sex trades either through coercion or the lack of any perceived viable alternatives for their personal survival.

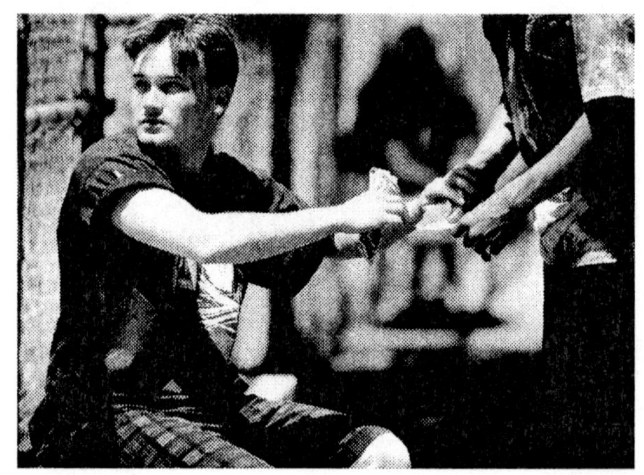

Male prostitutes, referred to as hustlers, account for more than a third of all prostitution arrests in the United States.

gigolo A male prostitute who is paid or otherwise compensated for providing sexual services to women.

male escort A man hired by women as a companion, not necessarily for sexual purposes.

hustler A male prostitute who services male clients and employs professional tactics similar to those of female streetwalkers.

Who Becomes a Prostitute?

The factors that combine to cause someone to turn to prostitution as a profession appear to be divided into two main categories. First are those that relate to a free choice some people make to become sex workers because they see it as a viable, beneficial profession that will allow for an adequate (or more than adequate) income and provide an opportunity to live a life of their choosing. In other words, these are the people who choose prostitution in much the same way as anyone chooses a particular job, career, or profession in any field. Second, however, are those who are forced into prostitution by the coercion of others or circumstances in their lives that they perceive leaving no other choice. An ongoing debate in this area relates to whether or not anyone truly chooses prostitution or if in all prostitutes' lives there are some elements of coercion or entrapment.

Prostitution by Choice

Would all prostitutes, given the opportunity to be self-sufficient in another career, choose to give up sex work? The answer is no. Some prostitutes are satisfied with the profession they have chosen.

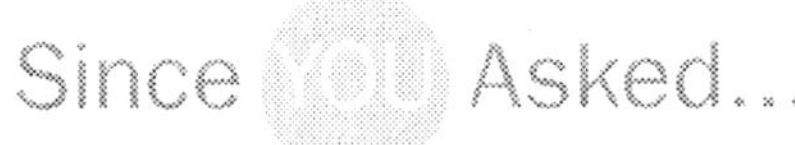

4. I cannot understand why any woman would ever become a prostitute. Is there something psychologically wrong with these women?

In the brothels in Nevada, for example, some prostitutes are able to choose their work hours and yearly schedules. Some will work four or five months out of the year and make enough money to live without working the rest of the time. Those women often say that they would be unable to have the life they want in any other profession and would not want to stop what they are doing. In other cases, especially among some highly paid call girls who are earning six-figure incomes, the women feel they could not make as much money in any other profession.

Some prostitutes say they enjoy their work. Most deny that they receive sexual pleasure from their interactions with clients, but some are pleased by the knowledge that they are helping and giving pleasure to others, as well as making a good living (Brewis & Linstead, 2000; Owens & Lopes, 2003). Prostitutes with such positive attitudes typically work in brothels or fall into the category of call girls or escorts. To get a feel for how someone might voluntarily enter into prostitution, see "Sexuality and Culture: A Personal Look at the Life of a Prostitute."

Involuntary Prostitution

The majority of prostitutes, especially streetwalkers and hustlers, are forced into a lifestyle they hate and from which they can see no escape. Many sex workers are pressured to engage in prostitution for any one or a combination of reasons, including (1) threats of bodily harm if they do not prostitute themselves to earn money for their husbands or boyfriends; (2) being coerced into streetwalking by pimps who "rescued" them from homelessness and who now maintain total financial control over them; (3) drug dependence or addiction, especially to crack cocaine (often initiated by a pimp), that can only be supported by exchanging sex for money or for the drugs themselves; (4) living in extreme poverty, often supporting children, and lacking the education or training to find other forms of work; and (5) being lured, sold, or kidnapped into the sex trades by international sex worker traffickers. These girls, boys, women, and men begin selling their bodies out of desperation or fear, but the lifestyle takes on a weight of its own, spiraling down to greater depths of poverty and addiction until escape feels literally impossible (McClelland, 2001).

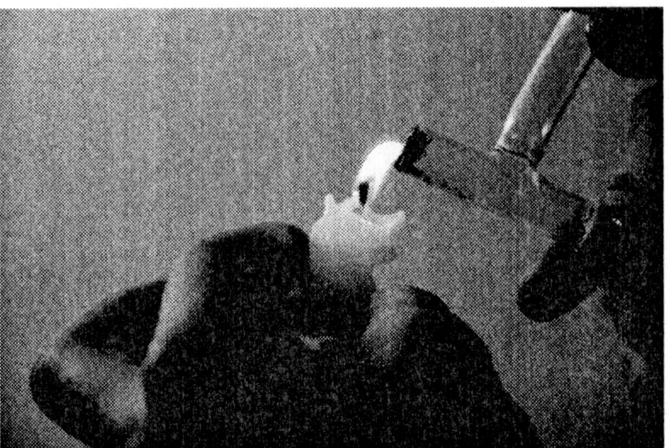

Many sex workers become addicted to drugs and see prostitution as the only way they can support their habit.

The illegal international trafficking of sex workers has become a major worldwide tragedy involving, by some estimates, as many as 4 million victims and an annual monetary exchange of as much as $15 billion (Smits, 2004). Children, mostly girls, as young as 9 or 10 years of age are lured, bought from their parents, or kidnapped from their homes in many of the less developed countries of the world, including Thailand, eastern Europe, China, and western Africa. These victims are often promised a good job, a better life, and other "dreams come true" in a Western country but instead are literally sold into sexual slavery and imprisonment (Power, Radcliff, & MacGregor, 2003). Some begin sex work as early as age

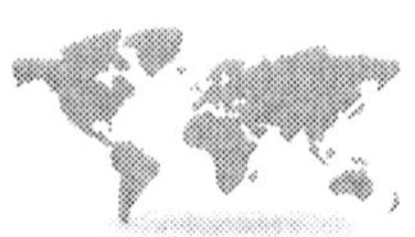

Sexuality and Culture

A Personal Look at the Life of a Prostitute

Dear Dr. Raj Persaud,

Please help me with this dilemma. I am 25, unemployed, a single mother with three children all under 8, and I desperately want to be able to buy them some proper clothes and take them on a short holiday. I could only afford to do this last year after dabbling in prostitution, and I am thinking of returning to it now. Could you give me any advice about whether I should?

Delia

Dr. R: *How did you get involved in prostitution the first time around?*

Delia: I saw an ad in a local newspaper for sauna staff, and the owner interviewed me in a pub—he asked whether I knew what kind of work it is and I answered I could take a good guess. I was desperate for the money, I felt so low and terrible at not being able to provide basics for my children. The girls at the sauna were really helpful—they ran though important safety tips, like you must always be on top as it is more difficult then for the man to turn aggressive or be in control than when he is on top of you, and never let him have sex from behind as then he could reach forward and strangle you. I found having sex surprisingly easy, and I really enjoyed the power—you are the one in control. I did three six-hour stints and earned over $300. But I stopped because it began to be difficult to explain to my parents, who were babysitting, where I had been. Also, I had split up with my boyfriend back then, and now we are together again and he is bound to be suspicious if I went out for so long again.

Dr. R: *Given these difficulties, how are you thinking of getting involved in prostitution again?*

Delia: This time I would advertise in phone booths and run it from home—seeing the men in local hotels. I would buy a mobile phone so they wouldn't call me on the home phone. If I did it that way, I would only be out of the house for around an hour, so my parents would think I was just visiting a friend. The problem with the sauna is you had to be there for too long; I could never organize babysitting for that period.

Dr. R: *Sounds as though you have it all pretty well thought out. What is stopping you from going ahead?*

Delia: I am worried that seeing men alone in hotel rooms might be less safe than seeing them at the sauna. I wondered, as you are a psychiatrist and see people from all walks of life, what your opinion is.

Dr. R: *It certainly doesn't sound very safe seeing men alone in a hotel room, particularly if it is a secret from everyone you know and no one else knows where you are. Have you discussed it with any prostitutes? What was their advice?*

Delia: No, the only prostitutes I know are the ones at the sauna, and I haven't been back there for a year. I suppose I could ask them. I did tell my two best friends about the escapade last year—they were really shocked and said if I was thinking of doing it again, I should discuss it with them first.

Dr. R: *And have you?*

Delia: No, I know they would disapprove and try to talk me out of it.

Dr. R: *Are you not worried about your parents or anyone else finding out? Could you not earn the money some other way?*

Delia: I would have to be very careful. Obviously, if the neighbors found out, I would have to move. The way my benefits are at the moment, there is no job I could get, even if there was work—which there isn't—that would leave me better off than I am at the moment. I am taking a course in secretarial skills, but even after that, I don't think I will earn as much as being a prostitute, particularly when you take the expense of child care into account.

Dr. R: *So it sounds like the only two issues that might stop you are your concerns about personal safety and other people finding out.*

Delia: But I don't think if I am careful anyone will find out.

Dr. R: *Well, that depends. But you still seem somehow very drawn to being a prostitute.*

Delia: Yes, I am. When I was there in the sauna, I was happy for the first time in a very long time. It was an escape for 12 hours—I had no contact with anyone from my neighborhood or home, no parents or anyone who knew me. It was an escape from reality of my life, where for a short period I had no responsibility or pressure.

Dr. R: *I get the feeling you really contacted me so that I might give you permission to do it. You really do seem to have made up your mind already. I am worried that you are naive about the downward spiral prostitutes get caught in.*

Dr. Persaud went on to comment on the potential pitfalls of prostitution, including the potential loss of self-respect and the dangers of drugs, violent pimps, and STIs. In addition, the stress of always being vigilant to keep her prostitution secret might affect Delia to the point that she was not as warm and loving with her children; and her attitude toward men might change to the point that she would find it difficult to form a loving long-term relationship with a man.

Dr. Raj Persaud's column, "The Session," appears monthly in *Cosmopolitan*.

Source: Text from http://www.stayingsane.com. Reprinted by permission of Dr. Raj Persaud, http://www.rajpersaud.com.

10, when they are marketed as virgins. One such victim's story makes the plight of these exploited sex workers abundantly clear:

> At 15 she accompanied [her pimp] and eight other pimps and their child prostitutes and drove to England. She spent the next few years working the length of the British Isles, servicing clients 18 hours a day, seven days a week. "Whatever they wanted they got," she says. (Power, Radcliff, & MacGregor, 2003, p. 34)

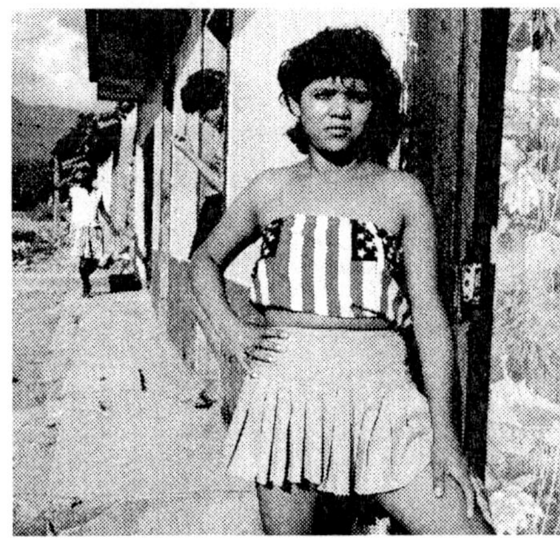

In what has become a worldwide tragedy, millions of young girls throughout the world have been coerced and forced into sexual slavery.

International laws protecting sex trafficking victims have been slow to keep pace with the scope of the problem. In the United States, the number of victims remains shockingly high, but prosecutions and punishments for traffickers, as well as help for victims, are increasing. In 2000, the U.S. Congress passed the Victims of Trafficking and Violence Prevention Act, which established new felony laws designed to combat sex trafficking and authorized a wide range of social services and protections for victims of trafficking. The law also provided for temporary U.S. visas allowing victims to remain in the United States for their protection and to help law enforcement officials capture and prosecute traffickers. In a statement made upon signing the legislation into law, President Clinton (2000) remarked:

> Traffickers who prey on vulnerable women and children should have no place to hide, and victims of trafficking must be treated with dignity and afforded vital assistance and protection. I expect this legislation to be of immense benefit in rooting out this despicable practice and in helping future Administrations carry on the vital work that this Administration has begun. (p. 2664)

U.S. legislation allows for pressure in the form of financial sanctions on other countries that fail to take steps to limit human trafficking, and many countries are attempting to control the practice (Mathews, 2005). However, for many countries, this problem is a low priority on their list of social problems, and human trafficking continues to increase internationally.

Prostitution and Drug Abuse

Drugs and the commercial sex trades often go hand in hand. Drug abuse plays a dominant role in the lives of most prostitutes. For many, it is the gateway into the trade and the primary force keeping them there. At first, prostitution may serve as a way for poor women and men to finance a drug habit. However, as they become trapped in a life of prostitution, drug use may become a coping mechanism to deal with the many stresses and anxieties encountered as a result of their occupation (Potterat et al., 1998). Some prostitutes report using drugs to enhance their perceptions of personal self-confidence and to decrease their feelings of guilt and lack of sexual intimacy in their lives (Young, Boyd, & Hubbell, 2000).

In addition to alcohol and marijuana, prostitutes frequently abuse cocaine, amphetamines, and heroin. However, one particular highly addictive drug places those involved in the commercial sex trades at the greatest risk: **crack**. Crack, a processed, more powerful form of cocaine, is smoked (or sometimes injected) rather than snorted. It is known for its intense but relatively short high and for its rapidly addictive qualities. Prostitutes who are addicted to crack therefore need more frequent fixes and are more willing to engage in a wide range of unsafe sexual practices in exchange for the drug or earn the money to buy it. Crack use thus increases these sex workers' risk and vulnerability to the most negative consequences of prostitution (Erickson et al., 2000). One large study by the National Institute on Drug Abuse found that among crack smokers and injectable drug users, over the previous 30 days, 80 percent had engaged in unprotected intercourse, 24 percent had exchanged sex for drugs, and 23 percent had had sex with an injectable drug user (Booth, Kwiatkowski, & Chitwood, 2000).

crack A powerful, processed form of cocaine that is smoked or sometimes injected, known for its intense but relatively short high and its highly addictive qualities.

Even if a prostitute were to decide to leave the trade, he or she would likely be unable to support an expensive drug habit and would be drawn inescapably back to prostitution. On the other hand, most prostitutes depend on the drugs to continue to do the work of prostitution and have little motivation to stop using drugs as long as they are continuing to work in the sex trades.

The Backgrounds of Prostitutes

In general, the personal and family lives of sex trade workers prior to becoming prostitutes are different in some significant ways from those of nonprostitutes. However, we must note that most men and women who have experienced the same life situations as sex workers do *not* become prostitutes. Life experiences do not by any means fully explain people's motivations toward prostitution. With that in mind, the three most salient factors associated with working in the commercial sex trades are poverty, early sexual experiences and abuse, and as we just discussed, drug addiction. These factors do not function separately but tend to be linked in important ways.

Throughout the world, commercial sex trade workers tend to come from the lowest economic levels of society (Bauerlein, 1995; Poudel, 1994). This makes a certain amount of sense in that choosing a profession generally fraught with great social stigma and the risks of disease, violence, and drug addiction would appear to imply a certain financial desperation. Some women feel that prostitution is their only option for financial and even physical survival. When we factor in drug abuse and addiction, the links between poverty and prostitution become even more compelling.

One question often asked in research on prostitution concerns the chronological sequence of drug use and prostitution. In other words, do poor young women and men generally become involved with drugs and then turn to prostitution to support their addiction? Or are girls living in poverty first introduced to sex work, which provides access to drugs and the drug culture, become addicted, and then remain in the profession to support the addiction?

One study that examined this issue produced some interesting findings (Potterat et al., 1998). The research revealed that the vast majority of prostitutes began using drugs prior to their first experience with prostitution. This finding is graphically illustrated in Figure 15.1. You will notice that age of first drug use among prostitutes was approximately 15, but the first prostitution experience was not until age 20.5. However, examining the data more closely, you can see that these women began their sex work within months, on average, after first using intravenous drugs and were regularly engaged in prostitution within 14 months after beginning regular use of IV drugs. We should note that the age of first drug use did not differ significantly among a matched group of nonprostitutes. This implies that women who later became prostitutes did not start using drugs sooner in life, but once they became addicted, they may have entered prostitution as a means of obtaining or buying the drugs.

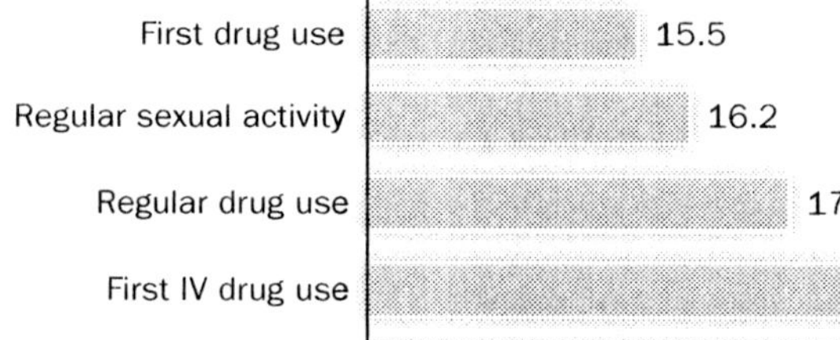

FIGURE 15.1 Age of Drug Use and Prostitution Onset among Sex Trade Workers
As shown in the data for one study, the age at which young women begin intravenous drug use corresponds closely to entry into prostitution.

Source: Data from Potterat et al. (1998), Table 3.

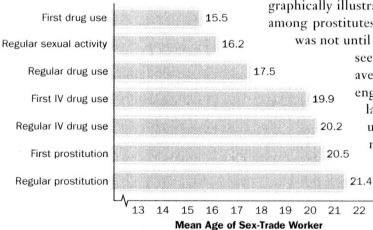

One stereotype of prostitutes depicts a teenager who becomes sexually active early and whose early sexual experience plays a role in the eventual entry into the sex trades. Thus precocious sexual activity is portrayed as a gateway to prostitution, either through the young person's initial enjoyment of sex or perhaps by desensitizing the youth to concerns about having sexual relations with many partners. However, do we have evidence that prostitutes do indeed experience sexual activity earlier than nonprostitutes? Some research does support this idea. In the same study by Potterat and colleagues (1998) cited earlier, the sexual histories of a sample of prostitutes was compared to a matched group of women seeking care at a free health clinic. These results are summarized in Figure 15.2. You can see that the age of first sexual intercourse, age of first consensual sex, and age of beginning regular sexual activity all differed significantly for the two groups. The prostitutes began all these activities 1.3 to 2.5 years earlier in life than the nonprostitutes. Similar findings have been reported for male prostitutes (Miller et al., 1997; West & de Villiers, 1993).

These are, of course, correlational findings, so we cannot assume that age of first sexual activity *caused* the women in the study to enter the sex trade. It may well be that these women were sexually precocious for other reasons in their lives that may have contributed to their eventual entry into prostitution. One possible cause that cannot be overlooked involves childhood sexual abuse. Looking at Figure 15.2, you probably noticed that "age of first penile penetration" was listed separately from "age of first consensual sex." The difference in age between first penile penetration and first consensual sex implies that many of these women were experiencing forced penile penetration earlier in their lives than consensual sex. "Forced sex" can only mean rape or childhood sexual abuse, or both, and this may imply being forced into prostitution as well.

Many studies leave little question that children who are abused sexually are at greater risk for various developmental difficulties as they grow into adults (this is discussed in greater detail in Chapter 13, "Sexual Aggression and Violence"). One of these risks involves sexual adjustment later in life. Prostitutes, on the whole, are significantly more likely to have been victims of childhood abuse or childhood sexual assault (Denenberg, 1997). This has been found to be true of both male and female prostitutes.

What conclusions can we draw from these factors in the lives of prostitutes? It is confusing, but probably the best interpretation is that no single variable can be isolated as a "cause" of a person's becoming a prostitute. All of the factors discussed here, along with others, probably play a role in a complex set of circumstances that determine how sex trade workers develop throughout their lives, how they view themselves, and how their experiences come together to move them along the path to prostitution. Childhood abuse, poverty, drug addiction, and sexual experiences in adolescence may form an interactive model, as shown in Figure 15.3, that explains some, but probably not all, of the forces at work in the development of a commercial sex trade worker.

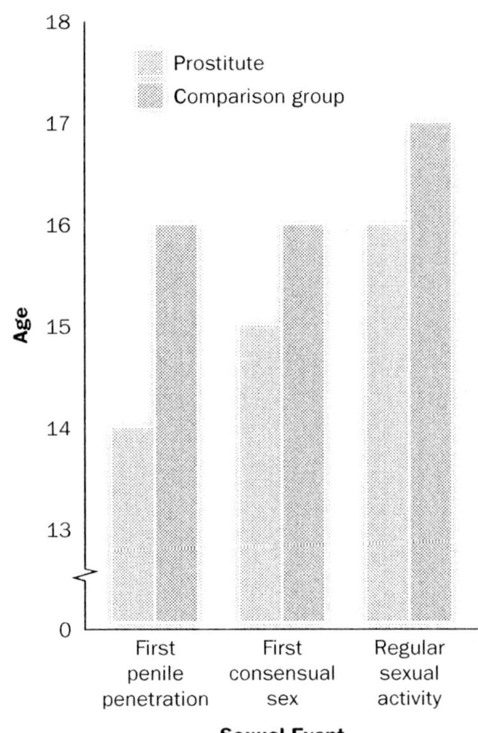

FIGURE 15.2 Age of Onset of Sexual Activity: Prostitutes versus Comparison Group
Age of first sexual intercourse, first consensual sex, and the beginning of regular sexual activity was significantly earlier for girls who entered prostitution.

Source: Data from Potterat et al., (1998), Table 2.

Prostitution and STIs

The commercial sex trade is often singled out as playing a major role in the spread of sexually transmitted infections, especially HIV/AIDS. It is true that prostitutes overall have significantly higher rates of sexually transmitted diseases than the population in general. However, the reasons behind this are more complicated than you may think. You are aware, of course, that one of the highest risks of contracting STIs is having multiple sexual partners, and prostitutes, obviously, have more sexual partners than virtually any other group of sexually active people. That factor alone places them at greater risk. Moreover, the other two highest-risk behaviors for the transmission of STIs are unprotected sexual activities (sex without a condom) and the sharing of drug paraphernalia, especially needles. In the world of the commercial sex trades, these risks tend to occur together.

Unprotected Sex, Drugs, and STIs

To the extent that a prostitute chooses to engage in unprotected oral, vaginal, or anal intercourse and abuses drugs, his or her risk of infection escalates accordingly. Furthermore, if a prostitute with an STI engages in unprotected intercourse with a client, the infection may transmit to the customer, who may in turn transmit it to other sexual partners; and those sexual partners may in turn spread the infection to additional partners.

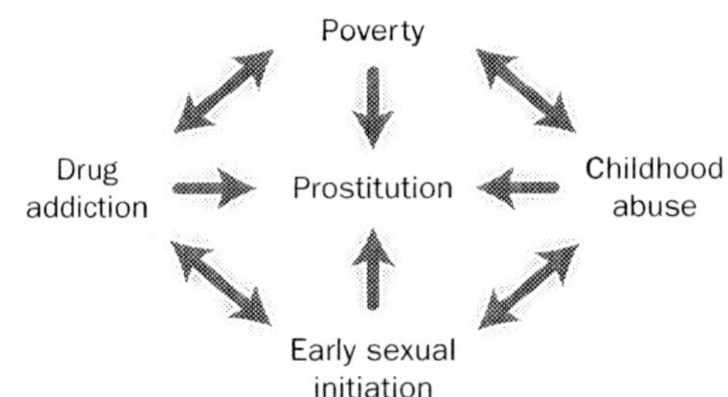

FIGURE 15.3 Factors Influencing the Evolution of a Prostitute
An interactive model may best illustrate the various factors that can lead a young person into prostitution.

One group of sex workers who are especially likely to spread STIs to the non-prostitute, heterosexual community are male transvestite prostitutes who impersonate women and engage in sexual interactions with male customers. "In Touch with Your Sexual Health: Male Transvestite Prostitutes and Sexually Transmitted Infections" describes the possibility for this exponential spreading of STIs to the general population. Moreover, many prostitutes are at increased risk of transmitting STIs among themselves if they share needles and other drug supplies, thereby exacerbating further the spread of these infections.

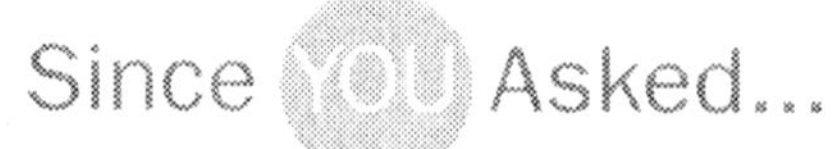

5. Is it true that AIDS and other diseases are spread mostly by prostitutes?

Streetwalkers and hustlers are among the groups with the highest rates of STIs worldwide (Decarlo, Alexander, & Hsu, 1996; Steen & Dallabetta, 2003). As we discussed earlier, these are the groups in the sex trades who are most likely to be drug abusers and to be struggling financially. Their often desperate need to make money to support their drug habit motivates them to agree to engage in high-risk sexual behaviors. The vast majority of crack-addicted prostitutes routinely agree to sexual acts without the use of a condom, usually for a higher price, and are especially likely to do so if business has been slow.

The widespread use of crack use among street-based sex workers also plays a role in higher rates of STI transmission. The reason for this appears to be that the frequent smoking of crack damages the lining of the mouth and gums. Street prostitutes are more likely to engage in unprotected fellatio than vaginal or anal intercourse due to the belief that it carries a lower risk of disease transmission and because it is the most common activity requested by clients of streetwalkers (Monto, 2001). However, the tissue damage in the mouth due to crack use may increase the risk for STI transmission more than commonly believed (Wallace, Weiner, & Bloch, 1996).

Brothel Workers and STIs

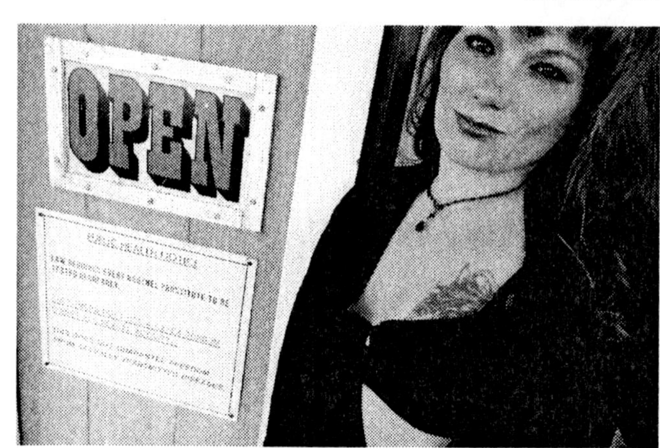

In brothels where prostitution is legal, condom use is usually strictly enforced. The text under the "Open" sign on this brothel says: "Customers must use a latex condom during all sexual activities."

Prostitutes who work in brothels, especially where they are legal, as in Nevada, or in countries where sex work has been decriminalized, appear to be at much less risk of STIs because they are less likely to be drug abusers and are much more likely to use condoms consistently. One study (Albert, Warner, & Hatcher, 1998) found that clients in Nevada brothels who were reluctant to use condoms (about 3 percent of all customers) ended up with one of three outcomes: They changed their mind and used them (72 percent), they chose a nonpenetrative sexual activity (12 percent), or they left "unfulfilled" (16 percent). If you do the math, that's 100 percent. With these kinds of statistics, we can assume that Nevada brothel workers' insistence on condom use is keeping both them and their clients better protected from STIs. Interestingly, however, the same study found that the brothel workers were far less likely to use condoms with their sexual partners *outside of the brothel*. It has been speculated that the reason for this is that not using a condom is one way that the women and their partners signal to each other the difference between a "real-life" personal relationship and a paid professional one.

On the other hand, women who work in noncontrolled houses, such as massage parlors, "saunas," or strip clubs, may be at an even greater risk of STIs than streetwalkers (Ibbison, 2002). In these venues, customers are more likely to request unprotected vaginal or anal intercourse because the sexual encounters are less hurried than on the streets and the prostitutes may agree more readily because they feel that repeat customers are more familiar and therefore present less risk. If there are no laws or house rules compelling them to use condoms and if prostitutes are able to charge significantly more money for these risky activities, they may also be more likely to comply. Consequently, these sex workers may be placing themselves at higher risk of some STIs than streetwalkers even without the added risk factor of drug abuse.

You can see that the link between the commercial sex trades and STIs is extremely complex. The simple fact of working as prostitutes does not automatically imply that they will contract STIs, nor does it necessarily mean that they will pass them on to their customers. The transmission of STIs in the sex trades depends on the very same behaviors that spread the infections in all populations. The relatively recent recognition of this fact is assisting public health efforts to reduce the incidence of

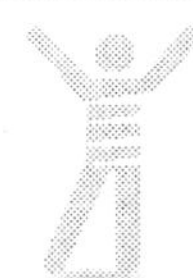

In Touch with Your Sexual Health

Male Transvestite Prostitutes and Sexually Transmitted Infections

One group of male sex workers is particularly susceptible to sexually transmitted infections: male transvestite prostitutes (MTPs). As the name implies, these are men who dress up as women and sell sexual services to other men. Although both male and female prostitutes, especially streetwalkers, are at a significantly increased risk of STIs, male transvestite hustlers face the greatest danger. Research has shown that over 60 percent of MTPs are HIV-positive, over 80 percent test positive for syphilis, and over 75 percent have contracted hepatitis B. Rates for these infections in nontransvestite male prostitutes are 27 percent, 22 percent, and 58 percent, respectively. What accounts for such an alarming difference?

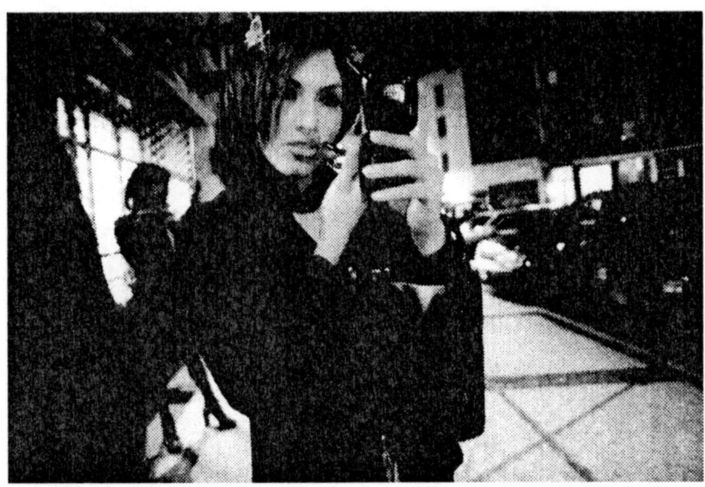

The risk is especially high for transvestite male prostitutes to spread STIs throughout the general nongay, nonprostitute population.

Several factors have been suggested to account for this. First, clients may be looking for and demanding to receive anal sex more frequently from MTPs than the clients of other male prostitutes. In an effort to obtain clients and to charge as much as possible, MTPs may be engaging more often in unprotected anal intercourse, which is known to be the easiest route of transmission for HIV and other STIs. Second, MTPs may experience emotional or psychological factors in their personal or professional lives that put them at greater risk of intravenous drug use, which also carries a high risk of bloodborne disease transmission. And third, the increased social stigma and prejudice experienced by MTPs may cause them to have less contact with public health care agencies and providers.

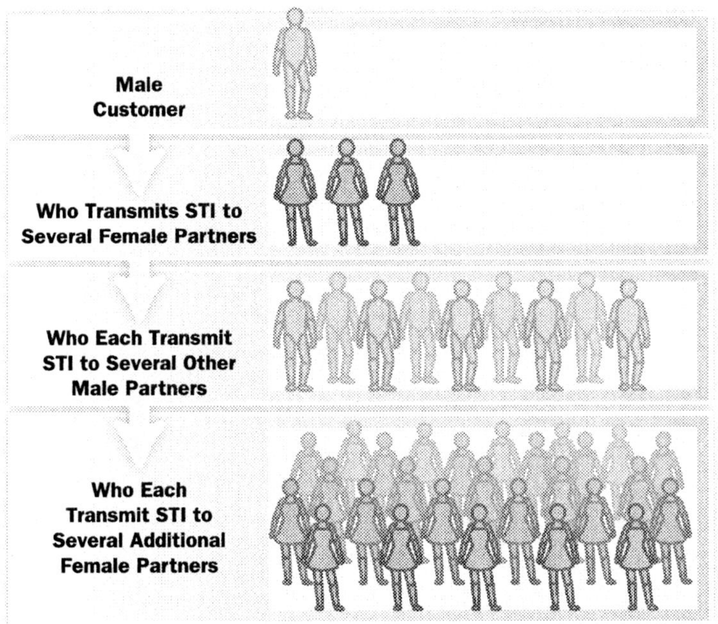

You may be wondering what this has to do with your sexual health. Perhaps nothing, but to the extent that MTPs are infected with STIs, they are also potentially transmitting those infections to their customers. Moreover, many of their customers self-identify as heterosexual and have intimate heterosexual relationships; if these customers keep their activities with MTPs secret and continue to have unprotected sex with their female partners, they are putting them at high risk for STIs. This is how the widespread STI infection among MTPs and other sex trade workers provides a vector for the spread of STIs throughout the general population. The diagram at the left illustrates the pervasiveness of the risk.

Sources: Elifson, Boles, and Sweat (1993); Elifson et al. (1993); Inciardi and Surratt (1997); and Morse et al. (1991).

STIs among prostitutes and nonprostitutes worldwide, without necessarily singling out one particular group as any more "at fault" than another.

Promoting Sexual Health among Sex Workers

During the 1980s and 1990s, as the HIV epidemic was expanding at an alarming rate, commercial sex workers (primarily streetwalkers and workers in unregulated brothels) were often the main focus of efforts to slow the spread of the deadly virus. Ibbison (2002) observed that the problem with those early approaches was that they generally took a "blame the prostitute" stance:

> Sex workers were generally perceived as "reservoirs of infection" who could potentially spread the virus into the "mainstream" heterosexual population. HIV prevention strategies developed not out of concern for the women themselves but rather out of their perceived role as "vectors of transmission" to male clients and their partners. Since then it has been broadly acknowledged that initiatives that are non-judgmental and empowering are more useful than those that stigmatize and blame. (Ibbison, 2002, p. 903)

Ibbison (2002) further discusses an outreach program undertaken in England in 1999 to assist women sex workers in reducing their risk of contracting or transmitting STIs. The goals of the program are as follows:

- To make contact and build trusting relationships with the women in the target group
- To provide a regular supply of condoms and lubricant
- To provide information and support to sex workers re sexual health issues including HIV prevention and prevention of sexually transmitted infections
- To reduce sexual risk-taking behavior among the target group
- To increase awareness of the needs of this group among healthcare professionals and to offer training to dispel myths and stereotyping about sex workers
- To conduct research, which will include needs identification, resource analysis and service review
- To work closely with local services to increase their flexibility to sex workers and to refer women to these services
- To develop with sex workers and for sex workers educational materials in relation to sexual health and general health (pp. 903–904).

When you read over the goals of this program, you can see how it might apply to virtually any group of people whose behavior might place them at risk of STIs. For example, try going back over the list and replace "sex workers" with "college students." It still sounds perfectly reasonable, doesn't it? That illustrates that the program is indeed nonjudgmental and avoids stigmatizing and stereotyping.

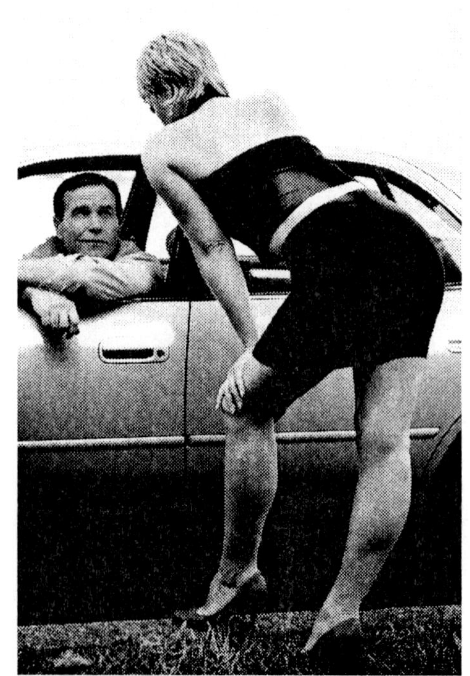

Increased attention is being paid to the clients of prostitutes in efforts to reduce demand for sex workers' services.

The Clients of Prostitutes

We have given quite a lot of attention to people who work in the sex trades, but what about the men who buy their services? As you probably know, the clients of prostitutes are usually called johns or tricks. In most places where selling sex is illegal, buying it is against the law too. Typically, soliciting the services of a prostitute is a misdemeanor and carries a possible sentence of 30 days in jail to years in prison. However, it is extremely rare that a male customer of a prostitute spends even one night in jail. Historically, prostitutes have been the ones who have been targeted by the criminal justice system with much more energy than their customers. The assumption behind these police tactics is that if the supply of prostitutes is reduced, the overall amount of illegal prostitution will decrease. However, this approach has proved to be ineffective, nearly universally, in areas where it has been attempted. If the demand for sex services remains constant, prostitutes will find a way to fill it. A crackdown on prostitution in one area of a city typically reduces sex work activity temporarily in that location while it moves to another neighborhood. After a while, the sex trade picks up once again in the previous location as police turn their attention elsewhere. Therefore, recently more attention is being paid to punishing and in some cases educating johns as a way of reducing prostitution through the demand side rather than the supply side.

Characteristics of Clients of Prostitutes

A study of more than 1,200 men arrested while attempting to buy the services of prostitutes (who, to the men's distress, turned out to be police decoys) in three major U.S. cities (San Francisco; Portland, Oregon; and Las Vegas) shed a great deal of light on the johns' characteristics (Monto, 2001). The myth that prostitutes' customers are depraved, deviant, drug-addicted men who are social outcasts with no other sexual outlets was soundly rejected. In fact, most johns are employed, middle- to upper-class, educated, heterosexual, married males. In other words, these are "normal," average, mainstream men. Table 15.1 summarizes the demographic findings for the men in the study. Looking them over, it is possible that if you were to randomly select 1,200 men from the same cities, their profiles would look fairly similar to the sample of johns, except that your random sample would probably have a higher percentage of non-heterosexuals and married men.

Twenty percent of these men claimed that this was the first time they had ever attempted to hire a prostitute, 59% reported having sex with a prostitute at least once

Table 15.1 DEMOGRAPHIC CHARACTERISTICS OF CLIENTS OF PROSTITUTES IN THE UNITED STATES

CHARACTERISTIC	PERCENTAGE
Ethnicity	
White	60
Hispanic, Chicano, or Latino	17
Asian	13
Black	5
Other or combination	5
Level of education	
Less than high school	9
High school	18
Some college	37
Bachelor's degree	25
Graduate degree	11
Marital status	
Married	42
Never married	35
Divorced	15
Separated	6
Widowed	2
Employment status	
Working full time	81
Working part time	6
Retired	2
Student	2
Other	9

CHARACTERISTIC	PERCENTAGE
Age	
18–21	4
22–25	9
26–35	33
36–45	31
46–55	17
56–65	4
66 or older	2
Sexual orientation	
Strictly heterosexual	94
Experienced with both	5
Strictly homosexual	1
Number of sexual partners past year	
0	9
1	38
2	16
3 or 4	17
5 to 10	13
11 or more	7

Source: Data from "Demographic Characteristics of Clients of Prostitutes in the U.S." from "Prostitution and Fellatio" by M. Monto in *Journal of Sex Research*, 38, (2000), pp. 140–145. Copyright © 2000. Reprinted by permission of The Society for the Scientific Study of Sex.

over the past year, and 10% admitted to buying sex from prostitutes at least once a month during the past 12 months (Monto, 2001).

What Do Prostitutes' Clients Want?

Many people believe that men seek out prostitutes for experiences that are strange, vastly different from the mainstream, or unlikely to be shared with their partner or wife. However, this appears not to be the case. As mentioned earlier, by far the most commonly purchased activity is fellatio. In Monto's study, 81 percent of the respondents had engaged in oral sex with prostitutes, compared to vaginal intercourse (55 percent), both oral and vaginal sex (36 percent), and manual masturbation (35 percent). Only 9 percent reported performing oral sex on the prostitute, and only 3 percent reported having anal sex or some other activity.

Since YOU Asked...

6. What are the main reasons men go to prostitutes? Is it usually because they can't get sex any other way?

Another common belief is that clients of prostitutes are dissatisfied with their sexual life with their partner or prefer the sex that they have with prostitutes over partner sex. This also appears to be a myth. Only 18 percent of the men studied said they strongly or somewhat preferred sex with a prostitute over sex in a conventional relationship. Moreover, nearly 60 percent of the men surveyed disagreed that the sexual activities they paid for were different from the activities engaged in with their regular partners. Finally, only 8 percent of the men in the study reported that their personal sexual interests were very different from those of their wife or partner. Table 15.2 summarizes the survey's findings in greater detail (Monto, 2001).

Why *do* men go to prostitutes? One reason often cited is that paying of sex allows men to experience a brief, uncomplicated sexual encounter and to avoid any emotional or relationship responsibilities that typically accompany sex in relationships. In other words, sex with a prostitute is self-serving for the customer both sexually and psychologically (Plumridge et al., 1997). Other common reasons offered by the johns themselves include loneliness, sexual problems at home, curiosity about sex with various women, desire for sexual behaviors refused by the primary sexual partner, lack of sex overall, and satisfying an overly strong sex drive (Lowman, Atchinson, & Fraser, 1997).

Whatever the true reasons behind people becoming sex workers and men paying them for sexual services, the fact remains that the "contract" that is agreed to and carried out between the sex worker and the client remains a major law enforcement issue in the United States and many other countries. Many people believe that enforcing laws against adults charging and paying for consensual sex is a futile exercise and a waste of tax revenues and police time and effort. This has led some people to question criminal approaches to reducing the prevalence of prostitution.

Prostitution and the Law

As mentioned early in this chapter, prostitution is illegal and carries criminal penalties in most countries and in most states in the United States. However, exceptions exist, as exemplified by the brothel business in Nevada and legalized prostitution in countries such as Germany and the Netherlands. One of the many heated controversies in the field of human sexuality and law enforcement is whether prostitution should be legalized or decriminalized. You may be wondering what the difference is between legalization and decriminalization. To those in the sex trades, the difference is an important one.

legalization of prostitution Regulation of prostitution by state laws, with statutes defining where, when, and how prostitution may take place.

decriminalization of prostitution Repeal of all laws against consensual adult sexual activity in both commercial and noncommercial contexts.

In simple terms, the result of **legalization of prostitution** would be similar to the current system of brothels in Nevada, where prostitution is limited and controlled by the state. **Decriminalization of prostitution** would equate the sex trade with any other commerce that a person chooses to pursue, as long as it adheres to the same laws

Table 15.2 SEXUAL ATTITUDES AND DESIRES OF CLIENTS OF PROSTITUTES

SURVEY ITEM	RESPONSE	PERCENTAGE OF RESPONDENTS
What kind of sexual activities have you ever engaged in with a prostitute?	Fellatio	81
	Vaginal sex	55
	Half and half (oral and vaginal sex)	36
	To be masturbated	35
	Anal sex	10
	Performing oral sex on her	9
What sexual activities did you engage in during your most recent encounter with a prostitute?	Fellatio	68
	Vaginal sex	43
	Manual masturbation	14
	Anal sex	4
	Performed oral sex on her	6
What kind of sexual activity do you engage in most often with a prostitute?	Fellatio	51
	Vaginal sex	12
	Half and half (oral and vaginal sex)	10
	Manual masturbation	6
	Anal sex	1
	Performing oral sex on her	0
	Selected two or more responses	18
	Other	2
I would rather have sex with a prostitute than have a conventional relationship with a woman.	Agree strongly	5
	Agree somewhat	13
	Disagree strongly	18
	Disagree somewhat	64
I want a different kind of sex than I have with my regular partner.	Agree strongly	12
	Agree somewhat	29
	Disagree somewhat	21
	Disagree strongly	38
Thinking about the sexual relationship with your wife or partner, how similar are your sexual interests?	Very similar	36
	Somewhat similar	39
	Somewhat different	17
	Very different	8

Source: Data from "Sexual Attitudes and Desires of Clients of Prostitutes" from "Prostitution and Fellatio" by M. Monto in *Journal of Sex Research*, 38, (2000), pp. 140–145.

governing all legal business practices. People arguing for legalizing or decriminalizing sex work contend that it is not the morality or immorality but the *illegality* of prostitution, that causes the drug abuse, violence, and STI problems related to street-level sex work. Some of the arguments that have been raised for the decriminalization of prostitution (C. Lee, 2005) contend that doing so would

- Reduce or eliminate the rampant victimization of prostitutes by pimps, johns, and the other criminal elements now associated with prostitution;
- Help control disease by requiring regular checkups and health certificates;
- Remove many prostitutes from street work and allow them to work in a safe, controlled environment;
- Redirect more of our limited law enforcement resources into fighting other, more serious crimes;
- Eliminate much of the motivation from pimps for addicting young women (and men) to drugs in order to prostitute and profit from them;
- Eradicate a significant source of income for criminal networks;
- Allow governments to receive tax benefits from the regulation of sex trade businesses.

On the other side of the debate are those who feel strongly that prostitution is fundamentally immoral and that removing it from criminal legal oversight would be a move in the wrong direction. The people on this side of the argument contend that prostitution invariably victimizes, exploits, and injures women in countless ways (Farley & Kelly, 2000) and that rather than encouraging it through legalization or decriminalization, we should be intensifying our efforts to eradicate it completely (Otchet, 1998).

The debate over the legal status of commercial sex trade work in the United States and elsewhere in the world is extremely contentious and hostile. Virtually no one believes that very much calming of these waters is likely to be seen in the near future. In the meantime, due in large part to the level of emotion generated by the debate, politicians completely avoid the issue whenever they can. Therefore, major changes in prostitution laws or in the overall business of prostitution any time soon are unlikely.

To sum up, studying prostitution, or the commercial sex trades, is a challenging task. Whether it is the world's oldest profession or not is far less important than the fact that it may be one of the world's *least understood* professions. It is safe to say that people will continue to study it, debate it, pass laws about it, work in it, and patronize it, regardless of whether or not we ever fully understand it.

Prostitution is connected to pornography, our next topic, in a way that surprises many people. The root of the word *pornography* actually means "writing about prostitutes." It derives from the Greek *porne*, meaning "prostitute" or "harlot," and *graphein*, "to write." Of course, as you will see, our current use of the word means substantially more than this formal etymological definition.

Pornography

Each semester, as a lead-in to class discussions on the topic of **pornography**, students in my human sexuality classes are asked to write down, anonymously, on 3-by-5-inch cards, the answer to the following question: "What is the most pornographic thing you've ever seen?" The cards are then collected and read aloud. The purpose of this exercise is threefold. First, because no further information is given with the question, it reveals how most people, at least most of the students in the classes, define pornography. Second, the range of answers given provides an excellent example of the variety of what is commonly perceived of as pornography. And third, it reminds the class of the diversity of personal experience with pornography that exists among their peers.

If students were each asked to write their own definition of pornography, the number of different definitions would probably equal the number of students in the class. Why? Because each of you, if asked to think critically about it, would likely draw the line differently between acceptable sexually explicit materials and those that you would call pornographic. Is *Playboy* magazine pornographic? How about R-rated movies (such as 2003's *Spider* or 1999's *American Pie*)? How about a book detailing the Michael Jackson scandal and trial? Many of you would disagree, perhaps forcefully, about this, primarily because you would disagree about the definition of the term. Our first task, then, is to determine what we mean when we talk about this vague abstraction we call pornography.

Searching for a Definition

pornography In legal terms, any sexually explicit work deemed obscene according to legal criteria and therefore exempt from freedom of speech protections.

One approach to a definition for pornography might be to turn to the dictionary. General dictionaries are generally not particularly useful for scientific definitions. However, for an idea of how a word is commonly used, they can at times be helpful. The problem here is that if you were to look up *pornography*, you would find yourself in one of those "dictionary scavenger hunts," looking up more and more words trying to understand the words used in each of the previous definitions. For example, your dictionary scavenger hunt might go something like this (feel free to try this yourself):

Pornography: *1. Written or graphic material intended to excite lascivious feeling.*

Lascivious: *1. Lewd. 2. Lecherous.*

Lewd: *1. Licentious. 2. Lustful 3. Obscene.*

Lecherous: *Given to inordinate sexual indulgence* (Inordinate: *Exceeding reasonable limits;* Indulgence: *Going unpunished for sinful acts*).

Lustful: *1. Excited by lust 2. Lecherous.*

Lust: *1. Intense or unbridled sexual desire* (Unbridled: *Freed from all restraint*). *2. Lasciviousness.*

Licentious: *1. Lacking moral discipline or sexual restraint 2. Lewd* (again!).

Obscene: *1. Disgusting to the senses. 2. Containing language regarded as taboo in polite usage. 3. Repulsive by reason of a crass disregard of moral or ethical principles. 4. Offensive to accepted standards of decency.*

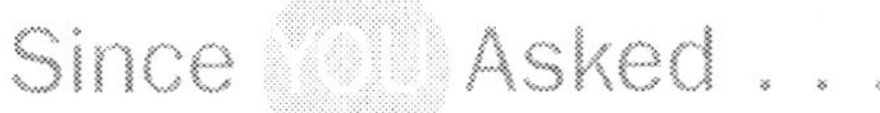

7. I like to look at magazines like *Playboy* and *Hustler*, but my girlfriend says they are pornographic trash. I think pornography refers to much worse kinds of magazines and videos. Who is right?

You get the idea. Clearly, pornography is not an easy word for anyone to define. However, our dictionary perseverance finally paid off somewhat in the last part of the exercise, as the word obscene comes closest to capturing the most formal definition of pornography developed thus far. It is called the "moral standard" and was not devised by sexuality researchers or psychologists but by judges sitting on the U.S. Supreme Court.

The Moral Standard

Throughout the history of the United States, a tension has existed between the First Amendment to the Constitution and citizens' rights to sell, distribute, look at, or otherwise participate in sexually explicit materials. The exact wording of the amendment is "Congress shall make no law . . . the freedom of speech, or of the press." The drafters of the Constitution saw this right as the most basic and most fundamental, along with freedom of religion, assembly, and the right to petition the government for change. Nothing, from the perspective of basic human rights in the United States, is considered more inviolate than the constitutional right to freedom of speech. However, several well-established exceptions exist to this basic right, including defamation of another's character; speech that causes panic, such as shouting "Fire!" in a crowded building; treasonous speech, such as advocating the overthrow of the government; and most pertinent to our discussion, **obscenity**, which has come to characterize certain sexually explicit works.

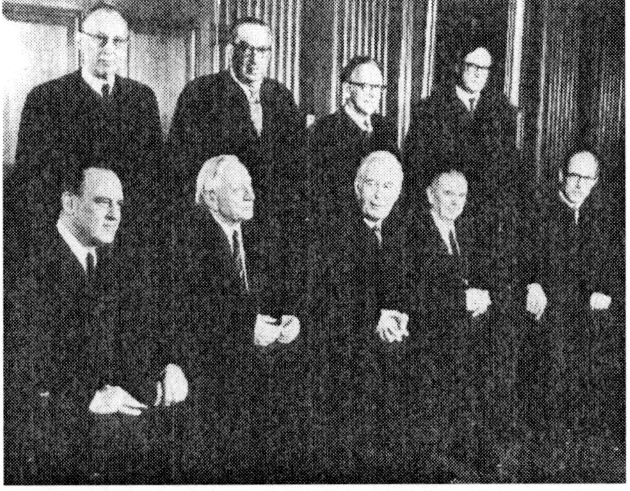

The Supreme Court led by Chief Justice Warren Burger drafted the 1973 definition of obscenity that continues to guide legal action on sexually explicit materials today.

Tension is bound to be created when something of a sexual nature, that some people may find offensive and immoral, is produced for public consumption. Those who produce the work and those who want access to it will invoke their First Amendment protections, while those who want to censor it or make it illegal will claim that the First Amendment does not protect and was never intended to protect that particular form of speech because, in their interpretation, it is obscene. Obviously, however, the problem lies in determining who will decide exactly what works should be labeled as obscene and allow them to be censored. Historically, where do you suppose these disagreements have gone for resolution? That's right: to the courts.

obscenity Sexually explicit works that meet specific legal criteria that may be censored and declared illegal.

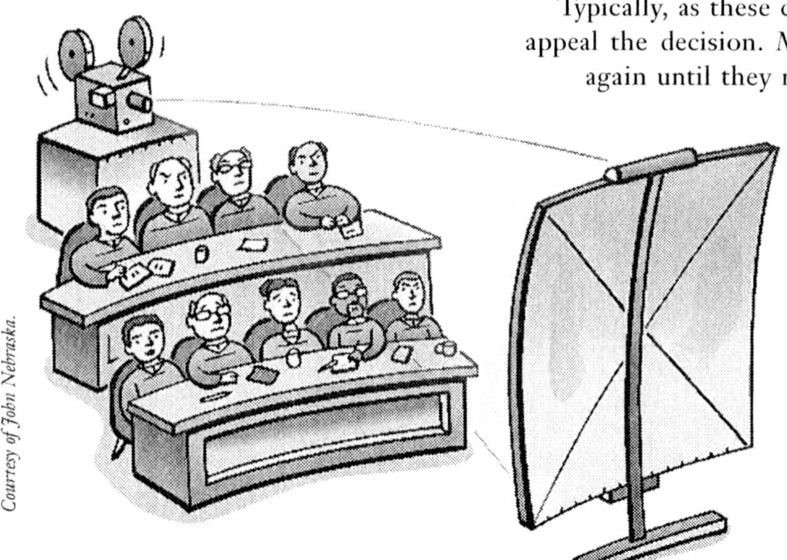
Courtesy of John Nebraska.

Typically, as these cases went through the lower courts, the losing side would appeal the decision. Many of those appealed cases were subsequently appealed again until they reached the U.S. Supreme Court, whose job is to interpret the legal meaning of the Constitution, in this case the limits of the First Amendment. As hundreds of obscenity cases relating to sexually explicit materials were heard and decided by the highest court over many years, the difficulty of this task became increasingly clear. How could one panel of nine justices, representing an entire nation, determine whether a particular sexually explicit work should be denied free-speech protection in one town or city when citizens in another town or city might have an entirely different set of standards? The answer is, it couldn't.

It was not that they didn't try. Here is how these three past justices' definitions have been described (Woodward & Armstrong, 2005):

> Justice Byron White: *No erect penises, no intercourse, no oral or anal sodomy.* For White, no erections and no insertions equaled no obscenity. Justice William J. Brennan: *No erections.* He was willing to accept penetration as long as the pictures passed what his clerks referred to as the "limp dick" standard. Oral sex was tolerable if there was no erection. Justice Potter Stewart: *I can't define it, but I know it when I see it.* Justice Stewart had "seen it" while serving in World War II as a Navy lieutenant. In Casablanca, as watch officer for his ship, he had seen his men bring back locally produced pornography. From this experience, he believed he knew the difference between true "hard core" materials and other, less extreme materials that came to the Court. He called it his "Casablanca Test." (p. 234)

Even among themselves, the Supreme Court justices could not agree on what was obscene and should be censored. In 1973, in a landmark case known as *Miller v. California*, the Court took a new approach. The case involved a mass mailing of sexually explicit brochures that were described in the Court's decision as follows:

> The brochures advertise four books entitled "Intercourse," "Man-Woman," "Sex Orgies Illustrated," and "An Illustrated History of Pornography," and a film entitled "Marital Intercourse." While the brochures contain some descriptive printed material, primarily they consist of pictures and drawings very explicitly depicting men and women in groups of two or more engaging in a variety of sexual activities, with genitals often prominently displayed. (Burger, 1973, p. 18)

In their opinion, the justices abandoned their long-standing attempts to separate obscene from nonobscene sexually oriented materials. Instead, they developed a test for obscenity to be applied nationally, but one that was, by its very nature, not intended to yield consistent results. That may sound strange, but it has been the law of the land for over a third of a century. Here is what they wrote. The Court provided three "basic guidelines," all of which must be met before a work may be deemed to be obscene and legally banned:

1. Whether the work depicts or describes, in a patently offensive way, sexual conduct specifically defined by the applicable state law
2. Whether the work, taken as whole, lacks serious literary, artistic, political, or scientific value
3. Whether an average person, applying contemporary community standards, would find that the work, taken as a whole, appeals to a **prurient interest** in sex.

prurient interest An excessive focus on exclusively sexual matters.

Remember, it is necessary, in applying this standard, that all three prongs of what has become known in legal circles as the *Miller* test must be present for a ruling of obscenity. In essence, these standards attempt to provide guidance for judging just the morality of a sexually explicit work.

Applying the Moral Standard

As you read through the three-pronged test of obscenity, you may have been thinking that it is still full of loaded, subjective wording that is open to individual interpretation: "offensive," "serious value," "community standards," "prurient interest." How, exactly, did this opinion by the Supreme Court fix that problem? It attempted to do so by developing the standards not for itself but to guide *local* governments and jurisdictions in resolving disputes before they ever leave the local community in which the complaint originated. As Chief Justice Burger (1973, p. 32) noted in his opinion:

> It is neither realistic nor constitutionally sound to read the First Amendment as requiring that the people of Maine or Mississippi accept public depiction of conduct found tolerable in Las Vegas or New York City. . . . People in different States vary in their tastes and attitudes, and this diversity is not to be strangled by the absolutism of imposed uniformity.

In essence, what the Court was saying was, "Please stop bringing these cases to us! We believe that no single, national standard of morality, as it relates to sexually explicit materials, can be determined or defended. You must decide for yourself, *in your own town*, whether offensive sexual works are obscene or not."

This legal standard for defining obscene sexually explicit materials has not been without its critics over the past three decades. Many of these critics' words echo Justice William O. Douglas (1973, p. 44) in his dissenting opinion in the *Miller* case: "The idea that the First Amendment permits punishment for ideas that are 'offensive' to the particular judge or jury sitting in judgment is astounding." This is the same criticism discussed earlier: that the language of the moral standard is too vague and subjective to allow any court, at any level, to find a work obscene while protecting the people's First Amendment rights.

Another criticism frequently raised to this moral standard relates not to whether the criteria are proper for defining obscenity but rather that the entire foundation on which the standard is based is misplaced. These critics maintain that the legal right to censor a sexually explicit work rests not on its morality but on the extent to which the work discriminates against a particular group of people—in this case, women.

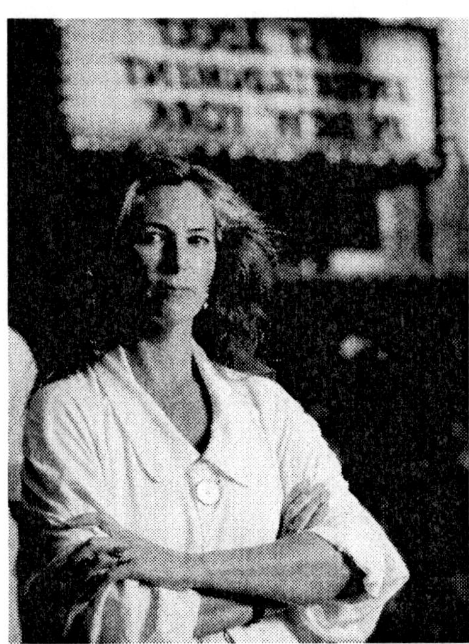

Catherine MacKinnon contends that pornography is a weapon that discriminates against women and justifies a culture of rape.

The Discrimination Standard

An alternative, if highly controversial, approach for dealing with the legality of sexually explicit materials is to view it from the perspective of discrimination rather than morality. That is, a sexually explicit work could be legally banned if proved to discriminate and victimize a particular group of people. Most of what is currently referred to as pornography is intended for male audiences, and much of it portrays women merely as sexual objects or "slaves" whose sole purpose is to provide sexual outlets for men, no matter what the women themselves may want. Some pornographic material depicts violence toward women in sexual contexts, glorifies rape, and may even show women being killed at the hands of their male oppressors. The discrimination standard for obscenity maintains that to the extent that these works victimize women in the making of the materials, in the viewing of them by men, and in the subsequent victimization of women by some of the men who view them, they are obscene and should be censored.

A leading proponent of this view is Catherine MacKinnon, who advocates the following basic ideas (MacKinnon, 1996; Richards, 2003):

1. Pornography, by its vary nature, is discrimination against women. The distinction between sexually explicit materials and the actions they depict is meaningless.

erotica Sexually explicit works expressing physical desire, passion, and attraction among people who freely choose to engage in sexual activities together.

2. Pornography reflects and constitutes male domination and dehumanization of women.
3. Pornography objectifies women by portraying women as nothing more than tools of male pleasure.
4. Pornography represents men's power over women in society and embodies the dehumanization of women in an already male-dominated world.
5. Pornography promotes discrimination against women, which in turn advocates and justifies rape.

These are fairly extreme views and are controversial in their own right. This approach to defining obscenity has not yet made its way into the legal statutes governing pornography in the United States. However, it does provide a provocative perspective for examining this highly charged issue. Moreover, this perspective begs the question as to whether extreme sexually explicit materials, such as those often referred to as pornography, can ever be seen as *not* discriminating against women. One argument that has been made in support of this possibility concerns the distinction between pornography and erotica.

Since YOU Asked...

8. Everybody's always saying how bad pornography is because it is violent toward women. But I've seen a lot of XXX videos that don't have any violence against women in them at all. So is that not pornography?

Pornography or Erotica?

Although people will never agree about issues relating to pornography and obscenity, most adults will allow that some sexually explicit materials, including those designed with the clear intent to be sexually arousing, are more acceptable than others and may even have desirable or beneficial effects. In Chapter 7, "Sexual Problems and Solutions," we discussed how sexually oriented materials can be useful in the treatment of certain sexual disorders in couples and individuals. However, if some people feel that pornography is obscene or that it discriminates against or victimizes women, how can we reconcile that belief with sexual materials that have positive effects?

One way this is done is by drawing a distinction between pornography and erotica. Some people may argue that this is simply a matter of semantics, and "one person's erotica is another's pornography." However, most researchers in this field see a clear difference between the two. **Erotica** is often applied to sexually explicit works, including films, books, and magazines, portraying expressions of physical desire, passion, and attraction among people who are freely and equally choosing to engage in sexual activities together. Erotica typically involves material that goes beyond "raw sex" and includes psychological and emotional factors as well. In others words, erotica is about *sexual sharing*, whereas pornography is about *sexual using*. This difference has been expressed in various ways by researchers in the field; for example:

> Pornography presents the coercion of a less powerful person by a more powerful one. Women are the slaves, the sexual playthings, for men to use and discard. Neither women nor men are accorded much compassion or empathy, but women, in particular, are degraded and demeaned. Erotica portrays nonaggressive sexual activity between willing, sensitive, caring partners. The partners share in the initiation and choice of activities, relatively free from the stereotyped pattern of male dominance and female subservience that characterizes much pornography. (Intons-Peterson & Roskos-Ewoldsen, 1989, p. 224)

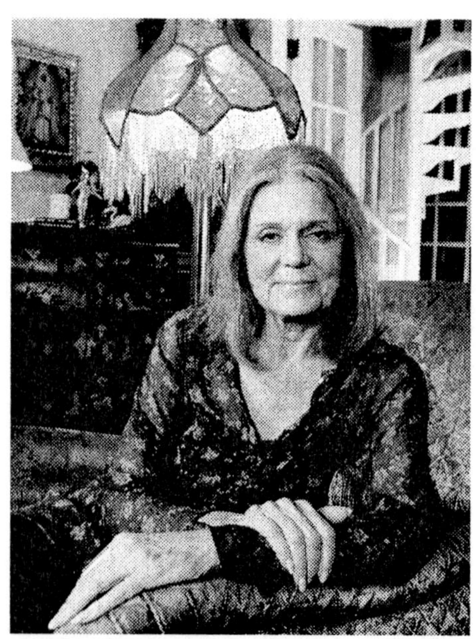

In the early 1980s, Gloria Steinem, a leading figure in the women's movement for the past 40 years, was among the first to suggest that pornography and erotica are fundamentally different.

Another cogent statement on the distinction between erotica and pornography was published in 1980 in an essay by Gloria Steinem, a former *Playboy* bunny who became one of the most influential and articulate founders of the women's movement. Her essay "*Erotica and Pornography: A Clear and Present Difference*" eloquently discriminated the differences between these two forms of sexual content as the following excerpt demonstrates:

> Sex as communication can send messages as different as life and death; even the origins of "erotica" and "pornography" reflect that fact. After all, "erotica" is rooted in "eros" or passionate love, and thus in the idea of positive choice, free will, the yearning for a particular person [the definition of erotica is not gender-specific]. "Pornography" begins with a root "porno," meaning "prostitution" or "female captives," thus letting us know that the subject is not mutual love, or love at all, but domination and violence against women. The message of pornography is one of violence, male dominance and conquest, of sex being used as a tool or weapon to create an inequality between men and women. . . . Erotica celebrates the equality of persons sharing the positive aura of sexuality and mutual pleasure. Erotica stresses freedom of choice. (Steinem, 1980, p. 50)

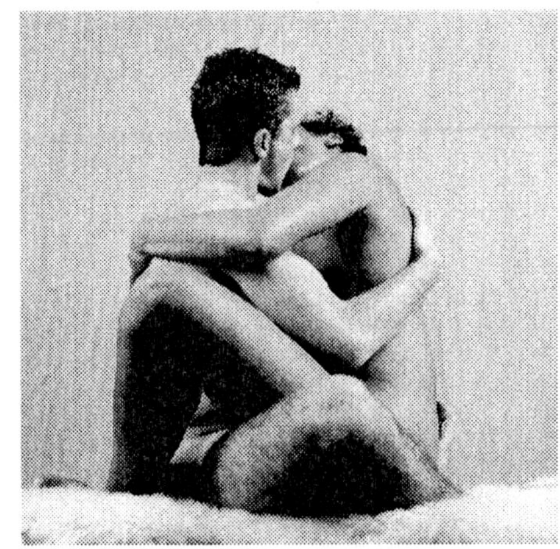

Most researchers today draw a distinction between pornography in which women are used and victimized by men, and erotica, which portrays mutual desire and equality in sexual activities, as shown above.

In the final analysis, everyone must decide individually where to draw the line between pornography and erotica, and some people may feel that such a line is unnecessary (because they feel that all sexually explicit materials are morally equal, good or bad). However, if consenting adults are to be allowed the freedom to view, read, or otherwise use sexual materials, and especially if the materials' effects on people and society and culture are to be studied, such a distinction is inescapable.

The Effects of Pornography

Beyond the issues involved in defining pornography, human sexuality researchers and other social scientists are interested in the effects sexually explicit materials have on the behaviors, attitudes, and feelings of the individuals who view it. Over the many decades of research in this area (often related to legal challenges about censorship), several questions have been of primary concern: Does pornography truly contribute to prejudice and discrimination against women? Does pornography lead to greater violence against women? Does pornography create attitudes conducive to rape? What is the relationship between sexually explicit materials and sexual arousal for men and women?

As you are undoubtedly aware, many people believe that the availability of these materials plays a significantly role in discrimination against and victimization of women in society. This is one of the central arguments in the frequent calls throughout the United States to criminalize all pornography. However, since public opinion is often based on emotions or myth and may bear little resemblance to the truth, researchers have attempted to determine what effects the viewing of pornography actually has on the viewer.

Pornography and Sexual Arousal

Does reading or viewing sexually explicit materials turn you on? Most of you probably answered with something along the lines of "Usually, but it depends on the material." In spite of all of the inherent flaws, problems, and controversies that we will discuss in the next sections, the fact remains that pornography and erotica exist primarily for the purpose of sexually arousing people. If these materials never turned anyone on, there would be little reason for their existence.

However, exactly what types of sexually explicit images or words arouse each individual is as varied as the real-life sexual activities people find exciting. You might be aroused by reading a certain passage in a sexually explicit book, seeing a sexy R-rated movie, or watching a specific pornographic video that another person might find repugnant. Interestingly, however, research has demonstrated that even when people are offended by sexual images, some sexual arousal may occur (Davis & McCormick, 1997; Laan et al., 1994). This is not surprising in that our sexual responses, as discussed in Chapter 3, are in part reflexive and not necessarily under our conscious control at all times. Also, the fact that something arouses a person sexually does not necessarily imply that the person likes the material or wants to imitate the behaviors involved (more on this in a moment).

Of course, people are aroused more by materials they find acceptable, pleasing to look at or read, and not offensive to their personal moral values. For example, people who tend to be religiously and politically conservative and have a strong authoritarian belief system feel more guilt and react more negatively to sexually explicit materials in general. Also, studies have found that men who score lower in intelligence and who exhibit greater anti-social and aggressive tendencies prefer more violent forms of pornography. But overall, the theme of the "insatiable female" is the most popular (Bogaert, 2001).

Interestingly, although men and women differ in some ways in their arousal reactions to sexually explicit materials, they are surprisingly similar in many ways. Some studies have found that upon viewing pornographic videos depicting degrading themes toward women, men reported more arousal and rated the videos as more acceptable and less degrading than women did overall (Gardos & Mosher, 1999). However, acceptance and enjoyment ratings decreased significantly as the level of degrading content increased. Another study compared pornographic videos made by men for men (pure explicit sex) with videos designed by women for women (explicit sex with more plot and partner interaction). The men in the study rated all the videos more positively than the women did, but as you might expect, the women rated the videos designed for female audiences significantly more positively than those made by men (Mosher & MacIan, 1994). In a similar vein, a study compared women's responses to sexually explicit videos designed for women or for couples versus standard videos aimed at male audiences (Pearson & Pollack, 1997). The women subjects rated their sexual arousal higher in response to the couples video than to the traditional male-oriented video.

On the other hand, some studies have failed to find this male-female difference. One study showed women erotic films made by women and erotic films made by men and measured sexual arousal using the vaginal plethysmographic device explained in Chapter 1 (Laan et al., 1994). Although sexual arousal was substantial, the level of physiological excitement did not differ between the two types of films. However, the women reported feeling more sexual arousal with the woman-made film and more feelings of shame, guilt, and aversion for the male-centered film. The contradictory findings among these studies probably reflect the fact that sexual feelings and arousal are complex reactions that involve both physical and psychological processes. Our bodies may react to sexual stimuli that emotionally and cognitively we may not find particularly arousing.

Before we condemn all men as emotionless, indiscriminate pornography lovers, some studies have uncovered a more romantic side in men's pornography preferences (see Table 15.3). For example, one study showed college men and women highly explicit sexual videos with either a romantic theme or a nonromantic theme

Table 15.3 SEXUAL AROUSAL IN RESPONSE TO EXPLICIT VIDEOS WITH AND WITHOUT ROMANTIC THEMES

	ROMANTIC CONTENT IN VIDEO*	
SEXUAL AROUSAL	LOW	HIGH
Males	3.22	4.07
Females	3.11	4.20

* Larger numbers indicate greater sexual arousal. The differences between men's and women's arousal were statistically significant.

Source: Data from "Romantic Themes in X-Rated Videos" from "Gender Effects of Romantic Themes in Erotica" by D. Quakenbush, D. Strassberg, and C. Turner in *Archives of Sexual Behavior*, 24, (2002), pp. 21–35. Copyright © 2002. Reprinted by permission of Springer Science+Business Media.

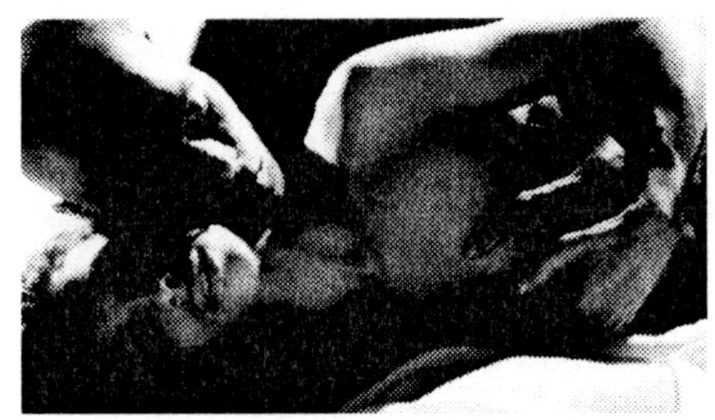

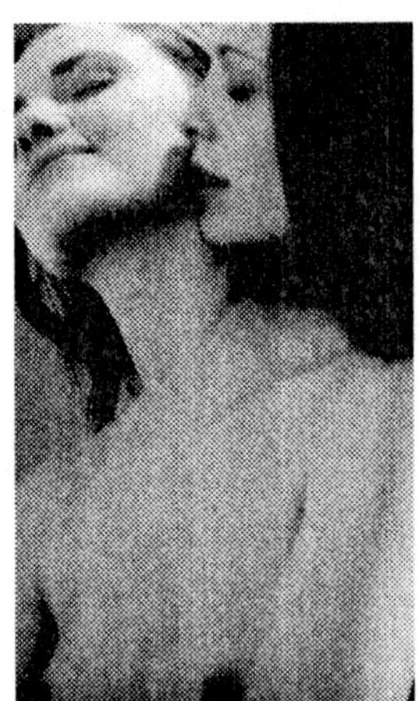

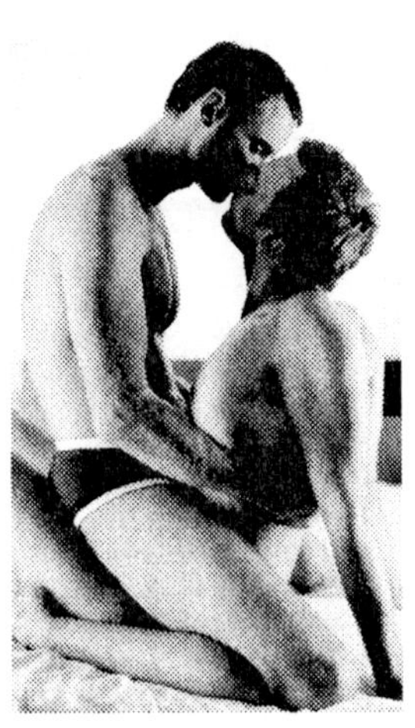

Research has shown that women tend to be sexually aroused by explicit sexual scenes of all sexual orientations, but men are primarily aroused by depictions of their personal sexual orientation.

(Quackenbush, Strassberg, & Turner, 1995, p. 21): "Results indicated that both male and female subjects rated the high explicit/high romantic vignette as significantly more arousing than the high explicit/low romantic vignette. The findings for males were contrary to expectations."

Finally, a recent study provided some evidence that the adult film industry may be targeting the entirely wrong audience in producing and marketing its products. Most of the materials that are considered pornographic are made for, bought by, and used primarily by men. If you ask most people who likes pornography more, they will nearly always say men. However, a 2003 study found that women are sexually aroused by a much wider variety of sexually explicit scenes (Dotinga, 2003). Using physiological devices to measure sexual arousal (see Chapter 1), researchers exposed self-identified heterosexual and homosexual men and women to pornographic videos showing sexual interactions between men and women, men and men, and women and women. Here is what they found:

> Women, no matter what their sexual orientation was, tended to respond to both male and female erotica, and even male-male erotica," Bailey says. "Straight men responded to female erotica, and gay men responded to male erotica. Nearly all the men responded more to videos featuring their preferred gender—men or women. But only 63 percent of women did. Judging by their arousal levels, heterosexual women were about equally turned on by male-male, female-female and male-female sex scenes. However, heterosexual men were much more excited by lesbian sex scenes than those featuring men and women. (Dotinga, 2003, p. 1)

Although both women and men are sexually turned on by some sexually explicit materials, there is widespread agreement that some forms of pornography may also have harmful and even dangerous effects on the viewers. Most of the concerns over pornography relate to the various negative, degrading, demeaning, and in some cases violent portrayals of women in sexually explicit materials on the market.

Pornography and Discrimination against Women

As we discussed earlier, most sexually explicit materials commonly referred to as pornography is made for, targeted at, and sold to men. Some of material (Davis & McCormick, 1997) demeans or victimizes women and portrays them as objects whose only reason for existence is to be used however men choose, for the men's sexual pleasure. It is estimated that 15 to 33 percent of pornographic materials depict men as having complete power over women and contain rape myths (such as that women enjoy being raped). However, less than 10 percent contains overt aggression, and only 1 to 3 percent involves actual physical violence or rape (Davis & McCormick, 1997). We discussed earlier that some researchers assert that pornography, in and of itself, is discrimination against women. The argument is that the presence of sexually explicit materials that glorify the subordination of and violence against women obscures any opportunity they may have of achieving equal rights with men. One of the leading writers promoting this view said, "If women are ever going to achieve civil equality in this country, we cannot have an 8-billion-dollar-a-year entertainment industry based on their brutalization" (quoted in Locayo, 1986, p. 67).

Encouraging violence against a particular group of people, in this case, women, is an indisputable example of discrimination. This specific form of discrimination will be discussed in the next two sections. Interestingly, little scientific research exists about the relationship between the availability of sexually explicit materials and overall social equality between men and women. What does exist appears to go counter to the pornography-equals-discrimination position. One study (Garcia, 1986) found that people who had greater lifetime experience with pornography expressed more liberal, less discriminatory attitudes toward women. The exception to this finding was that greater exposure to pornography with coercive (forced sex) or violent sexual content was associated with less tolerant views toward women. Another study from the late 1990s examined men's attitudes toward women as a function of the number of X-rated videos they rented (Davies, 1997). Results indicated the number of pornographic video rentals had no effect on the men's attitudes toward the Equal Rights Amendment, marital and date rape laws, or punishments for rape.

A provocative study examined 24 indicators of gender equality in politics, economics, and legal rights in all 50 states relative to the rates of circulation of sexually explicit magazines (Baron, 1990). This study set out to demonstrate that more widespread circulation of sexually explicit magazines such as *Playboy*, *Hustler*, and *Penthouse* leads to lower levels of gender social equality. However, the study found the opposite: that gender equality tends to be greater in states where the amount of pornography purchased is higher. The researchers concluded that such a correlation implies that where the political climate is more liberal and tolerant, both pornography and gender equality coexist.

Such a correlation may be explained by the fact that the effect of pornography, per se, when considered within overall societal influences on behavior, may be too small to have much of an impact. However, this does not necessarily mean that sexually explicit materials do not have a profound effect on individuals' attitudes and actions toward women.

Pornography, Violence, and Rape

To the extent that pornography contains depictions of victimization of and violence toward women, many people are convinced that pornography must also contribute in a causal way to real-world rape and other forms of violence against women. Many studies have been undertaken in an effort to demonstrate such a connection. All of these investigations employed either correlational or experimental laboratory methods, both of which contain important weaknesses in what we may conclude from the findings (this is discussed in greater detail in "Evaluating Sexual Research: The Lab Experiment–Correlation Trade-Off").

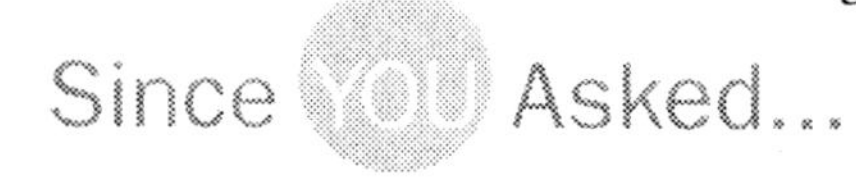

9. Can looking at pornography cause guys to want to do weird or sick things sexually?

It is important to note that most of the research in this area has drawn a distinction between pornography that portrays violence against or degradation of women and pornography that is equally explicit but without an overt degrading or violent component. Table 15.4 offers a wider view by summa-

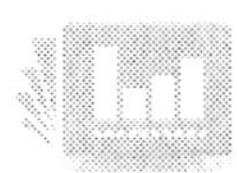

Evaluating Sexual Research

The Lab Experiment–Correlation Trade-Off

Research on the connection between pornography and violence against women provides an ideal example of the perplexing methodological difficulties often encountered in studying weighty social issues. Fundamentally, researchers only have two methods of study at their disposal, correlational research and experiments. Both are legitimate forms of scientific inquiry, yet either may lead us to erroneous conclusions.

As we have discussed elsewhere in this text, correlational research draws on existing data about the subjects being studied and attempts to find meaningful relationships among those data. To examine pornography and violence against women using correlational techniques, we might, for example, look for a link between convicted sex offenders and their exposure to pornography, compared to a similar group of nonoffenders (Langevin et al., 1988), or perhaps we could measure men's attitudes toward rape and their experiences with pornography to see if a predictable association exists (Davies, 1997). However, we must approach the findings of such studies with caution. Why? Because correlation does not imply causation. That is, the fact that sexually explicit materials may be associated with negative attitudes or violent behavior does not allow us to assume that the pornography *caused* the attitudes or behavior. Perhaps the causal link is in the entirely opposite direction: Men with more callous attitudes toward women are more drawn to pornography. Or maybe men who have more aggressive personalities are more likely to be violent toward women *and* read violent pornography. No matter how logical it may seem to make a causal connection, this is true for virtually any correlational finding. Results based on correlations may reflect a causal relationship between the two variables, but we cannot simply assume causation from a correlational finding.

If we wish to determine with some degree of confidence that one variable does indeed cause another, we would need to do an experiment. In an experiment, the researchers control what happens to the participants and the setting in which it happens. This is completely different from a correlational study, in which no control whatsoever is possible because the data are already "attached to" the participants. When we do an experiment, the data are gathered under controlled conditions, so we may draw cause-and-effect conclusions. An example would be to see if the effect of watching pornographic videos causes men to develop hostile attitudes or violent tendencies toward women (Donnerstein, 1980). In such an experiment, men would be divided randomly into two or more groups and shown different video programs over a specified amount of time. One group would be shown, say, violent pornography; another, nonviolent pornography; and perhaps another, nonpornographic videos. All other potential influences would be held constant for all the groups. Then the attitudes or behavioral tendencies of men from all three groups toward women would be measured. If the group exposed to the violent videos displayed significantly more negative attitudes or behaviors toward women, we could then conclude with reasonable certainty that the pornography was indeed the cause of the negative attitudes.

However, although we have now revealed a cause-and-effect relationship between pornography and negative reactions toward women, we cannot automatically assume that our findings can be applied to the real world outside of the controlled laboratory setting. It was a setting contrived by the experimenters and may not have resembled very accurately how pornography is used in the actual lives of men who are exposed to it. So we are left with a research conundrum: If we examine data from the real world, we cannot conclude cause and effect, but if we exert scientific control to reveal causal relationships, we give up some accuracy in applying our findings to the real world. What's a scientist to do?

Unfortunately, there is no ideal answer to that question. Obviously, we cannot go out and do a "real-world experiment" on the connection between pornography and violence (we would have to control people's real-life exposure to pornography, and we can't do that). All we can do is try to control for as many extraneous variables in our correlational research and try to make our experimental laboratory conditions as realistic as possible. And always, when we engage in or read about any research, we must be skeptical, think critically, and keep our minds open to other possibilities.

rizing a number of studies carried out since the early 1980s on the effects of pornography on violence and rape.

Correlational studies have generally come up with very mixed and confusing results when attempting to link pornography and violence toward women. For example, one study compared sex offenders with a matched control group of non-sex-offending men

Table 15.4 PORNOGRAPHY AND AGGRESSION TOWARD WOMEN: WHAT THE RESEARCH HAS SHOWN

STUDY	METHOD	MAIN FINDINGS
	CORRELATIONAL STUDIES	
Garcia (1986)	Gathered data from 115 undergraduate male college students	Subjects having greater exposure to violent sexual materials were found to express more negative attitudes toward women in the area of sexual behavior.
Smith and Hand (1987)	Presented a pornographic movie on a college campus; studied partner aggression reported by 230 college women during the week prior to and after the movie	No differences in reported aggression were found before versus after the showing or between males who viewed the movie and those who did not.
Demare, Briere, and Lips (1988)	Surveyed 222 male undergraduates on pornography use, attitudes toward women, and self-reported likelihood of rape or use of sexual violence	Use of sexually violent pornography combined with acceptance of interpersonal violence against women predicted greater self-reported likelihood of rape and sexual violence.
Padgett, Brislin-Slutz, and Neal (1989)	Assessed attitudes toward women of college students and patrons of X-rated theaters	Hours of viewing pornography did not predict attitudes toward women for either subject group.
	EXPERIMENTAL STUDIES	
Donnerstein (1980)	One hundred twenty college males saw either an aggressive pornographic film, a "slasher" film (nonsexual violence against woman), or a consensual sexually explicit film; were then angered by a female confederate, and aggression (level of "fake" shocks delivered to that female) was measured	Only aggressive pornography increased aggression toward the target female.
Donnerstein and Berkowitz (1981)	College males watched film of (1) a violent rape in which the victim was portrayed as "enjoying" the rape; (2) a rape in which the victim was not "enjoying" the rape; (3) a sexually explicit consensual sex; or (4) a nonsexual film; some subjects were insulted by a female confederate prior to seeing the films	Group 1 subjects displayed aggression to the female confederate whether insulted or not; group 2 displayed increased aggression to the insulting female; no aggression was found for the other groups.
Zillman and Bryant (1982)	Eighty men and 80 women were exposed to either 36 or 18 nonviolent pornographic films, nonsexual control films, or no films and then read a rape case, after which recommended punishment for rapists and support for the women's rights movement were measured	Subjects in the massive-exposure group (36 films) recommended half the prison sentence (5 years versus 10 years) for rapists and expressed half as much support for the women's movement compared to the low-exposure (18 files) group. (*Note:* This is the only study to find such results for *nonviolent* pornography.)
Fisher and Grenier (1994)	Seventy-nine undergraduate males were exposed to either violent pornography, nonviolent pornography, or neutral videos; then attitudes toward women were measured	No antiwoman aggression, fantasies, or attitudes were found.
Mullin and Linz (1995)	Subjects were exposed to a sequence of sexually violent films over several days; compared with a no-film group for sensitivity to victims of domestic violence	Three days following exposure to the final film, subjects were found to be less sensitive than the control group to domestic violence victims and rated their injuries as less severe. However, five days after the final film exposure, subjects' sensitivity to the domestic violence victims rebounded to control group levels.

from the same community in Canada (Langevin et al., 1988). The results indicated that the control group of men reported *greater* exposure to sexually explicit materials than the sex offenders, and the type of pornography both groups had been exposed to was about the same. A study comparing adolescent sexual offenders with matched nonoffenders found that the sexual offenders were more likely to have read pornographic *magazines*, but the nonoffenders were more likely to have viewed pornographic *videos* (Zgourides, Monto, & Harris, 1997). Another correlational study of more than 380 college men found that those who already harbored antiwomen attitudes and who had also viewed violent pornography scored higher on self-reported measures of likelihood to rape or use sexual force and were more likely to say they had used force or coercion to obtain sex in the past (Demare, Lips, & Briere, 1993). However, this same study found no association between nonviolent pornography and any measures of violence toward women, even among subjects with antiwomen attitudes.

Other correlational studies have focused on links between pornography laws and other sex offenses. One ambitious study looked at four states (Maine, North Carolina, Pennsylvania, and Washington) where pornography laws had at one time been strictly enforced but were later suspended (Winick & Evans, 1996). The rates of other sex crimes, including rape and prostitution, were compared for the periods of enforcement and nonenforcement of pornography statutes. The results indicated that the lifting of enforcement of antipornography laws in all four states had no significant effect on the rates of other sex crimes. Similar studies from other countries have produced comparable findings (i.e., Kutchinsky, 1991). We cannot conclude from this evidence that laws against pornography reduce sex-related crime. The study may actually suggest that laws have little effect on people who view pornography and who also tend to commit the crimes.

On the laboratory experimental side of the research on the effects of pornography, many studies have looked at how viewing various types of sexually explicit materials affects men's attitudes and behaviors toward women. Over the decades of research, the findings have become reasonably clear: Nonviolent sexually explicit materials, no matter how explicit they are, do not appear to produce negative effects on men's attitudes or behaviors toward women. However, when the pornography depicts violence toward or degradation of women, negative changes in men's attitude, behaviors, and intentions toward women do occur.

Variations on one investigation strategy have been employed by researchers in laboratory settings. This method exposes participants, usually college students, to differing types and amounts of sexually explicit materials and then measures the subjects on some response of interest, such as callous attitudes toward women, belief in rape myths, feelings of aggression toward women, appropriate punishment for a rapist, or willingness to punish a woman who had insulted them (for a review of these studies, Linz and Donnerstein, 1990, and C. Hunter, 2000). Two of the leading researchers in this field summarized the findings of these various studies as follows:

> To date [the research] clearly indicates that when males are exposed to violent pornography, they will display heightened levels of aggression against a woman in a laboratory setting . . . usually demonstrated by a subject's willingness to deliver electric shocks to a female victim in the laboratory (or at least to believe he is doing so). Given that, what does the research say about antisocial effects of pornography that fall short of actual violent behavior? Researchers have documented that men who view sexually *violent* materials in controlled situations may demonstrate increased callousness toward women. The men undergo several attitudinal and perceptual changes, tending to see a rape victim presented to them later as less injured and more responsible for her assault. The men also are more likely to endorse myths such as the idea that women secretly enjoy sexual assault. (Linz & Donnerstein, 1992, p. B3–4)

As noted earlier, these findings tend to disappear in nearly all studies when subjects are exposed to nonviolent pornography, even when the exposure is extreme. For example, one study exposed participants to five straight days of nonviolent pornography and then measured their attitudes toward women and rape. The results indicated no difference in subjects' attitudes before and after the "pornography-fest" and no difference between subjects who had viewed the pornography and a group of controls who viewed non–sexually explicit materials (Padgett & Brislin-Slutz, 1989). Again, it is important to keep in mind that regardless of whether laboratory research reveals a causal relationship between sexually explicit materials and negative attitudes, we still cannot assume that those findings signify such a relationship in the real world, outside of the controlled setting where the research took place.

Several reasons exist for the difficulty in generalizing laboratory results to real-life settings involving pornography and violence (Hunter, 2000). First, the subjects in most of the studies have been college students who have volunteered to participate to receive credit for their psychology classes. That these students accurately represent those in real life who view pornography is highly questionable. They are very likely different, on average, in age, education, and voluntary use of pornography from the population in general. Second, the laboratory setting is, by its very nature, artificial. In pornography experiments, students typically view pornography in groups, they know they are part of an experiment, and the methods of measuring their attitudes and behaviors toward women do not carry the weight of real-world limitations or freedoms. We cannot know to what extents these artificial conditions produce results that are different from events in real life. And finally, the sexually explicit materials shown in these studies are chosen by the experimenters, not by the subjects themselves, as would be the case in real life (Tsang, 1986). To the extent that pornography causes or fails to cause negative responses toward women may depend on other characteristics of the man viewing it and on the images he chooses to view. Linz and Donnerstein (1992) have summarized these problems as follows:

> Whether this [laboratory] aggression is representative of real-world aggression, such as rape, is a matter of great controversy among social scientists. Put simply, many behavioral scientists do not believe that it is reasonable to infer that because men are aggressive in the laboratory, where inhibitions against violence may be weak, they will behave violently in society, where there are (at least ostensibly) norms against sexual violence. We must be cautious when attempting to generalize from laboratory studies to behavior in the real world. Longitudinal field studies in which a group of men exposed to pornography would be monitored for aggressive behavior over a lengthy period of time would allow us to confirm experimental studies. To date, such very expensive investigations have not been undertaken, so the laboratory findings are best described as "suggestive" of a link between violent pornography and violence toward women. (p. B4)

The Violence-Not-Sex Hypothesis

As study after study continued to find a link between antisocial behavior and violent but not nonviolent pornography, some researchers began to wonder if the violence might be playing a larger role than the sexual content. Some research evidence exists to support this idea.

When the type of media found in the possession of violent sexual criminals is analyzed, it is often violent materials, such as detective magazines and violent nonpornographic movies that are found, not sexually explicit materials (Linz & Donnerstein, 1992).

As we have discussed previously, many studies have demonstrated a link between violent pornography and callousness or violent tendencies toward women, but some studies have found the same link for violent materials *without* the sexually explicit content. For example, in one study, three groups of subjects were each shown a different version of the same film (Donnerstein & Linz, 1986). The versions were as follows:

1. One group saw a film containing a sexual aggression scene in which a woman is violently tied up, threatened with a gun, and raped.
2. A second group saw the exact same film and the same scene, but only the violence was shown, and the sexually explicit rape sequence was removed.
3. A third group saw the same film with the same scene, but only the sexually explicit rape scene was shown, and the accompanying violence was deleted.

After all groups had viewed the films, the researchers measured the attitudes of the men toward rape. The members of group 2, who had seen the violence without the sexual content, were found to have the most insensitive attitudes about rape and the largest percentage of subjects who admitted some likelihood of raping (if they would not be caught) or using sexual force. Subjects in group 3 (sexual content only) were least callous or likely to rape, and those in group 1 (sexual and violent content) fell in between the other two groups.

The distinction between violent materials and violent pornography is becoming increasingly important as both violence and sex on TV, on DVDs, on the Internet, and in video and computer games becomes more prevalent and more easily accessible. Clearly, violence, whether in a sexual context or not, has the ability to influence men's attitudes toward women and may translate into greater violence toward, victimization of, and discrimination against women. However, as scientific research has made fairly clear, a free society must take great care in the limitations its institutions place on rights of free speech if clear, rational evidence fails to demonstrate harm convincingly.

One type of sexually explicit material, however, instead of inflaming controversy and debate over its harmful effects, brings forth solidarity in the fight against it: child pornography.

Child Pornography

When children are victimized for the sexual purposes of adults, whether involving prostitution, pornography, or sexual abuse, people stop worrying about defining it or arguing whether or not it should be stopped. Instead, the discussion turns to the horrors of such victimization of innocent children and how it can be stopped immediately. Child pornography is a huge business estimated at over $3 billion per year in the United States. The crimes of child sexual abuse are discussed in greater detail in Chapter 13, "Sexual Aggression and Violence," and Chapter 14, "Paraphilias."

During the 1980s, child pornography was a dying menace. Child pornographers were isolated, hunted individuals, and access to pornography involving children was relegated to the deepest, darkest recesses of society. In short, child pornography had been all but eradicated in most of the civilized world. But then along came the Internet, and the world of child pornography changed. Today, law enforcement around the world must fight a continuous and uphill battle to intervene and arrest individuals who produce and distribute child pornography on the Web. In addition, parents, schools, teachers, and public libraries are wrestling constantly with the problem of preventing access to child pornography (and all other pornography) on Internet-connected computers that have become an integral part of our lives. Anyone who wishes to can download 100,000 pornographic images of children, often engaged in unimaginable activities with other children or with adults, all of which have been produced in the past decade (P. Jenkins, 2002).

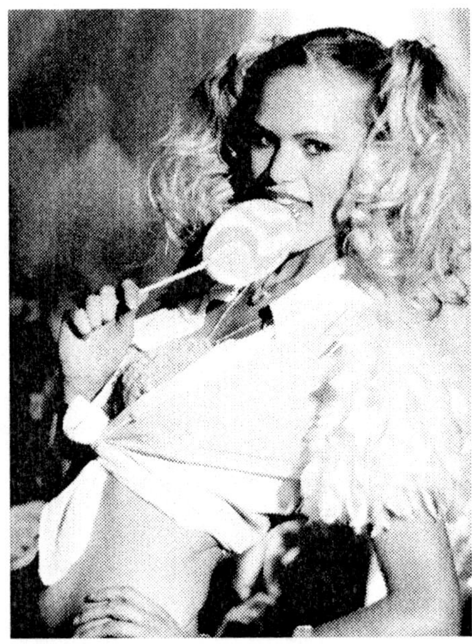

The availability of child pornography has exploded since the advent of the Internet in the 1980s, fueling an insidious worldwide industry. To circumvent child pornography laws, a common strategy in the pornography business is to use models of legal age posing as "children," as this photo depicts.

Child Pornography and the Law

Any use of child pornography, whether it involves producing it, looking at it, selling it, or distributing it, is illegal throughout the world. In the United States, the Supreme Court has developed guidelines for child pornography that make it for easier to find these materials obscene and ban them (Silver, 2001). Ten years after *Miller* v. *California*, the Court found that

> Recognizing and classifying child pornography as a category of material outside the protection of the First Amendment is not incompatible with our earlier decisions. . . . A trier of fact need not find that the material appeals to the prurient interest of the average person; it is not required that sexual conduct portrayed be done so in a patently offensive manner; and the material at issue need not be considered as a whole. (*New York* v. *Ferber*, 1982)

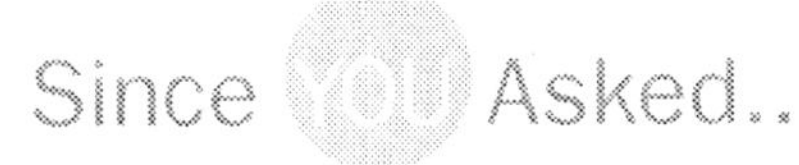

10. I read that child pornography is everywhere on the Internet. I think this is just so sick. What is being done to stop it?

Going after child pornography, pornographers, and users is a major endeavor throughout the world. International police agencies, FBI, Interpol, and other law enforcement organizations are becoming increasingly skilled at finding, tracing, and arresting adults who are engaged in child pornography practices online (see "Sexuality, Ethics, and the Law: The Child Pornography Fighters"). Moreover, criminal justice systems are attempting to keep pace by increasing penalties for these illegal activities. For example, in England, no distinction is drawn between downloading one pornographic child image or 10,000; the legal penalties are the same: a maximum of five years in jail. Similarly strict laws are being enacted in the United States. In Michigan, the maximum penalty for helping distribute child pornography is now seven years in prison and a $10,000 fine per violation; in Nebraska, possession of child pornography is punishable by a five-year prison term and a fine of $10,000; and in California, possession carries a three-year sentence and a $10,000 fine. All of these are recent increases to previous laws in those states.

However, despite some significant busts of major child pornography operations, these laws and penalties appear to be having little effect on the amount of child pornography available on the Internet. This is because as fast as law enforcement can

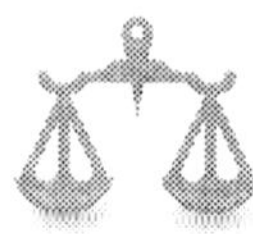

Sexuality, Ethics, and the Law

The Child Pornography Fighters

MARCH 19, 2002—Eighty-nine people, including two Catholic priests, two police officers, a foster parent and a nurse, have been charged in connection with an Internet-based child pornography ring that authorities have broken up, Justice Department officials announced. Numerous arrests have been made in a 14-month investigation, and 50 more arrests are expected later this week in the first phase of a nationwide crackdown on Internet-based child pornography. More than two dozen of those arrested have admitted to molesting 36 children, according to the FBI. The others were charged with possession of child pornography.

"It is clear a new marketplace for child pornography has emerged from the dark corners of cyberspace," Attorney General John D. Ashcroft said at a news conference at FBI headquarters, where he announced the sweep. "Innocent boys and girls have been targeted by offenders who view them as sexual objects. These individuals must be stopped."

The sting, known as "Operation Candyman," included more than 225 searches in more than 20 states. The ring has been disbanded and a Web site that allowed the suspects to send and receive pornography was shut down, FBI officials said.

FBI Director Robert S. Mueller III said in a statement that his agency will shut down "any and all Websites, e-groups, bulletin boards, and any other mediums that will foster the continued exploitation of our children."

"This extensive operation should serve as a warning to others that we will find and prosecute those who target and endanger our children," Ashcroft said.

"Operation Candyman" began in January 2001 when the FBI's Houston field office launched an investigation into three Internet groups involved in posting, downloading and sharing pornographic images of children. All 56 FBI field offices investigated 7,000 people who subscribed to the "Candyman" e-mail group, including 2,400 outside the United States.

Those charged include police officers in Pittsburgh and San Diego; a school bus driver from Albany, N.Y.; a therapist from Little Rock who later committed suicide; and a school guidance counselor from Philadelphia, FBI officials said.

It also includes the former associate pastor of the Cathedral of Mary Our Queen Catholic Church in Baltimore, according to Ray Kempisty, a spokesman with the Archdiocese of Baltimore. The priest was arrested four months ago and charged with possession of child pornography, Kempisty said. He was placed on administrative leave and is receiving inpatient treatment at St. Luke's Institute in Silver Spring, Kempisty said. FBI officials said they weren't sure where the other priest is from.

"Operation Candyman demonstrates both the scope of child pornography and the commitment of law enforcement to shut it down," Ashcroft said.

Bruce Gebhardt, the FBI's new executive assistant director in charge of cyber-crime, described the target of the operation as an "international ring of pedophiles" that the FBI is determined to dismantle.

"We're dealing with children," Gebhardt said. "I'd like to see a sweep a day until we get them all."

Source: C. Thompson (2002).

work to track down the perpetrators, the methods used to hide the operations throughout the world become increasingly sophisticated.

Technological Solutions to Child Pornography

In addition to criminal justice strategies to attempt to limit child pornography online or limit access or exposure to it, Internet filtering software has been developed, some of which can screen out most sexually explicit materials. The problem, however, is that while the program is blocking pornographic sites, it also restricts the user's access to nonpornographic sites that contain key words, phrases, or graphics that the software interprets as forbidden, such as some fine arts sites, legitimate sexuality education sites, and, perhaps most unfortunately, health-related sites. One study tested seven of the most popular pornography-filtering programs and found that at the most restrictive settings, out of 3,000 Internet health sites, more than 700 were blocked, and one of every three sexual health sites was blocked even at the least restrictive settings (R. Richardson et al., 2002). These were not minor Web-based sources of health information; they included sites from the Food and Drug Administration, the National Library of Medicine, and the Centers for Disease Control and Prevention (see Figure 15.4).

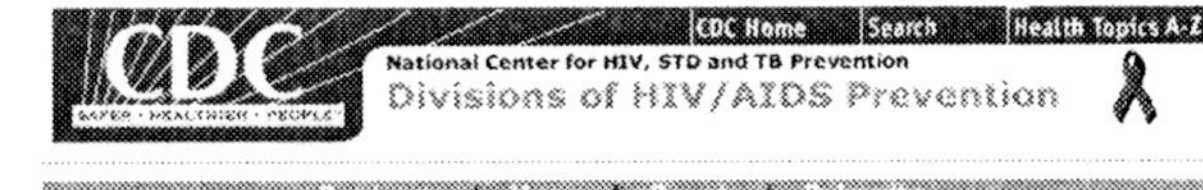

HIV and AIDS: Are You at Risk?

Esta página en español

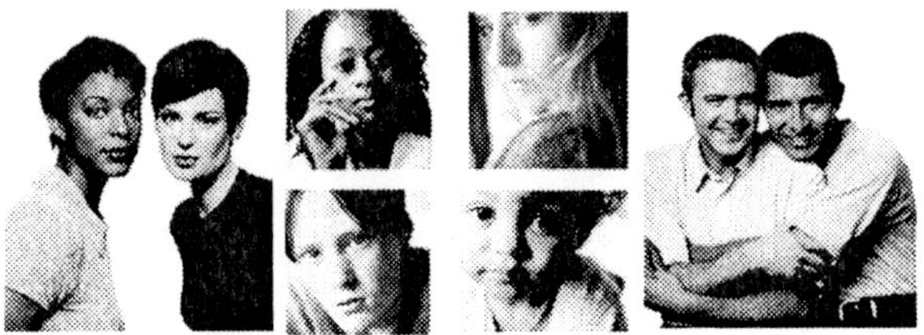

What is HIV and how can I get it?

HIV - the human immunodeficiency virus - is a virus that kills your body's "CD4 cells." CD4 cells (also called T-helper cells) help your body fight off infection and disease. HIV can be passed from person to person if someone with HIV infection has sex with or shares drug injection needles with another person. It also can be passed from a mother to her baby when she is pregnant, when she delivers the baby, or if she breast-feeds her baby.

What is AIDS?

AIDS - the acquired immunodeficiency syndrome - is a disease you get when HIV destroys your body's immune system. Normally, your immune system helps you fight off illness. When your immune system fails you can become very sick and can die.

What do I need to know about HIV?

The first cases of AIDS were identified in the United States in 1981, but AIDS most likely existed here and in other parts of the world for many years before that time. In 1984 scientists proved that HIV causes AIDS

Anyone can get HIV. The most important thing to know is how you can get the virus.

You can get HIV:

- By having unprotected sex- sex without a condom- with someone who has HIV. The virus can be in an infected person's blood, semen, or vaginal secretions and can enter your body through tiny cuts or sores in your skin, or in the lining of your vagina, penis, rectum, or mouth.
- By sharing a needle and syringe to inject drugs or sharing drug equipment used to prepare drugs for injection with someone who has HIV.

FIGURE 15.4 Software designed to filter out child pornography and other objectionable material may also filter out valuable Web-based sources of information such as this site from the Centers for Disease Control and Prevention.

Source: Courtesy of CDC.

This trade-off of filtering unwanted sites while losing access to legitimate Internet resources may be acceptable in some settings such as families with children who are on the Internet routinely. However, this is rarely acceptable for adults who rely on the World Wide Web to gather health-related and other information for their own purposes, and it is totally unacceptable for professionals who use the Internet for research or to augment information to their clients and patients.

On a related note, many communities have asked that public libraries be required by law to install these filters on their Web-ready computers, but many libraries have balked at this as a form of censorship over the materials they provide to the public. The U.S. Supreme Court, in *United States* v. *American Library Association* (2003), rejected librarians' claim of censorship and upheld the Children's Internet Protection Act, which allows withholding of government funding from libraries that refuse to install pornography filters on their computers (Holland, 2003).

One potential solution to this dilemma would change the Internet addresses of all pornographic Websites. In early 2006, the Internet Corporation for Assigned Names and Numbers (ICANN) that directs the operations of the Internet will consider adopting a new domain suffix, ".xxx" (Bergstein, 2005). If all Websites containing sexually explicit materials for "entertainment purposes" were to use this suffix, individuals and organizations wishing to filter them out would have a much easier time doing so. However, a great deal of controversy exists over this seemingly logical solution because, under current plans, the owners of the explicit Websites could keep their ".com" suffixes as well. Whether or not such sites would eventually be required to switch entirely to the ".xxx" domain remains undecided.

Fighting Child Pornography through *Greater* Accessibility?

One intriguing and courageous suggestion has been made by Philip Jenkins, professor of history and religious studies at Pennsylvania State University. Jenkins, a strong advocate of total elimination of child pornography on the Internet, suggests that the legal crackdown on child pornography, as ineffective as it is, prevents serious researchers from studying and uncovering how this illicit trade functions and how best to attack it. Although Jenkins estimates that only about one-tenth of 1 percent of

Internet child pornography distributors and users are ever caught, arrested, and prosecuted, no serious social scientist or legal scholar would ever want to take the risk of accessing the material for legitimate research purposes and then try to use their research goals as a defense if caught in a law enforcement action. As Jenkins states:

> Once I had found the child-porn culture on the Internet, the next question was how to study it, given a legal environment in which virtually any contact with the material can lead to a federal prison sentence. "Children," for legal purposes, means anyone below the age of 18, and "pornography" includes depictions that would be only mildly indecent if adult subjects were involved. Moreover, one "possesses" an electronic image merely by downloading it, by clicking on a Web link. (P. Jenkins, 2002, p. B16)

Jenkins is suggesting that we, as a society, think about making some sort of exception to the current laws to allow for legitimate access and study of the Internet child pornography subculture with the goal and intent of destroying it. The reason, Jenkins asserts, is that most people do not have the slightest notion of just how horrible and widespread the problem is:

> The absence of previous studies—journalistic or academic—explains why most writers have failed even to notice the existence of this burgeoning subculture. We search the literature in vain for references even to core child-porn newsgroups. If the public does not even know that the newsgroups and bulletin boards exist, then the police face no pressure to eradicate them, with all the complex international cooperation that such an effort would demand. . . . The main reason people don't fight child pornography is that most of them have never seen it. Actual exposure to this material would galvanize public opinion—and, incidentally, would make clear the huge difference in potential harm between child porn and even the hardest of hard-core adult images. . . . Opening this avenue would raise the possibility of better exposing the trade, creating public awareness about its key institutions, and pressuring politicians to act against major suppliers and trafficking institutions, rather than just hapless individual consumers. (P. Jenkins, 2002, p. B16)

Jenkins's ideas make sense but may be difficult to put into practice. Who would determine what constitutes "legitimate research"? How would a researcher go about obtaining such an exception from legal prosecution? How could we prevent abuse of such a system? These are all legitimate questions, but if, as a culture, we are to develop an effective defense against the victimization of children at the hands of Internet pornographers, bold new approaches will be necessary.

Although child pornography is of the utmost concern when we consider the availability of pornography on the Internet, it comprises only a small percentage of all the sexually explicit materials that are currently available online.

Cyberporn

If you have a computer, are connected to the Internet, and use e-mail, you probably already know just how rampant Internet pornography has become. Consider the following estimates of pornography online (Internet Filter Review, 2003):

Pornographic Web sites	4.2 million
Pornographic pages	372 million
Daily pornographic search engine requests	68 million (25 percent of total)
Daily pornographic e-mails	2.5 billion (8 percent of total)
Average daily pornographic e-mails per user	4.5
Monthly pornographic Internet downloads	1.5 billion (35 percent of total)

Many of the issues we discussed in relation to child pornography apply to adult pornography on the Web as well. The difference is that definitions and obscenity laws rear their heads once again when discussing X-rated adult Web sites. The problem of defining Internet-based pornography is that the notion of "contemporary community standards," mentioned earlier in our discussion of defining pornography, loses its meaning in cyberspace.

The U.S. Congress and legislatures around the world are attempting to write laws to control sexually explicit materials on the Internet. In the United States, such laws have invariably been struck down by the courts on the grounds that they violate the protections of the First Amendment and do not meet the three-pronged test for obscenity developed in *Miller* v. *California*, discussed earlier in this chapter. The main problem is that no single "community-standard" exists to use as a basis for judging whether or not sexually explicit material is offensive and should be deemed obscene. This is obviously a problem when nearly everything on the World Wide Web is available to anyone with an Internet connection, anywhere in the world. As one judge put it: "I believe that 'indecent' and 'patently offensive' are inherently vague, particularly in light of the government's inability to identify the relevant community by whose standards the material will be judged" (Sloviter, 1996, p. 854).

The debate on whether and how to control sexually explicit materials on the Internet is likely to proceed unabated for decades. One thing is clear, however: People are using the Internet to view sexually explicit materials. One study found that about half of all college students had used the Internet for sexual purposes of one kind or another (Boies, 2002). Tables 15.5 and 15.6 summarize how and why college students access sexual information on line.

Clearly, the use of the Internet for sexually explicit purposes is very common and will probably continue to grow as the number and variety of sites increase and more people begin to access them for their own personal reasons.

Table 15.5 ONLINE SEXUAL ACTIVITIES ENGAGED IN BY COLLEGE STUDENTS DURING THE PREVIOUS 12 MONTHS

	PERCENTAGE OF STUDENTS		
ONLINE SEXUAL ACTIVITY	MEN	WOMEN	TOTAL
Relationship-focused			
Sought new contacts*	48.2	38.6	41.8
Used online dating	18.0	9.7	12.5
Information-focused			
Sought sexual information or advice*	67.6	45.1	52.5
Entertainment-focused			
Viewed sexually explicit materials (SEM)*	72.0	24.1	40.1
E-mailed SEM to others*	52.2	35.8	41.2
Received SEM from others	87.8	86.1	86.9
Used sex chat rooms*	13.4	7.0	9.3
Masturbated while online*	71.6	22.1	38.5
Found online sex partners	9.9	7.3	8.2

* Items for which gender differences were statistically significant.

Source: Data from "Sexually-Related Online Activities of College Students" from "University Students' Uses of and Reactions to Online Sexual Information and Entertainment: Links to Online and Offline Sexual Behavior" by S. Boles from *The Canadian Journal of Human Sexuality*, 11, (2002), pp. 77–90. Copyright © 2002. Reprinted by permission of The Sex Information and Education Council of Canada.

Table 15.6 COLLEGE STUDENTS' REACTIONS TO SEXUAL MATERIALS VIEWED ONLINE

	PERCENTAGE OF STUDENTS	
REACTION TO SEXUALLY EXPLICIT MATERIALS VIEWED ONLINE	MALES	FEMALES
Sexually excited*	91.9	70.1
Satisfied curiosity*	71.1	57.8
Learned new sexual techniques*	71.0	54.5
Images were disturbing	54.0	61.0
Fulfilled sexual fantasies*	65.2	42.2
Improved personal sexual relationships offline*	50.8	36.4
Bored	36.5	43.2
Satisfied sexual need*	25.9	16.6

* Reactions for which gender differences were statistically significant.

Source: Data from "College Students' Reactions to Online Sexual Activities" from "University Students' Uses of and Reactions to Online Sexual Information and Entertainment: Links to Online and Offline Sexual Behavior" by S. Boles from *The Canadian Journal of Human Sexuality*, 11, (2002), pp. 77–90. Copyright © 2002. Reprinted by permission of The Sex Information and Education Council of Canada.

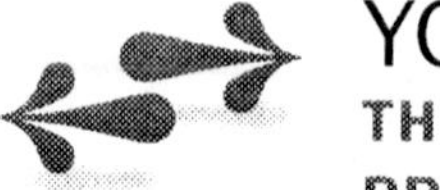

YOUR SEXUAL PHILOSOPHY

THE SEXUAL MARKETPLACE: PROSTITUTION AND PORNOGRAPHY

We have taken a fairly detailed look at two important ways human sexuality functions as a business: prostitution, in which sexual interactions between individuals are bought and sold; and pornography, in which various depictions of those interactions are bought and sold. Some would claim a world of difference exists between these two sexual marketplaces, while others would argue that they are in reality quite similar in terms of who sells, who buys, who profits, and who is victimized. Whether prostitution and pornography are distinct industries or represent two aspects of the same continuum of commercial sex, one point is clear: These are among the most controversial of sexually related issues worldwide.

You may be wondering why you would need to add the topics of prostitution and pornography to your developing sexual philosophy. After all, you are probably not planning to become a professional pornographer or a prostitute, right? Probably not. However, you should be aware that both of these issues *will* come up in your life, if they haven't already, in one way or another. This is just one more reason why it's easier and less stressful to have thought about such matters before they have a chance to cause a problem for you or your partner. As said before, your sexual philosophy is about knowing who you are, what you want and don't want, and planning accordingly.

As the debate about prostitution laws continues, it is possible that the lawmakers in your state, city, or town may at some point consider reducing legal control over commercial sex work. You may think it could never happen in *your* town, but that's what people said of lotteries, casinos, and other forms of legalized gambling only a couple of decades ago. So you never know. As an involved and concerned citizen, you will need to understand the issues relating to prostitution to participate intelligently in whatever controversy may arise. Furthermore, as discussed in this chapter, prostitution is here to stay. You are bound to see it, read about it, see ads for it (escort services, massage parlors, etc.), and maybe even be solicited by a prostitute. How will you react to these events if they occur to you or your partner? Chances are, after reading this chapter and thinking about the issues relating to prostitution and sex workers, you will be able to respond rationally and thoughtfully and avoid *overreacting* and creating more of a problem than might be necessary. In addition, now that you understand better the factors so often involved in the path to prostitution, you may one day want to become involved in helping young girls avoid the trap of prostitution or helping women already entangled find their way out.

Pornography is even more likely to be an issue in your life someday, and for some of you it may be already. A common problem in relationships is that one partner (usually the man, in heterosexual couples) becomes interested in viewing sexually explicit materials, but the other partner either is not interested or is offended and put off by the idea. This may raise difficult issues that the couple must address with knowledge and understanding to prevent them from threatening the relationship. Even more likely is the possibility that you will encounter sexually explicit materials yourself and you will need to analyze your feelings about them. Compared to several decades ago, access to sexually explicit materials has changed dramatically. Before VCRs and DVDs, the only way most people ever saw a pornographic film was to slip into an "adult theater" and hope no one they knew spotted them (or even worse, ran into them in the theater!). Today, however, it is a simple matter to walk into the local video store for a huge selection of X-rated videos, check some out, and watch them in the privacy of your own home. Furthermore, the Internet now makes readily accessible every kind of sexually explicit material imaginable—and you don't even have to leave the house to see it. In the information age, it has become more necessary than ever to understand what pornography is, what you want to view, and what you are unwilling to view. By understanding this now and planning ahead for situations in your life involving sexually explicit materials, you will be better equipped to handle these situations effectively, with confidence, control, and self-assurance when they arise.

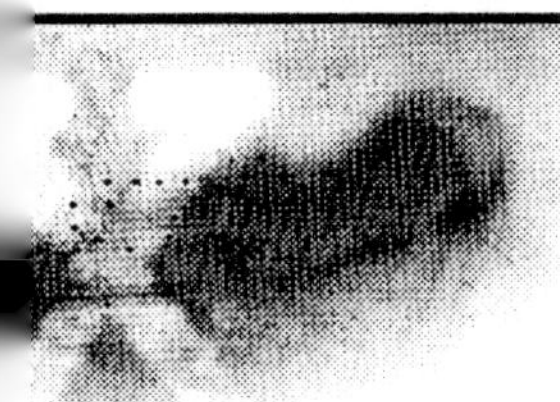

Summary

HISTORICAL PERSPECTIVES The Oldest Brothel?

- Archaeological findings reveal that prostitution is one of the oldest professions. While digging under the ruins of an ancient Roman forum in Greek Macedonia, scientists discovered a bathhouse and brothel from more than 2,000 years ago.

Prostitution

- Prostitution today, also termed the commercial sex trades, is defined as sexual acts exchanged for anything of value to the sex workers or their "managers" or pimps, including money, valued objects, personal property, drugs, shelter, or other services.
- Sex workers and their clients may be male or female and of the same or opposite sexes.
- Prostitution is illegal in most countries of the world and all U.S. states, with the exception of certain counties in Nevada, where prostitution is legal and controlled.
- Various types of prostitutes exist, the most common of which are referred to as streetwalkers, brothel workers, and call girls.
- Male prostitutes' customers are typically other men. When males are hired by women, they tend to function more as escorts, and their interaction may or may not include sex.
- Some women enter the profession of prostitution by choice, but most are forced into it through international human trafficking, drug abuse and addiction, or coercion by pimps. Studies show that most girls enter prostitution to pay for their addiction to crack or injectable drugs. Prostitutes' age at first intercourse, whether voluntary or not, is significantly younger than that of nonprostitutes.
- Rates of STIs are high among sex trade workers, due to the same risk factors faced by the general population: multiple sex partners, unprotected sex, and drug abuse. Rates of STIs among male prostitutes and transgender female prostitutes are particularly high.
- The profile of clients of prostitutes ("johns" or "tricks") does not differ significantly from males in general. The most common activity requested by clients is oral sex.
- The debate over the legalization or decriminalization of prostitution in the United States is often a heated one, but states show few signs of changing the legal status of prostitution.

Pornography

- Overall, college students have more experience with viewing pornography than is commonly believed.
- The current legal definition of pornography, called the "moral standard," was developed by the U.S. Supreme Court in 1973 and requires that local, contemporary community standards be applied to determine if a sexually explicit work should be deemed obscene and be exempt from First Amendment protections of freedom of expression. The sale, ownership, or viewing of material found to be obscene may be made illegal.
- Another position on defining pornography contends that sexually explicit materials that discriminate against a particular group of people, such as women, may be defined as obscene. This definition, however, is not used in current legal practice.
- Most researchers and writers draw a distinction between pornography and erotica. The term *erotica* is often applied to sexually explicit works expressing physical desire, passion, and attraction among people who freely choose to engage in sexual activities together. Erotica typically goes beyond "raw sex" and includes psychological and emotional factors as well. Erotica is seen as *sexual sharing*, whereas pornography is interpreted as *sexual using*.
- Research has demonstrated that women tend to be sexually aroused by a wider variety of sexually explicit images than men are.
- Studies show little effect of nonviolent pornography on men's attitudes toward women, but violent pornography appears to increase men's levels of callousness toward women. Violent pornography has also been shown to increase men's self-reported likelihood of rape. Overall, the violence may be more important than the sexual content in the effects of violent pornography on men's attitudes toward women.
- Child pornography is a huge business, estimated at over $3 billion a year in the United States alone. Child pornography was dying out in the 1980s as law enforcement was becoming increasingly effective in arresting and stamping out makers and users. However, today child pornography is growing at an alarming rate on the Internet, and worldwide attempts at controlling it are minimally effective.
- The Internet has made all forms of sexually explicit materials easily available to anyone, anywhere. Nearly 400 million pages of pornography exist on the Internet ("cyberporn"), and 35 percent of all downloads each month are from pornographic sites. That equals over 1.5 billion downloads.
- Much of the Internet use for sexually explicit materials is by college students. Students use the Internet to view pornography for a variety of reasons, ranging from seeking sexual excitement to satisfying their curiosity about pornography to learning new sexual techniques.

YOUR SEXUAL PHILOSOPHY: The Sexual Marketplace: Prostitution and Pornography

- If you have not already, you will encounter in your life, in one way or another, the main topics of this chapter: prostitution and pornography. Having thought about them and analyzed your feelings and attitudes will prevent them from catching you by surprise and causing discomfort for you or a problem for you and your partner. Remember, as we have discussed throughout this book, your sexual philosophy is about knowing who you are, what you want and don't want, and planning ahead.

Have You Considered?

1. Discuss three strategies that might be effective in helping women who are involved in street prostitution to find their way out of the business and into a healthier, happier life.
2. Do you believe that prostitution should be legalized or decriminalized? Explain your answer.
3. Discuss three reasons why you think male prostitutes for women customers are so rare.
4. Imagine that you are a social worker hired by a medium-size city to develop a program to prevent young girls from entering prostitution. List at least three strategies you might employ in your new job, and explain why you think they would be effective.
5. Prostitution is big business because there is big demand for the services of sex workers. One way to reduce prostitution (especially dangerous street prostitution) would be to reduce demand. Discuss at least three tactics that might be used to reduce the demand for the services of prostitutes.
6. Do you think some sexually explicit materials (other than child pornography) should be legally censored? If so, what materials and why? If not, why not?
7. Discuss your opinion about using the current "moral standard" in judging whether sexually explicit materials are obscene. Do you think it is effective? Why or why not?
8. Imagine that you have been very successful in your job discussed in item 4 on this list. Now the city council asks you to find ways of reducing the terrible problem of child pornography on the Internet. List at least three strategies you might employ in this assignment, and explain why you think they would be effective.

Companion Website Resources

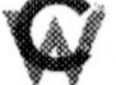
For further chapter resources go to **www.prenhall.com/hock**. This robust text website includes polling questions for you to vote on, regular news updates, quizzes, sample tests, suggested reading lists, and more.

SCENARIOS USA Also on the website are links to videos. *Scenarios USA's* films portray real-life narratives that explore the non-biological aspects of relationships and sexual health. The films will help you consider how the themes of the text affect your own life and the lives of those around you.

EPILOGUE

Human Sexuality:

Exploring Your Sexual Philosophy

Your sexual philosophy allows you to know who you are as a sexual person, to determine what you want or do not want throughout your sexual life, and to plan ahead so that *you* are in control of your life's sexual situations, rather than those situations controlling you.

Most people don't think enough about sex. You may find this statement surprising or even wonder if it's a joke. But it's neither. Although you probably do think about sex sometimes (or a lot of the time), when you do, you are probably fantasizing about sexual activities with a real or imaginary partner. However, "having sex," whatever that may mean to you, is only one small part—granted an important one—of the rich complexity of human sexuality.

This book is unique in many ways, the most important being that it deals with material about human sexuality that you truly need to "get"—both to incorporate into your base of sexual knowledge and to use in your life. If you are like most students, you've had many classes in which you learned the material well enough to pass tests and write papers, but then you've usually jettisoned most it from your brain when the class was over. Please, do not do that with the information you've learned from this text or this class! Each and every one of you will benefit from applying this information throughout your life.

A quick review of the chapters in this book reveals the wide range of topics included in a comprehensive understanding of humans as sexual beings. It is probably safe to say that you have given little thought to many of these topics, and yet nearly all of them will have an impact on your life—if they haven't already—in one way or another. People often give more thought and reflection to their education, their career goals, their overall lifestyle desires, and even their diet and wardrobe than they do to the complex issues relating to sexuality.

Now that you have come to the end of this text, focus for a moment on a major theme throughout: exploring *Your Sexual Philosophy*. Sexuality is essential to our basic nature as human beings. Therefore, incorporating the knowledge gained during your journey through this text into how you view yourself and the world around you is key to your overall philosophy of life—who you are as a sexual person, what you want and do not want sexually, and how you envision your sexual life now and in the future.

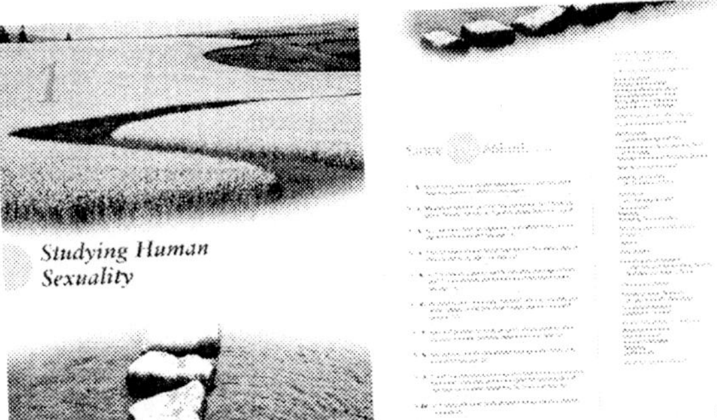

■ **Studying human sexuality** does not come naturally to most of us, and the information we need is not always acquired through personal experiences. It requires thought, reflection, accurate knowledge, and, perhaps most

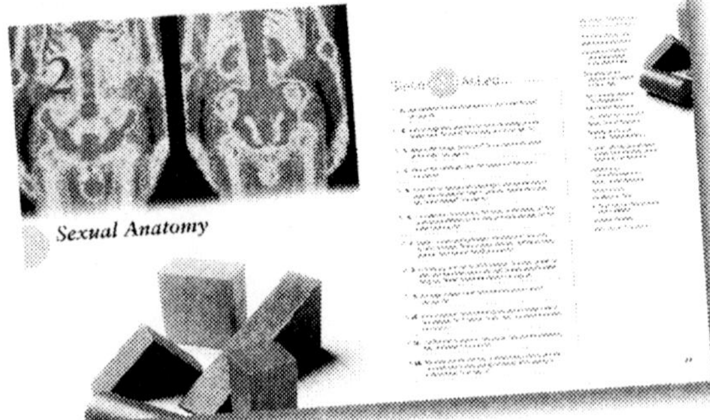

important, *planning ahead*. The worst time to try to figure out how you feel about any sexual situation or behavior is in the emotionally charged moment when it presents itself. That is why in this book we have explored human sexuality in ways that allow you not only to learn and understand it but also to make the information part of your life; to make smart sexual choices; to stay healthy, both physically and emotionally; and to incorporate this knowledge into your ever-changing, always growing sexual philosophy. The substance of every chapter, from the building blocks of sexual knowledge to the finer points of human sexuality, has a place in that philosophy.

A fundamental skill in the study of human sexuality is the ability to think critically about sexual research. With the media bombarding you with sexually related messages and images, your ability to filter out the factual from the distortions and myths is crucial to your healthy sexual development.

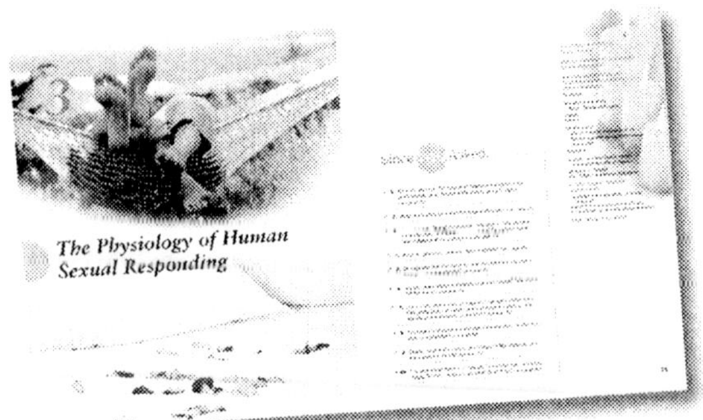

■ A working awareness of your own **sexual anatomy** and that of others will help you overcome any embarrassment some of you may have about your body. Not only can this enhance sexual satisfaction, but it can also help you stay sexually healthy by feeling less embarrassed about seeking medical attention if you notice any worrisome symptoms. Beyond having a working knowledge of sexual anatomy is understanding your **sexual physiology**, that is, how your body responds during sexual arousal. These are basic tools in your sexual philosophy. Using them will allow you to enrich your sexual life in many ways, both alone and with your present or future sexual partner or partners.

■ If you were to ask, most people will tell you that the most gratifying sexual interactions occur in the context of a **loving, intimate relationship**. These relationships are often among the closest connections we will ever experience with another person. As great as they may be, they sometimes pose challenges as well. Part of anyone's successful sexual philosophy is an understanding of how to establish and maintain a satisfying romantic relationship. Although many factors play a role, perhaps the most important is communication. And sex is one of the most important, though often the most difficult, topics of communication between partners. The expectation that sex is just something that "happens naturally" in an intimate relationship can move what might have been a good relationship into troubled waters. If you can learn to make effective intimate communication a high priority in your sexual philosophy, you and your relationships will be happier for it.

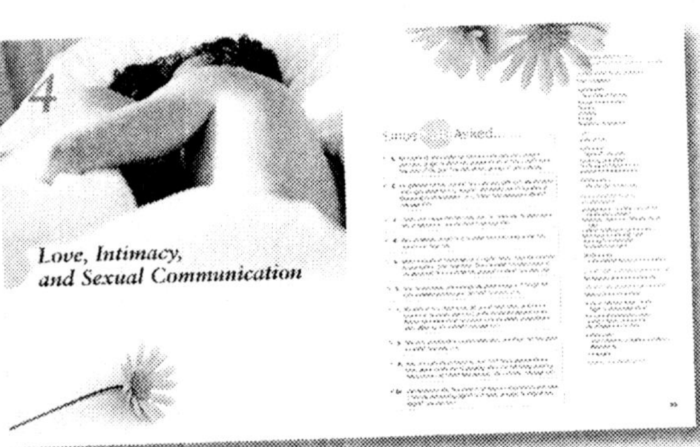

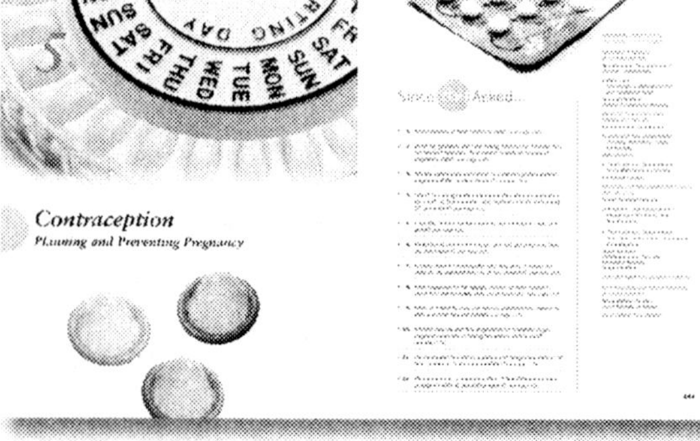

■ The topic of **contraception** obviously requires clear discussion early in a relationship, *before* you and your partner become sexual. We've discussed the most current information about the many forms of contraception available to you. It's up to you to reach an agreement with your partner about the consistent use of an effective contraception strategy. Determining the method that is best for you is the key to avoiding unintended pregnancies and sexually transmitted infections. You want to be certain about your own acceptable contraceptive choices (including abstinence) well in advance of the moment when you might need them. This text helps you do that.

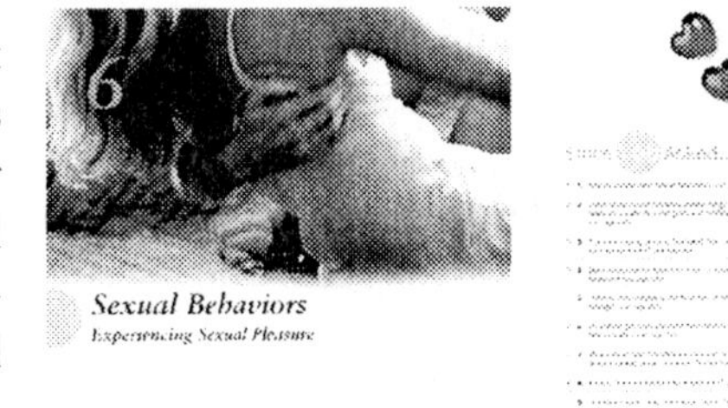

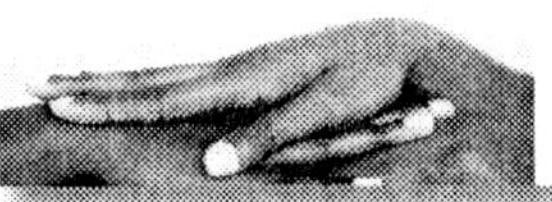

When it comes to sexual behavior, the emphasis is on pleasure. Sex should feel good, physically and mentally, and if it doesn't, something is wrong. Can you decide what is right and best for you without a working knowledge of various sexual activities? No. Think about your attitudes and feelings about the **sexual behaviors** discussed in this book, and make decisions as best you can about those behaviors now—not when confronted with them in the future. Adding this knowledge base to your sexual philosophy will prepare you if and when the moment arrives when you must make a choice in the heat of a sexual moment, when you might not be fully in control of your decision-making abilities. In moments like these, you are more likely to make bad choices if you have not already given some careful thought to what you want. Remember, your sexual philosophy is about knowing what you want and don't want, when (under what conditions) you want it, and planning ahead.

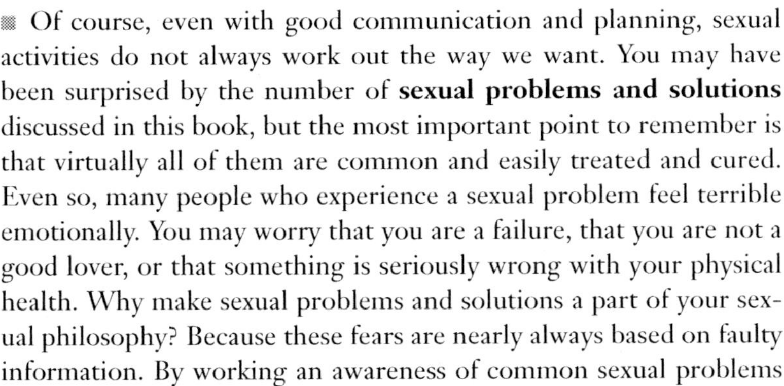

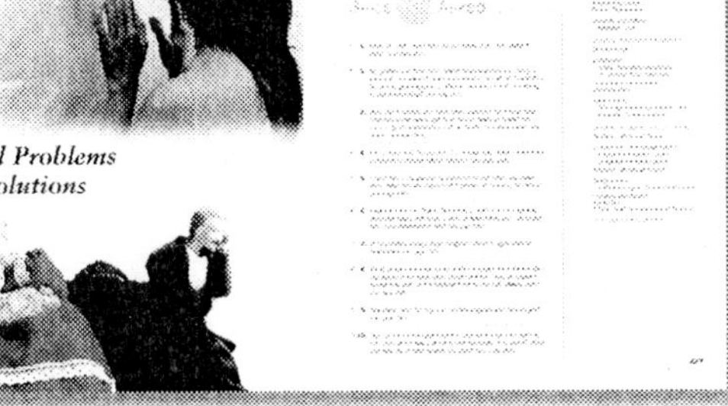

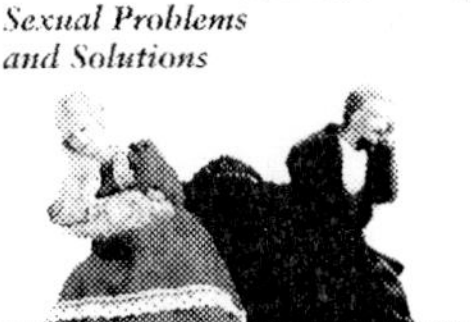

Of course, even with good communication and planning, sexual activities do not always work out the way we want. You may have been surprised by the number of **sexual problems and solutions** discussed in this book, but the most important point to remember is that virtually all of them are common and easily treated and cured. Even so, many people who experience a sexual problem feel terrible emotionally. You may worry that you are a failure, that you are not a good lover, or that something is seriously wrong with your physical health. Why make sexual problems and solutions a part of your sexual philosophy? Because these fears are nearly always based on faulty information. By working an awareness of common sexual problems and their solutions into your sexual philosophy, you will be better prepared and far less anxious (which typically only makes sexual problems worse) should you or your partner experience one. And if you're like most people, you probably will some day. But don't worry, you will be ready to deal with it.

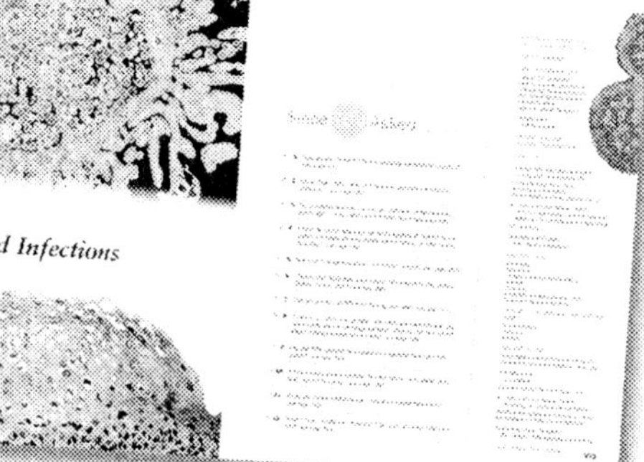

One potential outcome of sexual activities is the spread of **sexually transmitted infections**. STIs are the most common transmissible infections in the world, many of them are as yet incurable, and some can lead to serious health problems such as infertility and even death. If that sounds frightening to you, it should! The good news is that all STIs are avoidable—you never *have* to catch one. How can you avoid STIs? It's simple: Never have sexual contact with another person. OK; although that is indeed an effective strategy, let's get serious. Most of you have or will have one or more sexual partners during your life. Therefore, the best way to prevent contracting or transmitting STIs is by learning everything you can about them—how they are transmitted, the symptoms (if any), how to practice safe (or safer) sex, and the most up-to-date treatments and cures. With that knowledge as part of your working sexual philosophy, you will have the resources to avoid contracting an STI and to help prevent the spread of STIs.

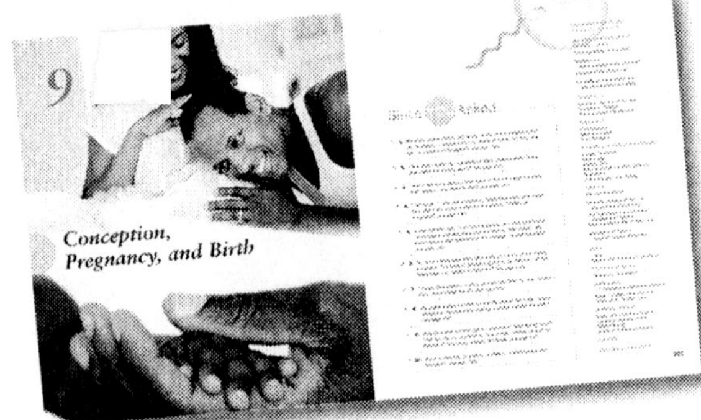

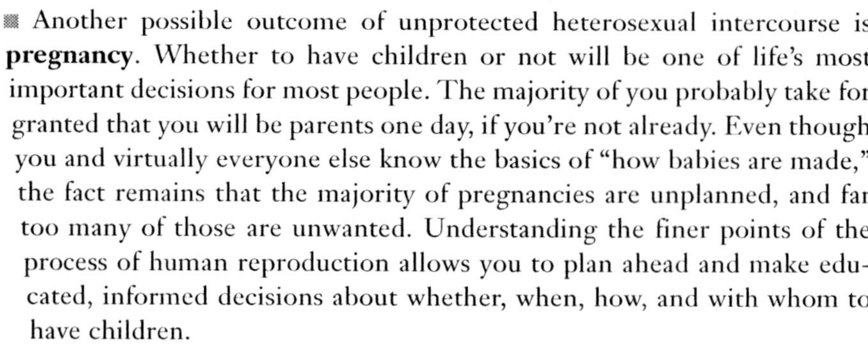

■ Another possible outcome of unprotected heterosexual intercourse is **pregnancy**. Whether to have children or not will be one of life's most important decisions for most people. The majority of you probably take for granted that you will be parents one day, if you're not already. Even though you and virtually everyone else know the basics of "how babies are made," the fact remains that the majority of pregnancies are unplanned, and far too many of those are unwanted. Understanding the finer points of the process of human reproduction allows you to plan ahead and make educated, informed decisions about whether, when, how, and with whom to have children.

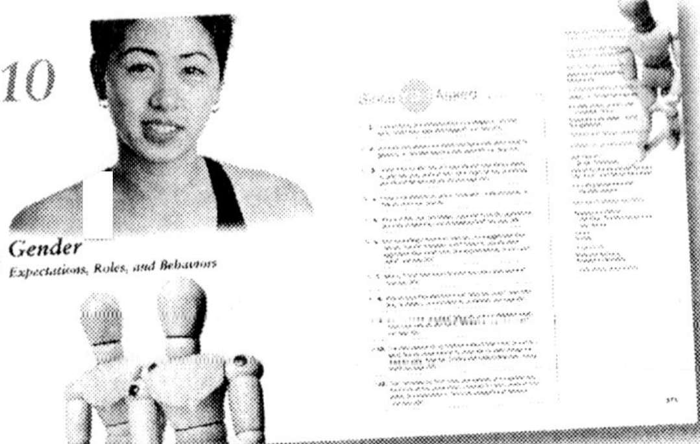

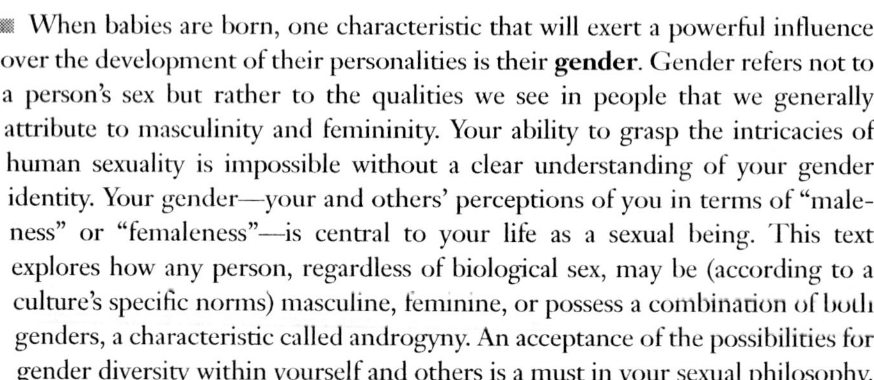

■ When babies are born, one characteristic that will exert a powerful influence over the development of their personalities is their **gender**. Gender refers not to a person's sex but rather to the qualities we see in people that we generally attribute to masculinity and femininity. Your ability to grasp the intricacies of human sexuality is impossible without a clear understanding of your gender identity. Your gender—your and others' perceptions of you in terms of "maleness" or "femaleness"—is central to your life as a sexual being. This text explores how any person, regardless of biological sex, may be (according to a culture's specific norms) masculine, feminine, or possess a combination of both genders, a characteristic called androgyny. An acceptance of the possibilities for gender diversity within yourself and others is a must in your sexual philosophy.

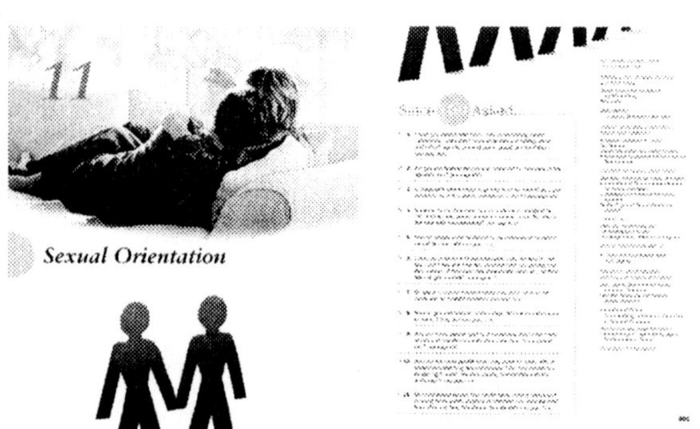

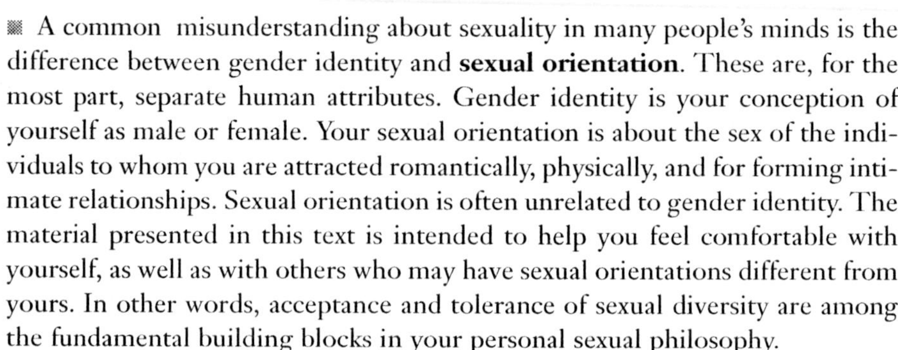

■ A common misunderstanding about sexuality in many people's minds is the difference between gender identity and **sexual orientation**. These are, for the most part, separate human attributes. Gender identity is your conception of yourself as male or female. Your sexual orientation is about the sex of the individuals to whom you are attracted romantically, physically, and for forming intimate relationships. Sexual orientation is often unrelated to gender identity. The material presented in this text is intended to help you feel comfortable with yourself, as well as with others who may have sexual orientations different from yours. In other words, acceptance and tolerance of sexual diversity are among the fundamental building blocks in your personal sexual philosophy.

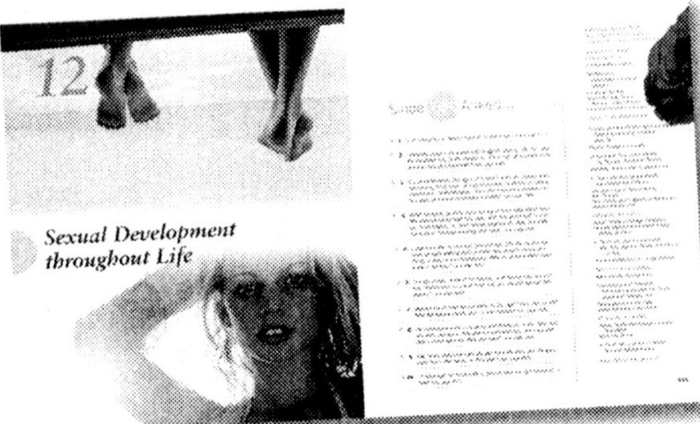

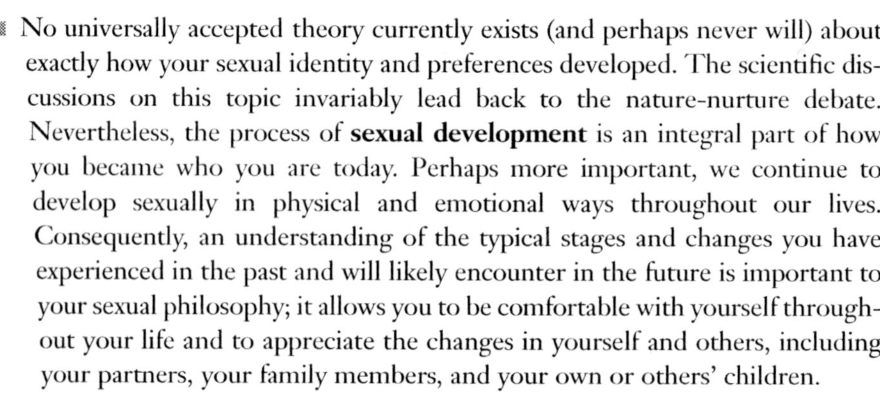

■ No universally accepted theory currently exists (and perhaps never will) about exactly how your sexual identity and preferences developed. The scientific discussions on this topic invariably lead back to the nature-nurture debate. Nevertheless, the process of **sexual development** is an integral part of how you became who you are today. Perhaps more important, we continue to develop sexually in physical and emotional ways throughout our lives. Consequently, an understanding of the typical stages and changes you have experienced in the past and will likely encounter in the future is important to your sexual philosophy; it allows you to be comfortable with yourself throughout your life and to appreciate the changes in yourself and others, including your partners, your family members, and your own or others' children.

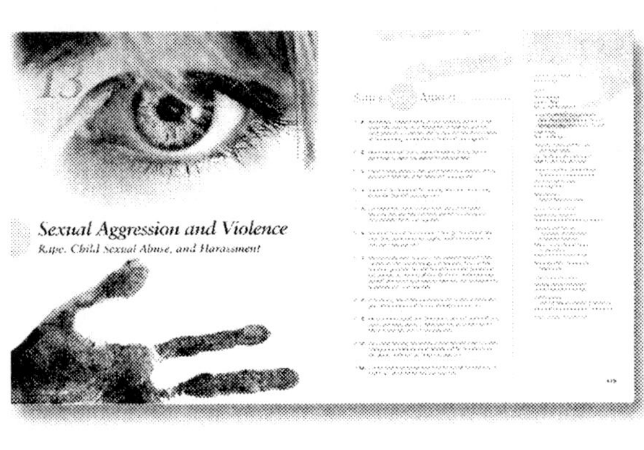

▪ Sexually-related behaviors such as **rape, childhood sexual abuse, and sexual harassment** represent the dark side of human sexuality. Unfortunately, these crimes are used as weapons to victimize, degrade, and harm others physically and emotionally. Although these actions may seem sexually motivated, for the perpetrators, they are typically less about sex and more about a twisted need to control, dominate, or humiliate their victims. The effects on the victims of rape, abuse, and harassment are psychologically (and sometimes physically) devastating and long-lasting. As unpleasant and uncomfortable as these topics may be, they are crucial to a comprehensive sexual philosophy for two primary reasons: one, to be able to recognize these acts and plan ahead helps minimize your personal risk of becoming a victim and to know what steps to take if you are; and two, to allow you to use your knowledge to help rid the world of these horrible crimes and offer assistance to victims whenever possible.

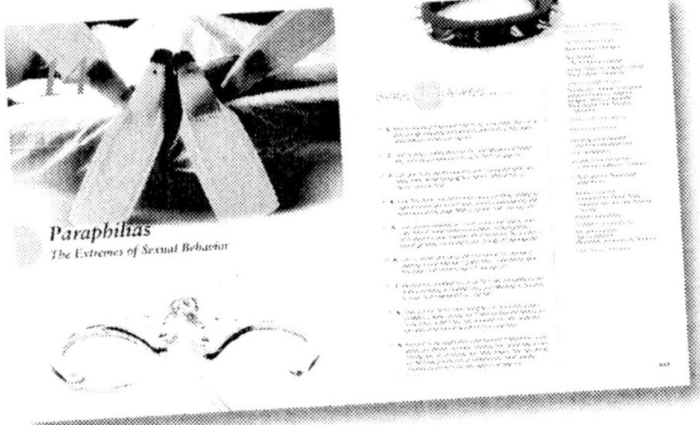

▪ Although most of this text is about what might be called mainstream sexual behaviors, a relatively small percentage of individuals or couples engage in sexual activities that most of you would consider somewhat (or very) strange or pathological (voyeurism, transvestism, pedophilia, or sadism, to name a few). These sexual activities are **paraphilias**, which roughly translates into "strange love." Paraphilias are included in this text because to recognize the full range of human sexual behaviors, you must go beyond the mainstream and explore the variations that exist on the fringes of what is considered socially acceptable by most members of a particular culture. Adding an awareness of paraphilias to your sexual philosophy may prove valuable one day if you or someone you care about is ever confronted with one of these behaviors.

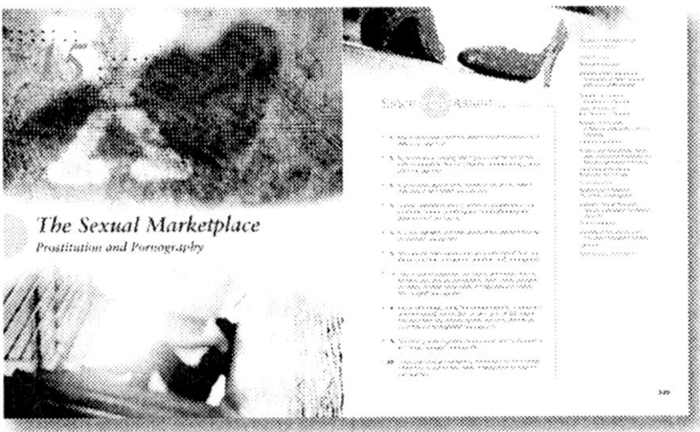

▪ You've heard the expression "sex sells." A slight variation on that theme is "sex sells sex." This text closes with a discussion of the businesses of **prostitution and pornography**. It's safe to say that many people, in most cultures, would prefer that these products and services didn't exist. However, they do exist; they always have and probably always will. How do you feel about them? After reading this text, you should have a better idea of how to answer that question. Why? Because your position on these topics is now part of your working sexual philosophy. And that's the point of this entire text—not just learning new and accurate information about sex, but putting all that information to good use and applying it in your life.

Glossary

Each entry is followed by the page number(s) on which discussion of the concept may be found.

abortion Termination of a pregnancy before week 37; in common usage, assumed to be the result of an intentional act as opposed to a miscarriage. (p. 343)

abstinence-only sex education Sexual education based on the assumption that adolescents will not engage in sexual activities until after marriage; may have the paradoxical effect of increasing teens' tendencies toward engaging in unhealthy sexual activities. (p. 460)

acceptable risk The level of risk one is willing to accept when making behavioral choices about one's health and well-being. (p. 314)

acquaintance rape Rape by an assailant the victim knows or is related to but is not dating. (p. 483)

acquired immune deficiency syndrome (AIDS) A gradual failure of the immune system, leading to serious infections and death. (p. 292)

adolescence The period of life between the ages of approximately 12 and 19 years, often a tumultuous, self-identity seeking stage of life. (p. 450)

afterglow The emotional and physical feeling of satisfaction, relaxation, and intimacy that follows the act of making love. (p. 82)

agape love A style of love focused on giving the partner whatever he or she may want or need without the expectation of receiving anything in return. (p. 109)

AIDS stigma Prejudice and discrimination against nonheterosexual individuals based on the erroneous belief that gay individuals are solely to blame for the AIDS epidemic and are the primary threat to the continuing spread of the disease. (p. 428)

alcohol myopia theory The belief that under the influence of alcohol, people are more likely to focus on immediate,"feel-good" behaviors (such as sexual arousal) and ignore future negative consequences. (p. 277)

amenorrhea Cessation of a woman's period. (p. 167)

anal intercourse A sexual position in which the penis is inserted through the partner's anus into the rectum. (p. 222)

androgynous Exhibiting both masculine and feminine traits. (p. 398)

anecdotal evidence Research information gathered through informal stories of people's experiences, which cannot be relied on to draw scientific conclusions. (p. 25)

anilingus Oral stimulation of the anus. (p. 222)

anonymous testing Tests administered without collecting any personal information about clients, who are identified only by an assigned code number. (p. 299)

antibiotic-resistant strain A strain of bacteria that has mutated and is no longer treatable with the current antibiotic therapy. (p. 311)

antiherpetics Medications developed to treat (reduce or prevent but not cure) outbreaks of the herpes virus. (p. 286)

anus The end of the digestive tract and outlet for bodily excretions. It is also a sexually stimulating area for some people. (p. 47)

APGAR score A test that analyzes infant health at birth on the basis of skin color, pulse, reflexes, movement, and breathing. (p. 352)

areola The darker skin encircling each nipple; actually part of the skin of the nipple. (p. 58)

assisted reproductive technology (ART) Various treatments to help infertile women or couples to become pregnant and have a child. (p. 364)

asymptomatic Having no noticeable symptoms despite the presence of an infectious agent. (p. 275)

asymptomatic shedding Release of infectious virus particles when no symptoms of infection are present. (p. 286)

autoerotic asphyxia Depriving the brain of oxygen, usually through some form of strangulation or hanging, during masturbation (also sometimes referred to as *sexual hypoxia* and *hypoxyphilia*) (p. 541)

aversion therapy Psychotherapy in which unwanted sexual behaviors and images are reduced by associating them with an unpleasant stimulus such as electric shocks or noxious odors. (p. 543)

barrier method Any contraceptive method that protects against pregnancy by preventing live sperm from entering the woman's reproductive tract and fertilizing the egg. (p. 170)

basal body temperature A fertility awareness method based on the woman's internal body temperature upon awakening in the morning. (p. 176)

BDSM Sexual activities that combine bondage, discipline, and sadomasochism. (p. 533)

birth defect A physical abnormality or metabolic dysfunction that is present at birth and may result in physical or mental deficits. (p. 341)

birthing center A hospital-like facility with basic medical care equipment, focusing on a natural, family-centered approach to the birth process in a homelike setting. (p. 354)

bisexual A person who is attracted romantically and sexually to members of both sexes. (p. 407)

blastocyst The developing zygote, with cells surrounding a fluid-filled core, upon entering the uterus and before implanting in the uterine wall. (p. 334)

bondage Being bound, tied up, or otherwise restrained during sexual activity; typically a consensual activity. (p. 536)

breech birth Delivery of a fetus emerging with buttocks or legs first rather than head first. (p. 351)

brothel worker A prostitute who works in a house of prostitution—such as a brothel, bordello, or massage parlor—and receives paying customers. (p. 555)

calendar method A minimally reliable method of ovulation prediction that requires a woman to keep a record of her menstrual cycle; her "window of fertility" is assumed to be from seven days before ovulation in her shortest recorded cycle to three days after ovulation in her longest recorded cycle; also referred to as the rhythm method. (p. 174)

call girl A prostitute who is contacted in private by clients when her services are desired and who generally charges more and provides a wider range of services than streetwalkers, such as serving as an escort or offering overnight stays. (p. 555)

case study An in-depth study and analysis of one person or group who demonstrates specific characteristics of interest to a researcher. (p. 23)

celibacy Abstinence from all sexual activities. (pp. 153, 318)

cervical cap A device similar to the diaphragm that fits more snugly over the cervix. (p. 171)

cervical mucus method A fertility awareness method of ovulation prediction that requires careful tracking of changes in the pattern of mucus that is secreted from the cervix into the vagina. (p. 175)

cervix The lower end of the uterus that connects it to the vagina. (p. 62)

cesarean section Removal of a fetus from the mother's uterus surgically, through an incision in her abdomen; also called a *C-section birth*. (p. 356)

chancre A sore that typically appears at the site of infection with syphilis. (p. 308)

chancroid A sexually transmitted bacterial infection causing one or more painful soft chancre sores in the genital or anal area. (p. 309)

chemical castration Blocking the production of testosterone in repeat sex offenders through the regular injection of female hormones. (p. 506)

child molestation Any sexual act performed with a child by an adult or a much older child. (p. 499)

child sexual abuse (CSA) The sexual victimization of a child by an adult or a significantly older child. (p. 498)

chlamydia A sexually transmitted bacterium, often causing a thick, cloudy discharge from the vagina or penis; may be asymptomatic, especially in women. (p. 303)

circumcision Removal of the foreskin of the penis. (p. 41)

cirrhosis of the liver A potentially serious liver disease that may lead to liver cancer. (p. 288)

civil union Another term used for domestic partnership. (p. 413)

clitoral glans The outer end or tip of the clitoris. (p. 52)

clitoral hood Tissue that partially or fully covers the clitoral glans. (p. 52)

clitoris An erectile sexual structure consisting of the clitoral glans and two shafts (*crura*) that is primarily responsible for triggering orgasm in most women. (p. 52)

coercive paraphilias Sexual activities involving an unsuspecting, nonconsenting, or unwilling victim who is the target of the atypical, compulsive behavior. (p. 528)

cognitive-behavioral therapy A therapeutic approach designed to gradually eliminate specific thoughts and associated behaviors that may be contributing to sexual problems. (pp. 247, 543)

cohabitation Living together as if married without legally marrying. (p. 465)

coitus Penis-vagina intercourse. (p. 217)

combination pill An oral contraceptive containing a combination of estrogen and progestin. (p. 160)

commercial sex trades Prostitution and related sexual activities for commercial purposes. (p. 551)

companionate love Love based on true intimacy and commitment but lacking passion; the couple are companions more than lovers. (p. 112)

complaining Expressing an unmet need, something a person desires but is not receiving from a partner. (p. 120)

complete androgen insensitivity syndrome (CAIS) A hormonal condition that results in babies who are genetically male but possess completely normal-appearing female external genitals and internal testicles. (p. 377)

comprehensive sex education Sexual education programs for adolescents that provide information about abstinence and about preventing STIs and unwanted pregnancy. (p. 460)

compulsive behavior Any behavior, sexual or otherwise, that a person is unable to control regardless of repeated attempts to do so. (p. 519)

confidential testing Medical test results that are kept confidential by the testing agency and not shared with anyone other than the patient and certain state record-keeping offices. (p. 299)

consensual A behavior entered into voluntarily by all parties. (p. 522)

consummate love Love that encompasses intimacy, passion, and commitment simultaneously. (p. 112)

contempt Disrespect, disgust, or hate expressed when the positive feelings partners once had for each other have dissipated. (p. 120)

contraception Any process or means used to prevent the fertilization of the ovum by a sperm cell. (p. 144)

contraceptive patch A pad that delivers a precise dose of two hormones into a woman's body through the skin, preventing ovulation. (p. 167)

contraceptive ring A colorless, flexible, transparent silicone ring about 2 inches in diameter that is inserted into the vagina and releases a continuous low dose of estrogen- and progestin-like hormones into the bloodstream. (p. 169)

contraceptive sponge A porous contraceptive device that releases spermicide when inserted into the vagina. (p. 172)

control group The participants in an experiment who receive no treatment and are allowed to behave as usual, for the purposes of comparison to an experimental group; also known as the *comparison group*. (p. 29)

corona The raised edge at the base of the penile glans. (p. 40)

corpora cavernosa Two parallel chambers that run the length of the penis and become engorged with blood during erection. (p. 41)

corpus spongiosum A middle chamber running the length of the penis into the glans that engorges with blood during erection. (p. 41)

correlational research A scientific research methodology that determines the extent to which two variables are systematically related to each other (how they "co-relate") (p. 27)

covert sensitization A type of aversion therapy in which instead of actual shocks or bad odors, the client repeatedly fantasizes the unwanted behavior and then adds an extremely aversive event to the fantasy. (p. 543)

Cowper's glands Small glands near the penile urethra that produce a slippery mucuslike substance during male sexual arousal (also referred to as the *bulbourethral glands*) (p. 50)

crack A powerful, processed form of cocaine that is smoked or sometimes injected, known for its intense but relatively short high and its highly addictive qualities. (p. 559)

criticism Verbal fault-finding, such as commenting on a character flaw in the partner. (p. 120)

cross-dressing Dressing in clothes traditionally associated with the opposite sex. (p. 539)

cultural gender stereotypes Beliefs about gender roles held by a majority of people in a given cultural setting. (p. 391)

cunnilingus Oral sex performed on a female. (p. 213)

cycle of violence The repetitive pattern of stages that define most abusive and violent relationships, cycling through the honeymoon stage, the tension-building phase, and the explosion of violence, followed by a return to the honeymoon stage, and the beginning of a new cycle. (p. 135)

date rape A rape that occurs in the context of a planned or spontaneous date. (p. 483)

date rape drugs Powerful sedatives that render a rapist's potential victim unconscious or otherwise unable to resist; also known as *club drugs*. (p. 489)

debriefing Explanations of the purpose and potential contributions of the findings given to participants at the end of a study. (p. 32)

decriminalization of prostitution Repeal of all laws against consensual adult sexual activity in both commercial and noncommercial contexts. (p. 566)

delusional jealousy Jealousy felt despite the fact that no threat to the relationship actually exists. (p. 130)

dependent variable The result of an experiment, evaluated to determine if the independent variable actually caused a change in the experimental group of participants. (p. 29)

diaphragm A flexible ring of latex or silicone inserted into the vagina that impedes conception by preventing sperm from getting past the cervix. (p. 170)

dilation and evacuation (D&E) A method of abortion commonly used when a pregnancy has progressed beyond the first trimester, involving scraping of the uterine walls and suctioning out of the contents. (p. 345)

directed masturbation A sex therapy strategy in which the therapist advises the client on how to use masturbation activities to help overcome a sexual problem. (p. 243)

domestic partnership A legal contract between two members of the same sex that imparts all or most of the legal benefits of marriage but is not socially or religiously equated with heterosexual marriage. (p. 413)

douching Washing the internal vagina with a stream of water or any other liquid solution (not usually medically recommended) (p. 148)

dyspareunia Painful sexual intercourse, usually experienced as pain in the vagina, the vaginal opening, or deeper in the abdominal cavity during or just after intercourse. (p. 264)

ectopic pregnancy A pregnancy complication in which a fertilized ovum attaches and begins to grow outside the uterus, most commonly in the fallopian tube, called a *tubal pregnancy*. (pp. 64, 338)

ejaculation Expulsion of semen through the penis. (p. 46)

ejaculatory duct A continuation of the tube that carries semen into the urethra for ejaculation. (p. 49)

ejaculatory inevitability In males, the sensation produced during the emission phase of ejaculation that expulsion of semen is imminent, reflexive, and cannot be stopped; often referred to as the "point of no return." (p. 82)

Electra complex A Freudian notion explaining how a young girl comes to identify with her mother. (p. 444)

embryo A blastocyst that has implanted in the uterine wall. (p. 334)

embryonic period The initial eight weeks of pregnancy following fertilization. (p. 335)

emergency contraceptive pills (ECPs) Hormonal pills concentrated enough to interrupt a woman's normal hormonal patterns and prevent pregnancy after unprotected intercourse has occurred. (pp. 169, 460)

emission In males, the buildup of sperm and semen in the urethral bulb just prior to being expelled through the urethra. (p. 82)

empty love Love based on commitment but lacking intimacy or real passion. (p. 112)

endometriosis A potentially painful and dangerous medical condition caused by endometrial cells migrating outside the uterus into the abdominal cavity. (p. 63)

endometrium The tissue lining the uterus that thickens in anticipation of pregnancy and is sloughed off and expelled during menstruation. (p. 63)

entry inhibitors A relatively new class of HIV medications that prevent the virus from entering immune system cells. (p. 300)

epididymis A crescent-shaped structure on each testicle where sperm cells are stored as they mature. (p. 46)

epididymitis A painful swelling and inflammation of the epididymis, the structure at the back of each testicle that stores maturing sperm; often caused by one or more untreated STIs. (p. 304)

episiotomy Surgical cutting of the perineum during childbirth, a procedure that was believed to allow for easier passage of the infant and less tearing of the vaginal opening. Found to be ineffective, it is rarely performed today. (p. 58)

EPOR model Masters and Johnson's approach to explaining the process of human sexual response, encompassing four arbitrarily divided phases: excitement, plateau, orgasm, and resolution. (p. 77)

erectile disorder (ED) Recurring or persistent difficulty in achieving or maintaining an erection. (p. 249)

erection Rigidity of the penis or clitoris resulting from an inflow of blood during sexual arousal. (p. 40)

eros love An erotic, passionate style of love often characterized by short-lived relationships. (p. 108)

Erotic Stimulus Pathway Theory A model of human sexual response based on the psychological and cognitive stages of seduction, sensations, surrender, and reflection. (p. 89)

erotic touch Intimate or sexual touching between partners, usually with the hands, for the purpose of sexual arousal and sharing sexual or sensual pleasure. (p. 208)

erotica Sexually explicit works expressing physical desire, passion, and attraction among people who freely choose to engage in sexual activities together. (p. 572)

erotophilia An attitude toward sexuality in which individuals are comfortable with sexual issues, seek out sexual information, enjoy sexual behavior, and respond with positive reactions to sexual topics. (p. 192)

erotophobia An attitude toward sexuality in which individuals are generally uncomfortable with sexual topics, respond negatively and uncomfortably to sexual issues, and tend to avoid sexual information and activities. (p. 192)

estrogen The female hormone responsible for regulating ovulation, endometrial development, and the development of female sexual characteristics. (p. 65)

excitement phase The first phase in the EPOR model, in which the first physical changes of sexual arousal occur. (p. 79)

exhibitionism Achieving sexual arousal and gratification by displaying one's genitals to others without their consent. (p. 529)

exotic becomes erotic (EBE) theory Psychologist Daryl Bem's explanation for the interaction of biology and environment in determining a person's sexual orientation. (p. 420)

experimental group The participants in an experiment who are subjected to a variable of research interest. (p. 29)

experimental method A type of scientific research in which variables of interest are changed while all other unrelated variables are held constant to determine cause-and-effect relationships among variables. (p. 29)

expulsion In males, the contraction of pelvic muscles that force semen through the urethra and out of the body through the penis. (p. 82)

fallopian tubes The tubes that carry the female ovum from the ovaries to the uterus and in which fertilization occurs. (p. 64)

fatuous love Love based on passion and commitment but lacking intimacy; a foolish, or pointless love. (p. 112)
fellatio Oral sex performed on a male. (p. 213)
female condom A tube or pouch of thin polyurethane with a flexible ring at each end. One end is sealed and the other is open. The condom is inserted into the vagina to protect against pregnancy and the transmission of STIs. (p. 158)
female genital mutilation (FGM) Removing part or most of the vulva to prevent sexual stimulation or pleasure; a cultural practice in many countries, especially in Africa. (p. 53)
female orgasmic disorder A sexual problem in which a woman rarely or never reaches orgasm or whose orgasms are delayed; also known as *inhibited female orgasm* or *anorgasmia*. (p. 257)
female sexual arousal disorder A woman's frequent or persistent inability to attain or maintain sexual arousal. (p. 249)
female-superior position A position for heterosexual intercourse in which the woman is sitting on or crouching over the male; this is the most common intercourse position throughout the world. (p. 218)
fertility awareness A method of contraception based on ovulation prediction and the viability of sperm; intercourse is timed to avoid fertile days or a barrier method is used during those days. (p. 173)
fetish A sexual preference for a nonhuman object or a body part that most members of a culture do not consider sexual. (p. 538)
fetus An embryo after eight weeks of pregnancy. (p. 335)
field of eligibles All the individuals who meet a person's criteria as a potential romantic partner. (p. 98)
flirting Subtle behaviors designed to signal sexual or romantic interest in another person. (p. 103)
follicle-stimulating hormone (FSH) A hormone that stimulates the development of a mature ovum. (p. 65)
follicular phase The early period during a woman's monthly fertility cycle when the pituitary gland secretes *follicle-stimulating hormone* to enhance ovum development. (p. 330)
foreskin A layer of skin covering the glans of the penis. (p. 40)
frenulum The band of tissue connecting the underside of the penile glans with the shaft of the penis. (p. 40)
frotteurism Rubbing one's genitals against a nonconsenting person for sexual arousal and, typically, orgasm. (p. 530)
gay Homosexual; often applied to both men and women. (p. 407)
gay bashing Criminal acts or violence, motivated by homophobia, committed against nonheterosexual individuals. (p. 435)
gender identification A developmental stage in children between the ages of 3 and 5 during which they begin to understand which sex they are. (p. 443)
gender The masculinity-femininity dimension of our basic nature as humans. (p. 372)
gender identity A person's view of himself or herself as a man or a woman. (pp. 6, 372, 540)
gender identity disorder A strong cross-gender identification characterized by the desire to be the other sex, combined with persistent discomfort about one's biological sex or culturally prescribed gender role. (p. 385)
gender roles The distinctive behaviors society expects and encourages its members to engage in, according to their sex. (p. 381)
gender stereotype An assumption about a person based solely on gender, without regard for his or her individuality as a person. (p. 388)
gender-conforming behavior Behavior that is consistent with traditional cultural expectations for a child's sex. (p. 421)
gender-nonconforming behavior Behavior that is inconsistent with traditional cultural expectations for a child's sex and considered more appropriate for children of the other sex. (p. 421)
genital herpes An STI caused by the herpes simplex virus (type 2) and characterized by painful sores and blisters, usually in the genital or anal area. (p. 284)
gigolo A male prostitute who is paid or otherwise compensated for providing sexual services to women. (p. 556)
gonadotropin A hormone released by the pituitary gland that signals the testes to release testosterone and the ovaries to release estrogen. (p. 452)
gonads Organs that produce cells (ova or sperm) for reproduction. (p. 46)
gonorrhea A sexually transmitted bacterium typically producing pain upon urination and a thick cloudy discharge from the penis or vagina; often asymptomatic, especially in women. (p. 305)
G-spot An especially sensitive area inside the vagina that some but not all women have identified and credit with enhancing sexual arousal. (pp. 62, 86)
hate crime laws Laws prescribing more stringent penalties for crimes motivated by bias or prejudice. (p. 435)
hate crimes Violent crimes motivated by prejudice and discrimination, targeting specific groups of individuals. (p. 435)
hepatitis B virus (HBV) A virus that may be sexually transmitted and may lead to inflammation and impaired functioning of the liver. (p. 287)
heterocentric The assumption of a universal heterosexual orientation. (p. 407)
heterosexual A person who is attracted romantically and sexually primarily to persons of the opposite sex. (p. 407)
highly active antiretroviral therapy (HAART) A combination of several medications prescribed for people who are HIV-positive to delay the onset of AIDS. (p. 300)
home birth Delivery of an infant in a private home setting, usually with necessary equipment and personnel provided by a professional service. (p. 355)
homophobia Extreme fear, discomfort, or hatred of nonheterosexual individuals. (p. 433)
homosexual A person who is attracted romantically and sexually primarily to persons of one's own sex. (p. 407)
hostile environment A distressing work or educational environment resulting from overt or covert sexually related activities or intrusions. (p. 508)
house prostitute A brothel worker. (p. 555)
human immunodeficiency virus (HIV) The virus that causes AIDS. (p. 292)
human papilloma virus (HPV) A sexually transmitted infection, some strains of which are believed to cause cervical cancer. (pp. 62, 289)
human sexuality An area of research and study focusing on all aspects of humans as sexual beings. (p. 4)
hustler A male prostitute who services male clients and employs professional tactics similar to those of female streetwalkers. (p. 556)
hymen A ring of tissue surrounding, partially covering, or fully screening the vaginal opening. (p. 56)

hymenorraphy A medical procedure, common in some cultures, to reconstruct or repair the hymen to allow a woman to appear "virginal"; also known as *hymenoplasty*. (p. 58)

hypoactive sexual desire A loss or lack of sexual desire; also known as *inhibited sexual desire*. (pp. 89, 245)

immune-based therapies Medications that are designed to help an infected person's immune system fight a virus, such as HIV, more effectively. (p. 300)

incest Molestation of a child by a blood relative such as a parent, aunt, uncle, grandparent, brother, or sister. (p. 499)

incidence The number of new cases of a disease in a given population over a specific time period. (p. 295)

incorporation therapy A treatment for paraphilias in which the paraphilic behavior is decreased or modified to acceptable levels but not completely abolished. (p. 542)

incubation period The time between infection and the appearance of physical symptoms of illness. (p. 288)

independent variable The variable of interest in an experiment that is allowed to change between or among groups while all other variables are held constant. (p. 29)

infatuation Love based on passion but lacking intimacy and commitment; usually very sexually charged but shallow and devoid of much meaning. (p. 111)

infertility A failure to conceive for 12 consecutive months despite persistent attempts. (p. 360)

informed consent Agreeing to participate in an experiment only after having been provided with complete and accurate information about what to expect in the study. (p. 32)

intersex Born with sexual anatomy that is neither completely male nor completely female but rather a combination with features of both. (p. 377)

intrauterine device (IUD) A small plastic device in the shape of a T that is inserted by a doctor into the uterus through the cervix via the vagina. It then remains in place one to ten years, during which time pregnancy is effectively prevented. (p. 177)

jaundice A symptom of hepatitis characterized by a deep yellowing of the skin and eyes. (p. 287)

Kaplan's Three-Stage Model An alternative to Masters and Johnson's EPOR model of human sexual response developed by Helen Singer Kaplan that features the three stages of desire, excitement, and orgasm. (p. 88)

Klinefelter syndrome A male genetic condition characterized by a rounded body type, lack of facial hair, breast enlargement in puberty, and smaller than normal testicles. (p. 376)

labia majora Folds of skin and fatty tissue that extend from the mons down both sides of the vulva, past the vaginal opening to the perineum. (p. 51)

labia minora The smooth, hairless, inner lips of the vulva. (p. 52)

laparoscopy A procedure whereby a viewing scope and surgical instruments are inserted through two very small incisions in the woman's abdomen in order to perform or reverse a tubal ligation. (pp. 179, 364)

Lea's Shield A relatively new vaginal barrier used much like a traditional diaphragm that does not require a prescription and does not need to be fitted by a health professional. (p. 172)

legalization of prostitution Regulation of prostitution by state laws, with statutes defining where, when, and how prostitution may take place. (p. 566)

lesbian A female with a homosexual orientation. (p. 407)

ludus love A style of love that focuses on the excitement of forming a relationship more than the relationship itself and typically moves rapidly from one relationship to another. (p. 108)

luteal phase The later period of a woman's monthly fertility when the lining of the uterus thickens in preparation for receiving a fertilized ovum if conception has occurred. (p. 331)

luteinizing hormone (LH) A hormone that acts in concert with follicle-stimulating hormone to stimulate ovulation and the release of estrogen and progesterone. (p. 65)

male condom A thin sheath of latex (rubber), polyurethane (plastic), or animal tissue that is placed over an erect penis prior to intercourse. (p. 154)

male escort A man hired by women as a companion, not necessarily for sexual purposes. (p. 556)

male orgasmic disorder A frequent or recurring delay or inhibition of orgasm and ejaculation; a relatively rare disorder. (p. 257)

mammogram Low dose X-ray of the breast to detect tumors. (p. 109)

mania love A possessive, dependent, and often controlling style of love. (p. 109)

masturbation Any sexual activity performed on oneself by oneself, typically focusing on manipulation of the genitals to orgasm. (p. 202)

matching hypothesis The theory that people tend to seek romantic and sexual partners who possess a level of physical attractiveness similar to their own. (p. 101)

medical abortion A method of abortion using drugs rather than surgery to terminate a pregnancy. (p. 346)

menarche In girls, the onset of the menstrual cycle in puberty. (pp. 65, 452)

menopause The time in a woman's life when menstruation and the reproductive cycle cease to occur. (p. 69)

menstrual cycle The hormone-controlled reproductive cycle in the human female. (p. 65)

mere exposure effect The psychological principle that humans appear to have a natural and usually unconscious tendency to grow fonder of a "novel stimulus" the more often they are exposed to it. (p. 102)

midwife A person (usually a woman) who has been trained in most aspects of pregnancy, labor, and delivery but who is not a physician or registered nurse. (p. 354)

midwifery The practice of assisting women through normal pregnancy and childbirth. (p. 325)

minipill An oral contraceptive containing progestin only. (p. 160)

miscarriage The loss, (without any purposeful intervention) of an embryo or fetus during the first 20 weeks of pregnancy; also called *spontaneous abortion*. (p. 338)

mons veneris A slightly raised layer of fatty tissue on the top of a woman's pubic bone, usually covered with hair in the adult. (p. 51)

multiple orgasms More than one orgasm at relatively short intervals as sexual stimulation continues without a resolution phase or refractory period in between orgasms. (p. 85)

mutual masturbation Partners' touching of each other's genitals, often to orgasm and enjoyed as a sexually intimate and satisfying activity. (p. 212)

neonate A newborn infant. (p. 352)

New view of women's sexual problems A model of female sexual response incorporating a larger variety of factors than previous models, including physical, cognitive, social, and relationships issues. (p. 90)
nocturnal penile tumescence (NPT) Erection of the penis while a man is asleep. (p. 253)
nongonococcal urethritis (NGU) A sexually transmitted bacterial infection of the urethra characterized by urethral inflammation and discharge, but not caused by the gonorrhea bacterium. (p. 307)
normal jealousy Jealousy based on a real threat to the relationship, as when one partner discovers that the other has been sexually unfaithful. (p. 130)
nurse-midwife A registered nurse who has completed an accredited midwifery program and has been certified by the state to deliver babies. (p. 354)
OB/GYN Short for obstetrician-gynecologist, a physician specializing in women's health care and childbirth. (p. 354)
obscenity Sexually explicit works that meet specific legal criteria that may be censored and declared illegal. (p. 569)
observational research Gathering behavioral data through direct or indirect observation using scientific techniques. (p. 25)
Oedipus complex A Freudian notion explaining how a young boy comes to identify with his father. (p. 443)
opportunistic infections Diseases that establish themselves in the human body when the immune system is weakened and incapable of fighting them off. (p. 294)
oral contraceptives Tablets containing female hormones that are ingested every day. They constitute the most popular reversible birth control method used by women in the United States; also known as birth control pills. (p. 160)
orgasm The peak of sexual arousal. (p. 50)
orgasmic phase The third stage in the EPOR model, during which sexual excitement and pleasure reach a climax. (p. 81)
orgasmic reconditioning A type of therapy for paraphilias in which a person is conditioned to become aroused and have orgasms in socially acceptable settings that bear no resemblance to the paraphilia. (p. 543)
os The very narrow passageway through the cervix from the vagina to the uterus. (p. 62)
outercourse A form of abstinence in which a couple chooses to engage only in sexual behaviors that are unlikely to result in pregnancy or infection and to avoid all others, such as vaginal or anal intercourse and oral sex. (p. 153)
ovaries The female organs that produce sex hormones such as estrogen and progesterone and where follicle cells are stored and mature into ova. (p. 64)
ovulation The release of an egg, or ovum, from the ovary into the fallopian tube. (p. 65)
ovum The female reproductive cell stored in the ovaries; usually, one ovum is released approximately every 28 days between menarche and menopause. The plural is *ova*. (p. 64)
pandemic A widespread epidemic. (p. 292)
Pap test A routine test in which cells from the cervix are examined microscopically to examine them for potentially cancerous abnormalities. (p. 62)
paraphilias Compulsive sexual activities that are practiced by a small percentage of people and that most members of a given culture would consider abnormal, deviant, or pathological. (p. 518)
partial androgen insensitivity syndrome (PAIS) A hormonal condition in which the fetus has a reduced reaction to androgens in the uterus, producing a baby with genitals that are not clearly male or female. (p. 377)
partner rape A rape that occurs in the context of an ongoing romantic and sexual relationship. (p. 483)
pedophile An adult, usually male, whose sexual focus is on children. (p. 534)
pedophilia Uncontrollable sexual compulsions involving children. (pp. 498, 534)
pelvic inflammatory disease (PID) A painful condition in women marked by inflammation of the uterus, fallopian tubes, and ovaries; typically caused by one or more untreated STIs. (p. 304)
penile glans The end or tip of the penis, its most sexually sensitive part. (p. 40)
penile plethysmograph An electronic device that records blood flow into the penis to detect sexual arousal. (p. 436)
penile shaft The area of the penis between the glans and the abdomen. (p. 40)
penis The primary male anatomical sexual structure. (p. 40)
perimenopausal changes The physical and psychological changes many women experience during the decade leading up to menopause. (p. 69)
perineum The area of skin in the female between the vulva and the anus and in the male between the scrotum and the anus. (p. 58)
personal gender stereotypes Beliefs about gender that are unique to each individual and may or may not agree with cultural stereotypes. (p. 391)
personal sexual philosophy A person's unique foundation of knowledge, attitudes, and actions relating to what the person wants and who he or she is as a sexual being. (p. 4)
pituitary gland A gland in the brain that at the onset of puberty releases hormones necessary for the physical changes of puberty. (p. 452)
placenta An organ that develops on the uterine wall during pregnancy joining the developing embryo to the mother's biological systems, transferring nourishment, oxygen and waste products between the fetus and the mother. (p. 335)
plateau phase The second phase in the EPOR model, during which sexual arousal levels off (reaches a plateau) and remains at an elevated level of excitement. (p. 79)
pornography In the legal terms, any sexually explicit work deemed obscene according to legal criteria and therefore exempt from freedom of speech protections. (p. 568)
postovulation method A fertility awareness method that has a couple limit unprotected intercourse in each cycle to a certain period of time after ovulation has occurred. (p. 176)
postpartum Literally, "following birth"; typically refers to the months or first year following the birth of a child. (p. 357)
postpartum depression (PPD) A psychological depressive disorder that begins within four weeks after childbirth. (p. 357)
postpartum psychosis A severe postpartum psychological disorder that may include delusions, hallucinations, and extreme mental disorganization. (p. 358)
pragma love A love style in which partners are selected in a businesslike way on the basis of rational, practical criteria. (p. 109)
pre-ejaculate The fluid produced by the Cowper's glands. (p. 50)
pregnancy The period of growth of the embryo and fetus in the uterus. (p. 334)

premature ejaculation (PE) A man's tendency to have an orgasm suddenly with little penile stimulation, typically just before, upon, or shortly after penetration of the penis into the vagina; also referred to as *rapid* or *early ejaculation*. (p. 257)
premenstrual dysphoric disorder (PMDD) A significantly more intense and debilitating form of PMS. (p. 69)
premenstrual syndrome (PMS) A set of symptoms that may occur during the days just before and during the start of a woman's period including irritability, depressed mood, and feelings of physical bloating or cramping. (p. 69)
preterm birth Birth of an infant less than 37 weeks after conception. (p. 339)
prevalence The total cumulative number of cases of a disease in a given population. (p. 295)
pro-choice The belief that a woman has the moral and legal right to choose freely to abort her pregnancy. (p. 344)
prodromal symptoms Warning signs, such as itching, burning, or pain, that an outbreak of an infection such as herpes may be impending. (p. 286)
progesterone The female hormone responsible for the release of ova and implantation of the fertilized egg in the uterine wall. (p. 65)
pro-life The belief that voluntary abortion is akin to murder, and that it should be illegal. (p. 344)
prostate gland A gland in males surrounding the urethra that produces the largest proportion of seminal fluid (ejaculate) (p. 49)
prostatitis An uncomfortable or painful inflammation of the prostate gland, usually caused by bacteria. (p. 49)
prostitution Providing or receiving sexual acts between a prostitute, a client, and sometimes the prostitute's employer ("pimp") in exchange for money or some other form of remuneration. (p. 552)
protected classes Specific groups of people protected under federal and state antidiscrimination laws, identified by race, religion, sex, age, or other characteristics. (p. 430)
proximity effect The theory that the closer we are to another person in geographical distance, the greater the probability that we will grow to like or even love the person. (p. 101)
prurient interest An excessive focus on exclusively sexual matters. (p. 570)
psychological defense mechanism Originally suggested by Freud, a psychological distortion of reality serving to defend against personally unacceptable thoughts or urges. (p. 436)
psychosexual stages Freud's theory that the development of human personality occurs in a series of stages during childhood. (p. 443)
pubic lice Small buglike parasites, usually sexually transmitted, that infest the genital area causing extreme itching; often referred to as "crabs," because of their resemblance to a sea crab. (p. 312)
quickening The first movement of the fetus that is felt by the mother. (p. 335)
quid pro quo Something given in exchange for a benefit or reward; with reference to sexual harassment, a situation in which a person in a position of power over another requires sexual favors in exchange of some beneficial outcome for the victim. (p. 508)
random sampling A method of selecting a sample of participants in such a way that each member of the population has an equal chance of being selected. (p. 19)
rape Nonconsensual sexual penetration of the body using physical force or the threat of bodily harm. (p. 483)
rape trauma syndrome A two-stage set of symptoms that follow the trauma of being raped, consisting of physical, emotional, and behavioral stress reactions. (p. 494)
reaction formation A type of defense mechanism in which a person engages in exaggerated behaviors in the *opposite* direction of internal urges felt to be unacceptable or intolerable. (p. 436)
rear-entry position A position for heterosexual intercourse in which the penis is inserted into the vagina while the man is behind the woman. (p. 219)
reciprocity of attraction The idea that someone you like or love likes or loves you back—reciprocates your feelings—with approximately the same degree of intensity. (p. 106)
refractory period A period of time following orgasm when a person is physically unable to become aroused to additional orgasms. (p. 85)
reliability The ability of any measuring instrument, such as a questionnaire or personality scale, to provide consistent responses over repeated administrations. (p. 17)
researcher expectancy effects The influence of the researchers' personal biases on participants' responses and consequently on the study's findings. (p. 24)
resolution phase The fourth and last stage in the EPOR model, during which sexual structures return to their unaroused state; also referred to as *detumescence*. (p. 84)
respondents Individuals selected to respond to a researcher's request for information. (p. 17)
retrovirus A type of virus, such as HIV, that survives by invading and destroying the DNA of normal body cells and then replicating its own DNA into the host cell's chromosomes. (p. 294)
romantic love Love based on intimacy and passion but lacking commitment. (p. 112)
sadomasochism Sexual activities that combine sadism and masochism. (p. 533)
safe sex fatigue A loss of tolerance for the necessity of always practicing safer sex behaviors. (p. 295)
sample A subset of the target population selected by researchers to represent the entire population under study. (p. 19)
scabies Microscopic parasitic mites, often sexually transmitted, that burrow under the skin on the hands, feet, and genitals and cause extreme itching. (p. 313)
scrotum The sac of thin skin and muscle containing the testicles in the male. (p. 45)
secondary sexual characteristics Physical changes not biologically related to reproduction that occur during puberty. (p. 452)
selective abstinence Choosing to engage in or avoid certain sexual behaviors on the basis of their risks of STIs or pregnancy. (p. 318)
self-disclosure Revealing personal, private, and intimate thoughts, feelings, and information to another person. (p. 116)
self-selection bias The effect of allowing members of a target population under study to volunteer to participate in the study; it may compromise the randomness and validity of the research. (p. 22)
semen The fluid produced primarily by the prostate gland and seminal vesicles that is ejaculated with the sperm cells by men during orgasm. (p. 48)

seminal vesicle A structure that produces fluid that becomes part of the semen that is expelled during ejaculation. (p. 49)

seminiferous tubules Tightly wound microscopic tubes that comprise the testicles in the male, where sperm cells are generated. (pp. 46, 332)

sensate focus A sex therapy technique that requires a couple to redirect emphasis away from intercourse and focus on their capacity for mutual *sensuality*. (p. 241)

sex flush A darkening or reddening of the skin of the chest area that occurs in some people during sexual arousal. (p. 79)

sex reassignment surgery Surgical procedures used to transform an individual from one sex to the other, commonly known as a "sex-change operation." (p. 385)

sexual abstinence Avoiding sexual behaviors that involve any risk of pregnancy or the spread of STIs. (p. 153)

sexual harassment A pattern of unwelcome sexual advances, requests for sexual favors, or other verbal and physical conduct that is coercive or create a hostile work or educational environment. (p. 508)

sexual health Overall physical and psychological health relating to sexuality. (p. 14)

sexual masochism Sexual arousal and gratification that is associated with acts or fantasies of being hurt, humiliated, or otherwise made to suffer. (p. 536)

sexual orientation A person's primary sexual, social, romantic, and emotional attraction with respect to gender. (pp. 6, 387, 407)

sexual sadism Inflicting pain, injury, or humiliation on another person for the sexual gratification of the person performing the action. (p. 530)

sexual self-disclosure Revealing private sexual thoughts and feelings to another person. (p. 125)

sexually transmitted infections (STIs) A group of viral, bacterial, and other infections that are spread primarily by sexual behaviors. (p. 272)

Skene's glands In the female, a pair of glands on either side of the urethra that in some women may produce a fluid that is expelled during orgasm; also known as the *paraurethral glands*. (p. 87)

social alienation A passive form of aggression that includes behaviors such as malicious gossip, spreading negative rumors, and shunning. (p. 392)

social desirability bias The tendency of individuals to answer survey questions in socially desirable and culturally approved ways. (p. 22)

sodomy laws Laws prohibiting specific sexual activities between adults, even in private and with their consent. (p. 431)

spectatoring Mentally observing and judging oneself during sexual activities with a partner; may cause sexual problems. (p. 250)

spermatic cords Supporting each testicle and encasing each vas deferens, nerves, and muscles. (p. 45)

spermicide Any substance containing a chemical (most commonly nonoxinol-9) that kills sperm cells, thereby preventing them from fertilizing an egg. (p. 170)

SSRIs Selective serotonin reuptake inhibitors, drugs administered to treat depression that may cause various sexual side effects, especially inhibited or delayed arousal or orgasm. (p. 235)

stage one labor The first stage of the birth process, involving the beginning of contractions of the uterus. (p. 350)

stage three labor The final stage of the birth process, when the placenta is expelled from the uterus with the umbilical cord attached. (p. 353)

stage two labor The stage of the birth process in which contractions occur closer together than in stage one, involve the muscles of the abdomen as well as the uterus, and continue until the infant has been expelled from the mother's body. (p. 351)

sterilization Any surgical alteration that prevents the emission of sperm or eggs; also referred to as *voluntary surgical contraception*. (p. 179)

stonewalling Relying on a passive form of power and aggression by being unresponsive (erecting a metaphorical "stone wall") when disagreements and disputes erupt. (p. 121)

storge love A love style characterized by caring and friendship. (p. 108)

straight Heterosexual. (p. 407)

stranger rape Rape by an assailant who is not known to the victim. (p. 483)

streetwalker A prostitute who sells her services on the street, typically to customers who are driving by, soliciting sexual acts. (p. 555)

styles of love Lee's theory that people follow individual psychological motifs or styles in relating to a love partner. (p. 106)

survey The scientific collection of data from a group of individuals about their beliefs, attitudes, or behaviors. (p. 17)

symptothermal method A fertility awareness method of predicting ovulation by combining various predictors, including the calendar, basal body temperature, and cervical mucus methods. (p. 176)

syphilis A sexually transmitted bacterium characterized by a sore, or chancre, at the point of infection; untreated, it may progress to more serious stages and even death. (p. 307)

target population The entire group of people to which a researcher is attempting to apply a study sample's findings. (p. 19)

tenting A widening of the inner two-thirds of the vagina during sexual arousal. (p. 81)

teratogen Any agent that has the potential to cause a fetal abnormality. (p. 342)

testicles Oval structures approximately 1.0 to 1.5 inches in length made up of microscopic tubes in which sperm cells and testosterone are produced in the male. (p. 46)

testosterone The male sex hormone responsible for male sexual characteristics and the production of sperm cells. (p. 46)

three-dimensional model of sexual problems A method of classifying or diagnosing sexual problems according to their duration, context, and frequency. (p. 232)

transgender persons Individuals who self-identify as the opposite gender from their biological sex; not considered a paraphilia. (p. 540)

transgendered Individuals whose gender identity is in conflict with their biological sex. (p. 384)

transsexual A transgender person who makes an effort to transition from his or her biological sex to his or her self-identified gender through dress, hormone therapy, or surgery. (pp. 385, 540)

transvestic fetishism The paraphilia engaged in by a transvestite. (p. 540)

transvestite A man who obtains sexual satisfaction by wearing female clothing. (p. 539)

treatment The action performed on or by a group in an experiment. (p. 29)

triangular theory of love Sternberg's theory that three fundamental components of love—intimacy, passion, and commitment—in various combinations, define the qualities of a relationship. (p. 111)

trichomoniasis A common sexually transmitted protozoan parasite causing symptoms in women, including genital irritation, painful urination, and a foul-smelling vaginal discharge; infected men are typically asymptomatic, yet contagious. (p. 312)

trimester One of three periods of about three months each that make up the phases of a full-term pregnancy. (p. 335)
tubal ligation Preventing eggs from passing through the fallopian tubes by tying, cutting, clipping, or otherwise blocking the tubes; also referred to as *tubectomy*. (p. 179)
Turner syndrome A female genetic condition characterized by short stature, slow or no sexual development at puberty, heart abnormalities, and lack of ovarian function. (p. 376)
two-dimensional model of gender An approach to defining gender suggesting that gender is not an either-or proposition but that people may manifest elements of both genders simultaneously. (p. 398)
umbilical cord A structure of approximately 22 inches in length, consisting of one large vein and two arteries, that transport nutrients, oxygen, and fetal waste products back and forth between the fetus and the placenta. (p. 335)
urethra The tube extending from the bladder to the urethral opening, which carries out of the body urine in women and men and semen as well in men. (p. 41)
urethral bulb The prostatic section of the urethra that expands with collected semen just prior to expulsion, creating the sensation of ejaculatory inevitability. (p. 50)
urethral opening An opening in the mid section of the vulva, between the clitoral glans and the vagina, that allows urine to pass from the body. (p. 53)
urethritis A painful inflammation of the urethra; often caused by one or more untreated STIs. (p. 304)
urinary tract infection An infection of the urethra, bladder, or other urinary structure, usually caused by bacteria. (p. 53)
uterus A very flexible organ with strong muscle fibers where a fertilized egg implants and an embryo and fetus grow from a few days after fertilization until birth. (p. 63)
vacuum aspiration A method of abortion in which a small tube is inserted through the cervix to extract the contents of the uterus, including the endometrium lining and embedded embryo. (p. 345)
vagina A flexible, muscular canal or tube, normally about 3 to 4 inches in length, that extends into the woman's body at an angle toward the small of the back, from the vulva to the cervix. (p. 61)
vaginismus Pain in a woman just prior to intercourse, due to involuntary contractions and spasms of the muscles controlling the opening to and outer third of the vagina. (p. 265)
validity The extent to which a measuring instrument is a true assessment of the characteristic it is intended to measure. (p. 18)
vas deferens A tube extending from the testicle (epididymis) into the male's body for the transport of mature sperm cells during ejaculation. (p. 46)
vasectomy Cutting and tying off or cauterizing (sealing) the vasa deferentia so that sperm produced by the testicles can no longer mix with semen in the ejaculate. (p. 179)
vasocongestion The swelling of erectile tissues due to increased blood flow during sexual arousal. (p. 79)
victimless Harming no one with the possible exception of the person performing the action. (p. 522)
viral shedding The release of virus particles that can potentially spread the infection to others. (p. 286)
voyeurism Secretly watching others undress or engage in sexual activities without their knowledge or consent for the purpose of achieving sexual arousal. (p. 528)
vulva The female external genitals. (p. 51)
withdrawal method Removing the penis from the vagina just prior to ejaculation—an unreliable method of contraception; also called *coitus interruptus* and "pulling out." (p. 148)
zygote A fertilized ovum (or egg) moving down the fallopian tube. (p. 334)

References

Abbey, A. (2002). Alcohol-related sexual assault: A common problem among college students. *Journal of Studies on Alcohol, 63*, S118–S128.

Abbey, A., McAuslan, P., & Ross, L. (1998). Sexual assault perpetration by college men: The role of alcohol, misrepresentation of sexual intent, and sexual beliefs and experiences. *Journal of Social and Clinical Psychology, 17*, 167–195.

Abbey, A., Saenz, C., & Buck, P. (2005). The cumulative effects of acute alcohol consumption and individual differences and situational perceptions on sexual decision making. *Journal of Studies on Alcohol, 66*, 82–90.

Abbey, A., Zawacki, T., Buck, P., Clinton, A., & McAuslan, P. (2001). Alcohol and sexual assault. *Alcohol Research and Health, 25*, 43–51.

Abouesh, A., & Clayton, A. (1999). Compulsive voyeurism and exhibitionism: A clinical response to paroxetine. *Archives of Sexual Behavior, 28*, 23–30.

About Lea's shield. (2004). Retrieved September 14, 2005, from **http://www.leasshield.com/about.htm**

Abramovitz, M. (2001, March). The knockout punch of date rape drugs. *Current Health*, pp. 18–21.

Abusharaf, R. (1998). Unmasking tradition: A Sudanese anthropologist confronts female "circumcision" and its terrible tenacity. *Sciences, 38*, 22–28.

Adams, H., Wright, L., & Lohr, B. (1996). Is homophobia associated with homosexual arousal? *Journal of Abnormal Psychology, 105*, 440–446.

Adler, A., David, H., Major, B., Roth, S., Russo, N., & Wyatt, G. (1990, April). Psychological responses after abortion. *Science*, pp. 41–44.

Adler., L. (2005). The future of sodomy. *Fordham Urban Law Journal, 32*, 197–229.

Administration on Aging. (2001). Summary table of age characteristics of the older population for the United States and for states, 2000. Retrieved July 14, 2003, from **http://www.aoa.gov/Census2000/stateprofiles/ageprofile-states.html**

Advanced Fertility Center of Chicago. (2004). Ectopic pregnancy. Retrieved May 4, 2004, from **http://www.advancedfertility.com/ectopic.htm**

Advocate. (2002, August 20). The *Advocate* Sex Poll: The 1800+ gays, lesbians, and bisexuals who took our online sex survey revealed both their passions and their weaknesses. *Advocate*, pp. 38–41.

Afriat, C., & Coustan, D. (1995). Birth. In D. Coustan, R. Haning, & D. Singer (Eds.), *Human reproduction: Growth and development* (pp. 307–326). Boston: Little, Brown.

Aggarwal, M., & Rein, J. (2003). Acute human immunodeficiency virus syndrome in an adolescent. *Pediatrics, 112*, 969.

Alan Guttmacher Institute. (2005). Induced abortion in the United States. Retrieved October 15, 2005, from **http://www.agi-usa.org/pubs/fb_induced_abortion.html**

Albaugh, J., & Kellogg-Spadt, S. (2002). Sensate focus and its role in treating sexual dysfunction. *Urologic Nursing, 22*, 402–403.

Albert, A. E., Warner, D. L., & Hatcher, R. A. (1998). Facilitating condom use with clients during commercial sex in Nevada's legal brothels. *American Journal of Public Health, 88*, 643–646.

Alfonso, V., Allison, D., & Dunn, G. (1992). Sexual fantasy and satisfaction: A multidimensional analysis of gender differences. *Journal of Psychology and Human Sexuality, 5*, 19–37.

Alien, H. H. (2001). Chancroid (sexually transmitted disease). *Contemporary OB/GYN, 46*, 126–127.

Allen, D. (2003, September 30). Sodomy laws still alive. *Advocate*, 15.

Allies Program. (2000). Sexual harassment and sexual assault. Retrieved August 30, 2002, from **http://www.udel.edu/ allies/resources/harass.html**

AllRefer.com. (2003a). Gonorrhea, male. Retrieved November 20, 2003, from **http://health.allrefer.com/health/gonorrhea-male.html**

AllRefer.com. (2003b). Pubic lice. Retrieved November 20, 2003, from **http://health.allrefer.com/health/pubic-lice-treatment.html**

Altman, C. (2000, February-March). Gay and lesbian seniors: Unique challenges of coming out in later life. *SEICUS Report*, pp. 14–17.

Altman, D., & Aggleman, P. (1999). *Men who sell sex: International perspectives on male prostitution and HIV/AIDS*. Philadelphia: Temple University Press.

Altman, I., & Taylor, D. (1973). *Social penetration: The development of interpersonal relationships*. New York: Holt, Rinehart and Winston.

American Academy of Pediatrics. (1999). Circumcision policy statement. *Pediatrics, 103*(3), 1–22.

American Association of University Women. (2002). A free resource for preventing sexual harassment in schools: The American Association of University Women (AAUW) Educational Foundation offers a new guide online. *Curriculum Review, 42*, 2–3.

American Cancer Society. (2004a). What are the key statistics for testicular cancer? Retrieved November 26, 2004, from **http://www.cancer.com**

American Cancer Society. (2004b). What are the risk factors for testicular cancer? Retrieved November 26, 2004, from **http://www.cancer.com**

American Civil Liberties Union. (1999, April 6). Overview of lesbian and gay parenting, adoption, and foster care. Retrieved June 13, 2002, from **http://www.aclu.org/issues/gay/parent.html**

American Civil Liberties Union. (2002). Lesbian and gay rights. Retrieved November 12, 2002, from **http://www.aclu.org/LesbianGayRights/LesbianGayRightsmain.cfm**

American Health Consultants. (2001). Organon launches NuvaRing, first combined contraceptive ring. Retrieved January 6, 2004, from **http://www.ahcpub.com/ahc_root_html/hot/archive/ctu122001.html**

American Psychiatric Association. (1994). *Diagnostic and statistical manual of mental disorders* (4th ed.) (DSM-IV). Washington, DC.

American Psychiatric Association. (2000). *Diagnostic and statistical manual of mental disorders* (4th ed., text revision) (DSM-IV-TR). Washington, DC.

American Psychological Association. (2004). Answers to your questions about sexual orientation and homosexuality. *PsychNet: APA Online*. Retrieved July 27, 2004, from **http://www.apa.org/pubinfo/answers.html#whatis**

American Society of Plastic Surgeons. (2002). Cosmetic and reconstructive patients: 2001 national plastic surgery statistics. Retrieved December 28, 2002, from **http://www.plasticsurgery.org/mediactr/2001_expanded_stats/national.pdf**

Amory, J., Anawalt, B., Paulson, A., & Bremmer, W. (2000). Klinefelter's syndrome. *Lancet, 356*, 333–335.

Anastasi, A., & Urbina, S. (1997). *Psychological testing* (7th ed.). New York: Macmillan.

Anderson, D. J. (2003). The impact on subsequent violence of returning to an abusive partner. *Journal of Comparative Family Studies, 34*, 93–125.

Anderson, M., Foster, C., McGuigan, M. R., Seebach, E., & Porcari, J. P. (2004). Training vs. body image: Does training improve subjective appearance ratings? *Journal of Strength and Conditioning Research, 18*, 255–259.

Anderson, R. A., & Walton, M. J. (2005) Contraceptive choices: is the future with men? Women's Health, 1, 183–189.

Angulo, J. M., & Espinoza, L. R. (1999). Gonococcal arthritis. *Comprehensive Therapy 25*, 155–162.

Annon, J. S. (1974). *The behavioral treatment of sexual problems*. Honolulu: Kapiolani Health Services.

Antibiotic for bacterial prostatitis. (2003). *Contemporary Urology, 15*, 81.

Apfelbaum, B. (2000). Retarded ejaculation: A much misunderstood syndrome. In S. Leiblum & R. Rosen (Eds.), *Principles and practice of sex therapy* (pp. 205–241). New York: Guilford Press.

Apostolides, M. (1999, September-October). The pleasure of pain: Why some people need S&M. *Psychology Today*, pp. 60–65.

Archer, D., & Ballagh, S. (2003). New research confirms efficacy of NuvaRing. *Time Contraceptive Technology Update, 24*, 68–69.

Arenofsky, J. (1996). In defense of DINKS. *Phoenix Magazine*. Retrieved March 3, 2002, from **http://www.members.aol.com/childfreeaz/a_in_defense.htm**

Arthur, J. (1997). Psychological aftereffects of abortion: The rest of the story. *Humanist, 57*, 7–9.

Aulette, J. (1994). *Changing families*. Belmont, CA: Wadsworth.

Australian Broadcasting Corp. (1998, October 22). *Body of knowledge* [Television broadcast]. Retrieved November 4, 2004, from **http://www.abc.net.au/quantum/scripts98/9825/clitoris.html**

Avert.com. (2004). Worldwide HIV/AIDS epidemic statistics. Retrieved December 27, 2004, from **http://www.avert.org/worlstatinfo.htm**

Axinn, W. G., & Barber, J. (1997) Living arrangements and family formation in early adulthood. *Journal of Marriage and the Family, 59*, 595–611.

Axinn, W. G., & Thornton, A. (1993). Mothers, children, and cohabitation: The intergenerational effects of attitudes and behavior. *American Sociological Review, 58*, 233–246.

Azam, S. (2000, August 15). What's behind retro virginity? *Toronto Star*. Retrieved December 27, 2002 from **http://www.psurg.com/star2000.html**

Baber, K., & Murray, C. (2001). A postmodern feminist approach to teaching human sexuality. *Family Relations, 50*, 23–33.

Baby Center. (2005). Evaluate your parenting readiness. Retrieved December 4, 2005, from **http://www.babycenter.com**

Bagarozzi, D. (1990). Marital power discrepancies and symptom development in spouses: An empirical investigation. *American Journal of Family Therapy, 18*, 51–65.

Bailey, J., & Benishay, D. (1993). Familial aggregation of female sexual orientation. *American Journal of Psychiatry, 150*, 272–277.

Bailey, J., & Pillard, R. (1991). A genetic study of male sexual orientation. *Archives of General Psychiatry, 48*, 1089–1096.

Baldwin, J., & Baldwin, J. (1997). Gender differences in sexual interest. *Archives of Sexual Behavior, 26*, 181–210.

Baldwin, J., & Baldwin, J. (2000). Heterosexual anal intercourse: An understudied high-risk behavior. *Archives of Sexual Behavior, 29*, 357–373.

Bancroft, J. (2002a). Biological factors in human sexuality. *Journal of Sex Research, 39*, 15–21.

Bancroft, J. (2002b). The medicalization of female sexual dysfunction: The need for caution. *Archives of Sexual Behavior, 31*, 451–455.

Bancroft, J., Loftus, J., & Long, S. (2003). Distress about sex: A national survey of women in heterosexual relationships. *Archives of Sexual Behavior, 32*, 193–208.

Barak, A., Fisher, W. A., Belfry, S., & Lashambe, D. (1999). Sex, guys, and cyberspace: Effects of Internet pornography and individual differences on men's attitudes toward women. *Journal of Psychology and Human Sexuality, 11*, 63–91.

Barbaree, H., Marshall, W., & McCormick, J. (1998). The development of deviant sexual behaviour among adolescents and its implications for prevention and treatment. *Irish Journal of Psychology, 19*, 1–31.

Barber, B. (2003). On the brink: Female circumcision. *World and I, 18*, 184.

Barinaga, M. (1991). Is homosexuality biological? *Science, 253*, 956–957.

Baron, L. (1990). Pornography and gender equality: An empirical analysis. *Journal of Sex Research, 27*, 363–380.

Barth, K., Cook, R., Downs, J., Switzer, G., & Fischhoff, B. (2002). Social stigma and negative consequences: Factors that influence college students' decisions to seek testing for sexually transmitted diseases. *Journal of American College Health, 50*, 153–159.

Bartlik, B., & Goldberg, J. (2000). Female sexual arousal disorder. In S. Leiblum & R. Rosen (Eds.), *Principles and practice of sex therapy* (pp. 85–117). New York: Guilford Press.

Bass, B. (1996). Short-term cognitive-behavioral treatment of hypoactive sexual disorder in an individual with a history of childhood sexual abuse. *Journal of Sex and Marital Therapy, 22*, 284–289.

Bauerlein, M. (1995). The borderless bordello. *Utne Reader, 72*, 30–31.

Baumeister, R. F. (1995, November-December). An inside look at S&M. *Psychology Today*, pp. 47–52.

BBC. (2003). China launches "sex Website." *BBC News World Edition*. Retrieved September 25, 2004, from **http://news.bbc.co.uk/2/hi/asia-pacific/3059267.stm**

Beatty, W. W. (1992). Gonadal hormones and sex differences in nonreproductive behaviors. In A. A. Gerall, H. Moltz, & I. L. Ward (Eds.), *Handbook of behavioral neurobiology*, Vol. 11: *Sexual differentiation* (pp. 85–128). New York: Plenum.

Beers, M. H. (Ed.). (2004). Nongonococcal urethritis and chlamydial cervicitis. In *Merck manual of medical information* (2d home ed.). Whitehouse Station, N.J.: Merck. Retrieved February 21, 2006, from **http://www.merck.com/mmhe/sec17/ch200/ch200d.html**

Bélanger, C., Laughrea, K., & Lafontaine, M. F. (2001). The impact of anger on sexual satisfaction in marriage. *Canadian Journal of Human Sexuality, 10*, 91–99.

Bell A., & Weinberg, M. (1978). *Homosexualities: A study of diversity among men and women*. New York: Simon & Schuster.

Bell, A., Weinberg, M., & Hammersmith, S. (1981). Sexual preference: Its development in men and women. Bloomington: Indiana University Press.

Belzer, E., Whipple, B., & Moger, W. (1984). On female ejaculation. *Journal of Sex Research, 20*, 403–406.

Bem, D. J. (1996). Exotic becomes erotic: A developmental theory of sexual orientation. *Psychological Review, 103*, 320–335.

Bem, D. J. (1997, August). *Exotic becomes erotic: Explaining the enigma of sexual orientation*. Address at the annual meeting of the American Psychological Association, Chicago.

Bem, D. J. (1998). Is EBE theory supported by the evidence? Is it androcentric? A reply to Peplau et al. *Psychological Review, 108*, 395–398.

Bem, D. J. (2000a). Exotic becomes erotic: Integrating biological and experiential antecedents of sexual orientation. In A. R. D'Augelli & C. J. Patterson (Eds.), *Lesbian, gay, and bisexual identities and youth: Psychological perspectives* (pp. 52–68). New York: Oxford University Press.

Bem, D. J. (2000b). Exotic becomes erotic: Interpreting the biological correlates of sexual orientation. *Archives of Sexual Behavior, 29*, 531–548.

Bem, S. (1974). The measurement of psychological androgyny. *Journal of Consulting and Clinical Psychology, 42*, 155–162.

Bem, S. (1994). *The lenses of gender*. New Haven, CT: Yale University Press.

Benedict, E. (1997, September). Please touch. *Esquire*, p. 138.

Bennett, H. (1998). APGAR scores for dads. *British Medical Journal, 317*, 1712.

Berenbaum, S. A., & Snyder, E. (1995). Early hormonal influences on childhood sex-typed activity and playmate preferences: Implications for the development of sexual orientation. *Developmental Psychology, 31*, 31–42.

Berer, M. (2002). Making abortions safe: A matter of good public health policy and practice. *Reproductive Health Matters, 10*(5), 31–44.

Bergen, R. (1999). Marital rape. Minnesota Center Against Violence and Abuse. Retrieved January 10, 2005 from **http://www.vaw.umn.edu/Vawnet/mrape.htm**

Bergstein, B. (2005, December 6). ICANN greenlights ".asia" domain, stalls again on red-light district. *InformationWeek*. Retrieved January 3, 2006, from **http://informationweek.com/story/showArticle.jhtml?articleID=174900995**

Berkowitz, C. (1998). Medical consequences of child sexual abuse. *Child Abuse and Neglect, 22*, 541–550.

Besharat, M. (2003). Relation of attachment style with marital conflict. *Psychological Reports, 92*, 1135–1140.

Best, K. (2000). New devices may be easier to use. *Network, 20* [Electronic version]. Retrieved January 10, 2002, from **http://www.fhi.org/en/fp/fppubs/network/v20-2/nt2023.html**

Bettencourt, A. B., & Miller, N. (1996). Gender differences in aggression as a function of provocation: A meta-analysis. *Psychological Bulletin, 119*, 422–448.

Bhugra, D. (2000). Disturbances in objects of sexual desire: Cross-cultural issues. *Sexual and Relationship Therapy, 15*, 67–78.

Billstein, S. (1999). Pubic lice. In K. K. Holmes, P. F. Sparling, P. March, S. M. Lemon, W. E. Stamm, P. Piot, & J. N. Wasserheit (Eds.), *Sexually transmitted diseases* (3d ed., pp. 641–644). New York: McGraw-Hill.

Billy, J. O. G., Tanfer, K., Grady, W. R., & Klepinger, D. H. (1993). The sexual behavior of men in the United States. *Family Planning Perspectives, 25*, 52–60.

Binder, R. (2001). Changing a culture: Sexual assault prevention and the fraternity and sorority community. In A. J. Ottens & K. Hotelling (Eds.), *Sexual violence on campus: Policies, programs, and perspectives* (pp. 121–140). New York: Springer.

Bing, E. (2001). Making love during pregnancy. Retrieved on Jun 12, 2002, from **http://www.lamaze.com/ pregnancy/relationships/articles**

Binik, Y., Mah, K., & Kiesler, S. (1999). Ethical issues in conducting sex research on the Internet. *Journal of Sex Research, 36*, 82–93.

Binik, Y., Reissing, E., Pukall, C., Flory, N., Payne, K., & Khalife, S. (2002). The female sexual pain disorders: Genital pain or sexual dysfunction? *Archives of Sexual Behavior, 31*, 425–429.

Bird, M. (1999, January 11) Glories that were Rome. *Time International*, p. 52.

Birken, R., Hill, A., & Berner, W. (2003). Pharmacotherapy of paraphilias with long-acting agonists of luteinizing hormone-releasing hormone. *Journal of Clinical Psychiatry, 64*, 890–897.

Blanc, A. (2001). The effect of power in sexual relationships on sexual and reproductive health: An examination of the evidence. *Studies in Family Planning, 32*, 189–213.

Blanchard, R., Cantor, J., Bogaert, A., Breedlove, S., & Ellis, L. (2006). Interaction of fraternal birth order and handedness in the development of male homosexuality. *Hormones and Behavior 49*: 405–414.

Bloom, M. (2005, March 27). Researchers pursue promising cervical cancer vaccine. *Scout News*. Retrieved March 29, 2005, from **http://www.healthcentral.com/news/NewsFullText.cfm?id=524502**

Blum, D. (1997). *Sex on the brain: The biological differences between men and women*. New York: Viking Press.

Blumstein, P., & Schwartz, P. (1983). *American couples*. New York: Morrow

Bobrow, R. (2002). Sexual orientation and suicide risk among teenagers. *Journal of the American Medical Association, 287*, 1265.

Bock, R. (1993, August). *Understanding Klinefelter syndrome: A guide for XXY males and their families*. NIH Publication No. 93-3202. Retrieved July 25, 2003, from **http://www.nichd.nih.gov/publications/pubs/klinefelter.htm**

Bode, N. (2000, November-December). Sexuality at hand. *Psychology Today*, p. 11.

Bogaert, A. (2001). Personality, individual differences, and preferences for sexual media. *Archives of Sexual Behavior, 30*, 29–53.

Bogaert, A., & Hershberger, S. (1999). The relation between sexual orientation and penile size. *Archives of Sexual Behavior, 28*, 213–221.

Bogart, L., Cecil, H., Wagstaff, D., Pinkerton, S., & Abramson, P. (2000). Is it sex? *Journal of Sex Research, 37*, 108–116.

Boies, S. (2002). University students' uses of and reactions to online sexual information and entertainment: links to online and offline sexual behavior. *Canadian Journal of Human Sexuality, 11*, 77–90.

Bolen, R., & Scannapieco, M. (1999). Prevalence of child sexual abuse: Corrective meta-analysis. *Social Science Review, 73*, 281–313.

Boles, J., & Elifson, K. (1994). Sexual identity and HIV: The male prostitute. *Journal of Sex Research, 31*, 39–46.

Bolton, R., & Nardi, P. (1993, June 1). The mysteries of sex-survey results. *Advocate*, p. 49.

Bonifazi, W. (2000). Somebody to love. *Contemporary Long-Term Care, 23*, 22–28.

Booth, R., Kwiatkowski, C., & Chitwood, D. (2000). Sex-related HIV risk behaviors. *Drug and Alcohol Dependence, 58*, 219–226.

Bornstein, R. (1989). Exposure and affect: Overview and meta-analysis of research. *Psychological Bulletin, 106*, 265–289.

Bortot, A., Risser, W., & Cromwell, P. (2004). Coping with pelvic inflammatory disease in the adolescent. *Contemporary Pediatrics, 21*, 33–40.

Boschert, S. (2001, September 1). Morning-after postcoital test offers best results. *OB/GYN News*, p. 18.

Boschert, S. (2002, April 1). Autoimmune woes more common with endometriosis: Increased prevalence of systemic lupus, multiple sclerosis, and rheumatoid arthritis—survey of 3,680 women. *OB/GYN News*, p. 32.

Bouchard, T. (1999). Genes, environment, and personality. In S. J. Ceci & W. M. Williams (Eds.), *The nature-nurture debate: The essential readings* (pp. 97–103). Malden, MA: Blackwell.

Bouchez, C. (2001, September 21). C-section by request. *USA Today*. Retrieved June 13, 2002, from **http://www.usatoday.com**

Bowen, J. (1999, March 4). Rub me tender: A reformed frotteurist explores the roots of his long-lost fetish. *Salon*. Retrieved December 7, 2004, from **http://www.salon.com/urge/feature/1999/03/04feature2.html**

Boy or girl? Best leave it to chance. (2004). *New Scientist, 182*, 3.

Boyd, M. (1997, June 24). Male bonding. *Advocate*, p. 11.

Bozdech, B. (1998). Fertility drugs for men. Retrieved June 9, 2002, from **http://blueprint.bluecrossmn.com/topic/4090**

Bozman, A., & Beck, J. (1991). Covariation of sexual desire and sexual arousal: The effects of anger and anxiety. *Archives of Sexual Behavior, 20*, 47–60.

Bradbury, T., Beach, S., Fincham, F., & Nelson, G. (1996). Attributions and behavior in functional and dysfunctional marriages. *Journal of Consulting and Clinical Psychology, 64*, 569–576.

Bradbury, T., & Fincham, F. (1992). Attributions and behavior in marital interaction. *Journal of Personality and Social Psychology, 63*, 613–628.

Bradford, J. M. W. (2001). The neurobiology, neuropharmacology, and pharmacology treatment of the paraphilias and compulsive sexual behavior. *Canadian Journal of Psychiatry, 46*, 26–34.

Bradford, J. M. W., & Greenberg, D. (1997). Pharmacological treatment of deviant sexual behavior. *Annual Review of Sex Research, 7*, 283–306.

Bradley, N. (1999). Sampling for Internet surveys. An examination of respondent selection for Internet research. *Journal of the Market Research Society, 41*, 387.

Brannon, G. (2002). Paraphilias. *eMedicine Journal, 3*. Retrieved July 2, 2002, from **http://www.emedicine.com/med/topic3127.htm**

Brehm, S. S., Kassin, S. M., & Fein, S. (1999). *Social psychology* (4th ed.). Boston: Houghton Mifflin.

Brents, B., & Hausbeck, K. (2001). State-sanctioned sex: Negotiating formal and informal regulatory practices in Nevada brothels. *Sociological Perspectives, 44*, 307–332.

Brett, J., & Austoker, J. (2002). Breast cancer awareness: Breast awareness is not widely accepted concept replacing the controversial breast self-examination. *Practice Nurse, 24*, 54–59.

Brewis, J., & Linstead, S. (2000). "The worst thing in the screwing": Context and career in sex work. *Gender, Work, and Organization, 7*, 168–180.

Bridgeland, W., Duane, E., & Stewart, C. (2001). Victimization and attempted suicide among college students. *College Student Journal, 35*, 63–76.

Brienza, J. (1997). California castration law greeted with skepticism. *Trial, 33*, 16–18.

Brocklehurst, P. (1999). Update on the treatment of sexually transmitted infections in pregnancy, 2. *International Journal of STDs and AIDS, 10*, 636–642.

Brody, J. (2004, June 1). Abstinence-only: Does it work? *New York Times*, p. F7.

Brody, S. (2003). Alexithymia is inversely associated with women's frequency of vaginal intercourse. *Archives of Sexual Behavior, 32*, 73–77.

Brooks, C. (1992, September 4). Hand jive. *Isthmus*, pp. 23–25.

Broussard, D., Leichliter, J., & Evans, A. (2002). Screening adolescents in a juvenile detention center for gonorrhea and chlamydia: Prevalence and infection rates. *Prison Journal, 82*, 8–18.

Brown, B. (2001). Sexual intercourse and orgasm during late pregnancy may have a protective effect against preterm delivery. *Family Planning Perspectives, 33*, 185–187.

Brown, K., Perlmutter P., & McDermott, R. (2000). Youth and tattoos: What school health personnel should know. *Journal of School Health, 70*, 355–360.

Brown, R., Sumner, K., & Nocera, R. (2002). Understanding sexual aggression against women: An examination of the role of men's athletic participation and related variables. *Journal of Interpersonal Violence, 17*, 937–952.

Brown, W. M., Finn, C. J., Cooke, B. M., & Breedlove, S. M. (2002). Differences in finger length ratios between self-identified "butch" and "femme" lesbians. *Archives of Sexual Behavior, 31*, 123–127.

Brunk, D. (2000, December 1). Sperm quantity, quality decline with age. *OB/GYN News*, p. 5.

Bryant, C. (2002). Psychological treatment of priest sex offenders. *America, 186*, 14–18.

Bulcroft, K., & O'Connor-Roden, B. (1986, June). Never too late: Single people over 65 who are dating and sexually active belie the notion that passion and romance are only for the young. *Psychology Today*, pp. 66–69.

Bull, C. (1999, April 13). The state of hate. *Advocate*, pp. 24–34.

Bullough, B., & Bullough, V. (1997). Are transvestites necessarily heterosexual? *Archives of Sexual Behavior, 26*, 1–11.

Bullough, V. (2001). Christine Jorgensen: A personal autobiography. *Journal of Sex Research, 38*, 379–380.

Bumpass, L., & Lu, H.-H. (2000). Trends in cohabitation and implications for children's family contexts in the United States. *Population Studies, 54*, 29–41.

Bunnell, R., Dahlberg, L., & Rolfs, R. (1999). High prevalence and incidence of sexually transmitted diseases in urban adolescent females despite moderate risk behaviors. *Journal of Infectious Diseases, 180*, 1624–1631.

Bureau of Justice Statistics. (2001). Criminal victimization in the United States, Table 38. Retrieved August 20, 2003, from **http://www.ojp.usdoj.gov/bjs/pub/pdf/cvus/current/cv0138.pdf**

Bureau of Labor Statistics. (2002). Wages by area and occupation. Retrieved August 15, 2003, from **http://www.bls.gov/bls/blswage.htm**

Burger, W. (1973). *Miller* v. *California*, 413 U.S. 15, 93 S.Ct. 2607, 37 L.Ed. 2d 419.

Burgess, A., & Holmstrom, L. (1974). Rape trauma syndrome. *American Journal of Psychiatry, 131*, 981–986.

Burk, R. D., Ho, G. Y., Beardsely, L., Lempa, M., Peters, M., & Bierman, R. (1996). Sexual behavior and partner characteristics are the predominant risk factors for genital human papillomavirus infection in young women. *Journal of Infectious Diseases, 174*, 679–689.

Burstein, G., Gaydos, C., Diener-West, M., Howell, M., Zenilman, J., & Quinn, T. (1998). Incident chlamydia trachomatis infections among inner-city adolescent females. *Journal of the American Medical Association. 280*, 521–526.

Burstein, G., Snyder, M., Conley, D., Boekeloo, B., Quinn, T., & Zenilman, J. (2001). Adolescent chlamydia testing practices and diagnosed infections in a large managed care organization. *Sexually Transmitted Diseases, 28*, 477–483.

Butcher, J. (1999). ABCs of sexual health: Female sexual problems II: Sexual pain and sexual fears. *British Medical Journal, 318*, 110–112.

Butcher, J. (2003, June 4). A psychosexual approach to managing dispareunia. *Practitioner*, pp. 484–487.

Buunk, B., & Hupka, R. B. (1987). Cross-cultural differences in the elicitation of sexual jealousy. *Journal of Sex Research, 23*, 12–22.

Byers, E. S., & Demmons, S. (1999). Sexual satisfaction and sexual self-disclosure within dating relationships. *Journal of Sex Research, 36*, 180–189.

Byers, E. S., & Grenier, G. (2003). Premature or rapid ejaculation: Heterosexual couples' perceptions of men's ejaculatory behavior. *Archives of Sexual Behaivor, 32*, 261–270.

Byers, E. S., Purdon, C., & Clark, D. A. (1998). Sexual intrusive thoughts of college students. *Journal of Sex Research, 35*, 359–369.

Byne, W. (1994). The biological evidence challenged. *Scientific American, 270*, 50–55.

Byne, W. (1997). Why we cannot conclude that sexual orientation is primarily a biological phenomenon. *Journal of Homosexuality, 34*, 73–80.

Byrd, J., Hyde, J., De Lamater, J., & Plant, E. (1998). Sexuality during pregnancy and the year postpartum. *Sexuality of Family Practice, 47*, 305–308.

Cabello Santamaría, F. (1997). Female ejaculation: Myth and reality. In J. J. Baras-Vass & M. Perez-Concillo (Eds.), *Sexuality and human rights: Proceedings of the 13th World Congress of Sexology* (pp. 325–333). Valencia, Spain: ECVSA. Retrieved August 16, 2005, from **http://www.doctorg.com/myth_reality1.htm**

Came, B. (1993, February 22). Young, gay, and alone. *Maclean's*, p. 34.

Camille, C. J., Kuo, R. L., & Wiener, J. S. (2002). Caring for the uncircumcised penis: What parents (and you) need to know. *Contemporary Pediatrics, 19*, 61–68.

Campaign for Our Children. (2003). Teen guide. Retrieved July 12, 2005, from **http://www.cfoc.org**

Can HPV Testing Replace Pap Smears in Primary Care? (2003). *Contemporary OB/GYN, 48*, 29–30.

Cannold, L. (2003). Do we need a normative account of the decision to parent? *International Journal of Applied Philosophy, 17*, 277–290.

Cantor, J. M., Blanchard, R., Paterson, A. D., & Bogaert, A. F. (2002). How many gay men owe their sexual orientation to fraternal birth order? *Archives of Sexual Behavior, 3*, 63–71.

Carey, M. (1998). Cognitive-behavioral treatment of sexual dysfunctions. In V. Caballo (Ed.), *International handbook of cognitive and behavioural treatments of psychological disorders*. Oxford: Pergammon/Elsevier.

Carlson, A. E., et al. (2003). CatSper1 required for evoked Ca^{2+} entry and control of flagellar function in sperm. *Proceedings of the National Academy of Sciences of the United States, 100*, 14864–14868.

Carr, J. L., & Van Deusen, K. M. (2004). Risk factors for male sexual aggression on college campuses. *Journal of Family Violence, 19*, 279–289.

Carr, R., & Grambling, L. (2004). Stigma: A health barrier for women with HIV/AIDS. *Journal of the Association of Nurses in AIDS Care, 15*, 30–39.

Caspi, A., Herbener, E. S., & Ozer, D. J. (1992). Shared experiences and the similarity of personalities: A longitudinal study of married couples. *Journal of Personality and Social Psychology, 62*, 281–291.

Caspi, A., & Silva, P. (1995). Temperamental qualities at age three predict personality traits in young adulthood: Longitudinal evidence from a birth cohort. *Child Development, 66*, 486–498.

Cass, V. (1984). Homosexual identity formation: Testing a theoretical model. *Journal of Homosexuality, 20*, 143–167.

Catania, J. A. (1999). A framework for conceptualizing reporting bias and its antecedents in interviews assessing human sexuality. *Journal of Sex Research, 36*, 25–38.

Cates, W., Jr. (1999a). Chlamydial infections and the risk of ectopic pregnancy. *Journal of the American Medical Association, 281*,117–118.

Cates, W., Jr. (1999b). Estimates of the incidence and prevalence of sexually transmitted diseases in the United States. *Sexually Transmitted Diseases, 26*(Suppl.), S2–S7.

Cates, W., Jr., & Ellertson, C. (1998). Abortion. In R. A. Hatcher, J. Trussell, F. Stewart, W. Cates Jr., G. K. Stewart, F. Guest, & D. Kowal (Eds.), *Contraceptive technology* (17th rev. ed., pp. 679–700). New York: Ardent Media.

Cates, W., Jr., Grimes, D., & Schulz, K. (2003). The public health impact of legal abortions: 30 years later. *Perspectives of Sexual and Reproductive Health, 35*, 25–28.

Cato, S., & Leitenberg, H. (1990). Guilt reactions to sexual fantasies during intercourse. *Archives of Sexual Behavior, 19*, 49–63.

The causes of homosexuality. (2001, September 11), *Advocate*, p. 6.

Centers for Disease Control and Prevention. (1997) Youth risk behavior surveillance: National college health risk behavior survey: United States, 1995. *Mortality and Morbidity Weekly Report, 46*, 1–54.

Centers for Disease Control and Prevention. (2000a). Gonorrhea: United States, 1998. *Morbidity and Mortality Weekly Report, 49*, 538–542.

Centers for Disease Control and Prevention. (2000b). HIV-related knowledge and stigma. *Morbidity and Mortality Weekly Report, 49*, 1062–1064.

Centers for Disease Control and Prevention. (2001a). The global HIV and AIDS epidemic, 2001. *Morbidity and Mortality Weekly Report, 50*, 434–439.

Centers for Disease Control and Prevention. (2001b). First report of AIDS. *Morbidity and Mortality Weekly Report, 50*, 429–445.

Centers for Disease Control and Prevention. (2002). Sexually transmitted disease treatment guidelines, 2002. *Mortality and Morbidity Weekly, 51*,1–80.

Centers for Disease Control and Prevention. (2003a). Advancing HIV preventions: New strategies for a changing epidemic, United States, 2003. *Morbidity and Mortality Weekly Report, 52*, 329–332.

Centers for Disease Control and Prevention. (2003b). Cases of HIV infection and AIDS in the United States, 2002. *HIV/AIDS Surveillance Report, 14*. Retrieved November 14, 2003, from **http://www.cdc.gov/hiv/stats/hasr1402.htm**

Centers for Disease Control and Prevention. (2003c). How safe is the blood supply in the United States? Retrieved June 12, 2004, from **http://www.cdc.gov/hiv/pubs/faq/faq15.htm**

Centers for Disease Control and Prevention. (2003d). Primary and secondary syphilis: United States, 2002. *Morbidity and Mortality Weekly Report, 52*, 1117–1120.

Centers for Disease Control and Prevention. (2004a). Assisted reproductive technology. Retrieved September 25, 2005, from **http://www.cdc.gov/reproductivehealth/art/index.htm**

Centers for Disease Control and Prevention. (2004b). Division of HIV/AIDS Prevention. Basic Statistics. Retrieved December 12, 2004 from **http://www.cdc.gov/hiv/stats.htm#hivest**.

Centers for Disease Control and Prevention. (2004c). 2002 assisted reproductive technology success rates. Retrieved January 8, 2005, from **http://www.cdc.gov/reproductivehealth/art.htm.**

Centers for Disease Control and Prevention (CDC) (2004c). Cases of HIV infection and AIDS in the United States, 2004. *HIV/AIDS Surveillance Report, 16*, 1–46.

Chase, C. (1998). Hermaphrodites with attitude: Mapping the emergence of intersex political activism. *GLQ: A Journal of Lesbian and Gay Studies, 4*, 189–211.

Chasen, S. T., Kalish, R. B., Gupta, M., Kaufman, J. E., Rashbaum, W. K., & Chatfield, J. (2001). FDA approves new monthly contraceptive. *American Family Physician, 64*, 1906.

Chesson, H., Harrison, P., & Stall, R. (2003). Changes in alcohol consumption and in sexually transmitted disease incidence rates in the United States, 1983–1998. *Journal of Studies on Alcohol, 64*, 623–630.

Chia, M., & Arava, D. A. (1997). *The multiorgasmic man: Sexual secrets every man should know.* San Francisco: HarperSanFrancisco.

Childless by choice. (2001, November 1). *American Demographics*, pp. 44–50.

Chillot, R. (2002). Overcome your greatest sexual fear. *Prevention, 54*, 144–149.

China rewards one-child families. (2005, February 28). *UPI NewsTrack*, p. 1.

Chlamydia, gonorrhea test. (2000, August 1). *Family Practice News*, p. 32.

Chopin-Marce, M. (2001). Exhibitionism and psychotherapy: A case study. *International Journal of Offender Therapy and Comparative Criminology, 45*, 626–633.

Christensen, C. (1995). Prescribed masturbation in sex therapy: A critique. *Journal of Sex and Marital Therapy, 21*, 87–96.

Chu, M., & Lobo, R. (2004). Formulations and use of androgens in women. *Journal of Family Practice, 53*, S3–S5.

Chumlea, W., Schubert, C., Kulin, H., Lee, P. Himes, J., & Sun, S. (2003). Age at menarche and racial comparisons in U.S. girls. *Pediatrics, 111*, 110–113.

Ciprofloxacin-resistant gonorrhea on the rise. (2002). *Contraceptive Technology Update, 23*, 64–66.

Clark, L., Jackson, M., &, Allen-Taylor, L. (2002). Adolescent knowledge about sexually transmitted diseases. *Sexually Transmitted Diseases, 29*, 436–443.

Clarke, V. (2001). What about the children? Arguments against lesbian and gay parenting. *Women's Studies International Forum, 24*, 555–570.

Clayton, A., Warnock, J., & Kornstein, S. (2004). Bupropion SR for SSRI-induced sexual dysfunction. *Psychopharmacological Update, 15*, 5–6.

Clement, U. (1990). Surveys of heterosexual behavior. *Annual Review of Sex Research, 1*, 45–74.

Clements, M., Stanley, S., & Markman, H. (2004). Before they said "I do": Discriminating among marital outcomes over 13 years. *Journal of Marriage and the Family, 66*, 613–626.

Clinton, W. J. (2000). Statement on signing the Victims of Trafficking and Violence Protection Act of 2000. Weekly Compilation of Presidential Documents, 36, 2662–2664.

Clottey, C., & Dallabetta, G. (1993). Sexually transmitted diseases and human immunodeficiency virus: Epidemiological synergy. *Infection Disease Clinics of North America, 7*, 753–777.

Cloud, J. (2002, April 29). Pedophilia. *Time*, pp. 42–46.

Cohen, K. M. (2002). Relationships among childhood sex-atypical behavior, spatial ability, handedness, and sexual orientation in men. *Archives of Sexual Behavior, 31*, 129–143.

Cohen, L. (2000, July 1). Antidepressants and breastfeeding. *Family Practice News*, p. 24.

Cohen, S. (1997). The role of contraception in reducing abortion. Retrieved June 12, 2002 from **http://www.guttmacher.org/pubs/ib19.html**

Colapinto, J. (2001). *As nature made him: The boy who was raised as a girl.* New York: Perennial Press.

Coleman, L., & Coleman, J. (2002). The measurement of puberty: A review. *Journal of Adolescence, 25*, 535–550.

Coleman, M., & Ganong, L. (1985). Love and sex role stereotypes. Do macho men and feminine women make better lovers? *Journal of Personality and Social Psychology, 49*, 170–176.

Collins, C., Alagiri, P., & Summers, T. (2002). *Abstinence only vs. comprehensive sex education: What are the arguments? What is the evidence?* San Francisco: AIDS Policy Research Center & Center for AIDS Prevention Studies, University of California.

Collins, N., & Miller, L. (1994). Self-disclosure and liking: A meta-analytic review. *Psychological Bulletin, 116*, 457–475.

Colombo, D. F. (2002). Predicting spontaneous preterm birth: Fetal fibronectin and ultrasonography help rule out labor, not rule it in. *British Medical Journal, 325*, 289–290.

Comer, R. (1998). *Abnormal psychology* (3d ed.). New York: Freeman.

Concern over AIDS grows internationally. (1983, May 24). *New York Times*. Retrieved October 30, 2003, from **http://www.nytimes.com/library/national/science/aids/052483sci-aids.html**

Condoms campaign planned in China. (2004, August 1). *UPI NewsTrack*, p. 1.

Conley, T. D., & Collins, B. E. (2005). Differences between condom users and condom nonusers in their multidimensional condom attitudes. *Journal of Applied Social Psychology, 35*, 603–620.

Connidis, I., & McMullin, J. (1999). Permanent childlessness: Percieved advantages and disadvantages. *Canadian Journal on Aging, 18*, 447–465.

Constantinople, A. (1973). Masculinity-femininity: An exception to a famous dictum? *Psychological Bulletin, 80*, 389–407.

Conway, L. (2003a). Basic TG/TS/IS information: Gender basics and transgenderism. Retrieved August 15, 2003, from **http://ai.eecs.umich.edu/people/conway/TS/TS-Ia.html**

Conway, L. (2003b). How many of us are there? Retrieved August 15, 2003, from **http://www.gendercentre.org.au/44article4.htm**

Cooper, A., McLoughlin, I., & Campbell, K. (2000). Sexuality in cyberspace: Update for the 21st century. *CyberPsychology and Behavior, 3*, 521–536.

Cooper, L. M. (2002). Alcohol use and risky sexual behavior among college students and youth: Evaluating the evidence. *Journal of Studies on Alcohol, 63*, S101–S117.

Cooper, L. M., & Orcutt, H. K. (2000). Alcohol use, condom use and partner type among heterosexual adolescents and young adults. *Journal of Studies on Alcohol, 61*, 413–419.

Corey, L., & Wald, A. (1999). Genital herpes. In K. K. Holmes, P. F. Sparling, P. March, S. M. Lemon, W. E. Stamm, P. Piot, & J. N. Wasserheit (Eds.), *Sexually transmitted diseases* (3d ed., pp. 285–586). New York: McGraw-Hill.

Cormier, S. (1993). *Am I normal? Your personal guide to understanding yourself and others.* New York: Carroll & Graf.

Cornforth, T. (2001). Vaginal douching: To douche or not to douche? The douche debate continues. Retrieved January 7, 2002 from **http://womenshealth.about.com/library/weekly/aa052901a.htm**

Cornforth, T. (2002). DES daughters and prenatal exposure. Retrieved February 21, 2006, from **http://womenshealth.about.com/library/weekly/aa122199a.htm**

Counseling Center for Human Development. (2001). Date rape. Retrieved February 24, 2006, from **http://www.rmit.usf.edu/counsel/self-hlp/daterape.htm**

Coustan, D., Haning, R., & Singer, D. (1995). *Human reproduction: Growth and development.* Boston: Little, Brown.

Cowan, G. (2000). Beliefs about the causes of four types of rape. *Sex Roles, 40*, 807–820.

Crawford, I., McLeod, A., Zamboni, B. D., & Jordan, M. B. (1999). Psychologists' attitudes toward gay and lesbian parenting. *Professional Psychology, Research and Practice, 30*, 394–401.

Creighton, S. (2004, April). Prevalence and incidence of child abuse: International comparisons. *NSPCC Information Briefings*, pp. 1–10.

Creinin, M., Potter, C., Holovanisin, M., Janczukiewicz, L., Pymar, H., & Schwartz, J. (2003). Mifepristone and misoprostol and methotrexate and misoprostol in clinical practice for abortion. *American Journal of Obstetrics and Gynecology, 188*, 664–669.

Crick, N., Casas, J., & Mosher, M. (1997). Relational and overt aggression in preschool. *Developmental Psychology, 33*, 579–588.

Crick, N., & Grotpeter, J. (1995). Relational aggression, gender, and social-psychological adjustment. *Child Development, 66*, 710–722.

Crombie, G., Pyke, S., Silverthorn, N., Jones, A., & Piccinin, S. (2003). Students' perceptions of their classroom participation and instructor as a function of gender and context. *Journal of Higher Education, 74*, 51–76.

Cunniff, C. (2004). Prenatal screening and diagnosis for pediatricians. *Pediatrics, 114*, 889–994.

Cusac, A. (1999). The promise of Stonewall. *Progressive, 6*, 10–13.

Dalla, R. L. (2002). Night moves: A qualitative investigation of street-level sex work. *Psychology of Women Quarterly, 26*, 63–73.

Dallager, C., and Rosen, L. (1993). Effects of a human sexuality course on attitudes toward rape and violence. *Journal of Sex Education and Therapy, 19*, 193–199.

Darling, C. A., Davidson, J., & Conway-Welch, C. (1990). Female ejaculation: Perceived origins, the Grafenberg spot, and sexual responsiveness. *Archives of Sexual Behavior, 19,* 29–47.

Darling, C. A., Davidson, J. K., & Jennings, D. A. (1991). The female sexual response revisited: Understanding the multiorgasmic experience in women. *Archives of Sexual Behavior, 20,* 527–540.

Darney, P. (1994). Hormonal implants: Contraception for a new century. *American Journal of Obstetrics and Gynecology, 170,* 1536–1542.

Davidson, J., & Moore, N. (1994). Masturbation and premarital sexual intercourse among college women: Making choices for sexual fulfillment. *Journal of Sex and Marital Therapy, 20,* 179–199.

Davidson, K., & Hoffman, L. (1986). Sexual fantasies and sexual satisfaction: An empirical analysis of erotic thought. *Journal of Sex Research, 22,* 184–205.

Davies, K. (1997). Voluntary exposure to pornography and men's attitudes toward feminism and rape. *Journal of Sex Research, 34,* 131–137.

Davis, C., Blank, J., Lin, H., & Bonillas, C. (1996). Characteristics of vibrator use among women. *Journal of Sex Research, 33,* 313–320.

Davis, C., & McCormick, N. (1997). What sexual scientists know about pornography. *Sexual Science, 3.* Retrieved June 25, 2003, from **http://www.sexscience.org/publications**

Davis, S. (2004). Clinical sequelae affecting the quality of life in the HIV-infected patient. *Journal of the Association of Nurses in AIDS Care, 15,* 23S–33S.

Davison, G. C. (2001). Conceptual and ethical issues in therapy for the psychological problems of gay men, lesbians, and bisexuals. *Journal of Clinical Psychology, 57,* 695–703.

Davison, G. C. (2005). Issues and nonissues in the gay-affirmative treatment of patients who are gay, lesbian, or bisexual. *Clinical Psychology: Science and Practice, 12,* 25–28.

Daw, J. (2002). Can psychology help a church in crisis? *Monitor on Psychology, 33.* Retrieved September 2, 2002, from **http://www.apa.org/monitor/jun02/church.html**

Daya, S. (1998). Definitions and factors affecting infertility. In O. Rodríguez-Armas (Ed.), *Infertility and contraception: A textbook for clinicians* (pp. 4–7). New York: Parthenon.

De Bro, S., Campbell, S., & Peplau, L. (1994). Influencing a partner to use a condom. *Psychology of Women Quarterly, 18,* 165–182.

Decarlo, P., Alexander, P., & Hsu, H. (1996) What are sex workers' HIV prevention needs? Retrieved June 6, 2003, from **http://www.caps.ucsf.edu/capsweb/prosttext.html**

De Lamiter, J., & Friedrich, W. (2002). Human sexual development. *Journal of Sex Research, 39,* 10–14.

Dell, D., Moskowitz, D., & Sondheimer, S. (2001). PMS and PMDD: Identification and treatment. *Contemporary OB/GYN, 46,* 15–30.

Delvin, D., & Webber, C. (2005). Sex after giving birth. Retrieved September 27, 2005, from **http://www.netdoctor.co.uk/sex_relationships/facts/sexdelivery.htm**

Demare, D., Briere, J., & Lips, H. (1988). Violent pornography and self-reported likelihood of sexual aggression. *Journal of Research in Personality, 22,* 140–153.

Demare, D., Lips, H., & Briere, J. (1993). Sexually violent pornography, antiwomen attitudes, and sexual aggression: A structural equation model. *Journal of Research in Personality, 27,* 285–300.

D'Emilio, J., & Freedman, E. (1988). *Intimate matters: A history of sexuality in America.* New York: Harper & Row.

Denenberg, R. (1997). Childhood sexual abuse as an HIV risk factor in women. *Treatment Issues, 11,* 7–8.

Depo-Provera bone loss. (2002, November 1). *Family Practice News,* p. 38.

Derlega, V. J., Metts, S., Petronio, S., & Marguilis, S. T. (1993). *Self-disclosure.* Thousand Oaks, CA: Sage.

Desiderato, L., & Crawford, H. (1995). Risky sexual behavior in college students: Relationships between number of sexual partners, disclosure of previous risky behavior, and alcohol use. *Journal of Youth and Adolescence, 24,* 55–68.

de Silva, P., & Pernet, A. (1992). Pollution in "Metroland": An unusual paraphilia in a shy young man. *Sexual and Marital Therapy, 7,* 301–306.

de Silva, W. (1999). Sexual variations. *British Medical Journal, 318,* 654–656.

Deu, N., & Edelmann, R. J. (1997). The role of criminal fantasy in predatory and opportunist sex offending. *Journal of Interpersonal Violence, 12,* 18–29.

De Witt, P. W., & Hamel, R. (1993). The birth business. *American Demographics, 15*(9), 44–50.

Dhawan, D., & Mayer K. H. (2006) Microbicides to prevent HIV transmission: overcoming obstacles to chemical barrier protection. *Journal of Infectious Diseases, 193,* 36–44.

Dickens, B. (2002). Can sex selection be ethically tolerated? *Journal of Medical Ethics, 28,* 335–336.

Dickenson, A. (1999, June 7). Sexual bullying: Schools are now required to protect kids from lewd harassment. *Time,* p. 86.

Diekman, A., & Murnen, S. (2004). Learning to be little women and little men: The inequitable gender identity in nonsexist children's literature. *Sex Roles, 50,* 373–385.

Dimitrov, D. (2001). Is Lunelle right for you? Retrieved January 8, 2002, from **http://www.plannedparenthood.org/bc/lunelle.html**

Dimmock, P., Wyatt, K., Jones, P., & O'Brien, S. (2000). Efficacy of selective serotonin-reuptake inhibitors in premenstrual syndrome: A systematic review. *Lancet, 356,* 1131–1136.

Discovery/Health.com. (2002). Hymen. Retrieved December 26, 2002, from **http://health.discovery.com/centers/sex/sexpedia/hymen.html**

Division of STD Prevention. (1998). *Sexually transmitted disease surveillance.* Atlanta: Centers for Disease Control and Prevention.

Division of STD Prevention. (1999). *National syphilis elimination plan.* Atlanta: Centers for Disease Control and Prevention.

Division of STD Prevention. (2000). *Sexually transmitted disease surveillance.* Atlanta: Centers for Disease Control and Prevention.

Division of STD Prevention. (2001). *Sexually transmitted disease surveillance.* Atlanta: Centers for Disease Control and Prevention.

Division of STD Prevention. (2004a). *STD Prevention.* Atlanta: Centers for Disease Control and Prevention. Retrieved June 24, 2004 from **http://www.cdc.gov/nchstp/dstd/disease_info.htm**

Division of STD Prevention. (2004b). *Tracking the hidden epidemics: Trends in STDs in the United States, 2000.* Atlanta: Centers for Disease Control and Prevention. Retrieved July 6, 2004, from **http://www.cdc.gov/nchstp/od/news/RevBrochure1pdf.htm**

Dlouhy, J. (2003). Senate panel moves to make video voyeurism a federal crime. *CQ Weekly, 61,* 1916.

Docter, R., & Prince, V. (1997). Transvestism: A survey of 1,032 cross-dressers. *Archives of Sexual Behavior, 26,* 589–606.

Dodson, B. (2002, December). Getting to know me: A primer on masturbation. *Ms.,* pp. 27–29. Reprinted from *Esquire,* August 1974, pp. 106–109.

Doherty, B. (2001, June 23). Evading blame. Retrieved June 6, 2002, from **http://reason.com/hod/bd062301.shtml**

Dolcini, M. (1993). Demographic characteristics of heterosexuals with multiple partners: The national AIDS behavioral surveys. *Family Planning Perspectives, 25,* 208–214.

Donnelly, D. (1993). Sexually inactive marriages. *Journal of Sex Research, 30,* 171–179.

Donnerstein, E. I. (1980). Aggressive erotica and violence against women. *Journal of Personality and Social Psychology, 39,* 269–277.

Donnerstein, E. I., & Berkowitz, L. (1981). Victim reactions in aggressive erotic films as a factor in violence against women. *Journal of Personality and Social Psychology, 41,* 710–724.

Donnerstein, E. I., & Linz, D. G. (1986, December). The question of pornography. *Psychology Today,* pp. 56–59.

Dotinga, R. (2003, June 19). Women's sexual arousal is all-encompassing. *Health Day.* Retrieved June 25, 2003, from **http://www.healthday.com/view.cfm?id=513724**

Dotinga, R. (2004, December 21). A pill to prevent AIDS? *Health Day.* Retrieved September 21, 2005, from **http://www.healthcentral.com/newsdetail/408/522964.html**

Douglas, W. O. (1973). *Miller* v. *California,* 413 U.S. 15, 93 S.Ct. 2607, 37 L.Ed. 2d 419.

Draper, E. S., Manktelow, B., Field, D. J., & James, D. (2003). Tables for predicting survival for preterm births are updated. *British Medical Journal, 327,* 872.

Driedger, S. (1996). Mystical passion: Tantric sex. *Macleans, 38,* 44–46.

Dryer, D., & Horowitz, L. (1997). When do opposites attract? Interpersonal complementarity versus similarity. *Journal of Personality and Social Psychology, 72,* 592–603.

Dugan, J. (2001). Kissin' cousins. *Colonial America*. Retrieved August 30, 2004, from **http://www.suite101.com/article.cfm/5871/61531**

Dugan, M. K., & Hock, R. R. (2006). *It's my life now: Starting over after an abusive relationship or domestic violence* (2d ed.). New York: Routledge.

Dunifon, R., & Kowaleski-Jones, L. (2002). Who's in the house? Race differences in cohabitation, single parenthood, and child development. *Child Development, 73*, 1249–1264.

Dunn, M. E., & Trost, J. (1989). Male multiple orgasms: A descriptive study. *Archives of Sexual Behavior, 18*, 377–387.

Dunn, M. S., Bartee, R. T., & Perko, M. A. (2003). Self-reported alcohol use and sexual behaviors of adolescents *Psychological Reports, 92*, 339–348.

Dunson, D. B., & Colombo, B. (2003). Bayesian modeling of markers of day-specific fertility. *Journal of the American Statistical Association, 98*, 28–37.

Dunson, D. B., Colombo, B., & Baird, D. (2002). Changes with age in the level and duration of fertility in the menstrual cycle. *Human Reproduction, 17*, 1399–1403.

Durex Corp. (2002a). Durex Global Sex Survey, 2002. Retrieved August 29, 2005, from **http://www.durex.com**

Durex Corp. (2002b). What is the average penis size? Retrieved August 29, 2005, from **http://www.durex.com**

Durex Corp. (2003). Frequency of sex. Durex Global Sex Survey, 2003. Retrieved August 29, 2005, from **http://www.durex.com**

Eagly, A. H., & Steffen V. J. (1986). Gender and aggressive behavior: A meta-analytic review of the social psychological literature. *Psychological Bulletin, 100*, 309–330.

Earl, D., & David, D. (1994). Depo-Provera: An injectable contraceptive. *American Family Physician, 49*, 891–894.

Early detection saves lives. (2002, November 14). *Women's Health Weekly*, p. 13.

Eccles, J. S., Jacobs, J. E., & Harold, R. D. (1990). Gender role stereotypes, expectancy effects, and parents' socialization of gender differences. *Journal of Social Issues, 46*, 183–202.

Ectopic pregnancy: United States, 1990–1992. (1995). *British Medical Journal, 273*, 533–534.

Edell, D. (2001). As big as that? Retrieved November 4, 2004 from **http://www.healthcentral.com/drdean/deanfulltexttopics.cfm?ID=50890**

Edwards, J., & Moore, A. (1999). Implanon: A review of clinical studies. *British Journal of Family Planning, 4*, 3–16.

Edwards, M. (2000). Adolescents would prefer parents as primary sexuality educators. *Families are talking*, special supplement to *Seicus Report, 1*. Retrieved July 3, 2003, from **http://www.siecus.org/pubs/families/Families_Newsletter.pdf**

Edwards, S. (1994). The role of men in contraceptive decision-making: Current knowledge and future implications. *Family Planning Perspectives, 26*, 77–82.

Ehrhardt, A., & Baker, S. (1974). Fetal androgens, central nervous system differentiation, and behavior sex differences. In R. Friedman, R. Richart, & R. Vandewiele (Eds.), *Sex differences in behavior* (pp. 33–51). New York: Wiley.

Eilers, G., & Swanson, T. (1994). Women's satisfaction with Norplant as compared with oral contraceptives. *Journal of Family Practice, 38*, 596–600.

Eisenberg, M. E. (2001). Differences in sexual risk behaviors between college students with same-sex and opposite-sex experience: Results from a national survey. *Archives of Sexual Behavior, 30*, 575–589.

Eisenberg, M. E., & Wechsler, H. (2003). Social influences on substance-use behaviors of gay, lesbian, and bisexual college students: Findings from a national study. *Social Science and Medicine, 57*, 1913–1923.

Eliason, M. J. (1997). The prevalence and nature of biphobia in heterosexual undergraduate students. *Archives of Sexual Behavior, 26*, 317–326.

Elifson, K., Boles, J., Posey, E, Sweat, M., Darrow, W., & Elsea, W. (1993). Male transvestite prostitutes and HIV risk. *American Journal of Public Health, 83*, 260–262.

Elifson, K., Boles, J., & Sweat, M. (1993). Risk factors associated with HIV infection among male prostitutes. *American Journal of Public Health, 83*, 79–83.

Elliot, V. (2001). Recent tragedies focus attention on postpartum depression. *American Medical News, 44*, 29–30.

Elliot, W. (2004). Valacyclovir reduces genital herpes transmission. *Infections Disease Alert, 23*, S1.

Ellis, B., & Symons, D. (1990). Sex differences in sexual fantasy: An evolutionary psychological approach. *Journal of Sex Research, 27*, 527–555.

Ellis, H. (1936). *Studies in the psychology of sex*. New York: Random House.

Engender Health. (2003a). Sexual response and aging. Retrieved January 5, 2003, from **http://www.engenderhealth.org/res/onc/sexuality/response/pg3.html**

Engender Health. (2003b). Signs and symptoms of HIV infection. Retrieved November 10, 2003, from **http://www.engenderhealth.org/res/onc/hiv/diagnosis/hiv4p2.html**

Engender Health. (2004). The sexual response cycle. Retrieved January 2, 2004, from **http://www.engenderhealth.org/res/onc/sexuality/response/pg2.html**

Epperson, C., Jatlow, P., Czarkowski, K., & Anderson, G. (2003). Maternal fluoxetine treatment in the postpartum period: Effects on platelet serotonin and plasma drug levels in breastfeeding mother-infant pairs. *Pediatrics, 112*, E425–E425.

Epstein, R., Klinkenberg, W., Wiley, D., & McKinley, L. (2001). Ensuring sample equivalence across Internet and paper-and-pencil assessments. *Computers in Human Behavior, 17*, 339–346.

Erickson, P. G., Butters, J., McGillicuddy, P., & Hallgren, A. (2000). Crack and prostitution: Gender, myths, and experiences. *Journal of Drug Issues, 30*, 767–788.

Erieden, J. (2003, January 15). Start Pap tests by age 21, consider ending by 70. *Family Practice News*, 32–33.

Evaluate your parenting readiness. (2005). Retrieved September 25, 2005, from **http://www.babycenter.com/refcap/preconception/gettingpregnant/7311.html**.

Evans, J. D. (1985). *Invitation to psychological research*. New York: Holt, Rinehart and Winston.

Evans, N. J., & Wall, V. A. (1993). *Beyond tolerance: Gays, lesbians, and bisexuals on campus*. Philadelphia: University Press of America.

Evans, W. (2003, September 6). Taboo topics: Where should line be drawn on cartoons? *Sacramento Bee*. Retrieved April 6, 2004, from **http://www.sacbee.com**

Everaerd, W. (1993). Male erectile disorder. In W. O'Donohue & J. Geer (Eds.), *Handbook of sexual dysfunctions* (pp. 201–224). Needham Heights, MA: Allyn & Bacon.

Eyre, S., Davis, E., & Peacock, B. (2001). Moral argumentation in adolescents' commentaries about sex. *Culture, Health, and Sexuality, 3*, 1–17.

Fackelmann, K. (1998). It's a girl! *Science News, 154*, 350–351.

Fairchild, A. L., & Bayer, R. (1999). Uses and abuses of Tuskegee. *Science, 284*, 919–921.

Family Health International. (1996). Reproductive health: How to use oral contraceptives. Retrieved December 21, 2003, from **http://www.fhi.org/en/rh/pubs/network/v16_4/nt1643.htm**

Family Health International. (2001). IUD mechanism affects sperm. Retrieved March 20, 2004, from **http://www.fhi.org**

Farley, M., & Kelly, V. (2000). Prostitution: A critical review of the medical and social sciences literature. *Women and Criminal Justice, 11*, 29–64.

Farr, G., Gabelnick, H., Sturgen, K., & Dorflinger, L. (1994). Contraceptive efficacy and acceptability of the female condom. *American Journal of Public Health, 84*, 1960–1964.

Farrington, J. (2002). Sexual myth or fact? Do you know what's true? *Current Health, 28*, SS1–SS3.

Faulkner, S. (2003). Good girl or flirt girl? Latinas' definitions of sex and sexual relationships. *Hispanic Journal of Behavioral Sciences, 25*, 174–205.

Fausto-Sterling, A. (1993). The five sexes: Why male and female are not enough. *Sciences, 33*(2), 20–27.

Fausto-Sterling, A., & Balaban, E. (1993). Genetics and male sexual orientation, *Science, 261*, 1257.

FDA approves Lea's. (2002). *Contraception Report, 13*, 4–5. Retrieved October 12, 2005, from **http://www.contraceptiononline.org/contrareport/pdfs/13_02.pdf**

FDA issues approval status for single rod implant. (2005). *Contraceptive Technology Update, 26*, 1–3.

Federal Bureau of Investigation. (2002). Crime in the United States. *Uniform Crime Reports*. Retrieved January 2, 2006, from **http://www.fbi.gov/ucr/cius_02/html/web/arrested/04-table42.html**

Federal Bureau of Investigation. (2004a). *Crime in the United States, 2003: Uniform crime reports*.

Retrieved October 7, 2005, from **http://www.fbi.gov/ucr/cius_03/pdf/03sec2.pdf**

Federal Bureau of Investigation. (2004b). *Uniform crime reports: Hate crime statistics.* Retrieved October 7, 2005, from **http://www.fbi.gov/ucr/ucr.htm**

Fedoroff, J. P., Fishell, A., & Fedoroff, B. (1999). A case series of women evaluated for paraphilic sexual disorders. *Canadian Journal of Human Sexuality, 8*, 127–140.

Feeney, J., Kelly, L., Gallois, C., Peterson, C., & Terry, D. (1999). Attachment style, assertive communication, and safer-sex behavior. *Journal of Applied Social Psychology, 29*, 1964–1983.

Fehr, B. (2004). Intimacy expectations in same-sex friendships: A prototype interaction-pattern model. *Journal of Personality and Social Psychology, 86*, 265–284.

Fehring, R., Lawrence, D., & Philpot, C. (1994). The effectiveness of the Creighton Model ovulation method of family planning. *Journal of Obstetric, Gynecologic, and Neonatal Nursing, 23*, 303–309.

Feigenbaum, R., Weinstein, E., & Rosen, E. (1995). College students' sexual attitudes and behaviors: Implications for sexuality education. *Journal of American College Health, 44*, 112–118.

Feingold, A. (1988). Matching for attractiveness in romantic partners: A meta-analysis and theoretical critique. *Psychological Bulletin, 104*, 226–235.

Feldman, M., Goldstein, I., Hatzichristou, D., Krane, R., & McKinlay, J. (1994). Impotence and its medical and psychosocial correlates: Results of the Massachusetts Male Aging Study. *Journal of Urology, 151*, 54–61.

Feldman, R., Eidelman, A., Sirota, L., & Weller, A. (2002). Comparison of skin-to-skin (kangaroo). and traditional care: Parenting outcomes and preterm infant development. *Pediatrics, 110*, 16–26.

Felitti, V. J. (1991). Long-term medical consequences of incest, rape, and molestation. *Southern Medical Journal, 84*, 328–331.

Female masturbation. (2005). Sexual Health Info Center. Retrieved September 17, 2005, from **http://www.sexhealth.org/masturbation/female-masturbation.shtml**

FemCAP method receives market approval from the FDA. (2003). *Contraceptive Technology Update, 24*, 61–65.

Feminist Women's Health Center. (2004). Fertility awareness: Basal body temperature chart. Retrieved August 24, 2005, from **http://www.fwhc.org/birth-control/fam.htm**

Fetal development: How your baby grows. (2005). Retrieved September 25, 2005, from **http://www.babycenter.com**

Figgs, S., Villani, L., Horjatschun, N., & Sepr-ish, S. (2001). Adolescence: Change and continuity. Retrieved July 3, 2003, from **http://inside.bard.edu/academic/specialproj/darling/adolesce.htm**

Fincham, F., & Beach, S. (1999). Conflict in marriage: Implications for working with couples. *Annual Review of Psychology, 1999*, 47–77.

Fincham, F., & Bradbury, T. (1992). Assessing attributions in marriage: The relationship attribution measure. *Journal of Personality and Social Psychology, 62*, 457–468.

Finer, L., & Henshaw, S. (2003). Abortion incidence and services in the United States in 2000. *Perspectives of Sexual and Reproductive Health, 35*, 6–15.

Finger, W., Lund, M., & Slagle, M. (1997). Medications that may contribute to sexual disorders. *Journal of Family Practice, 44*, 33–43.

Finkelhor, D., & Jones, L. (2004, January). Explanations for the decline in child sexual abuse. *Juvenile Justice Bulletin*, pp. 1–12.

Finkelhor, D., & Yllo, K. (1985). *License to rape: Sexual abuse of wives*. New York: Holt, Rinehart and Winston.

Finkelson, L., & Oswalt, R. (1995). College date rape: Incidence and reporting. *Psychological Reports, 77*, 526.

Finn, R. (2004, February 15). Better prenatal diagnostic accuracy with MRI over ultrasound for brain spine problems. *Family Practice News*, p. 79.

Fischer, G. (1986). College students' attitudes toward forcible date rape: Changes after taking a human sexuality course. *Journal of Sex Education and Therapy, 12*, 42–46.

Fisher, B. S., Cullen, F. T., & Turner, M. G. (2000, December). *The sexual victimization of college women*. Washington, DC: U.S. Department of Justice. Retrieved February 24, 2006, from **http://www.ncjrs.org/pdffiles1/nij/182369.pdf**

Fisher, W. A. (1988). The sexual opinion survey. In C. Davis, W. Yarber, and S. Davis (Eds.), *Sexually related measures: A compendium* (pp. 34–38). Lake Mills, IA: Graphic Publishing.

Fisher, W. A., Byrne, D., White, L. A., & Kelley, K. (1988). Erotophobia-erotophilia as a dimension of personality. *Journal of Sex Research, 25*, 123–151.

Fisher, W. A., & Grenier, G. (1994). Violent pornography, antiwoman thoughts, and antiwoman acts: In search of reliable effects. *Journal of Sex Research, 31*, 23–38.

Fissell, M. (1999a). The paradox of twilight sleep. *Women's Health in Primary Care, 2*, 972.

Fissell, M. (1999b). Removing the curse of Eve. *Women's Health in Primary Care, 2*, 908.

Fitzgerald, B. (1999). Children of lesbian and gay parents: A review of the literature. *Marriage and Family Review, 29*, 57–75.

Flanagan, L. (1990). Demystifying masturbation. *Nursing Times, 86*, 36–37.

Flannery, D., Ellingson, L., Votaw, K. S., & Schaefer, E. A. (2003). Anal intercourse and sexual risk factors among college women, 1993–2000. *American Journal of Health Behavior, 27*, 228–234.

Flores, S., & Hartlaub, M. (1998). Reducing rape-myth acceptance in male college students: A meta-analysis of intervention studies. *Journal of College Student Development*, 39 438–448.

Floyd, F., & Stein, T. (2002). Sexual orientation identity formation among gay, lesbian, and bisexual youths: Multiple patterns of milestone experiences. *Journal of Research on Adolescence, 12*, 167–191.

Food and Drug Administration. (2003a). Lea's shield—P010043. Retrieved March 15, 2004, from **http://www.fda.gov/cdrh/pdf/P010043.html**

Food and Drug Administration. (2003b, January-February). New female sterilization device. *FDA Consumer*. Retrieved August 24, 2005, from **http://www.fda.gov/fdac/departs/2003/103_udp.html**

Forbes, G., Adams-Curtis, L., Hamm, N., & White, K. (2003). Perceptions of the woman who breastfeeds: The role of erotophobia, sexism, and attitudinal variables. *Sex Roles, 49*, 379–388.

Ford, C. S., & Beach, F. (1951). *Patterns of sexual behavior*. New York: Harper Bros.

Ford, N. (2001). Tackling female genital cutting in Somalia. *Lancet, 358*, 1179–1180.

Formichelli, L. (2001, January-February). The male pill. *Psychology Today*, p. 16.

Fortenberry, J., McFarlane, M., Bleakley, A., Bull, S., Fishbein, M., & Grimley, D. (2002). Relationships of stigma and shame to gonorrhea and HIV screening. *American Journal of Public Health, 92*, 378–381.

Foubert, J. D., & McEwan, M. K. (1998). An all-male rape-prevention peer education program: Decreasing fraternity men's behavioral intent to rape. *Journal of College Student Development, 36*, 548–556.

Foubister, V. (2000). RU-486 approval redraws abortion practice. *American Medical News, 43*, 1–3.

Fox, K. (1997). Mirror, mirror: A summary of the findings on body image. Retrieved March 5, 2003, from **http://www.sirc.org/publik/mirror.html**

Fox, K. K., Whittington, W. L., Levine, W. C., Moran, J. S., Zaidi, A. A., & Nakashima, A. K. (1998). Gonorrhea in the United States, 1984–1996: Demographic and geographic trends. *Sexually Transmitted Diseases, 26*, 386–393.

Fox, M. (1994). Vasectomy reversal: Microsurgery for best results. *British Journal of Urology, 73*, 449–453.

Fraker, M. A., Brown, R. G., Gaunt, G. E., Kerr, J. A., & Pohajdak, B. (2002). Long-lasting, single-dose immunocontraception of feral fallow deer in British Columbia. *Journal of Wildlife Management, 66*, 1141–1147.

Francoeur, R. (1996). *Taking sides: Clashing views on controversial issues in human sexuality*. Guilford, CT: Dushkin.

Frank, M. L., Poindexter, A. N., III, Cornin, L. M., Cox, C. A., & Bateman, L. (1993). One-year experience with subdermal contraceptive implants in the United States. *Contraception, 48*, 229–243.

Franzini, L., & Sideman, L. (1994). Personality characteristics of condom users. *Journal of Sex Education and Therapy, 20*, 110–118.

French, D., Jansen, E., & Pidada, S. (2002). United States and Indonesian children's and adolescent's reports of relational aggression by disliked peers. *Child Development, 73*, 1143–1150.

Freud, S. (1965). New introductory lectures on psychoanalysis. New York: Norton.

Freund, K., Seto, M. C., & Kuban, M. (1996). Two types of fetishism. *Behaviour Research and Therapy, 34*, 687–694.

Friedman, J. (2002, June 15). FDA advisory panel back HPV test as Pap smear adjunct. *Family Practice News*, pp. 30–31.

Friedrich, W., Fisher, J., Broughton, D., Houston, M., & Shafran, C. (1998). Normative sexual behavior in children: A contemporary sample [Electronic version]. *Pediatrics, 101*, 9–16.

Friedrich, W., & Gerber, P. (1994). Autoerotic asphyxia: The development of a paraphilia. *Journal of the American Academy of Child and Adolescent Psychiatry, 33*, 970–974.

Friedrich, W., Grambsch, P., Broughton, D., Kuiper, J., & Beilke, R. (1991). Normative sexual behavior in children. *Pediatrics, 88*, 456–465.

Friis-Moller, N., et al. (2003). Combination antiretroviral therapy and the risk of myocardial infarction. *New England Journal of Medicine, 349*, 1993–2003.

Frishman, G. (1995a). Abortions, miscarriages, and ectopic pregnancies. In D. Coustan, R. Haning, & D. Singer (Eds.), *Human reproduction: Growth and development* (pp. 189–211). Boston: Little, Brown.

Frishman, G. (1995b). Gametogenesis, fertilization, and implantation. In D. Coustan, R. Haning, & D. Singer (Eds.), *Human reproduction: Growth and development* (pp. 15–26). Boston: Little, Brown.

Frontline. (2002, February 15). The life and death of Billy Jack Gaither. PBS, *Assault on Gay America*. Retrieved July 3, 2004 from **http://www.pbs.org/wgbh/pages/frontline/shows/assault/billyjack**

FSD Alert. (2000). A new view of women's sexual problems. Retrieved August 16, 2005, from **http://www.fsd-alert.org/manifesto.html**

Fuertes, M. (1998, November). Ruling out sexual harassment. *Techniques*, pp. 42–43.

Funderburk, J. (2001). Group counseling for survivors of sexual assault. In A. J. Ottens & K. Hotelling (Eds.), *Sexual violence on campus: Policies, programs, and perspectives* (pp. 254–282). New York: Springer.

Furman, W. (2002). The emerging field of adolescent romantic relationships. *Current Directions in Psychological Science, 11*, 177–181.

G-8 adopts plan to speed HIV vaccine development. (2004, June 30). *Vaccine Weekly*, p. 27.

Garbo, J. (2002). All about semen. *Gay Health*. Retrieved October 22, 2004, from **http://www.gayhealth.com/iowa-robot/sex?record=643**

Garcia, L. (1986). Exposure to pornography and attitudes about women and rape: A correlational study. *Journal of Sex Research, 22*, 378–385.

Garcia, L. (1999). The certainty of the sexual self-concept. *Canadian Journal of Human Sexuality, 8*, 263–270.

Garcia, S., Khersonsky, D., & Stacey, S. (1997). Self-perceptions of physical attractiveness. *Perceptual and Motor Skills, 84*, 242–248.

Gardos, P., & Mosher, D. (1999). Gender differences in reactions to viewing pornographic vignettes: Essential or interpretive? *Journal of Psychology and Human Sexuality, 11*, 65–83.

Gardos, S. (1999). Relationships and sex: Experts. Retrieved June 7, 2002, from **http://www.oxygen.com/experts/drgardos/drgardos_19991019_print.jhtml**

Garofalo, R., Wolf, C., Wissow, L. S., Woods, E. R., & Goodman, E. (1999). Sexual orientation and risk of suicide attempts among a representative sample of youth. *Archives of Pediatrics and Adolescent Medicine, 153*, 487–493.

Garrahy, D. A. (2001). Three third-grade teachers' gender-related beliefs and behavior. *Elementary School Journal, 102*, 81–94.

Gates, G., & Sonenstein, F. (2000). Heterosexual genital sexual activity among adolescent males. *Family Planning Perspectives, 32*, 295–297, 304.

Gazeteer for Scotland. (1995). Sir James Young Simpson. Retrieved September 25, 2005, from **http://www.geo.ed.ac.uk/scotgaz/people/famousfirst60.html**

Geerling, J. (1995). Natural family planning. *American Family Physician, 52*, 1749–1759.

Geiger, A., & Foxman, B. (1996). Risk factors of vulvovaginal candidiasis: A case-control study among university students. *Epidemiology, 7*, 182–187.

Geller, A. (1991, March). Sexual problems of the recovering alcoholic. *Medical Aspects of Human Sexuality*, pp. 56–59.

Gender makes a difference in risk of HIV transmission. (2001, October 22). *AIDS Weekly*, p. 3.

Genital piercing may increase HIV transmission through oral sex. (2003, December 22). *AIDS Weekly*, p. 29.

George, W. H., & Stoner, S. A. (2000). Understanding acute alcohol effects on sexual behavior. *Annual Review of Sex Research, 11*, 92–124.

Gerszberg. C. (1998, April). Pregnancy pleasures. *Parents*, pp. 89–90.

Gibbs, N. (2003, July 7). A yea for gays: The Supreme Court scraps sodomy laws, setting off a hot debate. *Time*, pp. 38–39.

Gibson, L., & Leitenberg, H. (2000). Child sexual abuse prevention programs: Do they decrease the occurrence of child sexual abuse? *Child Abuse and Neglect, 24*, 1115–1125.

Giles, G., Severi, G., English, D., McCredie, M., Borland, R., Boyle, P. & Hopper, J. (2003). Sexual factors and prostate cancer. *British Journal of Urology International, 92*, 211–216.

Giles, J. (1994). A theory of love and attraction. *Journal for the Theory of Social Behaviour, 24*, 339–357.

Gillespie, R. (2003). Childfree and feminine: Understanding the gender identity of voluntarily childless women. *Gender and Society, 17*, 122–136.

Gilman, S., Cochran, S., Mays, V., Hughes, M., Ostrow, D., & Kessler, R. (2001). Risk of psychiatric disorders among individuals reporting same-sex sexual partners in the National Comorbidity Survey. *American Journal of Public Health, 91*, 933–939.

Giovannucci, E., Ascherio, A., Rimm, E. B., Colditz, G. A., Stampfer, M. J., & Willett, W. C. (1993). A prospective cohort study of vasectomy and prostate cancer in U.S. men. *Journal of the American Medical Association, 269*, 873–877.

Giovannucci, E., Tosteson, T. D., Speizer, F. E., Ascherio, A., Vessey, M. P., & Colditz, G. A. (1993). A retrospective cohort study of vasectomy and prostate cancer in U.S. men. *Journal of the American Medical Association, 269*, 878–882.

Glasier, A., & Baird, D. (1998). The effects of self-administering emergency contraception. *New England Journal of Medicine, 339*, 1–4.

Glass, G. (1976). Primary, secondary and meta-analysis of research. *Educational Researcher, 5*, 3–8.

Glenn, D. (2004, April 30). A dangerous surplus of sons? *Chronicle of Higher Education*, pp. A14–A15.

Gliner, J., Morgan, G., & Harmon, R. (2000). Introduction to inferential statistics and hypothesis testing. *Journal of the American Academy of Child and Adolescent Psychiatry, 39*, 1568–1569.

Goldbaum, G. M., Yu, T., & Wood, R. W. (1996). Changes at a human immunodeficiency virus testing clinic in the prevalence of unsafe sexual behavior among men who have sex with men. *Sexual Transmission of Disease, 23*, 109–114.

Goldston, L., & Wong. N. (2003, June 13). Teens talk frankly about sex, themselves. *San Jose Mercury News*, p. B3.

Golombok, S., & Tasker, F. (1996). Do parents influence the sexual orientation of their children? Findings from a longitudinal study of lesbian families. *Developmental Psychology, 32*, 3–11.

Goodman, R. E. (2001). Beyond the enforcement principle: Sodomy laws, social norms, and social panoptics. *California Law Review, 89*, 643–740.

Goodson, P., Suther, S., Pruitt, B., & Wilson, K. (2003). Defining abstinence. *Journal of School Health, 73*, 91–96.

Goodstein, L. (2004, February 27). Two studies cite child sex abuse by 4% of priests. *New York Times*, p. A1.

Gorey, K., & Leslie, D. (1997). The prevalence of child sexual abuse: Integrative review adjustment for potential response and measurement biases. *Child Abuse and Neglect, 21*, 391–398.

Gorey, K., & Leslie, D. (2001). Working toward a valid prevalence estimate of child sexual abuse: A reply to Bolen and Scannapieco. *Social Science Review, 75*, 151–156.

Gosink, P. D., & Jumbelic, M. I. (2000). Autoerotic asphyxiation in a female. *American Journal Forensic Medicine and Pathology, 21*, 114–118.

Gottleib, S. (2003). Oral sex may transmit HIV. *British Medical Journal, 326*, 730.

Gottman, J. M. (1994, March-April). What makes marriage work? *Psychology Today, 27*, 38–43.

Gottman, J. M. (1998). Psychology and the study of marital processes. *Annual Review of Psychology, 49*, 169–197.

Gottman, J. M., & Levenson, R. W. (2001). 12-year study of gay and lesbian couples. Gottman Institute. Retrieved November 23, 2002, from **http://www.gottman.com/research/projects/gaylesbian**

Gottman, J. M., & Levenson, R. W. (2002). A two-factor model for predicting when a couple will divorce: Exploratory analyses using

14-year longitudinal data. *Family Process, 41*, 83–95.

Gottman, J. M., & Notarius, C. (2002). Marital research in the 20th century and a research agenda for the 21st century. *Family Process, 41*, 159–197.

Gottman, J., & Silver, N. (2000). *The seven principles for making marriage work*. New York: Three Rivers Press.

Gottman, J. M., et al. (2003). Correlates of gay and lesbian couples' relationship satisfaction and relationship dissolution. *Journal of Homosexuality, 45*, 23–40.

Goulder, P., & Walker, B. (2002). HIV-1 superinfection: A word of caution. *New England Journal of Medicine, 347*, 756–758.

Graber, B. (1993). Medical aspects of sexual arousal disorders. In W. O'Donohue & J. Geer (Eds.), *Handbook of sexual dysfunctions* (pp. 103–156). Needham Heights, MA: Allyn & Bacon.

Grady, W. R., Klepinger, D. H., Billy, J. O. F., & Tanfer, K. (1993). Condom characteristics: The perceptions and preferences of men in the United States. *Family Planning Perspectives, 25*(2), 67–73.

Graham, C. (2003). A new view of women's sexual problems. *Journal of Sex and Marital Therapy, 29*, 325–327.

Graham, R. (2001, November 21). College students shunning condoms. Retrieved January 13, 2004, from **http://www.intelihealth.com**

Grammatopoulos, D. K., & Hillhouse, E. W. (1999). Role of corticotropin-releasing hormone in onset of labor. *Lancet, 354*, 1546–1549.

Gray, R., et al. (2001). Probability of HIV-1 transmission per coital act in monogamous, heterosexual, HIV-1-discordant couples in Rakai, Uganda. *Lancet, 357*, 1149–1153.

Green, R. (2001). (Serious) sadomasochism: A protected right of privacy? *Archives of Sexual Behavior, 30*, 543–549.

Greenberg, J., Bruess, C., & Haffner, D. (2002). *Exploring the dimensions of sexuality*. Sudbury, MA: Jones & Bartlett.

Grenier, G., & Byers, E. S. (1995). Rapid ejaculation: A review of the conceptual, etiological, and treatment issues. *Archives of Sexual Behavior, 24*, 447–472.

Grenier, G., & Byers, E. S. (1997). The relationship among ejaculatory control, ejaculatory latency, and attempts to prolong sexual intercourse. *Archives of Sexual Behavior, 26*, 27–47.

Griffin, R. (2004). Living longer with HIV therapy. Retrieved July 10, 2004, from **http://www.intelihealth.com**

Griffing, S., Ragin, D., Sage, R., Madry, L., Bingham, L., & Primm, B. (2002). Domestic violence survivors' self-identified reasons for returning to abusive relationships. *Journal of Interpersonal Violence, 17*, 306–319.

Grimes, D., & Raymond, E. (2002). Emergency contraception. *Annals of Internal Medicine, 137*, 180–189.

Groopman, J. (1999, September 13). Contagion (HPV). *New Yorker*, pp. 34–39.

Grossman, H. (2004a). Currently approved drugs for HIV: A comparative chart. Retrieved July 10, 2004, from **http://www.aidsmeds.com/lessons/DrugChart.htm**

Grossman, H. (2004b). Opportunistic infections. Retrieved July 10, 2004, from **http://www.aidsmeds.com/lessons/StartHere8.htm**

Grunbaum, J., Kann, L., Kinchen, S., & Ross, J. (2002). Youth risk surveillance: United States, 2001. *Mortality and Morbidity Weekly Report, 51*, 1–64.

Guattery, D. (2002). Stages of labor: What to expect. Retrieved on June 2, 2002, from **http://www.expectantmothersguide.com/library/philadelphia/EPHlabor.htm**

Guha, S. K. (2005). RISUG (reversible inhibition of sperm under guidance)—an antimicrobial as male vas deferens implant for HIV free semen. Medical Hypotheses, 65, 61–64.

Guillebaud, J. (1985). *Contraception: Your questions answered*. New York: Pitman.

Guillette, E. (2002). Unambiguous results: When Mexico's Yaqui Indians split into two different agricultural camps in the 1950s, their children became an unusually perfect test group for the effects of pesticide exposure. *Alternatives Journal, 28*, 24–26.

Gunn, R., Podschun, G., Fitzgerald, S., Hovell, M., Farshy, C., Black, C. & Greenspan, J. (1998). Screening high-risk adolescent males for *Chlamydia trachomatis* infection: Obtaining urine specimens in the field. *Sexually Transmitted Diseases, 25*, 49–52.

Guzick, D. (2000). When infertility can't be explained. *Contemporary OB/GYN, 9*, 102–112.

Hackshaw, A., & Paul, E. (2003). Breast self-examination and death from breast cancer: A meta-analysis. *British Journal of Cancer, 88*, 1047–1053.

Hahn, J., & Blass, T. (1997). Dating partner preferences: A function of similarity of love styles. *Journal of Social Behavior and Personality, 12*, 595–610.

Halkitis, P. N., Parsons, J. T., & Wilton, L. (2003). Barebacking among gay and bisexual men in New York City: Explanations for the emergence of intentional unsafe behavior. *Archives of Sexual Behavior, 32*, 351–358.

Hall, D., & Zhao, J. (1995). Cohabitation and divorce in Canada: Testing the selectivity hypothesis. *Journal of Marriage and Family, 57*, 421–427.

Hall, J. A. (1978). Gender effects in decoding nonverbal cues. *Psychological Bulletin, 85*, 845–857.

Hall, J. A. (1998). How big are nonverbal sex differences? The case of smiling and sensitivity to nonverbal cues. In D. J. Canary & K. Dindia (Eds.), *Sex differences and similarities in communication: Critical essays and empirical investigations of sex and gender in interaction* (pp. 157–177). Mahwah, NJ: Erlbaum.

Halpern, C. J. T., Udry, J. R., Suchindran, C., & Campbell, B. (2000). Adolescent males' willingness to report masturbation. *Journal of Sex Research, 3*, 327–332.

Halpern-Felsher, B., Cornell, J., Kropp, R., & Tschann, J. (2005). Oral sex among adolescents: Perceptions, attitudes, and behavior. *Pediatrics, 115*, 845–851.

Halpert, S. C. (2002). Suicidal behavior among gay male youth. *Journal of Gay and Lesbian Psychotherapy*, 6, 53–79.

Hamer, D., Hu, S., Magnuson, V., Hu, N., & Pattatucci, A. (1993). A linkage between DNA markers and the X chromosome and male sexual orientation. *Science, 261*, 321–327.

Han, A. J. (2005 August 16). Ignoring *Lawrence*. *Advocate*, p. 60.

Hariton, E. (1973, March). The sexual fantasies of women. *Psychology Today*, pp. 39–44.

Harlap, S., Kost, K., & Forrest, J. (1991). *Preventing pregnancy, protecting health: A new look at birth control choices in the United States*. New York: Alan Guttmacher Institute.

Harmon, A. (2004, June 20). In new tests for fetal defects, agonizing choices for parents. *New York Times*, p. A1.

Harney, P. A., & Muehlenhard, C. L. (1991). Factors that increase the likelihood of victimization. In A. Parrot & L. Bechhofer (Eds.), *Acquaintance rape: The hidden crime* (pp. 159–175). New York: Wiley.

Harper, B. (2001). Where to have your baby: Home births. Retrieved June, 4, 2002, from **http://www.lamaze.com**

Hart, R. (2003). Unexplained infertility, endometriosis, and fibroids. *British Medical Journal, 327*, 721–723.

Hartmann, K., Palmieri, R., Gartlehner, G., Thorp, J., Lohr, K., & Viswanathan, M. (2005). Outcomes of routine episiotomy. *Journal of the American Medical Association, 293*, 2141–2148.

Harvard Medical School. (2004). Report: China to teach sex ed to teens. InteliHealth: Harvard Medical School. Retrieved September 24, 2004, from **http://www.intelihealth.com**

Hatcher, R. A. (1998). Depo-Provera, Norplant, and progestin-only pills (minipills). In R. A. Hatcher, J. Trussell, F. Stewart, W. Cates Jr., G. K. Stewart, F. Guest, & D. Kowal (Eds.), *Contraceptive technology* (17th rev. ed., pp. 467–509). New York: Ardent Media.

Hatcher, R. A., & Guillebaud, J. (1998). The pill: Combined oral contraceptives. In R. A. Hatcher, J. Trussell, F. Stewart, W. Cates Jr., G. K. Stewart, F. Guest, & D. Kowal (Eds.), *Contraceptive technology* (17th rev. ed., pp. 405–466). New York: Ardent Media.

Hatcher, R. A., & Nelson, A. L. (2004). Combined hormonal contraceptive methods. In R. A. Hatcher, J. Trussell, F. Stewart, W. Cates Jr., A. L. Nelson, F. Guest, & D. Kowal (Eds.), *Contraceptive technology* (18th rev. ed., pp. 391–460). New York: Ardent Media.

Hatcher, R. A., Trussell, J., Stewart, F., Cates, W., Jr., Stewart, G. K., Guest, F., & Kowal, D. (Eds.). (1998). *Contraceptive technology* (17th rev. ed.). New York: Ardent Media.

Hatcher, R. A., Trussell, J., Stewart, F., Nelson, A. L., Cates, W., Jr., Guest, F., & Kowal, D. (Eds.) (2004). *Contraceptive technology* (18th rev. ed.). New York: Ardent Media.

Hatcher, R. A., et al. (1994). *Contraceptive technology* (16th rev. ed.). New York, Irvington.

Havemann, E., & Lehtinen, M. (1990). *Marriages and families: New problems, new opportunities* (2nd ed.). Englewood Cliffs, NJ: Prentice Hall.

Hawaleshka, D. (2001, February 19). Peeping Toms go electronic: Cheap, tiny spy cameras make women increasingly vulnerable to digital voyeurs. *Maclean's*, p. 24.

Hawkins, D. (2001). Oral sex and HIV transmission. *Sexually Transmitted Infections, 77*, 307–308.

Hawkins, R. (1993). How does a course in the psychology of human sexuality affect one's values? *Australian Journal of Marriage and Family, 14*, 2–9.

Hawton, K., Catalan, J., & Fagg, J. (1992). Long-term outcome of sex therapy. *Behaviour Research and Therapy, 24*, 665–675.

Healthwise. (2004). Choices for an abortion. Retrieved June 12, 2004, from **http://my.webmd.com/hw/womens_conditions**

Heiman, J. (2002). Sexual dysfunction: Overview of prevalence, etiological factors, and treatments. *Journal of Sex Research, 39*, 73–78.

Heino, F. L., et al. (1995). Prenatal estrogens and the development of homosexual orientation. *Developmental Psychology, 31*, 12–21.

Helfgott, J. (1997). The relationship between unconscious defensive process and conscious cognitive style in psychopaths. *Criminal Justice and Behavior, 24*, 278–293.

Hendrick, C., & Hendrick, S. (1986). A theory and method of love. *Journal of Personality and Social Psychology, 50*, 392–402.

Hendrick, S. (2004). Close relationship research: A resource for couple and family therapists. *Journal of Marital and Family Therapy, 3*, 13–32.

Heneghan, A., Silver, E., Bauman, L., & Stein, R. (2000). Do pediatricians recognize mothers with depressive symptoms? *Pediatrics, 106*, 1367.

Henshaw, S. (1998). Unintended pregnancy in the United States. *Family Planning Perspectives, 30*, 24–29, 46.

Henshaw, S., & Singh, S. (1986). Sterilization regret among U.S. couples. *Family Planning Perspectives, 18*, 238–240.

Hepatitis C in crack users. (2003, July 15). *Family Practice News*, p. 15.

Herek, G. M., & Capitanio, J. P. (1999). AIDS stigma and sexual prejudice. *American Behavioral Scientist, 42*, 1126–1143.

Herek, G. M., Widaman, K. F., & Capitanio, J. P. (2005). When sex equals AIDS: Symbolic stigma and heterosexual adults' inaccurate beliefs about sexual transmission of AIDS. *Social Problems, 52*, 15–37.

Herndon, J., Strauss, L., Whitehead, S., Parker, W., Bartlett, L., & Zane, S. (2002). Abortion surveillance: United States, 1998. *Morbidity and Mortality Weekly Report, 51*, 1–32.

Herron, W., & Herron, M. (1996). The complexity of sexuality. *Psychological Reports, 78*, 129–130.

Hershberger, S. (1997). A twin registry study of male and female sexual orientation. *Journal of Sex Research, 34*, 212–221.

Hicks, T., & Leitenberg, H. (2001). Sexual fantasies about one's partner versus someone else: Gender differences in incidence and frequency. *Journal of Sex Research, 38*, 43–50.

Hill, C. (2002). Gender, relationship stage, and sexual behavior: The importance of partner emotional investment within specific situations. *Journal of Sex Research, 39*, 228–240.

Hines, M., Ahmed, F., & Hughes, I., (2003). Psychological outcomes and gender-related development in complete androgen insensitivity syndrome. *Archives of Sexual Behavior, 32*, 93–101.

Hines, T. (2001). The G-spot: A modern gynecologic myth. *American Journal of Obstetrics and Gynecology, 185*, 359–362.

Hippensteele, S., & Pearson, T. (1999). Responding effectively to sexual harassment. *Change, 31*, 48–53.

His and hers . . . and how to have them. (2001, November-December). *Psychology Today*, pp. 54–58.

Hite, S. (1976). *The Hite report*. New York: Macmillan.

Hite, S. (1981). *The Hite report on male sexuality*. New York: Random House.

Hite, S. (1987). *Women and love: A cultural revolution in progress*. New York: Knopf.

HIV puzzle cracked. (2003). *New Scientist, 178*, 22.

Hock, R. R. (2003). *Insights in human sexuality*. Boston: Pearson Custom Publishing.

Hock, R. R. (2005). *Forty studies that changed psychology: Explorations into the history of psychological research* (5th ed.). Upper Saddle River, NJ: Prentice Hall.

Hoff, T., Greene, L., & Davis, J. (2003). *National survey of adolescents and young adults: Sexual health knowledge, attitudes, and experiences*. Menlo Park, CA: Henry J. Kaiser Foundation.

Holland, G. (2003). U.S. Supreme Court approves of library filters. Retrieved June 25, 2003, from **http://story.news.yahoo.com/news**

Hollander, D. (2000). Most abortion patients view their experience favorably, but medical abortion gets a higher rating than surgical. *Family Planning Perspectives, 32*, 264.

Hollander, D. (2001a). Female condoms remain structurally sound after being washed and reused as many as seven times. *International Family Planning Perspectives, 27*, 155–156.

Hollander, D. (2001b). Once a victim, always a victim? *Family Planning Perspectives, 33*, 50.

Hollander, D. (2002). Medical abortions: Decisions, decisions. *Perspectives of Sexual and Reproductive Health, 34*, 177.

Hollander, D. (2003). Another early abortion option. *Perspectives of Sexual and Reproductive Health, 35*, 5.

Hollander, E., & Rosen, J. (2000). Impulsivity. *Journal of Psychopharmacology, 14*, S39-S44.

Holman, T., & Jarvis, M. (2003). Hostile, volatile, and validating couple-conflict types: An investigation of Gottman's couple-conflict types. *Personal Relationships, 10*, 267–282.

Hong, J. (1984). Survival of the fastest: On the origins of premature ejaculation. *Journal of Sex Research, 20*, 109–112.

Hook, E., & Handsfield, H. (1999). Gonococcal infections in the adult. In K. K. Holmes, P. F. Sparling, P. March, S. M. Lemon, W. E. Stamm, P. Piot, & J. N. Wasserheit (Eds.), *Sexually transmitted diseases* (3d ed., pp. 451–466). New York: McGraw-Hill.

Houston Area Women's Center. (2005). Personal safety awareness. Retrieved August 10, 2005, from **https://www.pageconcepts.net/HoustonAreaWomensCenter/teens.asp**

Howard, K., & Stevens, A. (2000). *Out and about campus: Personal accounts of lesbian, gay, bisexual, and transgendered college students*. Los Angeles: Alyson Publications.

Hsu, B., Kling, A., Kessler, C., Knapke, K., Diefenbach, P., & Elias, J. E. (1994). Gender differences in sexual fantasy and behavior in a college population: A ten-year replication. *Journal of Sex and Marital Therapy, 20*, 103–118.

Huang, A., Ring, A., Toich, S., & Torres, T. (1998, March 1). Gender inequalities in education. Gender relations in educational applications of technology. Retrieved July 8, 2003, from **http://www.stanford.edu/~ttorres/GREAT/index.htm**

Hubacher, D. (2002). The checkered history and bright future of intrauterine contraception in the United States. *Perspectives on Sexual and Reproductive Health, 34*, 98–103.

Hubler, D. (2004, December 1). New report finds abstinence-only programs mislead students. *Education Daily*, p. 3.

Hucker, S. J., & Blanchard, R. (1992). Death scene characteristics in 118 fatal cases of autoerotic asphyxia compared with suicidal asphyxia. *Behavioral Sciences and the Law, 10*, 509–523.

Huebner, D. M., Rebchook, G. M., & Kegeles, S. M. (2004). Experiences of harassment, discrimination, and physical violence among young gay and bisexual men. *American Journal of Public Health, 94*, 1200–1202.

Huffman, G. B. (2002). Is vasectomy associated with prostate cancer? *American Family Physician, 66*, 1762.

Human immunocontraceptive vaccine under development. (2000, December 27). *Vaccine Weekly*, p. 1.

Human Rights Campaign. (2004). Marriage/relationship recognition. Retrieved November 18, 2005, from **http://www.hrc.org**

Humphrey, S., & Kahn, A. (2000). Fraternities, athletic teams, and rape: Importance of identification with a risky group. *Journal of Interpersonal Violence, 15*, 1313–1322.

Hunt, M. (1974). *Sexual behavior in the 1970s*. Chicago: Playboy Press.

Hunter, C. (2000). The dangers of pornography? A review of the effects literature. Retrieved June 15, 2003, from **http://www.asc.upenn.edu/usr/chunter/porn_effects.html**

Hyde, J. S. (2005). The gender similarities hypothesis. *American Psychologist, 60*, 581–592.

Ibbison, M. (2002). Out of the sauna: Sexual health promotion with "off-street" sex workers. *Journal of Epidemiology and Community Health, 56*, 903–904.

Inaccurate data may sway choices when it comes to intrauterine devices: Push is on to dispel the myths surrounding IUDs. (2002). *Contraceptive Technology Update, 25*, 13–16.

Inciardi, J., & Surratt, H. (1997). Male transvestite sex workers and HIV in Rio de Janeiro, Brazil. *Journal of Drug Issues, 27*, 135–146.

Indman, P. (2000). What is hysteroscopy? Retrieved January 11, 2002, from **http://www.gynalternatives.com/hysteroscopy.htm**

Ingall, M. (1995, May). Sex in the USA: Wake us when it's over. *Ms.*, p. 93.

Ingrassia, M. (1989, May 5). In 1952 she was a scandal. *Newsday*, p. 2.

Initial results of phase III AIDS vaccine trial announced. (2003, March 24). *AIDS Weekly*, pp. 9–10.

InteliHealth. (2004a). Blood transfusions: Safer than ever. Retrieved June 12, 2004, from **http://www.intelihealth.com**

Inteli Health. (2004b). UN: HIV infections hit record high in '03. Retrieved July 10, 2003, from **http://www.intelihealth.com**

International Foundation for Gender Education. (2002). Transgender tapestry. Retrieved September 12, 2002, from **http://www.ifge.org**

Internet Filter Review. (2003). Internet statistics. Retrieved June 24, 2003, from **http://www.internetfilterreview.com/internet-pornography-statistics.html**

Intons-Peterson, M., & Roskos-Ewoldsen, B. (1987). Mitigating the effects of violent pornography. In S. Gubar & J. Hoff-Wilson (Eds.), *For adult users only: The dilemma of violent pornography* (pp. 220–228). Bloomington: Indiana University Press.

Irving, J. M. (1995). *Sexuality education across cultures: Working with differences*. San Francisco: Jossey-Bass.

Jacobson, G., Autry, A., Kirby, R., Liverman, E., & Motley, R. (2001). A randomized controlled trial comparing amoxicillin and azithromycin for the treatment of *Chlamydia trachomatis* in pregnancy. *American Journal of Obstetrics and Gynecology, 184*, 1352–1356.

Jancin, B. (2000, October 1). STD chemoprophylaxis reduces preterm birth. *Family Practice News*, pp. 24–25.

Jancin, B. (2004, January 15). High anal HPV prevalence in gay men of all ages: Unusual infection pattern. *Family Practice News*, p. 30.

Janus, S., & Janus, C. (1993). *The Janus report on sexual behavior*. New York: Wiley.

Jenike, M. A. (2004). Obsessive-compulsive disorder. *New England Journal of Medicine, 350*, 259–265.

Jenkins, A. P. (2000). When self-pleasuring becomes self-destruction: Autoerotic asphyxiation paraphilia. *International Electronic Journal of Health Education, 3*, 208–216.

Jenkins, A. P. (2004). *The autoerotic asphyxia pages*. Retrieved September 13, 2004, from **http://www.cwu.edu/~jenkinsa/Autoerotic_Asphyxia_Page.html**

Jenkins, P. (2002, March 1). Bringing the loathsome to light. *Chronicle of Higher Education*, pp. B16–B17.

Jennings, V., Lamprecht, V., & Kowal, D. (1998). Fertility awareness methods. In R. A. Hatcher, J. Trussell, F. Stewart, W. Cates Jr., G. K. Stewart, F. Guest, & D. Kowal (Eds.), *Contraceptive technology* (17th rev. ed., pp. 309–324). New York: Ardent Media.

Jenny, C., Roesler, T. A., & Poyer, K. (1994). Are children at risk of sexual abuse by homosexuals? *Pediatrics, 94*, 41–43.

Jensen, M. (1998). Heterosexual women have noisy ears. *Science News, 153*, 151.

Jick, S., Walker, A., & Jick, H. (1993). Oral contraceptives and endometrial cancer. *Obstetrics and Gynecology, 82*, 931–935.

Jobe, D. (2002). Helping girls succeed. *Educational Leadership, 60*, 64–66.

Johannsen, G. (2001). Can cranberry juice assist in the treatment of UTIs? *Health Observances, 9*. Retrieved December 26, 2002, from **http://med.usd.edu/family/hfactor/2001/01maypg8.htm**

Johns Hopkins University. (2001). Use of Norplant worldwide. Retrieved January 8, 2002, from **http://www.reproline.jhu.edu**

Johnson, F., & Young, K. (2002). Gendered voices in children's television advertising. *Critical Studies in Mass Communication, 19*, 461–480.

Johnson, J. (2005). The stages of development of puberty in girls. Retrieved February 22, 2006, from **http://www.coolnurse.com/puberty_stages.htm**

Johnson, K. (1996). The politics of the revival of infant abandonment in China. *Population and Development Review, 22*, 77–100.

Johnson, K. (2000a, February 1). Calcium channel blocker as a male contraceptive. *Family Practice News*, p. 49.

Johnson, K. (2000b, May 15). A half-dose ends ectopic pregnancy: Methotrexate. *Family Practice News*, p. 32.

Johnson, K. (2002, December 1). Sildenafil tackles women's sexual arousal disorder. *Family Practice News*, p. 40.

Johnson, K. (2004, December 15). Testosterone patch may relieve sexual dysfunction in surgically menopausal women. *Family Practice News*, p. 84.

Johnson, L. (2002). Sexuality after childbirth. *Baby Parenting*. Retrieved June 7, 2002, from **http://babyparenting.about.com/library/weekly/aa010999.htm**

Johnson, R. (2002). The changing face of AIDS. *AIDS Reader, 12*, 373–375.

Johnson, T. C. (2001, July). Understanding the sexual behavior of children. International Child and Youth Care Network. *CYC-Online*. Retrieved July 5, 2003, from **http://www.cyc-net.org/cyc-online/cycol-0701-toni1.html**

Jones, D. L., et al. (1998). The high-risk sexual practices of crack-smoking sex workers recruited from the streets of three American cities. *Sexually Transmitted Diseases, 25*, 187–195.

Jones, J., & Barlow, D. (1990). Self-reported frequency of sexual urges, fantasies, and masturbatory fantasies in heterosexual males and females. *Archives of Sexual Behavior, 19*, 269–279.

Jones, R. K., Darroch, J. E., & Henshaw, S. K. (2002). Contraceptive use among U.S. women having abortions in 2000–2001. *Perspectives in Sexual and Reproductive Health, 34*, 294–303.

Jordan, K., & Deluty, R. (1998). Coming out for lesbian women: Its relationship to anxiety, positive affectivity, self-esteem, and social support. *Journal of Homosexuality, 35*, 41–63.

Josefson, D. (2003). Unsafe sexual practices are common, say U.S. studies. *British Medical Journal, 327*, 10.

Jow, W., & Goldstein, M. (1994). No-scalpel vasectomy offers minimal invasiveness. *Contemporary OB/GYN, 39*, 83–96.

Jurand, S. H. (2004). Sexual privacy is not a right in Eleventh Circuit, despite Lawrence. *Trial, 40*, 87.

Kafka, M. P. (1997). A monoamine hypothesis for the pathology of paraphilia disorders. *Archives of Sexual Behavior, 26*, 343–358.

Kafka, M. P., & Hennen, J. (2003). Hypersexual desire in males: Are males with paraphilias different from males with paraphilia-related disorders? *Sex Abuse, 15*, 307–321.

Kagan, J. (1992). Behavior, biology, and the meanings of temperamental constructs. *Pediatrics, 90*, 510–513.

Kahn, J., Rosenthal, S., Succop, P., Ho, G., & Burk, R. (2002). Mediators of the association between age of first sexual intercourse and subsequent HPV infection. *Pediatrics, 109*, E5. Retrieved December 23, 2004, from **http://pediatrics.aappublications.org/cgi/content/full/109/1/e5**

Kaiser Family Foundation. (2001, May). *Condom fact sheet*. Menlo Park, CA.

Kalb, C. (2003, February 3). Farewell to 'Aunt Flo': A new version of the birth-control pill would limit menstruation to four times a year. Are women ready? *Newsweek*, 48.

Kalb, C., Nadeau, B., & Schafer, S. (2004, February 2). Brave new babies: Parents now have the power to choose the sex of their children. *Newsweek International*, pp. 38–40.

Kalick, S. (1988). Physical attractiveness as a status cue. *Journal of Experimental Social Psychology, 24*, 469–489.

Kalidad, R. (2001). We've come a long way, baby: The history of condoms. *Miscellany News* (Vassar College). Retrieved January 11, 2002, from **http://www.studentadvantage.lycos.com**

Kanin, E. (1982). Female rape fantasies: A victimization study. *Victimology, 7*, 114–121.

Kantrowitz, B., Roediger, H., & Elmes, D. (1994). *Experimental psychology*. Minneapolis, MN: West.

Kaplan, H. S. (1974). *The new sex therapy: Active treatment of sexual dysfunctions*. New York: Brunner/Mazel.

Kaplan, H. S. (1995). *The sexual desire disorders: Dysfunctional regulation of sexual motivation*. New York: Brunner/Mazel.

Kaplan, L. J. (1997). Clinical manifestations of the perverse strategy. *Journal of Psychoanalysis and Psychotherapy, 14*, 79–89.

Karney, B., Bradbury, T., Fincham, F., & Sullivan, K. (1994). The role of negative affectivity in the association between attributions and marital satisfaction. *Journal of Personality and Social Psychology, 66*, 413–424.

Karraker, K., Vogel, D., & Lake, M. (1995). Parents' gender-stereotyped perceptions of newborns: The eye of the beholder revisited. *Sex Roles, 33*, 687–701.

Kaschak, A., & Tiefer, L. (Eds.). (2002). *A new view of women's sexual problems*. Binghamtom, NY: Haworth Press.

Kass-Wolf, J. (2001). Bone loss in adolescents using Depo-Provera. *Journal of the Society of Pediatric Nurses, 6*, 21–31.

Katz, E. (2002). Biographical sketch: Mary Louise Higgins (Sanger). Retrieved February 16, 2004, from **http://www.nyu.edu/projects/sanger/msbio.htm**

Kaunitz, A. M. (2001). Choosing an injectable contraceptive. *Contemporary OB/GYN, 46*, 29–48.

Kay, D. S. G. (1992). Masturbation and mental health: Uses and abuses. *Sexual and Marital Therapy, 7*, 97–107.

Kaye, D. (2003). FDA approves rapid HIV-1 antibody test. *Clinical Infectious Diseases, 36*, i–ii.

Keller, M., von Sadovsky, V., Pankratz, B., & Hermsen, J. (2000). Self-disclosure of HPV infection to sexual partners. *Western Journal of Nursing Research, 22*, 285–302.

Kellogg, A. P. (2002, January 18). "Safe sex fatigue" grows among gay students: Health officials change their HIV-education strategies as condom use declines. *Chronicle of Higher Education*, pp. A37–A39.

Kelly, M., Strassberg, D., & Kircher, J. (1990). Attitudinal and experiential correlates of anorgasmia. *Archives of Sexual Behavior, 19*, 165–177.

Kelly, R. (2001). Sexual behavior of college students attending four universities in a southern state. *Research Quarterly for Exercise and Sport, 72*, A31.

Keltner, N., McAfee, K., & Taylor, C. (2002). Mechanisms and treatments of SSRI-induced sexual dysfunction. *Perspectives in Psychiatric Care, 38*, 111–116.

Kendall-Tackett, K. (2000). Physiological correlates of childhood abuse: Chronic hyperarousal in PTSD, depression, and irritable bowel syndrome. *Child Abuse and Neglect, 24*, 799–811.

Kendler, K., Thornton, L., Gilman, S., & Kessler, R. (2000). Sexual orientation in a U.S. national sample of twin and nontwin sibling pairs. *American Journal of Psychiatry, 157*, 1843–1844.

Kennedy, K., & Trussell, J. (1998). Postpartum contraception and lactation. In R. A. Hatcher, J. Trussell, F. Stewart, W. Cates Jr., G. K. Stewart, F. Guest, & D. Kowal (Eds.), *Contraceptive technology* (17th rev. ed., pp. 589–614). New York: Ardent Media.

Kerckhoff, A. (1962). Value consensus and need-complementarity in mate selection. *American Sociological Review, 27*, 295–303.

Kero, A., Hogmerg, U., Jacobsson, L., & Lalos, A. (2001). Legal abortion: A painful necessity. *Social Science and Medicine, 53*, 1481.

Kestleman, P., & Trussell, J. (1991). Efficacy of the simultaneous use of condoms and spermicide. *Family Planning Perspectives, 23*, 226–227.

Kimmel, S. (2002). Vaccine adverse effects: Separating myth from reality. *American Family Physician, 66*, 2113–2120.

King, B., Parisi, B., & O'Dwyer, K. (1993). College sexuality education promotes future discussions about sexuality between former students and their children. *Journal of Sex Education and Therapy, 19*, 285–293.

King, M., & Woolett, E. (1997). Sexually assaulted males: 115 men consulting a counseling service. *Archives of Sexual Behavior, 26*, 579–588.

Kinsey, A.C., Pomeroy, W. B., & Martin, C. E. (1948). *Sexual behavior in the human male*. Philadelphia: Saunders.

Kinsey, A. C., Pomeroy, W. B., Martin, C. E., & Gebhard, P. H. (1953). *Sexual behavior in the human female*. Philadelphia: Saunders.

Kirby, D. (2001). *Emerging answers: Research findings on programs to reduce teen pregnancy*. Washington, DC: National Campaign to Prevent Teen Pregnancy.

Kirn, T. F. (2001, October 1). Experts say IUD set for a rebound. *OB/GYN News*, pp. 15–16.

Klein, F., Sepekoff, B., & Wolf, T. J. (1985). Sexual orientation: A multivariable dynamic process. *Journal of Homosexuality, 11*, 35–49.

Klein, M. (1993, May). Am I sexually normal? *New Woman*, pp. 49–52.

Klein, M. (1997). Disorders of desire. In R. Charlton & I. Yalom (Eds.), *Treating sexual disorders* (pp. 201–236). San Francisco: Jossey-Bass.

Klitsch, M. (1988). The return of the IUD. *Family Planning Perspectives, 20*, 19–20.

Klitsch, M. (1994). Proportion of high school students receiving AIDS instruction increases, while risky behavior declines. *Family Planning Perspectives, 26*, 144–145.

Klohnen, E., & Mendelsohn, G. (1998). Partner selection for personality characteristics: A couple-centered approach. *Personality and Social Psychology Bulletin, 24*, 268–278.

Klotter, J. (2002, January). Pregnancy and older women. *Townsend Letter for Doctors and Patients*, pp. 17–18.

Knight, D. (2004). Health care screening for men who have sex with men. *American Family Physician, 69*, 2149–2156.

Knight, G. P., Fabes, R. A., & Higgins, D. A. (1996). Concerns about drawing causal inferences from meta-analyses: An example in the study of gender differences in aggression. *Psychological Bulletin, 119*, 410–421.

Knight, G. P., Guthrie, I. K., Page, M. C., & Fabes, R. A. (2002). Emotional arousal and gender differences in aggression: A meta-analysis. *Aggressive Behavior, 28*, 366–394.

Knowles, J., & Dimitrov, D. (2002). Medical abortion: Questions and answers. Retrieved June 12, 2004, from **http://www.plannedparenthood.org/abortion/medicalabortion.html**

Knox, D., Zusman, M. E., Mabon, L., & Shriver, L. (1999). Jealousy in college student relationships. *College Student Journal, 33*, 328–329.

Knudsen, D. (1991). Child sexual coercion. In E. Grauerholz & M. Koralewski (Eds.), *Sexual coercion: A sourcebook on its nature, causes, and prevention* (pp. 17–28). Lexington, MA: Lexington Books.

Koff, E., & Benavage, A. (1998). Breast size and satisfaction, body image, and psychological functioning in Caucasian and Asian college women. *Sex Roles, 38*, 655–673.

Kokish, R. (2001). Sex offender treatment: Does it work? Is it worth it? California Coalition on Sexual Offending. Retrieved September 15, 2002, from **http://www.ccoso.org/newsletter/worthit.html**

Komisaruk, B. R., & Whipple, B. (1995). The suppression of pain by genital stimulation in females. *Annual Review of Sex Research, 6*, 151–186.

Kopper, B., & Smith, S. (2001). Knowledge and attitudes toward infertility and childless couples. *Journal of Applied Social Psychology, 31*, 2275–2291.

Koutsky, L., & Kiviat, N. (1999). Genital human papillomavirus. In K. K. Holmes, P. F. Sparling, P. March, S. M. Lemon, W. E. Stamm, P. Piot, & J. N. Wasserheit (Eds.), *Sexually transmitted diseases* (3d ed., pp. 347–359). New York: McGraw-Hill.

Kovalevsky, G., & Polaneczky, M. (2004). An analysis of the Today sponge: Prepare for its return to the United States. *Contraceptive Technology Update, 25*, S1–S3.

Kowal, D. (1998a). Abstinence and the range of sexual expression. In R. A. Hatcher, J. Trussell, F. Stewart, W. Cates Jr., G. K. Stewart, F. Guest, & D. Kowal (Eds.), *Contraceptive technology* (17th rev. ed., pp. 297–302). New York: Ardent Media.

Kowal, D. (1998b). Coitus interruptus (withdrawal). In R. A. Hatcher, J. Trussell, F. Stewart, W. Cates Jr., G. K. Stewart, F. Guest, & D. Kowal (Eds.), *Contraceptive technology* (17th rev. ed., pp. 303–307). New York: Ardent Media.

Kowal, D. (2004). Abstinence and the range of sexual expression. In R. A. Hatcher, J. Trussell, F. Stewart, W. Cates Jr., A. L. Nelson, F. Guest, & D. Kowal (Eds.), *Contraceptive technology* (18th rev. ed., pp. 305–310). New York: Ardent Media.

Krafft-Ebing, R., von, & Klaf, F. (1998). *Psychopathia sexualis, with especial reference to the antipathic sexual instinct: A medico-forensic study*. New York: Arcade. (Originally published 1886)

Krahe, B., Waizenhofer, E., & Moller, I. (2003). Women's sexual aggression against men: Prevalence and predictors. *Sex Roles, 49*, 219–232.

Kreslin, D. (1993). Medical aspects of inhibited desire disorder. In W. O'Donohue & J. Geer (Eds.), *Handbook of sexual dysfunctions* (pp. 15–51). Needham Heights, MA: Allyn & Bacon.

Krueger, R. B., & Kaplan, M. S. (2001). Depot-leuprolide acetate for treatment of paraphilias: A report of twelve cases. *Archives of Sexual Behavior, 30*, 409–422.

Kruger, P. (2003, October 10). Catholic church accused of spreading bad advice on AIDS. Retrieved November 23, 2003, from **http://www.abc.net.au/worldtoday/content/2003/s964339.htm**

Kubetin, S. (2002). HPV-infected men need Pap smears to spot anal dysplasia. *Internal Medicine Review, 35*, 11.

Kunkel, A., & Burleson, B. (2003). Rational implications of communication skill evaluations and love-styles. *Southern Communication Journal, 68*, 181–197.

Kurdek, L. A. (2001). Differences between heterosexual nonparent couples and gay, lesbian, and heterosexual parent couples. *Journal of Family Issues, 22*, 727–754.

Kusseling, F., Wenger, N., & Shapiro, M. (1995). Inconsistent contraceptive use among female college students: Implications for intervention. *College Health, 43*, 191–195.

Kutchinsky, B. (1991). Pornography and rape: Theory and practice? Evidence from crime data in four countries where pornography is easily available. *International Journal of Law and Psychiatry, 14*, 47–64.

Laan, E., Everaerd, W., van Bellen, G., & Gerritt, H. (1994). Women's sexual and emotional responses to male- and female-produced erotica. *Archives of Sexual Behavior, 23*, 153–169.

Lab technique brings immune-based therapies closer to reality. (2003, May 14). *Immunotherapy Weekly*, pp. 93–94.

Lacy, R., Reifman, A., Pearson, J., Harris, S., & Fitzpatrick, J. (2004). Sexual-moral attitudes, love styles, and mate selection. *Journal of Sex Research, 41*, 121–128.

La Franiere, S. (2003, February 22). Russians feel abortion's complications. *Washington Post*, p. A16.

Lake Snell Perry & Associates. (2002). Lower-income parents on teaching and talking with children about sexual issues: Results from a national survey. *Sexuality Education and Information Council of the U.S. (SEICUS)*. Retrieved July 5, 2003, from **http://www.siecus.org/media/press/poll.pdf**

Lalumiere, M., Blanchard, R., & Zucker, K. J. (2000). Sexual orientation and handedness in men and women: A meta-analysis. *Psychological Bulletin, 126*, 575–592.

La Mastro, V. (2001). Childless by choice? Attributions and attitudes concerning family size. *Social Behavior and Personality, 29*, 231–243.

Lambda Legal Defense and Education Fund. (2005). State by state: Antidiscrimination laws. Retrieved October 6, 2005, from **http://www.lambdalegal.org/cgi-bin/iowa/states/antidiscrimi-map**

Lang, S. (1997). Childhood sexual abuse affects relationships in adulthood. *Human Ecology Forum, 25*, 3.

Langevin, R. (1992). Biological factors contributing to paraphilia behavior. *Psychiatric Annals, 22*, 309–314.

Langevin, R., Lang, R., Wright, P., Handy, L., Frenzel, R., & Black, E. (1988). Pornography and sexual offenses. *Annals of Sexual Research, 1*, 335–362.

Laqueur, T. W. (2004). *Solitary sex: A cultural history of masturbation*. Cambridge, MA: MIT Press.

Large clinican trial launced to test "male pill" in 14 European centers. (2004, February 9). *Clinical Trials Week*, p. 3.

Larsson, I., & Svedlin, C. (2002). Sexual experiences in childhood: Young adults' recollections. *Archives of Sexual Behavior, 31*, 263–273.

Lasker, J. N., & Toedter, L. J. (2003). The impact of ectopic pregnancy: A 16-year follow-up study. *Health Care for Women International, 24*, 209–220.

Laumann, E., Gagnon, J., Michael, R., & Michaels, S. (1994). *The social organization of sexuality: Sexual practices in the United States*. Chicago: University of Chicago Press.

Laumann, E., Paik, A., & Rosen, R. (1999). Sexual dysfunction in the United States: Prevalence and predictors. *Journal of the American Medical Association, 281*, 537–544.

Lawrence, A. (2003). Factors associated with satisfaction or regret following male-to-female sex reassignment surgery. *Archives of Sexual Behavior, 32*, 209–215.

Leaper, C. (1991). Influence and involvement in children's discourse: Age, gender, and partner effects. *Child Development, 62*, 797–811.

Leaper, C. (1994). Exploring the consequences of gender segregation on social relationships. In C. Leaper (Ed.), *New directions for child development, No. 65. Childhood gender segregation: Causes and consequences* (pp. 67–86). San Francisco: Jossey-Bass.

Lee, C. (2005). Common myths about prostitution. Retrieved June 6, 2005, from **http://www.internetcampus.com/prostitution.htm**

Lee, J., Jackson, H., Pattison, P., & Ward, T. (2002). Developmental risk factors for sexual offending. *Child Abuse and Neglect, 26*, 73–92.

Lee, J. A. (1973). *The colors of love: An exploration of the ways of loving*. Don Mills, Ontario: New Press.

Lee, J. A. (1977). A typology of styles of loving. *Personality and Social Psychology Bulletin, 3*, 173–182.

Lee, J. A. (1988). Love-styles. In R. J. Sternberg & M. L. Barnes (Eds.), *The psychology of love* (pp. 38–67). New Haven, CT: Yale University Press.

Leiblum, S. (2000). Vaginismus: A most perplexing problem. In S. Leiblum & R. Rosen (Eds.), *Principles and practice of sex therapy* (pp. 181–202). New York: Guilford Press.

Leiblum, S., & Rosen, R. (Eds.). (2000). *Principles and practice of sex therapy*. New York: Guilford Press.

Leitenberg, H., Detzer, M., & Srebnik, D. (1993). Gender differences in masturbation and the relation of masturbation experience in preadolescence and/or early adolescence to sexual behavior and sexual adjustment in young adulthood. *Archives of Sexual Behavior, 22*, 87–98.

Leitenberg, H., & Henning, K. (1995). Sexual fantasy. *Psychological Bulletin, 117*, 469–496.

Lemieux, R., & Hale, J. (2002). Cross-sectional analysis of intimacy, passion, and commitment: Testing the assumptions of the triangular theory of love. *Psychological Reports, 90*, 1009–1115.

Lemon, S. M., & Alter, M. J. (1999). Viral hepatitis. In K. K. Holmes, P. F. Sparling, P. March, S. M. Lemon, W. E. Stamm, P. Piot, & J. N. Wasserheit (Eds.), *Sexually transmitted diseases* (3d ed., pp. 361–384). New York: McGraw-Hill.

Letourneau, E., & O'Donohue, W. (1993). Sexual desire disorders. In W. O'Donohue & J. Geer (Eds.), *Handbook of sexual dysfunctions* (pp. 53–81). Needham Heights, MA: Allyn & Bacon.

Leung, A., & Robson, L. (1993). Childhood masturbation. *Clinical Pediatrics, 32*, 238–241.

LeVay, S. (1991). A difference in hypothalamic structure between heterosexual and homosexual men. *Science, 253*, 1034–1037.

LeVay, S. (1998). The knitting circle: Genetics. Retrieved February 22, 2006, from **http://myweb.lsbu.ac.uk/stafflag/simonlevay.html**

Levin, J. (2002). *Anal sex increases risk for heterosexual HIV transmission*. Conference report for the National AIDS Treatment Advocacy Project. Retrieved November 12, 2003, from **http://www.natap.org/2002/barcelona/day22.htm**

Levine, J., & Elders, J. M. (2002). Harmful to minors: The perils of protecting children from sex. Minneapolis, MN: University of Minnesota Press.

Li, Q. (1999). Teachers' beliefs and gender differences in mathematics: A review. *Educational Research, 41*, 63–76.

Li, Y., Cottrelli, D., Wagner, D., & Ban, M. (2004). Needs and preferences regarding sex education among Chinese college students: A preliminary study. *International Family Planning Perspectives, 30*, 1–11.

Lief, H., & Hubschman, L. (1993). Orgasm in the postoperative transsexual. *Archives of Sexual Behavior, 22*, 145–155.

Lin, K., & Kirchner, J. (2004). Hepatitis B. *American Family Physician, 69*, 75–82.

Linz, D. G., & Donnerstein, E. I. (1990, April-May). Sexual violence in the media. *World Health*, 26–27.

Linz, D. G., & Donnerstein, E. I. (1992, September 30). Research can help us explain violence and pornography. *Chronicle of Higher Education*, pp. B3–B4.

Liu, P. Y., Swerdloff, R. S., Christenson, P. D., Handelsman, D. J., Wang, C. (2006) Rate, extent, and modifiers of spermatogenic recovery after hormonal male contraception: an integrated analysis. The Lancet. 367, 1412–1420.

Locayo, R. (1986, March 10). Give-and-take on pornography. *Time*, p. 67.

Lockwood, C. J. (2000). Prediction of pregnancy loss. *Lancet, 355*, 1292–1293.

Loftus, E. (1980). *Memory: Surprising new insights into how we remember and why we forget*. Reading, MA: Addison-Wesley.

Long, H., Nelson, L., & Hoffman, R. (2002). Ketamine medication error resulting in death. *Journal of Toxicology: Clinical Toxicology, 40*, 614.

Longo, D., & Koehn, K. (1993). Psychosocial factors and recurrent genital herpes: A review of prediction and psychiatric treatment studies. *International Journal of Psychiatry in Medicine, 23*, 99–117.

Lopes, S. (2001). AIDS-related stigma. Retrieved November 23, 2002, from **http://www.asc.upenn.edu**

Lothstein, L. M. (1997). Pantyhose fetishism and self cohesion: A paraphilic solution? *Gender and Psychoanalysis, 2*, 103–121.

Lott, D. A., & Veronsky, F. (1999, January-February). The new flirting game. *Psychology Today*, pp. 42–45.

Lowman, J., Atchinson, C., & Fraser, L. (1997). Sexuality in the 1990s: Survey results: The Internet client sample. Retrieved June 28, 2003, from **http://users.uniserve.com/~lowman/ICSS/netcsamp.htm**

Lu, S. (2004, October). Vasectomy reversals work. *Prevention*, p. 139.

Lubman, S. (2000, March 17). Infanticide detailed in China. *San Jose Mercury News*, p. 1A.

Lucchetti, A. (1999). Deception in disclosing one's sexual history: Safe-sex avoidance or ignorance? *Communication Quarterly, 47*, 300–314.

Lunde, I., Larson, G. K., Fog, E., & Garde, K. (1991). Sexual desire, orgasm, and sexual fantasies: A study of 625 Danish women born in 1910, 1936, and 1958. *Journal of Sex Education and Therapy, 17*, 111–116.

Lyons, P. (1997). The rape: A physicians personal narrative of treating a rape survivor. *Journal of Family Practice, 45*, 457–458.

Maccoby, E. E. (1988). Gender as a social category. *Developmental Psychology, 24*, 755–765.

Maccoby, E. E., & Jacklin, C. N. (1987). Gender segregation in childhood. In E. H. Reese (Ed.), *Advances in child development and behavior* (Vol. 20, pp. 239–288). New York: Academic Press.

MacDonald, T. K., Zanna, M. P., & Fong, G. T. (1996). Why common sense goes out the window: Effects of alcohol on intentions to use condoms. *Personality and Social Psychology Bulletin, 22*, 763–775.

MacKinnon, C. (1996). *Just words*. Cambridge, MA: Harvard University Press.

MacNeil, S., & Byers, S. (1997). The relationships between sexual problems, communication, and sexual satisfaction. *Canadian Journal of Human Sexuality, 6*, 277–286.

MacReady, N. (2002, October 1). Norplant effective, but won't be back on market (called "real loss" for women). *Family Practice News*, p. 46.

Maes, M., De Vos, N., Van Hunsel, F., Van West, D., Westenberg, H., Cosyns, P., & Neels, H. (2001). Pedophilia is accompanied by increased plasma concentrations of catecholamines, in particular, epinephrine. *Psychiatry Research, 103*, 43–49.

Mah, K., & Binik, Y. (2002). Do all orgasms feel alike? Evaluating a two-dimensional model of the orgasm experience across gender and sexual context. *Journal of Sex Research, 39*, 104–113.

Mahalingam, R. (2003). Essentialism, culture, and beliefs about gender among the Aravanis of Tamil Nadu. *Sex Roles, 49*, 489–496.

Major, B., Cozzarelli, C., Cooper, M., Zubek, J., Richards, C., Wilhite, M., & Gramzow, R. (2000). Psychological responses of women after first-trimester abortion. *Archives of General Psychiatry, 57*, 777–784.

Male Infertility Specialists. (2002). What tests are included in a basic semen analysis? Retrieved May 5, 2002, from **http://www.maleinfertilitymds.com/faq_6.htm**

Mangan, D. (2003). New oral contraceptive means fewer menstrual periods. *RN, 66*, 95.

Marchell, T., & Cummings, N. (2001). Alcohol and sexual violence among college students. In A. J. Ottens & K. Hotelling (Eds.), *Sexual violence on campus: Policies, programs, and perspectives* (pp. 30–52). New York: Springer.

March of Dimes Perinatal Data Center. (2000). Leading categories of birth defects. Retrieved September 26, 2005, from **http://www.marchofdimes.com/aboutus/680_2164.asp**

March of Dimes Perinatal Data Center. (2004). Quick reference and fact sheets. Retrieved June 3, 2004, from **http://www.marchofdimes.com/professionals/681_1206.asp**

March of Dimes update: Taking action against prematurity. (2003). *Contemporary OB/GYN, 48*, 92–97.

Marcus, M. B. (2000, October 2). Don't let false alarms scare you off prenatal tests, but do get the facts first. *U.S. News and World Report*, pp. 69–71.

Marincovich, B., Castilla, J., Del Romero, J., Garcia, S., Hernando, V., Raposo, M., & Rodriguez, C. (2003). Absence of hepatitis C virus transmission in a prospective cohort of heterosexual serodiscordant couples. *Sexually Transmitted Diseases, 79*, 160–162.

Markman, H., Stanley, S., & Bloomberg, S. (2001). *Fighting for your marriage: Positive steps for preventing divorce and preserving a lasting love*. San Francisco: Jossey-Bass.

Marmor, J. (1998). Homosexuality: Is etiology really important? *Journal of Gay and Lesbian Psychotherapy, 2*, 19–28.

Marrazzo, J., Celum, C., Hillis, S., Fine, D., De Lisle, S., & Handsfield, H. (1997). Performance and cost-effectiveness of selective screening criteria for *Chlamydia trachomatis* infection in women. *Sexually Transmitted Diseases, 24*, 131–141.

Marsa, L. (2002). Don't let this drug trap you (GHB). *Health, 16*, 110–113.

Marston, C., & Cleland, J. (2003). Relationships between contraception and abortion: A review of the evidence. *International Family Planning Perspectives, 29*, 6–13.

Martin, W. E. (2001, September-October). A wink and a smile: How men and women respond to flirting. *Psychology Today*, pp. 26–27.

Martinson, F. (1994). *The sexual life of children*. Westport, CT: Bergin & Garvey.

Martz, D. (2003). Behavioral treatment for a female engaging in autoerotic asphyxiation. *Clinical Case Studies, 2*, 236–242.

Masters, W. H., & Johnson, V. E. (1966). *Human sexual response*. Boston: Little, Brown.

Masters, W. H., & Johnson, V. E. (1970). *Human sexual inadequacy*. Boston: Little, Brown.

Masters, W. H., & Johnson, V. E. (1974). *The pleasure bond*. Boston: Little, Brown.

Masters, W. H., & Johnson, V. E. (1979). *Homosexuality in perspective*. Boston: Little, Brown.

Masters, W. H., & Johnson, V. E. (1986). *Masters and Johnson on sex and human loving*. Boston: Little, Brown.

Masters, W. E., & Johnson, V. E. (1988). *Crisis: Heterosexual behavior in the age of AIDS*. New York: Grove Press.

Masters, W. H., Johnson, V. E., & Kolodny, R. C. (1977). *Ethical issues in sex therapy and research*. Boston: Little, Brown.

Masters, W. H., Johnson, V. E., & Kolodny, R. C. (1994). *Heterosexuality*. New York: HarperCollins.

Masters, W. H., Johnson, V. E., & Kolodny, R. C. (1995). *Human sexuality* (5th ed.). New York: HarperCollins.

Mastroianni, L., & Robinson, J. C. (1995, March 16). Hassle-free methods of contraception. *Patient Care*, pp. 46–58.

Mathews, S. (2005). International trafficking in children: Will new U.S. legislation provide an ending to the story? *Houston Journal of International Law, 27*, 649–703.

Maxwell, C., Robinson, A., & Post, L. (2003). The nature and predictors of sexual victimization and offending among adolescents. *Journal of Youth and Adolescence, 32*, 465–477.

Mayor, S. (2004). Pfizer will not apply for licence for sildenafil for women. *British Medical Journal, 328*, 542.

McBride, W. (1991). Spontaneous abortion. *American Family Physician, 43*, 175–183.

McCabe, M. P., & Cummins, R. A. (1998). Sexuality and quality of life among young people. *Adolescence, 33*, 761–766.

McCarthy, B. W. (1992). Erectile dysfunction and inhibited sexual desire: Cognitive-behavioral strategies. *Journal of Sex Education and Therapy, 18*, 22–34.

McCarthy, B. W. (1993). Relapse prevention strategies and techniques in sex therapy. *Journal of Sex and Marital Therapy, 19*, 142–147.

McCarthy, B. W. (1995). Bridges to sexual desire. *Journal of Sex Education and Therapy, 21*, 132–141.

McClelland, S. (2001, June 25). A way out. *Maclean's*, pp. 44–46.

McClure, E. (2000). A meta-analytic review of sex differences in facial expression processing and their development in infants, children, and adolescents. *Psychological Bulletin, 126*, 424–453.

McGarvey, R. (1998). Hands off! How do the latest Supreme Court decisions on sexual harassment affect you? *Entrepreneur, 26*, 85–87.

McKain, L. (2002). How long should we wait before having oral sex after childbirth? Retrieved June 7, 2002, from **http://www.babycenter.com/expert/baby/postpartumsex**

McNamara, D. (2004, February 15). HPV types, cancer link studied in young women: HPV 16, 18 implicated. *Family Practice News*, p. 69.

Mead, M. (1949). *Male and female: A study of the sexes in a changing world*. New York: Dell.

Meadows, B. (2004, March 1). Boy? Girl? You choose. *People*, pp. 68–73.

Mechcatie, E. (2002a, December 1). Manufacturer recalls prefilled Lunelle syringes. *Family Practice News*, p. 6.

Mechcatie, E. (2002b). Postpartum depression vastly undertreated despite prevalence. *Clinical Psychiatry News, 30*, 12.

Mechcatie, E. (2006). Data are mixed on thrombosis from Ortho Evra patch vs. pills. *Family Practice News, 36*, 5.

Medical Network. (2000). Bladder infections and *E. coli*. HealthAtoZ.com. Retrieved December 26, 2002, from **http://www.healthatoz.com**

Meraviglia, M., Becker, H., Rosenbluth, B., Sanchez, E., & Robertson, T. (2003). The expect respect project: Creating a positive elementary school climate. *Journal of Interpersonal Violence, 18*, 1347–1363.

Meston, C. (1997). Aging and sexuality. *Western Journal of Medicine, 167*, 285–290.

Meston, C., & Frohlich, P. (2002). Psychopharmacology of paraphilias with leuteinizing hormone–releasing agonists. *Archives of General Psychiatry, 59*, 469–470.

Meston, C., Heiman, J., & Trapnell, P. (1999). The relation between early abuse and adult sexuality. *Journal of Sex Research, 36*, 385–400.

Meyer-Bahlburg, H., Ehrhardt, A., & Gruen, R. (1995). Prenatal estrogens and the development of homosexual orientation. *Developmental Psychology, 31*, 12–21.

Michael, R., Gagnon, J., Laumann, E., & Kolata, G. (1994). *Sex in America: A definitive survey*. Boston: Little, Brown.

Michigan State University Counseling Center. (2003). *Sex and relationships: Establishing guidelines for decisions about sexual expression*. Retrieved August 15, 2005, from **http://www.couns.msu.edu/self-help/sexguide.htm**

Midwife-assisted deliveries good for mother and baby. (1997, June). *WIN News*, p. 27.

Miller, H., Cain, V., Rogers, S., Gribble, J., & Turner, C. (1999). Correlates of sexually transmitted bacterial infections among U.S. women in 1995. *Family Planning Perspectives, 31*, 4–9.

Miller, J. (2000). *What are paraphilias?* Retrieved December 7, 2004, from **http://www.athealth.com/Consumer/disorders/Paraphilias.html**

Miller, M. L., et al. (1997, October). *Characteristics of male sex trade workers enrolled in a prospective study of HIV incidence*. Paper presented at the Tenth Annual British Columbia AIDS Conference, Vancouver.

Miller, R., Klotz, D., & Eckholdt, H. (1998). HIV prevention with male prostitutes and patrons of hustler bars. *American Journal of Community Psychology, 26*, 97–132.

Mishell, D. (1985). Current status of intrauterine devices. *New England Journal of Medicine, 312*, 984–985.

Mishell, D. (2004). State of the art in hormonal contraception: An overview. *American Journal of Obstetrics and Gynecology, 190*, 1–3.

Mitchell, S. (2001, July 13). The Today sponge coming (back) soon. *WebMD*. Retrieved January 10, 2003, from **http://content.health.msn.com**

Mohler-Kuo, M., Dowdall, G. W., Koss, M. P., & Wechsler, H. (2004). Correlates of rape while intoxicated in a national sample of college women. *Journal of Studies on Alhobol, 65*, 37–45.

Monto, M. (2002). Prostitution and fellatio. *Journal of Sex Research, 38*, 140–145.

Moore, D. (2000). Postpartum depression. Retrieved December 6, 2004, from **http://www.drdonnica.com/display.asp?article=154**

Moore, K., & Sugland, B. (1999). Piecing together the puzzle of teenage childbearing. *Policy and Practice of Public Human Services, 57*, 36–42.

Moore, M. (2002). Courtship communication and perception. *Perceptual and Motor Skills, 94*, 97–104.

Moore, T., Eisler, R., & Franchina, J. (2000). Causal attributions and affective responses to provocative female partner behavior by abusive and nonabusive males. *Journal of Family Violence, 15*, 69–80.

Morantz, C., & Torrey, B. (2004). Progesterone to prevent preterm birth. *American Family Physician, 69*, 749.

More episiotomies performed by private practitioners and residents, hospital faculty. (2004, January 19). *OBGYN and Reproduction Week*, p. 5.

Morgenstern, J. (2004, May-June). Myths of bisexuality. *Off Our Backs*, pp. 46–48.

Morokoff, P. (1986). Volunteer bias in the psychophysiological study of female sexuality. *Journal of Sex Research, 22*, 35–51.

Morokoff, P. (1993). Female sexual arousal disorder. In W. O'Donohue & J. Geer (Eds.), *Handbook of sexual dysfunctions* (pp. 157–199). Needham Heights, MA: Allyn & Bacon.

Morris, R. (1996). The culture of female circumcision. *Advances in Nursing Science, 19*(2), 43–54.

Morse, E., Simon P., Osofsky H., Balson P., & Gaumer H. (1991). The male street prostitute: A vector for transmission of HIV infection into the heterosexual world. *Social Science and Medicine, 32*, 535–539.

Mosher, D. L., & MacIan, P. (1994). College men and women respond to X-rated videos intended for male of female audiences: Gender and sexual scripts. *Journal of Sex Research, 31*, 99–113.

Moster, D., Lie, R., & Markestad, T. (2002). Joint association of APGAR scores and early neonatal symptoms with minor disabilities at school age. *Archives of Disease in Childhood: Fetal and Neonatal Edition, 86*, 16–21.

Most resistance to anti-HIV drugs created by good pill-taking patients. (2003, September 8). *AIDS Weekly*, p. 2.

Motluk, A. (2003). The big brother effect: The more older brothers you have, the more likely you are to be gay. What's going on? *New Scientist, 177*, 44–47.

Mudur, G. (2002). India plans new legislation to prevent sex selection. *British Medical Journal, 324*, 385.

Mueller, K. A., & Yoder, J. D. (1999). Stigmatization of non-normative family size status. *Sex Roles, 41*, 901–919.

Mullin, C. R., & Linz, D. G. (1995). Desensitization and resensitization to violence against women: Effects of exposure to sexually violent films on judgments of domestic violence victims. *Journal of Personality and Social Psychology, 69*, 449–459.

Murdoch, J., & Price, D. (2001, July 9,). A sorry history of anti-gay bias. *National Law Journal, 23*, A24.

Murdock, M. (2004). Female fertility drug can be used for men with low sperm count. Retrieved June 12, 2004, from **http://www.hisandherhealth.com/articles**

Murphy, M., & Risser, N. (1999). Genital herpes recurrence rates. *Nurse Practitioner, 24*, 62.

Murray, J. B. (2000). Psychological profile of pedophiles and child molesters. *Journal of Psychology, 134*, 211–224.

Murray, S., & Miller, J. (2000). Birth control and condom usage among college students. *Research Quarterly for Exercise and Sport, 71*, A42.

Murray, S. L., Holmes, J. G., Bellavia, G., Griffin, D. W., & Dolderman, D. (2002). Kindred spirits? The benefits of egocentrism in close relationships. *Journal of Personality and Social Psychology, 82*, 563–581.

Murray, S. L., Holmes, J. G., Griffin, D. W., Bellavia, G., & Rose, P. (2001). The mismeasure of love: How self-doubt contaminates relationship beliefs. *Personality and Social Psychology Bulletin, 27*, 423–436.

The "M" word. (1995, April). *UC Berkeley Wellness Letter*, pp. 6–7.

MyDr. (2001, June 1). Essure PBC (permanent birth control). Retrieved August 19, 2005, from **http://www.mydr.com.au/default.asp?article=3223**

Nachmias, D., & Nachmias, C. (1987). *Research methods in the social sciences*. New York: St. Martin's Press.

Namnoum, A., & Hatcher, R. A. (1998). The menstrual cycle. In R. A. Hatcher, J. Trussell, F. Stewart, W. Cates Jr., G. K. Stewart, F. Guest, & D. Kowal (Eds.), *Contraceptive technology* (17th rev. ed., pp. 69–76). New York: Ardent Media.

Napoli, M. (2001, March). New long-acting contraceptive can also help women avoid hysterectomy. *Health Facts*. Retrieved February 21, 2006, from **http://www.zinkle.com**

Napoli, M. (2002, March). Spermicide gel is no protection against sexually transmitted diseases. *Health Facts*. Retrieved February 21, 2006, from **http://www.zinkle.com**

National Clearinghouse on Martial and Date Rape (2005). State law chart. Retrieved June 6, 2006 from **http://members.aol.com/ncmdr/state law chart.html**.

National Crime Victims Center. (2001). Statistics: Sexual assault. Retrieved August 7, 2003, from **http://www.ncvc.org/stats/sa.htm**

National Endometriosis Society. (2003). What is endometriosis? Retrieved December 12, 2003, from **http://www.endo.org.uk/info.html**

National Institute of Allergy and Infectious Diseases. (2002, September). HIV/AIDS statistics fact sheet. Retrieved November 20, 2002, from **http://www.niaid.nih.gov/factsheets/aidsstat.htm**

National Institute of Child Health and Human Development. (2003). Turner syndrome. Retrieved July 25, 2003, from **http://turners.nichd.nih.gov**

National Institutes of Health. (2000). Prostatitis. NIH Publication No. 00-4553. Retrieved January 2, 2003, from **http://www.niddk.nih.gov/health/urolog/summary/prostat/prostat.htm**

National Institutes of Health. (2003). Urinary tract infections in adults. NIH Publication No. 04-2097. Retrieved September 2, 2005, from **http://kidney.niddk.nih.gov/kudiseases/pubs/utiadult/#treatment**

National Women's Health Information Center, U.S. Department of Health and Human Services. (2002). Menstruation and the menstrual cycle. Retrieved December 9, 2003, from **http://www.4woman.gov/faq/menstru.htm?src=ng#1**

Nelson, A. (2000). The pink dragon is female: Halloween costumes and gender markers. *Psychology of Women Quarterly, 24*, 137–144.

Nelson, E., Heath, A., & Madden, P. (2002). Association between self-reported childhood sexual abuse and adverse psychosocial outcomes: Results from a twin study. *Archives of General Psychiatry, 59*, 139–146.

Nelson, T. S. (2003). *For love of country: Confronting rape and sexual harassment in the U.S. military*. New York: Haworth Maltreatment and Trauma Press.

New York v. *Ferber*, 458 U.S. 747 (1982).

Nguyen, C. (2001). Premenstrual dysphoric disorder (PMDD). Medem/American Psychiatric Association. Retrieved January 23, 2005, from **http://www.slwhc.yourmd.com**

Nichols, S. (1999). Gay, lesbian, and bisexual youth: Understanding diversity and promoting tolerance in schools. *Elementary School Journal, 99*, 505–518.

Nicollette, J. (1996). The female condom: Where method and user effectiveness meet. *Stanford Medical Student Clinical Journal*. Retrieved January 28, 2004, from **http://medworld.stanford.edu/features/review/nicolette.html#ref**

Nicolosi, J., & Byrd, D. (2002). A critique of Bem's "exotic becomes erotic" theory of sexual orientation development. *Psychological Reports, 90*, 931–945.

Nicolson, P., & Burr, J. (2003). What is "normal" about women's (hetero)sexual desire and orgasm? A report of an in-depth interview study. *Journal of Social Science and Medicine, 57*, 1735–1745.

Nimmons, D. (1994, March). Sex and the brain. *Discover*, pp. 64–70.

NOCIRC. (1997). Intact penis. Retrieved January 3, 2002, from **http://www.nocirc.org/publish/pam4.html**

Nordenberg, T. (2000). Escaping the prison of past trauma. *FDA Consumer, 34*, 21–27.

Norris, J. (1994). Alcohol and female sexuality: A look at expectancies and risks. *Alcohol and Research World, 18*, 197–201.

Notarius, C., & Markman, H. (1994, January-February). Six truths for couples. *Psychology Today*, pp. 24–25.

Nusbaum, M., Gamble, G., Skinner, B., & Heiman, J. (2000). The high prevalence of sexual concerns among women seeking routine gynecological care. *Journal of Family Practice, 49*, 229–232.

NZoom.com. (2003). Many women don't discuss STIs. Retrieved November 21, 2003, from **http://health.nzoom.com**

O'Brien, J. (2001). The MVP program: Focus on student-athletes. In A. J. Ottens & K. Hotelling (Eds.), *Sexual violence on campus: Policies, programs, and perspectives* (pp. 141–161). New York: Springer.

O'Brien, J. (2004). Unintended pregnancy. Retrieved June 3 2004, from **http://www.cdc.gov/reproductivehealth/prams_factsheet.htm**

O'Brien, M. (2003, March 21). Wrong messages: Your kids are casually experimenting with oral sex. Retrieved December 23, 2004, from **http://www.drsharonmaxwell.com/5parentsandkids.htm**

O'Connell, H., Hutson, J. Anderson, C., &. Plenter, R. (1998). Anatomical relationship between urethra and clitoris. *Journal of Urology, 159*, 1892–1897.

O'Connell, R. (2001). Implanon. Retrieved on January 9, 2002, from **http://www.unimed.co.uk/health/leaflets/implanon.htm**

O'Donohue, W. & Geer, J. (Eds.). (1993). *Handbook of sexual dysfunctions*. Needham Heights, MA: Allyn & Bacon.

O'Donohue, W., Letourneau, E., & Geer, J. (1993). Premature ejaculation. In W. O'Donohue & J. Geer (Eds.), *Handbook of sexual dysfunctions* (pp. 303–333). Needham Heights, MA: Allyn & Bacon.

Office of Health Education and Wellness. (2003). Safer sex, sexual health, and STDs. Arizona State University. Retrieved November 20, 2003, from **http://www.asu.edu/health/Safer_Sex_Health_STD.html**

Office of the Surgeon General. (2001). *The surgeon general's call to action to promote sexual health and responsible sexual behavior, 2001*. Rockville, MD.

Okami, P., Olmstead, R., & Abramson, P. (1997). Sexual experiences in early childhood: 18-year longitudinal data from the UCLA Family Lifestyles Project. *Journal of Sex Research, 34*, 339–347.

Oliver, M. (2002). HPV testing plus Pap smear every 2 years most cost-effective cervical cancer screen. *Journal of Family Practice, 51*, 677.

Ompad, D. C., Strathdee, S. A., Celentano, D. D., Latkin, C., & Poduska, J. M. (2006). Predictors of early initiation of vaginal and oral sex among urban young adults in Baltimore, Maryland. Archives of Sexual Behavior, 35, 53–65.

Oncale, R., & King, B. (2001). Comparison of men's and women's attempts to dissuade sexual partners from the couple using condoms. *Archives of Sexual Behavior, 30*, 379–397.

Oral fluid-based rapid HIV test approved. (2004). *AIDS Alert, 19*, 71–72.

Oral sex, masturbating—but not men—linked to recurrent infections. (2004, January 5). *OBGYN and Reproduction Week*, p. 12.

Oral sex: Tell teens it's not without risk. (2001). *Contraceptive Technology Update, 22*, 55–57.

Oral sex transmission rate is higher than expected. (2000). *AIDS Alert*, 15, 42–43.

O'Shea, P. (1995). The fetus and patient: Prenatal diagnosis and treatment. In D. Coustan, R. Haning, & D. Singer (Eds.), *Human reproduction: Growth and development* (pp. 247–264). Boston: Little, Brown.

Osman, A., & Al-Sawaf, M. (1995). Cross-cultural aspects of sexual anxieties and associated dysfunction. *Journal of Sex Education and Therapy, 21*, 174–181.

Otchet, A. (1998, December). Should prostitution be legal? *UNESCO Courier*, pp. 37–39.

Ottens, A. J. (2001). The scope of sexual violence on campus. In A. J. Ottens & K. Hotelling (Eds.), *Sexual violence on campus: Policies, programs, and perspectives* (pp. 1–29). New York: Springer.

Owen, P. R., & Laurel-Seller, E. (2000). Weight and shape ideals: Thin is dangerously in. *Journal of Applied Psychology, 30*, 979–990.

Owens, T., & Lopes, A. (2003). Recommendations for political policy on prostitution and the sex industry. International Union of Sex Workers. Retrieved June 28, 2003, from **http://www.iusw.org/policy**

Padgett, V. R., Brislin-Slutz, J. A., & Neal, J. A. (1989). Pornography, erotica, and attitudes toward women: The effects of repeated exposure. *Journal of Sex Research, 26*, 479–491.

Paglia, C. (1998, March 23). A call for lustiness: Just say no to the sex police. *Time*, p. 54.

Palmer, N. (2004). "Let's talk about sex, baby": Community-based HIV prevention work and the problem of sex. *Archives of Sexual Behavior, 33*, 271–275.

Palmquist, S. (2004, July-August). Handsome ambitions. *Psychology Today*, p. 33.

Pantly, E. (1999) *Perfect parenting*. New York: McGraw-Hill.

Parfitt, T. (2003). Russia moves to curb abortion rates. *Lancet, 362*, 968.

Parker, R., & Parrott, R. (1995). Patterns of self-disclosure across social support networks: Elderly, middle-aged and young adults. *International Journal of Aging and Human Development, 41*, 281–297.

Parsons, C. (2002). Medical encyclopedia: Gonorrhea—male. Retrieved February 21, 2006, from **http://www.nlm.nih.gov/medlineplus/print/ency/article/000623.htm**

Partner Therapy Group. (2003). Painful sex or dyspareunia in men. Retrieved April 25, 2004, from **http://www.minus1.com/165.html**

Paterson-Brown, S. (1998). Education about the hymen is needed. *British Medical Journal, 316*, 461–462.

Patrick, D., Althop, S., Pryor, J., & Rosen, R. (2005). Premature ejaculation: An observational study of men and their partners. *Journal of Sexual Medicine, 2*, 358–367.

Patton, W., & Mannison, M. (1994). Investigating attitudes towards sexuality: Two methodologies. *Journal of Sex Education and Therapy, 20*, 185–197.

Paul, J., et al. (2002). Suicide attempts among gay and bisexual men: Lifetime prevalence and antecedents. *American Journal of Public Health, 92*, 1338–1345.

Paulson, R. J., Milligan, R. C., & Sokol, R. Z. (2001). The lack of influence of age on male fertility. *American Journal of Obstetrics and Gynecology,184*, 818–824.

Pearson, S., & Pollack, R. (1997). Female responses to sexually explicit films. *Journal of Psychology and Human Sexuality, 9*, 73–88.

Pennachio, D. L. (2004). Norethindrone and ethinyl estradiol (Ovcon 35). *Patient Care, 38*, 12.

Peplau, L. (2003). Human sexuality: How do men and women differ? *Current Directions in Psychological Science, 12*, 37–40.

Peplau, L., Garnets, L., Spalding, R., Conley, D., & Veniegas, C. (1998). A critique of Bem's "exotic becomes erotic" theory of sexual orientation. *Psychological Review, 105*, 387–394.

Perper, T. (1986). *Sex signals: The biology of love*. Philadelphia: ISI Press.

Perper, T., & Fox, V. S. (1980, June). *Flirtation and pickup patterns in bars*. Paper presented at the Eastern Conference on Reproductive Behavior, Saratoga Springs, NY.

Perper, T., & Fox, V. S. (1981). *Flirtation behavior in public settings: Final report*. New York: Harry Frank Guggenheim Foundation.

Perper, T., & Weiss, D. (1987). Proceptive and rejective strategies of U.S. and Canadian college women. *Journal of Sex Research, 23*, 455–480.

Person, E. S., Terestman, N., Myers, W. A., Goldberg, E. L., & Salvadori, C. (1989). Gender differences in sexual behaviors and fantasies in a college population. *Journal of Sex and Marital Therapy, 15*, 187–198.

Petis, R. (2004, December 28). Hijras. In *GLBTQ: An Encyclopedia of Gay, Lesbian, Bisexual, Transgender, and Queer Culture*. Retrieved March 15, 2005, from **http://www.glbtq.com/social-sciences/hijras.html**

Pfaff, D., Frolich, J., & Morgan, M. (2002). Hormonal and genetic influences on arousal—sexual and otherwise. *Trends in Neurosciences, 25*, 45–50.

Pfizer Inc. (2005). Viagra: Rate your sexual health. Retrieved August 29, 2005, from **http://www.viagra.com/steps/fullShim.asp**

Pilcher, C. D. (2003, February 10–14). *Acute HIV infection*. Paper presented at the Tenth Conference on Retroviruses and Opportunistic Infections, Boston. Retrieved July 10, 2004, from **http://www.natap.org/2003/Retro/day20.htm**

Pilkinton, C., Kern, W., & Indest, D. (1994). Is safer sex necessary with a "safe" partner? Condom use and romantic feelings. *Journal of Sex Research, 31*, 203–210.

Pillard, R. (1998). Biologic theories of homosexuality. *Journal of Gay and Lesbian Psychotherapy, 2*, 75–85.

Pimenta, J., Gray, M., Hopwood, J., & Randall, S. (2000). Screening for genital chlamydial infection. *British Medical Journal, 321*, 629–631.

Pines, A. M., & Bowes, C. F. (1992, March). Romantic jealousy: The shadow of love. *Psychology Today*, pp. 48–55.

Pinkowish, M. (2000). Testicular cancer: Increasing in incidence and curability. *Patient Care, 34*, 18–38.

Pinto, L., Edwards, J., Castle, E., Harro, C., Lowy, D., & Schiller J. (2003). Cellular immune responses to human papillomavirus (HPV)-16 11 in healthy volunteers immunized with recombinant HPV-16 11 virus-like particles. *Journal of Infectious Diseases, 188*, 327–338.

Plante, T. (2004). Another aftershock: What have we learned from the John Jay Report? *America, 190*, 10–11.

Platts-Mills, T., & Rein, M. (1999). Scabies. In K. K. Holmes, P. F. Sparling, P. March, S. M. Lemon, W. E. Stamm, P. Piot, & J. N. Wasserheit (Eds.), *Sexually transmitted diseases* (3d ed., pp. 645–650). New York: McGraw-Hill.

Plumridge, E., Chetwynd, S., Reed, A., & Gifford, S. (1997). Discourses of emotionality in commercial sex: The missing client voice. *Feminism and Psychology, 7*, 165–181.

The politics of masturbation. (1994). *Lancet, 344*, 1714–1715.

Pollack, A. E., Carignan, C. S., & Jacobstein, R. (2004). Female and male sterilization. In R. A. Hatcher, J. Trussell, F. Stewart, W. Cates Jr., A. L. Nelson, F. Guest, & D. Kowal (Eds.), *Contraceptive technology* (18th rev. ed., pp. 531–574). New York: Ardent Media.

Polls and Surveys. (2004). Retrieved June 21, 2005 from **http://queendom.com/polls/sexapoll/masturbation**

Polonsky, D. (2000). Premature ejaculation. In S. Leiblum & R. Rosen (Eds.), *Principles and practice of sex therapy* (pp. 305–332). New York: Guilford Press.

Pomerleau, A., Bolduc, D., Malcuit, G., & Cossette, L. (1990). Pink or blue: Environmental gender stereotypes in the first two years of life. *Sex Roles, 22*, 359–367.

Pope, L., Adler, N., & Tschann, J. (2001). Postabortion psychological adjustment: Are minors at increased risk. *Journal of Adolescent Health, 29*, 2–11.

Popkin, J. (1994, December 19). A case of too much candor. *U.S. News and World Report*, p. 31.

Poppen, P. (1994). Adolescent contraceptive use and communication: Changes over a decade. *Adolescence, 29*, 503–515.

Potterat, J., Rothenberg, R., Muth, S., Darrow, W., & Phillips-Plummer, L. (1998). Pathways to prostitution: The chronology of sexual and drug abuse milestones. *Journal of Sex Research, 35*, 333–340.

Poudel, M. (1994). Poverty, prostitution, and women. *World Health, 47*, 10–12.

Powell, E. (1996). *Sex on your terms*. Needham Heights, MA: Allyn & Bacon.

Power, C., Radcliffe, L., & MacGregor, K. (2003, November 17). Preying on children. *Newsweek International*, pp. 34–35.

Predicting preterm births still nearly impossible. (2002, February 14). *Women's Health Weekly*, pp. 15–16.

Prentky, R., & Knight, R. (1991). Indentifying critical dimensions for discriminating among rapists. *Journal of Counseling and Clinical Psychology, 59*, 643–661.

Prentky, R., Lee, A., Knight, R., & Cerce, D. (1997). Recidivism rates among child molesters and rapists: A methodological analysis. *Law and Human Behavior, 21*, 635–659.

Previous *Chlamydia trachomatis* infections adversely affect male fertility. (2004, March 29). *OBGYN and Reproduction Week*, p. 35.

Preyde, M., & Ardal, F. (2003). Effectiveness of a parent "buddy" program for mothers of very preterm infants. *Canadian Medical Association Journal, 168*, 969–973.

Price, M., Gutheil, T., Commons, M., Kafka, M. P., & Dodd-Kimmey, S. (2001). Telephone scatalogia: Comorbidity and theories of etiology. *Psychiatric Annals, 31*, 226–232.

Pridal, D., & Lo Piccolo, J. (2000). Multielement treatment of desire disorders. In S. Leiblum & R. Rosen (Eds.), *Principles and practice of sex therapy* (pp. 57–81). New York: Guilford Press.

Prinstein, M., Meade, C., & Cohen, G. (2003). Adolescent oral sex, peer popularity, and perceptions of best friends' sexual behavior. *Journal of Pediatric Psychology, 28*, 243–249.

Project for Victims of Family Violence. (n.d.). *Signs to look for in an abusive personality*. Retrieved August 15, 2005, from **http://www.newbeginningsnh.org/html/signs.html**

Proust, J. (2004, March). Fewer periods, more questions. *Prevention*, p. 58.

Puente, S., & Cohen, D. (2003). Jealousy and the meaning (or nonmeaning) of violence. *Personality and Social Psychology Bulletin, 29*, 449–451.

Purdy, M. (2002). New contraceptive to block "sperm and germ." Retrieved January 11, 2002, from **http://www.jhu.edu/news_info/news/home02/jan02/germs.html**

Putnam, F. (2003). Ten-year research update review: Child sexual abuse. *Journal of the American Academy of Child and Adolescent Psychiatry, 42*, 269–278.

Quackenbush, D., Strassberg, D., & Turner, C. (2002). Gender effects of romantic themes in erotica. *Archives of Sexual Behavior, 24*, 21–35.

Quill, T., Sugden, S., Rossi, S., Doolittle, L., Hammer, R., & Garbers, D. (2003). Hyperactivated sperm motility driven by CatSper2 is required for fertilization. *Proceedings of the National Academy of Sciences, 100*, 14,869–14,874.

Quina, K., Harlow, L., Morokoff, P., Burkholder, G., &. Deiter, P. (2000). Sexual communication in relationships: When words speak louder than actions. *Sex Roles, 42*, 523–549.

Rahman, M., Da Vanzo, J., & Razzaque, A. (2001). Do better family planning services reduce abortion in Bangladesh? *Lancet, 358*, 1051–1056.

Ramisetty-Mikler, S., Caetano, R., Goebert, D., & Nishimura, S. (2004). Ethnic variation in drinking, drug use, and sexual behavior among adolescents in Hawaii. *Journal of School Health, 74*, 16–22.

Ramus, R., Sheffield, J., Mayfield, J., & Wendel, G. (2001). A randomized trial that compared oral cefixime and intramuscular ceftriaxone for the treatment of gonorrhea in pregnancy. *American Journal of Obstetrics and Gynecology, 185*, 629–632.

Randerson, J. (2003). Unique vaccine halts spread of herpes. *New Scientist, 178*, 23.

Ranke, M. B., & Saenger, P. (2001). Turner's syndrome. *Lancet, 358*, 309–314.

Raspa, R. (1993). Complications of vasectomy. *American Family Physician, 48*, 1264–1268.

Ray, S. (2001). Male survivors' perspectives of incest/sexual abuse. *Perspectives in Psychiatric Care, 37*, 49–59.

Read, J. (1999). Sexual problems associated with infertility, pregnancy, and aging. *British Medical Journal, 318*, 587–589.

Read, S., King, M., & Watson, J. (1997). Sexual dysfunction in primary medical care: Prevalence, characteristics, and detection by the general practitioner. *Journal of Public Health, 19*, 387–391.

Reddy, G. (2003). "Men" who would be kings: Celibacy, emasculation, and the reproduction of Hijras in contemporary Indian politics. *Social Research, 70*, 163–201.

Reinholtz, R., & Muehlenhard, C. (1995). Genital perceptions and sexual activity in a college population. *Journal of Sex Research, 32*, 155–165.

Reinisch, J. M. (1990). *The Kinsey Institute new report on sex: What you must know to be sexually literate*. New York: St. Martin's Press.

Reiss, I. (1995, November). *The new sex survey: Paradise lost or found?* Address at the annual meeting of the Society for the Scientific Study of Sexuality, San Francisco.

Reissing, E., Binik, Y., Khalifé, S., Cohen, D., & Amsel, R. (2004). Vaginal spasm, pain and behaviour: An empirical investigation of the diagnosis of vaginismus. *Archives of Sexual Behavior, 33*, 1–13.

Remafedi, G., French, S., & Story, M. (1998). The relationship between suicide risk and sexual orientation: Results of a population-based study. *American Journal of Public Health, 88*, 57–60.

Remez, L. (2000). Oral sex among adolescents: Is it sex or is it abstinence? *Family Planning Perspectives, 32*, 298–304.

Ren, D., et al. (2001). A sperm ion channel required for sperm motility and male fertility. *Nature, 413*, 603–609.

Renaud, C. A., & Byers, S. E. (1999). Exploring the frequency, diversity, and content of university students' positive and negative sexual cognitions. *Canadian Journal of Human Sexuality, 8*, 17–31.

Renaud, C. A., & Byers, S. E. (2001). Positive and negative sexual cognitions: Subjective experience and relationships to sexual adjustment. *Journal of Sex Research, 38*, 252–262.

Reproductive Health Technologies Project. (2000). Facts about fertility. Retrieved June 12, 2005, from **http://www.rhtp.org**

Reproductive Health Technologies Project. (2005). Manual vacuum aspiration. Retrieved June 12, 2005, from **http://www.rhtp.org/abortion/mva/default.asp**

Resnick, S. (2002). Sexual pleasure: The next frontier in the study of sexuality. *SEICUS Report, 30*, 6–11.

Ribner, D. (2003). Modifying sensate focus for use with Haredi (ultra-Orthodox) Jewish couples. *Journal of Sex and Marital Therapy, 29*, 165–171.

Ricciardelli, L., & Williams, R. (1995). Desirable and undesirable traits in three behavioral dimensions. *Sex Roles, 33*, 637–655.

Richards, M. (2003). Obscenity. Retrieved June 14, 2003, from **http://www4.gvsu.edu/richardm/PLS307/OBSCENITY.htm**

Richards, M. H., Crowe, P. A., Larson, R., & Swarr, A. (1998). Developmental patterns and gender differences in the experience of peer companionship during adolescence. *Child Development, 69*, 154–163.

Richardson, C. R., Resnick, P. J., Hansen, D. L., Derry, H. A., & Rideout, V. J. (2002). Does pornography-blocking software block access to health information on the Internet? *Journal of the American Medical Association, 288*, 2887–2894.

Richardson, J. (1995). Sexuality in the nursing home patient. *American Family Physician, 51*, 121–134.

Rietmeijer, C. A., Wolitski, R. J., Fishbein, M., Corby, N. H., & Cohn, D. L. (1998). Sex hustling, injection drug use, and non-gay identification by men who have sex with men: Associations with high-risk sexual behaviors and condom use. *Sexually Transmitted Diseases, 25*, 353–360.

Ringheim, K. (1995). Ethical issues in social science research with special reference to sexual behavior research. *Social Science and Medicine, 40*, 1691–1697.

RISUG has proved effective for preventing pregnancy in a clinical trial. (2003, March 17). *OBGYN and Reproduction Week*, p. 5.

Roberts, S. (1996). The sequelae of childhood sexual abuse: A primary care focus for adult female survivors. *Nurse Practitioner, 12*, 42–46.

Robinson, C. C., & Morris, J. T. (1986). The gender stereotyped nature of Christmas toys received by 36-, 48-, and 60-month-old children: A comparison between requested and nonrequested toys. *Sex Roles, 15*, 21–32.

Roche, T. (2002, January 20). The Yates odyssey. *Time*. Retrieved June 6, 2002, from **http://www.time.com**

Rodgers, J. E., & Veronsky, F. (1999, January-February). Flirting fascination. *Psychology Today*, pp. 36–41.

Rodriguez, J. (1990). It's never just a miscarriage. *RN, 53*(2), 19–22.

Rodriguez, M. (2004). Your first pregnancy. Obfocus. Retrieved October 20, 2004, from **http://www.obfocus.com/prenatal/firstpreg.htm**

Rodriguez, R. (1999, July 12). Axis One and Axis Two psychiatric disorders in pedophiles. *Impotence and Male Health Weekly*. Retrieved February 24, 2006, from **http://www.newsrx.com**

Roesler, T. A. (2000, October). Adult's reaction to child's disclosure of abuse will influence degree of permanent damage. *Brown University Child and Adolescent Behavior Letter*, pp. 1–2.

Rogoznica, J. (1997, September). Choices in childbirth. *Parents*, pp. 94–96.

Rokach, A. (1990). Content analysis of sexual fantasies of males and females. *Journal of Psychology 124*, 427–436.

Rosen, R., & Ashton, A. (1993). Prosexual drugs: Empirical status of the "new aphrodisiacs." *Archives of Sexual Behavior, 22*, 521–541.

Rosen, R., Lane, R., & Menza, M. (1999). Effects of SSRIs on sexual function: A critical review. *Journal of Clinical Pharmacology, 19*, 67–85.

Rosen, R., & Laumann, E. (2003). The prevalence of sexual problems in women: How valid are comparisons across studies? Commentary on Bancroft, Loftus, and Long's "Distress about sex: A national survey of women in heterosexual relationships." *Archives of Sexual Behavior, 32*, 209–211.

Rosen, R., & Leiblum, S. (1995). Treatment of sexual disorders in the 1990s: An integrated approach. *Journal of Consulting and Clinical Psychology, 63*, 107–121.

Rosen, R., Taylor, J., Leiblum, S., & Bachman, G. (1993). Prevalence of sexual dysfunction in women: Results of a survey study of 329 women in an outpatient gynecological clinic. *Journal of Sex and Marital Therapy, 19*, 171–188.

Rosenberg, M., & Phillips, R. (1992). Does douching promote ascending infection? *Journal of Reproductive Medicine, 37*, 930–938.

Rosen-Molina, M. (2001, April 2). Study provides insight into odd sexual kinks. *Daily Bruin Online*. Retrieved June 30, 2002, from **http://www.dailybruin.ucla.edu/db/articles.asp?ID'3458**

Rosler, A., & Witztum, E. (1998). Treatment of men with paraphilia with a long-acting analogue of gonadotropin-releasing hormone. *New England Journal of Medicine, 338*, 416–422.

Rosler, A., & Witztum, E. (2000). Pharmacotherapy of paraphilias in the next millennium. *Behavioral Science and the Law, 18*, 43–56.

Ross, M., & Williams, M. (2001). Sexual behavior and illicit drug use. *Annual Review of Sex Research, 12*, 290–310.

Ross, M., & Williams, M. (2002). Effective targeted and community HIV/STI prevention programs. *Journal of Sex Research, 39*, 58–62.

Rothenberger, J. (2001). The HPV/condom controversy provides opportunities for education. *SIECUS Report, 30*, 5–9.

Roumen, F., Apter, D., & Mulders, T. (2001). Efficacy, tolerability, and acceptability of a novel contraceptive vaginal ring releasing etonogestrel and ethinyl oestradiol. *Human Reproduction, 16*, 469–475.

Rubin, R. (2001, November 21). Weekly patch gets FDA approval as contraceptive device Ortho Evra is found as effective as pills. *USA Today*, pp. 13D–14D.

Rubin, Z., Hill, C., Peplau, L., & Dunkel-Schetter, C. (1980). Self-disclosure in dating couples: The ethic of openness. *Journal of Marriage and the Family, 42*, 499–506.

Rubin, Z., Provenzano, F., & Luria, Z. (1974). The eye of the beholder: Parents' views on sex of newborns. *American Journal of Orthopsychiatry, 44*, 512–519.

Russ, L., Simonds, C., & Hunt, S. (2002). Coming out in the classroom: An occupational hazard? The influence of sexual orientation on teacher credibility and perceived student learning. *Communication Education, 51*, 311–323.

Russell, C., & Keel, P. (2002). Homosexuality as a specific risk factor for eating disorders in men. *International Journal of Eating Disorders, 31*, 300–306.

Russell, D. E. H. (1990). *Rape in marriage*. Indianapolis: Indiana University Press.

Russell, L. (1990). Sex and couples therapy: A method of treatment to enhance physical and emotional intimacy. *Journal of Sex and Marital Therapy, 16*, 111–120.

Russell, S. (2005, October 7). Cervical cancer prevented in 2-year study: Experimental vaccine shows promise in halting early stages of disease. *San Francisco Chronicle*, p. A1.

Russell, S., & Joyner, K. (2001). Adolescent sexual orientation and suicide risk: Evidence from a national study. *American Journal of Public Health, 91*, 57–60.

Russo, N., & Dabul, A. (1997). The relationship of abortion to well-being: Do race and religion make a difference? *Professional Psychology: Research and Practice, 28*, 23–31.

Ryan, C., & Boxer, A. (1998). Coming out in prime time: The mental health impact of Ellen's "debut." *Cultural Diversity and Mental Health, 4*, 135–142.

Ryder, B., & Campbell, H. (1995). Natural family planning in the 1990s. *Lancet, 346*, 233–234.

Sadovsky, R. (2000a). Evidence-based review of contraception for adolescents. *American Family Physician, 62*, 1157–1158.

Sadovsky, R. (2000b). Management of dyspareunia and vaginismus. *American Family Physician, 61*, 2474–2476.

Sadovsky, R. (2001). Diagnosing and managing ecctopic pregnancy. *American Family Physician, 63*, 761–762.

Salerian, A., Deibler, W., Vittone, B., & Geyer, S. (2000). Sildenafil for psychotropic-induced sexual dysfunction in 31 women and 61 men. *Journal of Sex and Marital Therapy, 26*, 133–140.

Saltmarsh, N. (2001, September 11). BufferGel prevents pregnancy, STDs in animal models. *TB and Outbreaks Week*. Retrieved January 11, 2002, from the InfoTrac database.

Salzman, J. (1998, January 19). A cautionary campaign: Child-free couples need a group to fend off the persistent pressure of grandchildrenless parents. *Newsweek*, p. 14.

Sandberg, D., Meyer-Bahlburg, H., Ehrhardt, A., & Yager, T. (1993). The prevalence of gender-atypical behavior in elementary school children. *Journal of the American Academy of Child and Adolescent Psychiatry, 32*, 306–314.

Santelli, J., et al. (2003). The measurement and meaning of unintended pregnancy. *Perspectives of Sexual and Reproductive Health, 35*, 94–103.

Santos, D., & Nicholson, C. (2002, June 4). Anesthesia options for labor and delivery: What every expectant mother should know. Retrieved June 5, 2002, from **http://www.aana.com/patients/options.asp**

Santtila, P., Sandnabba, N., Alison, L., & Nordling, N. (2002). Investigating the underlying structure in sadomasochistically oriented behavior. *Archives of Sexual Behavior, 31*, 185–200.

Sardar, Z. (1999). The self-righteous gene. *New Statesman, 128*, 40–41.

Savage, T., & Neff, L. (1999, May 25). Costly trans-action. *Advocate*, p. 64.

Sax, L. (2002). How common is intersex? A response to Anne Fausto-Sterling. *Journal of Sex Research, 39*, 174–179.

Sayle, A. E., Savitz, D. A., Thorp, J. M., Hertz-Picciotto, I., & Wilcox, A. J. (2001). Sexual activity during late pregnancy and risk of preterm delivery. *Obstetrics and Gynecology, 97*, 283–289.

Scasta, D. (1998). Issues in helping people come out. *Journal of Gay and Lesbian Psychotherapy, 2*, 87–97.

Schaalma, H., Abraham, C., Gillmore, M. R., & Kok, G. (2004). Sex education as health promotion: What does it take? *Archives of Sexual Behavior, 33*, 259–269.

Schachter, D. L., Norman, K. A., & Koutstall, W. (1998). The cognitive neuroscience of constructive memory. *Annual Review of Psychology, 49*, 289–318.

Schaff, E., & Mawson, J. (2001). Contraceptive technology reports (mifepristone and misoprostol updates). *Contraceptive Technology Update, 22*, 1–14.

Schmidt, D. (2003). Universal sex differences in the desire for sexual variety: Tests from 52 nations, 6 continents, and 13 islands. *Journal of Personality and Social Psychology, 85*, 85–104.

Schmitt, D., et al. (2002). Is there an early-30s peak in female sexual desire? Cross-sectional evidence from the United States and Canada. *Canadian Journal of Human Sexuality, 11*, 1–17.

Schmitt, J., & Stuckey, C. (2004). AIDS: No longer a death sentence, still a challenge. *Southern Medical Journal, 97*, 329–330.

Schott, R. (1995). The childhood and family dynamics of transvestites. *Archives of Sexual Behavior, 24*, 309–337.

Schulman, A. (2000, April 13). Too much to swallow? *Boston Phoenix*. Retrieved September 14, 2005, from **http://www.bostonphoenix.com/archive**

Schuster, R., Bell, R., Berry, S., & Kanouse, D. (1998). Impact of a high school condom availability program on sexual attitudes and behaviors. *Family Planning Perspectives, 30*, 67–72.

Schwartz, I. M. (1999). Sexual activity prior to coital initiation: A comparison between males and females. *Archives of Sexual Beahvior, 28*, 63–69.

Scott and White Hospital, Department of Obstetrics and Gynecology. (2002). Assisted reproductive technology. Retrieved June 10, 2002, from **http://www.sw.org/depts/obgyn/clinical/rep_art1.htm**

Segraves, R., & Althof, S. (1998). Psychotherapy and pharmacotherapy of sexual dysfunctions. In P. Nathan & J. Gorman (Eds.), *A guide to treatments that work* (pp. 447–465). New York: Oxford University Press.

Seligman, L., & Hardenberg, S. (2000). Assessment and treatment of paraphilias. *Journal of Counseling and Development, 78*, 107–113.

Seppa, N. (2002, January 12). Suppressive drug therapy hinders herpes. *Science News*, p. 29.

Seth, W. (1997). The disavowal of desire: A relational view of sadomasochism. *Psychoanalysis and Psychotherapy, 14*, 107–123.

Seto, M. C., Lalumiere, M. L., & Kuban, M. (1999). The sexual preferences of incest offenders. *Journal of Abnormal Psychology, 108*, 267–272.

Severns, P. (2000, Summer). Doubting father: Resistance to home birthing. *Midwifery Today*, pp. 38–42.

Sex Info. (2003). Aging and the sexual response cycle. University of California–Santa Barbara, Department of Sociology. Retrieved July 10, 2005 from **http://www.soc.ucsb.edu/sexinfo/?article=anatomy&refid=008**

Sex trade workers. (2001). *Alberta Report, 28*, 41.

Sexual abuse. (2002). Retrieved July 5, 2003, from **http://www.counselingcorner.net/disorders/sexual-abuse.html**

Sexuality Information and Education Council of the United States (SIECUS). (2002). Teenage pregnancy, birth, and abortion. Retrieved October 22, 2005, from **http://www.siecus.org/pubs/fact/fact0010.html**

Seymour, R. (2000). Did you know? *Chatelaine, 73*, 32.

Shaw, M. (1998). Delight in the world: Tantric Buddhism as a path of bliss. *Parabola, 23*, 39–44.

Sheer, V., & Cline, R. (1994). Development and validation of a model explaining sexual behavior among college students. *Human Communication Research, 21*, 280–304.

Sheeran, P., Abraham, C., & Orbell, S. (1999). Psychosocial correlates of heterosexual condom use: A meta-analysis. *Psychological Bulletin, 125*, 90–93.

Shelby, L. (2003, February-March). Youth first: An integrated sexuality education program for preadolescents. *SIECUS Report*, pp. 31–32.

Shelton, J. D. (2001). Risk of clinical pelvic inflammatory disease attributable to an intrauterine device. *Lancet, 357*, 443.

Shima, T. (2002). Ectopic pregnancy. *Topics in Emergency Medicine, 24*, 12–20.

Shoskes, D., Katske, F., & Kim, S. (2001). Diagnosis and management of acute and chronic prostatitis. *Urologic Nursing, 21*, 255–262.

Shulman, S., & Kipnis, O. (2001). Adolescent romantic relationships: A look from the future. *Journal of Adolescence, 24*, 337–352.

Signorello, L. B., Harlow, B. L., Chekos, A. K., & Repke, J. T. (2001). Postpartum sexual functioning and its relationship to perineal trauma: A retrospective cohort study of primiparous women. *American Journal of Obstetrics and Gynecology, 184*, 881–990.

Silver, J. (2001). Movie day at the Supreme Court: "I know it when I see it." Retrieved June 13, 2003, from **http://www.coollawyer.com/webfront/pdf/Obscenity%20Article.pdf**

Silverman, J., & Peters, S. (2003,). Rapid HIV test. *Family Practice News*, p. 68.

Singer, D. (1995). Human embryogenesis. In D. Coustan, R. Haning, & D. Singer (Eds.), *Human reproduction: Growth and development* (pp. 27–37). Boston: Little, Brown.

Singer, H. S. (1979). *Disorders of sexual desire*. New York: Simon & Schuster.

Singer, L., Salvator, A., Guo, S., Collin, M., Lilien, L., & Baley, J. (1999). Maternal psychological distress and parenting stress after the birth of a very low-birth-weight infant. *Journal of the American Medical Association, 281*, 799–805.

Singh, D., Meyer, W., Zambrano, R., & Hurlburt, D. (1998). Frequency and timing of coital orgasm in women desirous of becoming pregnant. *Archives of Sexual Behavior, 27*, 15–29.

Sivin, I. (1989). IUDs are contraceptives, not abortifacients: A comment on research and beliefs. *Studies in Family Planning, 20*, 355–359.

Sked, A. (1999, June 5). The rehabilitation of Onan. *Spectator*, p. 12.

Skeen, D. (1991). *Different sexual worlds: Contemporary case studies of sexuality*. Lexington, MA: Lexington Books.

Skolnik, N., & Cohen, H. (2004). A short course on PMDD. *Contemporary OB/GYN, 49*, 56–61.

Slama, R., Werwatz, A., Boutou, O., Ducot, B., Spira, A., & Hardle, W. (2003). Does male age affect the risk of spontaneous abortion? An approach using semiparametric regression. *American Journal of Epidemiology, 157*, 815–824.

Slijper, F. (1997). Neither man nor women: The Hijras of India. *Archives of Sexual Behavior, 26*, 450–453.

Sloan, M. (2005, January 2). Concern over rising number of C-sections. *Santa Rosa Press Democrat*, pp. G1, G6.

Slob, A. K., van Berkel, A., & van der Werff ten Bosch, J. J. (2000). Premature ejaculation treated by local penile anaesthesia in an uncontrolled clinical replication study. *Journal of Sex Research, 37*, 244–251.

Sloviter, D. (1996). *Janet Reno* v. *American Civil Liberties Union*, 929 F. Supp. 824.

Smith, D. (2001). Harassment in the hallways. *Monitor on Psychology, 32*(8), 38–40.

Smith, G., Frankel, S., & Yarnell, J. (1997). Sex and death: are they related? Findings from the Caerphilly cohort study. *British Medical Journal, 315*, 1641–1645.

Smith, M. D., & Hand, C. (1987). The pornography-aggression linkage: Results from a field study. *Deviant Behavior, 8*, 389–399.

Smith, O. (1997). Age of sperm's owner irrelevant. *Physician's Weekly, 14*. Retrieved June 9, 2002, from **http://www.physweekly.com/archive/97/03_03_97/cu4.html**

Smith, S. (2004, March 10). Resistant form of gonorrhea gains foothold. *Boston Globe*, p. G8.

Smits, M. (2004, November 28). Sex slave's story told. *Sophia Echo*. Retrieved July 28, 2005, from **http://www.sofiaecho.com/article/sex-slaves-story-told/id_10416/catid_29**

Smock, P. (2000). Cohabitation in the United States: An appraisal of research themes, findings, and implications. *Annual Review of Sociology*, pp. 1–20.

Smotrich, D. (2002, April). Local medical center restores hope for San Diego couples. *San Diego Business Journal*, p. B7.

Smyth, A. (2002). Sexual problems overview. Retrieved March 6, 2004, from **http://www.nlm.nih.gov/medlineplus/ency/article/001951.htm**

Sodomy laws. (2005). *Laws around the world*. Retrieved October 6, 2005, from **http://222.sodomylaws.org/world/world.htm**

Solomon, S., Rothblum, E., & Balsam, K. (2004). Pioneers in partnership. Lesbian and gay male couples in civil unions compared with those not in civil unions and married heterosexual siblings. *Journal of Family Therapy, 18*, 275–286.

Somers, C., & Gleason, J. (2001). Does source of sex education predict adolescents' sexual knowledge, attitudes, and behaviors? *Education, 121*, 674–681.

Song, S., Downie, A., Gibson, H., Kloberdanz, K., & McDowell, J. (2004, April 19). Too posh to push? As more women schedule C-sections, doctors warn that the procedure is not risk-free. *Time*, pp. 58–59.

Sowell, T. (1994). Power plays. *Forbes, 154*, 233–235.

Sparks, S. (2005). Study casts new doubt on abstinence-only approach: Teens participating in Texas program found to be more sexually active, not less. *Education Daily*, pp. 4–5.

Spector, A. (2004). Psychological issues and interventions with infertile patients. *Women and Therapy, 27*, 91–105.

Spector, I., & Carey, M. (1990). Incidence and prevalence of the sexual dysfunctions: A critical review of the empirical literature. *Archives of Sexual Behavior, 19*, 389–408.

Splete, H. (2005, May 1). OraQuick test doubles HIV detection rates. *Family Practice News*, 31.

Sprecher, S. (2002). Sexual satisfaction in premarital relationships: Associations with satisfaction, love, commitment, and stability. *Journal of Sex Research, 39*, 190–197.

Starks, K., & Morrison, E. (1996). *Growing up sexual*. New York: HarperCollins.

Steele, C. M., & Josephs, R. A. (1990). Alcohol myopia: Its prized and dangerous effects. *American Psychologist, 45*, 921–933.

Steele, R. (2005). Masturbation: Is this normal for preschoolers? Retrieved September 14, 2005, from **http://parenting.ivillage.com/tp/tpbehavior/0,,lk45,00.html**

Steen, R. (2001). Eradicating chancroid. *Bulletin of the World Health Organization, 79*, 818–826.

Steen, R., & Dallabetta, G. (2003). Sexually transmitted infection control with sex workers: Regular screening and presumptive treatment augments efforts to reduce risk and vulnerability. *Reproductive Health Matters, 11*, 74–90.

Steinem, G. (1980). Erotica and pornography: A clear and present difference. In L. Lederer (Ed.), *Take back the night: Women on pornography* (pp. 35–39). New York: Morrow.

Stephenson, J. (2002). Experimental vaccine for recurrent UTIs. *Journal of the American Medical Association, 287*, 702–703.

Sternberg, R. J. (1986). A triangular theory of love. *Psychological Review, 93*, 119–135.

Sternberg, R. J. (1997). Construct validation of a triangular love scale. *European Journal of Social Psychology, 27*, 313–335.

Sternberg, R. J. (1998). *Cupid's arrow: The course of love*. New York: Cambridge University Press.

Stevens, L. (2002). Cesarian delivery. *Journal of the American Medical Association, 287*, 2738.

Stevens, L., & Glass, R. (2002). Postpartum depression. *Journal of the American Medical Association, 287*, 802.

Stewart, E. G. (2003). Dyspareunia: Five overlooked causes. *OBG Management, 15*, 50–68.

Stewart, F. (1998a). Intrauterine devices (IUDs). In R. A. Hatcher, J. Trussell, F. Stewart, W. Cates Jr., G. K. Stewart, F. Guest, & D. Kowal (Eds.), *Contraceptive technology* (17th rev. ed., pp. 511–543). New York: Ardent Media.

Stewart, F. (1998b). Vaginal barriers. In R. A. Hatcher, J. Trussell, F. Stewart, W. Cates Jr., G. K. Stewart, F. Guest, & D. Kowal (Eds.), *Contraceptive technology* (17th rev. ed., pp. 371–404). New York: Ardent Media.

Stewart, F., & Carignan, C. S. (1998). Female and male sterilization. In R. A. Hatcher, J. Trussell, F. Stewart, W. Cates Jr., G. K. Stewart, F. Guest, & D. Kowal (Eds.), *Contraceptive technology* (17th rev. ed., pp. 545–588). New York: Ardent Media.

Stewart, G. K. (1998). Impaired fertility. In R. A. Hatcher, J. Trussell, F. Stewart, W. Cates Jr., G. K. Stewart, F. Guest, & D. Kowal (Eds.), *Contraceptive technology* (17th rev. ed., pp. 653–678). New York: Ardent Media.

Stewart, G. K., & Carignan, C. S. (1998). Female and male sterization. In R. A. Hatcher, J. Trussell, F. Stewart, W. Jr. Cate, G. K. Stewart, F. Guest & D. Kowal, (Eds.), *Contraceptive* Technology (17th rev. ed., pp. 545–588). New York: Ardent Media.

Stimulants plus SSRIs used successfully to treat paraphilias in men. (2000). *Psychopharmacology Update, 11*, 1–2.

Stock, W. (1993). Inhibited female orgasm. In W. O'Donohue & J. Geer (Eds.), *Handbook of sexual dysfunctions* (pp. 253–277). Needham Heights, MA: Allyn & Bacon.

Stoddard, J. J., et al. (2000). Prevention of sexual harassment in the workplace and educational settings. *Pediatrics, 106*, 1498–1499.

Stolberg, M. (2003). A woman down to her bones: The anatomy of sexual difference in the sixteenth and early seventeenth centuries. *Isis, 94*, 274–300.

Stoler, M. (2000). Human papillomaviruses and cervical neoplasmia: A model for carcinogenesis. *International Journal of Gynecological Pathology, 19*, 16–28.

Stone, K. J., Viera, A. J., & Parman, C. L. (2003). Off-label applications for SSRIs. *American Family Physician, 68*, 498–504.

Stone, M., & Couch, S. (2004). Peer sexual harassment among high school students: Teachers' attitudes, perceptions, and responses. *High School Journal, 88*, 1–12.

Strassberg, D. S., & Lockerd, L. K. (1998). Force in women's sexual fantasies. *Archives of Sexual Behavior, 27*, 403–414.

Strassberg, D. S., & Lowe, K. (1995). Volunteer bias in sexuality research. *Archives of Sexual Behavior, 24*, 369–382.

Strauss, S. (1992). *Sexual harassment and teens: A program for positive change*. Minneapolis, MN: Free Spirit.

Striar, S., & Bartlik, B. (1999). Stimulation of the libido: The use of erotica in sex therapy. *Psychiatric Annals, 29*, 60–62.

Strough, J., Swenson, L. M., & Cheng, S. (2001). Friendship, gender, and preadolescents' representations of peer collaboration. *Merrill-Palmer Quarterly, 47*, 475–499.

Struckman-Johnson, C. (1988). Forced sex on dates: It happens to men, too. *Journal of Sex Research, 24*, 234–241.

Study finds vasectomy reversal highly effective, even after 15 years. (2004, March 15). *OBGYN and Reproduction Week*, p. 4.

Sue, D. (1979). Erotic fantasies of college students during coitus. *Journal of Sex Research, 15*, 299–305.

Sultan, S. (1995). The right of homosexuals to adopt: Changing legal interpretations of "parent" and "family." *Journal of the Suffolk Academy of Law, 10*, 1–58.

Sunger, M. (1999). Cultural factors in sex therapy: The Turkish experience. *Sexual and Marital Therapy, 14*, 165–171.

Suri, R. (2004). Postpartum depression: Risk factors and treatment options. *Psychiatric Times, 21*, 64–66.

Suriano, R. (2002, March 26). Medical experts struggle to pinpoint cause of pedophilia. *Orlando Sentinel*, p. E3.

Sutter Health Network. (2002). My baby's growth: Fetal development. Retrieved May 30, 2004, from **http://babies.sutterhealth.org/babygrowth/fetaldev/bg_fetaldev-3.html**

Swanson, J. M., Dibble, S. C., & Chenitz, C. W. (1995). Clinical features and psychosocial factors in young adults with genital herpes. *Journal of Nursing Scholarship, 27*, 16–22.

Sweeney, J., & Bradbard, M. (1988). Mothers' and fathers' changing perceptions of their male and female infants over the course of pregnancy. *Journal of Genetic Psychology, 149*, 393–404.

Szasz, T. (2000). Remembering Krafft-Ebing. *Ideas on Liberty, 50*, 31–32.

Talbot, M. (2001, May 6). Nip, tuck, and frequent flyer miles: How anything-goes plastic surgery became the latest thing in adventure travel. *New York Times Magazine*, p. 86.

Tanfer, K. (1993). National survey of men: Design and execution. *Family Planning Perspectives, 25*, 83–86.

Tanfer, K., Grady, W. R., Klepinger, D. H., & Billy, J. O. G. (1993). Condom use among U.S. men. *Family Planning Perspectives, 25*, 61–66.

Tannen, D. (1991). You just don't understand: Men and women in conversation. New York: Ballantine Books.

Tantleff-Dunn, S. (2001). Breast size and chest size: Ideals and stereotypes through the 1990s. *Sex Roles, 45*, 231–242.

Tay, J., & Walker, J. (2000). Ectopic pregnancy. *British Medical Journal, 320*, 916–923.

Taylor, M., & Hall, J. A. (1982). Psychological androgyny: Theories, methods, and conclusions. *Psychological Bulletin, 92*, 347–366.

Taylor, S. (1999). Harassment by kids: Are more lawsuits the answer? *National Journal, 231*, 1512–1513.

Teens cite alcohol, drugs as factors leading to sex. (2003, June 9). *Alcoholism and Drug Abuse Weekly*, p. 7.

Terris, M. (2003). Urethritis. Retrieved November 20, 2003, from **http://www.emedicine.com/med/byname/urethritis.htm**

Thomas, A., & Le Melle, S. (1995). The Norplant system: Where are we in 1995? *Journal of Family Practice, 40*, 125–128.

Thompson, C. W. (2002, March 19). FBI cracks child porn ring based on Internet: 89 charged so far in "Operation Candyman." *Washington Post*, p. A2.

Thompson, K. (2004). Experimental methods. Retrieved August 25, 2005, from **http://www.malecontraceptives.org**

Thys-Jacobs, S., Starkey, P., Bernstein, D., & Tian, J. (1998). Calcium carbonate and the premenstrual syndrome: Effects on premenstrual and menstrual symptoms. *American Journal of Obstetrics and Gynecology, 179*, 444–452.

Tiefer, L. (1998). Masturbation: Beyond caution, complacency, and contradiction. *Sexual and Marital Therapy, 13*, 9–14.

Tiefer, L. (2001). A new view of women's sexual problems: Why new? Why now? *Journal of Sex Research, 38*, 89–96.

Tiefer, L. (2004). *Sex is not a natural act* (2d ed.). Boulder, CO: Westview Press.

Timmerman, G. (2004). Adolescents' psychological health and experiences with unwanted sexual behavior at school. *Adolescence, 39*, 17–25.

Tjaden, P., & Thoennes, N. (2000). *Prevalence, incidence, and consequences of violence against women: Findings from the National Violence Against Women Survey*. Washington, DC: U.S. Department of Justice.

Todd, C., Soler, L., Castleman, M., Rogers, K., & Blumenthal, P. (2003). Manual vacuum aspiration for second-trimester pregnancy termination. *International Journal of Gynecology and Obstetrics, 83*, 5–9.

Toma, T. (2001). Unisex contraceptives. Retrieved on January 11, 2002, from **http://www.biomedcentral.com**

Tong, S., Marjono, B., Brown, D., Mulvey, S., Breitt, S, Manuelpillai, U., & Wallace, E. (2004). Serum concentrations of macrophage inhibitory cytokine 1 (MIC 1) as a predictor of miscarriage. *Lancet, 363*, 129–131.

Tough, S., Butt, J., & Sanders, G. (1994). Autoerotic asphyxial deaths: Analysis of nineteen fatalities in Alberta, 1978 to 1989. *Canadian Journal of Psychiatry, 39*, 157–160.

Travis, J. (2001). Sperm protein may lead to male pill. *Science News, 160*, 228.

Treatment options for trichomoniasis to grow? (2004). *Contraceptive Technology Update, 25*, 21–22.

Trends in sexual risk behaviors among high school students: United States, 1991–2001. (2002). *Mortality and Morbidity Weekly Report, 51*, 856–859.

Triandis, H. C. (1989). The self and social behavior in differing cultural contexts. *Psychological Review, 96*, 506–520.

Triandis, H. C., Bontempo, R., Villareal, M. J., Asai, M., & Lucca, N. (1988). Individualism and collectivism: cross-cultural perspectives on self-ingroup relationships. *Journal of Personality and Social Psychology, 54*, 323–338.

Troiden, R. (1989). The formation of homosexual identities. *Journal of Homosexuality, 17*, 43–71.

Troth, T., & Peterson, C. (2000). Factors predicting safe-sex talk and condom use in early sexual relationships. *Health Communication, 12*, 195–212.

Trudel, G., Marchand, A., Ravart, M., Aubin, S., Turgeon, L., & Fortier, P. (2001). The effect of a cognitive-behavioral group treatment on hypoactive sexual desire in women. *Sexual and Relationship Therapy, 16*, 145–164.

Trussell, J. (2004). The essentials of contraception. In R. A. Hatcher, J. Trussell, F. Stewart, W. Cates Jr., A. L. Nelson, F. Guest, & D. Kowal (Eds.), *Contraceptive technology* (18th rev. ed., pp. 221–252). New York: Ardent Media.

Trussell, J., & Kowal, D. (1998). The essentials of contraception. In R. A. Hatcher, J. Trussell, F. Stewart, W. Cates Jr., G. K. Stewart, F. Guest, & D. Kowal (Eds.), *Contraceptive technology* (17th rev. ed., pp. 211–247). New York: Ardent Media.

Trussell, J., Strickler, K., & Vaughan, B. (1993). Contraceptive efficacy of the diaphragm, sponge, and cervical cap. *Family Planning Perspectives, 25*, 101–105.

Tsang, A. (1986). Pornography as a cause or pornographic experience as constituted? *Bulletin of the Hong Kong Psychological Society, 16–17*, 29–32.

Tucker, M. E. (2001, January 1). Drug update: Chancroid. *Family Practice News*, p. 33.

Tucker, M. E. (2003, May 15). Trichomoniasis tricky to diagnose and treat: Better tests needed. *Family Practice News*, p. 30.

Tucker, M. E., & O'Grady, K. (1991). Effects of physical attractiveness, intelligence, age at marriage, and cohabitation on the perception of marital satisfaction. *Journal of Social Psychology, 131*, 253–269.

Tuller, D. (2003, November 25). Syphilis cases increase, raising fear of HIV rise. *New York Times*, p. F7.

Tun, W., Celentano, D., Vlahov, D., & Strathdee, S. (2003). Attitudes toward HIV transmission influence unsafe sexual and injection practices. *AIDS, 17*, 1953–1962.

Turnbull, D., et al. (1996). Randomised, controlled trial of efficacy of midwife-managed care. *Lancet, 347*, 213–218.

Turner, J., Garrison, C., Korpita, E., Waller, J., Addy, C., Hill, W., & Mohn, L. (1994). Promoting responsible sexual behavior through a college freshman seminar. *AIDS Education and Prevention, 6*, 266–277.

Two trials will examine capability of microbicide BufferGel. (2002). *Contraceptive Technology Update, 23*, 41–43.

UNAIDS. (2003, December). AIDS epidemic update. Retrieved July 16, 2004, from **http://www.unaids.org**

UNAIDS. (2004). UN agency calls for new approaches to fighting AIDS as infection rate increases. Retrieved July 13, 2004, from **http://www.un.org**

UNAIDS/WHO. (2005a). Global summary of the HIV and AIDS epidemic. Retrieved December 1, 2005, from **http://www.who.int/hiv/epiupdate2005/en/index.html**

UNAIDS/WHO. (2005b). UNAIDS fact sheet. Retrieved December 1, 2005, from **http://www.who.int/hiv/FS_SubSaharanAfrica_Nov05_en.pdf**

Unique contraceptive no longer available. (1995, September). *Consumer Reports*, p. 566.

United States v. *American Library Association*, 539 U.S. 194 (2003).

Ural, S. (2001). Birthing centers and hospital maternity centers. Retrieved June 4, 2004, from **http://kidshealth.org/parent/system/doctor/birth_centers_hospitals_p4.html**

U.S. Bureau of Justice Statistics. (2002). Homicide trends in the U.S. Retrieved September 5, 2004, from **http://www.ojp.usdoj.gov/bjs/homicide/intimates.htm**

U.S. Census Bureau. (2003). Married couple and unmarried households, 2000: Census 2000 special report. Retrieved July 12, 2005, from **http://www.census.gov/prod/2003pubs/censr-5.pdf**

U.S. Department of Health and Human Services. (2003). Pelvic inflammatory disease. Retrieved November 20, 2003, from **http://www.niaid.nih.gov/factsheets/stdpid.htm**

Vachss, A. (2002, July 14). The difference between sick and evil. *Parade*, pp. 4–5.

Vance, E. B., & Wagner, N. N. (1976). Written descriptions of orgasm: A study of sex differences. *Archives of Sexual Behavior, 5*, 87–98.

Vanfossen, B. (2002). Gender and aggression. Retrieved October 25, 2005, from **http://pages.towson.edu/itrow/research**

van Roosmalen, E., & McDaniel, S. (1998). Sexual harassment in academia: A hazard to women's health. *Women and Health, 28*, 33–43.

Vares, T., Potts, A., Gavey, N., & Grace, V. (2003). Hard sell, soft sell: Men read Viagra ads. *Media International Australia, 108*, 101–114.

Vasclip. (2005). Vasclip patient frequently asked questions, item 7. Retrieved August 24, 2005, from **http://www.vasclip.com/Webpage.asp?MID=275173**

Vasclip receives FDA clearance. (2003, May 26). *Clinical Trials Week*, p. 43.

Veniegas, R., & Conley, T. (2000). Biological research on women's sexual orientations: Evaluating the scientific evidence. *Journal of Social Issues, 56*, 267–282.

Venning, R., & Cavanah, C. (2003). *Sex toys 101: A playfully uninhibited guide*. New York: Fireside.

Ventura, S., Matthews, T., & Hamilton, B. (2001) Births to teenagers in the United States: State trends, 1991–2000. *National Vital Statistics Reports, 50*, 1–4.

Vernarec, E. (2002). Important news for Norplant users. *RN, 65*, 103.

Veseley, R. (2002, May 5). New Bay Area hotline offers postabortion counseling. Retrieved June 12, 2004, from **http://www.womensenews.org/article.cfm/dyn/aid/899/context/cover**

Victor, J. (1998). Moral panics and the social construction of deviant behavior: A theory and application to the case of ritual child abuse. *Sociological Perspectives, 41*, 541–565.

Vittinghoff, E., Douglas, J., Judson, F., McKirnan, D., MacQueen, K., & Buchbinder, S. (1999). Per-contact risk of human immunodeficiency virus transmission between male sexual partners. *American Journal of Epidemiology, 150*, 306–311.

Voeller, B. (1991). AIDS and heterosexual anal intercourse. *Archives of Sexual Behavior, 20*, 233–276.

von Sadovszky, V., Keller, M., & McKinney, K. (2002). College students' perceptions and practices of sexual activities in sexual encounters. *Journal of Nursing Scholarship, 34*, 133–138.

Vyas, K. (2004, September 12). Thais plan first live sex-change operation. Retrieved July 3, 2005, from **http://www.medicinenet.com/script/main/art.asp?articlekey=40972**

Wachter, K. (2005). Feds delay OTC decision for Plan B. Family *Practice News, 35*, 2.

Wagner, M. (1999). Episiotomy: A form of genital mutilation. *Lancet, 353*, 1977.

Wald, A. (1999). Genital herpes. *Western Journal of Medicine, 170*, 343–344.

Wald, A, Zeh, J., Selke, S., Warren, T., Ashley, R., & Corey, L. (2002). Genital shedding of HSV among men. *Journal of Infectious Diseases, 186*, S34–S39.

Waldinger, M., & Olivier, B. (1998). Selective serotonin reuptake inhibitor–induced sexual dysfunction. *International Clinical Psychopharmacology, 13*, S27–S33.

Waldo, C. (1998). Out on campus: Sexual orientation and academic climate in a university context. *American Journal of Community Psychology, 26*, 745–760.

Walen, S., & Roth, D. (1987). A cognitive approach. In J. H. Geer & W. T. O'Donohue (Eds.), *Theories of human sexuality* (pp. 335–362). New York: Plenum Press.

Wallace J., Weiner A., &, Bloch D. (1996, July). *Fellatio is a significant risk activity for acquiring AIDS in New York City streetwalking sex workers*. Paper presented at the Eleventh International Conference on AIDS, Vancouver, BC.

Walling, A. D. (1999). Etiology and management of cystitis. *American Family Physician, 59*, 1314.

Walling, A. D. (2000). Should an episiotomy be routine in childbirth? *American Family Physician, 62*, 1889.

Walling, A. D. (2002). Women's regret after sterilization procedures. *American Family Physician, 66*, 1326.

Walling, A. D. (2004). HAART and patients with HIV infection. *American Family Physician, 69*, 1797.

Walling, W. H. (1904). *Sexology*. Philadelphia: Puritan.

Walsh, N. (2003a, June 1). Over-the-counter access sought for emergency contraceptive pills: Prescription seen as barrier. *Family Practice News*, p. 38.

Walsh, N. (2003b). Tetravalent HPV vaccine now in phase III trials: Cervical cancer prevention. *Internal Medicine News, 36*(17), 38.

Warner, D. L., & Hatcher, R. (1998). Male condoms. In R. A. Hatcher, J. Trussell, F. Stewart, W. Cates Jr., G. K. Stewart, F. Guest, & D. Kowal (Eds.), *Contraceptive technology* (17th rev. ed., pp. 325–355). New York: Ardent Media.

Warner, D. L., Hatcher, R. A., & Steiner, M. J. (2004). Male condoms. In R. A. Hatcher, J. Trussell, F. Stewart, W. Cates Jr., A. L. Nelson, F. Guest, & D. Kowal (Eds.), *Contraceptive technology* (18th rev. ed., pp. 331–335). New York: Ardent Media.

Warshaw, R. (1994). *I never called it rape*. New York: HarperPerennial.

Washburn, P. (2003). Why me? Addressing the spiritual and emotional trauma of sexual assault. *Topics in Emergency Medicine, 25*, 236–241.

Washington State Medical Association. (2003). "Teen Dating Violence." Retrieved October 22, 2005, from **http://www.atg.wa.gov/violence/DVAC_brochure_10_2003.pdf**.

Washington State, Office of the Attorney General. (2004). Breaking the silence: Talking about dating violence. Retrieved February 24, 2006, from **http://www.atg.wa.gov/violence/points.shtml**.

Watanabe, M. (2004). Origins of HIV: The interrelationship between nonhuman primates and the virus. *BioScience, 54*, 810–814.

Waterman, A., Reid, J., Garfield, L., & Hoy, S. (2001). From curiosity to care: Heterosexual student interest in sexual diversity courses. *Teaching of Psychology, 28*, 21–26.

WebMD Health. (2002). Dilation and evacuation. Retrieved June 12, 2002, from **http://my.webmd.com/encyclopedia/article/1820.50530**

Weeks, G. R., & Gambescia, N. (2000). *Erectile dysfunction: Integrating couple therapy, sex therapy, and medical treatment*. New York: Norton.

Weeks, G. R., & Gambescia, N. (2002). *Hypoactive sexual desire: Integrating sex and couple therapy*. New York: Norton.

Weeks, R., & James, J. (1999). *Secrets of the superyoung: The scientific reasons some people look ten years younger than they really are—and how you can, too*. New York: Berkley.

Weiss, D., Rabinowitz, B., & Ruckstuhl, M. (1992). Individual changes in sexual attitudes and behavior within college-level human sexuality courses. *Journal of Sex Research, 29*, 43–59.

Wellesley Centers for Women. (1998). The wife rape information page: **http://www.ou.edu/womensoc/effects-of-rape.htm**. Retrieved August 7, 2005, from **http://www.wellesley.edu/WCW/mrape.html**

Well-Woman. (2001, October). Q&A. Retrieved August 13, 2005, from **http://www.barnard.columbia.edu/wwoman/qanda/sexuality/femejac.html**

Wendel, K., & Rompalo, A. (2002). Scabies and pediculosis pubis: An update of treatment regimens and general review. *Clinical Infectious Diseases, 35*, S146–S151.

Werner, N., & Crick, N. (1999). Relational aggression and social psychological adjustment in a college sample. *Journal of Abnormal Psychology, 108*, 615–623.

Wessells, L., & McAninch, J. (1996). Penile length in the flaccid and erect states: Guidelines for penile augmentation. *Journal of Urology, 156*, 995–997.

West, D., & de Villiers, B. (1993). *Male prostitution*. Binghamton, NY: Haworth Press.

Westphal, W. P. (2004, June 19). Dye method of sperm sorting appears safe. *New Scientist*, p. 13.

What happened to the wedding bells? Cohabitation is on the rise, new data from Census 2000 reveals. (2003). *Forecast, 23*, 1–3.

Wheeler, C. (1995). Labor: Normal and dysfunctional. In D. Coustan, R. Haning, & D. Singer (Eds.), *Human reproduction: Growth and development* (pp. 291–306). Boston: Little, Brown.

Whipple, B. (1999, November 4). *Beyond the G-spot: Where do we go from here?* Address delivered at the joint annual conference of the American Association of Sex Educators, Counselors, and Therapists and the Society for the Scientific Study of Sexuality, St. Louis, MO.

Whipple, B. (2000). Beyond the G-spot. *Scandinavian Journal of Sexology, 3*, 35–42.

Whipple, B. (2001). Women's sexuality in the 21st century. *Medical Aspects of Human Sexuality, 1*, 7–8.

Whipple, B. (2002). Review of Milan Zaviacic's book *The human female prostate: From vestigial Skene paraurethral glands and ducts to woman's functional prostate*. *Archives of Sexual Behavior, 31*, 457–458.

Whipple, B., Myers, B., & Komisaruk, B. (1998). Male multiple ejaculatory orgasms: A case study. *Journal of Sex Education and Therapy, 23*, 157–162.

Whipple, B., & Zaviacic, M. (1993). Update on the female prostate and the phenomenon of female ejaculation. *Journal of Sex Research, 30*, 148–152.

Wickelgren, I. (1999). Discovery of "gay gene" questioned. *Science, 284*, 571.

Wiederman, M. (1993). Demographic and sexual characteristics of nonresponders to sexual experience items in a national survey. *Journal of Sex Research, 30*, 27–35.

Wiederman, M. (1998). The state of theory in sex therapy. *Journal of Sex Research, 35*, 88–99.

Wiederman, M. (2001). "Don't look now!" The role of self-focus in sexual dysfunction. *Family Journal, 9*, 210–214.

Wight, D., Henderson, M., Raab, G., Abraham, C., Buston, K., Scott, S, & Hart, G. (2000). Extent of regretted sexual intercourse among young teenagers in Scotland: A cross-sectional survey. *British Medical Journal, 320*, 1243–1244.

Wilcox, A., Dunson, D., & Baird, D. (2000). The timing of the "fertile window" in the menstrual cycle: Day-specific estimates from a prospective study. *British Medical Journal, 321*, 1259–1262.

Wilcox, L. S., Chu, S. Y., Eaker, E. D., Zeger, S. L., & Peterson, H. B. (1991). Risk factors for regret after tubal sterilization: Five years of follow-up in a prospective study. *Fertility and Sterility, 55*, 927–933.

Williams, R. (1995). Breast-feeding best bet for babies. *FDA Consumer*, 29. Retrieved June 6, 2004, from **http://www.fda.gov/fdac/features/895_brstfeed.html**

Williams, S. P. (2001, August 12–15). *Living positively: A formative study of HIV+ seroconcordant heterosexual couples*. Presentation at the 2001 National HIV Prevention Conference, Atlanta.

Williamson, S., & Nowak, R. (1998). The truth about women: A new anatomical study shows there is more to the clitoris than anyone ever thought. *New Scientist, 159*, 34–36.

Wilson, B. (2003). Androgen insensitivity syndrome. Retrieved July 10, 2005, from **http://www.emedicine.com/ped/topic2222.htm**

Wilson, W. (1989). Brief resolution of the issue of similarity versus complementarity in mate selection using height preferences as a model. *Psychological Reports, 65*, 387–389.

Winick, C., & Evans, J. (1996). The relationship between nonenforcement of state pornography laws and rates of sex crime arrests. *Archives of Sexual Behavior, 25*, 439–453.

Winks, C., & Semans, A. (2002). *The good vibrations guide to sex*. Pittsburgh: Cleis Press.

Wisconsin Coalition Against Sexual Assault (2000). Campus sexual assault. Retrieved August 30, 2002, from **http://www.wcasa.org/pages/camp.html**

Wise, L., Zierler, S., Krieger, N., & Harlow, B. (2001). Adult onset of major depressive disorder in relation to early-life violent victimization: A case control study. *Lancet, 358*, 881–887.

Wise, T. (1985). Fetishism: Etiology and treatment: A review from multiple perspectives. *Comprehensive Psychiatry, 26*, 249–257.

Witt, S. (1997). Parental influence on children's socialization to gender roles. *Adolescence, 126*, 253–259.

Witt, S. (2000). The influence of television on childrens' gender role socialization. *Childhood Education, 76*, 322–324.

Wolchik, S., Spencer, S. L., & Lisi, I. (1983). Volunteer bias in research employing vaginal measures of sexual arousal. *Archives of Sexual Behavior, 12*, 399–408.

Women's Services and Gender Resource Center. (2005). Acquaintance rape. Retrieved February 24, 2006, from **http://www.plymouth.edu/psc/wsgr/acqaint.shtml**

Wood, E., Desmarias, S., & Guglia, S. (2002). The impact of parenting experience on gender-stereotyped toy play of children. *Sex Roles, 47*, 39–49.

Woodhill, B., & Samuels, C. (2003). Positive and negative androgyny and their relationship with psychological health and well-being. *Sex Roles, 48*, 555–565.

Woods, J. (2001). Hostile hallways. *Educational Leadership, 59*, 20–23.

Woods, L., & Emery, R. (2002). The cohabitation effect on divorce: Causation or selection? *Journal of Divorce and Remarriage, 37*, 101–122.

Woodward, B., & Armstrong, S. (2005). *The brethren: Inside the Supreme Court*. New York: Simon & Schuster. Originally published in 1979.

Woodward, C., & Fisher, M. A. (1999). Drug treatment of common STDs, Part 1: Herpes, syphilis, urethritis, chlamydia, and gonorrhea. *American Family Physician, 60*, 1387–1394.

Word, C., & Bowser, B. (1997). Background to crack cocaine addiction and HIV high-risk behavior: The next epidemic. *American Journal of Drug and Alcohol Abuse, 23*, 67–77.

World Health Organization. (1982). A randomized double-blind study of two combined and two progestin-only oral contraceptives. *Contraception, 25*, 243–252.

World Health Organization. (1996). Female genital mutilation. Report of a WHO Technical Working Group, Geneva, July 17–19, 1995. Document No. WHO/FRH/WHD/96.10. Geneva, Switzerland.

World Health Organization. (2003). Gender and HIV/AIDS. Retrieved November 14, 2003, from **http://www.who.int/gender/hiv_aids/en**

Worobey, J. (2001). Sex differences in associations of temperament with love-styles. *Psychological Reports, 89*, 25–27.

Xu, F., Schillinger, J., Sternberg, M., Johnson, R., Lee, F., Nahmias, A., & Markowitz, L. (2002). Seroprevalence and coinfection with herpes simplex virus type 1 and type 2 in the United States, 1988–1994. *Journal of Infectious Diseases, 185*, 1019–1024.

Yambo, C. M., McFee, R. B., Caraccio, T. R., & McGuigan, M. (2002). The case of the inkjet cleaner "hurricane": Another GHB recipe. *Journal of Toxicology: Clinical Toxicology, 40*, 688.

Yetter, J. (1998). Examination of the placenta. *American Family Physician, 57*, 1045–1054.

Yonkers, K. (2004). Management strategies for PMS/PMDD. *Journal of Family Practice, 53*, SS15–SS20.

Young, A. M., Boyd, C., & Hubbell, A. (2000). Prostitution, drug use, and coping with psychological distress. *Journal of Drug Issues, 30*, 789–800.

Young, M. (2001). PMS and PMDD: Identification and treatment. *Patient Care, 35*, 29–50.

Young, M., Luquis, R., Deny, G., & Young, T. (1998). Correlates of sexual satisfaction in marriage. *Canadian Journal of Human Sexuality, 7*, 115–127.

Zajonc, R. B. (1968). Attitudinal effects of mere exposure [Monograph]. *Journal of Personality and Social Psychology, 9*(Suppl.), 1–27.

Zajonc, R. B. (2001). Mere exposure: A gateway to the subliminal. *Current Directions in Psychological Science, 10*, 225–228.

Zaviacic, M. (2002a). Female urethral expulsions evoked by local digital stimulation of the G-spot: Differences in the response patterns. *Journal of Sex Research, 24*, 311–318.

Zaviacic, M. (2002b). *The human female prostate: From vestigial Skene paraurethral glands and ducts to woman's functional prostate*. Bratislavia, Slovakia: Slovak Academic Press.

Zaviacic, M., Zaviacicova, A., Holoman, I. K., & Molcan, J. (1988). Female urethral expulsions evoked by local digital stimulation of the G-spot: Differences in the response patterns. *Journal of Sex Research, 24*, 311–318.

Zepf, B. (2001). Sperm analysis values: Which indicate infertility? *American Family Physician, 65*, 1173–1174.

Zepf, B. (2003a). Adefovir for treatment of chronic hepatitis B infection. *American Family Physician, 68*, 1643–1645.

Zepf, B. (2003b). Watchful waiting or surgery for early prostate cancer? *American Family Physician, 67*, 599.

Zgourides, G., Monto, M., & Harris, R. (1997). Correlates of adolescent male sexual offense: Prior adult contact, sexual attitudes, and use of sexually explicit materials. *International Journal of Offender Therapy and Comparative Criminology, 41*, 272–283.

Zillman, D., & Bryant, J. (1982). Pornography, sexual callousness, and the trivialization of rape. *Journal of Communication, 32*, 10–21.

Zimmerman, T., Haddock, S., Current, L., & Ziemba, S. (2003). Intimate partnership: Foundation to the successful balance of family and work. *American Journal of Family Therapy, 31*, 107–114.

Zucker, K. J., Blanchard, R., & Siegelman, M. (2003). Birth order among homosexual men. *Psychological Reports, 92*, 117–118.

Zucker, K. J., Wilson-Smith, D., Kurita, J., & Stern, A. (1995). Children's appraisals of sex-typed behavior in their peers. *Sex Roles, 33*, 703–725.

Credits

Photos and Cartoons

Frontmatter

p. vii istockphoto.com/malcom romain; **p. viii (top)** GK Hart/Vikki Hart/Image Bank/Getty Images; **p. viii (bottom)** Kathleen Finlay/Masterfile Stock Image Library; **p. ix** istockphoto.com/Ole Jørgen Bratland and Gisele Jaquenod; **p. x (top)** istockphoto.com/Matthew Bowden; **p. x (bottom)** istockphoto.com; **p. xi** Keate/Masterfile Stock Image Library; **p. xii** Dr. David M. Phillips/Getty Images, Inc.; **p. xiii** istockphoto.com/Dana Spiropoulou; **p. xiv (top)** istockphoto.com/José Carlos Pires Pereira; **p. xiv (bottom)** istockphoto.com/Mike Bentley; **p. xv** Stock.xchng/Kathy McCallum; **p. xvi (top)** Stock.xchng; **p. xvi (bottom)** istockphoto.com/Todd Taulman; **p. xvii** Masterfile Stock Image Library; **p. xxviii** Roger R. Hock, Ph.D.

Chapter 1

p. 2 (top) and **p. 34** Ron Stroud/Masterfile Stock Image Library; **p. 2 (bottom)** and **p. 3** istockphoto.com/malcom romain; **p. 11** MGM/The Kobal Collection/Grobet, Lourdes; **p. 13** AP Wide World Photos; **p. 18 (left)** © Bettmann/CORBIS All Rights Reserved; **p. 18 (right)** Everett Collection; **p. 19 (top)** David Young-Wolff/PhotoEdit Inc.; **p. 19 (bottom)** Rachel Epstein/PhotoEdit Inc.; **p. 24** Imagination Photo Design; **p. 26** © CORBIS All Rights Reserved; **p. 27** © Bettmann/CORBIS All Rights Reserved; **p. 30 (left)** Behavioral Technology, Inc; **p. 30 (right)** Behavioral Technology, Inc., Salt Lake City, UT; **p. 32** David Young-Wolff/PhotoEdit Inc.

Chapter 2

p. 36 (top) and **p. 70** David Mendelsohn/Masterfile Stock Image Library; **p. 36 (bottom)** and **p. 37** GK Hart/Vikki Hart/Image Bank/Getty Images; **p. 39** Courtesy of the Library of Congress; **p. 40 (left)** Custom Medical Stock Photo, Inc.; **p. 40 (right)** Joel Gordon/Joel Gordon Photography; **p. 41** SuperStock, Inc.; **p. 44** Picture Desk, Inc./Kobal Collection; **p. 45** "erectionphotos.com"; **p. 46** Photo Researchers, Inc.; **p. 47 (top left)** AP Wide World Photos; **p. 47 (bottom right)** Joel Gordon/Joel Gordon Photograph; **p. 51 (left and right)** Tee A. Corinne; **p. 59 (top left and right, and bottom left)** Jules Selmes and Debi Treloar © Dorling Kindersley; **p. 59 (bottom right)** Joel Gordon Photography; **p. 60** Francoise Sauze/Science Photo Library; **p. 62** Photo Researchers, Inc.; **p. 63** Photo Researchers, Inc.

Chapter 3

p. 72 (top) and **p. 92** Eric Schmidt/Masterfile Stock Image Library; **p. 72 (bottom)** Kathleen Finlay/Masterfile Stock Image Library; **p. 73** Randy Allbritton/Getty Images, Inc.; **p. 74** Joel Gordon/Joel Gordon Photography; **p. 76** Ira Wyman/Corbis/Sygma; **p. 88** Helen Singer Kaplan, M.D., Ph.D.

Chapter 4

p. 94 (top) and **p. 140** Getty Images Inc.; **p. 94 (bottom)** and **p. 95** istockphoto.com/Ole Jørgen Bratland and Gisele Jaquenod; **p. 97** Corbis/Bettmann; **p. 98** Getty Images, Inc.; **p. 100 (left)** Hulton Archive/Getty Images; **p. 100 (right)** Globe Photos, Inc.; **p. 101** Getty Images/Digital Vision; **p. 102** Lisa Pines/Getty Images—Photonica Amana America, Inc.; **p. 104** Pictor International/Alamy Images; **p. 108** Art Resource, N.Y.; **p. 109 (top left)** Getty Images, Inc.; **p. 109 (top right)** Getty Images, Inc.; **p. 109 (bottom right)** © Jose Luis Pelaez/CORBIS All Rights Reserved; **p. 110** Art Resource, N.Y.; **p. 119 (top)** SuperStock, Inc.; **p. 119 (bottom)** Superstock Royalty Free; **p. 120** Alamy Images Royalty Free; **p. 124** © Paul Barton/CORBIS All Rights Reserved; **p. 128** © Michael Keller/CORBIS All Rights Reserved; **p. 129** Ghislain & Marie David de Lossy/Image Bank/Getty Images; **p. 132** Getty Images Inc.—Rubberball Royalty Free; **p. 137** Alamy Images Royalty Free.

Chapter 5

p. 142 (top) and **p. 186** Mark Wiens/Masterfile Stock Image Library; **p. 142 (bottom)** istockphoto.com/Hermann Danzmayr; **p. 143** istockphoto.com/Matthew Bowden; **p. 145** © Bettmann/CORBIS All Rights Reserved; **p. 153** Greg Ceo/Taxi/Getty Images; **p. 155** Jonathan A. Meyers/Photo Researchers, Inc.; **p. 156** James Darell/Getty Images Inc.—Stone Allstock; **p. 157 (left and right)** Joel Gordon/Joel Gordon Photography; **p. 159** Scott Camazine/Photo Researchers, Inc.; **p. 161** Joel Gordon/Joel Gordon Photography; **p. 165 (top and bottom)** Image reproduced with the permission of Organon USA Inc. and that Implanon™ is a trademark of N.V. Organon; **p. 167** Joel Gordon/Joel Gordon Photography; **p. 168** Joel Gordon/Joel Gordon Photography; **p. 169** Courtesy of John Nebraska; **p. 170 (top)** Joel Gordon/Joel Gordon Photography; **p. 170 (bottom)** Joel Gordon Photography; **p. 171** Joel Gordon/Joel Gordon Photography; **p. 172** Joel Gordon/Joel Gordon Photography; **p. 173** Joel Gordon/Joel Gordon Photography; **p. 178** Joel Gordon/Joel Gordon Photography.

Chapter 6

p. 188 (top) and **p. 224** Getty Images, Inc.; **p. 188 (bottom)** Dk & Dennies Cody/Masterfile Stock Image Library; **p. 189** istockphoto.com; **p. 191** Art Resource, N.Y.; **p. 200** Art Resource, N.Y.; **p. 203** MARY EVANS PICTURE LIBRARY; **p. 206 (left)** Joel Gordon/Joel Gordon Photography; **p. 206 (right)** Dion Ogust/The Image Works; **p. 208** Laurence Dutton/Getty Images Inc.—Stone Allstock; **p. 209** Getty Images, Inc.; **p. 210 (left)** Alamy Images Royalty Free; **p. 210 (right)** Getty Images, Inc.

Chapter 7

p. 226 (top) and **p. 268** Getty Images, Inc.; **p. 226 (bottom)** istockphoto.com/Diane Diederich; **p. 227** Keate/Masterfile Stock Image Library; **p. 234** Getty Images, Inc.; **p. 237** Alamy Images Royalty Free;

p. 240 Denis Poroy/AP Wide World Photos; **p. 247** Joel Gordon/Joel Gordon Photography; **p. 251** ©The New Yorker Collection 1999 Robert Mankoff from cartoonbank.com. All Rights Reserved; **p. 253** Joel Gordon/Joel Gordon Photography.

Chapter 8

p. 270 (top) and **p. 320** Getty Images, Inc.; **p. 270 (bottom)** Getty Images, Inc.; **p. 271** Getty Images, Inc.; **p. 273** Getty Images, Inc.; **p. 277** © Holger Scheibe/Zefa/CORBIS All Rights Reserved; **p. 279** ©The New Yorker Collection 2000 Barbara Smaller from cartoonbank.com. All Rights Reserved; **p. 284** Jeff Greenberg/PhotoEdit Inc.; **p. 285 (left)** Biophoto Associates/Photo Researchers, Inc.; **p. 285 (right)** Mediscan/Visuals Unlimited; **p. 288** Garry Watson/Photo Researchers, Inc.; **p. 291 (left)** Photo Researchers, Inc.; **p. 291 (right)** Bart's Medical Library/Phototake NYC; **p. 292** © Gideon Mendel/Action Aid/CORBIS All Rights Reserved; **p. 298** Getty Images, Inc.; **p. 304 (left)** ©Diepgen TL, Yihune G et al. Dermatology Online Atlas (www.dermis.net). Reprinted with permission; **p. 304 (right)** Courtesy, Director-General and Programme Manager Prevention of Blindness, World Health Organization; **p. 306** Centers for Disease Control & Prevention; **p. 307** Chris Bjornberg/Science Photo Library/Photo Researchers, Inc.; **p. 308 (left)** Photo Researchers, Inc.; **p. 308 (right)** C. James Webb/Phototake NYC; **p. 309** © Lester V. Bergman/CORBIS All Rights Reserved; **p. 310 (top)** CDC/Joe Miller/Centers for Disease Control and Prevention (CDC); **p. 310 (bottom)** Dr. M.A. Ansary/Photo Researchers, Inc.; **p. 311** Tony Freeman/PhotoEdit Inc.; **p. 312** David M. Phillips/The Population Control/Photo Researchers, Inc.; **p. 313 (top)** E. Gray/Photo Researchers, Inc.; **p. 313 (bottom)** Dr. P. Marazzi/Photo Researchers, Inc.; **p. 316** Noel Hendrickson/Getty Images—Digital Vision; **p. 317** Courtesy of John Nebraska; **p. 319** SuperStock, Inc.

Chapter 9

p. 322 (top) and **p. 368** Stockbyte/Getty Images, Inc.—Stockbyte; **p. 322 (bottom)** Getty Images, Inc.—Blend Images; **p. 323** istockphoto.com/Dana Spiropoulou; **p. 325** Getty Images, Inc.; **p. 331** From Tulandi's Atlas of Laparoscopy and Hysteroscopy Technique, W.B. Saunders, London, 1999 (Reproduced with permission); **p. 333 (top left)** Photo Researchers, Inc.; **p. 333 (top right)** Photo Researchers, Inc.; **p. 333 (bottom right)** Pascal Goetgheluck/Photo Researchers, Inc.; **p. 335 (top)** Petit Format/Photo Researchers, Inc.; **p. 335 (bottom)** © Petit Format/Nestle/Science Source/Photo Researchers, Inc.; **p. 336 (top)** Biophoto Associates/Photo Researchers, Inc.; **p. 336 (middle)** Ralph Hutchings/Visuals Unlimited; **p. 336 (bottom)** Lennart Nilsson; **p. 339** John Cole/Photo Researchers, Inc.; **p. 342** Dr. Najeeb Layyous/Photo Researchers, Inc.; **p. 344** Kevin Wolf/AP Wide World Photos; **p. 351 (top and bottom)** Michele Davidson/Pearson Education/PH College; **p. 355** Illini Hospital Operated by Genesis Health System; **p. 356** Medical-On-Line Ltd.; **p. 359** Masterfile Stock Image Library; **p. 360** © CORBIS All Rights Reserved; **p. 365 (top)** © Adrian Arbib/CORBIS All Rights Reserved; **p. 365 (bottom)** Mauro Fermariello/Photo Researchers, Inc.; **p. 366** Roger R. Hock, Ph.D.

Chapter 10

p. 370 (top) and **p. 402** Photodisc/Getty Images; **p. 370 (bottom)** and **p. 371** istockphoto.com/José Carlos Pires Pereira; **p. 373 (top left)** © CORBIS All Rights Reserved; **p. 373 (top right)** Fernando Aceves/Retna Ltd.; **p. 373 (bottom)** © Bettmann/CORBIS All Rights Reserved; **p. 374** © Bettmann/CORBIS All Rights Reserved; **p. 378** Dr. Samuel Freire da Silva/Samuel Freire da Silva; **p. 379** © CORBIS All Rights Reserved; **p. 381** Artiga Photo/Masterfile Stock Image Library; **p. 382 (top)** Aflo Foto Agency/Alamy Images; **p. 382 (bottom)** Tom & Dee Ann McCarthy © CORBIS All Rights Reserved; **p. 386 (top and bottom)** Courtesy of Gary J. Alter, M.D.; **p. 390** © Ariel Skelley/CORBIS All Rights Reserved; **p. 392** © The New Yorker Collection 1995 Donald Reilly from cartoonbank.com. All Rights Reserved; **p. 393** Big Cheese Photo/Superstock Royalty Free; **p. 397** Rob Elliott/Getty Images, Inc.; **p. 398 (top)** Kwame Zikomo/SuperStock, Inc.; **p. 398 (bottom)** Kevin Dodge/Masterfile Stock Image Library; **p. 399** Getty Images, Inc.

Chapter 11

p. 404 (top) and **p. 437** WireImageStock/Masterfile Stock Image Library; **p. 404 (bottom)** and **p. 405** istockphoto.com/Mike Bentley; **p. 407** Time Life Pictures/ Time Life Pictures/Time Magazine, Copyright Time Inc./Time Life Pictures/Getty Images; **p. 413** Dino Vournas/AP Wide World Photos; **p. 419** Getty Images, Inc.; **p. 421 (left)** Getty Images, Inc.; **p. 421 (right)** © Jennie Woodcock; Reflections Photolibrary/CORBIS All Rights Reserved; **p. 424** Andrew Brusso/Picture Desk, Inc./Kobal Collection; **p. 425** Jeremy O'Donnell/Getty Images, Inc.; **p. 426** Index Stock Imagery, Inc. Royaly Free; **p. 431** © Erich Schlegel/CORBIS All Rights Reserved; **p. 433** Corbis/Sygma.

Chapter 12

p. 440 (top) and **p. 476** David Nardini/Masterfile Stock Image Library; **p. 440 (bottom)** Getty Images/Digital Vision; **p. 441** Stock.xchng/Kathy McCallum; **p. 443 (top right)** Historical Pictures/Stock Montage, Inc./Historical Picures Collection; **p. 443 (bottom left)** Tony Freeman/PhotoEdit Inc.; **p. 443 (bottom right)** Daniel Boster/Photographer's Choice/Getty Images; **p. 447** Michael Newman/PhotoEdit Inc.; **p. 454** David Young-Wolff/PhotoEdit Inc.; **p. 455** Picturequest—Royalty Free; **p. 458** Elie Bernager/Photodisc Red/Getty Images; **p. 468** Corbis Royalty Free; **p. 472** © Norbert Schaefer/CORBIS All Rights Reserved; **p. 474** David Young-Wolff/PhotoEdit Inc.

Chapter 13

p. 478 (top) and **p. 514** Stock.xchng; **p. 478 (bottom)** and **p. 479** Stock.xchng; **p. 481** Ian Thraves/Alamy Images; **p. 485** Photodisc/Getty Images; **p. 486** © Roy Morsch/CORBIS All Rights Reserved; **p. 488** Superstock Royalty Free; **p. 491 (left and right)** David Hoffman/Alamy Images; **p. 502** Photodisc/Getty Images; **p. 507** Courtesy of National Alert Registry; **p. 512** Getty Images, Inc.

Chapter 14

p. 516 (top) and **p. 545** Getty Images, Inc.; **p. 516 (bottom)** istockphoto.com; **p. 517** istockphoto.com/Todd Taulman; **p. 525** Getty Images, Inc.; **p. 528** PhotoEdit Inc.; **p. 529** © Jutta Klee/CORBIS All Rights Reserved; **p. 530 (top)** ©2006 Bob Zahn from cartoonbank.com. All Rights Reserved; **p. 530 (bottom)** Digital Vision/Getty Images/Digital Vision; **p. 532 (top)** Private Collection/The Bridgeman Art Library; **p. 532 (bottom)** © Dorling Kindersley; **p. 535** Getty

Images, Inc.; **p. 538 (left)** Age Fotostock/SuperStock, Inc.; **p. 538 (middle)** Mark Leibowitz/Masterfile Stock Image Library; **p. 538 (right)** Getty Images, Inc.; **p. 539 (top)** Ron Kimball/Ron Kimball Photography; **p. 539 (bottom)** Getty Images, Inc.; **p. 540 (top)** Getty Images, Inc.; **p. 540 (bottom)** Getty Images, Inc.; **p. 541** Thinkstock.

Chapter 15

p. 548 (top) and **p. 587** Getty Images, Inc.; **p. 548 (bottom)** Green Project/Masterfile; **p. 549** Masterfile Stock Image Library; **p. 551** Archaeological Museum Tarquinia/Dagli Orti/Picture Desk, Inc./Kobal Collection; **p. 554** © John Van Hasselt/CORBIS All Rights Reserved; **p. 555 (top)** © Creasource/CORBIS All Rights Reserved; **p. 555 (bottom)** Getty Images, Inc.; **p. 556 (top)** © John Van Hasselt/CORBIS All Rights Reserved; **p. 556 (bottom)** Getty Images, Inc.; **p. 557** D.R/Corbis Sygma/Corbis/Sygma; **p. 559** © Bill Gentile/CORBIS All Rights Reserved; **p. 562** © John Van Hasselt/CORBIS All Rights Reserved; **p. 563** © Lynsey Addario/CORBIS All Rights Reserved; **p. 564** Corbis Digital Stock; **p. 569** AP Wide World Photos; **p. 570** Courtesy of John Nebraska; **p. 571** James Keyser/Time Life Pictures/Getty Images/Time Life Pictures; **p. 572** Getty Images, Inc.; **p. 573** © Red James/zefa/CORBIS All Rights Reserved; **p. 575 (left)** Ingram Publishing/Getty Images/Digital Vision; **p. 575 (middle)** Jean-Claude Marlaud/Getty Images/Digital Vision; **p. 575 (right)** ©Uwe Krejci/Zefa/CORBIS All Rights Reserved; **p. 581** Filippo Monteforte/Agence France Presse/Getty Images; **p. 583** Courtesy of CDC.

Figures and Tables

Chapter 1

Table 1.2 Adapted from King, Parisi, and O'Dwyer (1993); **Table 1.5** Adapted from Clement (1990); Morokoff (1986); Strassberg & Lowe (1995); Wiederman (1993); and Wolchik, Spencer, & Lisi (1983).

Chapter 2

Page 54 Map, p. 43 from *Female Genital Mutilation*: Integrating the Prevention and the Management of the Health Complications into the Curricula of Nursing and Midwifery, A Teacher's Guide, World Health Organization. (http://www.who.int/gender/other_health/en/teachersguide.pdf). Reprinted by permission of WHO.

Chapter 3

Figure 3.1 Adapted from Masters and Johnson (1966); **Figure 3.9** Based on data in Mah & Binik, 2002, p. 110; **Table 3.1** Adapted from Hock (2005b).

Chapter 4

Figure 4.1 Figure from *The Triangle of Love* by Robert J. Sternberg. Copyright © 1998. Published by Basic Books. Reprinted by permission of Dr. Robert J. Sternberg; **Figure 4.3** Based on *Social Penetration: The Development of Interpersonal Relationships* by I. Altman and D. Taylor, 1973, Holt; **Figure 4.4** Adapted from Brehm, Kassin, and Fein (1999), Fig. 9.10; **Table 4.2** "Warning Signs of a Potential Abuser" adapted from The Project for Victims of Family Violence, Inc. Reprinted by permission of The Project for Victims of Family Violence, Inc.

Chapter 5

Table 5.1 American Health Consultants (2001); Best (2000); Hatcher et al. (1994, 1998, 2004); Kirn (2001); Napoli (2001); Roumen, Apter, & Mulders (2001); R. Rubin (2001); **Table 5.2** "Strategies for Influencing a Resistant Partner to Use a Condom" from "Influencing a Partner to Use a Condom" by S. DeBro, S. Campbell, and L. Peplau, *Psychology of Women Quarterly*, 18, (1994), p. 176. Copyright © 1994. Reprinted by permission of Blackwell Publishing; **Figure 5.9** Adapted from Feminist Women's Health Center (2004).

Chapter 6

Table 6.1 Barak et al. (1999); Byers, Purdon, and Clark (1998); Fisher et al. (1988); Forbes et al. (2003); Garcia (1999); **Table 6.2** Hsu et al. (1994); Kelly (2001); von Sadovszky, Keller, & McKinney (2002); **Table 6.4** Alfonso, Allison, and Dunn (1992); Byers, Purdon, and Clark (1998); Cato and Leitenberg (1990); Davidson and Hoffman (1986); Leitenberg and Henning (1995); Masters, Johnson, and Kolodny (1995); Reinisch (1990); Renaud and Byers (1999); Striar and Bartlik (1999); **Table 6.5** Source: Adapted from Hsu et al. (1994); **Table 6.6** Davidson and Moore (1994); Kay (1992); Kelly, Strassberg, and Kircher (1990); Masters and Johnson (1974); "The Politics of Masturbation" (1994); Tiefer (1998); **Table 6.7** Table 8, p. 116 from *Sex in America* by R. Michael, J. Gagnon, E. Laumann, & G. Kolata. Copyright © 1994 by CSG Enterprises, Inc. Reprinted by permission of Little, Brown and Co., Inc. and Brockman, Inc.; **Table 6.8** Durex Corp. (2003).

Chapter 7

Table 7.2 Table, "Prevalence of Sexual Problems in the US" from *The Social Organization of Sexuality* by E. Laumann, J. Gagnon, R. Michael, and S. Michaels. Copyright © 1994. Reprinted by permission of The University of Chicago Press; **Table 7.4** Table, "Effects of Drug Abuse on Sexual Functioning" from "Medications That May Contribute to Sexual Disorders" by W. Finger, M. Lund and M. Slagle, *Journal of Family Practice*, 44, (1997), pp. 33–43. Copyright© 1997. Reprinted by permission of The Journal of Family Practice; **Table 7.6** Table, "Cognitive-Behavioral Approach to Hypoactive Sexual Desire" by B. McCarthy in *Journal of Sex Education & Therapy*, 21, (1995), pp. 132–141. Copyright ©1995. Reprinted by permission of American Association of Sex Educators, Counselors & Therapists; **Table 7.7** Table, "Understanding Male Arousal and Erections" from "Erectile Dysfunction and Inhibited Sexual Desire: Cognitive-Behavioral Strategies" by B. McCarthy in *Journal of Sex Education and Therapy*, 18, (1992), pp. 22–34. Copyright © 1992. Reprinted by permission of American Association of Sex Educators, Counselors & Therapists; **Table 7.8** Adapted from Kaplan, 1974; **Table 7.9** FSD Alert (2000); Kaschak and Tiefer (2002).

Chapter 8

Figure 8.1 DSTDP (2001), pp. 12, 20, and 32; **Page 293** Map, World Health Organization, (2005); **Table 8.4** CDC, (2004c). Cases of HIV infection and AIDS in the United States 2004. HIV/AIDS Surveillance Report, 16, 1–46; **Table 8.5** CDC (2001a); **Figure 8.5** Graph, "The Changing Face of AIDS" by R. Johnson from *Aids Read*, Vol. 12, No. 9, (2002), pp. 373–375. Copyright © 2002, The Aids Reader, Cliggott Publishing Group. All rights reserved; **Figure 8.6** Graph, "The Impact of HAART on Time from HIV Infection to AIDS" by R. Johnson from *Aids*

Read, Vol. 12, No. 9, (2002), pp. 373–375. Copyright © 2002, The Aids Reader, Cliggott Publishing Group. All rights reserved.

Chapter 9

Table 9.1 Arenofsky, 1996; "Childless by Choice, " 2001; Connidis and McMullen, 1999; Kopper and Smith, 2001; La Mastro, 2001; Morell, 2000; and Salzman, 1998; **Table 9.3** Adapted from Obstetrics-Gynecology and Infertility Group (2001); **Figure 9.11** "Predicted Survival Rates (%) for Preterm Infants by Weeks of Gestation" from "Tables for Predicting Survival for Preterm Births are Updated" by Draper, et al., in *British Medical Journal*, 327, (2003), p. 872. Copyright © 2003. Reprinted by permission from the BMJ Publishing Group; **Table 9.4** Adapted from March of Dimes Perinatal Data Center (2004); **Table 9.5** Cates and Ellerston, 1998; Healthwise, 2004; Hollander, 2000; and PregnancyOptions.info (2004); **Table 9.7** "'APGAR' Scores for New Dads" by H. Bennett in *British Medical Journal*, Vol. 317, p. 1712, (1998). Copyright © 1998. Reprinted by permission from the BMJ Publishing Group; **Table 9.8** Klotter (2002); G. Stewart (1998); **Figure 9.23** CDC (2004c), fig. 6.

Chapter 10

Table 10.2 Bureau of Labor Statistics (2002); **Figure 10.5** Graph, "Boys' and Girls' Aggressive Behavior, Grades 1–7" from "Gender and Aggression: The Baltimore Prevention Study", The Institute for Teaching and Research on Women, 2002. http://www.pages.towson.edu/itrow/research/current %20research%20projects/gender&agression.htm. Reprinted by permission of Institute for Teaching and Research on Women, Towson University; **Figure 10.6** Two Types of Aggression by Gender Among 7th Graders" based on data from The Institute for Teaching and Research on Women, 2002, http://www.pages.towson.edu/itrow/research/current% 20research%20projects/ gender&agression.htm. Reprinted by permission of Institute for Teaching and Research on Women, Towson University; **Figure 10.7** Table, Gender Differences in Types of Aggression (p. 1147) from "United States and Indonesian Children's and Adolescents' Reports of Relational Aggression by Disliked Peers" by D. French, E. Jansen, and S. Pidada, Child Development, 73, (2002), pp. 1143–1150. Copyright © 2002 Society for Research in Child Development. Reprinted by permission of the publisher; **Figure 10.8** Adapted from Baldwin and Baldwin (1997), p. 182; **Table 10.3** Adapted from Tannen (1991); **Table 10.4** Adapted from Ricciardelli and Williams (1995), pp. 644–645.

Chapter 11

Figure 11.1 "Kinsey's Sexual Orientation Rating Scale" from *Sexual Behavior in the Human Male* by A. Kinsey, W. Pomeroy, and C. Martin. Copyright 1948. Reprinted by permission of The Kinsey Institute for Research in Sex, Gender, and Reproduction, Inc.; **Table 11.2** Adapted from Gottman and Levinson (2001); **Figure 11.3** Bailey and Benishay (1993); Bailey and Pillard (1991); **Figure 11.4** "Bem's Exotic-Becomes-Erotic Theory of Sexual Orientation" from "Exotic Becomes Erotic: Interpretating the Biological Correlates of Sexual Orientation" by D. Bem in Archives of Sexual Behavior, 29, (2000), pp. 531–548. Copyright ©2000. Reprinted by Springer Science and Business Media; **Figure 11.5** Data from Remafedi (1998); **Figure 11.6** Lambda Legal Defense and Education Fund (2005); **Table 11.3** Myers (2005); **Figure 11.7** Federal Bureau of Investigation (2004b, 2005); **Table 11.4** Bureau of Investigation (2006), Table 1.

Chapter 12

Table 12.1 Adapted from Table #3 & #4 from "Normative Sexual Behavior in Children: A Contemporary Sample" by W. N. Friedrich, et al., in *Pediatrics*, April 1998, Vol. 101, No. 9. Copyright © 1998 by American Academy of Pediatrics. Reprinted by permission of The American Academy of Pediatrics; **Table 12.2** Adapted from Table, "Children's Sources of Sex Information" from "Does Source of Sex Information Predict Adolescents' Sexual Knowledge, Attitudes, & Behaviors?" by C. L. Somers and J. H. Gleason, *Education*, 121, (2001), pp. 674–681. Copyright © 2001. Reprinted by permission of Project Innovation, Mobile, AL and C. L. Somers; **Table 12.3** Grunbaum et al. (2002), p. 60; **Table 12.4** Table 1 from "Heterosexual Genital Sexual Activity Among Heterosexual Males: 1988 and 1995" by Gates & Sonenstein, *Family Planning Perspectives*, 2000, 32(6). Copyright © 2000. Reprinted by permission of The Alan Guttmacher Institute; **Figure 12.1** Martin et al. (2003), tab. 4; **Table 12.5** Table, "Sexual Behaviors of College Students" from "Gender Differences in Sexual Fantasy and Behavior in a College Population: A Ten-Year Replication" by Hsu, et al., in *Journal of Sex and Marital Therapy*, 20, (1994). Copyright © 1994. Reprinted by permission of Taylor & Francis Group, LLC., http://www.taylorandfrancis.com; **Figure 12.2** "Sexual Desire 'Peaks' for Men and Women by Age" from "Is There an Early-30s Peak in Female Sexual Desire? Cross-Sectional Evidence from the United States and Canada" by D. Schmitt et al., in *The Canadian Journal of Human Sexuality*, 11, (2002), pp. 1–17. Copyright © 2002. Reprinted by permission of The Sex Information and Education Council of Canada; **Figure 12.3** U.S. Census Bureau (2003); **Figure 12.4** Figure, "Factors Predicting Sexual Satisfaction in Marriage" by M. Young et al., in *The Canadian Journal of Human Sexuality*, 7, (1998), pp. 115–127. Copyright © 1998.Reprinted by permission of The Sex Information and Education Council of Canada; **Figure 12.5** Figure, "Emotional and Sexual Satisfaction among Married Couples" from *The Social Organization of Sexuality* by E. Laumann, J.Gagnon, R. Michael, and S. Michaels. Copyright ©1994. Reprinted by permission of The University of Chicago Press; **Figure 12.6** Figure, "Sexual Problems are Common" from *The Social Organization of Sexuality* by E. Laumann, J. Gagnon, R. Michael, and S. Michaels. Copyright © 1994. Reprinted by permission of The University of Chicago Press; **Table 12.6** Meston (1997) and Sex Info (2003).

Chapter 13

Figure 13.1 National Clearinghouse on Marital and Date Rape (2005); **Table 13.1** Based on FBI Uniform Crime Reports, 2004a; **Table 13.2** Counseling Center for Human Development (2001), Laumann et al., (1994), National Crime Victims Center (2001); **Figure 13.2** Data from Figure, "Relationships between Victims and Their Rapists" from *The Social Organization of Sexuality* by E. Laumann, J. Gagnon, R. Michael, and S. Michaels. Copyright © 1994. Reprinted by permission of The University of Chicago Press; **Figure 13.3** Data from Tjaden & Thoennes (2000), p. 36; **Table 13.3** Data from "Abusers' Relationships to Their Victims" from *The Social Organization of Sexuality* by E. Laumann, J. Gagnon, R. Michael, and S. Michaels. Copyright © 1994. Reprinted by permission of The University of Chicago Press; **Table 13.4** Data from "Percentage of Specific Contact Behaviors Among Survivors of Child Sexual Abuse" from *The Social Organization of Sexuality* by E. Laumann, J. Gagnon, R. Michael, and S. Michaels. Copyright © 1994. Reprinted by permission of The University of Chicago Press; **Table 13.5** Data from

Table, "Age at Which Sexual Abuse Occurred" from *The Social Organization of Sexuality* by E. Laumann, J. Gagnon, R. Michael, and S. Michaels. Copyright © 1994. Reprinted by permission of The University of Chicago Press.

Chapter 14

Table 14.2 Adapted from American Psychiatric Association (2000); **Figure 14.1** Data from "Adrenalin Levels in Pedophiles versus Normal Men" from "Pedophilia is Accompanied by Increased Plasma Concentrations of Catecholamines, in Particular, Epinephrine" by M. Maes et al., in *Psychiatry Research*, 103, (2001), pp. 43–49. Copyright © 2001. Reprinted by permission of Elsevier Ireland Ltd.; **Figure 14.2** Data from Finkelhor and Jones (2004).

Chapter 15

Figure 15.1 Data from Potterat et al. (1998), Table 3; **Figure 15.2** "Age of Onset Sexual Activity" from "Pathways to Prostitution: The Chronology of Sexual and Drug Abuse Milestones" by J. Potterat, et al., *Journal of Sex Research*, (1998), pp. 333–340. Copyright © 1998. Reprinted by permission of The Society for the Scientific Study of Sex; **Table 15.1** Data from "Demographic Characteristics of Clients of Prostitutes in the U.S." from "Prostitution and Fellatio" by M. Monto in *Journal of Sex Research*, 38, (2000), pp. 140–145. Copyright © 2000. Reprinted by permission of The Society for the Scientific Study of Sex; **Table 15.2** Data from "Sexual Attitudes and Desires of Clients of Prostitutes" from "Prostitution and Fellatio" by M. Monto in *Journal of Sex Research*, 38, (2000), pp. 140–145. Copyright © 2000. Reprinted by permission of The Society for the Scientific Study of Sex; **Table 15.3** Data from "Romantic Themes in X-Rated Videos" from "Gender Effects of Romantic Themes in Erotica" by D. Quakenbush, D. Strassberg, and C. Turner in *Archives of Sexual Behavior*, 24, (2002), pp. 21–35. Copyright ©2002. Reprinted by permission of Springer Science+Business Media; **Table 15.5** Data from "Sexually-Related Online Activities of College Students" from "University Students' Uses of and Reactions to Online Sexual Information and Entertainment: Links to Online and Offline Sexual Behavior" by S. Boles from *The Canadian Journal of Human Sexuality*, 11, (2002), pp. 77–90. Copyright © 2002. Reprinted by permission of The Sex Information and Education Council of Canada; **Table 15.6** Data from "College Students' Reactions to Online Sexual Activities" from "University Students' Uses of and Reactions to Online Sexual Information and Entertainment: Links to Online and Offline Sexual Behavior" by S. Boles from *The Canadian Journal of Human Sexuality*, 11, (2002), pp. 77–90. Copyright © 2002. Reprinted by permission of The Sex Information and Education Council of Canada.

Name Index

Subject Index